MANUAL of PERIOPERATIVE CARE in ADULT CARDIAC SURGERY

Sixth Edition

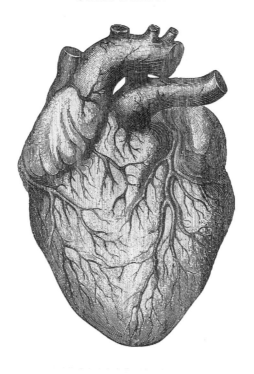

T0340689

MANUAL of PERIOPERATIVE CARE in ADULT CARDIAC SURGERY

Sixth Edition

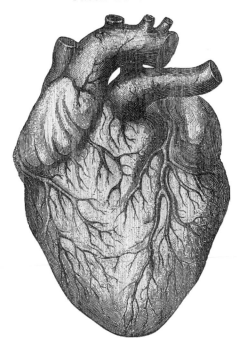

Robert M. Bojar, MD

Chief of Cardiothoracic Surgery
Saint Vincent Hospital
Worcester, Massachusetts, USA

WILEY Blackwell

This edition first published 2021
© 2021 John Wiley & Sons Ltd

Edition History
Robert M. Bojar (5e, 2011)

All rights reserved. No part of this publication may be reproduced, stored in a retrieval system, or transmitted, in any form or by any means, electronic, mechanical, photocopying, recording or otherwise, except as permitted by law. Advice on how to obtain permission to reuse material from this title is available at http://www.wiley.com/go/permissions.

The right of Robert M. Bojar to be identified as the author of this work has been asserted in accordance with law.

Registered Office(s)
John Wiley & Sons, Inc., 111 River Street, Hoboken, NJ 07030, USA
John Wiley & Sons Ltd, The Atrium, Southern Gate, Chichester, West Sussex, PO19 8SQ, UK

Editorial Office
9600 Garsington Road, Oxford, OX4 2DQ, UK

For details of our global editorial offices, customer services, and more information about Wiley products visit us at www.wiley.com.

Wiley also publishes its books in a variety of electronic formats and by print-on-demand. Some content that appears in standard print versions of this book may not be available in other formats.

Limit of Liability/Disclaimer of Warranty
The contents of this work are intended to further general scientific research, understanding, and discussion only and are not intended and should not be relied upon as recommending or promoting scientific method, diagnosis, or treatment by physicians for any particular patient. In view of ongoing research, equipment modifications, changes in governmental regulations, and the constant flow of information relating to the use of medicines, equipment, and devices, the reader is urged to review and evaluate the information provided in the package insert or instructions for each medicine, equipment, or device for, among other things, any changes in the instructions or indication of usage and for added warnings and precautions. While the publisher and authors have used their best efforts in preparing this work, they make no representations or warranties with respect to the accuracy or completeness of the contents of this work and specifically disclaim all warranties, including without limitation any implied warranties of merchantability or fitness for a particular purpose. No warranty may be created or extended by sales representatives, written sales materials or promotional statements for this work. The fact that an organization, website, or product is referred to in this work as a citation and/or potential source of further information does not mean that the publisher and authors endorse the information or services the organization, website, or product may provide or recommendations it may make. This work is sold with the understanding that the publisher is not engaged in rendering professional services. The advice and strategies contained herein may not be suitable for your situation. You should consult with a specialist where appropriate. Further, readers should be aware that websites listed in this work may have changed or disappeared between when this work was written and when it is read. Neither the publisher nor authors shall be liable for any loss of profit or any other commercial damages, including but not limited to special, incidental, consequential, or other damages.

Library of Congress Cataloging-in-Publication Data

Names: Bojar, Robert M., 1951– author.
Title: Manual of perioperative care in adult cardiac surgery / Robert M. Bojar.
Description: Sixth edition. | Hoboken, NJ : Wiley-Blackwell, 2020. | Includes bibliographical references and index.
Identifiers: LCCN 2020029687 | ISBN 9781119582557 (paperback) | ISBN 9781119582595 (adobe pdf) | ISBN 9781119582588 (epub)
Subjects: MESH: Cardiac Surgical Procedures | Perioperative Care–methods | Outline
Classification: LCC RD598 | NLM WG 18.2 | DDC 617.4/12–dc23
LC record available at https://lccn.loc.gov/2020029687

Cover Design: Wiley
Cover Image: © Jackie Niam/Getty Images

Set in 9/11pt Adobe Caslon by SPi Global, Pondicherry, India

SKY10079394_071024

Dedication

*In loving memory of my parents, who devoted their lives
to helping others and inspired me to do the same.*

Contents

Preface

Cardiac surgery has faced several challenges in this century. Advances in coronary stenting have allowed most patients with coronary disease to undergo percutaneous coronary intervention. This seems to leave only patients with nonstentable disease or failed stents for the surgeon. Transcatheter aortic valve replacements (TAVRs) have been performed more commonly than surgical AVRs for several years, and transcatheter mitral valve technology continues to evolve and should see wider applications. Descending thoracic aortic surgery has been all but replaced by endovascular stent grafting. Electrophysiologists have become more aggressive in ablating arrhythmias. Most of these technologies have evolved from the concept that a less invasive approach to treating structural heart disease is preferred by patients to reduce trauma, minimize complications, expedite recovery, and improve the quality of life – and this concept has become reality.

Although these approaches may be applicable to patients at both ends of the clinical spectrum, surgery will still remain the best approach for many patients, and invariably will require the use of cardiopulmonary bypass with its inherent morbidity. There is little doubt that surgical patient acuity will continue to increase, and excellence in perioperative care will remain essential to optimize outcomes, both for patients undergoing open-heart surgery and for the higher-risk patients undergoing transcatheter approaches.

The sixth edition of the *Manual* incorporates some of the newer guidelines, medications, and concepts that have evolved over the past nine years since the publication of the last edition. I have retained important references and added more current ones if they add new information. Online access to virtually all references should be available to the reader no matter how obscure the source may appear. I encourage the reader to review updated guidelines from the American College of Cardiology Foundation, the European Society of Cardiology, and the Society of Thoracic Surgeons as they become available online. As always, I am hopeful that this edition will provide a comprehensive, up-to-date review that will assist healthcare providers in delivering the best possible care to their cardiac surgical patients.

Robert M. Bojar, MD
Worcester, MA
October 2020

Acknowledgments

Cardiac surgery requires meticulous attention to detail to ensure the best possible outcomes. Decision-making in the perioperative period involves close cooperation and communication among all members of the healthcare team, including cardiac surgeons, anesthesiologists, cardiologists, physician assistants, nurse practitioners, perfusionists, respiratory therapists, and critical care and floor nurses. Identifying problems and seeking consultations with experts in other fields is important to optimize perioperative care. I am greatly appreciative of the efforts of many individuals who set aside valuable time to review sections of the manuscript in their areas of expertise. I would like to acknowledge the critiques and comments of Drs. Joseph Hannan, Arie Farji-Cisneros, Dharmender Chandok, Suzanne Martin, Rachel Kaplan, and Fady Marmoush. I would also like to thank Philip Carpino, PA-C, Bettina Alpert, CCP, Joshua Deisenroth, PA-C, and Wanda Reynolds, CCRT, for their reviews and suggestions. Lastly, I am indebted to my Chief Physician Assistant, Theresa Phillips, PA-C, who helps coordinate the care my patients receive, and who reviewed many sections of the manuscript to ensure their accuracy.

Notice: The indications and dosages of all drugs in this book have been recommended in the medical literature and conform to the practices of the general community. The medications described do not necessarily have specific approval by the Food and Drug Administration for use in the diseases and dosages for which they are recommended. The package insert for each drug should be consulted for use and dosage as approved by the FDA. Because standards for usage change, it is advisable to keep abreast of revised recommendations, particularly those concerning new drugs. Although the author has made every attempt to ensure the accuracy of drug dosages, it is the obligation of the reader to confirm drug dosages prior to prescribing any drug.

Abbreviations used through this book are typeset and easy to read. However, many hospitals have lists of approved abbreviations which initially were mandated to avoid medication errors caused by inability to interpret handwriting. Use of these abbreviations with computerized order writing within electronic medical records is recommended to avoid this problem.

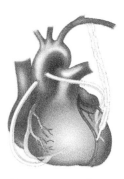

CHAPTER 1

Synopsis of Adult Cardiac Surgical Disease

♡ 1 Synopsis of Adult Cardiac Surgical Disease

It is essential that all individuals involved in the assessment and management of patients with cardiac surgical disease have a basic understanding of the disease processes that are being treated. This chapter presents the spectrum of adult cardiac surgical disease that is encountered in most cardiac surgical practices. The pathophysiology, indications for surgery, specific preoperative considerations, and surgical options for various diseases are presented. Diagnostic techniques and general preoperative considerations are presented in the next two chapters. Issues related to cardiac anesthesia and postoperative care specific to most of the surgical procedures presented in this chapter are discussed in Chapters 4 and 8, respectively. The most current guidelines for the evaluation and management of patients with cardiac disease can be obtained from the American College of Cardiology website (www.acc.org).

I. Coronary Artery Disease

A. **Pathophysiology.** Coronary artery disease (CAD) results from the progressive blockage of the coronary arteries by atherothrombotic disease. Significant risk factors include hypertension, dyslipidemia (especially high LDL, low HDL, elevated Lp(a) or apoB, or triglycerides), diabetes mellitus, obesity (a combination of the above being termed metabolic syndrome), cigarette smoking, and a family history of premature CAD. Clinical syndromes result from an imbalance of oxygen supply and demand resulting in inadequate myocardial perfusion to meet metabolic demand (ischemia). Progressive compromise in luminal diameter producing supply/demand imbalance usually produces a pattern of chronic stable angina, commonly referred to as "stable ischemic heart disease" (SIHD). Plaque rupture with superimposed thrombosis is responsible for most acute coronary syndromes (ACS), which include classic "unstable angina", non-ST-elevation myocardial infarctions (non-STEMI), and ST-elevation infarctions (STEMI). Paradoxically, plaque rupture more commonly occurs in coronary segments that are not severely stenotic. Endothelial dysfunction has become increasingly recognized as a contributing factor to worsening ischemic syndromes. Generalized systemic inflammation, indicated by elevated C-reactive protein levels, is usually noted in patients with ACS, and appears to be associated with adverse outcomes.

B. **Primary prevention** of cardiovascular disease entails control of modifiable risk factors. Notably, statins are generally not recommended for patients with normal cholesterol levels (unless there is a family history of premature CAD) or for patients at low risk for atherosclerotic cardiovascular disease (ASCVD) based on the ASCVD risk calculator (available at https://clincalc.com/cardiology/ascvd/pooledcohort.aspx).

Furthermore, aspirin, which had been widely utilized for primary prevention in the past, has received only a level IIb recommendation for patients age 40–70 with higher ASCVD risk but not at increased bleeding risk, and was considered contraindicated on a routine basis in patients >age 70 or in any patient with an increased risk of bleeding, according to a 2019 ACC report.[1]

C. **Management strategies in stable ischemic heart disease (SIHD)**

1. Symptomatic coronary disease is initially treated with medical therapy, including aspirin, nitrates, ß-adrenergic blockers, and calcium-channel blockers (CCBs). Ranolazine may be added as a second-line drug for symptomatic relief in patients with refractory angina. It inhibits inward sodium currents in the heart muscle, leading to a reduction in intracellular calcium levels, which reduces myocardial wall tension and oxygen requirements. It does not cause bradycardia and hypotension, which occasionally are limiting factors with the use of other antianginal drugs. Statins should be given to control dyslipidemias and are effective for plaque stabilization. Angiotensin-converting enzyme (ACE) inhibitors or angiotensin receptor blockers (ARBs) are given to patients with depressed left ventricular (LV) function (ejection fraction [EF] <40%) and to those with hypertension and diabetes. P2Y12 inhibitors (clopidogrel, ticagrelor) generally do not provide benefit to patients with SIHD.

2. Optimal medical therapy should be the initial management strategy for patients with SIHD, since studies have not shown that proceeding to percutaneous coronary intervention (PCI) reduces the risk of death, infarction or other major adverse cardiovascular events.[2] Thus, the decision to proceed with cardiac catheterization should be based on the rationale that the patient's symptoms are disabling enough or the degree of ischemia is significant enough to warrant an intervention to revascularize the heart. Risk stratification with noninvasive functional testing is important to provide objective evidence of inducible ischemia, using exercise stress testing, nuclear imaging, or dobutamine stress echocardiography.

3. The decision to proceed with an intervention must then take into consideration an angiographic assessment of the extent of coronary disease and an invasive assessment of its physiologic significance by fractional flow reserve (FFR)[3] or instantaneous flow reserve (iFR)[4], which is not dependent on the administration of adenosine. Additional critical information when considering PCI or coronary artery bypass grafting (CABG) includes the patient's comorbidities, particularly diabetes mellitus, and an assessment of LV function. Multiple studies comparing medical therapy with PCI for patients with SIHD have shown that PCI reduces the incidence of angina, may increase the short-term risk of myocardial infarction (MI), but does not lower the long-term risk of MI or improve survival.[5] However, PCI does reduce the need for urgent revascularization and may reduce the risk of MI in patients with a large ischemic burden. Superior clinical outcomes are achieved with complete revascularization, which in many patients is better accomplished with CABG than PCI.[6] Use of systematic anatomic assessments, such as with the SYNTAX score (see section C.4.a), has been accepted as an adjunct to this decision-making process.

4. Appropriate use criteria (AUC) with complex matrices have been set forth for coronary revascularization strategies in patients with SIHD.[7] These are subdivided by the number of diseased vessels (1–2–3), the presence of symptoms, the use of

antianginal therapy, and whether noninvasive testing indicates the patient is at low, intermediate, or high risk for a cardiac event, or in the absence of testing, by the results of FFR/iFr studies.

a. The SYNTAX score (http://www.syntaxscore.com) is also incorporated into the AUC guidelines and can be used to determine whether PCI or CABG is preferable for multivessel or left main (LM) disease. This provides an angiographic assessment of coronary disease with an additive score that evaluates the location and degree of stenosis in each vessel, the angiographic complexity of the lesion, vessel diameter and calcification. The SYNTAX trial divided patients into low risk (score of 0–22), intermediate risk (score of 23–32), and high risk (score >32) categories and used a primary end point of major adverse cardiac and cerebrovascular events (MACCE), which includes mortality, myocardial infarction (MI), stroke, and the need for repeat revascularization.

b. Five-year follow-up data from the SYNTAX trial showed that patients in the low-risk category had similar MACCE rates with PCI or CABG. However, CABG produced superior results in intermediate- to high-risk patients with three-vessel disease (score >22), and those at high risk with LM disease. In these cohorts, CABG was associated with less MACCE, more complete revascularization, reduced need for repeat revascularization, and improved long-term benefit.[8,9]

c. The FREEDOM trial showed that CABG was superior to PCI in diabetic patients with multivessel disease,[10,11] and the presence or absence of diabetes is specifically incorporated into the AUC guidelines for multivessel and LM disease. In these diabetic patients, the SYNTAX score was found to be a predictor of MACCE only with PCI, and therefore was not recommended to guide therapy.[12]

d. A "residual SYNTAX" score >8 after PCI for patients in the moderate- to high-risk cohorts, indicative of incomplete revascularization, had worse 30-day and one-year survival.[13] In fact, in the entire SYNTAX study, PCI resulted in a 10-fold increase in MI-related death compared with CABG, but this was mostly accounted for in patients with diabetes, multivessel disease, and high SYNTAX scores.[14]

e. One shortcoming of the SYNTAX score was that it correlated only an angiographic assessment with the best revascularization strategy. Because surgery might provide more benefit to patients with significant clinical comorbidities in addition to the anatomical complexity of disease, the SYNTAX II scoring system was devised. This included eight predictors – two anatomic (SYNTAX score and unprotected LM disease), and six clinical predictors (age, creatinine clearance, ejection fraction, female gender, peripheral vascular disease, and chronic obstructive pulmonary disease [COPD]). The SYNTAX II study used second-generation drug-eluting stents and intravascular ultrasound imaging with PCI. It showed that some patients with low SYNTAX scores had higher mortality rates with PCI and some with higher SYNTAX scores did better with PCI. Generally, the SYNTAX II score was a better predictor of four-year mortality rates than the original score.[15] To achieve similar four-year survival rates with PCI or CABG, it was found that young patients, females, and patients with reduced LVEF required lower SYNTAX scores, while older patients, those with COPD, and those with unprotected LM disease did well with PCI despite higher anatomical SYNTAX scores. The SYNTAX II score can be accessed at www.syntaxscore.com and it calculates the comparative four-year survival rates for PCI and CABG.

f. Although diabetes was not a discriminator using SYNTAX II scoring, other studies, including a subanalysis from the FREEDOM trial of diabetic patients with multivessel disease, found CABG superior to PCI in both insulin-treated and noninsulin-treated diabetics, but results were generally worse after either procedure in insulin-treated diabetics.[16]

g. Thus, the SYNTAX or SYNTAX II score might be used as part of the decision-making process for the preferable mode of revascularization, since, along with older age, female gender, smoking, and diabetes, it appears to be a strong predictor of mortality and MACCE in patients undergoing PCI for multivessel disease and unprotected left main stenosis. These scoring systems provide an evidence-based justification for selecting CABG as the treatment of choice for many patients with more complex multivessel disease.

5. **Indications for surgery in SIHD – symptom relief.** The primary indication for surgical revascularization is to improve symptoms. PCI is applicable to many of these patients, but CABG must be considered for diabetic patients and those with high SYNTAX scores and when satisfactory PCI cannot be accomplished.[5]

  a. Class I indications
  - ≥1 significant stenoses with unacceptable angina despite guideline-directed medical therapy (GDMT)

  b. Class IIa indications
  - ≥1 significant stenoses in patients who cannot implement GDMT
  - Complex three-vessel disease (SYNTAX score >22) with/without proximal left anterior descending (LAD) artery stenosis

  c. Class IIb indications
  - Redo CABG with ≥1 significant stenoses with ischemia and unacceptable angina despite GDMT

6. **Indications for surgery in SIHD – improvement in survival.** Although symptom relief is one objective of any revascularization procedure, an additional important benefit is an improvement in long-term survival compared with medical therapy. For example, CABG for LM disease >50% or for multivessel disease with extensive ischemia and/or impaired LV function can accomplish this, but there are limited data showing that PCI can do the same. It is also likely that CABG can prolong life by preventing MI, whereas the same may not be true for PCI.[17] The following recommendations for surgery represent slight modification from the randomized controlled trials of patients with primarily chronic stable angina in the early 1980s and were incorporated into the 2011 guidelines for CABG.[5] These are the anatomic subsets for which improved survival has been noted compared with medical therapy. Thus, for these patients, surgery can be justified even in the absence of disabling symptoms. PCI is often utilized for many of these indications, although a survival benefit has not necessarily been demonstrated.

  a. Class I indications
  - Unprotected left main stenosis >50%
  - Three-vessel disease with/without proximal LAD disease

- Two-vessel disease with proximal LAD disease
- Survivors of sudden death with presumed ischemic-mediated ventricular tachycardia (VT)

b. Class IIa indications
  - Two-vessel disease without proximal LAD disease with a large area of ischemic myocardium
  - One-vessel disease with proximal LAD disease (with a left internal thoracic artery [LITA] graft)
  - Proximal LAD or multivessel disease with EF 35–50% if viable myocardium in the region of intended revascularization

c. Class IIb indications
  - One-, two- or three-vessel disease except left main with EF <35%

7. The optimal strategy in patients with severe ischemic LV dysfunction is somewhat controversial. The STICH (Surgical Treatment for Ischemic Heart Failure) trial comparing CABG with optimal medical therapy in patients with ischemic LV dysfunction found an increased 30-day mortality but better 10-year survival with CABG, the crossover occurring at two years.[18]

a. There was no correlation of survival with the presence or absence of angina in the intention-to-treat analysis, but there was a prognostic benefit when crossover were included. Either way, angina relief was superior with surgery.[19]

b. Worse outcomes with medical management were noted with more extensive CAD, more LV dysfunction (EF <27%) and larger ventricles (LV end-systolic volume index >79 mL/m²), but these risk factors were not predictive of CABG mortality – thus a greater benefit with CABG was noted in these patients.

c. Another interesting finding of the STICH trial was that there was no difference in surgical outcomes whether viability was present or not, and in fact, this observation was irrespective of treatment strategy.[20] This seemed to contradict multiple studies and meta-analyses that have shown that viability testing is helpful in assessing which patients may benefit from surgery.[21] One potential limitation of this trial was the use of thallium stress imaging, which is not as discriminatory as PET (positron emission tomography) scanning in differentiating viable from nonviable myocardium. It was concluded that viability was predictive of a survival benefit in patients with moderate LV dysfunction, but lost its prognostic benefit when LV dysfunction became severe.[19]

d. Other studies comparing PCI with CABG in diabetic patients with LV dysfunction have confirmed that CABG is associated with a lower risk of death, MI, MACE, and repeat revascularization.[22]

D. **Management strategies in acute coronary syndromes**

1. **Non-STEMI** patients or those with unstable angina without a troponin leak usually have the substrate for recurrent ischemia and infarction. They should be treated with aspirin (162–325 mg) and unfractionated or low-molecular-weight heparin (LMWH), as well as standard therapies (e.g. nitrates, β-blockers, statins, ACE inhibitors).[23,24] A P2Y12 inhibitor, usually clopidogrel or ticagrelor, should be given in addition to aspirin to patients with non-STEMIs, but it is not necessarily indicated in patients with normal troponin levels. Initiation of dual antiplatelet therapy will provide a clinical benefit and will also provide adequate platelet inhibition for a

PCI which is feasible in most patients to relieve ischemia and prevent infarction. In patients who are considered intermediate–high risk for a clinical event or exhibit a large thrombus burden, the addition of a glycoprotein (GP) IIb/IIIa inhibitor may be considered (class IIb indication). If PCI is not feasible or is unsuccessful, a CABG is indicated for the anatomic findings listed in section C.6.

a. Low-risk patients may stabilize on medical therapy and can undergo risk stratification by noninvasive testing to assess the extent of inducible ischemia (the "ischemia-guided strategy"). Various scoring systems (GRACE or TIMI score for UA/NSTEMI) can be used to quantitate the patient's short-term risk of an ischemic event. The GRACE score provides estimates of in-hospital and six-month mortality and the TIMI score provides the 14-day risk of mortality, new or recurrent MI, or severe recurrent ischemia requiring urgent revascularization. Both of these scoring systems are available at a variety of sites on-line, including www.mdcal.com (search "GRACE" or "TIMI").[24]

b. In patients at intermediate–high risk, an "early invasive strategy" is used, which triages the patient to early catheterization. Although this strategy is considered to lead to improved outcomes compared with the ischemia-guided approach, some studies show that 10-year outcomes are comparable.[25] This approach provides an early definition of the patient's coronary anatomy and allows for early intervention to prevent myocardial damage. This strategy has been subdivided into immediate (<2 hours), early (<24 hours), or delayed (25–72 hours) catheterizations, depending on the patient's presentation. The immediate approach is applicable to patients with recurrent or refractory angina, ECG changes at rest, new-onset heart failure (HF), new-onset mitral regurgitation (MR), or hemodynamic instability. New ST depressions with rising troponins or a GRACE score >140 are an indication for an early approach, and patients with diabetes, chronic kidney disease, EF <40%, a GRACE score of 109–140, or a TIMI score ≥2 can have a delayed invasive approach.[24,26]

c. Since most patients are given a P2Y12 inhibitor upon hospital admission, when the extent of their coronary disease is not known, there will be patients undergoing catheterization in whom PCI is not feasible or in whom the benefits of CABG outweigh those of PCI (i.e. most diabetic patients with multivessel disease and patients with distal LM disease). An urgent CABG may then be recommended. A lower risk of renal dysfunction is noted for patients having on-pump CABG if surgery can be delayed for 24 hours after catheterization.[27] However, the timing of surgery must primarily balance the risk of a recurrent ischemic event vs. the risk of excessive bleeding. For patients requiring urgent, but not emergent, surgery who receive a P2Y12 inhibitor, surgery should be delayed at least 24 hours, if possible, and platelet aggregation testing obtained to elucidate whether the patient is sensitive or not to the P2Y12 inhibitor.[28,29] If inhibition is <30%, surgery can usually be done safely without resorting to platelet transfusions to control mediastinal bleeding.

2. **ST elevation infarctions (STEMIs)** are usually associated with coronary occlusions, and are preferentially treated by primary PCI, although thrombolytic therapy may be considered when PCI cannot be performed within a few hours. Clinical benefit is time-related ("time is myocardium"), and the best results are obtained with a "door to balloon" time of less than 90 minutes. However, PCI should still be considered up to 12 hours after the onset of symptoms, at 12–24 hours

if the patient has HF, persistent ischemic symptoms, or hemodynamic or electrical instability, or at any time if cardiogenic shock is present.[24] For the latter, emerging data suggest that improved survival may be achieved using mechanical circulatory support (MCS), such as an Impella (Abiomed, Danvers, MA) device, prior to PCI.[30,31] All patients presenting with a STEMI and with no contraindications to antiplatelet treatment should be given one dose of aspirin 325 mg, a load of either clopidogrel 600 mg or ticagrelor 180 mg, and either unfractionated heparin or bivalirudin upon presentation to the emergency room, if not sooner (i.e. in the ambulance).

a. If PCI of the culprit vessel can be accomplished in a patient with multivessel disease, it remains controversial as to whether stenting of other nonculprit stenotic vessels should be performed at the same time, even in patients with cardiogenic shock, although some observational studies do suggest a benefit.[32,33] However, if it is concluded that the other vessels would be better revascularized by surgery, the patient may be referred for CABG having received a P2Y12 inhibitor to prevent stent thrombosis. Once the culprit vessel has been opened, surgery is rarely required emergently. Thus, the oral P2Y12 inhibitor may be stopped and the patient given either a short-acting P2Y12 inhibitor (IV cangrelor) or a GP IIb/IIIa inhibitor as a bridge to surgery.

b. If PCI cannot be accomplished or is considered inadvisable due to extensive LM or multivessel disease, emergency surgery should be performed. Early surgical studies showed little myocardial salvage if CABG was not performed within six hours, with a significant increase in mortality for surgery performed between 7 and 24 hours, and then a lower mortality thereafter.[34] Thus, beyond six hours, surgery may be delayed in the absence of cardiogenic shock, active ischemia, or a significant area of myocardium at risk, although the latter is usually present. However, active ischemia with or without cardiogenic shock should usually be treated urgently by CABG, independent of the time since presentation. In a report from the STS database, the operative mortality rate for patients in cardiogenic shock was about 20%, but it was 37% in patients requiring intraoperative MCS and 58% in patients requiring postoperative MCS support.[35] Thus, if cardiogenic shock is present without active ischemia or with end-organ dysfunction, consideration might be given to use of MCS alone.[24]

c. If PCI cannot be performed or has failed, the ACC guidelines recommend emergency surgery for the following:

i. Class I

- Persistent ischemia or hemodynamic instability refractory to nonsurgical therapy (it is not stated if that includes an intra-aortic balloon pump [IABP])
- Cardiogenic shock irrespective of the time from MI to the onset of shock and the time from MI to CABG
- Mechanical complications of MI
- Life-threatening ventricular arrhythmias with LM or three-vessel disease

ii. Class IIb

- Multivessel disease with recurrent angina or MI within 48 hours of presentation
- Patients >age 75 with ST elevation or left bundle branch block (LBBB) regardless of time since presentation if in cardiogenic shock

E. CABG vs. PCI as a revascularization strategy – other comments

1. The ongoing debate about the relative merits and advantages of CABG or PCI has spawned innumerable studies, publications, and controversies. PCI is generally utilized for patients with a lesser extent of disease, as noted in the appropriate use criteria (AUC) guidelines, and should incorporate SYNTAX scores in the decision. However, PCI is also useful in patients at very high risk for surgery due to either very advanced "nonbypassable" coronary disease or significant comorbidities that make surgery a prohibitive risk. Mechanical circulatory-supported PCI procedures, primarily using the Impella devices, have been performed successfully in high-risk cases.[36]

2. Studies have shown that FFR-guided, rather than anatomy-guided, PCI produces superior outcomes in patients with SIHD, reducing the need for urgent revascularization.[37] In the 2011 ACC guidelines for CABG, there is no mention of using an FFR-guided approach to surgical revascularization. Some studies have shown that this approach results in less grafting, a higher graft patency rate, a lower rate of angina, and a significant reduction in MI and mortality out to six years.[38–40] Such information could be helpful in deciding which patients should undergo surgery and, in fact, which vessels need to be bypassed.

3. Second-generation drug-eluting stents (DES) have been associated with a lower risk of restenosis requiring repeat revascularization, lower rates of stent thrombosis, and fewer MIs than bare-metal stents (BMS), without a significant impact on mortality.[41] Although the risk of stent thrombosis may be greater in patients who are resistant to the antiplatelet effects of aspirin and/or a P2Y12 inhibitor, platelet function testing has not been that useful in adjusting treatment and influencing outcomes.[42] To minimize the risk of stent thrombosis, it is recommended that patients receiving a BMS take aspirin and a P2Y12 inhibitor for at least one month, and those receiving a DES take these medications for at least six months to one year.[43]

4. One should not consider either PCI or CABG an exclusive approach to a patient's CAD. For example, one hybrid approach is to perform a PCI of the culprit lesion causing a STEMI to achieve prompt myocardial salvage and then refer the patient for surgical revascularization of other lesions. If a patient does undergo PCI and urgent surgery is then recommended, a strategy must be devised to minimize the risk of stent thrombosis while minimizing the risk of perioperative bleeding. It has even been proposed that placing a LITA to the LAD in a patient with three-vessel disease provides the essential long-term benefit of a CABG and converts the patient's anatomy to two-vessel disease which can be managed medically or with PCI.[44,45] However, one study did suggest that the rate of mid-term reinterventions rates was higher using a hybrid approach.[46]

F. Preoperative considerations

1. A thorough history and physical examination is imperative when cardiac surgery is being contemplated. Whereas PCI specifically addresses the patient's cardiac issues with minimal impact on other organ systems except the kidneys, open-heart surgery can produce a significant number of potential morbidities, especially in patients with pre-existing problems, such as COPD, hepatic or renal dysfunction, cerebrovascular disease, diabetes, etc. Careful attention to and management of such issues prior to surgery may optimize surgical outcomes. These issues are discussed in detail in Chapter 3.

2. **Myocardial ischemia.** Aggressive management of ongoing or potential ischemia is indicated in patients with critical coronary disease to reduce surgical risk. This may include adequate sedation and analgesia, anti-ischemic medications to control heart rate and blood pressure (IV nitrates and β-blockers), antiplatelet and anticoagulant medications (aspirin, P2Y12 inhibitors, heparin, GP IIb/IIIa inhibitors), and/or placement of an IABP for refractory ischemia. It cannot be overemphasized that just because a patient has been catheterized and accepted for surgery does not mean that medical care should not be aggressive up to the time of surgery! If the patient has persistent ischemia despite all of these measures, emergency surgery is mandatory.

   a. All antianginal medications should be continued up to and including the morning of surgery. Studies have demonstrated the benefit of preoperative **β-blocker** therapy in lowering perioperative mortality in elective cardiac surgery patients, although this is probably limited to patients sustaining a remote infarction.[47,48] Patients being admitted the morning of surgery should be reminded to take their medications before coming to the hospital.

   b. **Unfractionated heparin** (UFH) is often used in patients with an ACS, left main coronary disease, or a preoperative IABP. The heparin may be stopped about four hours prior to surgery, but in patients at higher risk for ischemia, it may be continued up to the time of surgery without causing problems with central line insertion. Patients receiving heparin should have their platelet count rechecked daily to be vigilant for the development of heparin-induced thrombocytopenia (HIT). Note that preoperative assessment for HIT antibodies is not indicated in the absence of a clinical indication.

   c. **Low-molecular-weight heparin** (LMWH) is often used in patients presenting with an ACS and may be used in the cath lab as well. It must be stopped at least 24 hours prior to surgery to minimize the risk of perioperative bleeding. The **non-vitamin K antagonist oral anticoagulants** (NOACs) (dabigatran, apixaban, rivaroxaban, edoxaban) should be stopped 48 hours prior to surgery and probably longer in patients with renal dysfunction.[49–51] **Fondaparinux**, occasionally used for venous thromboembolism prophylaxis, has a half-life of 17–21 hours and must be stopped at least 60 hours prior to surgery.

   d. **Aspirin** is routinely used in patients with known coronary disease or is given upon presentation to the hospital. Aspirin 81 mg should be continued up to the time of surgery for virtually all patients undergoing CABG, since most studies have demonstrated improved outcomes without a significant increase in the risk of bleeding.[52–55]

   e. Preoperative use of **P2Y12 inhibitors** within a few days of surgery has been shown to significantly increase the risk of bleeding and re-exploration for bleeding. Thus, it has been recommended that clopidogrel and ticagrelor be stopped for five days and prasugrel for seven days before elective surgery.[55] Stopping the medication for only three days may be acceptable prior to off-pump surgery.[56] Platelet aggregation testing, more so than the duration of cessation prior to surgery, may dictate when surgery can be performed with a lower risk of bleeding.[28,29]

      i. In some cases, emergency balloon angioplasty and potential stenting of a culprit lesion causing an evolving infarction may be performed, with subsequent referral for urgent surgery to achieve complete revascularization.

In this situation, it is preferable to use a short-acting platelet inhibitor as a bridge to surgery to minimize the risk of stent thrombosis. IV cangrelor is preferable as it has a half-life of 3–6 minutes and need be stopped only 1–2 hours before surgery.[57] Alternatively, a GP IIb/IIIa inhibitor can be used and should be stopped four hours prior to surgery so that by the time surgery starts, 80% of platelet activity will have recovered.

ii. In patients requiring surgery who have had prior stenting (<1 month for a BMS and 6–12 months for a DES), there is an increased risk of stent thrombosis if the P2Y12 inhibitor is stopped. P2Y12 reaction units (PRU) testing may indicate the patient's sensitivity to the drug. It is best to avoid operating if the PRU suggests >30% inhibition. In the absence of such testing, stopping the medication for three days may leave some residual protective antiplatelet activity, yet hopefully cause less intraoperative bleeding.

f. **Anemia** is associated with worse clinical outcomes after surgery, but this may be related to its association with other risk factors, such as HF or chronic kidney disease. In fact, it has been reported that blood transfusions have a greater impact on risk-adjusted morbidity and mortality than the anemia itself.[58–61]

i. Most hospitalized patients suffer from hospital-acquired anemia, which results from repeated blood withdrawal for lab tests as well as the blood loss and hydration during a catheterization procedure. Guidelines recommend transfusion for a hemoglobin (Hb) <8 g/dL in patients with an ACS, although hemodynamically unstable patients may benefit from a Hb level between 8 and 10 g/dL.[58,61]

ii. Even in the stable patient awaiting surgery, it is not unreasonable to give a blood transfusion prior to surgery if the anticipated hematocrit (HCT) on pump will be <20%. Low hematocrits on pump will lower oncotic pressure and viscosity, increase fluid requirements, which contributes to extracellular edema, and make it more difficult to maintain an adequate blood pressure during and after cardiopulmonary bypass (CPB). A HCT below 20% has been associated with an increased risk of renal dysfunction, stroke, ischemic optic neuropathy, and mortality. Patients with profound anemia during surgery also tend to bleed more and require more blood component transfusions. Thus, preoperative transfusion to an adequate level may be considered to reduce patient morbidity, possibly reduce the overall number of transfusions required intra- and postoperatively, and potentially decrease mortality.

3. Other preoperative medications to be considered include the following:

a. **Amiodarone** is beneficial in reducing the incidence of postoperative atrial fibrillation (AF). Protocols that initiate amiodarone prior to or during surgery have been utilized successfully (see pages 623–624 in Chapter 11).[62]

b. **Statins** have been demonstrated to reduce operative mortality, the risks of stroke, delirium, AF, and arguably the risk of acute kidney injury.[63–66]

c. **Steroids** have been evaluated as a means of reducing the systemic inflammatory response to surgery and have been shown to improve myocardial function and possibly reduce the incidence of AF.[67] However, improvement in pulmonary function has not been clearly shown, and steroids do worsen postoperative hyperglycemia. Since the benefits are controversial, steroids have not seen widespread usage.

G. Surgical procedures

1. **Traditional coronary artery bypass grafting** is performed through a median sternotomy incision with use of CPB. Myocardial preservation is provided by cardioplegic arrest. The procedure involves bypassing the coronary blockages with a variety of conduits. The left internal thoracic (or mammary) artery (ITA) is usually used as a pedicled graft to the LAD and is supplemented by either a second ITA graft or radial artery graft to the left system and/or saphenous vein grafts interposed between the aorta and the coronary arteries (Figure 1.1).

   a. The saphenous vein should be harvested endoscopically to minimize patient discomfort, reduce the incidence of leg edema and wound healing problems, and optimize cosmesis. There are some concerns that endoscopic harvesting could produce endothelial damage that might compromise long-term patency and reduce long-term survival, but with more experience, this has not been found to be an issue.[68–70]

   b. Use of additional arterial conduits (bilateral ITAs, radial artery) can be recommended to improve event-free survival.[71–73] The radial artery can be harvested endoscopically using a tourniquet to minimize bleeding during the harvest with placement of a drain afterward to prevent blood accumulation within the tract. With radial artery grafting, use of a topical vasodilator, such as a combination of verapamil-nitroglycerin, is useful in minimizing spasm.[74] The STS guidelines suggest use of a systemic vasodilator during surgery, and IV diltiazem 0.1 mg/kg/h

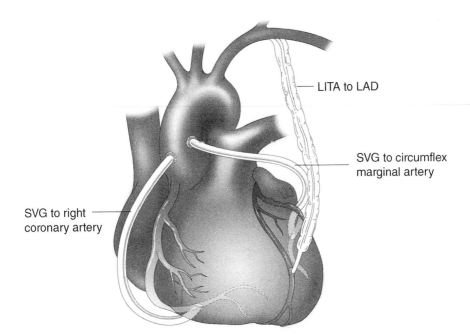

LITA to LAD

SVG to circumflex marginal artery

SVG to right coronary artery

Figure 1.1 • Coronary artery bypass grafting. A left internal thoracic artery (LITA) has been placed to the left anterior descending (LAD) artery with aortocoronary saphenous vein grafts (SVG) to the circumflex marginal and right coronary arteries.

(usually 5–10 mg/h) or IV nitroglycerin 10–20 µg/min (0.1–0.2 µg/kg/min) are commonly used.[71] This is continued in the intensive care unit and then converted to either amlodipine 5 mg po qd or Imdur 20 mg po qd for several months. The purported benefit of such pharmacologic management to prevent spasm has been universally accepted, although not rigorously studied, and routine use may not be indicated.[75]

2. Concerns about the adverse effects of CPB spurred the development of **"off-pump" coronary surgery (OPCAB)**, during which complete revascularization should be achieved with the avoidance of CPB. Deep pericardial sutures and various retraction devices are used to position the heart for grafting without hemodynamic compromise. A stabilizing platform minimizes movement at the site of the arteriotomy (Figure 1.2). Intracoronary or aortocoronary shunting can minimize ischemia after an arteriotomy is performed.

   a. Conversion to on-pump surgery may be necessary in the following circumstances:

      i. Coronary arteries are very small, severely diseased, or intramyocardial.

      ii. LV function is very poor, or there is severe cardiomegaly or hypertrophy that precludes adequate cardiac translocation without hemodynamic compromise or arrhythmias.

      iii. The heart is extremely small and vertical in orientation.

      iv. Uncontrollable ischemia or arrhythmias develop with vessel occlusion that persists despite distal shunting.

      v. Intractable bleeding occurs that cannot be controlled with vessel loops or an intracoronary shunt.

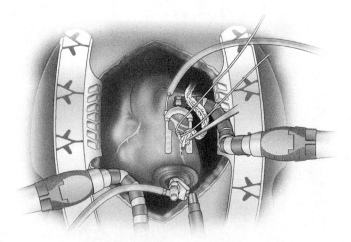

Figure 1.2 • Off-pump bypass grafting requires displacement of the heart using techniques to avoid hemodynamic compromise. These may include placement and elevation of deep pericardial sutures or the use of an apical suction device. A stabilizing device is used to minimize motion and a proximal vessel loop is placed to minimize bleeding at the site of the anastomosis.

b. OPCABs reduce transfusion requirements and the incidence of AF, but whether there is a reduction in the risk of stroke and renal dysfunction remains controversial.[76] OPCABs generally result in fewer grafts being placed, resulting in more incomplete revascularization and more repeat revascularization. Numerous long-term follow-up studies have shown inferior survival to on-pump surgery.[77–79] Enthusiasm for this technique is modest, and it is estimated that less than 20% of CABGs are performed off-pump. One randomized trial did show better outcomes with OPCABs when performed for a STEMI within six hours from the onset of symptoms or for patients in cardiogenic shock,[80] but most surgeons reserve its use for patients with limited disease. Its major advantage may be in the very high-risk patient with multiple comorbidities in whom it is critical to avoid CPB.

c. In some patients with severe ventricular dysfunction, the heart will not tolerate the manipulation required during off-pump surgery. In this circumstance, right ventricular (RV) assist devices can be used to improve hemodynamics. Alternatively, surgery can be done on-pump on an empty beating heart to avoid the period of cardioplegic arrest. This technique may be beneficial in patients with ascending aortic disease that prevents safe aortic cross-clamping, but does allow for safe cannulation and use of an aortic punch, such as the Heartstring proximal seal system (MAQUET Cardiovascular), to perform the proximal anastomoses.

3. **Minimally invasive direct coronary artery bypass (MIDCAB)** involves bypassing the LAD with the LITA without use of CPB via a short left anterior thoracotomy incision. Bilateral ITAs can be harvested under direct vision and an additional incision is made in the right chest to bypass the right coronary artery.[81,82] Combining a LITA to the LAD with stenting of other vessels ("hybrid" procedure) has also been described. A meta-analysis of the MIDCAB procedure found a lower risk of repeat revascularization compared with PCI of the LAD.[83]

4. **Robotic or totally endoscopic coronary artery bypass (TECAB)** can be used to minimize the extent of the surgical incisions and reduce trauma to the patient. Robotics can be used for both ITA takedown and grafting to selected vessels through small ports.[84] These procedures can be done without CPB or using CPB with femoral cannulation. Generally, TECAB is used for limited grafting, but wider applicability is certainly feasible. Anesthetic concerns during this procedure are discussed in Chapter 4, pages 265–266.

5. **Transmyocardial revascularization (TMR)** is a technique in which laser channels are drilled in the heart with CO_2 or holmium-YAG lasers to improve myocardial perfusion. Although the channels occlude within a few days, the inflammatory reaction created induces neoangiogenesis that may be associated with upregulation of various growth factors, such as vascular endothelial growth factor. This procedure is most commonly used as adjunct to CABG in viable regions of the heart where bypass grafts cannot be placed.[85,86] It can also be used as a sole procedure performed through a left thoracotomy or thoracoscopically for patients with inoperable CAD in regions of viable myocardium.[87] TMR has a level IIb indication to improve symptoms and may be reasonable to consider in patients with viable ischemic myocardium in areas that cannot be grafted.[5]

II. Left Ventricular Aneurysm

A. **Pathophysiology.** Occlusion of a major coronary artery may produce extensive transmural necrosis, which converts muscle into thin scar tissue. This results in formation of a left ventricular aneurysm (LVA) which exhibits dyskinesia during ventricular systole. Most LVAs occur in the anteroapical region due to occlusion of the LAD without collateralization, and are more likely to form in the absence of a patent infarct-related vessel. In contrast, early reperfusion of an occluded vessel by PCI or thrombolytic therapy may limit the extent of myocardial damage with preservation of epicardial viability, resulting in an area of akinesia. This will result in an ischemic cardiomyopathy with a dilated ventricle that remodels with altered spherical geometry but does not produce an aneurysm.

B. **Presentation.** The most common presentation of an LVA associated with an ischemic cardiomyopathy is heart failure (HF) due to systolic dysfunction. With LVAs, there is a reduction of forward stroke volume caused by geometric remodeling of the aneurysmal segment due to loss of contractile tissue and an increase in ventricular dimensions. This results in an increase in wall stiffness and an increase in the LV end-diastolic pressures. Angina may also occur due to the increased systolic wall stress of a dilated ventricle and the presence of multivessel CAD. Systemic thromboembolism may result from thrombus formation within the dyskinetic or akinetic segment, with thrombus being noted in over 50% of cases. Malignant ventricular arrhythmias or sudden death may result from either enhanced automaticity or triggered activity related to myocardial ischemia and increased myocardial stretch, or to the development of a macroreentry circuit at the border zone between scar tissue and viable myocardium.

C. **Indications for surgery.** Surgery is usually not indicated for the patient with an asymptomatic aneurysm, because of its favorable natural history. This is in contrast to the unpredictable prognosis and absolute indication for surgery in a patient with a false aneurysm, which is caused by a contained rupture of the ventricular muscle. Surgery may be beneficial in the asymptomatic or mildly symptomatic patient with significant volume overload causing LV dilatation and reduced ventricular function prior to the development of advanced HF symptoms. It may also be considered where there is extensive clot formation present within the aneurysm. However, surgery is most commonly indicated to improve symptoms and prolong survival when one of the four clinical syndromes (angina, HF, embolization, or arrhythmias) is present. Arrhythmias may be treated by a nonguided endocardial resection through the aneurysm with/without cryosurgery along with subsequent placement of a transvenous implantable cardioverter-defibrillator (ICD).

D. **Preoperative considerations**

1. Echocardiography is best for assessing ventricular size and dimensions, wall motion of the noninfarcted segments, the presence of thrombus, and mitral valve function, which is often abnormal with dilated cardiomyopathies. Biplane left ventriculography is helpful in identifying regions of akinesia and dyskinesia and assessing the function of noninfarcted segments. Cardiac CT angiography or cardiovascular magnetic resonance imaging (CT-MRI) are also helpful in making the diagnosis, and the latter can also be used to assess myocardial viability.[88]

2. Patients with LVAs with LV dysfunction are usually managed with an ACE inhibitor and ß-blocker. Anticoagulation may also be given during the early postinfarction period, but may not be necessary in chronic aneurysms with thrombus due to the low risk of embolism.[89] If the patient remains on warfarin, bridging to surgery with heparin can be recommended.

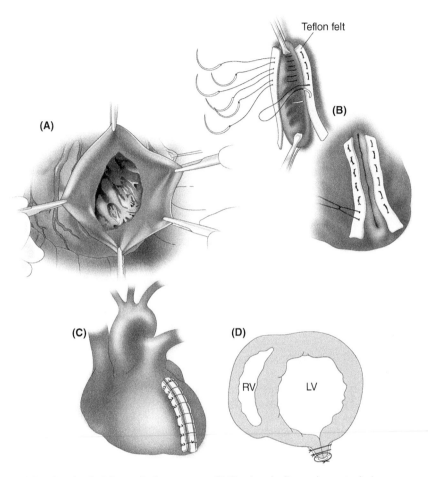

Figure 1.3 • Repair of a left ventricular aneurysm (LVA) using the linear closure technique. (A) The thinned-out scar tissue is opened and partially resected. Any LV thrombus is removed. (B) The aneurysm is then closed with mattress sutures over felt strips. (C) An additional over-and-over suture is placed over a third felt strip. (D) Cross-section of the final repair.

E. **Surgical procedures**

1. Standard aneurysmectomy ("linear repair") entails a ventriculotomy through the aneurysm, resection of the aneurysm wall, including part of the septum if involved, and linear closure over felt strips (Figure 1.3).[90,91]

2. Endoventricular reconstruction techniques are applicable to large aneurysms or akinetic segments with the intent of reducing ventricular volume and restoring an elliptical shape.

   a. The "endoaneurysmorrhaphy" technique is used for large aneurysms. A pericardial or Dacron patch is sewn to the edges of viable myocardium at the base of the aneurysm and the aneurysm wall is reapproximated over the patch

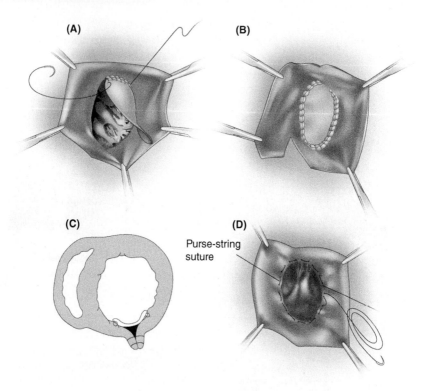

Figure 1.4 • Repair of a LVA using the endoaneurysmorrhaphy technique. (A, B) A pericardial patch is sewn at the base of the defect at the junction of the scar and normal myocardium to better preserve ventricular geometry. The resected edges of the LV are closed in a similar fashion to the linear technique. (C) Cross-section of the final repair. (D) The Dor procedure is a modification of this technique in which a circumferential pursestring suture is placed at the base of the defect to restore a normal orientation to the ventricle. A patch is then sewn over the defect.

(Figure 1.4). This preserves LV geometry and improves ventricular function to a greater degree than the linear closure method.

b. A slightly more elaborate endoventricular reconstruction involves the endoventricular circular patch plasty technique of Dor, which is termed "surgical ventricular restoration" (SVR). This can be applied to LVAs as well as cases of ischemic cardiomyopathy with anterior akinesis (Figure 1.4D).[92,93] The procedure involves placement of an encircling suture at the junction of the contracting and noncontracting segments, and then exclusion of the noncontracting segment with a patch. This produces an elliptical contour of the heart and results in significant improvement in ventricular size and function. This procedure is generally done on a beating heart to allow for better differentiation of akinetic and normal segments of the heart.

c. Although SVR is associated with a reduction in LV volume, clinical improvement is not uniform. Several studies have suggested that the addition of SVR to a CABG improves clinical status and long-term survival.[94–96] However, the

STICH trial of patients with CAD-related anterior akinesia or dyskinesia with an EF <35% was unable to demonstrate that reduction in LV size was associated with an improvement in symptoms or a reduction in mortality after four years.[97]

3. For patients with recurrent ventricular tachycardia, an endocardial resection with or without endocardial mapping may be performed with good results.[98,99]

4. Coronary bypass grafting of critically diseased vessels should be performed. Bypass of the LAD and diagonal arteries should be considered if septal reperfusion can be accomplished.

5. A mitral valve procedure is also indicated if the severity of MR is 2+ or greater. MR is usually related to apical tethering of the leaflets due to ventricular dilatation or may result from annular dilatation. Mitral valve repair with a complete annuloplasty ring may be successful when performed with ventricular restoration.

III. Ventricular Septal Rupture

A. **Pathophysiology.** Extensive myocardial damage subsequent to occlusion of a major coronary vessel may result in septal necrosis and rupture. This usually occurs within the first week of an infarction, more commonly in the anteroapical region (from occlusion of the LAD artery), and less commonly in the inferior wall (usually from occlusion of the right coronary artery). It is noted in less than 1% of acute MIs, and the incidence has declined because of early reperfusion therapy for STEMIs. The presence of a ventricular septal defect (VSD) is suggested by the presence of a loud holosystolic murmur that reflects the left-to-right shunting across the ruptured septum. The patient usually develops acute pulmonary edema and cardiogenic shock from the left-to-right shunt.[100]

B. **Indications for surgery.** Surgery is indicated on an emergency basis for nearly all postinfarction VSDs to prevent the development of progressive multisystem organ failure. A report from the STS database in 2012 noted an operative mortality rate of 54% if surgery was performed within seven days of an infarction, usually because the patient was hemodynamically unstable and often in cardiogenic shock. For surgery performed after seven days, the mortality rate decreased to 18.4%, most likely because these patients were more hemodynamically stable, had smaller VSDs and <2:1 shunts, and were naturally selected to have survived long enough to survive subsequent lower-risk surgery.[101] Risk factors for operative mortality included preoperative dialysis, older age, female gender, cardiogenic shock, use of an IABP, moderate–severe MR, redo operation, and emergency status.[102]

C. **Preoperative considerations**

1. Prompt diagnosis can be made using a Swan-Ganz catheter, which detects a step-up of oxygen saturation in the RV. Two-dimensional (2D) echocardiography can confirm the diagnosis of a VSD and differentiate it from acute MR, which can produce a similar clinical scenario.

2. Inotropic support and reduction of afterload, usually with an IABP, are indicated in virtually all patients with VSDs in anticipation of emergent cardiac catheterization and surgery.

3. Cardiac catheterization with coronary angiography should be performed to confirm the severity of the shunt and to identify associated CAD.

D. Surgical procedures

1. The traditional surgical treatment for postinfarct VSDs had been the performance of a ventriculotomy through the infarcted zone, resection of the area of septal necrosis, and Teflon felt or pericardial patching of the septum and free wall. This technique required transmural suturing and was prone to recurrence.

2. The preferred approach is to perform circumferential pericardial patching around the border of the infarcted ventricular muscle. This technique excludes the infarcted septum to eliminate the shunt and reduces recurrence rates, because suturing is performed to viable myocardium away from the area of necrosis (Figure 1.5).[103]

3. Coronary bypass grafting of critically diseased vessels should be performed. Early studies suggested this improved short- and long-term survival after surgery, but more recent data from the STS database did not corroborate this.[101,104]

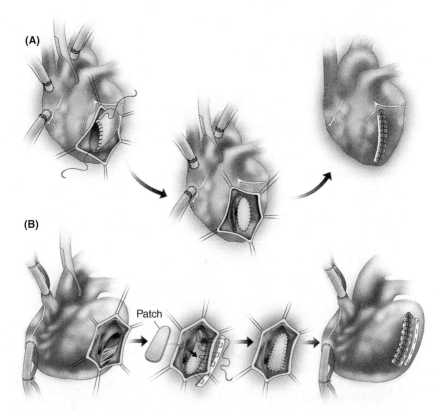

Figure 1.5 • Closure of a postinfarction ventricular septal defect (VSD) using the exclusion technique. (A) Anterior VSD. (B) Inferior VSD. The pericardial patch is anchored to viable myocardium away from the site of the defect, thus eliminating shunt flow across the septal defect. (Reproduced with permission from David et al., *Semin Thorac Cardiovasc Surg* 1998;10:105–10.)[103]

4. Consideration may be given to percutaneous VSD closure with the Amplatzer VSD closure device in patients with smaller VSDs or prohibitive surgical risks.[105] Use of MCS may also be considered in patients in cardiogenic shock to improve hemodynamics and organ system function, allowing for a lower-risk nonemergency procedure at a future date.

IV. Aortic Stenosis

A. **Pathophysiology.** Aortic stenosis (AS) results from thickening, calcification, and/or fusion of the aortic valve leaflets, which produce an obstruction to LV outflow.[106,107] In younger patients, AS usually develops on congenitally bicuspid valves, whereas in older patients, degenerative change in trileaflet valves is more common. Aortic sclerosis is a very common finding in elderly patients, and may be a manifestation of atherosclerosis, but usually does not progress to AS. Progression of AS may be related to endothelial cell activation and atherogenesis, as it is associated with the presence of cardiac risk factors, including hypertension, hyperlipidemia, and diabetes, but it has not been shown that statins or other medical therapy will slow the progression of degenerative AS.[108,109]

1. The impairment to cusp opening leads to pressure overload, compensatory left ventricular hypertrophy (LVH), and reduced ventricular compliance. The development of LVH maintains normal wall stress and a normal EF.

2. If the increase in wall thickness does not increase in proportion to the rise in intraventricular pressure, wall stress will increase and EF will fall. It is important to assess whether a reduced EF in patients with severe AS is the result of excessive afterload (i.e. inadequate hypertrophy to overcome the obstruction) or depressed contractility. If the latter is present, surgical risk is higher.

3. In patients with excessive and inappropriate degrees of LVH, wall stress is low and the heart will become hyperdynamic with a very high EF. This finding portends a worse prognosis after surgical correction.[110]

B. **Symptoms.** The classic symptoms associated with AS are angina, shortness of breath, and syncope. However, fatigue with limited activity appears to be one of the first symptoms described by most patients.

1. Angina may result from the increased myocardial oxygen demand caused by increased wall stress, from reduction in blood supply per gram of hypertrophied tissue, and/or from limited coronary vasodilator reserve. Hypertrophied hearts are more sensitive to ischemic injury, and exercise may induce subendocardial ischemia, inducing systolic or diastolic dysfunction. Thus, angina may occur with or without concomitant epicardial CAD.

2. Congestive HF results from elevation of filling pressures (LV end-diastolic pressure) with diastolic dysfunction and eventually by progressive decline in LV systolic function. This results in progressively worsening dyspnea on exertion.

3. Cardiac output is relatively fixed across the valve orifice and can lead to faintness, dizziness, or frank syncope in the face of peripheral vasodilation.

4. Palpitations may occur with the occurrence of AF, which, if persistent, leads to clinical deterioration, because the hypertrophied ventricle relies on atrial contraction to maintain a satisfactory stroke volume.

C. **Diagnosis.** Most patients do not become symptomatic until the degree of AS becomes severe (Table 1.1). The severity of AS is preferentially assessed by Doppler

Table 1.1 • Stages of Aortic Stenosis

Stage A: At risk for AS
Stage B: Progressive AS
Stage C: Asymptomatic severe AS (with AVA <1 cm²)
  C1: Asymptomatic with mean gradient >40 mm Hg
  C2: Asymptomatic with LV dysfunction
Stage D: Symptomatic severe AS (with AVA <1 cm²)
  D1: Symptomatic with high-gradient AS
  D2: Symptomatic with severe low flow/low gradient AS with reduced LVEF
  D3: Symptomatic with severe low flow/low gradient AS with normal LVEF
    (paradoxical low flow)[106]

Table 1.2 • Echocardiographic Assessment of the Severity of Aortic Stenosis

Indicator	Mild	Moderate	Severe
Jet velocity (m/s)	<3.0	3.0–4.0	>4.0
Mean gradient (mm Hg)	<25	25–40	>40
Aortic valve area (cm²)	>1.5	1.0–1.5	<1.0
Aortic valve area index (cm²/m²)			<0.6
Dimensionless index			<0.25

echocardiography, with evaluation by cardiac catheterization only indicated in equivocal cases. Performing a left heart catheterization and crossing the valve to measure gradients in a patient with known severe AS is considered a contraindication by the ACC guidelines (Level III indication) because of the increased risk of embolic stroke.[111] Coronary angiography is indicated before surgery to identify whether CAD is present.

1. Doppler echocardiography assesses the severity of AS by measuring the maximum instantaneous jet velocity and the mean transvalvular gradient, and allows for calculation of the aortic valve area (AVA) using the continuity equation (Tables 1.2 and 1.3, Figure 1.6). Because this calculation also includes the cross-sectional area of the left ventricular outflow tract (LVOT), it may indicate a very small valve area in a very small patient when severe stenosis may not be present. Using the ratio of the velocity time integral (VTI) of the LVOT to the aorta to eliminate the LVOT measurement provides a "dimensionless index". Echo imaging in the short-axis view can also measure the valve area directly by planimetry and can give an appreciation of the degree of calcification and cusp separation during systole.

Table 1.3 • Hemodynamics of Advanced Stages of Aortic Stenosis with Indications for AVR

Stage	Symptoms	AVA	Peak velocity (m/s)	Mean gradient (mm Hg)	Other considerations
C1	No	<1 cm²	>4	>40	Severe leaflet calcification or positive ETT
C2	No	<1 cm²	>4	>40	LV dysfunction (EF <50%)
D1	Yes	<1 cm²	>4	>40	
D2	Yes	<1 cm²	<4	<40	LV dysfunction (EF <50%)
D3	Yes	<1 cm²	<4	<40	SVI <35 mL/m²

SVI, stroke volume index

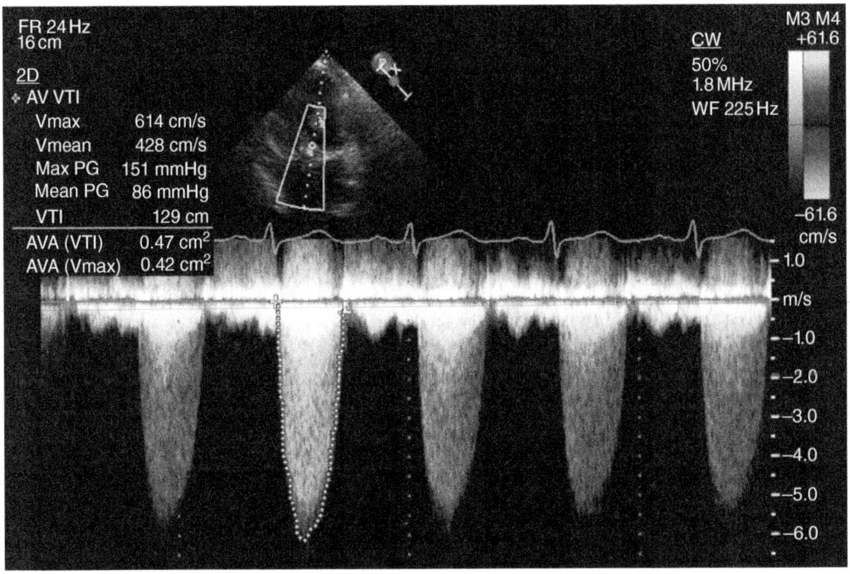

Figure 1.6 • Two-dimensional echocardiogram with continuous wave Doppler demonstrating very severe aortic stenosis.

2. Since the pressure gradient is related to both the orifice area and the transvalvular flow, low gradients may be noted with low stroke volumes despite an AVA of <1 cm². This issue of AVA-gradient discordance might create confusion as to which patients actually have severe AS and would benefit from an intervention versus those who might not.[112-114] Therefore, a critical measurement during echocardiography is calculation of the stroke volume index (SVI). A low-flow state (SVI

<35 mL/m²) can be seen in patients with reduced or preserved EF. This concept has led to a classification system incorporating SVI and EF.[115]

a. **Normal-flow, high gradient** (NF/HG), which fits the classic definition of severe AS (i.e. AVA <1 cm², peak velocity (Vmax) >4 m/s, or a mean gradient >40 mm Hg).

b. **Normal-flow, low gradient** (NF/LG), which in most cases is not severe AS. However, some studies have shown that NF/LG patients with an indexed AVA <0.6 cm²/m² have improved survival with aortic valve replacement (AVR).[113,114]

c. **Low-flow, high gradient** (LF/HG), which by virtue of gradient and AVA would be severe AS.

d. **Low-flow, low-gradient** (LF/LG), which can be seen with a normal EF, termed "paradoxical LF/LG" AS (stage D3 if symptomatic) or with a reduced EF (stage D2 if symptomatic). In the LF/LG patient, survival without surgery appears to be worse than in the other groups, and survival is markedly improved by AVR.[116]

3. Dobutamine stress echocardiography (DSE) is an important test in patients with LF/LG as well as NF/LG AS to corroborate the severity of AS. In patients with normal LV function, it has limited value except to indicate that the patient might have pseudo-severe AS. However, in patients with impaired LV function, it can be used to determine contractile reserve and assess whether the patient has true or pseudo-severe AS. The latter is present if dobutamine increases cardiac output without a concomitant increase in gradient, so the AVA increases to >1 cm². About one-third of patients with LF/LG, both with normal and reduced EF, are felt to have pseudo-severe AS.[113]

4. Quantification of aortic valve calcium has been recommended as a means of identifying severe AS in patients with LF/LG and NF/LG and has correlated with clinical outcomes.[117–119]

5. Assessment of the degree of AS is generally not indicated at the time of catheterization, except in equivocal cases. The AVA is calculated by most cath lab software programs and is derived from a measurement of transvalvular flow (essentially the cardiac output or stroke volume) and the peak and mean pressure gradients across the valve calculated from pressures obtained on a catheter pull-back from the LV into the aorta (Figure 2.4, page 136). The AVA may be manually calculated using the Gorlin formula:

$$AVA = \frac{CO/(SEP \times HR)}{44.3 \times \sqrt{mean\ gradient}}$$

where:

AVA = aortic valve area in cm² (normal = 2.5 − 3.5 cm²)

CO = cardiac output in mL/min

SEP = systolic ejection period/beat

HR = heart rate

Alternatively, the simplified Hakki formula calculates the AVA as follows:

$$AVA = \frac{CO \text{ (liters/min)}}{\sqrt{\text{peak-to-peak gradient}}}$$

6. If the above tests confirm the presence of severe AS, yet the patient is asymptomatic, exercise testing may be used to assess whether AVR may be indicated.[120,121] A meta-analysis reported that adverse cardiac events were three times more likely to occur in patients with an abnormal stress test, which was defined as the development of symptoms, a decrease in blood pressure or an increase in systolic pressure of <20%, <80% of normal exercise tolerance, ≥2 mm ST depression during exercise, or the development of complex ventricular arrhythmias. Thus, these findings were incorporated into the 2014 indications for AVR, such that a positive stress test was a level I indication for AVR.

7. Virtually all of the indications for AVR in the guidelines are for patients with severe AS, whether symptomatic or not. However, some patients with moderate AS and LV systolic dysfunction are symptomatic and at risk for adverse clinical events. It is not clear if earlier AVR may be beneficial to these patients.[122]

D. Natural history

1. It is estimated that approximately 40% of patients with asymptomatic severe AS will become symptomatic within two years and about 67% will be symptomatic by five years.[123,124] The rate of progression of AS is variable, and serial echocardiograms should be performed to assess for the rate of hemodynamic progression, which is predictive of clinical outcome. Patients with high jet velocities, LV hypertrophy, or severe valve calcification have a faster rate of progression of valve stenosis and a shorter symptom-free interval.

2. The presence of LV systolic dysfunction is an uncommon but ominous prognostic sign, as the long-term outlook is dismal. Although survival is generally improved by AVR for patients with LV dysfunction caused by afterload mismatch, a study from the Mayo Clinic reported a nearly 50% five-year mortality for asymptomatic patients with severe AS with an EF <50% with no survival benefit noted for AVR.[125] Another study of patients with moderate AS yet LV dysfunction found that most patients were symptomatic and were at high risk for clinical events.[122]

3. BNP (brain natriuretic peptide) levels in asymptomatic patients correlate with adverse events, including aortic valve-related deaths and HF admissions, so BNP or pro-BNP levels can serve as markers supporting early AVR.[126]

4. Once symptoms of AS are present, the prognosis for untreated AS is very poor with an average survival of one to two years and a less than 20% chance of surviving five years.[127] These data have been confirmed in the era of transcatheter aortic valve replacement (TAVR), with the PARTNER B cohort of "inoperable" patients having a 50% one-year mortality without AVR.[128] Patients with symptoms of heart failure (HF) have the worst survival, averaging only one year, whereas average survival is two years for patients with syncope and four years for patients with angina.

5. AVR has unequivocally been shown to improve survival, and in elderly patients has been found to restore a normal life expectancy. However, in younger patients (age <50), one study found a substantial loss in life expectancy.[129] It can be theorized that intervention prior to the development of myocardial fibrosis

might improve long-term results, thus justifying early intervention in asymptomatic patients with severe aortic stenosis.[130]

E. Indications for AVR per 2020 ACC Guidelines[131]

1. Class I indications ("AVR is recommended")

- Stage D1 – symptomatic patients with a peak velocity ≥4 m/s or a mean gradient >40 mm Hg; this also includes patients who may be asymptomatic at rest but have symptoms during an exercise tolerance test (ETT).

- Stage C2 – patients who are asymptomatic but have high gradients and depressed LV function (EF <50%). Survival will be improved by AVR if LV dysfunction is caused by afterload mismatch, but to a lesser degree if caused by impaired contractile reserve.

- Severe AS (any stage C or D) in a patient undergoing other cardiac surgery with a peak velocity ≥4 m/s or a mean gradient ≥40 mm Hg.

- Stage D2 – symptomatic patients with an AVA <1 cm² but a mean gradient <40 mm Hg with reduced EF. Since the gradient is conditional upon transvalvular flow, these patients are considered to have "low flow, low gradient" severe AS. A DSE should be performed to determine whether poor ventricular function with a low stroke volume is primarily related to afterload mismatch from true severe AS or is due to contractile dysfunction.

  i. If dobutamine produces an increase in stroke volume (or cardiac output) with little increase in gradient, the valve area may increase to >1 cm², suggesting this may be pseudo-severe AS. However, if both the gradient and cardiac output increase in tandem, the AVA will remain <1 cm², confirming severe AS. Patients in this category achieve a significant benefit from AVR.[132]

  ii. Confirmation of stage D2 generally requires an increase in the peak velocity to >4 m/s or a mean gradient to >40 mm Hg with dobutamine. However, the validity of the DSE may be limited if dobutamine fails to increase the stroke volume more than 20%. These patients have poor contractile reserve, suggesting that afterload mismatch is not the problem and inferentially that AVR may not improve LV function. However, studies have shown that both surgical aortic valve replacement (SAVR) and TAVR improve LV function independent of contractile reserve and improve long-term survival.[133,134] Interestingly, an elevated BNP level (>550) has been shown to be a very strong predictor of operative mortality, even more important than lack of contractile reserve documented by DSE.[135] Some studies have suggested that DSE has limited value in predicting the severity of AS and outcomes of AVR.[136] Use of the projected AVA (which estimates the AVA at a standardized normal flow rate) can better distinguish pseudo-severe from severe AS and correlates better with observed mortality in patients managed conservatively.[137,138]

- Stage D3 – symptomatic patients with an AVA <1 cm² (indexed AVA ≤0.6 cm²/m²), a low gradient, normotension, but a normal EF. In addition, a calcified valve with significantly reduced leaflet motion should be present. These patients are considered to have "paradoxical low flow/low gradient" severe AS if the SVI is <35 mL/m².[138] Reduced transvalvular flow may produce lower gradients despite the presence of a severely stenotic valve. This may be noted in patients with AF, concomitant MR, and impaired diastolic filling, and may be exacerbated in hypertensive patients with reduced arterial compliance or increased vascular resistance.[112]

The prognosis is poor with medical therapy, and both SAVR and TAVR have been shown to improve survival in these patients.[114,139,140] Nonetheless, one study found that the survival of LF/LG patients with normal EF was fairly similar to that of patients with mild–moderate AS and was not influenced by performing an AVR.[141]

- When the indication for AVR is met, the ascending aorta should be resected if ≥4.5 cm, whether with bicuspid or trileaflet valves.

2. Class IIa indications ("AVR is reasonable")

- Stage C1 – asymptomatic low-risk patients in whom exercise testing shows decreased exercise tolerance or a fall in systolic BP ≥10 mm Hg.
- Stage C1 – asymptomatic patients with very severe AS with a peak velocity ≥5 m/s. Nearly 50% of these patients will become symptomatic within 2 years and AVR has been shown to produce a significant survival benefit.[142]
- Stage C1 – asymptomatic patients with a BNP level > 3 times normal.
- Stage C1 – asymptomatic, high gradient patients in whom serial testing shows an increase in aortic velocity >0.3 m/s/yr.

3. Class IIb indications ("AVR may be considered")

- Stage C1 – asymptomatic patients with severe high-gradient AS with a progressive decrease in LVEF on 3 serial imaging studies to <60%.
- Stage B – asymptomatic patients with moderate AS undergoing other cardiac surgery. Most surgeons would consider performing an AVR with a cutoff around an AVA < 1.4 cm² to avoid another operation in the next few years. However, with the applicability of TAVR, the surgeon may consider not replacing the valve with an AVA >1.2 cm² with a mean gradient in the teens.

F. **Indications for AVR per 2017 appropriate use criteria.**[143] A 2017 publication from multiple societies reviewed the 2014 criteria noted above as well as the 2017 focused update and assessed the appropriateness of AVR for severe AS (AVA <1 cm²) in 95 different clinical scenarios, coding them as "appropriate", "may be appropriate", or "rarely appropriate". Assessments were made for patients corresponding to stages C1–2 and D1–3, those with comorbidities or frailty that might alter the procedural approach, and for patients requiring additional surgery (ascending aorta, valve, CABG) or undergoing reoperations. For certain categories, recommendations for surgical AVR (SAVR) or TAVR were made. Some differences from the 2014 criteria noted above include the following:

1. AVR "may be appropriate" for asymptomatic patients with high gradient AS (Vmax 4–4.9 m/s), a negative stress test, and no predictors of symptom onset or rapid progression, such as Vmax >0.3 m/s/yr, severe valve calcification, elevated BNP, or excessive LVH in the absence of hypertension. These stage C1 patients would not be candidates for AVR per the 2014 criteria unless the peak velocity was >5 m/s. However, AVR would be appropriate for these patients in the 2014 and AUC guidelines if the stress test were positive or these predictors were present.

2. AVR "may be appropriate" for asymptomatic patients with LF/LG severe AS with normal EF with a heavily calcified valve. As these patients would be stage C, not stage D3, AVR per the 2014 criteria would only be indicated if these patients were symptomatic and had an SVI <35 mL/m².

3. AVR is "appropriate" for symptomatic patients with preserved EF, NF/LG and an AVA <1 cm² if they have a heavily calcified valve, the latter being referred to as "a

calcified valve with significantly reduced leaflet motion" in the 2014 guidelines. However these guidelines also required a low SVI to qualify for an AVR.

4. AVR was "inappropriate" for patients with an EF of 20–49%, and LF/LG severe AS with no flow reserve on low-dose DSE. Although not specifically addressed in the 2014 guidelines, the literature does suggest that, despite the increased risk, SAVR or preferably TAVR may provide a hemodynamic and clinical benefit to these patients.[133,134]

5. AVR was "inappropriate" for patients with an EF <20% with a mean gradient <20 at rest and no flow reserve. The issue for these patients is whether there might be any clinical improvement after AVR despite lack of contractile reserve if the valve appeared severely stenotic on echo. Surgery would probably be contraindicated due to the high risk, but high risk "salvage" TAVR might be considered if the patient were severely symptomatic, had normal mental status, no other major comorbidities, and understood that the procedure might not provide any benefit.

G. Selection of procedure: TAVR vs. SAVR

1. The clinical trials of TAVR vs. medical therapy and TAVR vs. SAVR have confirmed excellent clinical outcomes for patients with progressively lower STS risk profiles, such that in 2019, TAVR was approved in the United States for use in low-risk patients.[144] Comparable results have been noted with the balloon-expandable valves (primarily the Edwards SAPIEN series) and self-expanding valves (primarily the Medtronic CoreValve/Evolut series). Consequently, calculation of the predicted operative risk using the STS risk model, which has been updated to reflect more comorbidities including frailty, has become less important in the selection of the appropriate procedure.

2. Not only have the hemodynamics of TAVR valves proven to be superior to surgically implanted valves with lower transvalvular gradients,[145] but the risk of mortality and morbidity with transfemoral TAVR procedures has been equivalent to if not better than SAVR. The risk of stroke is approximately 2% with the latest generation TAVR valves, and the need for a permanent pacemaker has gradually been declining, now estimated at around 5%, comparable to or perhaps slightly greater than SAVR. Patient recovery is expedited by the less-invasive nature of the procedure, and improvement in the quality of life is better as well. Remaining issues are those of long-term durability of the transcatheter valves if they are to be used in younger patients,[146] successful implantation within bicuspid valves, and use in patients with pure aortic regurgitation, which most likely will be feasible with newer valve designs.

3. AUC for TAVR continue to evolve, so any published recommendation is outdated. The STS-TVT registry tracks implantation data, and TAVR volumes have exceeded SAVRs for several years, and will only increase with the inclusion of more low-risk patients. TAVRs are indicated for the same reasons as SAVRs, but are preferable when the risk is high and the benefit is uncertain.

H. **Preoperative considerations**

1. Prior to SAVR or TAVR, coronary angiography should be performed in any patient over the age of 40 or in a younger patient with coronary risk factors, angina, or a positive stress test. TAVR can generally be performed in patients without an extensive ischemic burden, but preliminary or simultaneous PCI can be considered if TAVR is selected over SAVR + CABG.

2. Ischemic syndromes in patients with AS require judicious management. Medications that must be used very cautiously are those that can reduce preload

(nitroglycerin), afterload (calcium channel blockers), or heart rate (β-blockers), because they may lower cardiac output and precipitate cardiac arrest in a patient with critical AS. The ventricular response to AF must be controlled.

3. Some patients with AS have a history of gastrointestinal bleeding ascribed to colonic angiodysplasia (Heyde's syndrome). This has been associated with acquired type 2A von Willebrand syndrome.[147,148] This develops due to proteolysis of the largest multimers of von Willebrand factor by shear stress on the blood as it passes through the stenotic valve. Understandably, this is also noted with dysfunctional prosthetic valves.[149] These multimers are important for platelet-mediated hemostasis, so when reduced, they can cause bleeding. Use of preoperative desmopressin (0.3 μg/kg) given after the induction of anesthesia in patients with abnormal platelet function associated with this syndrome has been shown to significantly reduce perioperative blood loss.[150] AVR generally will resolve this hemostatic problem.

4. Dental work should be performed before surgery to minimize the risk of prosthetic valve endocarditis (PVE), unless it is felt to be a prohibitive risk. A study from the Mayo Clinic reported a 3% risk of death within 30 days after dental extraction in patients awaiting surgery.[151]

5. Selection of the appropriate procedure and valve type for surgical AVR depends on a number of factors, including the patient's age, contraindications to long-term anticoagulation, and the patient's desire to avoid anticoagulation. All mechanical valves require lifelong warfarin, as the NOACs do not appear to suffice. Structural valve deterioration of tissue valves is inversely related to patient age and is worse in the presence of renal failure (Figure 1.7). Improvements in

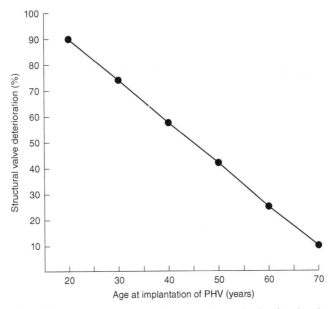

Figure 1.7 • Correlation of patient age with the risk of structural valve deterioration of tissue valves at 15–20 years. (Reproduced with permission from Rahimtoola, *J Am Coll Cardiol* 2010;55:2413–26.)

valve preservation techniques may improve valve longevity, supporting the use of tissue valves in younger patients. When either severe bioprosthetic stenosis or regurgitation occurs, it may be treated by reoperation or a valve-in-valve TAVR. The latter can often provide superior hemodynamics to even the original valve replacement because many tissue valve frames can be fractured allowing for better expansion of the transcatheter valve within the valve orifice.[152]

6. Selection of valve product for TAVRs is a matter of preference and experience, with potentially lower gradients in the small aortic root with the Medtronic CoreValve Evolut valves, which are constructed of porcine pericardium within a nitinol frame and lie more supra-annular than the Edwards valves.

I. Surgical procedures

1. Aortic valve procedures may be performed through a full median sternotomy incision or through a minimally invasive incision. These include an upper or lower sternotomy with a "J" or "T" incision into the third or fourth intercostal space, or an anterior right second or third interspace incision.[153–155] Cannulation for CPB for minimally invasive approaches can be performed either through the incision or using the femoral vessels. If the latter is planned, a preliminary abdominal-pelvic CT scan should be performed to assess for iliofemoral artery size, tortuosity, and calcification.

2. SAVR with either a tissue or mechanical valve has been the standard treatment for AS (Figure 1.8), but has been superseded by the use of transcatheter valves in most patients.

   a. Mechanical valves of bileaflet tilting disk design have virtually completely replaced single-leaflet tilting disk valves. They require lifelong anticoagulation with warfarin. Valve longevity is contingent on the development of complications such as thrombus formation or pannus ingrowth that impairs leaflet function, or the development of endocarditis.

   b. Tissue valves include porcine and bovine pericardial valves, all of which have various heat or chemical treatments to improve longevity. Rapid deployment valves are often considered to reduce cross-clamp times during complex operations or in older patients. These include the Sorin Perceval valve and the Edwards Intuity valves. They have similar valve leaflets but are designed for implantation with few sutures to expedite implantation. The lower segment of the valve frame may predispose to bundle branch blocks and complete heart block, the latter being noted in about 10% of patients.[156,157]

   c. A stentless valve may be selected to provide a larger effective orifice area and may be placed in the subcoronary position or as a root replacement. Its primary benefit may be noted in the small aortic root (Figure 1.9).[158,159]

   d. The Ross procedure, in which the patient's own pulmonary valve is used to replace the aortic root, with the pulmonary valve being replaced with a homograft (basically a double-valve operation for single-valve disease), is an even more complicated procedure generally reserved for patients younger than age 50 who wish to avoid anticoagulation (Figure 1.10).[160,161]

   e. Homografts are usually reserved for patients with aortic valve endocarditis, although other types of prostheses arguably provide comparable results.[162,163]

   f. An aortic root replacement, usually as a valved conduit, is indicated when the ascending aorta must also be replaced (Figure 1.11). If the sinuses of Valsalva are not dilated, replacing the aortic valve and using a supracoronary graft simplifies the procedure. In younger patients, a commercially available mechanical

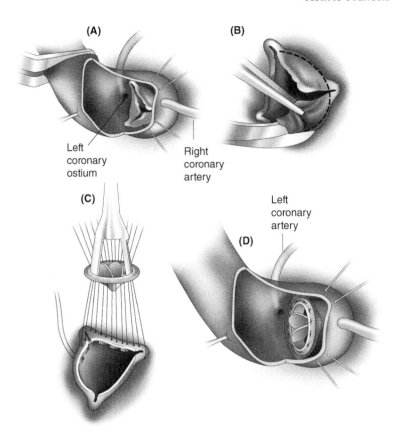

Figure 1.8 • Aortic valve replacement (AVR). (A) A transverse aortotomy incision is made and holding sutures are placed. (B) The valve is excised, and the annulus is debrided and sized. (C, D) Pledgeted mattress sutures are placed through the annulus and through the sewing ring of the valve, the valve is lowered to the annulus, and the sutures are tied. The aortotomy is then closed.

      valved conduit is selected. In older patients, a "bioroot" may be used to avoid anticoagulation. This is constructed by sewing a tissue valve into the proximal end of the Dacron graft.[164]

3. Transcatheter aortic valve replacement (TAVR) involves the endovascular placement of a tissue valve mounted on a catheter delivery system. Although numerous valves have been designed and are being evaluated, the two most popular ones are the Edwards SAPIEN series, which is a balloon-expandable bovine pericardial valve (Figure 1.12), and the Medtronic CoreValve/Evolut series, which has a porcine pericardial valve within a nitinol self-expanding valve frame delivered within a sheath (Figure 1.13). Both of these systems can be used for stenotic native valves as well as stenotic or regurgitant bioprosthetic valves ("valve-in-valve" procedure).

    a. A CT scan is an essential component of the preoperative evaluation. The chest imaging will assess the aortic annular area and perimeter to determine the appropriate-sized transcatheter heart valve. The distance from the annulus to the coronary ostia is measured to ensure that native valve displacement does

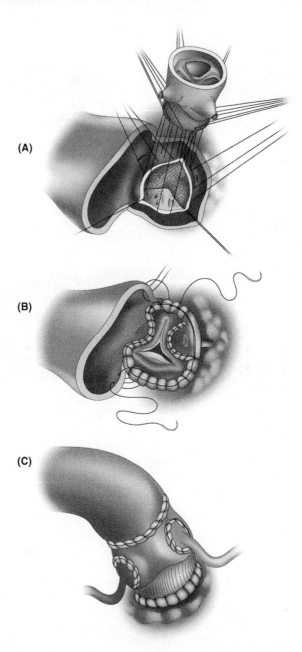

Figure 1.9 • Stentless valves have a larger effective orifice than stented valves, allowing for more regression of LV hypertrophy. (A) The proximal suture line sews the lower Dacron skirt of the prosthesis to the aortic annulus. (B) Subcoronary implantation of a Medtronic Freestyle valve. This requires scalloping of two sinuses with the distal suture line carried out below the coronary ostia. (C) A stentless valve can be used as a root replacement, requiring reimplantation of buttons of the coronary ostia. The distal suture line is an end-to-end anastomosis to the aortic wall.

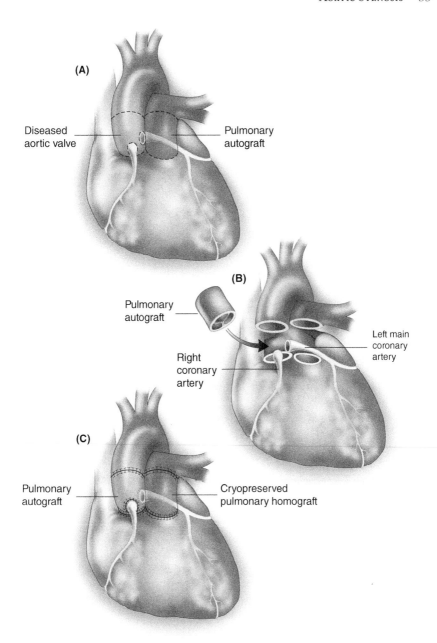

Figure 1.10 • Ross procedure. (A) The aorta is opened and the diseased aortic valve is removed. The pulmonic valve and main pulmonary artery are carefully excised and the coronary arteries are mobilized. (B) The pulmonary autograft is then transposed to the aortic root. (C) The coronary arteries are reimplanted and the RV outflow tract is reconstructed with a cryopreserved pulmonary valved homograft.

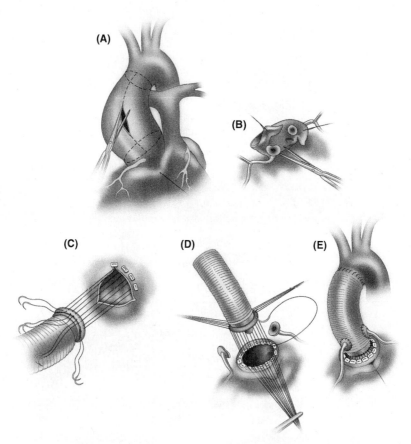

Figure 1.11 • Bentall procedure. (A) The aorta is opened and then divided proximally and distally. (B) Coronary ostial buttons are mobilized. (C, D) A valve incorporated into the proximal end of the conduit is sewn to the aortic annulus. (E) The coronary ostial buttons are reimplanted and the distal suture line is completed.

not obstruct the coronary ostia. This is especially important in valve-in-valve procedures. A BASILICA (Bioprosthetic Aortic Scallop Intentional Laceration to prevent Iatrogenic Coronary Artery obstruction) may be necessary in these procedures to avoid coronary ostial obstruction in patients with low coronary ostia. The abdominal-pelvic imaging assesses the size, tortuosity, and calcification of the iliofemoral vessels to determine whether a transfemoral approach is feasible (Figure 2.37, page 163).

b. The procedural risk is lower with a transfemoral approach. If not feasible, subclavian imaging should be evaluated to assess for axillary/subclavian access which can be achieved via cutdown or percutaneously. Additional alternative access sites include transcaval, transaortic through a limited upper sternotomy, transcarotid, and transapical approaches.[165–167] The latter was initially the approach of second choice, but was fraught with more complications, especially in elderly patients.

(A)   **(B)**

(C)   **(D)**

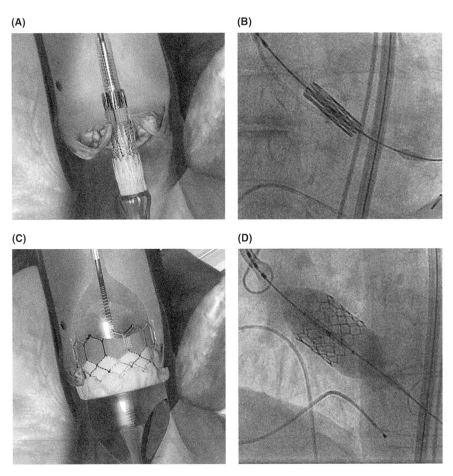

Figure 1.12 • Drawing and fluoroscopic images of a transcatheter aortic valve replacement (TAVR) with an Edwards SAPIEN 3 transcatheter heart valve. (A, B) Initial positioning across the native annulus. (C, D) Complete valve deployment by balloon inflation. (Image courtesy of Edwards Lifesciences (A and C)).

c. Transcatheter valves have less stent frame width than surgical valves and are designed for optimal opening of the leaflets. This produces superior hemodynamics to surgical valves, especially in the small aortic annulus. Clinical outcomes in patients at high, intermediate, and low surgical risk are equivalent, if not superior, to SAVR. The major risks are those of stroke, estimated at around 2%, which might be reduced by use of a cerebral protection device (SENTINEL cerebral protection systems [Boston Scientific Sentinel device]),[168–170] and the necessity for a permanent pacemaker for complete heart block. With less deployment in the LVOT, this risk has been substantially reduced to less than 5%. This risk is greater in patients with a pre-existing right bundle branch block and a left anterior hemiblock.

(A)

(B)

(C)

(D)

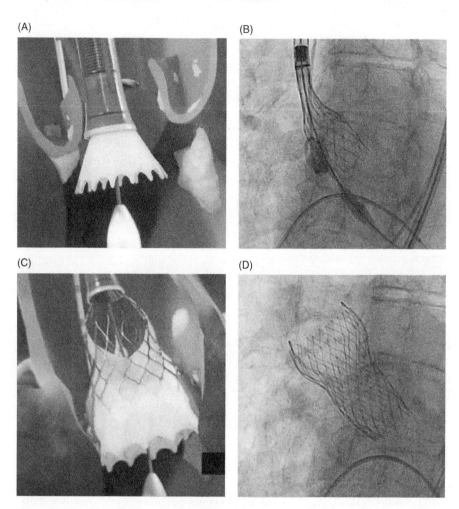

Figure 1.13 • Drawing and fluoroscopic images of a TAVR with a Medtronic Evolut Pro valve. (A, B) Partial self-expansion of the nitinol frame by withdrawal of the constraining sheath. (C, D) Complete valve deployment. (Image courtesy of Medtronic, Inc. (A and C)).

4. Reparative procedures, such as commissurotomy or debridement, have little role in the management of critical AS. However, debridement may be considered in the patient with moderate AS in whom the valve disease is not severe enough to warrant valve replacement, but in whom decalcification may delay surgery for a number of years.

V. Aortic Regurgitation

A. **Pathophysiology.** Aortic regurgitation (AR) results from abnormalities in the aortic valve leaflets (calcific degeneration, bicuspid valves, destruction from endocarditis) or from aortic root dilatation that prevents leaflet coaptation (idiopathic root dilatation causing annuloaortic ectasia, aortic dissection with cusp prolapse).[106]

Table 1.4 • Stages of Chronic Aortic Regurgitation

Stage A: At risk of AR (bicuspid valve, dilated sinuses, rheumatic heart disease)
Stage B: Progressive AR (mild–moderate AR, normal LV function and dimensions)
Stage C: Asymptomatic severe AR
    C1: Asymptomatic with EF ≥50% and LV-ESD ≤50 mm
    C2: Asymptomatic with EF ≤50% or LV-ESD >50 mm (indexed LVESD >25 mm/m^2)
Stage D: Symptomatic severe AR with any LVEF, moderate–severe LV dilatation

LV-ESD, left ventricular end-systolic dimension

1. Acute AR usually results from endocarditis or a type A dissection. The ventricle is unable to dilate acutely to handle the sudden increase in regurgitant volume, which increases the LV end-diastolic volume (LVEDV) and pressure (LVEDP), resulting in acute LV failure, cardiogenic shock, and pulmonary edema. Dramatic elevations in filling pressures may occur if acute AR is superimposed on a hypertrophied ventricle. Acute myocardial ischemia may result from increased afterload (LV dilatation), compensatory tachycardia, and a reduction in perfusion pressure as the LVEDP approaches the aortic diastolic pressure. As a result, sudden death may occur.

2. Chronic AR produces pressure and volume overload of the LV, resulting in progressive LV dilatation (increase in LVEDV) with an increase in wall stress, an increase in ventricular compliance, and progressive hypertrophy. Most patients remain asymptomatic for years, even with severe AR, because recruitment of preload reserve and compensatory hypertrophy maintain a normal EF despite the increased afterload. The increased stroke volume maintains forward output and is manifest by an increase in pulse pressure with bounding peripheral pulses. Eventually, increased afterload and impaired contractility lead to LV systolic dysfunction and a fall in EF. Usually at this point, the patient becomes symptomatic with dyspnea. Impairment of coronary flow reserve may cause angina (Table 1.4).

3. Generally, patients with advanced HF symptoms (NYHA class III–IV) or systolic dysfunction with a decreased EF and/or increased LV end-systolic dimension (LVESD) have a higher perioperative mortality rate and compromised long-term survival. Normalization of a depressed EF may occur after surgery when afterload excess is the cause of LV systolic dysfunction and when LV dysfunction is not long-standing. However, patients with prolonged LV dysfunction usually have depressed myocardial contractility and will have a suboptimal result from surgery with persistent LV dysfunction.

B. **Diagnosis.** Careful monitoring is essential to identify when patients become symptomatic, develop severe AR, and/or have evidence of incipient LV dysfunction. Echocardiography and aortic root aortography at the time of catheterization can delineate the degree of AR (Figure 2.8, page 138). Echo is valuable in assessing valve morphology, aortic root size, LV cavity dimensions, wall thickness, and systolic function. Color and pulsed wave Doppler findings can be used to assess the degree of AR (Table 1.5).

Table 1.5 • Echocardiographic Findings of Moderate and Severe Aortic Regurgitation

	Moderate	Severe
Doppler jet width	25–64% of LVOT	≥65% of LVOT
Vena contracta	0.3–0.6 cm	>0.6 cm
Diastolic flow reversal	no	yes
Regurgitant volume	0–59 mL/beat	≥60 mL/beat
Regurgitant fraction	30–49%	≥50%
ERO	0.1–0.29 cm²	≥0.3 cm²
LV dilatation	no	yes
Pressure half-time	200–500 ms	<200 ms

ERO, effective regurgitant orifice
Adapted with permission from Nishimura et al., *Circulation* 2014;129:e521–643.[107]

C. **Indications for surgery** (based on 2020 ACC guidelines)[131]

1. **Class I Indication** ("Surgery is recommended")

   a. Stage D – symptomatic severe AR, irrespective of LV systolic function. Once the heart becomes severely dilated, irreversible myocardial damage may already have occurred and the long-term results of surgery are suboptimal. The estimated mortality rate is >10%/year for patients with angina and >20%/year for patients with CHF without surgery.[106] Some patients are symptomatic with moderate AR when there is a reduced EF, LV dilatation, and a markedly elevated LVEDP.

   b. Stage C2 – asymptomatic severe AR with LVEF ≤55% at rest unless there is another cause for the decreased LVEF. These patients are already in a decompensated phase and develop symptoms at a rate of 25%/year. Prompt surgical intervention is indicated because long-term survival is compromised with a lower EF and LV dilatation (LVESD ≥40mm) due to more advanced remodeling.[171] If the etiology of the decreased EF is unrelated to the AR (i.e. a prior infarction, infiltrative disease, dilated cardiomyopathy), LV function may not improve and surgery may not be indicated.

   c. AVR is indicated for severe AR if cardiac surgery is being performed for another indication.

2. **Class IIa indication ("Surgery is reasonable")**

   a. Asymptomatic severe AR with an EF > 55% but LVESD >50 mm or indexed LVESD >25 mm/m². Evidence of LV dilatation also indicates a decompensated phase with a nearly 20% annual risk of developing systolic dysfunction once the LVESD exceeds 50 mm and a 25% risk once it exceeds 55 mm.

b. AVR is reasonable with moderate AR if other cardiac surgery is being performed for another indication.

3. **Class IIb indication ("Surgery may be considered")**

a. Stage C1 – Asymptomatic severe AR with normal EF (EF >55%), but with progressive severe LV dilatation (left ventricular end-diastolic dimension [LVEDD] >65 mm) or progressive decline in EF to the low-normal range (55-60%).These patients are at high risk for sudden death.

4. **Other comments**

a. Serial echocardiograms are important to identify early evidence of ventricular decompensation, since survival without surgery and the long-term prognosis after surgery are influenced by the degree of LV systolic dysfunction. Asymptomatic patients in stage C1 with an LVESD of 40–49 mm have about a 4% annual risk of developing symptoms, LV dysfunction or death, yet about 25% of patients may develop LV dysfunction or die before they become symptomatic. Thus, surgery is indicated at the first sign of ventricular decompensation, which is generally when the LVEF falls below 55% or the LVESD exceeds 50 mm.

b. The utility of stress testing in asymptomatic patients is not well defined. High-risk findings include development of symptoms, exercise capacity <85% of predicted, absence of contractile reserve with borderline hemodynamic indications for surgery (LVEF 50–55% or LVESD approaching 50 mm), and tricuspid valve annular plane systolic excursion <21 mm (a sign of RV dysfunction). These findings may identify patients who are truly not asymptomatic and those with subclinical LV dysfunction who might benefit from earlier surgery. A fall in ejection fraction during stress testing has unclear prognostic significance. None of these considerations was included in the 2014 guidelines.

c. Aortic valve endocarditis producing acute AR and hemodynamic compromise, or the presence of an annular abscess or conduction abnormalities are indications for urgent, if not emergent surgery (see section IX, pages 61–62). The presence of residual vegetations after an embolic event, large mobile vegetations, or persistent bacteremia are other indications for early surgery.

D. **Preoperative considerations**

1. Systemic hypertension may be treated with ACE inhibitors, ARBs, amlodipine, β-blockers, diuretics, and aldosterone receptor antagonists (spironolactone, eplerenone). Reducing the blood pressure may increase forward flow and reduce the degree of regurgitation, but excessive afterload reduction may reduce diastolic coronary perfusion pressure and exacerbate ischemia. β-blockers for control of ischemia must be used cautiously because a slow heart rate increases the amount of regurgitation. They are contraindicated in acute AR because they will block the compensatory tachycardia. ACE inhibitors and ARBs are usually held the morning of surgery to prevent vasoplegia, although this remains controversial.

2. Coronary angiography is indicated before surgery for virtually all patients to identify coronary dominance and potential stenoses that may need to be addressed.

3. Placement of an IABP for control of anginal symptoms is contraindicated.

4. As for all non-emergent valve patients, dental work should be completed before surgery.

5. Contraindications to warfarin should be identified so that the appropriate valve can be selected.

E. Surgical procedures

1. AVR has traditionally been the procedure of choice for adults with AR. This may involve use of a tissue or mechanical valve, the Ross procedure, or a cryopreserved homograft. Studies are underway to determine the feasibility of TAVR for pure AR.[172]

2. Aortic valve repair, involving resection of portions of the valve leaflets and re-approximation to improve leaflet coaptation (especially for bicuspid valves), often with a suture annuloplasty, has been performed successfully. This is valuable in the younger patient in whom any valve-sparing procedure is preferable to valve replacement.[173]

3. A valved conduit (Bentall procedure) is placed if an ascending aortic aneurysm ("annuloaortic ectasia") is also present (Figure 1.11). In younger patients, manufactured mechanical valved conduits are preferable, but if there is a strong indication for avoiding anticoagulation, a "bioroot" created by sewing a tissue valve into a graft can easily be accomplished.[174] Alternatively, a Medtronic Freestyle stentless valve can be placed with distal graft extension to replace an aortic aneurysm.[175]

4. Aortic valve-sparing root replacement is feasible in some patients with significant AR if adequate remodeling of the root can be accomplished, and it can be used successfully even in patients with bicuspid valves or Marfan syndrome (Figure 1.14). The aorta is resected, sparing the commissural pillars. A graft is then sewn at the subannular level, the aortic valve is resuspended within the graft, and the aortic remnants are sewn to the graft. Coronary ostial buttons are then sewn to the graft.[176–178]

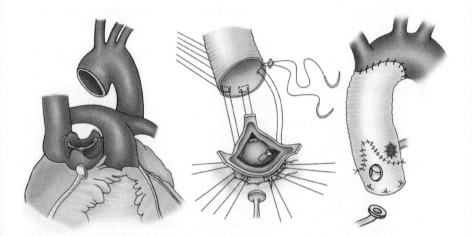

Figure 1.14 • Aortic valve-sparing root replacement. (A) The aortic root is resected, sparing the pillars that support the commissures and the coronary arteries are mobilized as buttons.
(B) Sutures are placed at the subannular level in a horizontal plane and passed through a tubular graft. (C) The graft is tied down and the aortic valve is resuspended by suturing the commissural posts and the base of the sinuses to the inside of the graft. The coronary buttons are reimplanted and the distal anastomosis is completed.

VI. Mitral Stenosis

A. **Pathophysiology.**[106] Mitral stenosis (MS) occurs nearly exclusively as a consequence of rheumatic fever. Thickening of the valve leaflets with commissural fusion and thickening and shortening of the chordae tendineae gradually reduce the size of the mitral valve orifice and the efficiency of LV filling. The increase in the diastolic transmitral gradient increases the left atrial and pulmonary venous pressures. Initially, left atrial size and compliance increase, and symptoms may be brought on by exercise or rapid heart rates, such as with AF. As the MS becomes severe, the left atrium remodels, and symptoms of heart failure, including dyspnea, orthopnea, and hemoptysis, may occur. An adaptive measure that can minimize symptoms is a decrease in pulmonary microvascular permeability and the development of pulmonary arteriolar vasoconstriction and thickening, which leads to pulmonary hypertension (PH). This may then lead to right-sided HF and functional tricuspid regurgitation (TR). As the severity of MS and PH worsen, the cardiac output is compromised at rest and fails to increase with exercise. The development of AF further increases LA pressures, decreases ventricular filling, and compromises cardiac output. It may predispose to left atrial thrombus formation and systemic thromboembolism (Table 1.6).

B. **Natural history.** MS is a slowly progressive process which may not produce symptoms for several decades. The minimally symptomatic patient has an 80% 10-year survival, but once symptoms develop, survival is very poor with a 10-year survival in some of the early natural history studies of only 33% and 0% for patients in NYHA classes III and IV, respectively.[179] Severe PH (pulmonary artery [PA] pressure >80 mm Hg) is associated with a mean survival of less than three years. Therefore, intervention should be considered when the patient develops class II–III symptoms.

C. **Diagnosis.** The severity of MS is determined primarily by echocardiography and can also be defined by cardiac catheterization (Table 1.7).

1. Echocardiography measures the mean diastolic gradient and, by the continuity equation, determines the mitral valve area (MVA). Echo also measures the diastolic pressure half-time, estimates the PA pressure from the tricuspid velocity jet, and can evaluate valve morphology using an echo score (Table 1.7).[180] This assesses leaflet mobility, thickening, calcification, and subvalvular thickening and can be used to determine whether the valve is amenable to balloon valvuloplasty.

2. Cardiac catheterization allows for calculation of the MVA from the cardiac output and the transvalvular mean gradient (pulmonary capillary wedge pressure [PCWP] minus the LV mean diastolic pressure). The PA pressure is measured by right-heart catheterization.

Table 1.6 • Stages of Mitral Stenosis

Stage A: At risk of MS (mitral valve doming during diastole)
Stage B: Progressive MS (rheumatic valve changes, mitral valve area [MVA] >1.5 cm², normal PA pressures, mild–moderate LA enlargement, pressure half-time <150 ms
Stage C: Asymptomatic severe MS
Stage D: Symptomatic severe MS – decreased exercise tolerance, exertional dyspnea

Table 1.7 • Echocardiographic and Hemodynamic Abnormalities in Severe Mitral Stenosis
Commissural fusion and diastolic doming of leaflets
MVA ≤1.5 cm² (≤1.0 cm² = very severe MS)
Pressure half-time ≥150 ms (≥220 ms = very severe MS)
Severe LA enlargement
PA systolic pressure >30 mm Hg
Note that gradients are utilized to measure the MVA, but are not that useful in the determination of severity.
Right heart catheterization can quantitate mean pulmonary artery pressures:

mild PAH:	mean PAP >25–40 mm Hg
moderate PAH:	mean PAP 41–55 mm Hg
severe PAH:	mean PAP ≥55 mm Hg

PAP, pulmonary artery pressure; PAH, pulmonary artery hypertension
Adapted with permission from Nishimura et al., *Circulation* 2014;129:e521–643.[107]

$$MVA = \frac{CO/(DFP \times HR)}{37.7 \times \sqrt{\text{mean gradient}}}$$

where:

MVA = mitral valve area in cm² (normal = 4–6 cm²)
DFP = diastolic filling period/beat
mean gradient = PCWP − LV mean diastolic pressure

3. Exercise stress echocardiography is helpful in assessing the physiologic severity of disease in patients whose symptoms appear inconsistent with the degree of MS.[181] Exercise will increase the heart rate and decrease the diastolic filling time. In patients with significant MS, this will increase the mean gradient and/or pulmonary artery pressures. Hemodynamically significant MS, an indication for intervention, includes an exercise-induced increase in the mean gradient to >15 mm Hg (>18 mm Hg if a dobutamine stress echo is performed), or an increase in the PCWP to >25 mm Hg. Another high-risk finding is a rise in the RV systolic pressure to >60 mm Hg at peak exercise, although that is not included in the guidelines.

D. **Indications for intervention**[107,131]

1. **Percutaneous** mitral balloon commissurotomy (PMBC) is the procedure of choice for patients with an indication for intervention if valve morphology is favorable by echo score. This procedure generally results in a doubling of the valve area and a 50% reduction in the mean gradient, with excellent long-term results. Mitral valve surgery is indicated when PMBC is contraindicated or not feasible due to unfavorable valve morphology, left atrial thrombus, or 3-4+ MR.[182,183]

2. **Class I indications**

   a. Stage D – PMBC is recommended for symptomatic patients with severe MS (MVA <1.5 cm^2) and favorable anatomy with less than 2+ MR and no LA thrombus.

   b. Stage D – mitral valve surgery is indicated in NYHA class III–IV patients with severe MS (MVA <1.5 cm^2) who are not candidates for PMBC, have failed a prior PMBC, or require other cardiac procedures.

   c. Stage C or D – concomitant mitral valve surgery is indicated for severe MS when cardiac surgery is performed for another indication.

3. **Class IIa indications**

   a. Stage C – PMBC is reasonable for asymptomatic patients with very severe MS (MVA <1.5 cm^2), favorable anatomy with less than 2+ MR, no LA thrombus, and a PA systolic pressure > 50 mm Hg).

4. **Class IIb indications**

   a. Stage C – PMBC may be considered for asymptomatic patients with severe MS (MVA <1.5 cm^2) and favorable anatomy with new onset of AF.

   b. Stage B/D – PMBC may be considered for symptomatic MS with a mitral valve >1.5 cm^2 if there is hemodynamically significant MS during exercise stress testing (PCWP > 25 mm Hg or mean mitral gradient > 15 mm Hg).

   c. Stage D – PMBC may be considered for NYHA class III-IV patients with severe MS with suboptimal anatomy for PMBC when surgery is considered too high risk.

   d. Mitral valve surgery with excision of the left atrial appendage may be considered for any patient in stage C or D who has had recurrent embolic events on adequate anticoagulation.

E. **Preoperative considerations**

1. Hemodynamic performance is frequently compromised by a low cardiac output state, which can be worsened by the presence of AF. A rapid ventricular response will shorten the diastolic filling period, reduce LV preload, and elevate LA pressures. Thus, the ventricular response to AF is best controlled in the perioperative period by β-blockers or calcium channel blockers. There is usually a delicate balance between fluid overload, which can precipitate pulmonary edema, and hypovolemia from aggressive diuresis, which can compromise renal function when the cardiac output is marginal. Thus, preload must be adjusted judiciously to ensure adequate LV filling across the stenotic valve.

2. Many patients with long-standing MS are cachectic and at increased risk for developing respiratory failure. Aggressive preoperative diuresis and nutritional supplementation may reduce morbidity in the early postoperative period.

3. Warfarin used for AF, left atrial thrombus, or a history of systemic embolism should be stopped four days before surgery. Since most patients with MS and AF are considered at high risk for embolization, outpatient LMWH may be prescribed as a bridge, but must be stopped 24 hours before surgery. Admission for unfractionated heparin the day before surgery may be considered once the international normalized ratio (INR) falls below the therapeutic range. The NOACs (dabigatran, apixaban, rivaroxaban) should not be used in patients with rheumatic MS.

F. Surgical procedures

1. Closed mitral commissurotomy has been supplanted by PMBC, which produces superior results. Either should be considered in the pregnant patient with critical MS in whom CPB should be avoided.

2. Open mitral commissurotomy is performed if PMBC is not considered feasible or there is evidence of left atrial thrombus. It produces better hemodynamics than either a PMBC or a closed commissurotomy and is associated with improved long-term event-free survival, especially in patients with high echo scores or AF.[182-185] Although recurrent symptoms are noted in 60% of patients after nine years, most symptoms are related to the development of MR or CAD, and not to recurrent MS.[106]

3. Mitral valve replacement (MVR) is indicated if the valve leaflets are calcified and fibrotic or there is significant subvalvular fusion (Figure 1.15).

4. Transcatheter treatment of MS is in its infancy. Transcatheter "valve-in-valve" procedures using aortic transcatheter heart valves have been used to treat bioprosthetic MS or regurgitation.[186,187] If imaging suggests that leaflet displacement may produce LVOT obstruction, a LAMPOON procedure (Laceration of the Anterior Mitral leaflet to Prevent lvOt ObstructioN) may be necessary. Use of these valves for MS associated with very heavy mitral annular calcification ("valve-in-MAC") has been performed, but with high mortality rates.[188] Routine transcatheter MVR with specifically designed valves has been accomplished and may eventually see more widespread use.[186]

5. Patients with a duration of AF exceeding six months will most likely remain in that rhythm postoperatively. Therefore, a Maze procedure should be considered in a patient with either paroxysmal or persistent AF. This should also include exclusion of the left atrial appendage by various techniques. The "cut and sew" Cox-Maze procedure has been replaced by use of energy sources (usually radio-frequency and cryoablation) that can be applied to create transmural ablation lines in well-described patterns to ablate this arrhythmia with fairly good success rates (see section XIII, pages 84–89). It is less likely to be successful when the left atrial dimension exceeds 6 cm.[189,190]

6. Functional TR usually improves after left-sided surgery due to a reduction in pulmonary vascular resistance, but is more likely to persist or progress in patients with AF, large atria, or moderate TR. Since moderate TR often progresses to severe TR, which may compromise long-term survival, tricuspid valve repair is recommended for patients with moderate or severe TR or tricuspid annular dilatation.[191,192] Further comments on TV repair during surgery for MR are noted on pages 57–58.

VII. Mitral Regurgitation

A. **Pathophysiology.** Mitral regurgitation (MR) has been classified as primary (degenerative) or secondary (functional) depending on the pathologic changes involved.[106,107,193]

1. Primary MR usually results from myxomatous change or fibroelastic deficiency of the valve leaflets causing redundancy, along with chordal elongation or rupture. This results in leaflet prolapse and flail and is also commonly associated with annular dilatation. Rheumatic changes can cause leaflet distortion and chordal damage. Endocarditis is usually associated with the formation of vegetations, leaflet deformity, or perforation.

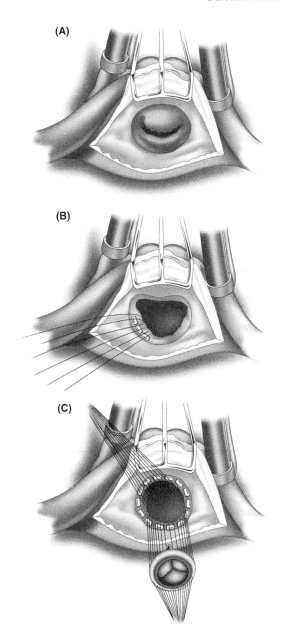

Figure 1.15 • Mitral valve replacement (MVR) via the posterior approach. (A) The left atrium is opened behind the intra-atrial groove and the retractor arms are positioned. Although both leaflets may be retained, the anterior leaflet is usually resected. (B) The posterior leaflet should be retained and is imbricated into the suture line. (C) Pledgeted mattress sutures are placed through the annulus, through or around the valve tissue, and into the sewing ring. The valve is then tied into position. The left atrial appendage may be oversewn from inside the left atrium.

2. Secondary or functional MR is associated with LV dysfunction, most commonly following an infarction, but also in association with dilated or hypertrophic cardiomyopathies. LV remodeling with a change in LV geometry and papillary muscle displacement may cause apical leaflet tethering as well as annular dilatation resulting in failure of the mitral leaflets to coapt properly, resulting in MR. The prognosis is worse with secondary MR because the MR is the result of a ventricular problem rather than a primary leaflet or chordal problem.

   a. The term "ischemic MR" has been applied to most cases of secondary MR caused by coronary disease. The spectrum of "ischemic MR" includes acute MR from infarct-related acute papillary muscle rupture or ischemic dysfunction of the ventricular wall below the papillary muscles as well as chronic secondary MR from prior myocardial damage.

   b. Patients with long-standing AF and those with restrictive cardiomyopathies (amyloid) may develop "atrial functional MR" when severe LA dilatation causes pure annular dilatation.[193]

B. Clinical presentation

1. Acute MR usually results from myocardial ischemia, an acute MI with papillary muscle rupture, endocarditis, or from idiopathic chordal rupture. Acute LV volume overload develops with a reduction in forward output and new-onset regurgitant flow into a small noncompliant left atrium. This may result in both cardiogenic shock and acute pulmonary edema.

2. Chronic MR is a condition of volume overload that is characterized by a progressive increase in compliance of the left atrium and ventricle, followed by a progressive increase in LVEDV as the LV dilates. Some degree of hypertrophy accompanies LV dilatation to normalize LV systolic wall stress. The increase in preload increases overall stroke volume and maintains forward cardiac output. At the same time, there is a decrease in afterload due to ventricular unloading into the left atrium which will normalize systolic wall stress. In the compensated phase, the ejection fraction will usually increase as contractility is also maintained. Patients are usually asymptomatic at this point and may remain so even as ventricular decompensation occurs. An EF in the low–normal range usually reflects some degree of contractile dysfunction. Eventually, prolonged volume overload causes more LV dilatation, significant contractile dysfunction, and an increase in afterload, which lowers the ejection fraction. This results in an increase in end-systolic volume with less forward output, and elevated filling pressures which worsen symptoms of HF.

C. Diagnostic considerations. The progression of MR and assessment of LV dimensions and function should be followed by serial echocardiograms to identify when an intervention should be undertaken to optimize the clinical outcome.

1. Transesophageal echocardiography (TEE) with 3D imaging is the best technique to quantitate the severity of MR and identify its mechanism, and it also assesses LV function and provides an estimate of PA pressure. It can define whether MR is primary (degenerative) with leaflet prolapse from chordal prolongation or rupture, or secondary (functional) on the basis of a dilated annulus or enlarged LV with apical tethering of the leaflets. Generally, single-leaflet prolapse or tethering produces eccentric jets (Figures 2.22 and 2.23), whereas annular dilatation causes central MR (Figure 2.24). TEE assessment is invaluable to the surgeon in helping to determine whether a valve can be repaired, what type of repair may be necessary, or whether replacement is indicated from the outset (Tables 1.8 and 1.9).

Table 1.8 • Stages of Primary Mitral Regurgitation

Stage A: At risk of MR
Stage B: Progressive MR
1. Severe prolapse with normal coaptation
2. Rheumatic changes with leaflet restriction and loss of central coaptation
3. Prior infective endocarditis
4. Central jet MR 20–40% of LA or late systolic eccentric jet of MR
5. VC <0.7 cm, RV <60 mL, RF <50%, ERO <0.4 cm^2
6. Mild LA enlargement, no LV enlargement, normal PA pressures

Stage C: Asymptomatic severe MR
Stage C1 – LVEF >60% and LVESD <40 mm
Stage C2 – LVEF ≤60% and LVESD ≥40 mm
1. Severe prolapse with loss of coaptation or flail leaflet
2. Rheumatic changes with leaflet restriction and loss of central coaptation
3. Prior IE
4. Central jet MR >40% of LA or holosystolic eccentric jet of MR
5. VC ≥0.7 cm, RV ≥60 mL, RF ≥50%, ERO ≥0.4 cm^2
6. Moderate to severe LA enlargement
7. LV enlargement
8. Pulmonary hypertension at rest or with exercise

Stage D: Symptomatic severe MR - same findings as stage C with HF symptoms (decreased exercise tolerance, exertional dyspnea)

IE, infective endocarditis; VC, vena contracta; RV, regurgitant volume; RF, regurgitant fraction; ERO, effective regurgitant orifice; LVESD, left ventricular end-systolic dimension
Adapted with permission from Nishimura et al., *Circulation* 2014;129:e521–643.[107]

Table 1.9 • Stages of Secondary Mitral Regurgitation

Stage A: At risk of MR
Stage B: Progressive MR
1. RWM abnormalities with mild mitral leaflet tethering
2. Annular dilatation with mild loss of central coaptation
3. RWM abnormalities, LV dilatation, and systolic dysfunction due to primary myocardial disease
4. ERO <0.4 cm^2, RV <60 mL, RF <50%

Stage C: Asymptomatic severe MR
1. RWM abnormalities and/or LV dilatation with severe mitral leaflet tethering
2. Annular dilatation with severe loss of central coaptation
3. RWM abnormalities, LV dilatation, and systolic dysfunction due to primary myocardial disease
4. ERO ≥0.40 cm^2, RV ≥60 mL, RF ≥50%

Stage D: Symptomatic severe MR – same findings as stage C with HF symptoms (decreased exercise tolerance, exertional dyspnea) that persist after revascularization and appropriate medical therapy

Hemodynamic parameters to define severe MR were modified in the 2017 AHA/ACC focused update to be identical to those of severe primary MR.
Adapted with permission from Nishimura RA, Otto CM, Bonow RO, Carabello BA, Erwin III JP, Fleisher LA, Jneid H, Mack MJ, McLeod CJ, O'Gara PT, Rigolin VH, Sundt III TM, Thompson A. 2017 AHA/ACC focused update of the 2014 AHA/ACC guideline for the management of patients with valvular heart disease. *J Am Coll Cardiol* 2017, doi: 10.1016/j.jacc.2017.03.011.

a. Both color flow Doppler and quantitative parameters, such as calculation of the effective regurgitant orifice area (EROA), regurgitant fraction (RF), and regurgitant volume (RV) are important to appropriately assess the severity of MR.[193]

b. The presence of LV or LA dilatation in primary MR is consistent with severe MR, whereas lack of LA or LV dilatation suggests that the MR is not severe.

c. The degree of MR can be difficult to determine in some cases of secondary MR, because findings such as a dilated LA and LV and systolic blunting of pulmonary venous flow may be related to an underlying cardiomyopathy. Furthermore, the shape of the regurgitant orifice in secondary MR is crescentic and may lead to an underestimation of the EROA.[193]

d. A discrepancy is often noted between the degree of MR identified preoperatively in the awake patient and that assessed under general anesthesia, which alters systemic resistance and loading conditions. Thus, a preoperative TEE is important to quantitate the degree of MR and define the precise anatomic mechanism for the MR. However, the use of sedation for a preoperative TEE may also lessen the degree of MR to some extent.

2. Cardiac magnetic resonance (CMR) imaging is helpful in determining the severity of MR when TEE is inconclusive. It is considered more accurate for quantitating the RV and RF as well as LV volumes and LVEF.[193]

3. Left ventriculography may be used to assess LV function and the degree of MR, but it is frequently insensitive in assessing its severity, which may depend on catheter position, the amount and force of contrast injection, the size of the left atrium or ventricle, and the presence of arrhythmias or ischemia.

D. **Indications for intervention for acute MR**

1. Acute MR due to papillary muscle rupture usually produces the picture of HF or cardiogenic shock and mandates emergency surgery prior to the development of multisystem organ failure.

2. Active infective endocarditis producing severe MR with hemodynamic compromise is a class I indication for urgent surgery.

E. **Indications for intervention in chronic primary MR**[107,131,193–195]

1. Class I indications
   - Stage D – symptomatic, severe MR, irrespective of LVEF
   - Stage C2 – asymptomatic, severe MR, LVEF ≤60% and/or LVESD ≥40 mm
   - Mitral valve repair is preferable to MVR if feasible in both of these categories

2. Class IIa indications
   - Stage C1 – mitral valve repair is reasonable if asymptomatic, severe MR, LVEF >60%, and LVESD ≤40 mm if there is a 95% likelihood of successful repair. This recommendation recognizes numerous reports that have demonstrated that mitral valve repair in asymptomatic patients with severe MR improves long-term survival.[196–199] However, it also implies that if a mitral valve repair may not be feasible, these patients should be followed with periodic monitoring for clinical symptoms or hemodynamic deterioration prior to offering surgery. It is noteworthy that indications for repair noted in the 2014 guidelines,[107] such as new onset of AF or a resting PA systolic pressure >50 mm Hg, were removed from the 2020 guidelines.[131]

- Stage D – transcatheter edge-to-edge repair (TEER), such as with the Mitraclip device (Abbott), is reasonable for symptomatic patients with severe primary MR who are at high surgical risk and have favorable anatomy for repair.[200]

3. Class IIb indications

- Stage C1 – mitral valve surgery (repair or replacement) is reasonable in asymptomatic patients with LVEF >60% and LVESD <40 mm if there is a progressive increase in LV size or decrease in EF on serial studies. This recommendation was based on concern that LV systolic dysfunction may already be present despite documentation of "normal" LV function, and earlier surgery may optimize outcomes.[193]
- Symptomatic patients with severe primary MR due to rheumatic valve disease may be considered for mitral valve repair in experienced centers.

F. **Indications for intervention for secondary MR**[131]

1. The ACC/AHA guidelines do not provide any class I indications for surgery for secondary MR, because most studies have not shown a survival benefit of surgery in these patients despite symptomatic improvement.[131,201] Multiple studies comparing CABG with CABG + mitral valve repair for moderate ischemic MR have not shown any improvements in survival or LV reverse remodeling out to two years with either approach.[202–205] In the Cardiothoracic Surgical Trials Network Trial (CTSN) study comparing mitral valve repair and replacement for severe ischemic MR (which usually also included CABG), the two-year mortality was about 20% (19% after mitral valve repair and 23.2% after MVR),[206] and this comparable mortality between groups was confirmed in a meta-analysis.[207] Other studies of patients with HF from nonischemic severe MR with impaired LV function have shown that mitral valve repair may improve symptoms without any survival benefit compared with medical therapy.[208,209] Thus, the presence of secondary MR carries a poor prognosis whether surgery is performed or not.

2. Class IIa indications

- Stage D – TEER is reasonable for symptomatic patients with chronic severe secondary MR (EROA ≥30 mm² and/or RV ≥45 mL) on optimal guideline-directed medical therapy (GDMT) who have an LVEF of 20-50%, LVESD ≤70 mm, a PA systolic pressure ≤70 mm Hg, and appropriate anatomy. The Mitraclip device was approved for use in patients with functional MR in the United States in 2019. Only one of the two supporting trials showed a survival benefit, which was evident in patients with more severe MR but less advanced LV dysfunction.[210,211] MitraClip was found to reduce HF readmissions and mortality if applied to patients with persistent ≥ NYHA class II symptoms on GDMT with ≥3+ MR with an LVEF of 20–50% and LVESD <70 mm.[212]
- Mitral valve surgery is reasonable for chronic severe secondary MR during CABG performed for ischemia. Most surgeons would certainly correct severe MR during such operations, as it will predictably improve symptoms. However, despite a reduction in late MR, no survival benefit to performing a mitral valve procedure for moderate or severe MR has been demonstrated in such cases.

3. Class IIb indications

- Stage D – mitral valve surgery may be considered for patients with chronic severe secondary MR from atrial annular dilatation with an LVEF ≥50% or for those with an LVEF <50% who have persistent class III–IV HF symptoms on GMDT. In these patients, mitral valve repair and replacement have comparable long-term survival rates, but the risk of recurrence is significantly higher with mitral valve repair.[206,213] In the CTSN trial, the two-year recurrence rate of MR was 58.8% for repairs vs. 3.8% for replacement. Therefore, a chordal-sparing MVR has been suggested.

- 2014 guidelines suggested that mitral valve repair may be considered for stage B patients with moderate MR undergoing CABG.[107] This may result in a lower risk of moderate MR at follow-up, but the rate of adverse events was similar to CABG alone with comparable two-year survival. This recommendation was absent in the 2020 guidelines.[131]

4. It should be noted that in the 2020 ACC guidelines, surgery has a class Ia indication for patients with symptomatic severe primary MR regardless of LV function, and TEER is only recommended for severely symptomatic high-risk surgical patients. In contrast, TEER has a higher level of recommendation than surgery (IIa vs. IIb) for patients with severe secondary MR and reduced LV function, independent of surgical risk.[131]

G. Other comments

1. Atrial fibrillation (AF) is very common in patients with mitral valve disease, and persistence of AF after mitral valve surgery alone is more likely when LA size exceeds 5.5–6 cm or AF has been present over six months.[106] Postoperative AF is associated with reduced survival, worse late cardiac function, and less freedom from late stroke in patients with nonischemic MR and should be addressed by a Maze procedure with obliteration of the left atrial appendage at the time of mitral valve surgery.[189,190,214,215] It should also be considered in patients with AF and ischemic MR, primarily to reduce the risk of stroke. Reducing the size of a dilated left atrium may improve atrial mechanical function and improve the results of a Maze procedure.[216] A report from the Mayo Clinic found that there was a greater risk of developing late AF after mitral valve repair in patients with a left atrial size >50 mm or more than mild TR, although repairing the TR did not influence the risk of AF. This led to a proposal to perform a Maze procedure in these patients even in the absence of preexisting AF.[217]

2. In patients undergoing AVR who have moderate functional MR, the severity of MR improves in about 70% of patients following the AVR, with comparable survival to those in whom mitral valve repair is performed. The likelihood of improvement is greater in patients with a small left atrium, preoperative HF, lesser degrees of TR or MR, a lower ejection fraction and larger LV size, the presence of AR, and lower RV systolic pressures.[218–220] If degenerative MR is present with single-leaflet prolapse and eccentric jets, it is unlikely that the MR will improve after relief of the outflow tract obstruction, and consideration should be given to repairing 2–3+ MR.

H. Preoperative considerations

1. Patients with acute MR are susceptible to pulmonary edema and multisystem organ failure from reduced forward cardiac output. Use of inotropes, vasodilators, and often an IABP can transiently improve myocardial function and forward flow in anticipation of urgent cardiac catheterization and surgery. Intubation and mechanical ventilation are frequently required for progressive hypoxia or hypercarbia. Diuretics must be used judiciously to improve pulmonary edema while not creating prerenal

azotemia. Some patients with chordal rupture who present with acute pulmonary edema may stabilize and develop chronic MR, which can be treated electively.

2. Patients with chronic MR are managed with diuretics or aldosterone antagonists (spironolactone, eplerenone) to reduce preload, and with vasodilators, such as the ACE inhibitors and ARBs, to improve forward flow. However, ACE inhibitors are usually beneficial only if the patient is symptomatic and has hypertension or systolic dysfunction. ACE inhibitors should not be given the morning of surgery, because of concerns about perioperative hypotension associated with their use.

3. Adequate preload must be maintained to ensure forward output while carefully monitoring the patient for evidence of HF. Systemic hypertension should be avoided because it will increase the amount of regurgitant flow. If the patient has ischemic MR or a borderline cardiac output, use of systemic vasodilators or an IABP generally improves forward flow.

I. **Surgical procedures**

1. Mitral valve reconstruction is applicable to more than 90% of patients with degenerative MR, although success rates are greater for posterior than anterior leaflet repairs. Techniques include annuloplasty rings, leaflet repairs, neochords, and chordal transfers (Figures 1.16 and 1.17).[107,221,222] Some of these reparative

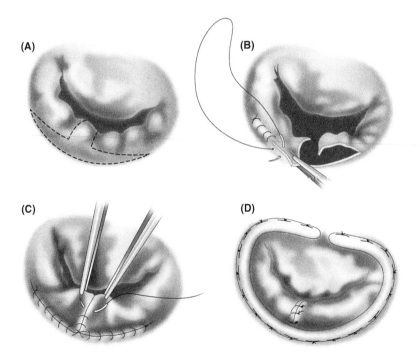

Figure 1.16 • Mitral valve repair. The most common pathology involves a flail posterior mitral leaflet. (A) A quadrangular excision is made as indicated by the dotted lines and the flail segment is resected. The remaining leaflet tissue may be incised along the annulus. (B) It is then advanced and reattached to the annulus ("sliding plasty"). (C) The leaflet tissue is then approximated, and (D) an annuloplasty ring is placed.

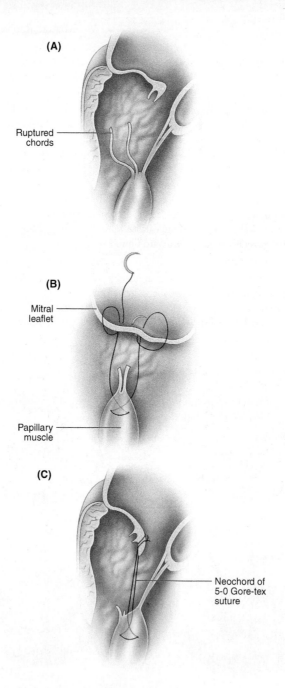

(A)

Ruptured
chords

(B)

Mitral
leaflet

Papillary
muscle

(C)

Neochord of
5-0 Gore-tex
suture

Figure 1.17 • Mitral valve repair with creation of PTFE neochords, used primarily for anterior leaflet prolapse. (A) Torn chords to one leaflet. (B) A figure-of-eight suture is placed through the head of the papillary muscle and each end of the suture is passed twice around the free edge of the leaflet. The suture is tied down to approximate the length of a normal length chord. (C) The final result after the suture is tied. (Image courtesy of Kaiser et al. *Mastery of Cardiothoracic Surgery*, Lippincott Williams and Wilkins 1st and 2nd editions.)

techniques can also be applied to patients with mitral valve endocarditis.[223,224] Mitral valve repair gives a survival advantage over mitral valve replacement (MVR) in patients with degenerative MR and coexisting CAD, but replacement appears superior for ischemic MR because of a lower recurrence rate despite equivalent survival.[206,210]

2. MVR is indicated when satisfactory repair cannot be accomplished. Acute MR from papillary muscle rupture usually requires MVR. Patients with ischemic MR have comparable clinical results and survival with MVR and repair, but a significantly lower rate of recurrence at two years with MVR. Chordal preservation of at least the posterior leaflet should be considered for all MVRs performed for MR. This improves ventricular function and will minimize the risk of LV rupture.

3. Traditional mitral valve operations have been performed through a median sternotomy incision, but other "minimal access" approaches have also been utilized successfully. An upper or lower sternotomy incision can be used and a right anterolateral thoracotomy or robotic approach through the right chest provide excellent visualization of the mitral valve. With experience, these procedures have comparable success rates of mitral valve repair and are associated with less blood loss, a lower rate of AF, and better cosmesis.[225–228] The latter two approaches do require femoral cannulation for bypass with its inherent complications.

4. A concomitant Maze procedure should be performed in patients with either paroxysmal or persistent AF. Whether a biatrial Maze procedure is superior to a left atrial Maze for these patients is controversial.[190,215,229]

5. The presence of TR or a dilated tricuspid annulus may affect long-term outcome and should be addressed at the time of mitral valve repair or replacement (see page 57).

6. Percutaneous approaches to MR continue to evolve and appear to be applicable to patients with both degenerative and functional MR.[212,230] The MitraClip mimics the "Alfieri stitch" in grasping both leaflets with a nitinol clip producing edge-to-edge approximation (Figure 1.18). Transapical off-pump mitral valve repairs with neochords have also been used succesfully.[231,232]

   a. The EVEREST II trial comparing MitraClip to surgical repair for degenerative MR found that the MitraClip was successful in reducing the degree of MR and improving clinical symptoms in high-risk patients, although the degree of MR reduction was inferior to that achieved with surgery. However, after a 30% conversion rate to surgery, most of which occurred during the first year, the MitraClip repair appeared durable. Owing to the high-risk population, the five-year mortality was comparable at about 20–25%.[200]

   b. As part of the EVEREST II trial, patients with functional MR underwent MitraClip placement. This was successful in reducing the degree of MR, reducing LV dimensions, improving symptoms, and reducing HF hospitalizations. The one-year survival for high-risk patients was only 74%, but was 86.4% for non-high-risk patients.[200]

   c. Subsequent studies have shown controversial benefits using the MitraClip device for functional MR. Data from the COAPT trial in 2018 showed that

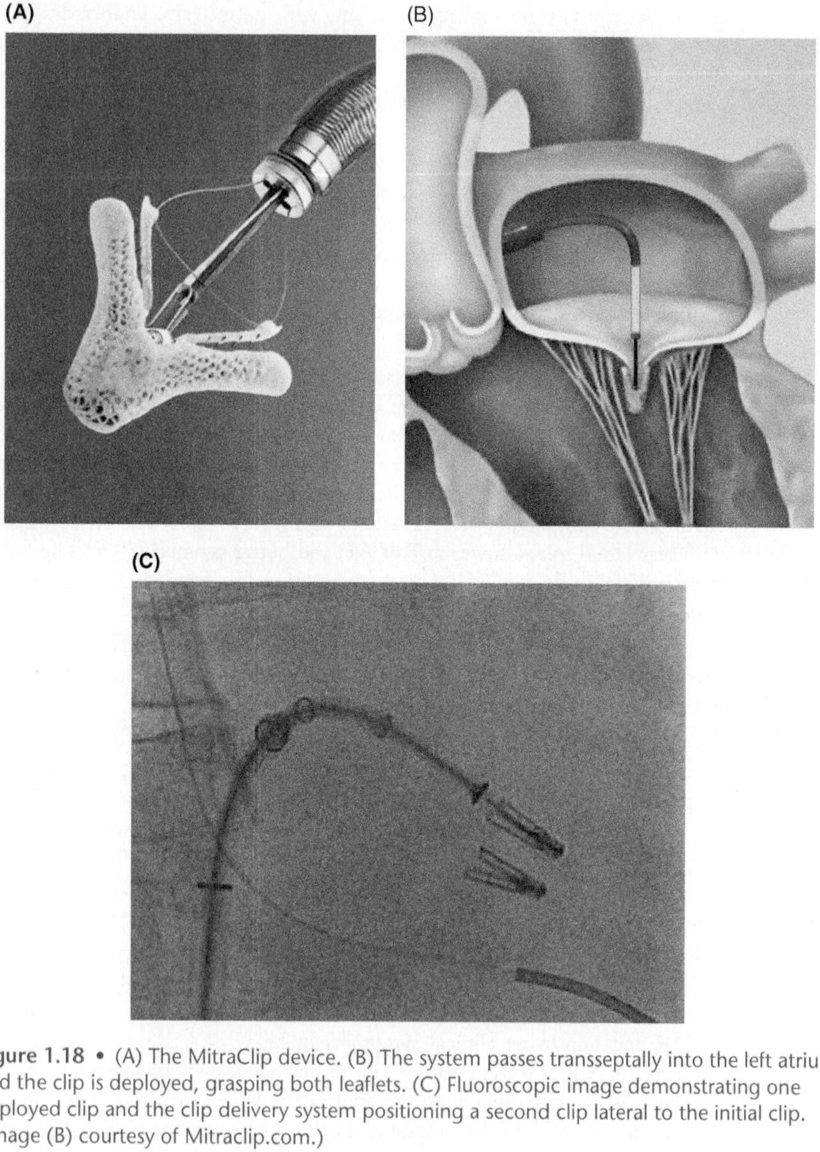

Figure 1.18 • (A) The MitraClip device. (B) The system passes transseptally into the left atrium and the clip is deployed, grasping both leaflets. (C) Fluoroscopic image demonstrating one deployed clip and the clip delivery system positioning a second clip lateral to the initial clip. (Image (B) courtesy of Mitraclip.com.)

percutaneous repair of severe secondary or functional MR in patients who remained symptomatic on optimal medical therapy had a lower rate of hospitalization and death at two years, although the combined endpoint was still quite significant (46% vs. 68%).[211] However, the Mitra-FR study published at the same time failed to show any difference in one-year survival comparing these two modalities, although the patients were not quite as ill as in the COAPT trial, yet had advanced disease with higher LVESVs.[212] The conclusion of the COAPT trial was that MitraClip could be recommended only after patients had truly failed a course of optimal medical therapy and cardiac resynchronization therapy (CRT) if appropriate. The appropriate candidates had an LVEF of 20–50% and LVESD <70 mm.[213]

    d. These studies confirmed the dismal prognosis of patients with secondary MR and LV dysfunction with one-year mortality rates of 22–24% (with/without intervention in the Mitra-FR study) and two-year mortality rates of 29% and 46% with and without interventions (COAPT).

VIII. Tricuspid Valve Disease

A. Pathophysiology[106]

    1. Tricuspid stenosis (TS) is very rare, usually developing as a result of rheumatic heart disease in association with MS. It is invariably associated with the presence of TR.

    2. TR is "functional" about 80% of the time, usually occurring as a consequence of left-sided heart disease which leads to PH and then pressure and volume overload of the RV. It may result from PH of any etiology. These conditions cause RV dilatation and remodeling with the subsequent development of tricuspid annular dilatation and leaflet tethering. Other common causes of TR include endocarditis (usually with IV drug abuse or hemodialysis) or valve distortion and damage from transvenous pacemaker leads.[233] RV systolic dysfunction leads to further elevation in right atrial (RA) and systemic venous pressures, producing signs of right-sided HF. Forward output may be reduced, resulting in fatigue and a low output state. AF is common.

B. Diagnosis

    1. Tricuspid stenosis. Signs of systemic venous congestion are present (jugular venous distention, ascites, hepatomegaly, peripheral edema) with abnormal liver function tests from hepatic congestion. Echocardiography of severe TS will show a pressure half-time ≥190 ms with a valve area of ≤1 cm^2 and the right atrium and inferior vena cava (IVC) will be dilated. The presence of associated TR will further increase the diastolic gradient across the valve and increase the RA pressure.

    2. TR produces a systolic murmur that increases with inspiration, prominent jugular venous pulsations, and, occasionally, a pulsatile liver. The diagnosis is confirmed by echocardiography, which can assess the tricuspid valve anatomy, the severity of TR, RV size and function, provide estimates of PA and RV pressures, and identify associated contributing pathology (Table 1.10).

C. Indications for Surgery[107,131]

    1. Tricuspid stenosis (TS)

        a. Class I

          • Tricuspid valve (TV) surgery is recommended for severe TS at the time of operation for left-sided valve disease. TV replacement (TVR) is recommended for patients at low surgical risk, especially if TR is moderate to severe.

          • TV surgery is recommended for symptomatic, isolated severe TS. These patients may have class III–IV symptoms, including hepatic congestion, ascites, and peripheral edema, that are refractory to salt restriction and diuretics. TVR is usually performed.

Table 1.10 • Stages of Functional Tricuspid Regurgitation

Stage A: At risk of TR
Stage B: Progressive TR: echo findings of mild–moderate TR (see Table 1.11)
Stage C: Asymptomatic severe TR: echo findings of severe TR (see Table 1.11)
Stage D: Symptomatic severe TR: same as stage C but with fatigue, palpitations, dyspnea, abdominal bloating, anorexia, peripheral edema

Adapted with permission from Nishimura et al., *Circulation* 2014;129:e521–643.[107]

Table 1.11 • Echocardiographic Findings in Functional TR

	Mild	Moderate	Severe
Central jet area	<5 cm²	5–10 cm²	>10 cm²
CW jet density	soft/parabolic	dense, variable contour	dense, triangular with early peak
Vena contracta width	not defined	<0.7 cm	>0.7 cm
Hepatic vein flow	mostly systolic	systolic blunting	systolic reversal
TV annular dilatation	early	early	>40 mm or >21 mm/m²
RA/RV/IVC size	normal	normal to mildly enlarged	dilated with decreased IVC respirophasic variation
RA pressure	normal	normal	elevated
RV function	normal	normal	reduced in late phase
Leaflet tethering	mild	moderate	marked
Other			diastolic interventricular septal flattening

Adapted with permission from Nishimura et al., *Circulation* 2014;129:e521–643.[107]

    b. Class IIb. Percutaneous balloon tricuspid commissurotomy might be considered in patients with isolated, symptomatic severe TS without accompanying TR who are at high surgical risk.

  2. Tricuspid regurgitation[131,234]

    a. Class I: Stage C–D: TV surgery is recommended when severe TR is present during left-sided valve surgery. This must be undertaken after careful deliberation if severe RV dysfunction is present.

b. Class IIa

- Stage B – TV repair is beneficial for patients with progressive TR at the time of left-sided valve surgery when tricuspid annular dilatation (>40 mm or >21 mm/m²) is present or there is prior evidence of right HF. Failure to reduce annular dilatation may subsequently lead to RV dysfunction, which will adversely affect functional outcome.

- Stage D – TV surgery can be beneficial for patients with signs and symptoms of right-sided HF due to primary TR or severe isolated secondary TR due to annular dilatation (in the absence of pulmonary hypertension or left-sided disease) that is unresponsive to medical therapy.

c. Class IIb

- Stage C – TV surgery may be considered for asymptomatic or minimally symptomatic patients with severe primary TR and progressive RV dilatation and/or systolic dysfunction. However, operative risk is high when there is evidence of RV systolic dysfunction prior to TV repair.

- Reoperation may be considered for symptomatic patients with isolated severe TR following prior left-sided valve surgery in the absence of significant PH or significant RV systolic dysfunction, since the latter two conditions significantly increase the operative risk.

d. Persistent sepsis in a patient with TV endocarditis (see pages 63–64).

3. Comments on management of TR: the adverse effects of the dilated annulus and degree of TR.

a. Severe TR has a very poor prognosis if untreated, with a 64% one-year survival, and therefore should always be addressed during left-sided heart procedures.[235] Concomitant mitral valve repair should theoretically reduce pulmonary artery pressures, RV dilatation, and the degree of TR. However, the reduction in TR is unpredictable because the dilated annulus will usually not return to its normal size and configuration despite relief of elevated RV afterload. Severe preop TR may increase operative mortality rates, but severe late postop TR reduces long-term survival. Thus, a competent, long-lasting repair is important in these patients.

b. Moderate TR also reduces patient survival, estimated at 79% at one year.[235] Since improvement in TR after left-sided repair is unpredictable, TV repair should also be considered in these patients to prevent the progression of TR and the development of RV dysfunction and HF symptoms.[236–238]

c. Numerous risk factors for the persistence or progression of TR after left-sided valve surgery have been identified, several of which can be addressed by TV repair.[107] These include tricuspid annular dilatation (>40 mm or >21 mm/m² on echo or >70 mm measured intraoperatively), RV dysfunction, leaflet tethering height (the distance between the leaflet coaptation point and the annular plane in midsystole) >5 mm, PH, AF, and presence of an endovascular lead across the TV valve.[239]

d. Studies have shown that a dilated annulus is a predictor of progressive TR, and TV repair for a dilated annulus, irrespective of the degree of TR, is associated with less subsequent progression in the degree of TR, improved RV remodeling, and better functional outcomes, although survival may not be improved.[240–242]

One study found that a dilated annulus, even in patients with mild or no TR, may lead to worsening of TR if not repaired, although functional outcomes or survival may not be affected by performing the repair.[243] Although RV systolic function tends to be worse with severe TR, one study suggested that RV dysfunction, but not significant TR, was the reason for compromised long-term survival.[244]

D. Preoperative considerations

1. Passive congestion of the liver resulting from elevated right-heart pressures frequently leads to coagulation abnormalities, which should be treated aggressively before and during surgery. Frequently, these patients have uncorrectable INRs before surgery.

2. Salt restriction and diuretics may improve hepatic function, but significant improvement in liver function tests may not be possible until after surgery.

3. Maintenance of an elevated central venous pressure is essential to achieve satisfactory forward flow. A normal sinus mechanism provides better hemodynamics than AF, although the latter is frequently present. Slower heart rates are preferable for TS, and faster heart rates for TR.

E. Operative procedures

1. Tricuspid commissurotomy (balloon or under direct vision) can be performed for rheumatic TS.

2. Tricuspid annuloplasty with a ring (Carpentier) or suture technique (De Vega) should reduce annular dilatation and restore annular geometry (Figure 1.19). An undersized annuloplasty ring (26–28 mm) has been recommended by some surgeons for functional TR.[245] Ring annuloplasties appear to produce superior outcomes with less recurrence, but some studies have still noted a fairly high recurrence rate with rings (about 16%) at five years.[246–249] If the patient has severe TV tethering (tethering distance >0.76 mm or a tethering area >1.63 cm), adjunctive techniques may be necessary to achieve a satisfactory result from repair.[250]

3. A variety of techniques have been used to repair the tricuspid valve. Because most dilatation occurs at the posterior annulus, bicuspidization involving a mattress suture extending from the anteroposterior to the posteroseptal commissure along the posterior annulus can correct most cases of functional TR (Figure 1.20).[251] This technique can also be used when there is destruction of either the posterior or septal leaflet by endocarditis and can avoid TVR in many cases.[252,253]

4. Tricuspid valve replacement (TVR) is necessary when leaflet shrinkage and poor coaptation prevent an annuloplasty technique from eliminating the TR. There is no particular preference for valve selection.[254,255] Tissue valves have a lower risk of thromboembolism than mechanical valves when placed in the right heart, and valve survival may be better due to lower stress on the valve leaflets. Tissue valves may also be preferable because long-term survival after TVR is somewhat limited, most likely because it is associated with RV dysfunction and with more advanced multivalvular disease. The overall mortality rate for TVR, whether performed as an isolated procedure or in combination with left heart surgery, has been reported to be in the 20% range,[254–257] although reports from the STS database have indicated that it was around 9%.[258,259]

5. Percutaneous tricuspid valve repair has been accomplished using the MitraClip system.[260] Bicuspidizing the valve may reduce the degree of TR to some degree,

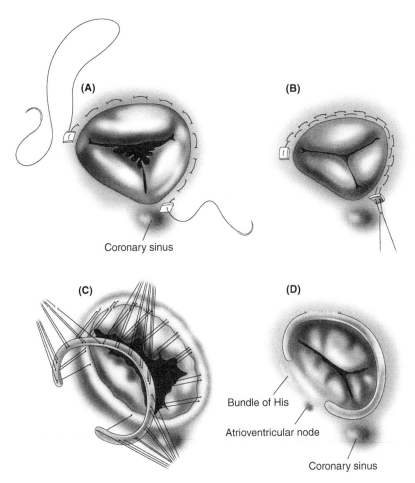

Coronary sinus

Bundle of His

Atrioventricular node

Coronary sinus

Figure 1.19 • Tricuspid valve repair involves reduction of annular dilatation to correct functional TR. (A, B) The circumferential suturing technique (De Vega repair). (C, D) Placement of an annuloplasty ring. Note the location of the coronary sinus and the proximity of the conduction system to the repair.

but this fails to reduce annular dilatation. Other devices are being investigated to improve leaflet coaptation and provide annular remodeling.[261,262]

6. Owing to the necessity of placing sutures near the conduction system, patients are more prone to developing heart block after tricuspid valve surgery. If there are concerns that permanent pacing may be required, epicardial pacing leads should be placed on the RV, pacing and sensing thresholds determined, and the pacing leads buried in a subcutaneous pocket for later attachment to a permanent pacemaker. In one report, more than 20% of patients undergoing TV surgery required postoperative permanent pacemakers.[263]

7. The management of tricuspid valve endocarditis is noted in the next section.

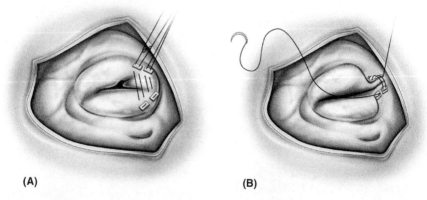

(A)   **(B)**

Figure 1.20 • Bicuspidization of the tricuspid valve for functional TR. (A) Two pledgeted mattress sutures are placed from the anteroposterior commissure to the posteroseptal commissure along the posterior annulus. (B) Tying down the sutures produces a "bicuspid" valve and should eliminate the TR.

IX. Infective Endocarditis

A. **Pathophysiology.** Infective endocarditis (IE) can result in the destruction of valve leaflets, invasion of surrounding myocardial tissue, systemic embolization of valve vegetations, or persistent systemic sepsis. Embolization is more likely with mitral than aortic valve involvement, staphylococcal organisms, and large (>10–15 mm) or mobile vegetations. Native valve endocarditis (NVE) is most commonly caused by *Streptococcus viridans, Staphylococcus aureus*, or coagulase-negative staphylococcal organisms. Tricuspid valve endocarditis is usually caused by IV drug abuse, although less than 50% of intravenous drug abusers (IVDAs) have isolated tricuspid valve involvement.[264,265] The incidence of prosthetic valve endocarditis (PVE) is approximately 0.5–1% per patient-year for most mechanical and tissue valves. It is most commonly caused by staphylococcal organisms.

B. **Diagnosis**

1. The modified Duke criteria are used to diagnose endocarditis.[106,107] These include two major criteria (positive blood culture and echocardiographic findings consistent with endocarditis) and several minor criteria (a predisposing condition, fever, vascular or immunologic manifestations).

2. Transthoracic echo (TTE) can usually identify vegetations, valve pathology, and anterior prosthetic valve abscesses, but its overall sensitivity for NVE is 50–90% with a specificity of 90%. Sensitivity is only 40–70% for PVE.[266]

3. Transesophageal echo (TEE) is usually more sensitive and specific in identifying complex problems, such as perforations, abscesses, and fistulas. It should be performed if the TTE is positive or nondiagnostic, if complications are present, and if surgery is to be performed (Figures 2.25 and 2.26).

4. When there are indeterminate findings on TTE or TEE, which is quite common with PVE or with pacemaker or defibrillator lead involvement, nuclear imaging studies, including metabolic imaging ([18]FDG PET-CT scanning) and radiolabeled leukocyte scintigraphy using single-photon emission CT (SPECT) may be useful.[266–268]

5. Cardiac CT is helpful in identifying paravalvular complications and should be considered to rule out coronary pathology since it is important to avoid catheter manipulation in the aortic root when aortic valve endocarditis is present.[269]

6. Routine brain CT scanning is essential in patients sustaining a neurologic complication, especially to identify hemorrhage, which usually contraindicates early surgery. Brain MRI may detect subclinical cerebral complications, including embolism, abscesses, or hemorrhage, in upwards of 80% of patients,[266] although such findings may not influence decisions regarding early surgery. CT cerebral angiography has identified small intracranial mycotic aneurysms in more than 30% of patients as well.[266] This may account for the finding of small ectopic hemorrhagic strokes in many patients after surgery.[270]

C. **Indications for surgery in native and prosthetic valve endocarditis.** Although medical therapy is often successful in the treatment of IE, certain pathologic problems portend an ominous prognosis for which urgent surgery is indicated. These conditions are HF due to valvular regurgitation, cardiac invasion, and large vegetations with an increased risk of systemic embolization. ACC/AHA guidelines noted below do not differentiate between right- and left-sided endocarditis.[107,131] The European Society of Cardiology (ESC) guidelines do make that distinction, and also provide the recommended timing for surgery (Table 1.12).[271] Indications for early surgery before completion of a full course of antibiotics per the ACC/AHA guidelines are:

1. Class I indications

   a. Valve dysfunction causing symptoms of HF. Despite its high risk, surgery should not be delayed if cardiogenic shock or pulmonary edema is present unless the likelihood of recovery from complications (severe stroke) is remote. Otherwise, the patient will develop multisystem organ failure and likely die without surgical intervention.

   b. IE caused by *S. aureus*, fungal, or other highly resistant organisms. These are aggressive organisms that are associated with large vegetations, embolization, cardiac invasion, and persistent infection.

   c. Evidence of local extension resulting in heart block, aortic or annular abscesses, or destructive penetrating lesions (intracardiac fistulae, mitral leaflet perforation from aortic valve endocarditis). For prosthetic valves, this may produce valve dehiscence with a paravalvular leak or rocking on echo.

   d. Persistent infection manifested by persistent bacteremia or fevers after 5–7 days of appropriate antibiotic therapy.

   e. For PVE, a relapsing infection after completion of a course of antibiotics during which blood cultures are negative.

2. Class IIa: recurrent embolization with persistent vegetations despite antibiotic treatment. The risk of embolization is highest during the first week of antibiotic therapy and occurs in up to 50% of patients, then rapidly declines to very low levels after two weeks.[271-274] Thus, very early intervention can be recommended to avoid recurrent embolization. Embolization risk correlates with older age, diabetes, AF, previous embolization, vegetation length, and *S. aureus* infection.[274]

3. Class IIb: mobile vegetations >10 mm in diameter even in the absence of documented embolization. These vegetations, especially on the mitral valve and with *Staph.* organisms, have an increased risk of embolization. Early surgery has been shown to reduce embolic events and improve survival.[275,276]

Table 1.12 • Indications for Surgery for Left-Sided Valve Infections per the European Society of Cardiology

	Heart Failure	
Class	**Timing**	
I	Emergent	NVE or PVE with severe AR or MR, obstruction, or fistula causing refractory pulmonary edema or cardiogenic shock
I	Urgent	NVE or PVE with severe AR or MR or obstruction with symptoms of CHF or echo signs of poor hemodynamic tolerance causing heart failure symptoms (high LVEDP, PH, high LA pressures)
	Uncontrolled Infection	
I	Urgent	Locally uncontrolled infection (abscess, false aneurysm, fistula, enlarging vegetation) – i.e. persistent positive blood cultures after 7–10 days of antibiotics; perivalvular abscess is noted in 10–40% of aortic NVE and 56–100% of PVE
I	Urgent/elective	Infection with fungal or multiresistant organism
IIa	Urgent	Persistent positive blood culture on appropriate antibiotics and adequate control of septic metastatic foci
IIa	Urgent/elective	PVE with *Staph.* or HACEK gram-negative organism
	Prevention of Embolism	
I	Urgent	Aortic or mitral NVE or PVE IE with persistent vegetations >10 mm after ≥1 embolic episode on antibiotics
IIa	Urgent	Aortic or mitral NVE with vegetations >10 mm with severe valve stenosis or regurgitation and low surgical risk
IIa	Urgent	Aortic or mitral NVE or PVE with very large vegetations >30 mm
IIb	Urgent	Aortic or mitral NVE or PVE with isolated vegetation >15 mm and no other indication for surgery

Adapted with permission from Habib et al., *Eur Heart J* 2015;36:3075–128.[271]

D. **Specific issues**

1. **Neurologic complications.** Approximately 15–30% of patients manifest overt neurologic complications from IE and another 35–60% may develop clinically silent cerebral embolization.[266,267,271] Concerns that early surgery will exacerbate a neurologic deficit due to heparinization and hypotension have not been substantiated, and urgent surgery is recommended to prevent recurrent embolization in the absence of cerebral hemorrhage on CT scan (class IIb). If there is evidence of intracerebral bleeding, surgery should be delayed at least four weeks (class IIb).

However, microbleeds noted on MRI scanning should not be considered equivalent to intracerebral hemorrhage and should not contraindicate urgent surgery.[271] Ectopic intracranial hemorrhage has been noted postoperatively in over 10% of patients regardless of the timing of surgery and may be related to mycotic angiopathy or small undetected mycotic aneurysms.[276] In most patients, the indication for surgery will be HF, uncontrolled infection, large mobile vegetations with high embolic risk and less commonly, a perivalvular abscess. Intracranial infectious aneurysms may be identified by CT or MR angiography prior to surgery.

2. **Tricuspid valve infective endocarditis** (TVIE) comprises 5–10% of all cases of IE and is usually noted in IVDAs, as well as patients with hemodialysis catheters and pacing/defibrillator leads.[277,278] *S. aureus* is the most common organism. These patients usually present with fever, bacteremia, and septic pulmonary emboli, and most eventually develop TR. Fortunately, IV antibiotics can successfully treat 70–85% of these patients, with a fairly low mortality. The threshold for recommending surgery is fairly high in IVDAs because of concerns about the influence of IV drug recidivism on recurrent endocarditis and survival.[278-283]

a. A meta-analysis of patients with TVIE (41% with IVDA) found comparable four-year survivals with TV repair and TVR, but repair was associated with more residual moderate–severe TR, less recurrent IE, fewer reoperations, and a reduced need for a permanent pacemaker.[278]

b. A study from the Cleveland Clinic of TVIE also found that a significant percentage of patients (44%) undergoing TV repair were left with moderate–severe TR, but this did not worsen with time, and TV repair produced significantly better survival out to seven years than TVR. Five-year survival was about the same for TVIE resulting from IVDA and cardiac implantable devices, but was only 18% in patients on dialysis.[280]

c. Another study from the Cleveland Clinic of IE in IVDA patients, independent of valve location, reported a 10-fold increase in the risk of death or reoperation between three and six months after surgery, most likely due to recurrent IV drug abuse.[281]

d. A study from Boston reported a nearly fourfold increase in valve-related complications in IVDAs, usually attributable to valve reinfection.[265] That study found no difference in 10-year survival between IVDA patients and non-IVDA patients (about 70% survival), but a 60% reinfection rate at eight years for IVDA. Other studies suggest that 10-year survival for IVDAs was much worse at 40%.[282]

e. Early surgery for TVIE is indicated when the standard indications for concomitant left-sided endocarditis are present, and when there is an infected pacemaker lead or PVE. The association of left-sided endocarditis with TVIE compromises survival. However, a conservative approach has been recommended in IVDAs with isolated TVIE, such that persistent bacteremia but not recurrent septic pulmonary emboli should be the only strong indication for early surgery. However, in other patients with severe TR, early surgery might permit tricuspid repair before extensive destruction of tricuspid valve tissue has occurred since repair is highly protective against recurrent TVIE.[281] The Cleveland Clinic data support this concept of trying to repair the TV at all costs, but it is not clear if this approach and the results achieved at this world-class institution are reproducible by less experienced surgeons. Indications for surgery may include:

- Worsening right HF from severe TR with poor response to diuretic therapy.
- Persistent vegetations >20 mm with bacteremia (and possibly recurrent septic pulmonary emboli).
- Difficult to eradicate organisms (fungus).
- Bacteremia for at least seven days despite adequate antibiotics (especially if *Staph.* or *Pseudomonas*).

3. **Cardiac implantable electronic device-related infective endocarditis (CDRIE)** from pacemakers and defibrillator implants can be difficult to identify, but must be suspected in any patient with positive blood cultures. This is to be differentiated from local device infection which involves the device and implantation pocket without lead involvement. TEE is more sensitive than TTE in identifying lead-associated vegetations, but differentiation from clot or adherent tissue is not always possible. Use of intracardiac echocardiography (ICE), [18]FDG-PET/CT or radiolabeled leukocyte scintigraphy may be helpful.[271] Complete hardware removal, including the device and leads, is indicated when CDRIE is suspected.[266,271]

   a. Percutaneous transvenous lead extraction is preferable to avoid an open-heart procedure, but has moderate risk and requires expertise. Extraction may result in embolization of vegetations, but this is usually not clinically significant.

   b. Open extraction should be considered if percutaneous removal is unsuccessful or there is severe destructive TVIE or very large vegetations >20 mm.

   c. If the patient is pacer-dependent, temporary transvenous pacing leads may be necessary, but they are a risk factor for subsequent cardiac device infection. Use of active fixation leads connected to external devices produces secure leads until another permanent pacing system can be implanted.[284]

   d. When there is evidence of NVE or PVE and no evidence of CDRIE, it may be possible to leave the system behind, so the European guidelines assigned a level IIb indication to removing the device and leads.

4. **Hemodialysis** patients have a high risk of bloodborne infections and are more prone to NVE and PVE. Hospital mortality rates for patients on hemodialysis who present with endocarditis were 23.5 and 37% in two studies.[285,286] In fact, US national data showed that only 10–15% of these patients survived three years.[285] In surgical studies, operative mortality rate has been quite high (42% in one study of AVRs)[287] with recurrent PVE in 50% of patients by five years and an overall five-year survival of around 20%.[280,288,289] Thus, it is predictable that these patients will do very poorly even following appropriate guidelines.

5. **Transcatheter valve** infections occur at a rate of 1–2%/year (comparable to surgical valves), and tend to occur in the first six months following the procedure.[290,291] They are usually associated with other surgical procedures, chronic vascular access (hemodialysis), or peripheral vascular disease. There is limited experience in dealing with this complication, but the hospital mortality rate with medical management approaches 50%. Because many patients have undergone TAVR because of high surgical risk, an operative approach to remove the transcatheter valve may also carry high risk. With lower-risk patients now undergoing TAVR, this is

surely going to become a more common problem that will need to be managed with similar indications as for surgical prosthetic valve endocarditis, but may require more complex aortic root procedures.

E. **Preoperative considerations**

1. **Antibiotic therapy.** Ideally, the patient should receive a six-week course of antibiotics prior to surgery, which should reduce the risk of PVE from about 10% down to 2%. However, hemodynamic deterioration, intracardiac invasion, and risk of embolization are compelling indications for earlier surgery. Attempts should be made to optimize hemodynamic and renal status before operation in patients with hemodynamic compromise, but surgery should not be delayed if there is evidence of progressive organ system deterioration, especially with acute AR or MR. The appropriate antibiotics should be given for a total perioperative course of six weeks, although a shorter course may be feasible if complete extirpation of the infection is achieved and microbiology suggests very sensitive organisms, such as *Streptococcus*.

2. Patients with aortic valve endocarditis may have evidence of heart block from involvement of the conduction system by periannular infection. This may require preoperative placement of a transvenous pacing wire.

3. Coronary angiography should be avoided, if possible, when mobile aortic valve vegetations are identified. Cardiac CT angiography can be performed to identify potential coronary stenoses.

F. **Surgical procedures**

1. Surgery entails excision of all infected valve tissue, drainage and debridement of abscess cavities, and repair or replacement of the damaged valves.[292] An aortic valve homograft is arguably the valve of choice for aortic valve IE because of its increased resistance to infection and adaptability to disrupted tissue in the aortic root.[162,293] However, homograft replacement is technically quite complex and the operative mortality may be greater when performed by surgeons without extensive experience with these conduits. AVR with either mechanical or tissue valves is a satisfactory alternative with a comparable rate of complications and late mortality to homografts in several studies.[294,295] The risk of PVE on tissue or mechanical valves is fairly comparable.

2. Mitral valve endocarditis can frequently be repaired, especially if leaflet perforation is the primary pathology, and there are proponents of earlier surgery in mitral valve endocarditis to preserve the patient's native valve.[296] More advanced stages of endocarditis usually require valve replacement.

3. Tricuspid valve endocarditis should usually be treated more conservatively, especially in IVDAs who remain at increased high risk of developing PVE.

   a. When surgery is indicated, tricuspid valve repair is usually recommended and should be attempted aggressively in these patients.[280–282] Bicuspidization after resection of infected tissue is often successful. Otherwise, the tricuspid valve should be replaced, accepting the higher risk of recurrence. Again, the Cleveland Clinic data recommended a TV repair even if it leaves the patient with a significant amount of TR, and the authors recommended avoiding a TVR if at all possible.[280]

b. Although most surgeons believe that a valvectomy should only be performed in extreme cases and in the absence of PH, a single center study comparing valvectomy with TVR and TV repair found similar 30-day mortality rates and a lower readmission rate at one year with valve excision than TVR (although 60% of patients were lost to follow-up).[297] The readmission rate after TVR was 23% and was usually associated with recurrent infection. Apparently, since many patients already have severe TR, they appear to tolerate valve excision well without developing severe HF. Generally, if TV repair cannot be successfully performed, TVR should be considered if the patient is undergoing left-sided valve surgery, has PH, and is not an IVDA. However, valvectomy may be a reasonable option if IVDA recidivism is highly likely and the valve cannot be repaired.

X. Hypertrophic Obstructive Cardiomyopathy

A. **Pathophysiology.** Hypertrophic obstructive cardiomyopathy (HOCM) is characterized by diastolic dysfunction and varying degrees of dynamic LVOT obstruction. The latter most commonly results from hypertrophy of the basal septum with mitral–septal apposition from systolic anterior motion (SAM) of the mitral valve. This also leads to MR from incomplete leaflet apposition. A variety of anomalies of the mitral valve and papillary muscles may contribute to these problems, including elongated anterior and posterior mitral leaflets (AML and PML), anterior and basilar displacement of the anterolateral papillary muscle, and the insertion of the anterolateral papillary muscle or anomalous chords into the middle of the AML.[298–302]

B. **Clinical presentations.** Several different clinical patterns may be noted with HOCM.

1. Patients generally become symptomatic with congestive HF, which is related to diastolic dysfunction, left ventricular outflow tract (LVOT) obstruction, and the presence of MR. About 70% of patients have either resting or provoked LVOT obstruction, with 25% having a significant resting gradient. LVOT obstruction with a gradient >30 mm Hg at rest or with exercise is an independent predictor of the development of HF and carries a poor prognosis. Syncope may occur due to hemodynamic compromise from LVOT obstruction.

2. Angina from microvascular ischemia may develop because of abnormal coronary microvasculature and inadequate capillary density for the degree of hypertrophy.

3. Supraventricular and ventricular arrhythmias are noted with HOCM, and the risk of sudden death is estimated at 0.5–1.5%/year, being more common in patients <age 30 and rare in patients >age 60. This risk is increased in patients with any of the following major risk factors:[302]
   - History of cardiac arrest
   - Family history of HOCM-related sudden death
   - Sustained ventricular tachycardia (VT) or repetitive prolonged bursts of nonsustained VT
   - Massive LVH >30 mm
   - LV apical aneurysm
   - Late gadolinium enhancement (LGE) >15% of LV mass
   - End-stage HOCM with an EF <50% and an LV apical aneurysm

4. Advanced HF may develop with remodeling and systolic dysfunction that may require heart transplantation.

5. Atrial fibrillation (AF) may develop due to left atrial enlargement in 20% of patients and is not uncommon in patients with advanced HF and systolic dysfunction. Because of impaired LV filling due to the lack of atrial "kick" with severe LVH, cardiac output may be compromised. AF is generally poorly tolerated and is a predictor of adverse outcomes. Management may involve amiodarone for rhythm control, anticoagulation to minimize the risk of stroke, potential catheter ablation if the rhythm is not well-tolerated, and possibly a Maze procedure at the time of surgical myectomy.

6. Patients with nonobstructive hypertrophic cardiomyopathy generally have a benign course with only 10% progressing to class III/IV symptoms. Their survival is comparable to age-matched controls.[303]

C. Diagnosis

1. Echocardiography at rest and with exercise will demonstrate the anatomic variant of HOCM (most commonly upper septal hypertrophy), the resting outflow tract gradient, the provocable gradient, and the degree of MR and its mechanism (usually SAM). TEE is essential to identify abnormalities of the mitral valve leaflets and papillary muscles so that they can be addressed at the time of surgery.

2. During left heart catheterization, the Brockenbrough–Braunwald–Morrow sign may be noted. This occurs when a post-PVC beat results in a reduction rather than an increase in the arterial pulse pressure despite increasing diastolic filling time, increased LVEDP, and an increase in LV systolic pressure. The increase in cardiac stretch increases cardiac contractility and accentuates the outflow tract gradient, reducing the blood pressure.

3. Risk stratification for sudden death may be improved by use of contrast-enhanced CMR using gadolinium. The risk of sudden death is proportional to the degree of LGE, which reflects areas of myocardial fibrosis (Figure 2.40). Patients with absent LGE are at low risk for sudden death, whereas those with LGE >15% of LV mass are at higher risk, even in the absence of other risk factors. The extent of LGE correlates with adverse LV remodeling and the progression to end-stage HOCM with LV systolic dysfunction.[302, 304, 305]

D. Indications for intervention

1. No pharmacologic regimen has been shown conclusively to reduce the risk of sudden death. However, β-blockers decrease cardiac inotropy, are effective in blunting gradients provoked by exercise, and generally improve symptoms. They are recommended for patients with or without obstruction. Verapamil is a second alternative, and disopyramide can be added when there is outflow tract obstruction as it will decrease SAM and the outflow gradient.

2. Dual-chamber pacing and biventricular pacing might be useful in reducing the gradient, but these modalities are only indicated if a dual chamber implantable cardioverter-defibrillator (ICD) is implanted or if the patient is not a candidate for an ablative procedure.

3. Further intervention is indicated in patients with a gradient >50 mm Hg at rest or with provocation who have persistent symptoms despite medications or have syncope due to LVOT obstruction. Intervention may also be considered in asymptomatic patients considered at high risk for sudden death, including younger patients and those with a peak gradient >80 mm Hg.

E. Preoperative considerations

1. Measures that produce hypovolemia or vasodilatation must be avoided because they increase the outflow tract gradient. Volume infusions should be used to maintain preload, with the use of α-agonists to maintain systemic resistance.

2. Use of β-blockers and calcium channel blockers to reduce heart rate and contractility are the mainstay of the medical management of HOCM and should be continued up to the time of surgery.

F. Interventional procedures[306]

1. The traditional surgical approach of a LV septal myectomy entailed resection of a 1.5 × 4 cm wedge of septum below the right coronary aortic leaflet through an aortotomy incision.

2. With further understanding of the mechanism of SAM, the current operation is more elaborate and involves performing an extended septal myectomy to the base of the papillary muscles, mobilization and partial excision of the papillary muscles off the ventricular wall to allow the papillary muscles to assume a more posterior position in the LV, and AML plication if there is any redundancy. This reduces chordal and leaflet slack that can produce SAM (Figure 1.21). Surgery can successfully treat patients with massive LVH and other subvalvular issues that contribute to LVOT obstruction or MR that cannot be addressed by alcohol septal ablation.

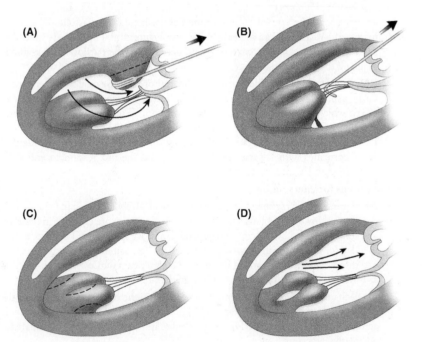

Figure 1.21 • (A) Hypertrophic obstructive cardiomyopathy is characterized by septal hypertrophy, which orients the outflow jet into the anterior leaflet of the mitral valve, producing SAM. An extensive septal myectomy is performed, often requiring a midventricular resection. (B, C) Using a nerve hook to provide traction, the atypical attachments of hypertrophied anomalous papillary muscles are partially detached from the ventricular wall and trimmed. (D) After this procedure, the outflow jet is directed more anteriorly.

a. The concept of "resect-plicate-release" should be applied depending on the degree of septal thickness (resect if >18 mm), AML height (plicate AML if >30 mm or >17 mm/m^2), and anterior displacement of the anterolateral papillary muscle (release/resection of the papillary muscle by extending the resection laterally into the free wall above the base of the papillary muscle). Resection of midventricular obstruction or anomalous chords and relief of papillary muscle fusion may be necessary.[298]

b. A successful operation dramatically reduces the gradient, eliminates MR, improves functional status, and may reduce the risk of sudden death. This procedure is also successful in reducing the gradient in patients with significant LVOT obstruction or MR but less basal septal hypertrophy by "plication" and "release" without septal resection.

c. A comprehensive extended myectomy and subvalvular procedure should eliminate SAM and MR in patients without intrinsic mitral valve disease or elongated chords.[307] Only if these problems are present should an MVR be necessary.[308]

3. Alcohol septal ablation of the upper septal perforator branch of the LAD produces an infarct of the upper septum. This should reduce basal septal thickness (which may take up to three months), which enlarges the LV outflow tract and reduces SAM in appropriately selected patients. It has been shown to produce a substantial reduction in gradient with improvement in symptoms, exercise tolerance, and possibly survival.[309]

a. Although comparative studies suggest that septal myectomy produces a lower gradient and reduces the need for permanent pacemaker implantation (3% vs.10%) than alcohol septal ablation, no significant difference in long-term survival, functional class, or ventricular arrhythmias has been noted, except perhaps better symptom relief in patients <age 65.[309]

b. Nonetheless, because open-heart surgery allows the surgeon to address papillary muscle pathology, massive LVH, and perform a concomitant cardiac procedure (for coronary disease or AF), and, because it avoids the long-term concerns of creating an arrhythmogenic focus with alcohol ablation, myectomy is the preferred procedure, reserving alcohol septal ablation for older patients and those considered high risk for surgery.

4. Transcatheter mitral valve repair using the MitraClip device has seen limited use in HOCM, but may be considered in patients with severe MR and systolic anterior motion who are at prohibitive risk for surgical myectomy or have coronary anatomy not amenable to alcohol septal ablation. It can reduce the LVOT gradient and the degree of MR.[310]

5. ICD placement should be considered in patients at high risk for sudden death (as noted above) and has been the only modality demonstrated to reduce that risk and prolong life.

XI. Aortic Dissections

A. **Pathophysiology.** An aortic dissection results from an intimal tear that allows passage of blood into the media, creating a false channel. This channel is contained externally by the outer medial and adventitial layers of the aorta. With each cardiac contraction, the dissected channel can extend proximally or distally, potentially causing branch artery compromise or rupture as the outer wall weakens. Dissections involving the

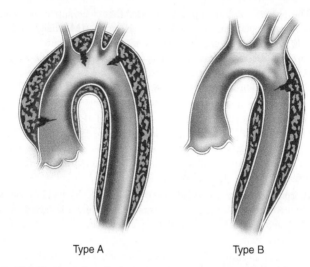

Type A   Type B

Figure 1.22 • Classification of aortic dissection. Type A dissections involve the ascending aorta. Type B dissections usually originate distal to the left subclavian artery and do not involve the ascending aorta. If they do extend retrograde, they are then considered type A dissections.

ascending aorta are classified as Stanford type A (DeBakey type I–II, or proximal) dissections, whereas those not involving the ascending aorta are called Stanford type B (DeBakey type III, or distal) dissections (Figure 1.22). In the past, a dissection was termed "acute" when diagnosed within two weeks of its onset; otherwise, it was termed "chronic". The International Registry of Acute Aortic Dissections (IRAD) has reclassified dissections as the following: hyperacute (<24 hours from symptom onset), acute (2–7 days), subacute (8–30 days) and chronic (>30 days) from symptom onset.[311] Either cystic medial degeneration or increased aortic wall stress (usually hypertension) is present in most patients with aortic dissection.[312,313] A variant of an acute dissection is an intramural hematoma in the absence of an intimal tear, which is usually treated in the same manner.

B. **Presentation**

1. **Type A dissection.** This is a life-threatening condition that must be considered in any patient presenting to the emergency room with the acute onset of chest pain. Failure to be aware of the various presentations of type A dissections has led to a misdiagnosis in up to 40% of patients.[314] Early suspicion and evaluation are critical to expedite surgery since the estimated mortality rate for medically managed type A dissections is about 15–30% during the first 24 hours (about 1–2%/h), then 10–20% in the next 24 hours, before decreasing.[315]

   a. The traditional notion is that patients develop tearing, ripping chest pain that radiates to the back, and have severe hypertension, a widened mediastinum on chest x-ray, and a normal ECG on admission. However, IRAD data have reported this classic presentation to be uncommon. In an IRAD report from 2015 that looked at trends in demographic data, the most recent three-year interval found tearing, ripping chest pain to be present in only 23.8% of patients, hypertension on admission in 27%, a widened mediastinum in 52.2%

with a normal chest x-ray in 28.6%, and a normal ECG in 40.7%.[316] The key symptoms that had not changed over time were the presence of **the acute onset of severe pain,** whether neck, chest, back, or abdominal, which is usually the worst pain the patient has ever experienced. The pain is caused by tearing of the aortic wall and its extension; it often abates and may wax and wane – this may be deceptive to the clinician if this fact is not appreciated.

b. An "aortic dissection risk score" (ADD) based on IRAD data was published in 2011 and is very helpful in prioritizing the work-up of patients presenting with chest pain.[317] This assessed three clinical categories and assigned one point to each. In this study, nearly 96% of patients with dissections had an ADD score of 1–3. It was recommended that expedited imaging be performed for scores of 2–3 and for an ADD score of 1 if there was no specific alternative diagnosis. Expedited imaging was also recommended for an ADD score of 0 in patients with unexplained hypotension or a widened mediastinum. Even if these findings were not present, aortic imaging should still be considered in patients presenting with syncope or with other risk factors for dissection (for example hypertension) if no clear alternative diagnosis is present.

  i. High-risk conditions – Marfan syndrome, family history of aortic disease, known aortic valve disease or thoracic aneurysm, or prior aortic manipulation.

  ii. High-risk pain features – chest, back, or abdominal pain that is abrupt in onset, severe in intensity, or ripping, tearing. It should be noted that the original publication states that any of these features had to be present, not all three.

  iii. High-risk exam features – pulse deficit, blood pressure differential, focal neurologic deficit in conjunction with pain, murmur of AR, hypotension or shock.

c. Depending on the location of the intimal tear and the extent of the dissection, potential complications include cardiac tamponade from hemopericardium (the most common cause of death), AR, MI, stroke, and branch artery compromise causing malperfusion. The latter may involve the brachiocephalic vessels, causing syncope, a stroke, or a discrepancy in upper-extremity blood pressures; the intercostal vessels perfusing the spinal cord, causing paraplegia; the mesenteric or renal vessels, compromising blood flow to the bowel or the kidneys; or the iliofemoral vessels, reducing distal blood flow to the legs. Surgical mortality rates increase approximately 10% for each organ system involved with malperfusion.[318]

d. An elevation in D-dimer levels is usually, but not always, noted in acute dissections and may be useful in supporting suspicion of the diagnosis.[319,320] However, an ADD of 0 combined with a negative D-dimer essentially rules out the presence of an aortic dissection.[321] Another biomarker that is being studied is smooth muscle myosin heavy chain protein that is released from damaged aortic medial smooth muscle.

2. **Type B dissection.** This classically presents with back pain that may radiate into the abdomen. However, IRAD data reported that 78% of patients with type B dissections presented with anterior chest pain, so pain location does not reliably correlate with the site of the dissection.[316] Potential rupture into the mediastinum, pleural spaces, or abdomen may occur. Malperfusion from branch artery compromise from the descending thoracic and abdominal aorta may occur as noted above.

C. Indications for surgery

1. **Type A dissection.** Surgery is indicated for all patients unless it is considered to carry a prohibitive risk because of patient age, overall medical condition and comorbidities, or the development of extensive renal, myocardial, or bowel infarction or massive stroke. In selected cases of mesenteric malperfusion, fenestration and/or stenting may be indicated prior to surgical repair of the site of the dissection.[322,323] Surgery is also indicated for virtually all patients with chronic type A dissections.

2. **Type B dissections.** Patients with uncomplicated type B dissections are usually treated medically with mortality rates of 2–6%.[324–327] Interventional (endovascular) or surgical procedures have traditionally been reserved for patients with complicated dissections. This has been defined as persistent pain, uncontrollable hypertension, evidence of aneurysmal expansion or rupture, or visceral, renal, or lower-extremity vascular compromise. However, the long-term prognosis of medically treated type B dissections is not ideal, with a 30–40% likelihood of developing subsequent aneurysmal expansion or a complicated dissection. This is more likely if the patient's heart rate and blood pressure are not well controlled, the false lumen remains patent, the initial aortic diameter is >40 mm, the false lumen diameter is >22 mm, or the proximal entry tear is >10 mm.[327] Because of this concern, it has been proposed that patients with uncomplicated dissections but high-risk features for increased growth rate should undergo elective endovascular procedures to optimize their survival. Chronic type B dissections should be operated upon when they reach 6 cm in diameter.

D. Preoperative considerations and diagnostic testing

1. **Medical management**

   a. Upon suspicion of the diagnosis, all patients must be treated pharmacologically to reduce the blood pressure (to about 110 mm Hg systolic), the heart rate (to 60–70 bpm), and the force of cardiac ejection (dp/dt). The patient should be carefully monitored and must undergo diagnostic testing as soon as possible to establish or exclude the diagnosis.

   b. Recommended antihypertensive regimens include a β-blocker (esmolol, metoprolol, or labetalol) with or without addition of sodium nitroprusside (see Table 11.8, page 576, for doses). Clevidipine is also helpful. Aggressive management up to the time of surgery is essential to prevent rupture.

2. **Examination**

   a. A careful pulse examination may indicate the extent of the dissection. Particular attention should be paid to the carotid, radial, and femoral pulses. Differential upper-extremity blood pressures in a young patient with chest pain is a strong clue to the presence of a dissection. Cardiac evaluation may reveal the presence of an AR murmur.

   b. A detailed preoperative neurologic examination is essential because a deficit recognized postoperatively may have been present at the time of presentation. A change in neurologic status may indicate progressive compromise of cerebral perfusion that can resolve with emergency surgery. However, cerebral malperfusion during CPB may also cause a significant cerebral insult. Evidence of renal dysfunction (rising BUN or creatinine, oliguria) or bowel ischemia (abdominal pain, acidosis) may necessitate modification of the surgical approach. Recurrent chest or back pain usually indicates extension, expansion, or rupture of the dissection.

3. **Diagnostic tests**

   a. The chest x-ray will usually demonstrate either a widened mediastinum or irregularity of the aortic contour, but may be normal in up to 30% of patients with a type A dissection (Figure 2.1).[316] Mediastinal width can be difficult to assess on a portable chest x-ray obtained in the emergency room, so the clinical presentation should take precedence in determining the need to obtain more definitive imaging.

   b. In a patient with severe chest pain, one might suspect that an abnormal ECG would be more consistent with an ACS, and a normal ECG would suggest the diagnosis of dissection. However, IRAD data showed that only 30–40% of patients with type A dissections had a normal ECG. Nonspecific ST changes were noted in about 40% of patients and about 20% had ischemic changes, possibly related to coronary ostial involvement with the dissection.

   c. In most hospitals, a **CT scan with contrast** is performed first. It has about 90% sensitivity and specificity in identifying an intimal flap and differential flow into true and false lumens (Figures 2.32 and 2.33). Volume-rendered imaging can provide beautiful images of aortic dissections (Figure 2.34) and can demonstrate branch artery compromise as well.

   d. **TEE** is the best procedure for identifying intimal flaps, evidence of tamponade, and AR (Figure 2.27).

      i. If the diagnosis of a type A dissection is unequivocal on CT scanning, TEE is best deferred until the patient is anesthetized in the operating room. If the diagnosis is in doubt, TEE should be performed very **cautiously** because sedation may lead to hypotension in a patient with a pericardial effusion, and acute hypertension in an inadequately sedated patient could precipitate rupture. A TTE may be valuable in ruling out a significant pericardial effusion before proceeding with a TEE.

      ii. Note that a pericardial effusion identified by CT scanning or echo usually indicates oozing of blood through the adventitia and not a free rupture. The accumulated blood under mild pressure may tamponade small bleeding sites through the aortic wall. It is generally recommended that pericardiocentesis should not be performed in this situation due to the fear of precipitating free rupture by increasing the pressure gradient between the aorta and pericardial space. Nonetheless, in salvage situations, especially in smaller hospitals without cardiac surgical availability, a controlled pericardiocentesis could prove life-saving.[328,329]

   e. **Magnetic resonance imaging (MRI)** may be the most sensitive and specific diagnostic technique to identify a dissection, but only rarely can it be obtained on an emergency basis (Figure 2.39). Furthermore, there are usually limitations to its performance in a patient requiring careful monitoring and IV drug infusions.

   f. There is little role for aortography in the evaluation of an acute dissection. Malperfusion of visceral vessels in the abdomen can be identified by CT angiography.

   g. Coronary angiography is usually not indicated in cases of acute aortic dissection, because of the necessity for emergent surgical repair. However, evidence of significant ECG changes may sometimes lead to coronary angiography as the initial diagnostic test, only to find that coronary ostial compromise is caused by an aortic dissection. In contrast, coronary angiography is helpful in planning surgical strategy in patients with chronic dissections.

E. Surgical procedures

1. Type A dissections

a. Repair involves resuspension or replacement of the aortic valve (if AR is present), resection of the intimal tear, and placement of an interposition graft to reapproximate the aortic wall (Figure 1.23). BioGlue (CryoLife) can be used to improve tissue integrity for grafting. If the root is destroyed and cannot be reconstructed, a Bentall procedure (valved conduit) is performed. If the tear extends across the arch or the tear originates in the descending thoracic aorta, consideration should be given to replacing the entire arch, often with a frozen elephant trunk (endograft) placed distally, using standard techniques of cerebral perfusion to protect the brain.[330] In experienced centers, a "total aortic repair" does not appear to increase mortality and should improve long-term outcomes by reducing the need for subsequent intervention.[331,332] Patients with visceral malperfusion have a high mortality rate and may benefit from a fenestration procedure prior to repair of the ascending aorta.[333] Iliofemoral malperfusion may require an additional revascularization procedure after the ascending aorta is replaced.

b. Repair of type A dissections should usually be performed during a period of deep hypothermic circulatory arrest (DHCA), but performing the distal anastomosis with a clamp on the distal aorta is feasible in selected cases.[334] A variety of cannulation sites for bypass have been described, most commonly using the axillary or femoral artery. Although there is a potential risk of cerebral malperfusion with initial femoral cannulation, results have been comparable with both of these approaches.[335,336] If the patient has cardiac tamponade, cannulation for and even initiation of CPB prior to opening the pericardium may be indicated, because release of tamponade could trigger free rupture and exsanguination before going on bypass.

c. Dissections with arch tears but no ascending aortic involvement are often treated as type B dissections with medical management alone. IRAD data suggest that surgical mortality exceeds medical mortality in this group of patients because the operation is more complex.[337]

d. Tears in the arch or descending aorta that extend retrograde to involve the ascending aorta are challenging. They should be managed by an ascending aorta and arch repair via a median sternotomy and placement of a frozen elephant trunk in the descending aorta.[330,338]

e. A retrograde dissection occurring after placement of an endovascular stent for a type B dissection is a difficult problem that may be managed by total arch replacement and placement of a frozen elephant trunk with partial preservation of the previous thoracic endovascular aortic repair (TEVAR) stent.[339]

2. Type B dissections

a. The traditional surgical approach to complicated type B dissections involves resection of the intimal tear and interposition graft replacement to reapproximate the aortic wall. The risk of paraplegia is greater than in patients with atherosclerotic aneurysms because less collateral flow is present. Thus, measures to reduce spinal cord ischemia by maintaining distal perfusion should be taken (see pages 81–82). Visceral malperfusion may improve with restoration of flow into the true lumen. Otherwise, a percutaneous fenestration procedure to produce a communication between the true and false lumen or additional grafting may be necessary to improve organ system or distal limb perfusion.

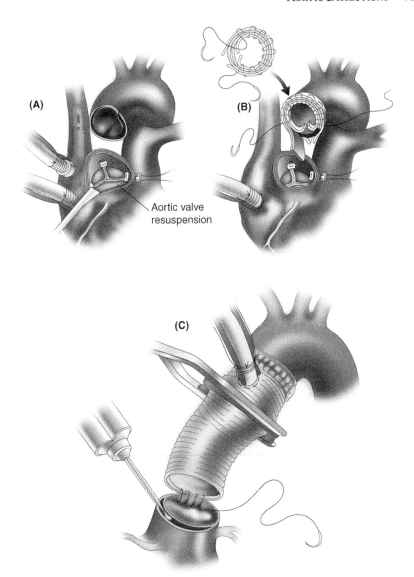

Figure 1.23 • Repair of a type A aortic dissection. (A) The aorta is opened and the entry site is resected. The aortic valve is resuspended. (B) The proximal and distal suture lines are fragile and are reinforced. During circulatory arrest with the aorta unclamped, two felt strips are shown for the distal suture line, being placed inside the true lumen and outside the adventitia. (C) After the distal suture line is completed, the graft is cannulated to reestablish antegrade cardiopulmonary bypass flow with proximal application of a cross-clamp. BioGlue may be injected to stabilize the distal and proximal (shown here) suture lines, and the proximal graft anastomosis is performed, again using felt reinforcement.

    b. Owing to the substantial morbidity and mortality associated with surgical repair, endovascular stenting (TEVAR) is the recommended approach for complicated type B dissections, if feasible.[324-327] This procedure should seal the entry site to allow for thrombosis of the false lumen. Additional fenestration and stenting may be required if reconstitution of true channel flow does not correct malperfusion. Because of the high rate of progression of uncomplicated type B dissections to malperfusion and aneurysm formation (up to 50% in IRAD studies), TEVAR is recommended for patients with "high-risk" uncomplicated dissections to promote false lumen thrombosis and aortic remodeling. The aorta tends to retain adequate plasticity to achieve adequate remodeling for three months, so the best results are achieved with a TEVAR within that timeframe.[325]

XII. Thoracic Aortic Aneurysms

    A. Pathophysiology. Ascending aortic (AAo) aneurysms usually result from medial degeneration whereas those in the distal arch, descending thoracic, and thoracoabdominal aorta are generally atherosclerotic in nature. Aneurysms in any location may result from expansion of chronic dissections. Although progressive enlargement may result in compression of adjacent structures, most deaths result from aneurysm rupture or dissection.[312,313]

    B. Indications for surgery: Ascending aortic aneurysms

      1. Guidelines for prophylactic resection of ascending aortic aneurysms are based on natural history studies which have primarily correlated aortic size with the risk of adverse aortic events (AAEs), which include rupture, dissection, or death. The latter is a confusing endpoint because death from non-aortic causes may be considered an AAE, and patients who die from dissections or rupture are included twice. These studies have not included other potentially relevant contributory factors, such as aortic stiffness or distensibility. Nonetheless, there are concerns that size criteria may not be applicable to all adult patients and should be modified based on either the patient's body surface area (the indexed aortic size) or, preferably, just the patient's height.

      2. The published risk of rupture or dissection differs only slightly in the literature, and suggests that these risks are quite low in aortas measuring <5.5 cm (Figure 1.24).

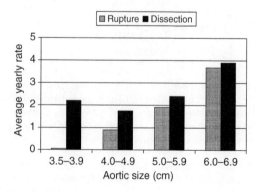

Figure 1.24 • Risk of aortic dissection or rupture based on the initial aortic size. (Adapted from Davies et al., *Ann Thorac Surg* 2002;73:17–27.)

A 2018 report from the Aortic Institute at Yale-New Haven Hospital of 780 patients with ascending aortic aneurysms showed that the annual dissection rates were 1.2, 2.0, and 1.8% for aneurysms measuring 4.0–4.4, 4.5–4.9, and 5–5.4 cm in size, respectively, with rupture alone being very rare.[340] Similarly, a study from Boston reported that the five-year risks were 0.4, 1.1, and 2.9% for aortas measuring 4.5, 5.0, and 5.5 cm, respectively.[341] Surgery was recommended when the estimated risk of adverse events exceeded the surgical risk, which may vary depending on the experience of the surgical team. Notably, it was found in the latter study that these risks were independent of whether the patient had a bicuspid valve or not.

3. Indications for surgery per ACC guidelines are based solely on aortic size.

   a. Class I indications

- Aortic root or ascending aorta >5.5 cm.[342] Although these guidelines are provided for patients with bicuspid valves, they should apply to those with trileaflet valves as well. This recommendation differs from a prior joint committee class I recommendation to perform surgery for an aorta >5.5 cm if there is no genetic disease, but for an aorta >5 cm for genetically associated disorders, including a bicuspid valve.[343]

- Aorta ≥4.5 cm in Marfan syndrome

- Aorta ≥4.2 cm in Loeys–Dietz syndrome (2010 recommendation)

- Acute type A aortic dissections

   b. Class IIa indications

- Aortic root ≥5 cm if there is a family history of aortic dissection, an aortic growth rate >0.5 cm/year, or for patients with a low surgical risk (<4%) operated on by an experienced surgical team.[344] Again, although written for patients with bicuspid valves, this should also apply to patients with trileaflet valves.[345] It has been noted that familial cases of dissection tend to occur at younger ages and have faster aortic growth rates with a threefold greater risk of dissection. Thus, it is not unreasonable to consider prophylactic aortic replacement at smaller sizes than recommended in the ACC guidelines in these patients.[346]

- Aneurysms ≥4.5 cm if an operation is indicated for aortic valve pathology. One study showed that the risk of developing an aortic dissection following AVR was more than 25% if the aortic size exceeded 5 cm at the time of AVR, but current recommendations are to replace an aorta ≥4.5 cm, probably for both bicuspid and trileaflet valves.[347]

4. Acceptance of these guidelines is confounded by IRAD data showing that 60% of aortic dissections were noted to occur in aortas measuring <5.5 cm and 40% occurred when the aorta was <5 cm in diameter.[348] Furthermore, studies have shown that aortic dimensions tend to be 7 mm larger after a dissection occurs, suggesting that surgery for smaller aortas may be justifiable.[340]

   a. Using the "one size fits all" guidelines for resection, independent of the patient's size, may not provide an accurate assessment of risk. The Yale group initially introduced the concept of the aortic size index (ASI), which was the aortic diameter divided by the body surface area (BSA) (Appendix 17).[349] They found that the risk of adverse events was low for an ASI <2.75 cm/m^2, moderate for an ASI of 2.75–4.25 cm/m^2, and significant once the ASI exceeded 4.25 cm/m². For short women with Turner's syndrome, an ASI >2.5 cm/m² is considered significant and an indication for surgery.[350]

b. However, further analysis suggested that height, rather than BSA, was a more accurate predictor of AAE. The aortic cross-sectional area/height ratio (πr^2/ht in meters) was proposed in 2002, with a value >10 producing a higher risk for dissection, and this became a level IIa indication for surgery in the 2010 and 2013 STS guidelines.[343,351] Although this was initially applied to patients with Marfan syndrome and bicuspid valves,[352,353] it was later found to be applicable to patients with trileaflet valves as well.[345] Of interest was that 42% of patients with trileaflet valves with aortas measuring 4.5–5.5 cm in diameter, which was below the 5.5 cm resection guidelines, had a height ratio >10.[345]

c. Subsequently, the Yale group reported that the aortic height index (AHI) was found to have a better correlation with AAE than the ASI.[340] The AHI was the aortic size in centimeters divided by the patient's height in meters. The risk was greater when the AHI exceeded 2.43 cm/m² (Appendix 18). Notably, the low-risk patients in this study had a composite 4%/year risk of dissection, rupture, and death, but the latter also included nonaortic deaths.

d. The Yale group then reported that ascending aortic length (AAL), which measured the centerline distance between the aortic annulus and the innominate artery, strongly correlated with the risk of AAE.[354] They derived a new metric termed the length height index (LHI) that indexed the AAL to the patient's height. They found that the risk of AAE was five times greater with an AAL ≥13 cm compared with an AAL <9 cm, and was also five times greater when the LHI was ≥7.5 cm/m compared with <5.5 cm/m. In their latest report, they renamed the AHI as the diameter height index (DHI) and redefined the AHI as the DHI + LHI to incorporate the concept of aortic length (Appendix 19). Utilizing this concept depends on an accurate measurement of aortic length, which is not routinely measured on CT angiograms in most hospitals. They found that the risk of AAE was low for an AHI <9.33, and then increased progressively for AHIs of 9.38–10.81, 10.86–12.50 and ≥12.57 cm/m.[354]

C. Indications for surgery: arch and descending aortic aneurysms

1. Arch aneurysms – all are class IIb indications per the joint guidelines.[343]

- Ascending aortic aneurysms that warrant surgery with extension into the arch. This should entail resection of the ascending aorta and partial arch replacement using DHCA with axillary inflow to allow for antegrade cerebral perfusion (ACP). It should be noted that the "aortopathy" associated with bicuspid valves tends to involve the arch in 75% of patients, and hemiarch or arch replacement should be considered in these patients.[355] A growth rate >0.5 cm/year or the development of symptoms is an indication for surgery.

- Replacement of the entire arch is reasonable for an acute dissection with an intimal tear in the arch, or when there is evidence of arch expansion, extensive tissue destruction, leakage, or rupture.[330–332] It is also reasonable for chronic dissections with arch enlargement and distal arch aneurysms extending into the descending thoracic aorta. Note that the presence of an arch tear with ascending aortic involvement mandates surgery, but medical therapy can be considered if the ascending aorta is not involved.[337]

- Isolated degenerative or atherosclerotic aneurysms >5.5 cm in diameter.

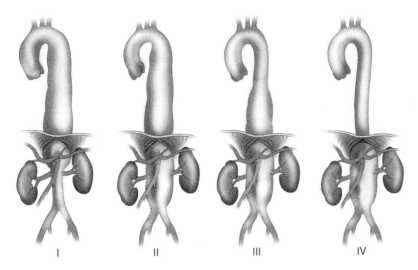

Figure 1.25 • Crawford classification of thoracoabdominal aneurysms.

2. **Descending thoracic (DAo) and thoracoabdominal aneurysms** (see Figure 1.25 for classification) – all of the below are class I indications for intervention; endografting is preferable when feasible.

- Symptomatic aneurysms
- Thoracic aneurysms ≥5.5 cm in diameter (atherosclerotic or chronic dissections) and thoracoabdominal aneurysms >6.0, but smaller in patients with connective tissue disorders.
- Complicated acute type B dissections and uncomplicated type B dissections at high risk for distal expansion.[325]

D. **Preoperative considerations**

1. Preoperative risk assessment is very important in patients undergoing resection of aortic aneurysms, especially descending aneurysms which carry higher risk.

2. Coronary angiography should be performed prior to all elective surgery in patients over age 40. It should also be performed on all patients prior to ascending aortic and arch surgery to identify coronary dominance and anatomy, since coronary button implantation is necessary in most procedures.

3. A careful preoperative baseline neurologic evaluation is important because of the risks associated with circulatory arrest (stroke, seizures) and aortic cross-clamping for surgery (the risk is highest for type II aneurysms) or with endograft coverage of intercostal arteries (paraplegia). A detailed informed-consent discussion with the patient about these devastating complications is essential and must be documented.

4. Pulmonary status must be optimized prior to surgery. Many patients with descending aortic aneurysmal disease have concomitant COPD, and the use of a thoracotomy incision, lung manipulation during surgery, anticoagulation, and multiple blood transfusions may have a detrimental effect on pulmonary function.

5. Renal function must be monitored carefully after angiography, especially in diabetic patients. The creatinine should be allowed to return to baseline before surgery to reduce the risk of renal dysfunction associated with aortic cross-clamping. Preoperative hydration may be beneficial.

6. CT angiography is essential to identify the extent of the aneurysm and potential landing zones. An assessment of aortoiliac disease is essential prior to any endovascular stenting procedure. Severe stenosis, tortuosity, or extensive atherosclerotic disease may necessitate an alternative site for arterial access or may lead to abandonment of the proposed procedure.

E. Surgical procedures

1. Ascending aortic aneurysms

a. Supracoronary interposition graft placement is performed if the aneurysm develops above the sinotubular junction, thus sparing the segment from which the coronary arteries arise.

b. If the sinuses are aneurysmal, they should be resected and replaced. For patients with moderate–severe aortic valve pathology, a valved conduit (Bentall procedure, Figure 1.11), using either a mechanical valved conduit, a manually constructed bioroot (sewing a tissue valve into a tube graft), or a stentless miniroot can be performed (Figure 1.9).[356,357] However, if there is minimal valve pathology or valve repair is feasible, an aortic valve-sparing operation should be considered, even in patients with Marfan syndrome or bicuspid valves (Figure 1.14).[358,359] The design of this procedure depends on the extent of the aneurysm and the pathophysiology of AR.

c. CPB is required for repair of AAo aneurysms. Depending on the site of the distal anastomosis, simple aortic cross-clamping or a period of DHCA may be necessary. Arterial access for CPB can be achieved through the aneurysm if DHCA is to be used, since that section of the aorta will subsequently be resected. Antegrade perfusion is then reinitiated either through a side arm limb of the graft or with direct cannulation through the graft. Alternatively, femoral or axillary artery cannulation can be used. The latter can provide ACP during a period of circulatory arrest and avoids potential retrograde embolization of atherosclerotic debris that may occur with retrograde femoral flow.

d. For DHCA, the central core temperature should be lowered to 18–20 °C, at which time there is presumed to be electroencephalographic silence. This should provide 45 minutes of safe arrest with minimal risk of neurologic insult. Adjuncts to improve cerebral protection during a period of DHCA include methylprednisolone 30 mg/kg, packing the head in ice, and either continuous retrograde cerebral perfusion (RCP) through the superior vena cava (SVC) or preferably antegrade cerebral perfusion (ACP) directly or through the axillary artery.[360-365] With the latter approach, the operation can be done at moderate systemic hypothermia.[363]

2. Transverse arch aneurysms

a. Hemiarch repair using DHCA with RCP or ACP is performed if the ascending aorta and proximal arch are involved. A graft is sewn to the undersurface of the arch leaving the brachiocephalic vessels attached to the native aorta.

b. Extended arch repair involves placement of an interposition graft sewn to the proximal descending aorta with reimplantation of a brachiocephalic island during a period of circulatory arrest. Alternatively, a debranching operation

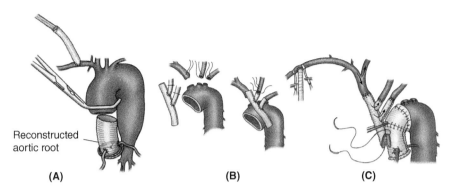

Reconstructed
aortic root

(A)   (B)   (C)

Figure 1.26 • Aortic arch replacement using a trifurcation graft (TG). (A) Using axillary cannulation for CPB, the aorta is clamped and the proximal root reconstruction is performed. (B) During DHCA, the arch vessels are divided 1 cm from their origins, and individual anastomoses are sequentially performed to the arch vessels with side limbs off the TG. (C) Flow is then restored to the brain with a clamp on the proximal segment of the TG. The distal arch anastomosis is constructed and the two aortic grafts are reapproximated. Finally, the TG is sewn to the proximal portion of the aortic graft.

with use of individual trifurcation grafts to the arch vessels may be performed. This should reduce the duration of DHCA and improve cerebral protection, potentially reducing neurologic morbidity (Figure 1.26).[366,367]

c. Distal arch repair can be performed via a left thoracotomy without cardiopulmonary bypass, but left heart bypass or CPB are commonly used. A period of DHCA may be useful when clamping is not feasible for the proximal anastomosis or for more complex operations. Endografting with carotid or subclavian artery bypass grafting can be considered in select cases.

d. If it is anticipated that a surgical descending aortic repair may be necessary in the future, a piece of graft material is left dangling from the distal anastomosis and can be retrieved at a subsequent operation through the left chest (the "elephant trunk" procedure).[368] The frozen elephant trunk procedure places a stent graft distally at the time of the arch repair, and distal stenting may be performed later.[369]

3. **Descending thoracic aorta**

a. Open graft replacement of the diseased aorta is performed with reimplantation of intercostal vessels at the level of T8–T12 for more extensive aneurysms. This is performed through a left thoracotomy or thoracoabdominal incision with use of one-lung anesthesia.

b. Consideration should be given to the use of adjuncts (medications, cerebrospinal fluid [CSF] drainage, shunting) to prevent spinal cord ischemia during the period of aortic cross-clamping or during extensive endograft placement to reduce the risk of paraplegia.[370–372] During surgical procedures, shunting can be accomplished by draining blood from a site proximal to the aortic cross-clamp (inferior pulmonary vein/left atrium/proximal aorta) and returning it distally (distal aorta/femoral artery) to perfuse the spinal cord and kidneys. A Biomedicus centrifugal pump, which actively returns blood to the patient at a designated rate, can be used with or without oxygenation. Left heart bypass alone has been shown to reduce the incidence of paraplegia during surgery for thoracoabdominal aneurysms, but not necessarily for more limited descending thoracic aneurysms.[373]

c. Because of the inherent risk of descending aortic clamping, TEVAR has become popularized for the treatment of descending thoracic and thoraco-abdominal aneurysms. This requires careful evaluation of the aorta by CT or MR imaging for landing zones and is performed using transfemoral access. Although paraplegia remains a risk of this procedure, TEVAR may reduce the risk of early death and postoperative complications, including acute kidney injury, bleeding, pneumonia, and cardiac morbidity.[374–376]

d. Femorofemoral bypass can be used to provide distal protection. It can also be used along with DHCA when clamping is not possible due to extensive disease or calcification. This technique also provides visceral and spinal cord protection.

e. Arterial monitoring lines are inserted in the right radial and femoral arteries to monitor proximal and distal pressures during the period of aortic cross-clamping, especially if left heart bypass is used.

XIII. Atrial Fibrillation

A. Pathophysiology[190]

1. Atrial fibrillation (AF) results from the presence of multiple reentrant circuits that prevent the synchronous activation of adequate atrial tissue to generate mechanical contraction. Focal triggers promote sustained reentry. Atrial distention may predispose to this arrhythmia, which then promotes progressive atrial dilatation and remodeling, leading to permanent AF. AF can lead to:

   a. Loss of atrioventricular (AV) synchrony, which reduces ventricular filling and stroke volume. This can produce dizziness, fatigue, and shortness of breath, especially in hypertrophied hearts and when the ventricular rate is high.

   b. Thrombus formation in the left atrial appendage with a predisposition to thromboembolism and stroke

   c. Symptoms of an irregular heartbeat (palpitations)

   d. A cardiomyopathy if the rate is not controlled

   e. Long-term cognitive dysfunction

2. AF may occur as an isolated entity ("lone AF") in patients with no structural heart disease or in patients with underlying heart disease. It is more common in older patients and those with hypertension, valvular heart disease, or coronary disease. It is categorized as:

   a. Paroxysmal: recurrent AF (two or more episodes) that terminates spontaneously or with an intervention within seven days. In these patients, the atrial foci that serve as the trigger are usually located in the tissue surrounding the pulmonary veins as they enter the left atrium.

   b. Persistent: lasts >7 days and responds to pharmacologic or electrical cardioversion. The reentrant circuits usually originate in the left atrium.

   c. Long-standing persistent or permanent: fails to respond to medications or cardioversion and lasts over one year.

B. **Management considerations and indications for surgery**

1. AF is managed with medications to control the ventricular rate (β-blockers, calcium channel blockers, amiodarone), potentially convert the patient to sinus rhythm, and prevent thromboembolism (warfarin or a non-vitamin K antagonist oral anticoagulant [NOAC]). When surgery is being considered, rate-control medications should be continued up to the time of surgery. NOACs should be stopped 36–48 hours prior to surgery and warfarin should be stopped five days prior to surgery. Bridging anticoagulation is indicated in patients at high risk for embolic stroke, including those with a CHA_2DS_2-VASc score ≥ 5 (see Appendix 10 A), stroke or systemic embolism within three months, or rheumatic MS.

2. When the ventricular rate cannot be controlled, symptoms are disabling, or anticoagulation cannot be tolerated or is not desirable, an ablative procedure should be considered.[377,378] Catheter ablations are very successful in ablating paroxysmal AF arising from the pulmonary veins, and with adequate mapping, reasonable success (60%) can be achieved in patients with persistent AF. In patients with long-standing persistent AF in whom anticoagulation is high risk or not desirable, a transcatheter procedure to exclude the left atrial appendage (Watchman device, Lariat) can be considered (Figure 1.27).[379,380] This may

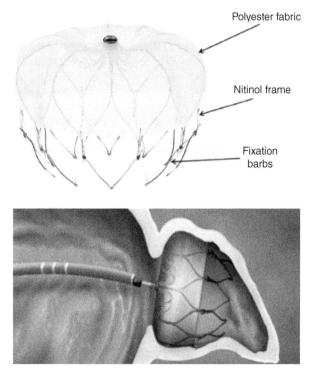

Figure 1.27 • The Watchman device is positioned at the orifice of the left atrial appendage to prevent formation of left atrial appendage thrombus. It endothelializes fairly quickly, but short-term use of warfarin is recommended. (Image courtesy of Boston Scientific Corporation (A), http://azheartrhythmcenter.com/resources/procedure-instructions/watchman-device/ (B).)

allow the patient to be off long-term anticoagulation, although a short course of warfarin is indicated after placement of a Watchman device.

3. The ability to restore sinus rhythm with an ablation performed as a stand-alone procedure or during concomitant cardiac surgery improves symptoms, quality of life, and long-term survival, and may reduce the incidence of stroke.[378] Stroke risk is also reduced by more than 50% simply by excluding the left atrial appendage without performance of an ablation procedure. Numerous societies have provided recommendations for ablative procedures. The 2017 STS practice guidelines make the following recommendations for surgical ablation:[190]

   a. Class I – As a concomitant procedure during CABG, aortic, or mitral valve surgery.

   b. Class IIa

      • As a stand-alone procedure for symptomatic AF in the absence of structural heart disease that is refractory to class I/III antiarrhythmic drugs or catheter ablation.

      • As a stand-alone Cox-Maze IV procedure for symptomatic persistent or long-standing AF in the absence of structural heart disease.

      • Left atrial appendage excision during surgical ablation or without ablation in the patient undergoing other cardiac operations.

C. **Surgical procedures**

1. In 1987, Cox designed a technically complex "cut-and-sew" operation called the "Maze" procedure that was designed to ablate AF, restore AV synchrony, and preserve atrial transport function. Subsequent iterations led to the Cox-Maze III operation, which included incisions that not only interrupted the micro-reentrant circuits but also allowed the sinus node to function, and directed propagation of the sinus impulse through both atria. AF was eliminated in about 90% of patients, but about 10% of patients required pacemakers.

2. Ablation technologies, primarily using cryoablation and radiofrequency, have been developed to mimic the suture lines of the Cox-Maze III lesion set, then called the Cox-Maze IV.[381–383] To achieve success, the lesions created must achieve transmurality.

   a. Since the left atrium is usually the primary focus of reentry, a left-sided Maze is most commonly performed, but most studies suggest that a biatrial Maze procedure is more successful in eliminating AF.[384–386] However, it is associated with more bleeding and a higher rate of pacemaker implantation, related primarily to sinus node dysfunction.[386]

   b. Success rates are lower with large left atria, advanced patient age, and pre-existing long durations of AF, although use of cryoablation rather than radiofrequency may mitigate failure rates.[190,387,388] One study found that the two-year risk of recurrence of AF was 20% greater for each one-year increase in preoperative AF duration due to more advanced tissue remodeling.[388] The likelihood of recurrence progressively increases when the left atrial size exceeds 5 cm.[389]

   c. Although these techniques have virtually completely supplanted the "cut and sew" Maze, a comparative study found that they had higher failure rates.[390]

3. For patients with paroxysmal AF, bilateral pulmonary vein isolation (PVI) with obliteration of the left atrial appendage is usually successful. This can be

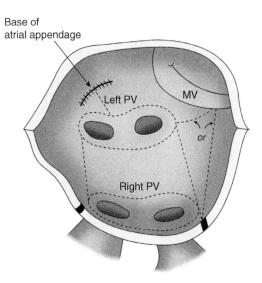

Base of
atrial appendage

Figure 1.28 • The left-sided Maze involves ablation lines that encircle and connect the right and left pulmonary veins and one that extends from the inferior box lesion near the right or left inferior pulmonary vein to the mitral valve annulus. The left atrial appendage is amputated and an additional ablation line is placed from the base of the appendage to the left pulmonary veins. The base of the left atrial appendage is then oversewn.

achieved with endocardial catheter ablation, bilateral thoracoscopic approaches with epicardial ablation, or concomitantly with other cardiac operations. Bilateral PVI is more successful after AVR than mitral valve surgery, often because the left atrium is smaller.[190]

4. For patients with persistent AF undergoing mitral valve surgery, the optimal lesion set for surgical ablation is somewhat controversial. Meta-analyses have suggested that freedom from AF is greater with a biatrial Maze than a left atrial Maze, but some studies found equivalent benefit.[384–386,391,392] One study reported that the freedom from AF (about 60–65%) was comparable with bilateral PVI and biatrial Maze procedures, but the requirement for a permanent pacemaker was 21.5% with an ablation procedure.[393] Although bilateral PVI is generally considered an inadequate operation for persistent AF, this report would seem to justify performing bilateral PVI with LA appendage excision during AVR or CABG, although better success rates can be achieved with a full left atrial Maze.[394,395]

5. **Left atrial Maze.** Persistent AF should generally be treated at a minimum by a left atrial Maze procedure (Figure 1.28). This is most commonly performed in association with mitral valve surgery, since 30–50% of these patients have preoperative AF.[393] This procedure produces ablation lines that encircle and connect the right and left pulmonary veins ("box lesion"), and one that extends from the inferior pulmonary vein ablation line to the mitral valve annulus. The left atrial appendage is amputated and an ablation line is placed through the base of the appendage to the left pulmonary vein encircling line. Left atrial volume reduction may be helpful when the LA dimension exceeds 6 cm.[396] Use of ganglionic plexi mapping and ablation with confirmation of

conduction block by pacing may improve results.[397] With use of radiofrequency ablation, the freedom from AF at two years with antiarrhythmic drugs (AAD) ranges from 65 to 85% and without drugs from 55 to 75%.[382,383,390]

6. **Right atrial Maze.** The right-sided maze includes amputation of the RA appendage (or an ablation line across its base) and an incision into the right atrium from the septum toward the AV groove. Through this incision, ablation lines are extended up the SVC and down to the IVC, across the fossa ovalis down to the coronary sinus, from the IVC to the coronary sinus, and from the sinus to the tricuspid annulus (isthmus lesions). Additional ablation lines extend from the anterior tricuspid leaflet to the base of the excised RA appendage and from the posterior tricuspid leaflet to the AV groove (Figure 1.29).

7. Exclusion of the left atrial appendage (LAA) by resection and oversewing is an integral element of any Maze procedure.[398] It has a level IIa indication in patients with AF undergoing a PVI or other cardiac procedure without an ablation.

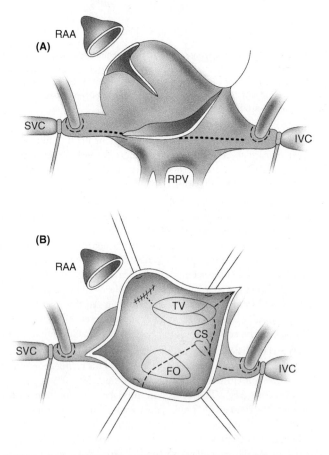

Figure 1.29 • (A) The right-sided Maze includes ablation of the base of the right atrial appendage and an incision in the right atrial wall through which multiple bipolar and unipolar ablation lines can be carried out. (B) Sites for endocardial ablation are shown by the dotted lines (see text).

a. Despite evidence that LAA resection significantly reduces the risk of thromboembolic stroke, the risk still persists even if sinus rhythm has been restored and there has been satisfactory obliteration of the LAA. One study found that, even with a return to sinus rhythm, lack of LA mechanical contraction was noted in 30% of patients after a Maze procedure and increased the risk of stroke fivefold. In addition, a large left atrium (LA volume index $\geq$33 mL/m²) increased the risk of stroke threefold. Therefore, it was recommended that anticoagulation should be utilized if either of these two findings was identified, even if sinus rhythm has been restored.[399]

b. Resection of the LAA along with a Maze procedure has even been proposed for patients in sinus rhythm undergoing mitral valve surgery with a large left atrium or more than mild TR in whom there is an increased long-term risk of developing AF.[217] It is not clear if LAA resection alone can be justified for routine open-heart operations just because of the 25% incidence of postoperative AF, which is usually self-limited.

8. For patients with "lone" persistent AF and indications for an ablation, minimally invasive surgical approaches are often considered when catheter ablation has failed. Among the various procedures that have been described are the following:

a. **Bilateral thoracoscopic approaches** generally allow for epicardial PVI using radiofrequency ablation and resection of the left atrial appendage.

b. **Dallas lesion** set (Figure 1.30). This is an epicardial procedure performed through minimal access incisions that isolates and interconnects the pulmonary

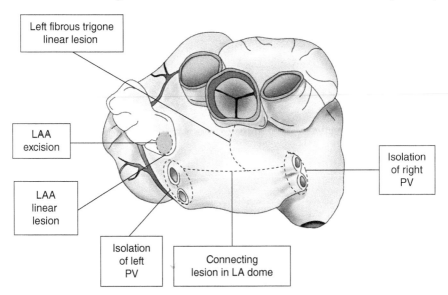

Left fibrous trigone linear lesion

LAA excision

LAA linear lesion

Isolation of left PV

Connecting lesion in LA dome

Isolation of right PV

LAA = left atrial appendage; PV = pulmonary veins

Figure 1.30 • Epicardial lesion set for a thoracoscopic approach to atrial fibrillation. Bilateral pulmonary vein isolation and a connecting lesion between the right- and left-sided pulmonary veins are performed. In addition, a linear lesion over the dome of the left atrium is created extending from the left fibrous trigone at the anterior mitral valve annulus to the base of the junction of the left and noncoronary cusps to mimic the mitral isthmus lesion performed endocardially.

veins and places an ablation line from the left fibrous trigone across the dome of the left atrium to the base of the aortic valve, mimicking the mitral isthmus lesion of the left atrial Cox-Maze III.[400] Partial autonomic denervation and excision of the left atrial appendage can also be performed.[401]

c. **Convergent procedure** (Figure 1.31). With recognition that chronic atrial stretch and structural remodeling can cause conduction abnormalities in the posterior left atrium, a hybrid approach termed the "convergent" procedure was developed. This combined partial bilateral PVI and multiple epicardial radiofrequency posterior left atrial lesions performed through a subcostal

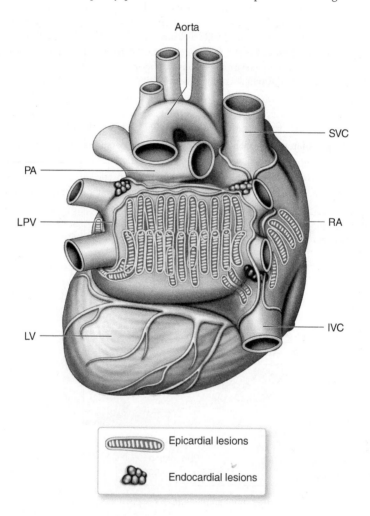

Epicardial lesions

Endocardial lesions

Figure 1.31 • Convergent procedure. Through a subxiphoid incision, bilateral pulmonary vein isolation is performed along with multiple interconnecting ablation lesions across the posterior left atrium. Subsequently, additional endocardial ablation over the pulmonary veins is performed. (Reproduced with permission of Gersak et al. *Ann Thorac Surg* 2016;102:1550–7.)[402]

approach with endocardial ablation lines performed by an electrophysiologist to complete the PVI.[402] This procedure has been recommended in symptomatic patients who fail medical therapy or catheter ablation and was given a level IIb indication by an expert consensus panel in 2017.[377]

XIV. Advanced Heart Failure

A. **Pathophysiology.** Advanced heart failure (HF) is a clinical syndrome that develops due to progressive deterioration in LV function associated with LV remodeling. It is most commonly the result of multiple infarctions from CAD (ischemic cardiomyopathy), but may result from a dilated cardiomyopathy or end-stage valvular heart disease. As ventricular function deteriorates, the LV dilates and changes from an elliptical to a spherical shape. This increases wall stress, which then increases oxygen requirements, causes pathologic cardiomyocyte hypertrophy that further compromises contractile function, and induces functional MR. These changes lead to intractable HF. In addition, ventricular remodeling increases the tendency to develop ventricular arrhythmias.[403]

1. Neurohormonal activation may contribute to remodeling. Elevation of various hormones increases sodium retention and produces peripheral vasoconstriction, increasing hemodynamic stress. There are also direct toxic effects on myocardial cells, stimulating the development of fibrosis. This relationship between neurohormonal activation and worsening of HF forms the basis of the medical approach to HF.

2. The prognosis for patients with advanced HF is quite poor, with a 50% mortality rate within one year of diagnosis. For patients in stage D, the estimated mortality rate is 80% at five years.[403]

B. **Classification and treatment considerations**

1. HF patients are generally divided into those with preserved ventricular function (HFpEF) and those with reduced ventricular function (HFrEF). The former usually develop diastolic HF from long-standing hypertension and the latter are associated with ischemic cardiomyopathies from MI, advanced valvular disease, or other nonischemic dilated cardiomyopathies. Systolic and diastolic components coexist in many patients.

2. The NYHA classification (Appendix 1B) assesses the patient's functional capacity and symptoms, progressing from no limitations of physical activity to more significant limitations with less and less activity and eventually at rest (stage IV).

3. The ACC/AHA guidelines have defined four stages in the progression of HF:

   a. **Stage A:** high risk for development of HF. These patients should have their risk factors (primarily hypertension) aggressively managed.

   b. **Stage B:** structural heart disease with LVH and reduced EF without HF. These patients need more aggressive medical therapy with ß-blockers, ACE inhibitors, or ARBs for hypertension, diuretics for volume overload, and an ICD for asymptomatic ischemic cardiomyopathy with an EF ≤30% at least 40 days post infarction.

   c. **Stage C:** structural heart disease with HF. These patients can be in NYHA class I–IV with preserved or reduced EF. Treatment includes ß-blockers, ACE inhibitors, or ARBs, and diuretics for fluid retention. CABG may be considered for angina or extensive myocardial ischemia, and valve procedures should be offered for significant valve pathology. In patients with HFrEF who have persistent class II–IV symptoms and are in stage C or D, additional considerations include:[404]

- Addition of an aldosterone receptor antagonist (spironolactone or eplerenone)
- Substitution of an ARNI (angiotensin-receptor neprilysin inhibitor [valsartan/sacubitril]) for the ACE inhibitor or ARB
- ICD for an EF ≤35% and >40 days post MI (see page 92).
- Cardiac resynchronization therapy (CRT) if EF ≤35%, normal sinus rhythm, and QRS interval >150 ms with LBBB; this is a class I indication with several class IIa and IIb indications for patients with shorter QRS intervals and non-LBBB patterns
- Ivabradine if heart rate remains >70 in sinus rhythm on ß-blockers

   d. Stage D: refractory HF requiring specialized intervention. These patients are usually in NYHA class IV and may require assist devices as a bridge to cardiac transplantation or for destination therapy.[405]

4. The INTERMACS (Interagency Registry for Mechanically Assisted Circulatory Support) profile identifies seven levels of advanced HF for patients who are in stage D with NYHA class IV (see Table 1.13 and Appendix 1D). The ROADMAP study showed that ventricular assist devices improved

Table 1.13 • INTERMACS Classification of Heart Failure

IM	Description	NYHA Class	ACC Stage	Recommended Time to MCS
1	Cardiogenic shock ("crash and burn")	IV	D	Within hours
2	Progressive decline on inotropic medications ("sliding fast")	IV	D	Within a few days
3	Stable on inotropic support ("dependent stability")	IV	D	Within a few weeks
4	Recurrent advanced HF; resting symptoms at home on oral meds ("frequent flyer")	Ambulatory IV	D	Within a few weeks–months
5	Exercise intolerance "housebound"	Ambulatory IV	D	Variable
6	Exercise limited "walking wounded"	Ambulatory IV	C–D	Variable
7	Advanced NYHA class III	IIIB	C–D	Variable

MCS, mechanical circulatory support

survival in patients with INTERMACS profile 4 and 5–7, but fewer clinical benefits were shown in profiles 5–7.[406]

C. **Indications for surgery and surgical procedures.** A variety of surgical procedures can be utilized to treat the patient with advanced HF, depending upon the pathology present and the degree of ventricular dysfunction.

1. Coronary bypass surgery should be performed in patients with an ischemic cardiomyopathy to reduce anginal symptoms, possibly improve ventricular function, alleviate symptoms of HF, lower the risk of sudden death, and improve survival. ACC/AHA guidelines recommend revascularization for the following:[403,404]

   a. Class I – angina and bypassable or stentable anatomy, especially LM or LM equivalent disease.

   b. Class IIa
      - Mild–moderate LV systolic dysfunction and significant LAD or multivessel disease with viable myocardium to increase survival. This recommendation is consistent with vast literature suggesting that CABG will improve survival in the patient with multivessel disease and impaired LV function. Furthermore, this benefit is more likely to occur when there is demonstration of viable myocardium in the area subtended by stenotic or occluded vessels.
      - CABG or medical therapy is reasonable to improve morbidity and mortality in patients with significant CAD, an EF <35%, and HF symptoms. Long-term follow-up data from the STICH trial did show improved 10-year survival in such patients compared with medical therapy.[18–20]

   c. Class IIb – CABG may be considered with ischemic heart disease, severe LV systolic dysfunction (EF <35%), and operable anatomy whether or not viable myocardium is present. A substudy of the STICH trial found that outcomes were not affected by whether myocardium was viable or not, especially in patients with severe LV dysfunction, for whom viability lost prognostic significance.[19]

2. Aortic valve surgery. Patients with symptomatic AS, especially with HF symptoms, have an average survival of 1–2 years.[127] TAVR and SAVR produce comparable long-term results in most patients, but TAVR is a less invasive procedure with rapid recovery and may be preferable in patients with advanced HF symptoms.

3. Mitral valve surgery

   a. Ischemic MR is an important predictor of the development of HF and of poor survival. Revascularization alone may be beneficial in reducing the degree of MR with acute ischemia, but is less likely with chronic ischemic MR. Whether there is any survival benefit to addressing MR with a restrictive mitral annuloplasty at the time of CABG in patients with moderate–severe LV dysfunction remains controversial, although there may be some improvement in symptoms.[202–209,407]

   b. The 2013 ACCF/AHA guidelines for management of HF considered mitral valve surgery or percutaneous mitral repair as class IIb indications in stage D patients due to uncertain benefit.[403] For patients with dilated cardiomyopathies, placement of a small restrictive annuloplasty ring has been shown to promote reverse remodeling (usually a reduction in end-systolic volume index >15%), restore normal geometric relationships, and may alleviate symptoms of HF. Improvement in long-term survival is less evident, but has been demonstrated in some studies.[407–411] Results may depend on ventricular size, since poor results have been noted with severely dilated ventricles (LV end-diastolic dimension >65 mm) and in many patients with nonischemic cardiomyopathies.[412]

c. Studies comparing mitral valve repair and replacement for patients with severe ischemic MR showed comparable two-year survival rates of about 80%, but a high rate of recurrence with mitral valve repair (58% vs. 3%). There was a significantly higher risk of HF-related adverse events with mitral valve repair as well (58% vs. 3%). These studies did not use medical therapy as a control arm and patients did not undergo CABG.[206]

d. Although the MitraClip was initially approved for patients with degenerative MR, several studies have demonstrated benefits in patients with advanced HF from functional MR. As discussed in the section on MR (pages 49–50 and 53–55), two trials published in 2018 found improvement in symptoms and reduced rehospitalization compared with medical therapy, but only one of the two supporting trials showed a survival benefit, which was evident in patients with more severe MR but less advanced LV dysfunction.[210,211] Therefore, it was concluded that MitraClip could reduce HF readmissions and mortality if applied to patients with persistent NYHA class II–IV on GDMT, including CRT, if appropriate, with ≥3+ MR (EROA ≥30 mm^2 and/or RV ≥45 mL) with an LVEF of 20–50% and LVESD <70 mm.[212]

4. Cardiac resynchronization therapy (CRT) (atrial-synchronized biventricular pacing) has been demonstrated to improve HF symptoms and exercise tolerance and promote reverse remodeling. In patients with a QRS duration >120 m/s, ventricular dyssynchrony produces suboptimal ventricular filling, a reduction in contractility, paradoxical septal wall motion, and worsening MR. By activating both ventricles in a synchronized manner, CRT is able to increase LV filling time, decrease septal dyskinesis, and reduce MR. CRT is most applicable to patients with stage C–D HF with an EF ≤35% and a QRS duration ≥120 msec. However, studies have shown a survival benefit compared with an ICD even for patients in stage B (asymptomatic HF).[413]

5. An ICD is indicated in many patients with stage B–D HF because of the frequent association of a dilated dysfunctional ventricle with ventricular tachyarrhythmias. These may be placed transvenously or subcutaneously.[414]

a. Class I indications
   • For primary prevention if EF ≤35% (NYHA class II–III) or EF ≤30% (NYHA class I) at least 40 days post MI or 90 days post revascularization on GDMT if anticipated survival >1 year
   • For nonsustained VT due to prior MI, EF <40%, inducible VT/VF by EP study

b. Class IIa indication: patients with NYHA class IV symptoms who are candidates for a left ventricular assist device (LVAD) or transplantation[415]

6. Surgical ventricular restoration (SVR) can be used for patients who develop regional akinesia or dyskinesia subsequent to a single-territory MI and have class III–IV HF symptoms.[416] Combining a CABG with resection of nonfunctioning tissue to decrease ventricular size, restore geometry, and decrease wall stress should improve ventricular function. Cardiac MR is recommended to detect myocardial scar (LGE) and assess the function of remaining viable myocardium prior to considering SVR.

a. The LV end-systolic volume index (LVESVI) is a major determinant of survival in patients with ischemic cardiomyopathy. One study found that medical therapy, CABG, or mitral repair alone had limited benefit in patients with an LVESVI >60 mL/m².[417] However, in the STICH trial, a CABG + SVR was able to produce a reduction in LV volumes and a survival benefit if the initial LVESVI was <70 mL/m², although no improvement in symptoms or exercise tolerance was achieved.[418,419] Other studies reported a better reduction in LVESVI if a viable anterior wall could be revascularized,[420] with improved survival at follow-up if the residual LVESVI after SVR was <60 mL/m².[421]

b. In patients with large ventricular dimensions and moderate MR, CABG + SVR may reduce MR by reducing sphericity of the LV, thus reducing the longitudinal and transverse dimensions of the LV that increase the interpapillary muscle distance and cause apical tethering of the leaflets.[422] However, in patients with 3–4+ MR, mitral repair should be considered in addition to SVR, and has been shown to improve five-year survival.[416]

7. When the patient has advanced HF and is not a candidate for any of the above procedures, or remains severely symptomatic despite them, more advanced interventional therapy may be required.

a. Ventricular assist devices (VADs) have been recommended on an urgent basis for patients in INTERMACS class 1–2. However, the ROADMAP study suggested that survival was also improved with VADS for ambulatory patients in profile 3–4 compared with profiles 5–7.[406]

b. Cardiac transplantation should be considered in patients with advanced HF who have an EF <15% and a peak VO₂ <10–15 mL/min/m² with maximal exercise testing. Patients in lower INTERMACS categories can be managed medically until a transplant becomes available, but sicker patients may requiring bridging with a VAD.

c. VADs can be considered for destination therapy in patients who are not considered transplant candidates. The HeartMate III (Abbott) and HeartWare (Medtronic) systems are the most commonly used VADs for destination therapy.[423]

XV. Pericardial Disease

A. **Pathophysiology and diagnostic techniques.** The pericardium may become involved in a variety of systemic disease processes that produce either pericardial effusions or constriction. The most common causes of effusions are idiopathic (probably viral), postcardiotomy, malignant, uremic, pyogenic, and tuberculous. The most common causes of constriction are idiopathic or viral, postcardiotomy, radiation, and tuberculous. Early and late postoperative cardiac tamponade due to hemopericardium are discussed on pages 446–447 and 757–761.

1. Large effusions result in tamponade physiology with progressive low output states. They are best documented by 2D echocardiography, which delineates their size and provides hemodynamic evidence of tamponade.[424] Findings include:

a. RA and ventricular diastolic collapse

b. Exaggerated ventricular interdependence (enlarged RV and smaller LV dimensions during inspiration and vice versa during expiration with increased septal bounce toward the left during inspiration)

    c. Abnormal respirophasic flow: a >20% reduction in mitral valve flow (peak E wave velocity) with inspiration and a >40% reduction in TV flow during expiration

    d. Increased reversal of flow in the hepatic veins during atrial systole

    e. A dilated IVC to >20 mm with lack of inspiratory collapse

    f. Equilibration of intracardiac pressures (RVEDP = PCWP = LVEDP) by cardiac catheterization

2. Constriction can also produce a low output state despite preserved systolic function.

    a. Cardiac catheterization will demonstrate a "square-root sign" in the RV tracing, indicating rapid early filling and a diastolic plateau caused by severe impairment to RV filling (Figure 1.32). There is equilibration of end-diastolic pressures and opposing changes in RV and LV filling during respiration.

    b. Echocardiographic findings may mimic those of cardiac tamponade, but there is no respiratory variation of the dilated IVC.

    c. Cardiovascular CT and MRI scanning can be done to assess the thickness of the pericardium, and MRI can identify pericardial inflammation.

    d. The differentiation of constriction, which is surgically correctable, from restriction, which is not, can be difficult because they have many findings in common. Although restrictive pathology is associated with diastolic dysfunction, it may or

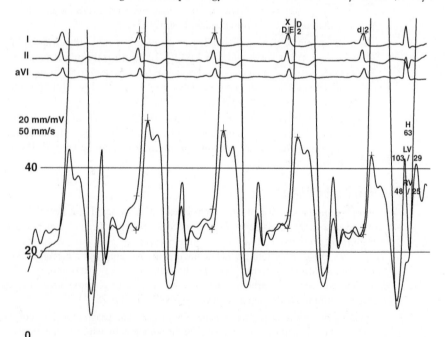

Figure 1.32 • Simultaneous right and left ventricular pressure tracings in constrictive pericarditis. Note the "dip-and-plateau" pattern as diastolic filling of the ventricular chambers is abruptly truncated by the constriction. Note also the equilibration of diastolic ventricular pressures. (Reproduced with permission from Myers et al., *Am Heart J* 1999;138:219–32.)

may not be associated with systolic dysfunction. However, the presence of significant PH suggests a restrictive process, since it is rarely seen with constriction. A number of echocardiographic methods are helpful in differentiating constriction from restriction, including septal bounce and respirophasic transvalvular flow variations, which are noted with constriction but not with restriction.[424–428]

B. **Indications for surgery**

1. Large effusions that fail to respond to noninvasive measures (dialysis for uremia, antibiotics for infection, radiation or chemotherapy for malignancy, thyroid replacement for myxedema) may be treated initially by a percutaneous drainage procedure (either pericardiocentesis with catheter drainage or balloon pericardiostomy).[429] Echocardiography is helpful in localizing the effusion and determining whether it is easily accessible to a percutaneous needle or not. Evidence of significant stranding of an effusion often suggests that percutaneous drainage will not be effective. If these procedures cannot be performed or the effusion recurs, surgical drainage should be performed.

2. Constriction that produces a refractory low output state, hepatomegaly, or peripheral edema should be treated by a pericardiectomy. Lesser degrees of constriction may resolve spontaneously or respond to a course of nonsteroidal anti-inflammatory medications or steroids.

C. **Preoperative considerations**

1. The subacute development of cardiac tamponade increases systemic venous pressures with eventual compromise in organ system perfusion from a low cardiac output syndrome. Patients frequently develop oliguric renal dysfunction, worsening respiratory status, and hepatic congestion. None of these will improve until drainage is accomplished. Fresh frozen plasma should be available if there is a pre-existing coagulopathy.

2. Both tamponade and constriction are associated with low cardiac output states. Intrinsic compensatory mechanisms to maintain blood pressure and cardiac output include a tachycardia and increased sympathetic tone. Maintenance of adequate preload is essential to increase cardiac output. β-blockers and vasodilators must be avoided. Patients with low output states from severe constriction may benefit from a few days of inotropic support prior to surgery. Patients with abnormal LV contractility and relaxation before surgery have a higher inotropic requirement after surgery with a higher mortality rate and worse long-term outcome. They might benefit the most from preoperative support.[430]

3. Preliminary pericardiocentesis for a very large effusion improves the safety of anesthetic induction, which can produce vasodilation, a fall in filling pressures, and profound hypotension.

4. Prepping and draping the patient prior to the induction of anesthesia may be a prudent maneuver in patients with an extremely tenuous hemodynamic status.

D. **Surgical procedures**

1. **Pericardial effusions.** If percutaneous drainage is inadequate or contraindicated, surgery should be performed.

   a. A subxiphoid pericardiostomy opens the pericardium, drains the pericardial space, allows for obtaining a small biopsy specimen, and obliterates the pericardial space by promoting the formation of adhesions with several days of chest

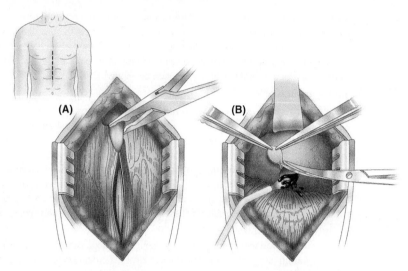

(A)

(B)

Figure 1.33 • The subxiphoid approach to pericardial disease. (A) An incision is made over the xiphisternal junction, extending inferiorly for 5 cm. The rectus fascia is incised and the xiphoid process is removed. (B) With upward traction on the distal sternum, the preperitoneal fat is swept away. The pericardium is grasped and incised and a small specimen may be removed. A finger is insinuated to break up any loculations, and pericardial fluid is aspirated with a suction catheter. A posterior chest tube is then placed below the heart.

tube drainage (Figure 1.33). It is the safest approach in the unstable patient and the best for patients with malignancies and a limited lifespan. Recurrence rate is lower with this procedure than with percutaneous catheter drainage.[431]

b. A pericardial window, created by a videothoracoscopic approach (VATS) or a limited thoracotomy, can be used to drain the effusion into the pleural space and obtain a biopsy specimen. These procedures require general anesthesia and are best utilized when there is suspicion of underlying pleuropulmonary pathology. One study suggested that a VATS approach produced a lower recurrence rate than a subxiphoid drainage procedure.[432]

2. **Constrictive pericarditis**

a. Pericardiectomy is best performed through a median sternotomy approach with pump standby, reserving a thoracotomy approach for cases of suspected infection. The pericardium is removed to within 2 cm of the phrenic nerves on either side, or at least as far as exposure allows. Dissection of the aorta and pulmonary arteries should be performed first, followed by the left and then the right ventricle to avoid pulmonary edema.

b. When the dissection plane between the thickened pericardium and the epicardium is difficult to achieve, the operation can be quite tedious. When dense calcific adhesions are present without a cleavage plane, use of CPB may allow for a safer dissection, although bleeding may be increased by heparinization. It is frequently prudent to leave heavily calcified areas adherent to the heart to minimize bleeding and pericardial damage.

    c. Rarely, patients will develop epicardial constriction with a severe inflammatory response postoperatively, anecdotally noted in some patients with prior mediastinal radiation. This problem is approached using a "waffle" procedure, which entails multiple crisscrossing incisions in the scar tissue to optimize ventricular expansion and filling.

    d. The operative mortality for pericardiectomies is 5–10%. Factors that compromise the long-term results of pericardiectomy include higher NYHA class, radiation-induced constriction, higher PA pressures, worse LV systolic function, and the presence of hyponatremia or renal dysfunction.[430,433]

XVI. Congenital Heart Disease: Atrial Septal Abnormalities

A. Pathophysiology

1. The atrial septum is composed embryologically of two separate septa which form a flap-like orifice that permits right-to-left blood flow as part of the fetal circulation. After birth, the septum seals, producing an intact atrial septum. In 25% of patients, it remains patent and is called a "patent foramen ovale" or PFO. The risk of a PFO is that of paradoxical embolism associated with right-to-left shunting when the RA pressure exceeds the LA pressure. This may be noted during straining, heavy lifting, and coughing, but can be present in more than half of patients at rest.

2. An atrial septal aneurysm (ASA) reflects redundant tissue in the area of the fossa ovalis that produces excessive mobility of the septum. This promotes adherence of platelet–fibrin debris to the left atrial side which can embolize into the systemic circulation, most commonly when there is a right-to-left shunt, which is present in 50–80% of patients with these aneurysms. The shunting may occur if there is a PFO or perforations developing within the aneurysm. Aneurysms are present in only 2% of patients with PFOs, but when present, the likelihood of sustaining a stroke is four times greater than with PFOs alone. Overall, PFOs are noted in 40% of patients with cryptogenic stroke, with 10% having both an ASA and a PFO.[434–436]

3. A small percentage of patients born with congenital atrial septal defects (ASDs) will reach adult life with a persistent left-to-right communication that may remain asymptomatic for decades. The increased shunt flow results in RA and RV enlargement, eventually leading to PH, AF, and TR. An untreated large ASD will eventually cause reversal of shunt flow, which is an inoperable situation.

B. Clinical presentation

1. **PFO.** Most patients with a PFO are asymptomatic. Clinical presentation is usually a transient ischemic attack (TIA) or stroke, or migraine-like headaches. In one study, a PFO and/or ASA could be identified in about 30% of patients <age 55 and 40% >age 55 who were diagnosed with a cryptogenic stroke.[437] Shunting through a PFO is believed to be the mechanism in platypnea–orthodeoxia syndrome (dyspnea and deoxygenation when sitting or standing up from a recumbent position).

2. **ASDs.** Depending on the size of the ASD, the degree of shunt flow, and the presence of partial anomalous pulmonary venous drainage (noted with sinus venosus defects), a patient may develop shortness of breath, fatigue, exercise

intolerance, frequent pulmonary infections, and palpitations from atrial arrhythmias. Although the flow is predominantly left-to-right, paradoxical embolism is noted in about 15% of patients.[438]

C. Evaluation

1. TEE with agitated saline injection should be performed in patients with cryptogenic stroke to detect right-to-left shunting through a PFO. A transcranial Doppler study with agitated saline is also helpful. Noninvasive lower-extremity venous studies tend to be negative because the embolus usually arises from the heart or consists of platelet-fibrin particles that are too small to detect.

2. **ASDs.** An echocardiogram can define the location and size of the septal defect, which can determine whether percutaneous closure is feasible. It should also quantitate the degree of left-to-right shunting, and assess RA and RV dilatation, RV dysfunction, and the degree of PH.

D. Indications for intervention

1. There is no indication for a prophylactic intervention in an asymptomatic patient with a PFO, because as an isolated entity, it is not an independent risk factor for stroke.[434]

2. There has been some interest in PFO closures in patients with migraine headaches and documented ischemic cerebral events.[439] However, a trial of patients undergoing percutaneous PFO closure for migraines failed to reach the study endpoint of a 50% reduction in migraine attacks.[440]

3. The optimal treatment for patients with a prior TIA or cryptogenic stroke associated with a PFO is controversial. Medical therapy with aspirin and/or warfarin can be recommended, because the risk of recurrent stroke is fairly low (about 2.5% at four years).[441] However, after several studies suggested that there was no benefit to PFO closure for secondary stroke prevention, a growing body of evidence suggested that use of a PFO percutaneous closure device, such as the Amplatzer PFO occluder device, is more efficacious than antiplatelet therapy in reducing the risk of subsequent stroke in selected patients.[436,441] One long-term follow-up study showed a 1% stroke rate out to 10 years.[442] Closure can be recommended for patients with coexistent PFO and ASA, in whom the risk of recurrent stroke is significantly greater (15% at four years).[443]

4. An ASD associated with symptoms, RA and RV enlargement (even if asymptomatic), or shunt flow exceeding 1.5:1 should be closed. Surgery can improve the patient's functional status with a reduction in RV volumes and pressures, although with no improvement in RV systolic function. ASD closure may also cause a slight reduction in LV volumes with an improvement in the LV EF. However, it has only a weak benefit in improving survival, and does not reduce the incidence of AF.[444] Patients over age 30–40 tend to have more preoperative AF and higher PA pressures, with the latter being predictive of late death from arrhythmias or HF.[445–447] An intervention can be offered as long as the PA pressure is less than 2/3 systemic or responds to vasodilators; irreversible PH contraindicates closure.

E. Interventions

1. Percutaneous closure can be performed for PFOs and secundum ASDs that are less than 38 mm in size and have a satisfactory tissue rim. Anticoagulation with antiplatelet therapy (aspirin +/- clopidogrel) is indicated for six months after placement of the device (Amplatzer).

2. Surgical closure, usually with a patch, is indicated for large secundum ASDs not amenable to percutaneous closure and for all nonsecundum ASDs, including sinus venosus defects close to the SVC with associated anomalous pulmonary venous drainage, and ostium primum defects. This can frequently be done through a right minithoracotomy incision.[448]

XVII. Adults with Other Congenital Heart Disease

For the management of adults with all other forms of congenital heart disease, the reader is referred to the ACC/AHA guidelines available at www.acc.org.[449]

References

1. Arnett DK, Blumenthal RS, Albert MA, et al. ACC/AHA guideline on the primary prevention of cardiovascular disease: executive summary: a report of the American College of Cardiology/American Heart Association task force on clinical practice guidelines. *J Am Coll Cardiol* 2019;74:1376–414.

2. Boden WE, O'Rourke RA, Teo KK. Optimal medical therapy with or without PCI for stable coronary disease. *N Engl J Med* 2007;356:1503–16.

3. De Bruyne B, Fearon WF, Pijls NHJ. Fractional flow reserve-guided PCI for stable coronary artery disease. *N Engl J Med* 2014;371:1208–17.

4. Gotberg M, Christiansen EH, Gudmundsdottir IJ, et al. Instantaneous wave-free ratio versus fractional flow reserve to guide PCI. *N Engl J Med* 2017;376:1813–23.

5. Hillis LD, Smith PK, Anderson JL. 2011 ACCF/AHA guideline for coronary artery bypass graft surgery. *J Am Coll Cardiol* 2011;58:e123–210.

6. Weiss S, Weintraub W. Revascularization vs. medical therapy in stable ischemic heart disease. *Prog Cardiovasc Dis* 2015;58:299–305.

7. Patel MR, Calhoon JH, Dehmer JH, Grantham JA, Maddox TM, Maron DJ, Smith PK. ACC/AATS/AHA/ASE/ASNC/SCAI/SCCT/STS 2017 appropriate use criteria for coronary revascularization in patients with stable ischemic heart disease. *J Am Coll Cardiol* 2017;69:2212–41.

8. Mohr FW, Morice MC, Kappetein AP, et al. Coronary artery bypass graft surgery versus percutaneous intervention in patients with three-vessel disease and left main disease: 5-year follow-up of the randomized clinical SYNTAX trial. *Lancet* 2013;381:629–38.

9. Mack M, Baumgarten H, Lytle BS. Why surgery won the SYNTAX trial and why it matters. *J Thorac Cardiovasc Surg* 2016;152:1237–40.

10. Farkouh ME, Domanski M, Dangas GD, et al. on behalf of the FREEDOM follow-on study investigators. Long-term survival following multivessel revascularization in patients with diabetes (FREEDOM follow-on study). *J Am Coll Cardiol* 2019;73:629–38.

11. Farkouh ME, Domanski M, Sleeper LA, et al. Strategies for multivessel revascularization in patients with diabetes. *N Engl J Med* 2012;367:2375–84.

12. Esper RB, Farkouh ME, Riberio EE, et al. SYNTAX score in patients with diabetes undergoing coronary revascularization in the FREEDOM trial. *J Am Coll Cardiol* 2018;72:2826–37.

13. Généreux P, Palmerini T, Caixeta A. Quantification and impact of untreated coronary artery disease after percutaneous coronary intervention: the residual SYNTAX (Synergy Between PCI with Taxus and Cardiac Surgery) score. *J Am Coll Cardiol* 2012;59:2165–74.

14. Milojevic M, Head SJ, Parasca CA, et al. Causes of death following PCI versus CABG in complex CAD: 5-year follow-up of SYNTAX. *J Am Coll Cardiol* 2016;67:42–55.

15. Farooq V, van Klaveren D, Steyerberg EW, et al. Anatomical and clinical characteristics to guide decision making between coronary artery bypass surgery and percutaneous coronary intervention for individual patients: development and validation of SYNTAX score II. *Lancet* 2013;381:639–50.

16. Dangas GD, Farkouh ME, Sleeper LA, et al. Long-term outcome of PCI versus CABG in insulin and non-insulin treated diabetic patients: results from the FREEDOM trial. *J Am Coll Cardiol* 2014;64:1189–97.

17. Doenst T, Haverich A, Serruys P, et al. PCI and CABG for treating stable coronary artery disease. *J Am Coll Cardiol* 2019;73:964–76.

18. Velaquez EJ, Lee KL, Deja MA, et al. for the STICH investigators. Coronary-artery bypass surgery in patients with left ventricular dysfunction. *N Engl J Med* 2011;364:1607–16.

19. Michler RE. A decade after the Surgical Treatment for Ischemic Heart Failure (STICH) trial: weaving firm clinical recommendations from lessons learned. *J Thorac Cardiovasc Surg* 2019;157:950–7.

20. Bonow RO, Maurer G, Lee KL, et al. Myocardial viability and survival in ischemic left ventricular dysfunction. *N Engl J Med* 2011;364:1617–25.

21. Allman KC, Shaw LJ, Hachamovitch R, Udelson JE. Myocardial viability testing and impact of revascularization on prognosis in patients with coronary artery disease and left ventricular dysfunction: a meta-analysis. *J Am Coll Cardiol* 2002;39:1151–8.

22. Nagendran J, Bozso SJ, Norris CM, et al. Coronary artery bypass surgery improves outcomes in patients with diabetes and left ventricular dysfunction. *J Am Coll Cardiol* 2018;71:819–27.

23. Amsterdam EA, Wenger NK, Brindis RG, et al. 2014 AHA/ACC guideline for the management of patients with non-ST-elevation acute coronary syndromes. *Circulation* 2014;130:3349–426.

24. Anderson JL, Morrow DA. Acute myocardial infarction. *N Eng J Med* 2017;376:2053–64.

25. Hoedemaker NPG, Damman P, Woudstra P, et al. Early invasive versus selective strategy for non-ST-segment elevation acute coronary syndrome: the ICTUS trial. *J Am Coll Cadiol* 2017;69:1883–93.

26. Patel MR, Calhoon JH, Dehmer JH, Grantham JA, Maddox TM, Maron DJ, Smith PK. 1: ACC/AATS/AHA/ASE/ASNC/SCAI/SCCT/STS: 2016 appropriate use criteria for coronary revascularization in patients with acute coronary syndromes. *J Am Coll Cardiol* 2017;69:570–91.

27. Hu Y, Zhiping L, Chen J, Shen C, Song Y, Zhong Q. The effect of the time interval between coronary angiography and on-pump cardiac surgery on risk of postoperative acute kidney injury: a meta-analysis. *J Cardiothorac Surg* 2013;8:178.

28. Kwak YL, Kim JC, Choi YS, Yoo KJ, Song Y, Shim JK. Clopidogrel responsiveness regardless of the discontinuation date predicts increased blood loss and transfusion requirement after off-pump coronary artery bypass graft surgery. *J Am Coll Cardiol* 2010;56:1994–2002.

29. Mahla E, Suarez TA, Bliden KP, et al. Platelet function measurement-based strategy to reduce bleeding and waiting time in clopidogrel-treated patients undergoing coronary artery bypass graft surgery: the timing based on platelet function strategy to reduce clopidogrel-associated bleeding related to CABG (TARGET-CABG) Study. *Circ Cardiovasc Interv* 2012;5:261–9.

30. Basir MB, Schreiber T, Grines CL, et al. Effect of early initiation of mechanical circulatory support on survival in cardiogenic shock. *Am J Cardiol* 2017;119:845–51.

31. Flaherty MP, Khan AR, O'Neill WW. Early initiation of Impella in acute myocardial infarction complicated by cardiogenic shock improves survival: a meta-analysis. *JACC Cardiovasc Interv* 2017;10:1805–6.

32. McCann GP, Khan JN, Greenwood JP, et al. Complete versus lesion-only primary PCI. The Cardiovascular MR CvLPRIT Substudy. *J Am Coll Cardiol* 2015;66:2713–24.

33. Thiele H, Akin I, Sandri S, et al. One-year outcomes after PCI strategies in cardiogenic shock. *N Engl J Med* 2018;379:1699–710.

34. Caceres M, Weiman DS. Optimal timing of coronary artery bypass grafting in acute myocardial infarction. *Ann Thorac Surg* 2013;95:365–72.

35. Acharya D, Gulack BC, Loyaga-Rendon RY, et al. Clinical characteristics and outcome of patients with myocardial infarction and cardiogenic shock undergoing coronary artery bypass surgery: data from The Society of Thoracic Surgeons national database. *Ann Thorac Surg* 2016;101:558–66.

36. Dangas GD, Kini AS, Sharma SK, et al. Impact of hemodynamic support with Impella 2.5 versus intra-aortic balloon pump on prognostically important clinical outcomes in patients undergoing high-risk percutaneous coronary intervention (from the PROTECT II randomized trial). *Am J Cardiol* 2014;113:222–8.

37. Tonino PA, De Bruyne B, Piljls NH, et al. Fractional flow reserve versus angiography for guiding percutaneous coronary intervention. *N Eng J Med* 2009;360:213–24.

38. Shah T, Geleris JD, Zhong M, Swaminathan R, Kim LK, Feldman DN. Fractional flow reserve to guide surgical coronary revascularization. *J Thorac Dis* 2017;9 (Suppl 4): S317–26.

39. Toth G, De Bruyne B, Casselman F, et al. Fractional flow reserve-guided versus angiography-guided coronary artery bypass graft surgery. *Circulation* 2013;128:1405–11.

40. Fournier S, Toth GG, De Bruyne B, et al. Six-year follow-up of fractional flow reserve-guided versus angiography-guided coronary artery bypass graft surgery. *Circ Cardiovasc Interv* 2018;11:e06368.

41. Mahmoud AN, Shah NH, Elgendy IY, et al. Safety and efficacy of second-generation drug-eluting stents compared with bare-metal stents: an updated meta-analysis and regression of 9 randomized clinical trials. *Clin Cardiol* 2018;41:151–8.

42. Ng VG, Lansky AJ. Platelet function testing: a research tool with limited clinical utility. www.acc.org/latest-in-cardiology/articles/2016/05/10/07/22.

43. Misumida N, Abo-Aly M, Kim SM, Ogunbayo GO, Abdel-Latif A, Ziada KM. Efficacy and safety of short-term dual antiplatelet therapy (≤6 months) after percutaneous coronary intervention for acute coronary syndrome: a systematic review and meta-analysis of randomized controlled trials. *Clin Cardiol* 2018;41:1455–62.

44. Puskas JD, Halkos ME, DeRose JJ, et al. Hybrid coronary revascularization for the treatment of multivessel coronary artery disease: a multicenter observational study. *J Am Coll Cardiol* 2016;68:356–65.

45. Rosenblum JM, Harskamp RE, Hoedemaker N, et al. Hybrid coronary revascularization versus coronary artery bypass surgery with bilateral or single internal mammary artery grafts. *J Thorac Cardiovasc Surg* 2016;151:1081–9.

46. Xia Y, Katz AN, Forest SJ, Pyo RT, Greenberg MA, DeRose JJ Jr. Hybrid coronary revascularization has improved short-term outcomes but worse mid-term reintervention rates compared to CABG: a propensity matched analysis. *Innovations (Phila)* 2017;12:174–9.

47. Thaper A, Kulik A. Rationale for administering beta-blocker therapy to patients undergoing coronary artery bypass surgery: a systematic review. *Expert Opin Drug Saf* 2018;17:805–13.

48. Brinkman W, Herbert MA, O'Brien S, et al. Preoperative ß-blocker use in coronary artery bypass grafting surgery: national database analysis. *JAMA Intern Med* 2014;174:1320–7.

49. Doherty JU, Gluckman TJ, Hucker WJ, et al. 2017 ACC Expert consensus decision pathway for periprocedural management of anticoagulation in patients with nonvalvular atrial fibrillation. *J Am Coll Cardiol* 2017;69:871–92.

50. Renda G, Ricci F, Giugliano RP, De Caterina R. Non-vitamin K antagonist oral anticoagulants in patients with atrial fibrillation and valvular heart disease. *J Am Coll Cardiol* 2017;69:1363–71.

51. Hassan K, Bayer N, Schlingloff F, et al. Bleeding complications after use of novel oral anticoagulants in patients undergoing cardiac surgery. *Ann Thorac Surg* 2018;105:702–8.

52. Aboul-Hassan SS, Stankowski T, Marczak J, et al. The use of preoperative aspirin in cardiac surgery: a systematic review and meta-analysis. *J Card Surg* 2017;32:758–74.

53. Hastings S, Myles PA, McIlroy DM. Aspirin and coronary artery surgery: an updated meta-analysis. *Br J Anaesth* 2016;116:716–7.

54. Myles PS, Smith JA, Forbes A, et al. Stopping vs. continuing aspirin before coronary artery surgery. *N Engl J Med* 2016;374:728–37.

55. Ferraris VA, Saha SP, Oestreich JH, et al. 2012 Update to The Society of Thoracic Surgeons guideline on use of antiplatelet drugs in patients having cardiac and noncardiac operations. *Ann Thorac Surg* 2012;94:1761–81.

56. Maltais S, Perrault LP, Do QB. Effect of clopidogrel on bleeding and transfusions after off-pump coronary artery bypass graft surgery: impact of discontinuation prior to surgery. *Eur J Cardiothorac Surg* 2008;34:127–31.

57. Angiolillo DJ, Firstenberg MS, Price MJ, et al. Bridging antiplatelet therapy with cangrelor in patients undergoing cardiac surgery: a randomized controlled trial. *JAMA* 2012;307:265–74.

58. Stucchi M, Cantoni S, Piccinelli E, Savonitto S, Morici N. Anemia and acute coronary syndrome: current perspectives. *Vasc Health Risk Manag* 2017;14:109–18.

59. Carson JL, Stanworth SJ, Alexander JH, et al. Clinical trials evaluating red blood cell transfusion thresholds: an updated systematic review and with additional focus on patients with cardiovascular disease. *Am Heart J* 2018;200:96–101.

60. Williams ML, Rankin JS, Slaughter MS, Gammie JS. Preoperative hematocrit is a powerful predictor of adverse outcomes in coronary artery bypass graft surgery: a report from the Society of Thoracic Surgeons adult cardiac surgery database. *Ann Thor Surg* 2013;96:1628–34.

61. LaPar DJ, Hawkins RB, McMurry TL, et al. Preoperative anemia versus blood transfusion: which is the culprit for worse outcomes in cardiac surgery? *J Thorac Cardiovasc Surg* 2018;156:66–74.

62. Bagshaw SM, Galbraith PD, Mitchell LB, Suave R, Exner DV, Shali WA. Prophylactic amiodarone for prevention of atrial fibrillation after cardiac surgery: a meta-analysis. *Ann Thorac Surg* 2006;82:1927–37.

63. Liaopoulos OJ, Choi YH, Kuhn EW, et al. Statins for prevention of atrial fibrillation after cardiac surgery: a systematic literature review. *J Thorac Cardiovasc Surg* 2009;138:678–86.

64. Curtis M, Deng Y, Lee VV, et al. Effect of dose and timing of preoperative statins on mortality after coronary artery bypass surgery. *Ann Thorac Surg* 2017;104:782–9.

65. Katznelson R, Djaiani GN, Borger MA, et al. Preoperative use of statins is associated with reduced early delirium rates after cardiac surgery. *Anesthesiology* 2009;110:67–73.

66. Wang J, Gu C, Gao M, Yu W, Yu Y. Preoperative statin therapy and renal outcomes after cardiac surgery: a meta-analysis and meta-regression of 59,771 patients. *Can J Cardiol* 2015;31:1051–60.

67. Whitlock RP, Chan S, Devereaux PJ, et al. Clinical benefit of steroid use in patients undergoing cardiopulmonary bypass: a meta-analysis of randomized trials. *Eur Heart J* 2008;29:2592–600.

68. Rousou LJ, Taylor KB, Lu XG, et al. Saphenous vein conduits harvested by endoscopic technique exhibit structural and functional damage. *Ann Thorac Surg* 2009;87:62–70.

69. Kroeze VJ, Lam KY, van Straten AHM, Houterman S, Soliman-Hamad, MA. Benefits of endoscopic vein harvesting in coronary artery bypass grafting. *Ann Thorac Surg* 2019;108:1793–800.

70. Zenati MA, Bhatt DL, Bakaeen FG, et al. Randomized trial of endoscopic or open-vein harvesting for coronary-artery bypass. *N Engl J Med* 2019;380:132–41.

71. Aldea GS, Bakaeen FG, Pal J, et al. The Society of Thoracic Surgeons Clinical Practice Guidelines on arterial conduits for coronary artery bypass grafting. *Ann Thorac Surg* 2016;101:801–9.

72. Gaudino M, Taggart D, Suma H, Puskas JD, Crea F, Massetti M. The choice of conduits in coronary artery bypass surgery. *J Am Coll Cardiol* 2015;66:1729–37.

73. Samadashvili Z, Sundt TM III, Wechsler A, et al. Multiple versus single arterial coronary bypass graft surgery for multivessel disease. *J Am Coll Cardiol* 2019;74:1275–85.

74. Yoshizaki T, Tabuchi N, Toyama M. Verapamil and nitroglycerin improves the patency rate of radial artery grafts. *Asian Cardiovasc Thorac Ann* 2008;16:396–400.

75. He GW, Taggart DP. Antispastic management in arterial grafts in coronary artery bypass grafting surgery. *Ann Thorac Surg* 2016;102:659–68.

76. Puskas KD, Stringer A, Hwang SN, et al. Neurocognitive and neuroanatomic changes after off-pump versus on-pump coronary artery bypass grafting: long-term follow-up of a randomized trial. *J Thorac Cardiovasc Surg* 2011;141:1116–27.

77. Shroyer AL, Hattler B, Wagner TH, et al. Five-year outcomes after on-pump and off-pump coronary-artery bypass. *N Engl J Med* 2017;377:623–32.

78. Smart NA, Dieberg G, King N. Long-term outcomes of on- versus off-pump coronary artery bypass grafting. *J Am Coll Cardiol* 2018;71:983–91.

79. Chikwe J, Lee T, Itagaki S, Adams DH, Egorova NN. Long-term outcomes after off-pump versus on-pump coronary artery bypass grafting by experienced surgeons. *J Am Coll Cardiol* 2018;72:1478–86.

80. Fattouch K, Guccione F, Dioguardi P, et al. Off-pump versus on-pump myocardial revascularization in patients with ST-segment myocardial infarction: a randomized trial. *J Thorac Cardiovasc Surg* 2009;137:650–7.

81. Kikuchi K, Mori M. Minimally invasive coronary artery bypass grafting: a systematic review. *Asian Cardiovasc Thorac Ann* 2017;25:364–70.

82. Kikchi K, Chen X, Mori M, Kurata A, Tao L. Perioperative outcomes of off-pump minimally invasive coronary artery bypass grafting with bilateral internal thoracic arteries under direct vision. *Interact Cardiovasc Thorac Surg* 2017;24:696–701.

83. Deppe AC, Liakopoulos OJ, Kuhn EW, et al. Minimally invasive direct coronary bypass grafting versus percutaneous intervention for single-vessel disease: a meta-analysis of 2885 patients. *Eur J Cardiothorac Surg* 2015;47:397–406.

84. Kofler M, Stastny L, Reinstadler SJ, et al. Robotic versus conventional coronary artery bypass grafting: direct comparison of long-term clinical outcome. *Innovations (Phila)* 2017;12:239–46.

85. Allen KB, Dowling RD, Angell WW, et al. Transmyocardial revascularization: 5 year follow-up of a prospective, randomized multicenter trial. *Ann Thorac Surg* 2004;77:1228–34.

86. Aaberge L, Rootwelt K, Blomhoff S, Saatvedt K, Abdelnoor M, Forfang K. Continued symptomatic improvement three to five years after transmyocardial revascularization with CO(2) laser: late clinical follow-up of the Norwegian randomized trial with transmyocardial revascularization. *J Am Coll Cardiol* 2002;39:1588–93.

87. Allen GS. Mid-term results after thoracoscopic transmyocardial laser revascularization. *Ann Thorac Surg* 2005;80:553–8.

88. Heatlie GJ, Mohiaddin R. Left ventricular aneurysm: comprehensive assessment of morphology, structure and thrombus using cardiovascular magnetic resonance. *Clin Radiol* 2005;60:687–92.

89. Lapeyre AC 3rd, Steele PM, Kazmier FJ, Chesebro JH, Vlietstra RE, Fuster V. Systemic embolism in chronic left ventricular aneurysm: incidence of and the role of anticoagulation. *J Am Coll Cardiol* 1985;6:534–8.

90. Doss N, Martens S, Sayour S, Hemmer W. Long term follow up of left ventricular function after repair of left ventricular aneurysm: a comparison of linear closure versus patch plasty. *Eur J Cardiothorac Surg* 2001;20:783–5.

91. Shapira OM, Davidoff R, Hilkert RJ, Aldea GS, Fitzgerald CA, Shemin RJ. Repair of left ventricular aneurysm: long-term results of linear repair versus endoaneurysmorrhaphy. *Ann Thorac Surg* 1997;63:701–5.

92. Dor V, Di Donato M, Sabatier M, Montiglio F, Civaia F, RESTORE Group. Left ventricular reconstruction by endoventricular circular patch plasty repair: a 17-year experience. *Semin Thorac Cardiovasc Surg* 2001;13:435–7.

93. Athanasuleas C, Buckberg GD, Stanley AW, et al. Surgical ventricular restoration in the treatment of congestive heart failure due to post-infarction ventricular dilatation. *J Am Coll Cardiol* 2004;44:1439–45.

94. Di Donato M, Castelvecchio S, Kukulski T, et al. Surgical ventricular restoration: left ventricular shape influence on cardiac function, clinical status, and survival. *Ann Thorac Surg* 2009;87:455–62.

95. Dzemali O, Risteski P, Bakhtiary F, et al. Surgical ventricular remodeling leads to better long-term survival and exercise tolerance than coronary artery bypass grafting alone in patients with moderate ischemic cardiomyopathy. *J Thorac Cardiovasc Surg* 2009;138:663–8.

96. Di Donato M, Sabatier N, Dor V, Toso A, Maioli M, Fantini F. Akinetic versus dyskinetic postinfarction scar: relation to surgical outcome in patients undergoing endoventricular circular patch plasty repair. *J Am Coll Cardiol* 1997;29:1569–75.

97. Jones RH, Velazquez EJ, Michler RE, et al. Coronary bypass surgery with or without surgical ventricular reconstruction. *N Engl J Med* 2009;360:1705–17.

98. Dor V, Sabatier M, Montiglio F, et al. Results of nonguided subtotal endocardiectomy associated with left ventricular reconstruction in patients with ischemic ventricular arrhythmias. *J Thorac Cardiovasc Surg* 1994;107:1301–7.

99. Sosa E, Jatene A, Kaeriyama JV, et al. Recurrent ventricular tachycardia associated with post infarction aneurysm: results of left ventricular reconstruction. *J Thorac Cardiovasc Surg* 1992;103:855–60.

100. Birnbaum Y, Fishbein MC, Blanche C, Siegel RJ. Ventricular septal rupture after acute myocardial infarction. *N Engl J Med* 2002;347:1426–32.

101. Arnaoutakis GJ, Zhao Y, George TJ, Sciortino CM, McCarthy PM, Conte JV. Surgical repair of ventricular septal defect after myocardial infarction: outcomes from The Society of Thoracic Surgeons national database. *Ann Thorac Surg* 2012;94:436–44.

102. Lundblad R, Abdelnoor M, Geiran OR, Svennevig JL. Surgical repair of postinfarction ventricular septal rupture: risk factors of early and late death. *J Thorac Cardiovasc Surg* 2009;137:862–8.

103. David TE, Armstrong S. Surgical repair of postinfarction ventricular septal defect by infarct exclusion. *Semin Thorac Cardiovasc Surg* 1998;10:105–10.

104. Muehrcke DD, Daggett WM Jr, Buckley MJ, Akins CW, Hilgenberg AD, Austen WG. Postinfarct ventricular septal defect repair: effect of coronary artery bypass grafting. *Ann Thorac Surg* 1992;54:876–83.

105. Sabiniewicz R, Huczek Z, Zbronski K, et al. Percutaneous closure of post-infarction ventricular septal defects: an over decade-long experience. *J Interv Cardiol* 2017;30:63–71.

106. Bonow RO, Carabello BA, Chatterjee K, et al. 2008 focused update incorporated into the ACC/AHA 2006 guidelines for the management of patients with valvular heart disease: a report of the American College of Cardiology/American Heart Association Task Force on Practice Guidelines (Writing

committee to revise the 1998 guidelines for the management of patients with valvular heart disease): endorsed by the Society of Cardiovascular Anesthesiologists, Society for Cardiovascular Angiography and Interventions, and Society of Thoracic Surgeons. *J Am Coll Cardiol* 2008;52:1–142.

107. Nishimura, RA, Otto CM, Bonow RO, et al. 2014 AHA/ACC Guideline for the management of patients with valvular heart disease: a report of the American College of Cardiology/American Heart Association Task Force on Practice Guidelines. *Circulation* 2014;129:e521–643.

108. Yan AT, Koh M, Chan KK, et al. Association between cardiovascular risk factors and aortic stenosis: the CANHEART aortic stenosis study. *J Am Coll Cardiol* 2017;69:1523–32.

109. Rossebø AB, Pedersen TR, Boman K, et al. Intensive lipid lowering with simvastatin and ezetimibe in aortic stenosis. *N Engl J Med* 2008;359:1343–56.

110. Bartunek J, Sys SU, Rodrigues AC, Schuerbeeck EV, Mortier L, de Bruyne B. Abnormal systolic intracavity flow velocities after valve replacement for aortic stenosis: mechanisms, predictive factors, and prognostic significance. *Circulation* 1996;93:712–9.

111. Omran H, Schmidt H, Hackenbroch M, et al. Silent and apparent cerebral embolism after retrograde catheterisation of the aortic valve in valvular stenosis: a prospective, randomised study. *Lancet* 2003;361:1241–6.

112. Pibarot P, Dumesnil JG. Paradoxical low-flow, low-gradient aortic stenosis: new evidence, more questions. *Circulation* 2013;128:1729–32.

113. Pibarot P, Clavel MA. Management of paradoxical low-flow, low-gradient aortic stenosis: need for an integrated approach, including assessment of symptoms, hypertension, and stenosis severity. *J Am Coll Cardiol* 2015;65:67–71.

114. Eleid MF, Sorajja P, Michelena HI, Malouf JF, Scott CG, Pellikka PA. Flow-gradient patterns in severe aortic stenosis with preserved ejection fraction: clinical characteristics and predictors of survival. *Circulation.*2013;128:1781–9.

115. Dumesnil JG, Pibarot P, Carabello B. Paradoxical low flow and/or low gradient severe aortic stenosis despite preserved left ventricular ejection fraction: implications for diagnosis and treatment. *Eur Heart J* 2010;31:281–9.

116. Ozkan A, Hachamovitch R, Kapadia SR, Tuzcu EM, Marwick TH. Impact of aortic valve replacement on outcome of symptomatic patients with severe aortic stenosis with low gradient and preserved left ventricular ejection fraction. *Circulation* 2013;128:622–31.

117. Pawade T, Clavel MA, Tribouilloy C, et al. Computed tomography aortic valve calcium scoring in patients with aortic stenosis. *Circ Cardiovasc Imaging* 2018;111:e007146.

118. Clavel MA, Burwash IG, Pibarot P. Cardiac imaging for assessing low-gradient severe aortic stenosis. *JACC Cardiovasc Imaging* 2017;10:185–202.

119. Clavel MA, Pibarot P, Messika-Zeitoun D, et al. Impact of aortic valve calcification, as measured by MDCT, on survival in patients with aortic stenosis: results of an international registry study. *J Am Coll Cardiol* 2014;64:1202–13.

120. Rafique AM, Biner S, Ray I, et al. Meta-analysis of prognostic value of stress testing in patients with asymptomatic aortic stenosis. *Am J Cardiol* 2009;104:972–7.

121. Magne J, Lancelotti P, Piérard LA. Exercise testing in asymptomatic aortic stenosis. *JACC Cardiovasc Imaging* 2014;7:188–99.

122. van Gils L, Clavel MA, Vollema EM, et al. Prognostic implications of moderate aortic stenosis in patients with left ventricular systolic dysfunction. *J Am Coll Cardiol* 2017;69:2383–92.

123. Pellikka PA, Nishimura RA, Bailey KR, Tajik AJ. The natural history of adults with asymptomatic, hemodynamically significant aortic stenosis. *J Am Coll Cardiol* 1990;15:1012–7.

124. Pellikka PA, Sarano ME, Nishimura RA, et al. Outcome of 622 adults with asymptomatic, hemodynamically significant aortic stenosis during prolonged follow-up. *Circulation* 2005;111:3290–5.

125. Henkel DM, Malouf JF, Connolly HM, et al. Asymptomatic left ventricular systolic dysfunction in patients with severe aortic stenosis. *J Am Coll Cardiol* 2012;60:2325–9.

126. Nakatsuma K, Taniguchi T, Morimoto T, et al. B-type natriuretic peptide in patients with asymptomatic severe aortic stenosis. *Heart* 2019;105:384–90.

127. Horstkotte D, Loogen F. The natural history of aortic valve stenosis. *Eur Heart J* 1988;9(Suppl E): 57–64.

128. Leon MB, Smith CR, Mack M, et al. Transcatheter aortic-valve implantation for aortic stenosis in patients who cannot undergo surgery. *N Engl J Med* 2010;36:1597–607.

129. Glaser N, Persson M, Jackson V, Holzmann MJH, Franco-Cereceda A, Sartipy U. Loss in life expectancy after surgical aortic valve replacement: SWEDEHEART study. *J Am Coll Cardiol* 2019;74:26–33.

130. Shirai S, Taniguchi T, Morimoto T, et al. Five-year clinical outcome of asymptomatic vs. symptomatic severe aortic stenosis after aortic valve replacement. *Circ J* 2017;81:485–94.

131. Otto CM, Nishimura RA, Bonow RO, et al. 2020 ACC/AHA guideline for the management of patients with valvular heart disease: a report of the American College of Cardiology/American Heart Association Joint Committee on Clinical Practice Guidelines. *J Am Coll Cardiol* 2021;77:e25–197.

132. Levy F, Laurent M, Monin JL, et al. Aortic valve replacement for low-flow/low-gradient aortic stenosis: operative risk stratification and long-term outcome: a European Multicenter study. *J Am Coll Cardiol* 2008;51:1466–72.

133. Tribouilloy C, Lévy F, Rusinaru D, et al. Outcome after aortic valve replacement for low-flow/low-gradient aortic stenosis without contractile reserve on dobutamine stress echocardiography. *J Am Coll Cardiol* 2009;53:1865–73.

134. Maes F, Lerakis S, Barbosa Ribeiro H, et al. Outcomes from transcatheter aortic valve replacement in patients with low-flow, low-gradient aortic stenosis and left ventricular ejection fraction less than 30%: a substudy from the TOPAS-TAVI Registry. *JAMA Cardiol* 2018;4:64–70.

135. Bergler-Klein J, Mundigler G, Pibarot P, et al. B-type natriuretic peptide in low-flow, low-gradient aortic stenosis: relationship to hemodynamics and clinical outcome: results from the Multicenter Truly or Pseudo-Severe Aortic Stenosis (TOPAS) study. *Circulation* 2007;115:2848–55.

136. Annabi MS, Touboul E, Dahou A, et al. Dobutamine stress echocardiography for management of low-flow, low-gradient aortic stenosis. *J Am Coll Cardiol* 2018;71:475–85.

137. Clavel MA, Ennezat PV, Marechaux S, et al. Stress echocardiography to assess stenosis severity and predict outcome in patients with paradoxical low-flow, low-gradient aortic stenosis and preserved LVEF. *JACC Cardiovasc Imaging* 2013;6:175–83.

138. Hachicha Z, Dumesnil JG, Bogaty P, Pibarot P. Paradoxical low-flow, low-gradient severe aortic stenosis despite preserved ejection fraction is associated with higher afterload and reduced survival. *Circulation* 2007;115:2856–64.

139. Herrmann HC, Pibarot T, Hueter I, et al. Predictors of mortality and outcomes of therapy in low-flow severe aortic stenosis: a Placement of Aortic Transcatheter Valves (PARTNER) trial analysis. *Circulation* 2013;127:2316–26.

140. Pai RG, Varadarajan P, Razzouk A. Survival benefit of aortic valve replacement in patients with severe aortic stenosis with low ejection fraction and low gradient with normal ejection fraction. *Ann Thorac Surg* 2008;86:1781–90.

141. Tribouilloy C, Rusinaru D, Marechaux S, et al. Low-gradient, low-flow severe aortic stenosis with preserved left ventricular ejection fraction: characteristics, outcome, and implications for surgery. *J Am Coll Cardiol* 2015;65:55–66.

142. Kang DH, Park SJ, Lee SA, et al. Early surgery or conservative care for asymptomatic aortic stenosis. *N Engl J Med* 2020;382:111–9.

143. Bonow RO, Brown AS, Gillam LD, Kapadia SR, Kavinsky CJ, Lindman BR, Mack MJ, Thourani VH. ACC/AATS/AHA/ASE/EACTS/HVS/SCA/SCAI/SCCT/SCMR/STS 2017 Appropriate Use Criteria for the Treatment of Patients With Severe Aortic Stenosis. A Report of the American College of Cardiology Appropriate Use Criteria Task Force, American Association for Thoracic Surgery, American Heart Association, American Society of Echocardiography, European Association for Cardio-Thoracic Surgery, Heart Valve Society, Society of Cardiovascular Anesthesiologists, Society for Cardiovascular Angiography and Interventions, Society of Cardiovascular Computed Tomography, Society for Cardiovascular Magnetic Resonance, and Society of Thoracic Surgeons. *J Am Coll Cardiol* 2017;70:2566–92 and doi: 10.1016/j.jacc.2017.09.018

144. Mack MJ, Leon MB, Thourani V, et al. Transcatheter aortic-valve replacement with a balloon expandable valve in low-risk patients. *N Engl J Med* 2019;380:1695–705.

145. Clavel MA, Webb JG, Pibarot P, et al. Comparison of the hemodynamic performance of percutaneous and surgical bioprostheses for the treatment of severe aortic stenosis. *J Am Coll Cardiol* 2009;53:1883–91.

146. Blackman DJ, Saraf S, MacCarthy PA, et al. Long-term durability of transcatheter aortic valve prostheses. *J Am Coll Cardiol* 2019;73:537–45.

147. Vincentelli A, Sisen S, Le Tourneau T, et al. Acquired von Willebrand syndrome in aortic stenosis. *N Engl J Med* 2003;349:343–9.

148. Van Belle E, Vincent F, Rauch A, et al. von Willebrand factor and management of heart valve disease. *J Am Coll Cardiol* 2019;73:1078–88.

149. Blackshear JL, McRee CW, Safford R, et al. von Willebrand factor abnormalities and Heyde syndrome in dysfunctional heart valve prostheses. *JAMA Cardiol* 2016;1:198–204.

150. Steinlechner B, Zeidler P, Base E, et al. Patients with severe aortic valve stenosis and impaired platelet function benefit from preoperative desmopressin infusion. *Ann Thorac Surg* 2011;91:1420–6.

151. Smith MM, Barbara DW, Mauermann WJ, Viozzi CF, Dearani JA, Grim KJ. Morbidity and mortality associated with dental extraction before cardiac operation. *Ann Thorac Surg* 2014;97:838–44.

152. Allen KB, Chhatriwalla AK, Cohen DJ, et al. Bioprosthetic valve fracture to facilitate transcatheter valve-in-valve implantation. *Ann Thorac Surg* 2017;104:1501–8.

153. Salenger R, Gammie JS, Collins JA. Minimally invasive aortic valve replacement. *J Card Surg* 2015;31:38–50.

154. Glauber M, Miceli A, Gilmanov D, et al. Right anterior minithoracotomy versus conventional aortic valve replacement: a propensity score matched study. *J Thorac Cardiovasc Surg* 2013;145:1222–6.

155. Stoliński J, Plicner D, Grudzień G, et al. A comparison of minimally invasive and standard aortic valve replacement. *J Thorac Cardiovasc Surg* 2016;152:1030–9.

156. Ensminger S, Fujita B, Bauer T, et al. Rapid deployment versus conventional bioprosthetic valve replacement for aortic stenosis. *J Am Coll Cardiol* 2018;71:1417–28.

157. Liakopoulos OJ, Gerfer S, Weider S, et al. Direct comparison of the Edwards Intuity Elite and Sorin Perceval S rapid deployment aortic valves. *Ann Thorac Surg* 2018;105:108–14.

158. Harky A, Wong CHM, Hof A, et al. Stented versus stentless aortic valve replacement in patients with small aortic root: a systematic review and meta-analysis. *Innovations (Phila)* 2018;13:404–16.

159. Ennker JAC, Albert AA, Rosendahl UP, Ennker IC, Dalladaku F, Florath I. Ten-year experience with stentless aortic valves: full-root versus subcoronary implantation. *Ann Thorac Surg* 2008;85:445–53.

160. Maxine A, El-Hamamsy I, Verma S, et al. Ross procedure in adults for cardiologists and cardiac surgeons: JACC state-of-the-art review. *J Am Coll Cardiol* 2018;72:2761–77.

161. Weymann A, Sabashnikov A, Popov AF. The Ross procedure: suitable for everyone? *Expert Review Cardiovasc Therapy* 2014;12:549–56.

162. Avierinos JF, Thuny F, Chalvignac V, et al. Surgical treatment of active aortic endocarditis: homografts are not the cornerstone of outcome. *Ann Thorac Surg* 2007;84:1935–42.

163. Gaudino M, De Filippo C, Pennestri F, Possati G. The use of mechanical prostheses in native aortic valve endocarditis. *J Heart Valve Dis* 1997;6:79–83.

164. McCarthy FH, Bavaria JE, Pochettino A, et al. Comparing aortic root replacements: porcine bioroots versus pericardial versus mechanical composite roots: hemodynamic and ventricular remodeling at greater than one-year follow-up. *Ann Thorac Surg* 2012;94:1975–82.

165. Young MN, Singh V, Sakhuja R. A review of alternative access for transcatheter aortic valve replacement. *Curr Treat Options Cardiovasc Med* 2018;20:62.

166. Greenbaum AB, Babaliaros VC, Chen MY, et al. Transcaval access and closure for transcatheter aortic valve replacement: a prospective investigation. *J Am Coll Cardiol* 2017;69:511–21.

167. Mathur M, Krishnan SK, Levin D, Aldea G, Reisman M, McCabe JM. A step-by-step guide to fully percutaneous transaxillary transcatheter aortic valve replacement. *Structural Heart* 2017;1:209–15.

168. Seeger J, Kapadia SR, Kodali S, et al. Rate of peri-procedural stroke observed with cerebral embolic protection during transcatheter aortic valve replacement: a patient-level propensity-matched analysis. *Eur Heart J* 2019;40:1334–40.

169. Kapadia SR, Kodali S, Makkar R, et al. Protection against cerebral embolism during transcatheter aortic valve replacement. *J Am Coll Cardiol* 2017;69:367–77.

170. Bagur R, Solo K, Alghofaili S, et al. Cerebral embolic protection devices during transcatheter aortic valve implantation: systematic review and meta-analysis. *Stroke* 2017;48:1306–15.

171. Murashita T, Schaff HV, Suri RM, et al. Impact of left ventricular systolic function on outcome of correction of severe aortic valve regurgitation: implications for timing of surgical intervention. *Ann Thorac Surg* 2017;103:1222–8.

172. Yoon SH, Schmidt T, Bleizifger S, et al. Transcatheter aortic valve replacement in pure native aortic valve regurgitation. *J Am Coll Cardiol* 2017;70:2752–63.

173. Pettersson GB, Crucean AC, Savage R, et al. Toward predictable repair of regurgitant aortic valves: a systematic morphology-directed approach to bicommissural repair. *J Am Coll Cardiol* 2008;52:40–9.

174. Etz CD, Homann TH, Rane N, et al. Aortic root reconstruction with a bioprosthetic valved conduit: a consecutive series of 275 procedures. *J Thorac Cardiovasc Surg* 2007;133:1455–63.

175. Zannis K, Deux JF, Tzvetkov B, et al. Composite freestyle stentless xenograft with Dacron graft extension for ascending aortic replacement. *Ann Thorac Surg* 2009;87:1789–94.

176. Boodhwani M, de Kerchove L, El Khoury G. Aortic root replacement using the reimplantation technique: tips and tricks. *Interact Cardiovasc Thorac Surg* 2009;8:584–6.

177. Sareyyupoglu B, Suri RM, Schaff HV, et al. Survival and reoperation risk following bicuspid aortic valve sparing root replacement. *J Heart Valve Dis* 2009;18:1–8.

178. David TE, Armstrong S, Maganti M, Colman J, Bradley TJ. Long-term results of aortic valve-sparing operations in patients with Marfan syndrome. *J Thorac Cardiovasc Surg* 2009;138:859–64.

179. Olesen KH. The natural history of 271 patients with mitral stenosis under medical treatment. *Brit Heart J* 1962;24:349–57.

180. Wilkins GT, Weyman AE, Abascal VM, Block PC, Palacios IF. Percutaneous balloon dilatation of the mitral valve: an analysis of echocardiographic variables related to outcome and the mechanism of dilatation. *Br Heart J* 1988;60:299–308.

181. Gentry JL III, Phelan D, Desai MY, Griffin BP. The role of stress echocardiography in valvular heart disease: a current appraisal. *Cardiology* 2017;137:137–150.

182. Passeri JJ, Dal-Bianco JP. Percutaneous mitral valvuloplasty: echocardiographic eligibility and procedural guidance. *Interv Cardiol Clinics* 2018;7:405–13.

183. Song JK, Kim MJ, Yun SC, et al. Long-term outcome of percutaneous mitral balloon valvuloplasty versus open cardiac surgery. *J Thorac Cardiovasc Surg* 2010;139:103–10.

184. Farhat MB, Bussadia H, Ganaddjbakhch I, et al. Closed versus open mitral commissurotomy in pure noncalcific mitral stenosis: hemodynamic studies before and after operation. *J Thorac Cardiovasc Surg* 1990;99:639–44.

185. Choudhury SK, Dhareshwar J, Govli A, Airan B, Kumar AS. Open mitral commissurotomy in the current era: indications, techniques, and results. *Ann Thorac Surg* 2003;75:41–6.

186. Eleid MF. Mitral valve-in-valve/ring and other percutaneous treatments of surgical failures. *Prog Cardiovasc Dis* 2017;60:415–21.

187. Urena M, Himbert D, Brochet E, et al. Transseptal transcatheter mitral valve replacement using balloon-expandable transcatheter heart valves: a step-by-step approach. *JACC Cardiovasc Interv* 2017;10:1905–19.

188. Guerrero M, Eleid M, Foley T, Said S, Rihal C. Transseptal transcatheter mitral valve replacement in severe mitral annular calcification (transseptal valve-in-MAC). *Ann Cardiothorac Surg* 2018;7:830–3.

189. Ad N, Holmes SD, Massimiano PS, Rongione AJ, Fornaresio LM. Long-term outcome following concomitant mitral valve surgery and Cox maze procedure for atrial fibrillation. *J Thorac Cardiovasc Surg* 2018;155:983–94.

190. Badhwar V, Rankin JS, Damiano RJ Jr, et al. The Society of Thoracic Surgeons 2017 Clinical Practice Guidelines for the surgical treatment of atrial fibrillation. *Ann Thorac Surg* 2017;103:329–41.

191. Benedetto U, Melina G, Angeloni E, et al. Prophylactic tricuspid annuloplasty in patients with dilated tricuspid annulus undergoing mitral valve surgery. *J Thorac Cardiovasc Surg* 2012;143:632–8.

192. Chan V, Burwash IG, Lam BK, et al. Clinical and echocardiographic impact of functional tricuspid regurgitation repair at the time of mitral valve replacement. *Ann Thorac Surg* 2009;88:1209–15.

193. Bonow RO, O'Gara PT, Adams DH, Badhwar V, Bavaria JE, Elmariah S, Hung JW, Lindenfeld J, Morris AA, Satpathy R, Whisenant B, Woo JY. 2020 focused update of the 2017 ACC expert consensus decision pathway on the management of mitral regurgitation. *J Am Coll Cardiol* 2020;75:2236–70.

194. Nishimura RA, Otto CM, Bonow RD, et al. 2017 AHA/ACC focused update of the 2014 AHA/ACC guidelines for the management of patients with valvular heart disease: a report of the American College of Cardiology American Heart Association Task Force on Clinical Practice Guidelines. *Circulation* 2017;135:e1159–1193.

195. Coutinho GF, Antunes MJ. Mitral valve repair for degenerative mitral valve disease: surgical approach, patient selection and long-term outcomes. *Heart* 2017;103:1663–9.

196. Zhou T, Li J, Lai H, et al. Benefits of early surgery on clinical outcomes after degenerative mitral valve repair. *Ann Thorac Surg* 2018;106:1063–70.

197. Montant P, Chenot F, Robert A, et al. Long-term survival in asymptomatic patients with severe degenerative mitral regurgitation: a propensity score-based comparison between an early surgical strategy and a conservative treatment approach. *J Thorac Cardiovasc Surg* 2009;138:1339–48.

198. Tomšič A, Hiemstra YL, van Hout FMA, et al. Long-term results of mitral valve repair for severe mitral regurgitation in asymptomatic patients. *J Cardiol* 2018;72:473–9.

199. Nishimura RA, Vahanian A, Eleid MF, Mack MJ. Mitral valve disease: current management and future challenges. *Lancet* 2016;387:1324–34.

200. Feldman T, Kar S, Elmariah S, et al. Randomized comparison of percutaneous repair and surgery for mitral regurgitation: 5-year results of EVEREST II. *J Am Coll Cardiol* 2015;66:2844–54.

201. Pierard LA, Carabello BA. Ischaemic mitral regurgitation: pathophysiology, outcomes, and the conundrum of treatment. *Eur Heart J* 2010;31:2996–3005.

202. Michler RE, Smith PK, Parides MK, et al. Two-year outcomes of surgical treatment of moderate ischemic mitral regurgitation. *N Engl J Med* 2016;374:1932–41.

203. Kopjar T, Gasparovic H, Mestres CA, Milicic D, Biocina B. Meta-analysis of concomitant mitral valve repair and coronary artery bypass surgery versus isolated coronary artery bypass surgery in patients with moderate ischaemic mitral regurgitation. *Eur J Cardiothorac Surg* 2016;50:212–22.

204. Narayanan MA, Aggarwal S, Reddy YNV, et al. Surgical repair of moderate ischemic mitral regurgitation: a systematic review and meta-analysis. *Thorac Cardiovasc Surg* 2017;65:447–56.

205. Virk SA, Tian DH, Sriravindrarajah A, et al. Mitral valve surgery and coronary artery bypass grafting for moderate-severe ischemic mitral regurgitation: meta-analysis of clinical and echocardiographic outcomes. *J Thorac Cardiovasc Surg* 2017;154:127–36.

206. Goldstein D, Moskowitz AJ, Gelijns AC, et al. Two-year outcome of surgical treatment of severe ischemic mitral regurgitation. *N Engl J Med* 2016;374:344–53.

207. Wang X, Zhang B, Zhang J, Ying Y, Zhu C, Chen B. Repair or replacement for severe ischemic mitral regurgitation: a meta-analysis. *Medicine (Baltimore)* 2018;97:e11546.

208. Di Salvo TG, Acker MA, Dec GW, Byrne JG. Mitral valve surgery in advanced heart failure. *J Am Coll Cardiol* 2010;55:271–82.

209. Gorman JH 3rd, Gorman RC. Mitral valve surgery for heart failure: a failed innovation? *Semin Thorac Cardiovasc Surg* 2008;18:135–8.

210. Stone GW, Lindenfeld JA, Abraham WT, et al. Transcatheter mitral-valve repair in patients with heart failure. *N Engl J Med* 2018;379:2307–18.

211. Obadia JF, Messika-Zeitoun D, Leurent G, et al. Percutaneous repair or medical treatment for secondary mitral regurgitation. *N Engl J Med* 2018;279:2297–306.

212. Pibarot P, Delgado V, Bax JJ. MITRA-FR vs. COAPT: lessons from two trials with diametrically opposed results. *Eur Heart J* 2019;20:620–4.

213. Dayan V, Soca G, Cura L, Mestres CA. Similar survival after mitral valve replacement or repair for ischemic mitral regurgitation: a meta-analysis. *Ann Thorac Surg* 2014;97:758–66.

214. Bando K, Kasegawa H, Okada Y, et al. Impact of preoperative and postoperative atrial fibrillation on outcome after mitral valvuloplasty for nonischemic mitral regurgitation. *J Thorac Cardiovasc Surg* 2005;129:1032–40.

215. Gillinov AM, Gelijns AC, Parides MK, et al. Surgical ablation of atrial fibrillation during mitral-valve surgery. *N Engl J Med* 2015;372:1399–409.

216. Marui A, Saji Y, Nishina T, et al. Impact of left atrial reduction concomitant with atrial fibrillation surgery on left atrial geometry and mechanical function. *J Thorac Cardiovasc Surg* 2008; 135:1297–305.

217. Stulak JM, Suri RM, Dearani JA, Sundt TM III, Schaff HV. When should prophylactic Maze procedure be considered in patients undergoing mitral valve surgery? *Ann Thorac Surg* 2010; 89:1395–401.

218. Wan CKN, Suri RM, Li Z, et al. Management of moderate functional mitral regurgitation at the time of aortic valve replacement: is concomitant mitral valve repair necessary? *J Thorac Cardiovasc Surg* 2009;137:635–40.

219. Waisbren EC, Stevens LM, Avery EG, Picard MH, Vlahakes GJ, Agnihotri AK. Changes in mitral regurgitation after replacement of the stenotic aortic valve. *Ann Thorac Surg* 2008;86:56–63.

220. Joo HC, Chang BC, Cho SH, Youn YN, Yoo KJ, Lee S. Fate of functional mitral regurgitation and predictors of persistent mitral regurgitation after isolated aortic valve replacement. *Ann Thorac Surg* 2011;92:82–7.

221. Foster E. Mitral regurgitation due to degenerative mitral-valve disease. *N Engl J Med* 2010;363:156–65.

222. Glower DD. Surgical approaches for mitral regurgitation. *J Am Coll Cardiol* 2012;60:1315–22.

223. Shang E, Forrest GN, Chizmar T, et al. Mitral valve infective endocarditis: benefit of early operation and aggressive use of repair. *Ann Thorac Surg* 2009;87:1728–34.

224. Shimokawa T, Kawegawa H, Matsuyama S, et al. Long-term outcome of mitral valve repair for infective endocarditis. *Ann Thorac Surg* 2009;88:733–9.

225. Tang P, Onatis M, Gaca JG, Milano CA, Stafford-Smith M, Glower D. Right minithoracotomy versus median sternotomy for mitral valve surgery: a propensity matched analysis. *Ann Thorac Surg* 2015;100:575–81.

226. Moscarelli M, Fattouch K, Gaudino M, et al. Minimal access versus sternotomy for complex mitral valve repair: a meta-analysis. *Ann Thorac Surg* 2020;109:737–44.

227. Mihaljevic T, Jarrett CM, Gillinov AM, et al. Robotic repair of posterior mitral valve prolapse versus conventional approaches: potential realized. *J Thorac Cardiovasc Surg* 2011;141:72–80.

228. Murphy DA, Moss E, Binongo J, et al. The expanding role of endoscopic robotics in mitral valve surgery: 1257 consecutive procedures. *Ann Thorac Surg* 2015;100:1675–82.

229. Yang S, Mei B, Feng K, et al. Long-term results of surgical atrial fibrillation radiofrequency ablation: comparison of two methods. *Heart Lung Circ* 2018;27:621–8.

230. Feldman T, Fernandes E, Levisay JP. Transcatheter mitral valve repair/replacement for primary mitral regurgitation. *Ann Cardiothorac Surg* 2018;7:755–63.

231. Savic V, Pozzoli A, Gülmez G, et al. Transcatheter mitral valve chord repair. *Ann Cardiothorac Surg* 2018;7:731–40.

232. Kiefer P, Meier S, Noack T, et al. Good 5-year durability of transapical beating heart off-pump mitral valve repair with neochordae. *Ann Thorac Surg* 2018;106:440–6.

233. Chang JD, Manning WJ, Ebrille E, Zimetbaum PJ. Tricuspid valve dysfunction following pacemaker or cardioverter-defibrillator implantation. *J Am Coll Cardiol* 2017;69:2331–41.

234. Taramasso M, Vanermen, H, Maisano F, Guidotti A, La Canna G, Alfieri O. The growing clinical importance of secondary tricuspid regurgitation. *J Am Coll Cardiol* 2012;59:703–10.

235. Nath J, Foster E, Heidenreich PA. Impact of tricuspid regurgitation on long-term survival. *J Am Coll Cardiol* 2004;43:405–9.

236. De Bonis M, Lapenna E, Pozzoli A, et al. Mitral valve repair without repair of moderate tricuspid regurgitation. *Ann Thorac Surg* 2015;100:2206–12.

237. Kara I, Koksal C, Erkin A, et al. Outcomes of mild to moderate functional tricuspid regurgitation in patients undergoing mitral valve operations: a meta-analysis of 2488 patients. *Ann Thorac Surg* 2015;100:2398–407.

238. Navia JL, Brozzi NA, Klein AL, et al. Moderate tricuspid regurgitation with left-sided degenerative heart disease: to repair or not to repair? *Ann Thorac Surg* 2012;93:59–69.

239. Mazine A, Bouchard D, Moss E, et al. Transvalvular pacemaker leads increase the recurrence of regurgitation after tricuspid valve repair. *Ann Thorac Surg* 2013;96:816–22.

240. Benedetto U, Melina G, Angeloni E, et al. Prophylactic tricuspid annuloplasty in patients with dilated tricuspid annulus undergoing mitral valve surgery. *J Thorac Cardiovasc Surg* 2012;143:632–8.

241. Chikwe J, Itagaki S, Anyanwu A, Adams DH. Impact of concomitant tricuspid annuloplasty on tricuspid regurgitation, right ventricular function, and pulmonary artery hypertension after repair of mitral valve prolapse. *J Am Coll Cardiol* 2015;65:1931–8.

242. Dreyfus GD, Corbi PJ, Chan KM, Bahrami T. Secondary tricuspid regurgitation or dilatation: which should be the criteria for surgical repair? *Ann Thorac Surg* 2005;79:127–32.

243. Chan V, Burwash IG, Lam BK, et al. Clinical and echocardiographic impact of functional tricuspid regurgitation repair at the time of mitral valve replacement. *Ann Thorac Surg* 2009;88:1209–15.

244. Kammerlander AA, Marzluf BA, Graf A, et al. Right ventricular dysfunction, but not tricuspid regurgitation, is associated with outcome late after left heart valve procedure. *J Am Coll Cardiol* 2014;64:2633–42.

245. Ghoreishi M, Brown JM, Stauffer CE, et al. Undersized tricuspid annuloplasty rings optimally treat functional tricuspid regurgitation. *Ann Thorac Surg* 2011;92:89–96.

246. Parolari A, Barili F, Pilozzi A, Pacini D. Ring or suture annuloplasty for tricuspid regurgitation: a meta-analysis review. *Ann Thorac Surg* 2014;98:2255–63.

247. Huang X, Gu C, Men X, et al. Repair of functional tricuspid regurgitation: comparison between suture annuloplasty and rings annuloplasty. *Ann Thorac Surg* 2014;97:1286–93.

248. Ren WJ, Zhang BG, Liu JS, Qian YJ, Guo YQ. Outcomes of tricuspid annuloplasty with and without prosthetic rings: a retrospective follow-up study. *J Cardiothorac Surg* 2015;10:81.

249. McCarthy PM, Bhudia SK, Rajeswaran J, et al. Tricuspid valve repair: durability and risk factors for failure. *J Thorac Cardiovasc Surg* 2004;127:674–85.

250. Meng H, Pan SW, Hu SS, Pang KJ, Hou JF, Wang H. Surgical treatment of secondary tricuspid regurgitation: insight derived from annulus sizes and tethering distances. *Ann Thorac Surg* 2015;100:1238–44.

251. Ghanta RK, Chen R, Narayanasamy N, et al. Suture bicuspidization of the tricuspid valve versus ring annuloplasty for repair of functional tricuspid regurgitation: midterm results of 237 consecutive patients. *J Thorac Cardiovasc Surg* 2007;133:117–26.

252. Russo CF, Cannata A, Lanfranconi M, Martinelli L. Destruction of the tricuspid septal leaflet: correction by bicuspidization. *Ann Thorac Surg* 2010;90:1028–9.

253. Isidro AB, Kalra KG, Reis GJ, Pentz WH, Patel VA, Bridges CR. Bicuspidization of the tricuspid valve for the treatment of posterior leaflet endocarditis: a case report. *Heart Surg Forum* 2007;10:e129–30.

254. Garatti A, Nano G, Bruschi G, et al. Twenty-five year outcomes of tricuspid valve replacement comparing mechanical and biologic prostheses. *Ann Thorac Surg* 2012;93:1146–53.

255. Hwang HY, Kim KH, Kim KB, Ahn H. Propensity score matching analysis of mechanical versus bioprosthetic tricuspid valve replacements. *Ann Thorac Surg* 2014;97:1294–9.

256. Filsoufi F, Anyanwu AC, Salzberg SP, Frankel T, Cohn LH, Adams DH. Long-term outcomes of tricuspid valve replacement in the current era. *Ann Thorac Surg* 2005;80:845–50.

257. Civelek A, Ak K, Akgün S, Isbir SC, Arsan S. Tricuspid valve replacement: an analysis of risk factors and outcomes. *Thorac Cardiovasc Surg* 2008;56:456–60.

258. Kilic A, Saha-Chaudhuri P, Rankin JS, Conte JV. Trends and outcomes of tricuspid valve surgery in North America: an analysis of more than 50,000 patients from the Society of Thoracic Surgeons database. *Ann Thorac Surg* 2013;96:1546–52.

259. LaPar DJ, Likosky DS, Zhang M, et al. Development of a risk prediction model and clinical risk score for isolated tricuspid valve surgery. *Ann Thorac Surg* 2018;106:129–37.

260. Nickenig G, Kowalski M, Hausleiter J, et al. Transcatheter treatment of severe tricuspid regurgitation with the edge-to-edge MitraClip technique. *Circulation* 2017;135:1802–14.

261. Perlman G, Praz F, Puri R, et al. Transcatheter tricuspid valve repair with a new transcatheter coaptation system for the treatment of severe tricuspid regurgitation: 1-year clinical and echocardiographic results. *JACC Cardiovasc Interv* 2017;10:1994–2003.

262. Campelo-Parada F, Perlman G, Philippon F, et al. First-in-man experience of a novel transcatheter repair system for treating severe tricuspid regurgitation. *J Am Coll Cardiol* 2015;66:2475–83.

263. Jokinen JJ, Turpeinen AK, Pitkänen O, Hippeläinen MJ, Hartikainen JEK. Pacemaker therapy after tricuspid valve operations: implications on mortality, morbidity, and quality of life. *Ann Thorac Surg* 2009;87:1806–14.

264. Pericàs JM, Liopis J, Athan E, et al. Prospective cohort study of infective endocarditis in people who inject drugs. *J Am Coll Cardiol* 2021;77:544–55.

265. Kim JB, Ejiofor JI, Yammine M, et al. Surgical outcomes of infective endocarditis among intravenous drug users. *J Thorac Cardiovasc Surg* 2016;152:832–41.

266. Cahill TJ, Baddour LM, Habib G, et al. Challenges in infective endocarditis. *J Am Coll Cardiol* 2017;69:3235–44.

267. Alberto San Román J, Vilacosta I, López J, Sarriá C. Critical questions about left-sided infective endocarditis. *J Am Coll Cardiol* 2015;66:1068–76.

268. Tanis W, Scholtens A, Habets J, et al. CT angiography and ^{18}F-FDG-PET fusion imaging for prosthetic heart valve endocarditis. *JACC Cardiovasc Imaging* 2013;6:1008–13.

269. Feuchtner GM, Stolzmann P, Diehtl W, et al. Multislice computed tomography in infective endocarditis: comparison with transesophageal echocardiography and operative findings. *J Am Coll Cardiol* 2009;53:436–44.

270. Yashioka D, Toda K, Okazaki S, et al. Anemia is a risk factor for new intraoperative hemorrhagic stroke during valve surgery for endocarditis. *Ann Thorac Surg* 2015;100:16–23.

271. Habib G, Lancellotti P, Antunes MJ, et al. 2015 ESC guidelines for the management of infective endocarditis: the Task Force for the management of infective endocarditis of the European Society of Cardiology (ESC). *Eur Heart J* 2015;36:3075–128.

272. Vilacosta I, Graupner C, San Román A, et al. Risk of embolization after institution of antibiotic therapy for infective endocarditis. *J Am Coll Cardiol* 2002;39:1489–95.

273. Dickerman SA, Abrutyn E, Barsic B, et al. The relationship between the initiation of antimicrobial therapy and the incidence of stroke in infective endocarditis: analysis from the ICE prospective cohort study (ICS-PCS). *Am Heart J* 2007;154:1086–94.

274. Hubert S, Thuny F, Resseguier M, et al. Prediction of symptomatic embolism in infective endocarditis: construction and validation of a risk calculator in a multicenter cohort. *J Am Coll Cardiol* 2013;62:1384–92.

275. Kang DH, Kim YJ, Kim SH, et al. Early surgery versus conventional treatment for infective endocarditis. *N Engl J Med* 2012;366:2466–73.

276. Yoshioka D, Sakaguchi T, Yamauchi T, et al. Impact of early surgical treatment on postoperative neurologic outcome for active infective endocarditis complicated by cerebral infarction. *Ann Thorac Surg* 2012;94:489–96.

277. Hussain ST, Witten J, Shreshtha NK, Blackstone EH, Pettersson GB. Tricuspid valve endocarditis. *Ann Cardiothorac Surg* 2017;6:255–61.

278. Yanagawa B, Elbatarny M, Verma S, et al. Surgical management of tricuspid valve infective endocarditis: a systematic review and meta-analysis. *Ann Thorac Surg* 2018;106:708–15.

279. Prendergast BD, Tornos P. Surgery for infective endocarditis: who and when? *Circulation* 2010;121:1141–52.

280. Witten JC, Hussain ST, Shreştha NK, et al. Surgical treatment of right-sided infective endocarditis. *J Thorac Cardiovasc Surg* 2019;157:1418–27.

281. Shrestha NK, Jue J, Hussain ST, et al. Injection drug use and outcomes after surgical intervention for infective endocarditis. *Ann Thorac Surg* 2015;100:875–83.

282. Rabkin DG, Mokadam NA, Miller DW, Goetz RR, Verrier ED, Aldea GS. Long-term outcome for the surgical treatment of infective endocarditis with a focus on intravenous drug users. *Ann Thorac Surg* 2012;93:51–8.

283. Dawood MY, Cheema FH, Ghoreishi M, et al. Contemporary outcomes of operations for tricuspid valve infective endocarditis. *Ann Thorac Surg* 2015;99:539–46.

284. Braun MU, Rauwolf T, Bock M, et al. Percutaneous lead implantation connected to an external device in stimulation dependent patients with systemic infection: a prospective and controlled study. *Pacing Clin Electrophysiol* 2006;29:875–9.

285. Shroff GR, Herzog CA, Ma JZ, Collins AJ. Long-term survival of dialysis patients with bacterial endocarditis in the United States. *Am J Kidney Dis* 2004;44:1077–82.

286. Nori US, Manoharan A, Thornby JI, Yee J, Parasuraman R, Ramanathan V. Mortality risk factors in chronic haemodialysis patients with infective endocarditis. *Neph Dialysis Transplant* 2006;21:2184–90.

287. Dohmen PM, Binner C, Mende M, et al. Outcome of aortic valve replacement for active infective endocarditis in patients on chronic hemodialysis. *Ann Thorac Surg* 2015;99:532–8.

288. Farrington DK, Kilgo PD, Thourani VH, Jacob JT, Steinberg JP. High risk of prosthetic valve endocarditis and death after valve replacement operations in dialysis patients. *Ann Thorac Surg* 2016;101:2217–23.

289. Herzog CA, Ma JZ, Collins AJ. Long-term survival of dialysis patients in the United States with prosthetic heart valves: should ACC/AHA practice guidelines on valve selection be modified? *Circulation* 2002;105:1336–41.

290. Ando T, Ashraf S, Villablanca PA, et al. Meta-analysis comparing the incidence of infective endocarditis following transcatheter aortic valve implantation versus surgical aortic valve replacement. *Am J Cardiol* 2019;123:827–32.

291. Butt JW, Ihlemann N, De Backer O, et al. Long-term risk of infective endocarditis after transcatheter aortic valve replacement. *J Am Coll Cardiol* 2019;73:1646–55.

292. Byrne JG, Rezai K, Sanchez JA, et al. Surgical management of endocarditis: the Society of Thoracic Surgeons Clinical Practice Guidelines. *Ann Thorac Surg* 2011;91:2012–9.

293. Sultan I, Bianco V, Kilic A, Chu D, Navid F, Gleason TG. Aortic root replacement with cryopreserved homograft for infective endocarditis in the modern North American opioid epidemic. *J Thorac Cardiovasc Surg* 2019;157:45–50.

294. Jassar AS, Bavaria JE, Szeto WY, et al. Graft selection for aortic root replacement in complex active endocarditis: does it matter? *Ann Thorac Surg* 2012;93:480–8.

295. Toyoda N, Itagaki S, Tannous H, Egorova NN, Chikwe J. Bioprosthetic versus mechanical valve replacement for infective endocarditis: focus on recurrence rates. *Ann Thorac Surg* 2018;106:99–106.

296. Rostagno C, Carone E, Stefano PL. Role of mitral valve repair in active infective endocarditis: long-term results. *J Cardiothorac Surg* 2017;12:29.

297. Protos AN, Trivedi JR, Whited WM, et al. Valvectomy versus replacement for the surgical treatment of tricuspid endocarditis. *Ann Thorac Surg* 2018;106:664–9.

298. Sherrid MV, Balaram S, Kim B, Axel L, Swistel DG. The mitral valve in obstructive hypertrophic cardiomyopathy: a test in context. *J Am Coll Cardiol* 2016;67:1846–58.

299. Maron BJ, Ommen SR, Semsarian C, Spirito P, Olivotto I, Maron MS. Hypertrophic cardiomyopathy: present and future, with translation into contemporary cardiovascular medicine. *J Am Coll Cardiol* 2014;64:83–99.

300. Maron BJ, Rowin EJ, Udelson JE, Maron MS. Clinical spectrum and management of heart failure in hypertrophic cardiomyopathy. *JACC Heart Failure* 2018;6:653–63.

301. Geske JB, Ommen SR, Gersh BJ. Hypertrophic cardiomyopathy: clinical update. *JACC Heart Failure* 2018;6:364–75.

302. Maron BJ. Clinical course and management of hypertrophic cardiomyopathy. *N Engl J Med* 2018;379:655–68.

303. Maron MS, Rowin EJ, Olivotto I, et al. Contemporary natural history and management of nonobstructive hypertrophic cardiomyopathy. *J Am Coll Cardiol* 2016;67:1399–409.

304. Chan RH, Maron BJ, Olivotto I, et al. Prognostic value of quantitative contrast-enhanced cardiovascular magnetic resonance for the evaluation of sudden death risk in patients with hypertrophic cardiomyopathy. *Circulation* 2014;130:484–95.

305. Weng Z, Yao J, Chan RH, et al. Prognostic value of LGE-CMR in HCM: a meta-analysis. *JACC Cardiovasc Imaging* 2016;9:1392–1402.

306. Price J, Clarke N, Turer A, et al. Hypertrophic obstructive cardiomyopathy: review of surgical treatment. *Asian Cardiovasc Thorac Ann* 2017;25:594–607.

307. Parry DJ, Raskin RE, Poynter JA, et al. Short and medium term outcomes of surgery for patients with hypertrophic obstructive cardiomyopathy. *Ann Thorac Surg* 2015;99:1213–9.

308. Hong JH, Schaff HV, Nishimura RA, et al. Mitral regurgitation in patients with hypertrophic obstructive cardiomyopathy: implications for concomitant valve procedures. *J Am Coll Cardiol* 2016;68:1497–504.

309. Liebreghts M, Vriesendorp PA, Majmoodi BK, Schinkel AE, Michels M, ten Berg JM. A systematic review and meta-analysis of long-term outcomes after septal reduction therapy in patients with hypertrophic cardiomyopathy. *JACC Heart Fail* 2015;3:896–905.

310. Gupta S, Slater M, Heitner S, Wei K. TCT-810 percutaneous mitral valve repair for management of systolic anterior motion and mitral regurgitation associated with hypertrophic cardiomyopathy. *J Am Coll Cardiol* 2016;68: doi: 10.1016/j.jacc.2016.09.842.

311. Evangelista A, Isselbacher EM, Bossone, E, et al. Insights from the International Registry of Acute Aortic Dissection: a 20-year experience of collaborative clinical research. *Circulation* 2018;137:1846–60.

312. Goldfinger JZ, Halperin JL, Marin ML, Stewart AS, Eagle KA, Fuster V. Thoracic aortic aneurysm and dissection. *J Am Coll Cardiol* 2014;64:1725–39.

313. Elefteriades JA, Farkas EA. Thoracic aortic aneurysm: clinical pertinent controversies and uncertainties. *J Am Coll Cardiol* 2010;55:841–57.

314. Hansen MS, Nogareda GJ, Hutchison FJ. Frequency of and inappropriate treatment of misdiagnosis of acute aortic dissection. *Am J Cardiol* 2007;99:852–6.

315. Bonser RS, Ranasinghe AM, Loubani M, et al. Evidence, lack of evidence, controversy, and debate in the provision and performance of the surgery of acute type A aortic dissection. *J Am Coll Cardiol* 2011;58:2455–74.

316. Pape LA, Awais M, Woznicki EM, et al. Presentation, diagnosis, and outcomes of acute aortic dissection: 17-year trends from the International Registry of Acute Aortic Dissection. *J Am Coll Cardiol* 2015;66:350–8.

317. Rogers AM, Hermann LK, Booher AM, et al. Sensitivity of the aortic dissection detection risk score, a novel guideline-based tool for identification of acute aortic dissection at initial presentation: results from the International Registry of Acute Aortic Dissection. *Circulation* 2011;123:2213–8.

318. Czerny M, Schoenhoff F, Etz C, et al. The impact of pre-operative malperfusion on outcome in acute type A aortic dissection: results from the GERAADA Registry. *J Am Coll Cardiol* 2015;65:2628–35.

319. Suzuki T, Distante A, Zizza A, et al. Diagnosis of acute aortic dissection by D-Dimer: the International Registry of Acute Aortic Dissection substudy on biomarkers (IRAD-Bio) experience. *Circulation* 2009;119:2702–7.

320. Paparella D, Malvindi PG, Scrascia G, et al. D-dimers are not always elevated in patients with acute dissection. *J Cardiovasc Med (Hagerstown)* 2009;10:212–4.

321. Nazerian P, Mueller C, Soeiro AM, et al. Diagnostic accuracy of the Aortic Dissection Detection Risk Score plus D-Dimer for acute aortic syndromes: The ADvISED Prospective Multicenter Study. *Circulation* 2018;137:1846–60.

322. Patel HJ, Williams DM, Dasika NL, Suzuki Y, Deeb GM. Operative delay for peripheral malperfusion syndrome in acute type A aortic dissection: a long-term analysis. *J Thorac Cardiovasc Surg* 2008;135:1288–96.

323. Yagdi T, Atay Y, Engin C, et al. Impact of organ malperfusion on mortality and morbidity in acute type A aortic dissections. *J Card Surg* 2006;21:363–9.

324. Fattori R, Cao P, De Rango P, et al. Interdisciplinary expert consensus document on management of type B aortic dissection. *J Am Coll Cardiol* 2013;61:1661–78.

325. Nauta AJH, Trimarchi S, Kamman AV, et al. Update in the management of type B aortic dissection. *Vasc Med* 2016;21:251–63.

326. Moulakakis KG, Mylonas SN, Daleinas I, Kakisis J, Kotsis T, Liapis CD. Management of complicated and uncomplicated acute type B dissection: a systematic review and meta-analysis. *Ann Cardiothorac Surg* 2014;3:234–46.

327. Tadros ROI, Tang GHL, Barnes JH, et al. Optimal treatment of uncomplicated type B aortic dissection. *J Am Coll Cardiol* 2019;74:1494–504.

328. Cruz I, Stuart B, Caldeira D, et al. Controlled pericardiocentesis in patients with cardiac tamponade complicating aortic dissection: experience of a centre without cardiothoracic surgery. *Eur Heart J Acute Cardiovasc Care* 2015;4:112–22.

329. Hayashi T, Tsukube T, Yamashita T, et al. Impact of controlled pericardial drainage on critical cardiac tamponade with acute type A aortic dissection. *Circulation* 2012;126(11 Suppl 1):S97–S101.

330. Tagagi H, Uemoto T, ALICE Group. A meta-analysis of total arch replacement with frozen elephant trunk in acute type A aortic dissection. *Vasc Endovascular Surg* 2016;50:33–46.

331. Poon SS, Theologou T, Harrington D, Kuduvalli M, Oo A, Field M. Hemiarch versus total aortic arch replacement in acute type A dissection: a systematic review and meta-analysis. *Ann Cardiothorac Surg* 2016;5:15–73.

332. Masalanis G, Ip S. A new paradigm in the management of acute type A aortic dissection: total aortic repair. *J Thorac Cardiovasc Surg* 2019;157:3–11.

333. Geirsson A, Szeto WY, Pochettino A, et al. Significance of malperfusion syndromes prior to contemporary surgical repair for acute type A dissection: outcomes and need for additional revascularization. *Eur J Cardiothorac Surg* 2007;32:255–62.

334. Geirsson A, Shioda K, Olsson C, et al. Differential outcomes of open and clamp-on distal anastomotic techniques in acute type A aortic dissection. *J Thorac Cardiovasc Surg* 2019;157:1750–8.

335. Abe T, Usui A. The cannulation strategy in surgery for acute type A dissection. *Gen Thorac Cardiovasc Surg* 2017;65:1–9.

336. Stamou SC, Gartner D, Kouchoukos NT, et al. Axillary versus femoral arterial cannulation during repair of type A aortic dissection? An old problem seeking new solutions. *Aorta (Stamford)* 2016;4:115–123.

337. Trimarchi S, de Beaufort HWL, Tolenaar JL, et al. Acute aortic dissections with entry tear in the arch: a report from the International Registry of Acute Aortic Dissection. *J Thorac Cardiovasc Surg* 2019;157:66–73.

338. Sun L, Qi R, Chang Q, et al. Surgery for acute type A dissection with the tear in the descending aorta using a stented elephant trunk procedure. *Ann Thorac Surg* 2009;87:1177–81.

339. Chen Y, Zhang S, Liu L, Qingsheng L, Zhang T, Jing Z. Retrograde type A aortic dissection after thoracic endovascular aortic repair: a systematic review and meta-analysis. *J Am Heart Assoc* 2017;6:e004649.

340. Zafar MA, Li Y, Rizzo JA, et al. Height alone, rather than body surface area, suffices for risk stratification in ascending aortic aneurysm. *J Thorac Cardiovasc Surg* 2018;155:1938–50.

341. Kim JB, Spotnitz M, Lindsay ME, MacGillivray TE, Isselbacher EM, Sundt TM, III. Risk of aortic dissection in the moderately dilated ascending aorta. *J Am Coll Cardiol* 2016;68:1209–19.

342. Nishimura RA, Ott CM, Bonow RO, et al. 2014 AHA/ACC guideline for the management of patients with valvular heart disease: a report of the American College of Cardiology/American Heart Association Task Force Practice Guideline. *J Am Coll Cardiol* 2014;63:e57–185.

343. Hiratzka LF, Bakris FL, Beckmann JA, et al. 2010 ACCF/AHA/AATS/ACR/ASA/SCAI/SIR/STS/SVM guidelines for the diagnosis and management of patients with thoracic aortic disease: a report of the American College of Cardiology Foundation/American Heart Association Task Force on Practice Guidelines, American Association of Thoracic Surgery, American College of Radiology, American Stroke Association, American Society of Cardiovascular Anesthesiologists, Society for Cardiovascular Angiography and Interventions, Society of Interventional Radiology, Society of Thoracic Surgeons, and Society for Vascular Medicine. *Circulation* 2010;121:1544–79.

344. Hiratzka LF, Creager MA, Isselbacher EM, Svensson LG. Surgery for aortic dilatation in patients with bicuspid aortic valves. A statement of clarification from the American College of Cardiology/American Heart Association Task Force on Clinical Practice Guidelines. *J Am Coll Cardiol* 2016;67:724–31.

345. Masri A, Kalahasti V, Svensson G, et al. Aortic cross-sectional area/height ratio and outcomes in patients with a trileaflet aortic valve and a dilated aorta. *Circulation* 2016;134:1724–37.

346. Ziganshin BA, Zafar MA, Elefteriades JA. Descending threshold for ascending aortic aneurysmectomy: is it time for a "left-shift" in guidelines? *J Thorac Cardiovasc Surg* 2019;157:37–42.

347. Prenger K, Pieters F, Cheriex E. Aortic dissection after valve replacement: incidence and consequences for strategy. *J Card Surg* 1994;9:495–8.

348. Pape LA, Tsai TT, Isselbacher EM, et al. Aortic diameter > or = 5.5 cm is not a good predictor of type A aortic dissection: observations from the International Registry of Acute Aortic Dissection (IRAD). *Circulation* 2007;116:1120–7.

349. Davies RR, Gallo A, Coady MA, et al. Novel measurement of relative aortic size predicts rupture of thoracic aortic aneurysms. *Ann Thorac Surg* 2006;81:169–77.

350. Matura LA, Ho VB, Rosing DR, Bondy CA. Aortic dilatation and dissection in Turner syndrome. *Circulation* 2007;116:1663–70.

351. Svensson LF, Adams DH, Bonow RO, et al. Aortic valve and ascending aorta guidelines for management and quality measures: executive summary. *Ann Thorac Surg* 2013;95:1491–505.

352. Svensson LG, Khitin L. Aortic cross-sectional area/height ratio timing of aortic surgery in asymptomatic patients with Marfan syndrome. *J Thorac Cardiovasc Surg* 2002;123:360–1.

353. Svensson LG, Kim KH, Lytle BW, Cosgrove DM. Relationship of aortic cross-sectional area to height ratio and the risk of aortic dissection in patients with bicuspid aortic valves. *J Thorac Cardiovasc Surg* 2003;126:892–3.

354. Wu J, Zafar MA, Li Y, et al. Ascending aortic length and risk of aortic adverse events: the neglected dimension. *J Am Coll Cardiol* 2019;74:1883–94.

355. Fazel SS, Mallidi HR, Lee RS, et al. The aortopathy of bicuspid aortic valve disease has distinctive patterns and usually involves the transverse aortic arch. *J Thorac Cardiovasc Surg* 2008;135:901–7.

356. Mookhoek A, Korteland NM, Arabkhani B, et al. Bentall procedure: a systematic review and meta-analysis. *Ann Thorac Surg* 2016;101:1684–9.

357. Bianco V, Kilic A, Gleason TG, et al. Aortic root replacement with stentless xenografts in patients with aortic stenosis. *J Thorac Cardiovasc Surg* 2019;158:1021–7.

358. Price J, Magruder JT, Young A, et al. Long-term outcomes of aortic root operations for Marfan syndrome: a comparison of Bentall versus aortic valve-sparing procedures. *J Thorac Cardiovasc Surg* 2016;151:330–6.

359. Ouzounian M, Feindel CM, Manlhiot C, David C, David TE. Valve-sparing root replacement with bicuspid versus tricuspid aortic valves. *J Thorac Cardiovasc Surg* 2019;158:1–9.

360. Tian DH, Weller J, Hasmat S, et al. Adjunct retrograde cerebral perfusion provides superior outcomes compared with hypothermic circulatory arrest alone: a meta-analysis. *J Thorac Cardiovasc Surg* 2018;156:1339–48.

361. Fan S, Li H, Wang D, et al. Effects of four major brain protection strategies during proximal aortic surgery: a systematic review and network meta-analysis. *Int J Surg* 2019;63:8–15.

362. Perreas K, Samanitis G, Thanopoulos A, et al. Antegrade or retrograde cerebral perfusion in ascending aorta and hemiarch surgery? A propensity-matched analysis. *Ann Thorac Surg* 2018;101:146–52.

363. Numata S, Tsutsumi Y, Monta O, et al. Aortic arch repair with antegrade selective cerebral perfusion using mild to moderate hypothermia of more than 28 °C. *Ann Thorac Surg* 2012;94:90–6.

364. Itagaki S, Chikwe J, Sun E, Chu E, Toyoda N, Egorova N. Impact of cerebral perfusion on outcomes of aortic surgery: the Society of Thoracic Surgeons adult cardiac surgery database analysis. *Ann Thorac Surg* 2020;109:428–36.

365. Lau C, Gaudino M, Iannaconne EM, et al. Retrograde cerebral perfusion is effective for prolonged circulatory arrest in arch aneurysm repair. *Ann Thorac Surg* 2018;105:491–7.

366. Pérez MA, Coto JML, del Castro Madrazo JA, Prendes CF, Gay MG, Al-Sibbai AZ. Debranching aortic surgery. *J Thorac Dis* 2017;9(suppl 6):S465–S477.

367. Spielvogel D, Etz CD, Silovitz D, Lansman SL, Griepp RB. Aortic arch replacement with a trifurcated graft. *Ann Thorac Surg* 2007;83:S791–5.

368. Etz CD, Plestis KA, Kari FA, et al. Staged repair of thoracic and thoracoabdominal aortic aneurysms using the elephant trunk technique: a consecutive series of 215 first stage and 120 complete repairs. *Eur J Cardiothorac Surg* 2008;34:605–14.

369. Koizumi S, Nagasawa A, Koyama T. Total aortic arch replacement using frozen elephant trunk technique with J Graft Open Stent Graft for distal aortic arch aneurysm. *Gen Thorac Cardiovasc Surg* 2018;66:91–4.

370. Estrera AL, Miller CC III, Chen EP, et al. Descending thoracic aortic aneurysm repair: a 12-year experience using distal aortic perfusion and cerebrospinal fluid drainage. *Ann Thorac Surg* 2005;80:1290–6.

371. Estrera AL, Sheinbaum R, Miller CC, et al. Cerebrospinal fluid drainage during thoracic aortic repair: safety and current management. *Ann Thorac Surg* 2009;88:9–15.

372. Tanaka A, Safi HJ, Estrera AL. Current strategies of spinal cord protection during thoracoabdominal aortic surgery. *Gen Thorac Cardiovasc Surg* 2018;66:307–14.

373. Coselli JS, LeMaire SA, Conklin LD, Adams GJ. Left heart bypass during descending thoracic aortic aneurysm repair does not reduce the incidence of paraplegia. *Ann Thorac Surg* 2004;77:1298–303.

374. Cheng D, Martin J, Shennib H, et al. Endovascular aortic repair versus open surgical repair for descending thoracic aortic disease: a systematic review and meta-analysis of comparative studies. *J Am Coll Cardiol* 2010;55:986–1001.

375. Chiu P, Goldstone AB, Schaffer JM, et al. Endovascular versus open repair of intact descending thoracic aneurysms. *J Am Coll Cardiol* 2019;73:643–51.

376. Hnath JC, Mehta M, Taggert JB, et al. Strategies to improve spinal cord ischemia in endovascular thoracic aortic repair: outcomes of a prospective cerebrospinal fluid drainage protocol. *J Vasc Surg* 2008;48:836–40.

377. Calkins H, Hindricks G, Cappato R, et al. 2017 HRS/EHRA/ECAS/APHRS/SOLAECE expert consensus statement on catheter and surgical ablation of atrial fibrillation. *Heart Rhythm* 2017;14:e275–444. and *Europace* 2018;20:e1–160.

378. Ad N, Damiano RJ Jr, Badhwar V, et al. Expert consensus guidelines: examining surgical ablation for atrial fibrillation. *J Thorac Cardiovasc Surg* 2017;153:1330–54.

379. Khawar W, Smith N, Masroor S. Managing the left atrial appendage in atrial fibrillation: current state of the art. *Ann Thorac Surg* 2017;104:2111–9.

380. Turagam K, Velagapudi P, Kar S, et al. Cardiovascular therapies targeting left atrial appendage. *J Am Coll Cardiol* 2018;72:448–63.

381. Barnett SD, Ad N. Surgical ablation as treatment for the elimination of atrial fibrillation: a meta-analysis. *J Thorac Cardiovasc Surg* 2006;131:1029–35.

382. Gillinov M, Soltsz E. Surgical treatment of atrial fibrillation: today's questions and answers. *Semin Thorac Cardiovasc Surg* 2013;25:197–205.

383. Philpott JM, Zemlin CW, Cox JL, et al. The ABLATE trial: safety and efficacy of Cox Maze-IV using a bipolar radiofrequency ablation system. *Ann Thorac Surg* 2015;100:1541–8.

384. Churyla A, Iddriss A, Andrei AC, et al. Biatrial or left atrial lesion set for ablation during mitral surgery: risks and benefits. *Ann Thorac Surg* 2017;103:1858–65.

385. Kim JB, Bang JH, Jung SH, Choo SJ, Chung CH, Lee JW. Left atrial ablation versus biatrial ablation in the surgical treatment of atrial fibrillation. *Ann Thorac Surg* 2011;92:1397–405.

386. Cappabianca G, Ferrarese S, Tutino C, et al. Safety and efficacy of biatrial vs left atrial surgical ablation during concomitant cardiac surgery: a meta-analysis of clinical studies with a focus on the causes of pacemaker implantation. *J Cardiovasc Electrophys* 2019;30:2150–63.

387. Geidel S, Krause K, Boczor S, Kuck KH, Lass M, Ostermeyer J, Schmoeckel M. Ablation surgery in patients with persistent atrial fibrillation: an 8-year clinical experience. *J Thorac Cardiovasc Surg* 2011;141:377–82.

388. Ad N, Holmes SD, Shuman DJ, Pritchard G. Impact of atrial fibrillation duration on the success of first-time concomitant Cox maze procedures. *Ann Thorac Surg* 2015;100:1613–9.

389. Ad N, Holmes SD. Prediction of sinus rhythm in patients undergoing concomitant Cox maze procedure through a median sternotomy. *J Thorac Cardiovasc Surg* 2014;148:881–7.

390. Stulak JM, Dearani JA, Sundt TM III, Daly RC, Schaff HV. Ablation of atrial fibrillation: comparison of catheter-based techniques and the Cox-Maze III operation. *Ann Thorac Surg* 2011;91:1882–9.

391. Damiano RJ Jr, Badhwar V, Acker MA, et al. The CURE-AF trial: a prospective, multicenter trial of irrigated radiofrequency ablation for the treatment of persistent atrial fibrillation during concomitant cardiac surgery. *Heart Rhythm* 2014;11:39–45.

392. Ad N, Holmes SD, Massimiano PS, Rongione AJ, Fornaresio LM. Long-term outcome following concomitant mitral valve surgery and Cox maze procedure for atrial fibrillation. *J Thorac Cardiovasc Surg* 2018;155:983–94.

393. Gillinov AM, Gelijns AC, Parides MK, et al. Surgical ablation of atrial fibrillation during mitral-valve surgery. *N Engl J Med* 2015;372:1399–409.

394. Henn MC, Lawrance CP, Sinn LA, et al. Effectiveness of surgical ablation in patients with atrial fibrillation and aortic valve disease. *Ann Thorac Surg* 2015;100:1253–9.

395. Al-Atassi T, Kimmaliardjuk DM, Dagenais C, Bourke M, Lam BK, Rubens FD. Should we ablate atrial fibrillation during coronary artery bypass grafting and aortic valve replacement? *Ann Thorac Surg* 2017;104:515–22.

396. Marui A, Saji Y, Nishina T, et al. Impact of left atrial reduction concomitant with atrial fibrillation surgery on left atrial geometry and mechanical function. *J Thorac Cardiovasc Surg* 2008;135:1297–305.

397. Doll N, Pritzwald-Stegmann P, Czesla M, et al. Ablation of ganglionic plexi during combined surgery for atrial fibrillation. *Ann Thorac Surg* 2008;86:1659–63.

398. Tsai YC, Phan K, Munkholm-Larsen S, Tian DH, La Meir M, Yan TD. Surgical left atrial appendage occlusion during cardiac surgery for patients with atrial fibrillation: a meta-analysis. *Eur J Cardiothorac Surg* 2015;47:847–54.

399. Buber J, Luria D, Sternik L, et al. Left atrial contractile function following a successful modified Maze procedure at surgery and the risk for subsequent thromboembolic stroke. *J Am Coll Cardiol* 2011;58:1614–21.

400. Edgerton JR, Jackman WM, Mack MJ. A new epicardial lesion set for minimal access left atrial Maze: the Dallas lesion set. *Ann Thorac Surg* 2009;88:1655–7.

401. Edgerton JR, Brinkman WT, Weaver T, et al. Pulmonary vein isolation and autonomic denervation for the management of paroxysmal atrial fibrillation by a minimally invasive surgical approach. *J Thorac Cardiovasc Surg* 2010;140:823–8.

402. Gersak B, Jan M. Long-term success from the convergent atrial fibrillation procedure: 4-year outcome. *Ann Thorac Surg* 2016;102:1550–7.

403. Yancy CW, Jessup M, Bozkurt, et al. 2013 ACCF/AHA guidelines for the management of heart failure. *J Am Coll Cardiol* 2013;62:e147–239.

404. Yancy CW, Jessup M, Bozkurt B, et al. 2017 ACC/AHA/HFSA focused update of the 2013 ACCF/AHA guidelines for the management of heart failure. *J Am Coll Cardiol* 2017;70:776–803.

405. Mancini D, Colombo PC. Left ventricular assist devices: a rapidly evolving alternative to transplant. *J Am Coll Cardiol* 2015;65:2542–55.

406. Shah KB, Starling RC, Rogers JG, et al. Left ventricular assist devices versus medical management in ambulatory heart failure patients: an analysis of INTERMACS Profiles 4 and 5 to 7 from the ROADMAP study. *J Heart Lung Transplant* 2018;37:706–14.

407. Diodato MD, Moon MR, Pasque MK. Repair of ischemic mitral regurgitation does not increase mortality or improve long-term survival in patients undergoing coronary artery revascularization: a propensity analysis. *Ann Thorac Surg* 2004;78:794–9.

408. Fattouch K, Guccione F, Sampognaro R, et al. POINT: efficacy of adding mitral valve restrictive annuloplasty to coronary artery bypass grafting in patients with moderate ischemic mitral valve regurgitation: a randomized trial. *J Thorac Cardiovasc Surg* 2009;138:278–85.

409. Onarati G, Rubino AS, Marturano D, et al. Mid-term clinical and echocardiographic results and predictors of mitral regurgitation recurrence following restrictive annuloplasty for ischemic cardiomyopathy. *J Thorac Cardiovasc Surg* 2009;138:654–62.

410. Braun J, van de Veire NR, Klautz RJ, et al. Restrictive mitral annuloplasty cures ischemic mitral regurgitation and heart failure. *Ann Thorac Surg* 2008;85:430–6.

411. Samad Z, Shaw LK, Phelan M. Management and outcomes in patients with moderate or severe functional mitral regurgitation and severe left ventricular dysfunction. *Eur Heart J* 2015;36: 2733–41.

412. ten Brinke EA, Klautz RJ, Tulner SA, et al. Clinical and functional effects of restrictive mitral annuloplasty at midterm follow-up in heart failure patients. *Ann Thorac Surg* 2010;90:1913–21.

413. Kutyifa V, Quesada B, Klein H, et al. Long-term outcomes of cardiac resynchronization therapy in asymptomatic heart failure patients. *J Am Coll Cardiol* 2018;71 (suppl):10–2.

414. Al-Ghamdi B. Subcutaneous implantable cardioverter defibrillators: an overview of implantation techniques and clinical outcomes. *Current Cardiology Reviews* 2019;15:38–48.

415. Al-Khalib SM, Stephenson WG, Ackerman MJ, et al. 2017 AHA/ACC/HRS guideline for management of patients with ventricular arrhythmias and the prevention of sudden death: a report of the American College of Cardiology/American Heart Association Task Force on Clinical Practice Guidelines and the Heart Rhythm Society. *Circulation* 2018;138:e272–391.

416. Castelvecchio S, Garatti A, Gagliardotto PV, Menicanti L. Surgical ventricular reconstruction for ischaemic heart failure: state of the art. *Eur Heart J* 2016;18:e8–14.

417. Buckberg G, Athanasuleas C, Conte J. Surgical ventricular restoration for the treatment of heart failure. *Nat Rev Cardiol* 2012;9:703–16.

418. Ribeiro GA, da Costa CE, Lopes M, et al. Left ventricular reconstruction benefits patients with ischemic cardiomyopathy and non-viable myocardium. *Eur J Cardiothorac Surg* 2006;29:196–201.

419. Jones RH, Velazquez EJ, Michler RE, et al. Coronary bypass surgery with or without ventricular reconstruction. *N Engl J Med* 2009;360:1705–17.

420. Michler RE, Rouleau J, Al-Khalidi HR, et al. Insights from the STICH trial: change in left ventricular size after coronary artery bypass grafting with and without surgical ventricular restoration. *J Thorac Cardiovasc Surg* 2013;146:1139–45.

421. Witkowski TG, ten Brinke EA, Delgado V, et al. Surgical ventricular restoration for patients with ischemic heart failure: determinants of two-year survival. *Ann Thorac Surg* 2011;91:491–8.

422. Prucz RB, Weiss ES, Patel ND, Nwakanma LU, Shah AS, Conte JV. The impact of surgical ventricular restoration on mitral valve regurgitation. *Ann Thorac Surg* 2008;86:726–34.

423. Fukunaga N, Rao V. Left ventricular assist device as destination therapy for end stage heart failure: the right time for the right patients. *Curr Opin Cardiol* 2018;33:196–201.

424. Pérez-Casares, Cesar S, Brunet-Garcia L, Sanchez-de-Toledo J. Echocardiographic evaluation of pericardial effusion and cardiac tamponade. *Front Pediatr* 2017;5:79.

425. Depboylu BC, Mootoosamy P, Vistarini N, Testuz A, El-Hamamsy I, Cikirikcioglu M. Surgical treatment of constrictive pericarditis. *Tex Heart Int J* 2017;44:101–6.

426. Miranda WR, Oh JK. Constrictive pericarditis: a practical clinical approach. *Prog Cardiovasc Dis* 2017;59:369–79.

427. Geske JB, Anavekar NS, Nishimura RA, Oh JK, Gersh B. Differentiation of constriction and restriction: complex cardiovascular hemodynamics. *J Am Coll Cardiol* 2016;68:2329–47.

428. Rajagopalan N, Garcia MJ, Rodriguez L, et al. Comparison of new Doppler echocardiographic methods to differentiate constrictive pericardial disease and restrictive cardiomyopathy. *Am J Cardiol* 2001;87:86–94.

429. Ziskind AA, Pearce AC, Lemmon CC, et al. Percutaneous balloon pericardiotomy for the treatment of cardiac tamponade and large pericardial effusions: description of technique and report of the first 50 cases. *J Am Coll Cardiol* 1993;21:1–5.

430. Ha HW, Oh JK, Schaff HV, et al. Impact of left ventricular function on immediate and long-term outcomes after pericardiectomy in constrictive pericarditis. *J Thorac Cardiovasc Surg* 2008;136: 1136–41.

431. Allen KB, Faber LP, Warren WH, Shaar CJ. Pericardial effusion: subxiphoid pericardiostomy versus percutaneous catheter drainage. *Ann Thorac Surg* 1999;67:437–40.

432. O'Brien PK, Kucharczuk JC, Marshall MB, et al. Comparative study of subxiphoid versus video-thoracoscopic pericardial "window". *Ann Thorac Surg* 2005;80:2013–9.

433. Bertog SC, Thambidorai SK, Parakh K, et al. Constrictive pericarditis: etiology and cause-specific survival after pericardiectomy. *J Am Coll Cardiol* 2004;43:1445–52.

434. Meissner I, Khandheria BK, Heit JA, et al. Patent foramen ovale: innocent or guilty? Evidence from a prospective population-based study. *J Am Coll Cardiol* 2006;47:440–5.

435. Lamy C, Giannesini C, Zuber M, et al. Clinical and imaging findings in cryptogenic stroke patients with and without patent foramen ovale: the PFO-ASA study: atrial septal aneurysm. *Stroke* 2002;33:706–11.

436. Mojadidi MK, Zaman MO, Elgendy IY, et al. Cryptogenic stroke and patent foramen ovale. *J Am Coll Cardiol* 2018;71:1035–43.

437. Handke M, Harloff A, Olschewski M, Hetzel A, Geibel A. Patent foramen ovale and cryptogenic stroke in older patients. *N Engl J Med* 2007;357:2262–8.

438. Bannan A, Shen R, Silvestry FE, Herrmann HC. Characteristics of adult patients with atrial septal defects presenting with paradoxical embolism. *Catheter Cardiovasc Interv* 2009;74:1066–9.

439. Papa M, Gaspardone A, Fracasso G, et al. Usefulness of transcatheter patent foramen ovale closure in migraineurs with moderate to large right-to-left shunt and instrumental evidence of cerebrovascular damage. *Am J Cardiol* 2009;104:434–9.

440. Tobis JM, Charles A, Silberstein SD, et al. Percutaneous closure of patent foramen ovale in patients with migraine: the PREMIUM trial. *J Am Coll Cardiol* 2017;70:2766–74.

441. Shah R, Nayyar M, Jovin IS, et al. Device closure versus medical therapy alone for patent foramen ovale in patients with cryptogenic stroke: a systematic review and meta-analysis. *Ann Intern Med* 2018;168:335–42.

442. Wintzer-Wehekind J, Alperi A, Houde C, et al. Long-term follow-up after closure of patent fora-men ovale in patients with cryptogenic embolism. *J Am Coll Cardiol* 2019;73:278–87.

443. Mas JL, Arquizan C, Lamy C, et al. Recurrent cerebrovascular events associated with patent foramen ovale, atrial septal aneurysm, or both. *N Engl J Med* 2001;345:1740–6.

444. Oster MA, Bhatt AB, Zaragoza-Macias E, Dendukuri N, Marelli A. Interventional therapy versus medical therapy for secundum atrial septal defect: a systematic review (Part 2) for the 2018 AHA/ACC guideline for the management of adults with congenital heart disease: a report of the American College of Cardiology/American Heart Association Task Force on Clinical Practice Guidelines. *J Am Coll Cardiol* 2019;73:1579–95.

445. Hörer J, Müller S, Schreiber C, et al. Surgical closure of atrial septal defect in patients older than 30 years: risk factors for late death from arrhythmia or heart failure. *Thorac Cardiovasc Surg* 2007;55:79–83.

446. Gatzoulis MA, Freeman MA, Siu SC, Webb GD, Harris L. Atrial arrhythmia after surgical closure of atrial septal defects in adults. *N Engl J Med* 1999;340:839–46.

447. Ghosh S, Chatterjee S, Black E, Firmin RK. Surgical closure of atrial septal defects in adults: effect of age at operation on outcome. *Heart* 2002;88:485–7.

448. An G, Zhang H, Zheng S, Wang W, Ma L. Mid-term outcomes of common congenital heart defects corrected through a right subaxillary thoracotomy. *Heart Lung Circ* 2017;26:376–382.

449. Stout KK, Daniels CJ, Valente AM, et al. 2018 AHA/ACC guideline for the management of adults with congenital heart disease: executive summary: a report of the American College of Cardiology/American Heart Association Task Force on Clinical Practice Guidelines. *J Am Coll Cardiol* 2019;73:1494–563.

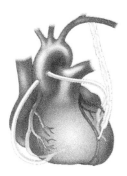

CHAPTER 2

Diagnostic Techniques in Cardiac Surgery

2 Diagnostic Techniques in Cardiac Surgery

Although the general nature of a patient's cardiac disease can usually be ascertained from a thorough history and physical examination, diagnostic tests are essential to define the pathology and extent of cardiac disease more precisely. A variety of noninvasive and invasive modalities can be used to identify the presence and severity of cardiovascular abnormalities that may require surgery. This chapter briefly reviews the basic types of diagnostic tests available to the clinician and defines their role in preoperative evaluation. In-depth discussions of several of these modalities with extensive references can be found on medical websites, including www.uptodate.com and www.emedicine.medscape.com.

I. Chest Radiography

A. PA and lateral chest x-ray should be obtained on all patients before surgery. It should be consistent with the patient's cardiac diagnosis and can provide a wealth of potential information to the surgeon (Figure 2.1).

1. Compatibility with the clinical diagnosis:

   a. Left ventricular (LV) enlargement in patients with volume overload (aortic regurgitation or mitral regurgitation) or a dilated cardiomyopathy

   b. Left ventricular hypertrophy (LVH) (aortic stenosis, hypertension)

   c. Enlarged cardiac silhouette (pericardial effusion)

   d. Large left atrium or calcified mitral valve or annulus (mitral valve disease)

   e. Wide superior mediastinum (aortic dissection or aortic aneurysm)

   f. Pulmonary vascular redistribution (congestive heart failure)

2. Identify other potentially relevant abnormalities:

   a. Pulmonary: emphysema, pneumonia, parenchymal nodules, interstitial disease, previous pulmonary resection

   b. Pleural space: effusions, pneumothorax

   c. Mediastinum: tumors or widened mediastinum consistent with aortic disease

   d. Bone: pectus excavatum, rib resection from a previous thoracotomy

   e. Foreign bodies: sternal wires from a previous sternotomy, type of prosthetic heart valve, pacemaker wires, central venous catheters, position of an intra-aortic balloon pump (IABP)

B. The chest x-ray can also provide important information that may influence operability or operative technique.

Manual of Perioperative Care in Adult Cardiac Surgery, Sixth Edition. Robert M. Bojar.
© 2021 John Wiley & Sons Ltd. Published 2021 by John Wiley & Sons Ltd.

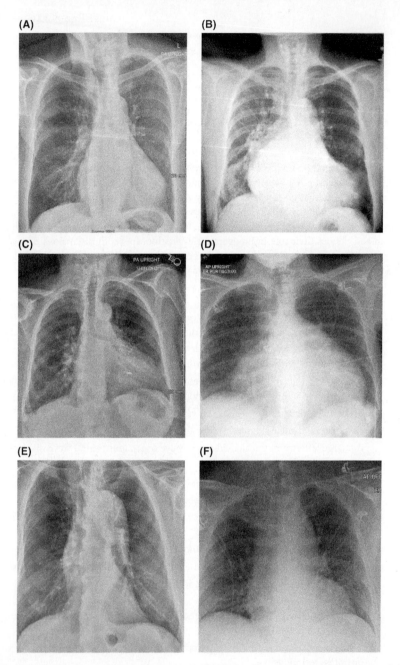

Figure 2.1 • Chest x-rays obtained preoperatively. (A) Aortic regurgitation (AR) showing left ventricular (LV) enlargement from volume overload. (B) Advanced mitral stenosis (MS) demonstrating marked enlargement of the left atrium projecting to the right of the cardiac silhouette. (C) LV enlargement from volume overload in a patient with chronic mitral regurgitation (MR). (D) A markedly enlarged cardiac silhouette in a patient with a large pericardial effusion. (E) A wide mediastinum in a patient with an ascending aortic aneurysm. (F) A wide mediastinum in a patient with an acute type A aortic dissection.

1. Calcification of the ascending aorta or arch is an important finding that may increase the risk of stroke. This may require an alternative cannulation site (femoral or axillary artery), avoidance of aortic cross-clamping (beating or fibrillating heart surgery), or avoidance of both cannulation and aortic cross-clamping (off-pump surgery). It may necessitate the use of deep hypothermic circulatory arrest to perform an aortic valve replacement or resection of the ascending aorta. The presence of significant ascending aortic calcification in a patient with symptomatic severe AS is usually an indication for a transcatheter aortic valve replacement (TAVR). Epiaortic echocardiography may be indicated during surgery to evaluate for ascending aortic atherosclerosis. Suspicion of ascending aortic calcification by chest x-ray (usually on the lateral film) or fluoroscopy during cardiac catheterization may be further defined by noncontrast CT scanning (see Figure 2.10). Calcification of the aortic knob alone is a common finding on chest x-ray but is usually of little significance.

2. An elevated hemidiaphragm on one side might deter the surgeon from using the contralateral internal thoracic artery (ITA), especially in diabetic patients, who arguably are more prone to phrenic nerve paresis.[1,2]

3. Mitral annular calcification in patients with MR makes mitral valve repair or replacement more difficult and may necessitate creative surgical techniques.

4. For patients undergoing reoperation, PA and lateral films are essential. The PA film may identify the proximity of the ITA pedicle (identified by metallic clips) to the midline, although this usually requires a selective ITA angiogram to detect its true course. However, the lateral film will demonstrate the proximity of an aortic aneurysm, the right ventricle (RV), and occasionally the ITA to the posterior sternal table. If there is a concern about potential damage to any of these structures with a sternotomy, femoral or axillary cannulation and even initiation of cardiopulmonary bypass (CPB) prior to sternotomy may be indicated. Alternatively, a thoracotomy incision should be considered, especially for redo mitral valve surgery (right chest) or redo coronary surgery to the left-sided vessels (left chest).

5. The location and orientation of the heart (craniocaudal as well as relationship to the midline) should be considered when selecting the appropriate incision for minimally invasive surgery. For example, in thin patients and those with emphysema, the heart has a vertical orientation and lies quite caudal in the chest. Thus, for aortic valve surgery, a more distal intercostal space incision may be necessary with either a partial upper sternotomy incision or anterior thoracotomy approach to obtain appropriate exposure.

6. The patient with congestive heart failure may benefit from aggressive diuresis prior to surgery or hemofiltration during CPB.

II. Electrocardiography

A. A 12-lead ECG must be reviewed prior to surgery because it can yield valuable information about the nature of the patient's disease, the urgency of surgery, the appropriate management of arrhythmias, and other considerations in perioperative management.

B. **Common disorders of rate and rhythm**

1. The presence of sinus tachycardia in a patient with coronary disease suggests that the patient is inadequately ß-blocked. This may predispose the patient to the development of ischemia preoperatively and to atrial fibrillation (AF) after surgery. Most patients undergoing CABG should be managed preoperatively with ß-blockers.

2. Patients with sinus bradycardia usually require temporary postoperative pacing and may not tolerate ß-blockers or amiodarone that might otherwise be used prophylactically to prevent postoperative AF. Patients with sick sinus or tachycardia/bradycardia syndrome are more likely to require a permanent pacemaker postoperatively.

3. A rapid ventricular response to AF must be controlled pharmacologically. It can precipitate myocardial ischemia in patients with coronary artery disease (CAD) and can compromise the cardiac output in patients with significant LVH. If long-standing persistent AF has been present, the use of prophylactic medications to prevent postoperative AF is usually of little benefit, but postoperative anticoagulation is indicated to prevent a thromboembolic stroke. A Maze procedure may be considered as an adjunct to other cardiac operations in patients with either paroxysmal or persistent AF.

4. Ventricular tachyarrhythmias may result from active ischemia or remote myocardial infarction. If revascularization is indicated, a postoperative electrophysiology study should be considered in patients with sustained ventricular tachycardia (VT). An implantable cardioverter-defibrillator (ICD) should be inserted if VT is inducible or if the ejection fraction (EF) remains <35% 90 days after revascularization.

C. **Conduction problems**

1. Ischemic ECG changes are difficult to assess in the patient with a bundle branch block. Early catheterization may be indicated in patients with acute coronary syndromes considered at high risk based on clinical criteria.

2. The presence of a left bundle branch block (LBBB) increases the risk of asystole during insertion of a Swan-Ganz pulmonary artery (PA) catheter. This should be deferred until after the sternotomy has been performed so that immediate epicardial pacing can be achieved.

3. Patients with a right bundle branch block (RBBB) and a first degree block are more prone to the development of complete heart block after TAVR and may require placement of a permanent pacemaker.

4. The development of conduction abnormalities in a patient with aortic valve endocarditis suggests annular extension of the infection, which is an indication for urgent surgery.

5. Patients sustaining an inferior infarction may develop heart block and require temporary pacing preoperatively.

D. **Evidence of ischemia and infarction**

1. ST and T wave changes consistent with ischemia require aggressive management. This may entail use of intravenous nitrates, antiplatelet agents (aspirin, P2Y12 inhibitors [clopidogrel, ticagrelor, prasugrel], and/or glycoprotein IIb/IIIa inhibitors), unfractionated heparin or low molecular weight heparin, and/or placement of an IABP. An early invasive strategy with urgent percutaneous coronary intervention (PCI) or surgery is usually indicated. Evidence of recent infarction may influence the timing and risk of surgery. Waiting several days may lower the

surgical risk in stable patients, but is inadvisable if the patient develops recurrent chest pain, ischemia, or cardiogenic shock, or has threatening coronary anatomy.

2. In patients with depressed LV function, an ECG with Q waves is more consistent with transmural infarction, but the absence of Q waves suggests that the myocardium may be chronically ischemic and hibernating, rather than infarcted. Further evaluation with viability studies may be indicated to determine whether surgery will prove beneficial in improving LV function and survival.

E. **Transvenous pacemaker and ICD issues**

1. The function of a permanent transvenous pacing system can be disrupted by use of electrocautery at the time of surgery. A magnet must be available to convert the pacemaker to a fixed pacing mode.

2. ICD units should be inactivated prior to surgery.

3. Because the right atrial lead of a dual-chamber pacemaker may be displaced during surgery or the pulse generator may be damaged by electrocautery, all permanent pacemaker systems must be interrogated immediately after surgery to ensure appropriate sensing and pacing.

III. Stress Testing and Myocardial Perfusion Imaging in Coronary Disease

A. Stress testing plays a major role in detecting the potential presence and functional significance of CAD. In addition to basic exercise stress testing, rest and stress myocardial perfusion imaging (MPI) have greater sensitivity and specificity in identifying viable and ischemic myocardium that will benefit from an interventional procedure. The technology has become very sophisticated, and only the salient features are presented.[3-5]

B. **Exercise ECG (exercise tolerance test or ETT).** In patients who can exercise, stress testing to maximal exercise (or at least >85% of maximal predicted heart rate to optimize sensitivity) is performed on a treadmill with a graded protocol (Figure 2.2). ECG changes of ischemia can be difficult to detect in patients with a LBBB, ventricular-paced rhythms, significant LVH, or ST changes on baseline ECG, so for these patients, an imaging study is preferable. The ECG leads that demonstrate ST depressions during exercise testing do not necessarily correlate with the site of ischemia, but this can be determined more precisely with imaging studies.

1. It is recognized that the sensitivity and specificity of ETTs are not ideal and the proper interpretation of a stress test depends on the pretest probability of CAD.[6,7] For example, a positive ETT in an asymptomatic nondiabetic patient may be a false positive, and a negative ETT in a patient with symptoms and multiple risk factors does not exclude CAD. Therefore, exercise ECG testing is most useful for the patient with an intermediate probability of disease based on clinical criteria.

2. Exercise testing is of value in that it mimics the clinical circumstances during which the patient becomes symptomatic and can determine the workload level at which symptoms occur. The latter correlates with the likelihood of more severe coronary disease and also correlates with prognosis.

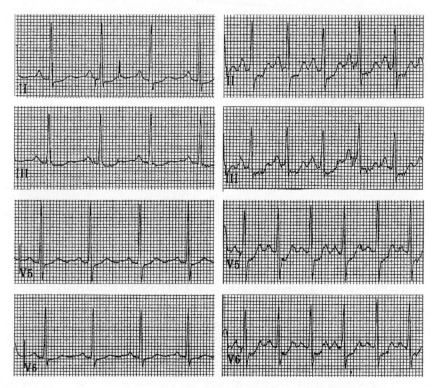

Figure 2.2 • Positive exercise stress test. (Left) baseline ECG before exercise (leads II, III, V5, V6). (Right) exercise ECG after four minutes of stage 2. At a heart rate of 157 bpm, note the presence of 3 mm of ST depression in these leads, suggesting inferolateral ischemia.

3. The following findings are consistent with multivessel coronary disease and an adverse prognosis, especially when they occur at a low workload (<6 METs):

   a. Development of anginal symptoms

   b. More than 2 mm ST depression in multiple leads that persists more than five minutes into recovery

   c. ST segment elevation

   d. Failure to increase blood pressure to higher than 120 mm Hg or a sustained decrease in blood pressure greater than 10 mm Hg or below rest levels

   e. Sustained ventricular tachycardia

C. **Radionuclide myocardial perfusion imaging (rMPI).**[8–11] Use of rest and stress imaging can assess myocardial perfusion, viability, global myocardial function and regional wall motion abnormalities. Stress may be induced either as part of an exercise protocol, pharmacologically using a coronary vasodilator, or with an inotrope (dobutamine) to increase myocardial oxygen demand with mild vasodilatation. Perfusion distal to a stenosis is maintained at rest by autoregulatory dilatation of resistance vessels that maintains distal flow despite a reduced perfusion pressure.

Exercise or use of vasodilators elicits regional differences in coronary flow reserve, as blood flow may increase three- to fivefold in normal arteries, but much less so beyond coronary stenoses. This discrepancy allows for the identification of ischemic zones and, inferentially, coronary stenosis.

1. rMPI is more sensitive and specific than exercise stress testing in detecting CAD and is more effective in determining the severity and location of ischemia. It is most useful when the patient has baseline ECG changes that preclude adequate interpretation of an ECG exercise test or when the patient cannot adequately exercise. Single-photon emission CT (SPECT) imaging and positron emission tomography (PET) scanning can be used, the former being more widely available. Radioactive tracers commonly used for SPECT MPI include Tc-99m tetrofosmin (Myoview) and Tc-99m sestamibi (Cardiolite), which have essentially supplanted the use of thallium-201.

2. If the patient can exercise, a treadmill or bicycle is used, and at peak exercise or when symptoms develop, a radioisotope is injected, exercise is continued for a minute, and SPECT imaging is obtained. Low-level treadmill exercise combined with vasodilator stress imaging can give an assessment of exercise capacity, provides excellent images, and is associated with fewer noncardiac side effects.[12]

3. If the patient cannot exercise, pharmacologic stress is generally induced with a vasodilator, most commonly regadenoson (Lexiscan), which is a selective adenosine A2A receptor agonist, and, less commonly, adenosine or dipyridamole. For purely stress imaging, regadenoson 400 µg is given intravenously (IV), flushed with saline, and is followed 10–20 seconds later by an injection of a radioisotope, and imaging is obtained 15–45 minutes later. These medications produce coronary vasodilation with a fourfold increase in myocardial blood flow above baseline in normal arteries (coronary flow reserve being the ratio of hyperemic to baseline coronary flow). With flow-limiting coronary stenosis, there is less coronary flow reserve and less tracer uptake in the myocardium subtended by those vessels.[13] At peak stress, lack of tracer update ("cold spot") may be consistent with either irreversible infarction or ischemia.

4. In patients with contraindications to vasodilators, such as hypotension, sick sinus syndrome, high-degree AV block, bronchospastic lung disease, or use of theophylline, dobutamine can be used for MPI.[14] This is given in five three-minute stages at increasing doses, starting at 5 µg/kg/min, followed by doses of 10, 20, 30, and eventually 40 µg/kg/min. Dobutamine will increase heart rate (chronotropy) and myocardial contractility (inotropy), producing an increase in oxygen demand and, consequently, myocardial blood flow. Once target heart rate is achieved (occasionally with the use of atropine) or the patient becomes symptomatic, the radionuclide is injected over 10 seconds, allowed to circulate for a minute, and then imaging is obtained.

5. Rest/stress protocols are most commonly used because they can assess the presence of viability and ischemia. A common protocol involves infusion of the radioactive tracer for rest images (e.g. 9 µg of tetrofosmin), then injection of the vasodilator followed by re-administration of a three-times-higher dose of tracer, with imaging obtained 15–60 minutes later (Figure 2.3).

6. Stress/redistribution studies may be performed using thallium-201, either given after exercise or after the administration of dipyridamole. After the tracer is

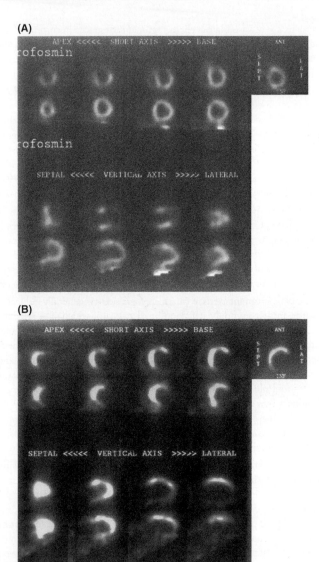

Figure 2.3 • Stress imaging studies with Tc-99m tetrofosmin. (A) Short-axis (upper two rows) and vertical long-axis views (lower two rows) at stress (top image of each pair) and redistribution (lower image of each pair). The stress images demonstrate reduced tracer uptake in the anteroapical region that improves during the redistribution phase, consistent with anteroapical ischemia. (B) Similar views demonstrating a defect in the inferolateral region in the stress images that does not improve with redistribution. This is consistent with infarction.

injected, the initial stress imaging is obtained within 10 minutes and then repeated 2.5–4 hours later for the redistribution imaging. If there is still a residual imaging defect, delayed reimaging is performed 18–24 hours later after a small reinjection of thallium-201. The latter will improve sensitivity in determining myocardial viability.[15] Alternatively, a rest-only image may be obtained along with initial and delayed redistribution images to assess for viability.[9]

D. **Stress MRI scanning** has excellent spatial and temporal resolution and is very effective in assessing regional wall motion abnormalities and in detecting, localizing, and quantifying the degree of ischemia.[11] Various applications include rest/stress perfusion imaging and dobutamine cine stress cardiac magnetic resonance (CMR), which has >80% sensitivity and specificity in identifying significant coronary stenosis. Some consider nuclear imaging the gold standard for assessing myocardial perfusion and recommend it as a noninvasive approach to assess intermediate- to high-risk patients with equivocal stress tests. This approach entails a cardiac CT scan to assess for anatomic stenosis and, if present, a subsequent stress MRI to assess the hemodynamic significance of the lesion. Delayed gadolinium enhancement on cardiac MR can be used to identify areas of viability and nonviability (see section F.3.e).

E. **Stress echocardiography** is based on the principle that stress-induced ischemia caused by coronary artery stenosis will produce regional wall motion abnormalities.[16] This may be performed using bicycle or treadmill exercise (ESE). An alternative to exercise is the use of **dobutamine** to increase myocardial oxygen demand (dobutamine stress echocardiogram, or DSE). If the demand cannot be met by an increase in blood flow, ischemia will produce regional wall motion abnormalities in the distribution of the stenotic coronary artery. Thus, this can determine the location and extent of ischemia. Stress echoes are more sensitive and specific than exercise ECG testing and provide comparable results to those of exercise nuclear imaging.

F. **Viability studies.**[17] Myocardial viability studies are useful in patients with severe LV dysfunction to distinguish areas of myocardial necrosis from "hibernating myocardium" that may recover function after revascularization. The clinical utility of these studies has been called into question and may not be as useful as previously thought.

1. Revascularization of viable areas generally improves LV function and symptoms in patients with CHF with or without angina, although in some patients, symptoms will improve without any improvement in global or regional function.[18,19] Extensive remodeling and high end-systolic volumes are associated with less improvement in LV function.

2. Numerous meta-analyses have reported a strong association between viability and improvement in survival with CABG.[20] However, other important studies suggest this may not be the case. In a 10-year follow-up of the STICH (Surgical Treatment for Ischemic Heart Failure) trial, which is discussed on page 7, the presence of viability was associated with an improvement of LV function with both medical and surgical therapy, but this did not translate into improved survival.[21] Another analysis of STICH data indicated that viability was predictive of a survival benefit in patients with moderate LV dysfunction but lost its prognostic benefit when LV dysfunction became severe.[22]

3. Among the modalities available to detect viability are the following:

a. **SPECT imaging with Tc-99m tracers** (tetrofosmin or sestamibi) is based on intact mitochondrial function reflecting viability. Gated SPECT scanning allows for the assessment of ventricular function as well as viability using routine rest/stress imaging.

b. **SPECT imaging with thallium** provides a comparable assessment of viability.[23] Thallium uptake reflects cell membrane integrity, so that viable zones, whether ischemic or not, will perfuse and retain thallium at rest. With rest-redistribution imaging, nonischemic viable tissue will retain thallium at rest. However, if there is rest ischemia, a defect may be evident initially but show redistribution four hours later, indicating viability. With stress-redistribution imaging, an area of ischemia that produces a defect at stress may demonstrate redistribution either with reinjection of thallium or on delayed imaging up to 18–24 hours later.[15]

c. **^{18}F-deoxyglucose (FDG) uptake** using PET or SPECT imaging is a very sensitive test of viability. FDG is a marker of glucose uptake by the myocardium, thus assessing metabolism and cell viability. An assessment of perfusion is made with ^{13}N-ammonia or rubidium-82, and then ^{18}FDG is injected to assess metabolism. Zones with matching perfusion and metabolism are either not ischemic or are infarcted. Evidence of preserved metabolic activity in zones of reduced perfusion indicates viable, hibernating myocardium. These studies may detect viability in zones considered nonviable by thallium imaging.[24]

d. **Dobutamine stress echo (DSE)** can be used to identify contractile reserve, which suggests viability.[15] Low doses of dobutamine are administered during echocardiography to assess any change in global and regional wall motion. A biphasic response during dobutamine echocardiography (improvement in function at low dose and worsening of function at peak stress from high doses of dobutamine) is highly predictive of recovery of regional contractile function in patients with LV dysfunction.[25]

e. **Delayed enhancement magnetic resonance imaging (MRI)** is indexed on cell membrane integrity and uses gadolinium-based contrast as a means of assessing viability and nonviability. Normal myocardium has a very low concentration of gadolinium after its injection and will appear black on imaging, whereas abnormal myocardial tissue will accumulate gadolinium and appear hyper-enhanced and bright.[26] Late gadolinium enhancement (LGE) is noted in regions of transmural nonviability. LGE >15% has been found to correlate with the risk of sudden death in patients with hypertrophic obstructive cardiomyopathy.[27] MRI-defined diastolic wall thickness >5.5 mm is predictive of contractile recovery after CABG. MRI provides excellent image quality with a precise identification of epicardial and endocardial borders to allow for the assessment of wall motion and thickening.[28]

IV. Stress Echocardiography in Valvular Heart Disease

A. **General comments.**[29,30] Exercise stress echo (ESE) is very useful in assessing the physiologic and hemodynamic severity of valvular heart disease in patients without significant symptoms and can be used to assess prognosis (see section VII for discussion of non-stress echo imaging). The patient should have a resting and then stress echocardiogram for the assessment of valve gradients, degree of regurgitation, stroke volume, PA and right ventricular systolic pressures (RVSP), and RV and LV size and function. The test is abnormal if:

- Symptoms occur at lower than expected workload
- Exercise capacity is <85% of predicted
- Blood pressure falls or increases <20 mm Hg
- RVSP rises to >60 mm Hg

- Degree of valvular regurgitation worsens
- EF falls or regional wall motion abnormalities develop
- Sustained ventricular arrhythmias occur

B. **Aortic stenosis (AS)** is a progressive process, and patients often limit their activities and deny symptoms. Because of the adverse impact of symptoms on survival (mean survival of only 1–2 years), stress testing is recommended in "asymptomatic" stage C patients with severe AS. Studies have shown that an abnormal symptom-limited ESE is associated with an eightfold higher risk of major adverse cardiac events (MACE) and a 5.5 times higher risk of sudden death.[29] In addition, an increase in mean gradient of >20 mm Hg or development of exercise-induced pulmonary hypertension is associated with a higher risk of MACE. Therefore, both ACC/AHA and European Society of Cardiology (ESC) guidelines recommend aortic valve replacement (AVR) for patients who develop symptoms (class I) or an abnormal blood pressure response (class IIa) with exercise stress testing.

1. DSE is very useful in the assessment of patients with stage D2 low-flow, low-gradient AS with depressed LV function. DSE can differentiate true AS from pseudo-severe AS, the latter being present if the aortic valve area (AVA) increases with dobutamine due to an increase in cardiac output without an increase in gradient.

   a. In stage D2 patients, the diagnosis of severe AS is confirmed by an increase in the mean gradient to >40 mm Hg with dobutamine, but often the AVA will calculate to <1.0 cm^2 even though the gradient does not reach that level. This AVA-gradient discordance may occur when inadequate contractile reserve is present, i.e. when the stroke volume increases <20% or the EF falls. This suggests intrinsic myocardial dysfunction, not just afterload mismatch, as the cause of poor LV function. Even though the results of AVR (either surgical or TAVR) are suboptimal in these patients with a much higher mortality, AVR still improves upon the poor natural history of AS if left untreated.

   b. In patients with poor contractile reserve, it may be difficult to differentiate true from pseudo-severe AS. It has been proposed that a "projected AVA" based on a normal transvalvular flow rate be used to more appropriately assess the severity of AS.[31]

2. The role of DSE is not clear-cut in patients with stage D3 AS, which is termed paradoxical low-flow, low gradient AS with normal EF. The diagnosis is usually made because of a low stroke volume index <35 mL/m^2. If that is not present, one might presume that severe AS is not present. Again, use of the projected AVA may be helpful, but assessment of aortic valve calcium by CT scanning may be more suggestive of severe AS.[32]

C. **Aortic regurgitation (AR).** The progression to symptomatic AR is fairly slow, and patients often remain asymptomatic despite the onset of progressive LV dysfunction. ESE can be used to elicit symptoms or assess contractile reserve, the absence of which correlates with potentially irreversible LV dysfunction even after AVR. An exercise-induced fall in EF may also prompt early consideration of surgery. Other subtle changes, such as early RV systolic dysfunction or measurements approaching the guideline recommendations for surgery (EF 50–55% or LVESD approaching 50 mm) are considered high-risk findings.

D. **Mitral stenosis (MS).** ESE or DSE is useful in assessing the physiologic significance of MS when there is discordance between clinical symptoms and hemodynamics. Some patients appear asymptomatic with severe MS, while others are symptomatic with moderate MS. With exercise, the heart rate increases with less diastolic filling time, and the mitral gradient increases along with an increase in left atrial (LA) and PA pressures. Nearly 50% of patients with asymptomatic moderate–severe MS have been shown to develop symptoms during exercise.[30] Other high-risk features include an increase in the mean gradient to >18 mm Hg with DSE or >15 mm Hg with exercise and an RVSP >60 mm Hg at peak exercise, with dyspnea more likely to develop if there is a rapid rise in RV systolic pressure with less exercise.[33]

E. **Mitral regurgitation (MR).** Stress echo is helpful in assessing exercise-induced changes in MR when there is a discordance between symptoms and the severity of MR. For patients with primary degenerative MR, an increase in RVSP to >60 mm Hg, exercise capacity <85% of predicted, latent LV dysfunction, AF, or abnormal heart rate recovery are high-risk features. For patients with secondary (functional or ischemic) MR, ESE may reveal subclinical LV dysfunction due to ischemia and is suggestive of severe MR if the patient develops pulmonary edema, ischemic wall motion abnormalities, or an increase in the effective regurgitant orifice area of >13 mm.

V. Cardiac Catheterization

A. The gold standard for the diagnosis of most forms of cardiac disease remains cardiac catheterization.[34] It is indicated in most patients whose clinical presentation and diagnostic testing suggest that an interventional procedure (PCI or cardiac surgery) may be indicated. The exceptions are acute type A aortic dissections, which are surgical emergencies, and aortic valve endocarditis with vegetations, with which catheter manipulation in the root may cause embolization.

B. **Techniques** (Tables 2.1 and 2.2; Figures 2.4–2.6)

1. **Right-heart catheterization** is performed in patients with valve disease and those with coronary disease and LV dysfunction. It involves placement of a Swan-Ganz PA catheter to obtain intracardiac pressures and measure oxygen saturations from each chamber to detect intracardiac shunts (atrial or ventricular septal defects). The mixed venous oxygen saturation from the PA port indirectly reflects the cardiac output. A thermodilution cardiac output is obtained and can be used along with pressure gradients obtained from right- and left-heart catheterization to calculate valve areas using the Gorlin formula (see page 24).

2. **Left-heart catheterization** involves advancing a catheter from the aorta through the aortic valve into the LV. This allows for the measurement of the left ventricular end-diastolic pressure (LVEDP), obtaining a left ventriculogram to assess the EF (end-diastolic volume minus end-systolic volume divided by the end-diastolic volume) (Figure 2.7), and identification of MR (Figure 2.8). A Fick cardiac output can be calculated. The aortic valve gradient can be measured during pullback of the catheter, but in patients with AS, crossing the valve has been reported to increase the risk of stroke.[35] Therefore, this should not be performed if severe AS is confirmed by echocardiography.

3. Evaluation of both left- and right-heart pressures is invaluable in making the diagnosis of constrictive pericarditis (see Figure 1.32).[36,37]

4. An **aortogram** ("root shot") may be performed in patients with aortic valve disease to assess the degree of AR (Figure 2.9). Excessive whip of an angiographic catheter may suggest the presence of a dilated aortic root. An aortogram can provide an estimate of aortic size that might necessitate replacement of the ascending aorta, but a CT scan or echocardiogram can assess the size of the aorta more precisely.

Table 2.1 • Information Obtained from Right- and Left-Heart Catheterization

Elevated RA pressure	Tricuspid stenosis (large "a" wave) Tricuspid regurgitation (large "v" wave) RV dysfunction (pulmonary hypertension, RV infarction) Constrictive pericarditis/tamponade/restrictive disease
Elevated RV pressure	RV dysfunction (pulmonary hypertension, RV infarction) Constrictive pericarditis (square root sign; rapid "x" and "y" descent) Restrictive disease Cardiac tamponade (absent "y" descent)
Elevated PA pressure	Mitral stenosis/regurgitation LV systolic or diastolic dysfunction (ischemic, dilated cardiomyopathy, aortic stenosis/regurgitation) Pulmonary hypertension of other etiologies Constrictive pericarditis/tamponade/restrictive disease
Elevated PCW pressure	Mitral stenosis (large "a" wave if sinus rhythm) Mitral regurgitation (large "v" wave) LV systolic or diastolic dysfunction (ischemic, dilated cardiomyopathy, aortic stenosis/regurgitation) Constrictive pericarditis/tamponade
Elevated LVEDP	LV systolic or diastolic dysfunction (ischemic, dilated cardiomyopathy, aortic stenosis/regurgitation) Constrictive pericarditis/tamponade

RA, right atrial; RV, right ventricular; PA, pulmonary artery; LV, left ventricular; PCW, pulmonary capillary wedge; LVEDP, left ventricular end-diastolic pressure.

Table 2.2 • Hemodynamic Norms for Intracardiac Pressures

Location	Pressures (mm Hg)
Right atrium	Mean 3–8
Right ventricle	Systolic 15–30 Diastolic 3–8
Pulmonary artery	Systolic 15–30 Diastolic 5–12 Mean 9–16
Pulmonary capillary wedge	5–12
Left atrium	5–12
Left ventricle	Systolic 90–140 End-diastolic 5–12
Aorta	Systolic 90–140 Diastolic 60–90 Mean 70–105

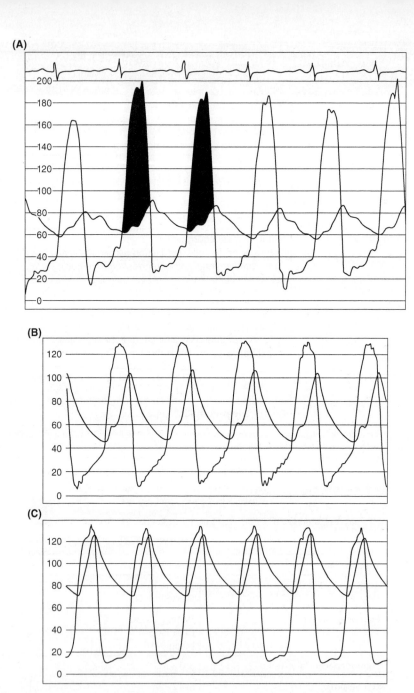

Figure 2.4 • Left heart catheterization performed during a TAVR procedure. (A) Simultaneous LV and aortic root pressures are measured with a peak gradient of 100 mm Hg and a mean gradient of 78 mm Hg calculated by the software program. (B) Hemodynamic tracing of another patient with moderate aortic stenosis (AS), but severe AR. Note that the left ventricular end-diastolic pressure (LVEDP) is nearly equivalent to the low aortic diastolic pressure. (C) Following a TAVR in this patient, there is a substantial increase in the aortic diastolic pressure and a significant reduction in LVEDP.

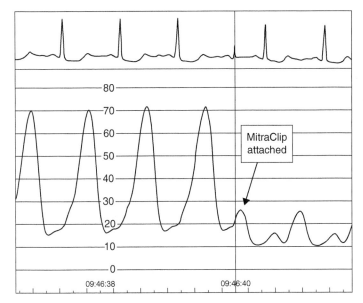

Figure 2.5 • Direct measurement of the left atrial "v" wave during a MitraClip procedure indicating severe MR with a "v" wave up to 70 mm Hg.

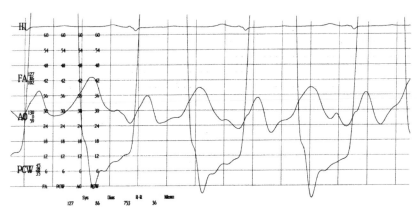

Figure 2.6 • Left-heart catheterization of MS. There is a pressure difference (gradient) of approximately 20 mm Hg between the pulmonary capillary wedge pressure and the mean LV diastolic pressure.

5. **Fluoroscopy** can yield valuable information, including:

   a. Calcification of the ascending aorta that may require further evaluation by non-contrast CT scanning (Figure 2.10)

   b. Severe coronary calcification or extensive coronary stenting that may make bypass grafting virtually impossible

   c. The location of intravascular catheters or assist devices, or the position of an intra-aortic balloon pump (IABP)

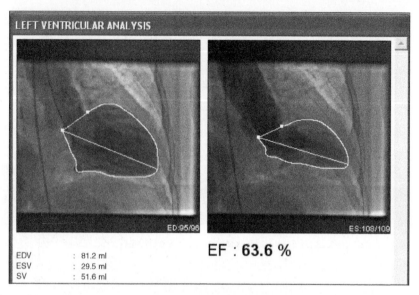

Figure 2.7 • Left ventriculogram. The ejection fraction (EF) is calculated by dividing the end-diastolic volume (left) minus the end-systolic volume (right) by the end-diastolic volume.

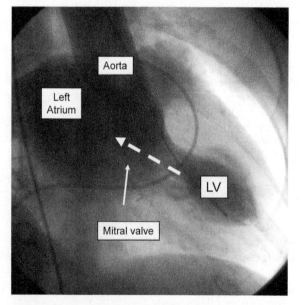

Figure 2.8 • Left ventriculogram obtained at end-systole, demonstrating severe MR into a dilated left atrium.

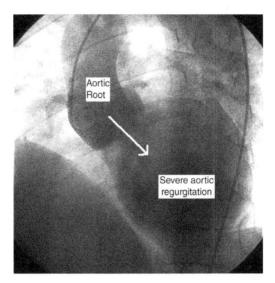

Figure 2.9 • A "root shot" with a pigtail catheter in the proximal aorta will demonstrate the size of the aorta and the degree of AR, which in this patient was severe.

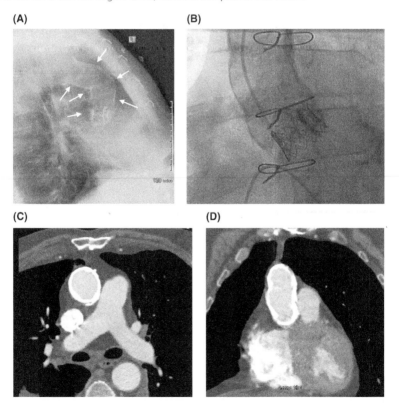

Figure 2.10 • (A) Lateral chest x-ray demonstrating severe ascending aortic calcification. (B) Using fluoroscopy prior to injection of contrast, significant calcification can be seen in the wall of the ascending aorta. A noncontrast CT scan in the transverse (C) and coronal (D) cuts further defines the degree of calcification, which produced essentially a "porcelain" aorta. This patient received a transcatheter heart valve because of the high risk of surgery.

    d. Severe mitral annular calcification that can make mitral valve repair or replacement technically challenging (Figure 2.11)

    e. "Rocking" of a prosthetic valve suggestive of endocarditis with annular invasion and possible dehiscence

    f. Limitation of movement of prosthetic valve discs, consistent with valve thrombosis or restriction by pannus ingrowth (Figure 2.12)

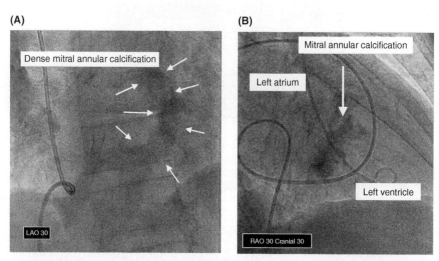

Figure 2.11 • Dense horseshoe-shaped mitral annular calcification seen by fluoroscopy in (A) the left anterior oblique (LAO) 30° and (B) the right anterior oblique (RAO) 30° cranial 30° projections during cardiac catheterization.

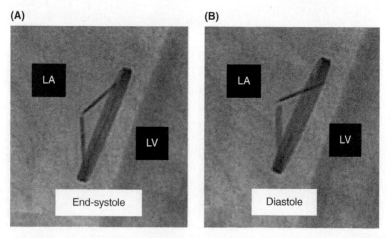

Figure 2.12 • Fluoroscopy of a patient with a St. Jude Medical valve in the mitral position. (A) At end-systole, the leaflets are closed preventing MR. (D) During diastole, the leaflets barely open due to valve thrombosis, preventing filling of the left ventricle and leading to elevated left atrial pressures.

VI. Coronary Angiography

A. Coronary angiography is performed as part of the cardiac catheterization procedure by placing special preformed catheters directly into the coronary ostia and injecting contrast into the coronary arteries (Figures 2.13 and 2.14). Angiography will assess whether the circulation is right or left dominant (i.e. whether the posterior descending artery arises from the right or left system), and will define the location, extent, and degree of coronary stenoses (Figure 2.15). This information is then used to determine if an interventional procedure is indicated and whether PCI or CABG is preferable. The SYNTAX and SYNTAX II scores (see pages 5–6) are often used to

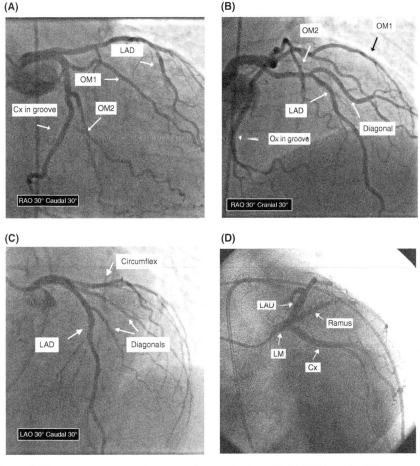

Figure 2.13 • Left coronary angiograms in four projections. (A) RAO 30° caudal 30° angulation nicely demonstrates the multiple branches of the circumflex (Cx) marginal system. (B) RAO 30° cranial 30° angulation best demonstrates the left anterior descending (LAD) artery and the origin of its diagonal branches. (C) LAO 30° caudal 30° projection provides a good view of the LAD system and the origin of the circumflex. (D) LAO caudal "spider" view shows the left main giving rise to three vessels in another patient, including a large ramus intermedius. LM, left main; OM, obtuse marginal artery.

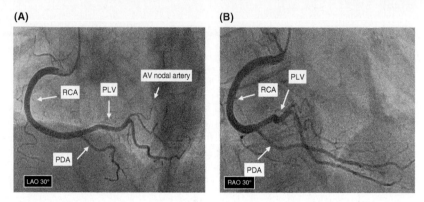

Figure 2.14 • Right coronary angiograms in the (A) LAO and (B) RAO projections. The right coronary artery (RCA) divides at the crux into the posterior left ventricular (PLV) branch, best seen in the LAO view, and the posterior descending artery (PDA), best seen in the RAO projection.

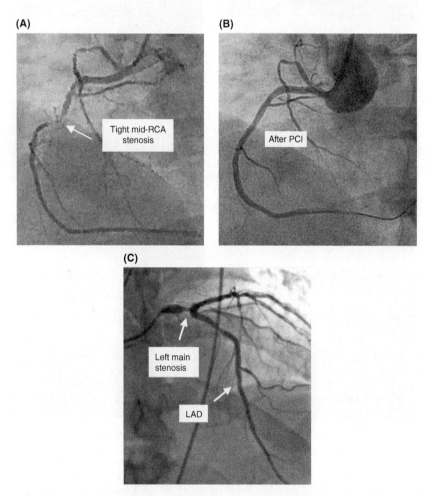

Figure 2.15 • Significant coronary stenosis. (A) A 99% stenosis of the mid-RCA. (B) PCI of this stenosis. (C) An 80% left main stenosis.

make that determination. Among the anatomic factors to be considered when contemplating surgery are the quality and bypassability of the target vessels based on their size and the extent of distal disease.

B. Anteroposterior (AP), right anterior oblique (RAO), and left anterior oblique (LAO) views are obtained at varying degrees of cranial and caudal angulation to optimally visualize each of the coronary arteries. For re-operative procedures, imaging of the ITA pedicle in a true AP projection is indicated to identify whether the ITA pedicle is very close to the midline (Figure 2.16). A lateral projection can identify its relationship to the posterior sternal table. Occasionally, a very unique finding may be noted with angiography, such as a tumor blush (Figure 2.17).

C. Coronary angiography is still considered the gold standard for the identification of CAD, but it has limitations that need to be understood when interpreting the significance of stenoses and making a decision to proceed with an interventional approach.

1. Lesions can be concentric or eccentric. For a purely concentric stenosis, the correlation of diameter and loss of cross-sectional area (CSA) is estimated as follows:
   • 50% diameter = 75% loss of CSA
   • 67% diameter = 90% loss of CSA

   Thus, >50% diameter stenosis is considered significant.

2. The calculation of % diameter stenosis with contrast injection is based upon a comparison of the luminal diameter of a narrowed segment to that of the largest segment of an artery, unless the artery is ectatic. In patients with diffuse CAD, the

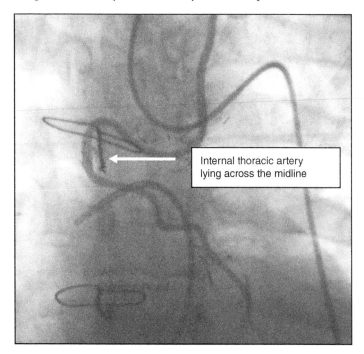

Internal thoracic artery lying across the midline

Figure 2.16 • Selective coronary angiogram of the left internal thoracic artery (ITA) in the anteroposterior (AP) projection. The pedicle has been pushed medially by the lung and extends to the midline, risking damage during a midline redo sternotomy.

(A)

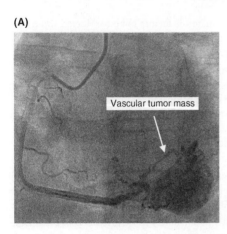

(B)

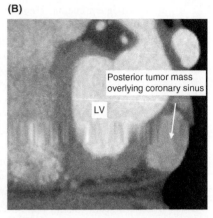

Figure 2.17 • (A) A right coronary angiogram demonstrating a tumor blush at the terminal end of the LV branch. (B) Both CT and MRI scanning (shown here) demonstrated this mass to overlie the coronary sinus near the AV groove, which was found to be a paraganglioma.

larger segment may not reflect normal vessel diameter if the entire vessel is diseased and narrowed, and thus angiography will underestimate the extent of disease.

3. **Intravascular ultrasound** (IVUS) can visualize the entire vessel wall and give a more precise calculation of the true extent of narrowing, measured as a "minimal luminal area" (MLA) in mm^2 (Figure 2.18). IVUS can be used to identify a stenosis that may benefit from stenting, and it is particularly helpful in indeterminate left main stenosis. A left main MLA <7 mm^2 in a symptomatic patient or <5.5–6 mm^2 in an asymptomatic patient is considered significant.[38,39] An MLA <4 mm^2 in the other proximal arteries is considered significant. **Optical coherence tomography** (OCT) is an optical analog of IVUS which has a tenfold higher resolution than IVUS. It is beneficial in assessing plaque burden in native arteries, but is most often used to assess the result of coronary stenting, as it can identify dissections, thrombus, and incomplete stent apposition.[40,41]

4. The correlation of the degree of stenosis and its functional significance is imprecise. **Fractional flow reserve (FFR)** measurements using a pressure wire can help to determine whether an intervention is indicated.[42–44] This basically assesses the maximal myocardial flow that can be achieved beyond a stenosis relative to what it would be for a normal artery. Hyperemic flow decreases significantly when there is a >50% stenosis. To calculate the FFR, a catheter is placed through the stenosis in the coronary artery, and proximal and distal pressure measurements are obtained after inducing a hyperemic response with either intracoronary or IV adenosine. If the distal/proximal pressure ratio (FFR) is ≤0.8, the lesion is considered functionally significant, and revascularization will provide a clinical benefit; otherwise, intervention is generally not indicated. This is also beneficial in sorting out the significance of left main lesions.[45]

5. The **instantaneous wave-free ratio fractional flow reserve (iFR)** is a non-hyperemic pressure-based index of stenosis severity.[46,47] It uses the wave-free period of diastole to measure the physiologic impact of the stenosis on the distal coronary bed. Although conceptually more complex, an iFR ≤0.89 is considered functionally significant, has excellent correlation with an FFR ≤0.8, and provides a comparable outcome in guiding PCI.

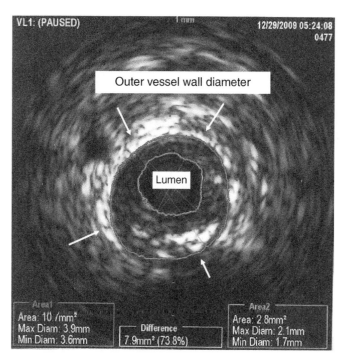

Figure 2.18 • Intravascular ultrasound (IVUS) study of the left main coronary artery. A 2 Fr echo probe is introduced into the vessel, producing images of the lumen and the surrounding vessel wall. This allows for the calculation of a minimal luminal area (MLA). In this case, the MLA was <4 mm², consistent with severe left main stenosis.

6. An FFR-guided approach to surgical revascularization is uncommon. However, studies have shown that this approach results in less grafting, a higher graft patency rate, a lower rate of angina, and a significant reduction in myocardial infarction and mortality out to six years. Such information could be helpful in deciding which patients should undergo surgery and, in fact, which vessels need to be bypassed.[48-50]

7. Occluded vessels that are underfilled via collateral flow may represent large vessels that are good surgical targets (but not always). Symptomatic patients with viable myocardium subtended by occluded vessels may benefit from PCI of the chronically occluded vessel or from CABG.

D. Important indications for coronary angiography include:

1. Any patient with suspected CAD in whom an interventional procedure might be indicated on a clinical basis. This includes patients presenting with ST-elevation myocardial infarctions (STEMIs), acute coronary syndromes (non-ST elevation infarction [non-STEMI] or unstable angina), stable ischemic heart disease with positive stress tests, or ischemic pulmonary edema.

2. Patients >age 40 who require open-heart surgery for other reasons. Angiography should also be considered in younger patients with multiple risk factors for premature CAD.

3. Annual follow-up of the cardiac transplant patient to detect the development of silent allograft CAD.

E. Coronary angiography is preferably performed through a transradial approach, which avoids the risk of a groin hematoma, or even worse a retroperitoneal hematoma. Bleeding complications are more likely to occur in patients undergoing PCI, since they should receive aspirin and a P2Y12 inhibitor prior to the procedure, might also receive a glycoprotein IIb/IIIa inhibitor, and may also receive heparin or bivalirudin during the procedure in the cath lab. Patients with critical left main disease may not tolerate catheter manipulation in the coronary ostium, and are more prone to develop a myocardial infarction, arrhythmias, hemodynamic compromise, or death. However, outcomes after catheterization are usually related to the patient's clinical status and preexisting comorbidities, especially renal dysfunction.

1. Patients taking metformin for diabetes should withhold this medication starting the day before their catheterization.

2. The efficacy of numerous medications to reduce the risk of contrast-induced acute kidney injury (AKI) has not been consistently demonstrated. Thus, most protocols involve hydration prior to, during, and following catheterization to dilute contrast in the kidneys. However, excessive hydration can contribute to heart failure and venous hypertension, which can prove deleterious to renal function as well.[51–53] Using hemodynamically-guided hydration, based on either the central venous pressure[54] or LVEDP[55], has been shown to reduce the risk of contrast-induced AKI, and is especially important in patients with HF and chronic kidney disease. A commonly used protocol from the POSEIDON study[55] involves giving fluid before, during, and after the procedure as follows:

- Pre-procedure: 3.5 mL/kg/h × 4 h

- 5 mL/kg/h for LVEDP <13 mm Hg
- 3 mL/kg/h for LVEDP of 13–18 mm Hg
- 1.5 mL/kg/h for LVEDP >18 mm Hg

- Post-procedure: 1.5 mL/kg/h for 1 h

VII. Echocardiography

A. Echocardiography provides real-time two- and three-dimensional (2D and 3D) imaging of the thoracic aorta and cardiac structures. It is an invaluable noninvasive means of evaluating RV and LV size and function, with use of color, continuous wave, and pulsed Doppler recordings to assess valve function before, during, and after surgery.[56] Although adequate information can be ascertained from a transthoracic study in the preoperative patient (Figures 2.19 and 2.20), transesophageal echocardiography (TEE) provides superior imaging because of the proximity of the probe to the heart. Both 2D and 3D imaging are extremely helpful in assessing the nature of mitral valve pathology and the results of surgical or percutaneous mitral valve repair. A further discussion of TEE with images of the most important views in the surgical patient is presented in Chapter 4.

B. TEE is very important in the preoperative evaluation of MR because it provides an assessment of the nature and degree of MR, which may be different from an intraoperative evaluation due to altered loading conditions. Two-dimensional imaging will delineate the presence of leaflet prolapse, torn chords, a ruptured papillary muscle, and/or annular dilatation (Figure 2.21–2.24). Color flow analysis can

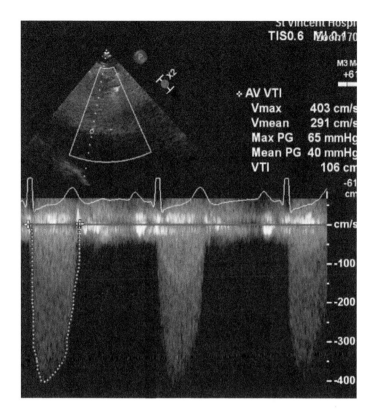

Figure 2.19 • Transthoracic echocardiogram with continuous wave Doppler to determine the severity of AS. This patient has severe AS with a peak velocity of 4 m/s and a mean gradient of 40 mm Hg.

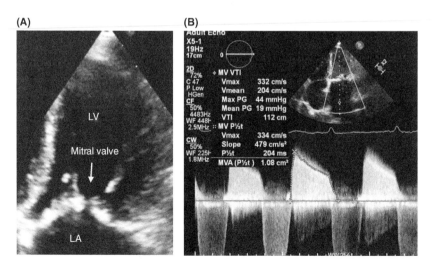

Figure 2.20 • (A) Transthoracic echocardiogram of a patient with severe MS showing very thickened leaflets with limited opening during diastole. (B) Continuous wave Doppler showing a mean mitral gradient of 19 mm Hg.

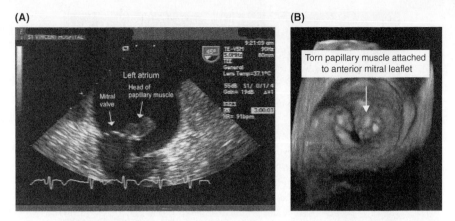

Figure 2.21 • Transesophageal echocardiograms of mitral valve pathology. (A) Papillary muscle rupture producing acute MR. Note the flail anterior leaflet with the attached papillary muscle head. (B) 3D image of the head of the papillary muscle attached to the anterior mitral leaflet.

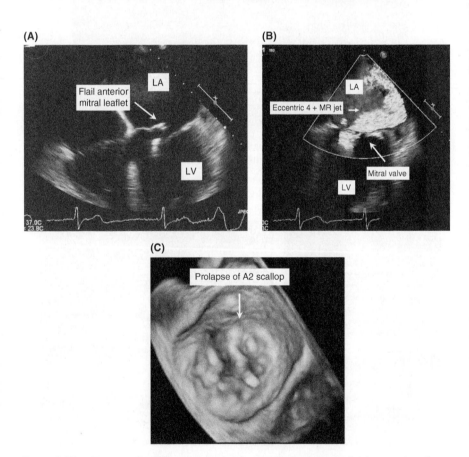

Figure 2.22 • Degenerative MR with torn chordae. (A) Flail anterior leaflet from ruptured chordae with calcified chords. (B) Color flow Doppler showing a posteriorly directed jet with 4+ MR (a bright mosaic yellow/green jet on the color image). (C) 3D image of A2 prolapse.

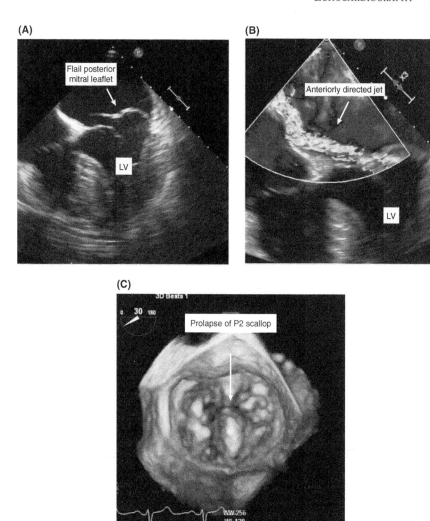

Figure 2.23 • (A) Flail posterior leaflet from ruptured chordae. (B) Color flow Doppler showing an anteriorly directed jet with 4+ MR. (C) 3D image of P2 prolapse.

provide an estimate of the degree of regurgitant flow, and the nature of the pathology (eccentric jets from leaflet prolapse or tethering, or a central jet from annular dilatation). Several methodologies can be used to calculate the regurgitant fraction, the regurgitant volume, and the effective orifice area of the valve, which are often necessary to confirm the severity of MR (see page 47 in Chapter 1).[57] Three-dimensional imaging is very helpful in identifying the location of pathology, especially prior to MitraClip procedures.[58,59]

(A)   **(B)**

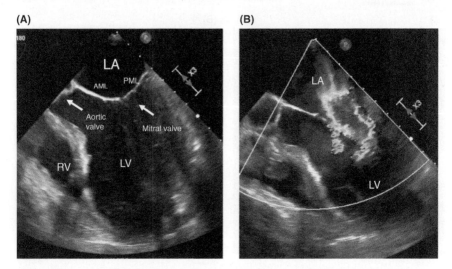

Figure 2.24 • Transesophageal echocardiogram in the five-chamber view of a patient with severe functional MR. (A) End-systolic image shows a high end-systolic volume (EF is 25%) and no evidence of leaflet prolapse. (B) Color Doppler shows a jet of severe functional central MR.

1. TEE also provides excellent images of vegetations in patients with endocarditis (Figure 2.25), which may result in severe valvular regurgitation (Figure 2.26). It is better than TTE in identifying periannular abscesses, vegetations on prosthetic heart valves, and involvement of endocardial pacing or defibrillator leads.

2. Although most patients with suspected dissections undergo a CT scan with contrast as the initial imaging modality, TEE has very high sensitivity and specificity in identifying dissections, noting the intimal flap and its origin, potential differential flow in the true and false lumens, the degree of AR, and the presence of a pericardial effusion. The study is usually performed intraoperatively but may be performed preoperatively in indeterminate cases (Figure 2.27).

3. TEE is usually the best technique to identify the location and site of attachment of a cardiac tumor (Figures 2.28 and 2.29).

4. TEE is invaluable in identifying pericardial effusions and tamponade when transthoracic imaging is not adequate.

C. DSE can be used to identify ischemia and myocardial viability and to determine contractile reserve and the severity of AS in patients with low-flow, low-gradient AS, primarily with decreased LV function (stage D2) and occasionally with normal LV function (stage D3).[16,29,30]

D. A summary of information that can be derived from preoperative and postoperative echocardiography is noted in Tables 2.3 and 2.4. The utility of TEE in the operating room is noted in Table 4.1 (page 225).

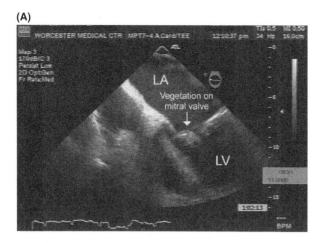

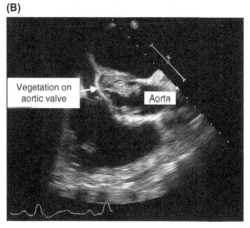

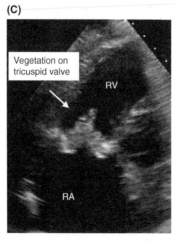

Figure 2.25 • Echocardiograms of patients with endocarditis. (A) TEE showing a vegetation on the anterior mitral valve leaflet. (B) TEE showing a vegetation on the aortic valve seen in the long-axis view. (C) Transthoracic echocardiogram showing a tricuspid valve vegetation in an IV drug abuser.

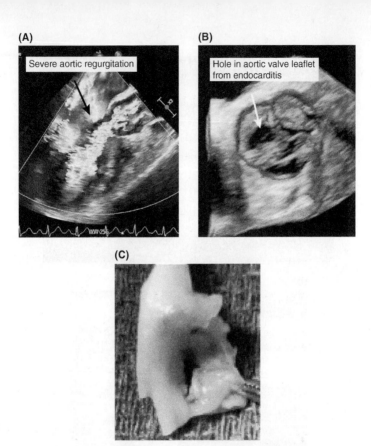

Figure 2.26 • (A) Transesophageal echocardiogram showing severe central AR from endocarditis. (B) The 3D short-axis view shows a hole in one of the leaflets. (C) Photograph of the resected aortic leaflet.

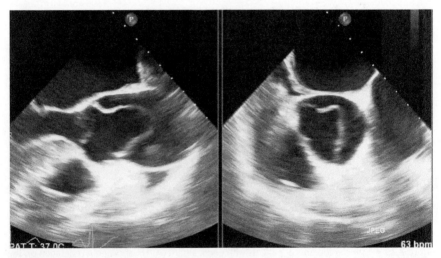

Figure 2.27 • Transesophageal echocardiogram of the ascending aorta in a type A aortic dissection. Note the intimal flap separating the true and false lumens which was very mobile with each systolic contraction.

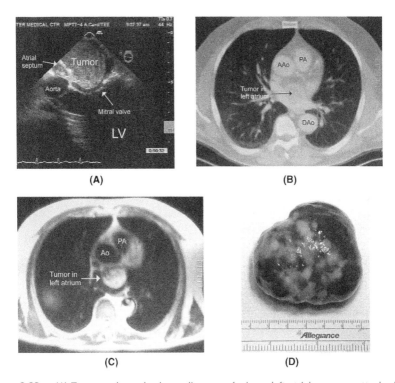

Figure 2.28 • (A) Transesophageal echocardiogram of a large left atrial myxoma attached to the superior aspect of the atrial septum. Before the TEE was performed, both a CT scan (B) and an MRI scan (C) demonstrated the mass. (D) A photograph of the resected myxoma.

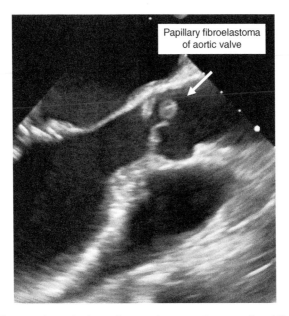

Figure 2.29 • Transesophageal echocardiogram demonstrating a small mobile mass attached to the aortic valve in a patient who presented with a stroke. This was a papillary fibroelastoma attached to the noncoronary cusp of the aortic valve.

Table 2.3 • Information Obtained from Preoperative Echocardiography

All patients	Global and regional wall motion abnormalities Signs of diastolic dysfunction Valve function Aortic atherosclerosis Pericardial fluid and thickening Presence of an intracardiac shunt
Coronary artery disease	Global and regional wall motion abnormalities Signs of diastolic dysfunction Left ventricular mural thrombus Presence of mitral regurgitation Stress imaging for ischemic zones
Aortic stenosis	Gradient calculation from flow velocity Planimetry of valve area Annular diameter (root enlargement, selection of homograft size) Stress imaging if low-flow/low-gradient stenosis Presence of mitral regurgitation
Aortic regurgitation	Severity of regurgitation Annular diameter (selection of homograft size)
Ascending aortic aneurysm	Size of sinuses, ascending aorta and proximal arch
Aortic dissection	Location of intimal flap Detection of aortic regurgitation Presence of pericardial effusion
Mitral stenosis	Size of left atrium Mean diastolic gradient Planimetry of valve area Presence of left atrial thrombus
Mitral regurgitation	Size of left atrium Severity of regurgitation Nature of pathology (annular dilatation, anterior or posterior leaflet prolapse, elongated or torn chords, papillary muscle rupture)
Tricuspid valve disease	Calculation of pulmonary artery pressure from tricuspid regurgitation jet velocity ($4v^2$) Gradient (stenosis) or severity of regurgitation
Endocarditis	Vegetations Annular abscesses Valvular regurgitation
Cardiac masses	Location and relationship of tumors, thrombus, and vegetations to cardiac structures
Pericardial tamponade	Diastolic collapse of atrial or ventricular chambers Location of fluid around heart

Table 2.4 • Indications for Postoperative Echocardiography

Low output states	LV or RV systolic dysfunction LV diastolic dysfunction Cardiac tamponade Hypovolemia
New/persistent murmur (recurrent congestive heart failure)	Paravalvular leak Inadequate valve repair Outflow tract gradient from small valve or systolic anterior motion (SAM) of anterior mitral valve leaflet Recurrent ventricular septal defect
Evaluation of ventricular recovery after assist device insertion	LV or RV systolic function

VIII. Noninvasive Coronary Angiography

A. Technological advances in noninvasive imaging have led to the use of CT and MRI scanning for the evaluation of coronary anatomy. The temporal and spatial resolution is quite good in evaluating the proximal coronary arteries, although there are limitations to each modality. They are generally recommended for patients with equivocal stress tests, intermediate coronary risk, or atypical symptoms, but not as a screening tool in asymptomatic patients or for patients with typical symptoms that may warrant PCI or CABG.

B. **Multidetector row or multislice CT scanning** (MDCT or MSCT) that can acquire at least 64 slices per gantry rotation (and preferably 256 or 320 slices) provides adequate imaging of arteries with little motion artifact when the heart rate is slowed to less than 70 bpm with β-blockers.[60–62]

1. Coronary CT angiography (CCTA) provides excellent imaging of native coronary arteries and bypass grafts with a sensitivity and specificity of about 80–90% (Figure 2.30).[63,64] It is able to detect clinically significant lesions (>50% stenosis) quite accurately. It does require contrast and radiation and produces suboptimal imaging with an irregular heart rhythm, severe coronary calcification or the presence of stents, or very small vessels <1.5 mm in size. Although stents do interfere with imaging, CCTA is quite accurate in assessing in-stent stenosis.[64] It is contraindicated in patients with renal dysfunction or an allergy to contrast.

2. CCTA is also beneficial in identifying the proximal course of the coronary arteries near the great vessels in patients with coronary anomalies. However, since this is usually a concern in younger patients, cardiac MRI is preferable to avoid radiation.

3. The ability to assess physiologic significance simultaneously with anatomic findings can be achieved using combined technologies. CCTA combined with SPECT MPI has improved the accuracy of CCTA.[65] FFR derived from CCTA using special software is very accurate in detecting hemodynamically significant lesions in patients with multivessel disease, and was found to be superior to standard CTA, SPECT, or PET scanning in doing so.[66–69]

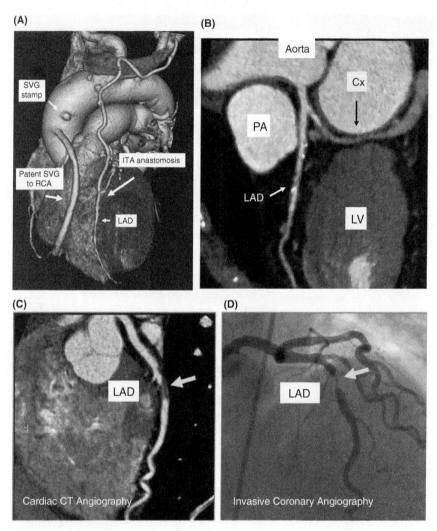

Figure 2.30 • (A) Coronary CT angiogram (CCTA) obtained on the Toshiba Aquilion scanner. This patient with prior surgery had a patent LITA to the LAD and a patent saphenous vein graft (SVG) to the right coronary artery (RCA). A nubbin of occluded SVG is noted on the aorta. (B) Native coronary arteries can be evaluated more extensively in one view using multiplanar reconstruction. Here, the LAD has diffuse calcific disease. (C) Tight stenosis of the LAD on CCTA. (D) Corresponding stenosis noted on invasive coronary angiography. Adapted with permission from Cury, et al. *J Am Coll Cardiol Img* 2016;9:1099-113 (C & D).[70]

C. **Cardiovascular magnetic resonance (CMR) imaging** is able to visualize the proximal portions of coronary arteries, but it is not quite as sensitive and specific as CCTA and therefore is not recommended for the routine identification of coronary disease (Figure 2.31A and B).[71,72]

1. The advantages of CMR are the lack of irradiation or contrast, less interference from coronary calcification, and less motion artifact at higher heart rates. However, suboptimal images will be obtained in patients with stents, arrhythmias, or irregular breathing patterns.

2. The primary indications for CMR imaging in the assessment of CAD are:

   a. Coronary anomalies, by identifying their proximal course (especially in young patients) (Figure 2.31C)

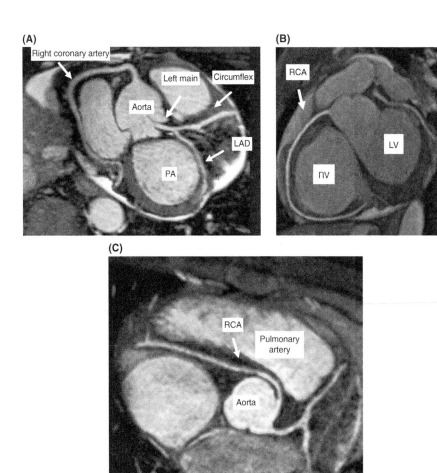

Figure 2.31 • Cardiovascular magnetic resonance (CMR) images showing (A) the origin of the right and left coronary arteries in a transverse image at the base of the aorta. (B) The anterior course of the right coronary artery on a sagittal image. (C) An anomalous right coronary artery arising from the left main artery and coursing between the aorta and pulmonary artery. (Image courtesy of AD Elster, ELSTER LLC. (A), Siemens Medical Solutions USA, Inc., (B), Public Domain (C).)

  b. Coronary aneurysms

  c. Saphenous vein graft stenosis or internal thoracic artery graft stenosis. CMR has a sensitivity and specificity >90% in identifying significant lesions.[72] However, if the patient is symptomatic and may require an intervention, CMR is usually not indicated unless the graft cannot be selectively cannulated by routine angiography. CMR and CCTA have similar accuracy in assessing bypass grafts.

3. CMR can provide important information about myocardial flow and function, and thus is preferentially used for the functional assessment of coronary disease (see section IX).

4. Newer pacemakers and ICDs are considered MRI-conditional and allow for performance of MRI scans. Older systems, termed "legacy devices", initially considered to contraindicate performance of an MRI, have been shown to be MRI safe using a field strength of up to 1.5 tesla.[73]

IX. Evaluation of Aortic and Cardiac Disease by CT and MR Scanning

A. **Computerized tomography (CT) scanning** is used primarily for the evaluation of aortic disease, but it has several other potential uses in identifying chest pathology in addition to CCTA. Sixty-four or greater slice CT angiography with color volume-rendered multiplanar reformation provides excellent angiographic images. Indications include:

1. Identification of an aortic dissection in a patient with a typical or atypical presentation (Figures 2.32–2.34). This requires a CT scan with contrast and can also simultaneously rule out a pulmonary embolism with appropriate gating. CT scans can also be used for postoperative follow-up to identify distal aneurysmal disease.

2. Assessment of aortic size

  a. A contrast CT scan with 3D reconstruction can provide transverse, sagittal, and coronal cuts as well as a rotational 3D image (Figure 2.35). These can provide an exact measurement of aortic diameter, since an obliquely coursing structure (such as a tortuous or ectatic segment of aorta) will give a spuriously increased measurement on transverse cuts which will not reflect the true diameter of the aorta. Software programs can provide centerline analysis to overcome these shortcomings. They are usually applied to patients with descending thoracic aneurysms in anticipation of endografting.[74] However, centerline analysis has also been used in models to predict the risk of aortic dissection.[75] The volume-rendered image often gives a better assessment of the distal extent of the aneurysm and is helpful in deciding whether the distal anastomosis will need to be sewn using circulatory arrest. If the aneurysm tapers proximal to the arch, it may be possible to sew a distal anastomosis with a cross-clamp in place.

  b. Descending thoracic aneurysms (Figure 2.36). The proximal and distal extent of the aneurysm and vessel tortuosity are important elements in devising a strategy for thoracic endografting (TEVAR).

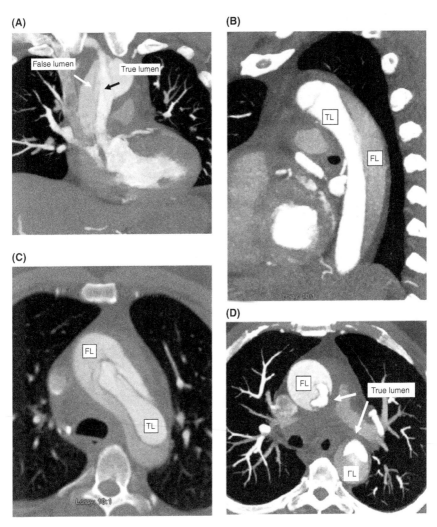

Figure 2.32 • CT scan with contrast demonstrating a type A aortic dissection visualized in (A) coronal, (B) sagittal, and (C) transverse cuts across the arch and (D) at the mid-heart level. Note the intimal flap separating the true lumen (TL) and false lumen (FL), with opacification of the TL, which is significantly compressed by the FL as the dissection extends into the descending aorta.

3. Evaluation of ascending aortic calcification suggested by chest x-ray or fluoroscopy (see Figure 2.10). This should be done without contrast.
4. Location of the RV, aorta, saphenous vein grafts, or ITA graft relative to the sternum in the planning of re-operative surgery.[76] This is also applicable to patients undergoing minimally invasive surgery to select the proper incision site and is useful for transaortic TAVR planning as well.

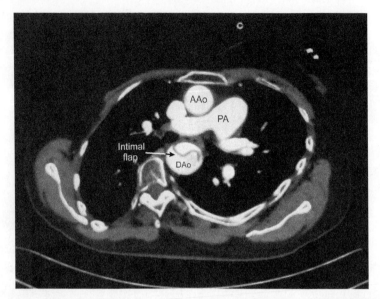

Figure 2.33 • CT scan with contrast of a type B dissection which starts just distal to the left subclavian artery without any involvement of the ascending aorta. Note the intimal flap separating the true and false lumens. AAo, ascending aorta; DAo, descending aorta; PA, pulmonary artery.

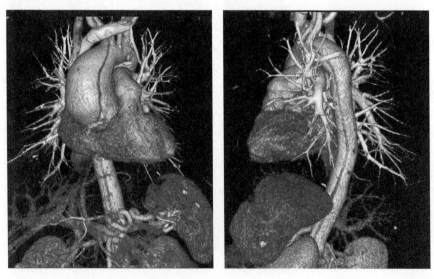

Figure 2.34 • Volume-rendered image of a type A aortic dissection shown in (A) coronal and (B) sagittal cuts.

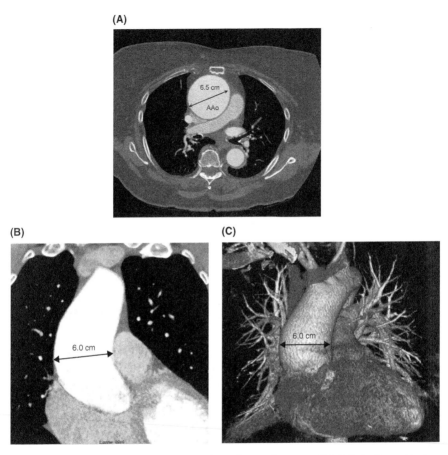

Figure 2.35 • CT scan demonstrating an enlarged ascending aorta (AAo) that will need to be replaced. (A) The axial slice may not provide an accurate size assessment if the measurement is not coaxial. (B) The coronal (and sagittal) slices are helpful in defining the precise diameter of the aorta from the root to the arch. (C) A 3D volume-rendered reconstruction image of the same patient can be rotated to give a better appreciation of the aortic diameter near the arch.

5. Identification of pericardial (and pleural) effusions or the thickness of the pericardium in cases of constrictive pericarditis.

6. Identification of intracardiac masses (see Figure 2.28B).

7. Evaluation of the abdominal aorta and iliofemoral systems. This is essential prior to minimally invasive cases during which femoral arterial cannulation is to be utilized. Diffusely diseased vessels may dissect during retrograde perfusion, and atherosclerotic disease can embolize retrograde to the brain. Prior to TAVR procedures, the iliofemoral systems are assessed for size, calcification, and tortuosity and, if markedly abnormal, may mandate an alternate site for access (Figure 2.37).

8. Evaluation for a retroperitoneal hematoma which may occur after percutaneous femoral vessel cannulation (Figure 2.38).

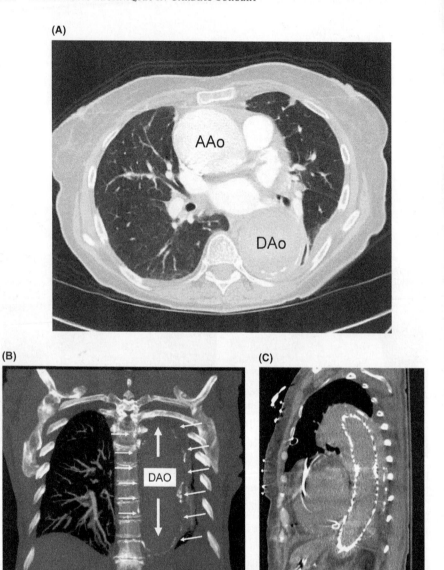

Figure 2.36 • (A) CT scan of ascending and descending thoracic aneurysms. (B) The coronal cut demonstrates the large descending thoracic aneurysm (no contrast present). (C) An endovascular stent has been placed to repair the aneurysm.

(A)   **(B)**

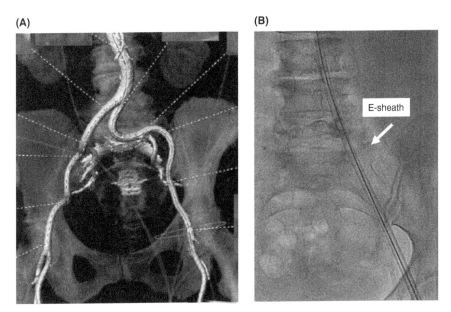

Figure 2.37 • (A) 3Mensio analysis (Pie Medical Imaging BV, the Netherlands) of a CT scan demonstrating moderate tortuosity of the iliofemoral vessels. (B) In the absence of calcification, the iliofemoral system can usually be straightened out nicely with a Super Stiff or Lunderquist wire, allowing for placement of the Edwards E-sheath (arrow).

(A)   **(B)**

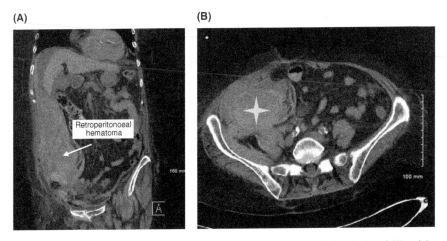

Figure 2.38 • A retroperitoneal bleed identified on a CT scan in (A) abdominal and (B) pelvic images following a transfemoral catheterization.

9. Identification of pulmonary or mediastinal abnormalities noted on preoperative chest x-ray. Obtaining a baseline CT scan prior to cardiac surgery eliminates the potential distortion of pulmonary pathology by postoperative changes.

B. **Cardiovascular magnetic resonance (CMR) imaging** is useful in the identification of ischemic and nonischemic myocardial disease, imaging of the aorta and its branches, analyzing congenital heart disease, and providing images of coronary arteries and bypass grafts.[77-81]

1. CMR can be performed in patients with coronary stents (fields <3 tesla), current-generation mechanical prosthetic heart valves (note that most bileaflet valves are composed of carbon and silicone and not metal), and retained epicardial pacing wires.[82,83] It is safe for patients with legacy pacemakers and defibrillators using a field <1.5 tesla.[73]

2. The major advantage of MRI is the avoidance of radiation, and therefore it is preferable in the young patient. Contraindications to MRI are noted on multiple websites under a search for this topic.

3. Pharmacologic stress CMR with dobutamine or coronary vasodilators can identify areas of myocardial ischemia and may be more sensitive than DSE in detecting coronary disease and predicting functional recovery after revascularization.[84,85] Myocardial viability may be evaluated using gadolinium (to distinguish viable from infarcted myocardium) or dobutamine (systolic wall thickening >2 mm being predictive of functional recovery).

4. CMR is the most sensitive and specific test for detection of an aortic dissection (Figure 2.39). It can demonstrate differential flow velocities in the true and

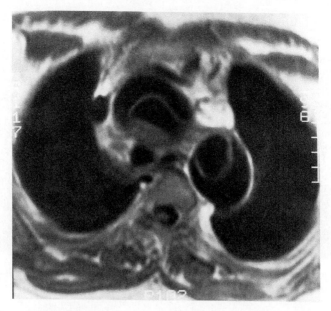

Figure 2.39 • MRI scan demonstrating the intimal flap separating the true and false lumens in a patient with an extensive aortic dissection involving both the ascending and the descending thoracic aorta.

false channels and can identify branch artery compromise. However, it generally cannot be performed in the unstable patient requiring careful monitoring and often IV infusions. However, it should be considered when the clinical suspicion of a dissection is very high, yet other tests have been inconclusive. Most commonly, it is used in the follow-up of patients who have had repair of an aortic dissection to assess the status of the false channel or distal aneurysmal expansion.

5. Late gadolinium enhancement (LGE) identifies areas of focal myocardial fibrosis and infarction and thus can be used to assess for viability and the likelihood of improvement in contractility after revascularization. Greater degrees of LGE correlate with a higher risk of sudden death in patients with hypertrophic cardiomyopathy (HCM).[27] CMR can identify variations in the pathology within the LV in patients with HOCM. It is very useful in identifying other types of nonischemic cardiomyopathies (Figure 2.40).

6. Aortic and cerebrovascular diseases can be defined by magnetic resonance angiography (MRA) using time-of-flight (TOF) MRA and gadolinium-enhanced MRA (Figure 2.41). Spin-echo and cine steady-state free precession (SSFP) CMR can also be used to provide excellent 3D images of aortic disease, including true and false aneurysms and periaortic abscesses or perigraft fluid collections.

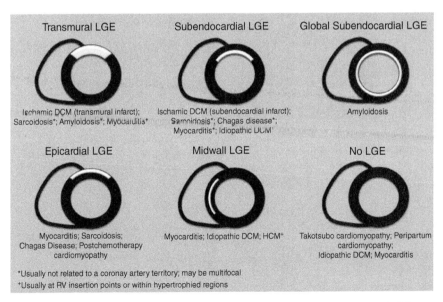

Figure 2.40 • The various patterns of late gadolinium enhancement (LGE) seen with different types of cardiomyopathies. Typical patterns include transmural, subendocardial (regional and global), epicardial, and midwall LGE. These may differentiate between ischemic (subendocardial and transmural) and nonischemic cardiomyopathies, HOCM, myocarditis, sarcoidosis, and amyloidosis. (Image courtesy of Silva Marques et al., *Heart* 2015;101:565–72.)

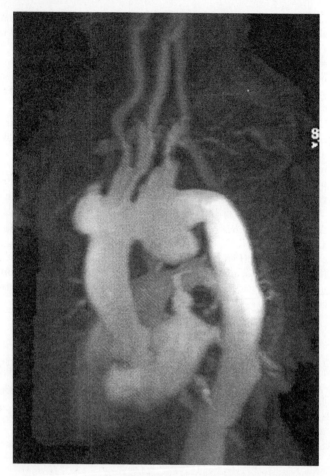

Figure 2.41 • MRA with gadolinium demonstrating aneurysms of the aortic arch on a rotational image that were poorly delineated in transverse images.

7. Cine CMR allows for differentiation of blood (bright images) from cardiac tissue (dark images). It is useful in the assessment of ventricular function, valvular pathology, and intracardiac masses (see Figure 2.28C).

8. CMR is useful in the assessment of pericarditis or tumor invasion into the pericardium. It can differentiate restrictive from constrictive pathology.

References

1. Yamazaki K, Kato H, Tsujimoto S, Kitamura R. Diabetes mellitus, internal thoracic artery grafting, and the risk of an elevated hemidiaphragm after coronary artery bypass surgery. *J Cardiothorac Vasc Anesth* 1994;8:437–40.

2. Merino-Ramirez MA, Juan G, Ramón M, et al. Electrophysiologic evaluation of phrenic nerve and diaphragm function after coronary bypass surgery: prospective study of diabetes and other risk factors. *J Thorac Cardiovasc Surg* 2006;132:530–6.

3. Garber AM, Hlatky MA, Chareonthaitawee P, Askew JW. Stress testing for the diagnosis of obstructive coronary heart disease. www.uptodate.com 2020.

4. Garner KK, Pomeroy W, Arnold JJ. Exercise stress testing: indications and common questions. *Am Fam Physician* 2017;96:293–9.

5. Gibbons RJ, Balady GJ, Bricker JT, et al. ACC/AHA 2002 guidelines for exercise testing: summary article: a report of the American College of Cardiology/American Heart Association Task Force on Practice Guidelines (Committee to Update the 1997 Exercise Testing Guidelines). *J Am Coll Cardiol* 2002;40:1531–40.

6. Wolk MJ, Bailey SR, Doherty JU, et al. American College of Cardiology Foundation Appropriate Use Criteria Task Force: ACCF/AHA/ASE/ASNC/HFSA/HRS/ SCAI/SCCT/SCMR/STS 2013 multimodality appropriate use criteria for the detection and risk assessment of stable ischemic heart disease: a report of the American College of Cardiology Foundation Appropriate Use Criteria Task Force, American Heart Association, American Society of Echocardiography, American Society of Nuclear Cardiology, Heart Failure Society of America, Heart Rhythm Society, Society for Cardiovascular Angiography and Interventions, Society of Cardiovascular Computed Tomography, Society for Cardiovascular Magnetic Resonance, and Society of Thoracic Surgeons. *J Am Coll Cardiol* 2014;63:380–406.

7. Qaseem A, Fihn SD, Williams S, et al. Diagnosis of stable ischemic heart disease: summary of clinical practice guidelines from the American College of Physicians/American College of Cardiology Foundation/American Heart Association/American Association for Thoracic Surgery/Preventive Cardiovascular Nurses Association/Society of Thoracic Surgeons. *Ann Intern Med* 2012;157:729–34.

8. Chareonthaitawee P, Askew JW. Overview of stress radionuclide myocardial perfusion imaging. www.uptodate.com 2019.

9. Henzlova MJ, Duvall WL, Einstein AJ, Travin MI, Verberne HJ. ASNC imaging guidelines for SPECT nuclear cardiology procedures: stress, protocols, and tracers. *J Nucl Cardiol* 2016;23:606–39.

10. Dorbala S, Ananthasubramaniam K, Armstrong IS, et al. Single photon emission computed tomography (SPECT) myocardial perfusion imaging guidelines: instrumentation, acquisition, processing, and interpretation. *J Nucl Cardiol* 2018;25:1784–6.

11. Daly C, Kwong RY. Cardiac MRI for myocardial ischemia. *Methodist Debakey Cardiovasc J* 2013;9:123–31.

12. Cabrera R, Husain Z, Palani G, et al. Comparison of hemodynamic and stress testing variables in patients undergoing regadenoson stress myocardial perfusion imaging to regadenoson with adjunctive low-level exercise myocardial perfusion imaging. *J Nucl Cardiol* 2013;20:336–43.

13. Gould KL. Coronary flow reserve and pharmacologic stress perfusion imaging: beginnings and evolution. *JACC Cardiovasc Imaging* 2009;2:664–9.

14. Elhendy A, Bax JJ, Poldermans D. Dobutamine stress myocardial perfusion imaging in coronary artery disease. *J Nucl Med* 2002;43:1634–46.

15. Dilsizian V, Rocco TP, Freedman NM, Leon MB, Bonow RO. Enhanced detection of ischemic but viable myocardium by the reinjection of thallium after stress-redistribution imaging. *N Engl J Med* 1990;323:141–6.

16. Pellikka PA, Nagueh SF, Elhendy AA, Kuehl CA, Sawada SG. American Society of Echocardiography recommendations for performance, interpretation, and application of stress echocardiography. *J Am Soc Echocardiogr* 2007;20:1021–41.

17. Patel H, Mazur W, Williams KA Sr, Kalra DK. Myocardial viability: state of the art: is it still relevant and how to best assess it with imaging? *Trends Cardiovasc Med* 2018;28:24–37.

18. Di Carli MF, Hachamovitch R, Berman DS. The art and science of predicting postrevascularization improvement in left ventricular (LV) function in patients with severely depressed LV function. *J Am Coll Cardiol* 2002;40:1744–7.

19. Schinkel AF, Poldermans D, Rizzello V, et al. Why do patients with ischemic cardiomyopathy and a substantial amount of viable myocardium not always recover in function after revascularization? *J Thorac Cardiovasc Surg* 2004;127:385–90.

20. Allman KC, Shaw LJ, Hachamovitch R, Udelson JE. Myocardial viability testing and impact of revascularization on prognosis in patients with coronary artery disease and left ventricular dysfunction: a meta-analysis. *J Am Coll Cardiol* 2002;39:1151–8.

21. Panza JA, Ellis AM, Al-Khalidi HR, et al. Myocardial viability and long-term outcomes in ischemic cardiomyopathy. *N Engl J Med* 2019;381:739–48.

22. Michler RE. A decade after the Surgical Treatment for Ischemic Heart Failure (STICH) trial: weaving firm clinical recommendations from lessons learned. *J Thorac Cardiovasc Surg* 2019;157:950–7.

23. Marzullo P, Parodi O, Reisenhofer B, et al. Value of rest thallium-201/technetium-99m sestamibi scans and dobutamine echocardiography for detecting myocardial viability. *Am J Cardiol* 1993;71:166–72.

24. Schinkel AF, Bax JJ, Biagini E, et al. Myocardial technetium-99m-tetrofosmin single-photon emission computed tomography compared with 18F-fluorodeoxyglucose imaging to assess myocardial viability. *Am J Cardiol* 2005;95:1223–5.

25. Cornel JH, Bax JJ, Elhendy A, et al. Biphasic response to dobutamine predicts improvement of global left ventricular function after surgical revascularization in patients with stable coronary artery disease: implications of time course of recovery on diagnostic accuracy. *J Am Coll Cardiol* 1998;31:1002–10.

26. Van Assche LMR, Kim HW, Kim RJ. Cardiac MR for the assessment of myocardial viability. *Methodist Debakey Cardiovasc J* 2013;9:163–8.

27. Mantias A, Raeisi-Giglou P, Smedira NG. Late gadolinium enhancement in patients with hypertrophic cardiomyopathy and preserved systolic function. *J Am Coll Cardiol* 2018;72:857–70.

28. Shan K, Constantine G, Sivananthan M, Flamm SD. Role of cardiac magnetic resonance imaging in the assessment of myocardial viability. *Circulation* 2004;109:1328–34.

29. Lancellotti P, Pellikka PA, Budts W, et al. The clinical use of stress echocardiography in non-ischaemic heart disease: recommendations from the European Association of Cardiovascular Imaging and the American Society of Echocardiography. *J Am Soc Echocardiogr* 2017;30:101–38 and *Eur Heart J Cardiovasc Imaging* 2016;17:1191–1229.

30. Gentry JL III, Phelan D, Desai MY, Griffin BP. The role of stress echocardiography in valvular heart disease: a current appraisal. *Cardiology* 2017;137:137–50.

31. Clavel MA, Burwash IG, Mudingler G, et al. Validation of conventional and simplified methods to calculate projected valve area at normal flow rate in patients with low flow, low gradient aortic stenosis: the multicenter TOPAS (True or PseudoSevere Aortic Stenosis) study. *J Am Soc Echocardiogr* 2010;23:380–6.

32. Pawade T, Clavel MA, Trivouilloy C, et al. Computed tomography aortic valve calcium scoring in patients with aortic stenosis. *Circ Cardiovasc Imaging* 2018;11:e007146.

33. Brochet E, Détaint D, Fondard O, et al. Early hemodynamic changes versus peak values: what is more useful to predict occurrence of dyspnea during stress echocardiography in patients with asymptomatic mitral stenosis? *J Am Soc Echocardiogr* 2011;24:392–8.

34. Moscucci M. *Grossman & Baim's Cardiac Catheterization, Angiography, and Intervention*, 8th edition. Philadelphia: Lippincott, Williams & Wilkins, 2013.

35. Meine TJ, Harrison JK. Should we cross the valve?. The risk of retrograde catheterization of the left ventricle in patients with aortic stenosis. *Am Heart J* 2004;148:41–2.

36. Doshi S, Ramakrishnan S, Gupta SK. Invasive hemodynamics of constrictive pericarditis. *Indian Heart J* 2015;67:175–82.

37. Geske JB, Anavekar NS, Nishimura RA, Oh JK, Gersh B. Differentiation of constriction and restriction: complex cardiovascular hemodynamics. *J Am Coll Cardiol* 2016;68:2329–47.

38. Tobis J, Azarbal B, Slavin L. Assessment of intermediate severity coronary lesions in the catheterization laboratory. *J Am Coll Cardiol* 2007;49:839–48.

39. Saito Y, Kobayashi Y, Fujii K, et al. Clinical expert consensus documentation standards for measurements and assessment of intravascular ultrasound from the Japanese Association of Cardiovascular Intervention and Therapeutics. *Cardiovasc Interv Ther* 2020;35:1–12.

40. Terashima M, Kaneda H, Suzuki T. The role of optical coherence tomography in coronary intervention. *Korean J Intern Med* 2012;27:1–12.

41. Gerbaud E, Weisz G, Tanaka A, et al. Plaque burden can be assessed using intravascular optical coherence tomography and a dedicated automated processing algorithm: a comparison study with intravascular ultrasound. *Eur Heart J Cardiovasc Imaging* 2020;21:640–52.

42. Toth GG, Johnson NP, Jeremias A, et al. Standardization of fractional flow reserve measurements. *J Am Coll Cardiol* 2016;68:742–53.

43. Tonino PA, Fearon WF, De Bruyne B, et al. Angiographic versus functional severity of coronary artery stenoses in the FAME study: fractional flow reserve versus angiography in multivessel evaluation. *J Am Coll Cardiol* 2010;55:2816–21.

44. Tonino PA, De Bruyne B, Piljls NH, et al. Fractional flow reserve versus angiography for guiding percutaneous coronary intervention. *N Eng J Med* 2009;360:213–24.

45. Courtis J, Rodés-Cabau J, Larose E, et al. Usefulness of coronary fractional flow reserve measurements in guiding clinical decisions in intermediate or equivocal left main coronary stenoses. *Am J Cardiol* 2009;103:943–9.

46. Götberg M, Cook CM, Sen S, et al. The evolving future of instantaneous wave-free ratio and fractional flow reserve. *J Am Coll Cardiol* 2017;70:1379–402.

47. Götberg M, Christiansen EH, Gudmundsdottir IJ, et al. Instantaneous wave-free ratio versus fractional flow reserve to guide PCI. *N Engl J Med* 2017;376:1813–23.

48. Shah T, Geleris JD, Zhong M, Swaminathan R, Kim LK, Feldman DN. Fractional flow reserve to guide surgical coronary revascularization. *J Thorac Dis* 2017;9(Suppl 4): S317–26.

49. Toth G, De Bruyne B, Casselman F, et al. Fractional flow reserve-guided versus angiography-guided coronary artery bypass graft surgery. *Circulation* 2013;128:1405–11.

50. Fournier S, Toth GG, De Bruyne B, et al. Six-year follow-up of fractional flow reserve-guided versus angiography-guided coronary artery bypass graft surgery. *Circ Cardiovasc Interv* 2018;11:e06368.

51. Liu Y, Li H, Chen S, et al. Excessively high hydration volume may not be associated with a decreased risk of contrast-induced acute kidney injury after percutaneous coronary intervention in patients with renal insufficiency. *J Am Heart Assoc* 2016;5:e003171.

52. Gupta R, Moza A, Cooper CJ. Intravenous hydration and contrast-induced acute kidney injury: too much of a good thing? *J Am Heart Assoc* 2016;5:e003777.

53. Bei WJ, Wang K, Li HL. Safe hydration to prevent contrast-induced acute kidney injury and worsening heart failure in patients with renal insufficiency and heart failure undergoing coronary angiography or percutaneous coronary intervention. *Int Heart J* 2019;60:247–54.

54. Qian G, Fu Z, Guo J, Cao F, Chen Y. Prevention of contrast-induced nephropathy by central venous pressure-guided fluid administration in chronic kidney disease and congestive heart failure patients. *JACC Cardiovasc Interv* 2016;9:89–96.

55. Brar SS, Aharonian V, Mansukhani P, et al. Hemodynamic-guided fluid administration for the prevention of contrast-induced acute kidney injury: the POSEIDON randomised controlled trial. *Lancet* 2014;383:1814–23.

56. Oh JK, Seward JB, Tajik AJ. *The Echo Manual*, 3rd edition. Philadelphia: Lippincott Williams & Wilkins, 2012.

57. Bonow RO, O'Gara PT, Adams DH, Badhwar V, Bavaria JE, Elmariah S, Hung JW, Lindenfeld J, Morris AA, Satpathy R, Whisenant B, Woo WJ. 2020 focused update of the 2017 ACC expert consensus decision pathway on the management of mitral regurgitation. *J Am Coll Cardiol* 2020;75:2236–70.

58. Quader N, Rigolin VH. Two and three dimensional echocardiography for pre-operative assessment of mitral valve regurgitation. *Cardiovasc Ultrasound* 2014;12:42.

59. Gripari P, Muratori M, Fuisini L, Tamborini G, Pepi M. Three-dimensional echocardiography: advancements in qualitative and quantitative analyses of mitral valve morphology in mitral valve prolapse. *J Cardiovasc Echocardiogr* 2014;24:1–9.

60. Hoffmann U, Manning WJ. Cardiac imaging with computed tomography and magnetic resonance in the adult. www.uptodate.com 2020.

61. Budoff MJ, Dowe D, Jollis JG, et al. Diagnostic performance of 64-multidetector row coronary computed tomographic angiography for evaluation of coronary artery stenosis in individuals without known coronary artery disease: results from the prospective multicenter ACCURACY (Assessment by Coronary Computed Tomographic Angiography of Individuals Undergoing Invasive Coronary Angiography) Trial. *J Am Coll Cardiol* 2008;52:1724–32.

62. Villines TC. Coronary CTA should be the initial test in most patients with stable chest pain. www.acc.org/latest-in cardiology/articles/2018/05/21/06/37/coronary-cta-pro.

63. Jones CM, Athanasiou T, Dunne N, et al. Multi-detector computed tomography in coronary artery bypass graft assessment: a meta-analysis. *Ann Thorac Surg* 2007;83:341–8.

64. Ehara M, Kawai M, Surmely JF, et al. Diagnostic accuracy of coronary in-stent stenosis using 64-slice computed tomography: comparison with invasive coronary angiography. *J Am Coll Cardiol* 2007;49:951–9.

65. Rispler S, Keidar Z, Ghersin E, et al. Integrated single-photon emission computed tomography and computed tomography coronary angiography for the assessment of hemodynamically significant coronary artery lesions. *J Am Coll Cardiol* 2007;49:1059–67.

66. Collet C, Miyazaki Y, Ryan N, et al. Fractional flow reserve derived from computed tomographic angiography in patients with multivessel CAD. *J Am Coll Cardiol* 2018;71:2756–69.

67. Tesche C, De Cecco CN, Albrecht WH, et al. Coronary CT angiography-derived fractional flow reserve. *Radiology* 2017;285:17–33.

68. Nørgaard BL, Jensen JM, Blanke P. Coronary CT angiography derived fractional flow reserve: the game changer in noninvasive testing. *Curr Cardiol Rep* 2017;19:112.

69. Driessen RS, Danad I, Stuijfzand WJ, et al. Comparison of coronary computed tomography angiography, fractional flow reserve, and perfusion imaging for ischemia diagnosis. *J Am Coll Cardiol* 2019;73:171–3.

70. Cury RC, Abbara S, Achenbach S, et al. Coronary artery disease- reporting and data system (CAD-RADs) *J Am Coll Card Img* 2016;9:1099–113.

71. Schuijf JD, Bax JJ, Shaw LJ, et al. Meta-analysis of comparative diagnostic performance of magnetic resonance imaging and multislice computed tomography for noninvasive coronary angiography. *Am Heart J* 2006;151:404–11.

72. Langerak SE, Vliegen HW, Jukema JW, et al. Value of magnetic resonance imaging for the noninvasive detection of stenosis in coronary bypass grafts and recipient coronary arteries. *Circulation* 2003;107:1502–8.

73. Nazarian S, Hansford R, Rahsepar AA, et al. Safety of magnetic resonance imaging in patients with cardiac devices. *N Engl J Med* 2017;377:2555–64.

74. Müller-Eschner M, Rengier F, Partovi S, et al. Accuracy and variability of semiautomatic centerline analysis versus manual aortic measurement techniques for TEVAR. *Eur J Vasc Endovasc Surg* 2013;45:241–7.

75. Wu J, Zafar MA, Li Y, et al. Ascending aortic length and risk of aortic adverse events: the neglected dimension. *J Am Coll Cardiol* 2019;74:1883–94.

76. Kamdar AR, Meadows TA, Roselli EE, et al. Multidetector computed tomographic angiography in planning of reoperative cardiothoracic surgery. *Ann Thorac Surg* 2008;85:1239–46.

77. Saeed M, Van TA, Hetts SW, Wilson MW. Cardiac MR imaging: current status and future direction. *Cardiovasc Diagn Ther* 2015;5:290–310.

78. Fuisz AR, Pohost GM. Clinical utility of cardiovascular magnetic resonance imaging. www.uptodate.com 2020.

79. Lopez-Mattei JC, Shah DJ. The role of cardiac magnetic resonance in valvular heart disease. *Methodist Debakey Cardiovasc J* 2013;9:142–8.

80. Kassi M, Nabi F. Role of cardiac MRI in the assessment of nonischemic cardiomyopathies. *Methodist Debakey Cardiovasc J* 2013;9:149–55.

81. Partington SL, Valente AM. Cardiac magnetic resonance in adults with congenital heart disease. *Methodist Debakey Cardiovasc J* 2013;9:156–162.

82. Kaya MG, Okyay K, Yazici H, et al. Long-term clinical effects of magnetic resonance imaging in patients with coronary artery stent implantation. *Coron Artery Dis* 2009;20:138–42.

83. Syed MA, Carlson K, Murphy M, Ingkanisorn WP, Rhoads KL, Arai AE. Long-term safety of cardiac magnetic resonance imaging performed in the first few days after bare-metal stent implantation. *J Magn Reson Imaging* 2006;24:1056–61.

84. Baer FM, Theissen P, Crnac J, et al. Head to head comparison of dobutamine-transesophageal echocardiography and dobutamine-magnetic resonance imaging for the prediction of left ventricular functional recovery in patients with chronic coronary disease. *Eur Heart J* 2000;21:981–91.

85. Wellnhofer E, Olariu A, Klein C, et al. Magnetic resonance low-dose dobutamine test is superior to SCAR quantification for the prediction of functional recovery. *Circulation* 2004;109:2172–4.

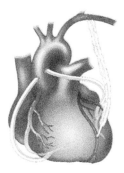

CHAPTER 3

General Preoperative Considerations and Preparation of the Patient for Surgery

3 General Preoperative Considerations and Preparation of the Patient for Surgery

I. General Considerations

A. When a patient is considered a potential candidate for cardiac surgery, a comprehensive evaluation of their overall medical condition and comorbidities is essential. This includes a detailed history and physical examination, which may identify cardiac and noncardiac problems that may need to be addressed perioperatively to minimize postoperative morbidity (Table 3.1). On occasion, the presence of multiple comorbidities and/or a compromised quality of life may contraindicate a surgical procedure that might otherwise seem to be indicated from a cardiac perspective. Attention should also be paid to identifying new cardiac abnormalities that may have arisen since the initial cardiac evaluation that may warrant further work-up. Baseline laboratory tests, if not recently performed, are also obtained, and further evaluation and consultation are performed, if indicated.

B. Evaluation of demographic factors, cardiac disease, and noncardiac comorbidities can provide the surgeon, the patient, and the patient's family an insight into the risk of surgery. The Society of Thoracic Surgeons (STS) operative risk calculator is available online at www.sts.org and is updated every few years with an increasing number of data entry fields. This provides a reliable computerized assessment of mortality for most types of cardiac surgical procedures and also quantitates the risk of important postoperative morbidities, such as re-exploration for bleeding, stroke, prolonged ventilation, and renal failure. In other countries, the additive and logistic EuroSCORE, available at www.euroscore.pil-media.com), is used for similar purposes. The cardiac surgeon can use this information when discussing the proposed operative plan with the patient, during which an informed consent discussion detailing potential complications is essential. Data entry into software programs compatible with the STS database allows surgeons to obtain an extensive analysis of their hospital's unadjusted and risk-adjusted results and a comparison with national norms.

C. A cardiac anesthesiologist should interview and examine the patient and discuss issues related to sedation, anesthetic medications, monitoring lines, awakening from anesthesia, and mechanical ventilation. The anesthesiologist should also carefully review the patient's medications and make recommendations (in conjunction with the surgeon's policies)

Manual of Perioperative Care in Adult Cardiac Surgery, Sixth Edition. Robert M. Bojar.
© 2021 John Wiley & Sons Ltd Published 2021 by John Wiley & Sons Ltd.

Table 3.1 • Preoperative Evaluation for Open-Heart Surgery

History (concerns in parentheses)

1. Smoking (COPD, bronchospasm, oxygenation)
2. Alcohol (cirrhosis, postoperative withdrawal)
3. Diabetes (wound infections, use of bilateral ITAs, risk of protamine reaction)
4. Neurologic symptoms (transient ischemic attacks, remote stroke, previous carotid endarterectomy)
5. Vein stripping (alternative conduits)
6. Distal vascular reconstruction (alternative conduits)
7. Urologic symptoms (antibiotics for UTI, catheter placement problems)
8. Ulcer disease/GI bleeding (stress prophylaxis)
9. Active infections (urinary tract, leg ulcerations)
10. Coagulation issues (need for bridging off warfarin, cessation of medications)
11. Current medications, especially antiplatelet drugs and anticoagulants
12. Drug allergies
13. Previous cardiothoracic surgery or interventions (pleural adhesions during ITA takedown)

Physical Examination

1. Skin infections/rash
2. Dental caries (valve surgery)
3. Vascular examination: carotid bruits (stroke), abdominal aneurysm and peripheral pulses (IABP placement, groin cannulation for minimally invasive procedures or aortic surgery)
4. Differential arm blood pressures (use of pedicled ITA grafts)
5. Heart/lungs (congestive heart failure, new murmur)
6. Varicose veins (alternative conduits)

Laboratory Tests

1. Hematology: CBC, PT, PTT, platelet count
2. Chemistry: electrolytes, BUN, creatinine, blood glucose, liver function tests (baseline for use of statins)
3. Arterial blood gases if room air O_2 saturation <90%
4. TSH (if amiodarone to be used)
5. Hemoglobin A1c level (assessment of diabetic control or to capture undiagnosed diabetes)
6. BNP/pro-BNP level
7. Urinalysis
8. Chest x-ray PA and lateral
9. Electrocardiogram
10. Vein mapping (varicosities, prior vein stripping)
11. Pulmonary function tests with room air blood gas (quantitate COPD in smokers)

about whether certain medications should be modified or discontinued preoperatively.

D. Providing patients with information booklets related to their cardiac disease and proposed procedure is invaluable in alleviating some of the stress and anxiety of having to undergo cardiac surgery. If possible, nurses or physician assistants with experience in postoperative care should discuss a clinical care pathway so that the patient has a realistic expectation of what will transpire during the hospital stay. Informing the patient of what procedures will take place and when, what is expected of them on each day, when discharge should be anticipated, and what the options are for posthospital discharge care (home healthcare, rehabilitation facility, or skilled nursing facility) is extremely beneficial in enhancing the patient's involvement in their own care and promoting a prompt recovery from surgery and early hospital discharge.

II. History

A. The nature, duration, and pattern of the patient's cardiac symptoms should be briefly summarized to allow for symptomatic classification using either the Canadian Classification System (for angina) or the New York Heart Association (NYHA) system (for both angina and heart failure symptoms) (see Appendices IB and IC). The latter is included in the STS risk model. A careful history of medical problems and a complete "review of systems" for noncardiac issues could influence care and draw attention to issues that may need to be addressed perioperatively.

B. **Chronic obstructive pulmonary disease** (COPD) is a term often applied to patients with a significant smoking history independent of the degree of respiratory impairment. However, the degree of COPD is best defined by pulmonary function testing (PFTs). Although this is not essential in patients without functional limitations, there is a significant discrepancy between clinical symptoms and spirometric values in 30–40% of patients.[1,2] Thus, failure to perform spirometry testing may lead to underreporting of COPD and thus an underestimation of the risk of adverse outcomes in the STS database.

1. The definitions of chronic lung disease in version 2.40 (2020) of the STS database specifications are as follows:

a. Mild: forced expiratory volume in the first second (FEV_1) 60–75% of predicted and/or on chronic inhaled or oral bronchodilator therapy

b. Moderate: FEV_1 50–59% of predicted and/or on chronic steroid therapy

c. Severe: FEV_1 <50% predicted and/or room air PO_2 <60 torr or PCO_2 >50 torr

2. Although there are reports that the severity of COPD does not correlate with the risk of respiratory failure or mortality after coronary artery bypass grafting (CABG),[3,4] most studies have shown that patients with severe COPD have higher risks of pneumonia, prolonged ventilation, atrial fibrillation (AF), deep sternal wound infection, length of stay, and an increased operative mortality.[2,5–8] These complications may be more prevalent in elderly patients and those on steroids. Because of the association of COPD with other risk factors, such as hypertension, peripheral vascular disease (PVD), and poor left ventricular (LV) function, patients with COPD have compromised long-term survival following CABG.[3] One study found a higher, yet comparable, incidence of respiratory complications in patients with COPD after off-pump and on-pump coronary surgery.[9]

3. The patient's physiologic reserve and functional status, including the ability to walk up a flight of stairs or several hundred feet on a level surface, are sometimes as important, if not more important, than spirometric values in determining whether the patient can tolerate a surgical procedure. However, markedly abnormal PFTs, including an FEV_1 <0.6 or less than 50% predicted, a FEV_1/FVC ratio <70% predicted, and a diffusion capacity <50% predicted, are associated with greater morbidity and mortality after cardiac surgery.[2,4–10]

4. The differential diagnosis of worsening dyspnea includes both exacerbation of COPD and congestive heart failure (HF). The chest x-ray may be helpful in differentiating between these two entities, but they are often present concomitantly. It can be difficult to quantitate the cardiac contribution to abnormal PFTs or a low diffusion capacity, especially in patients with mitral valve disease. In this situation, careful clinical judgment must be used in deciding whether surgery will improve the patient's pulmonary status or will leave the patient a pulmonary cripple.

   a. B-type natriuretic peptide (BNP) is secreted by the atria and ventricles in patients with systolic and diastolic dysfunction, with levels generally correlating with the patient's age and ejection fraction (EF).[11] BNP levels are helpful in differentiating whether dyspnea is primarily of cardiac or pulmonary origin. A BNP level <100 pg/mL indicates that a patient's dyspnea is most likely related to a primary pulmonary process, such as exacerbation of COPD. In contrast, dyspnea in a patient with a BNP level >500 pg/mL is usually caused by decompensated heart failure. Intermediate values may be associated with LV dysfunction without decompensation, but a pulmonary process must also be considered in the differential diagnosis.[12]

   b. An elevated preoperative BNP level (>385 pg/mL in two studies) is a predictor of postoperative LV dysfunction, the requirement for inotropic or intra-aortic balloon pump support, and is associated with greater perioperative, one- and five-year mortality after cardiac surgery.[13–16]

   c. Some hospitals measure pro-BNP levels, which are interpreted in a similar fashion to the BNP. Values may vary depending on the hospital's reference range and also differ with age. A normal pro-BNP is <125 pg/mL for patients <age 75 and <450 pg/mL for patients >age 75. Levels >450 pg/mL under age 50, >900 pg/mL for ages 50–75, and >1800 pg/mL for patients over age 75 are consistent with acute heart failure.[17]

5. Baseline pulse oximetry on room air should be obtained on every patient, and if the oxygen saturation is less than 90%, arterial blood gases (ABGs) on room air should be obtained. If the patient has significant COPD or interstitial lung disease, ABGs can be valuable for comparison with postoperative values when weaning the patient from the ventilator. An elevated PCO_2 (>50 torr) is a significant marker for postoperative pulmonary morbidity and mortality. Additionally, patients on home oxygen or with a baseline PO_2 <60 torr are extremely borderline operative candidates.

6. In addition to significant COPD, pulmonary complications are more common in patients who actively smoke, as they often have a productive cough or lower respiratory colonization. Other risk factors include advanced age, obesity, diabetes, preoperative cardiac instability, pulmonary hypertension, emergency surgery, and a history of cerebrovascular disease.[18–20] A logistic risk model in patients undergoing

valve surgery found respiratory failure to be more common with age >70, diabetes, prior myocardial infarction (MI), congestive HF, reoperations or emergency operations, surgery for endocarditis, complex operations, and for bypass times over three hours (see Figure 10.2, p. 471).[21]

7. Actively smoking patients should be advised to terminate smoking at least four weeks (and preferably two months) before surgery to decrease the volume of airway secretions and improve mucociliary transport.[22] Actively smoking patients are more prone to postoperative hypoxemia, more obstructive and restrictive abnormalities in pulmonary function, more coughing that can lead to sternal dehiscence, increased fibrinogen levels and platelet aggregation leading to more thrombotic complications, and an increased risk of sternal wound infection.[20,22,23] Use of medications to assist smokers to quit, such as varenicline (Chantix) or bupropion HCL (Zyban), should be recommended as soon as possible once the patient understands the adverse influence of smoking on the perioperative course and the long-term results of surgery. However, some patients have extreme difficulty stopping smoking due to their nicotine addiction and simply cannot stop prior to surgery. Unfortunately, not smoking for just a few days before surgery is probably of little benefit and may increase airway secretions. If a patient indicates that they have stopped smoking, further inquiry as to when this occurred is important, because being off of cigarettes for a few days ("Yes, I quit") while hospitalized still places the patient at increased risk of pulmonary complications.

8. An active pulmonary or bronchitic process (evidenced by a productive cough) should be resolved before surgery using antibiotics. Bronchospastic disease should be treated with bronchodilators and, if severe, with steroids. Pulmonary consultation may be indicated in this situation. Short-term pulmonary rehabilitation is effective in improving perioperative pulmonary function in patients with significant COPD and can reduce the risk of pulmonary complications.[24]

9. Some patients on chronic high-dose amiodarone therapy are prone to the development of pulmonary toxicity and adult respiratory distress syndrome (ARDS) after surgery. This is manifested by dyspnea, hypoxia, radiographic infiltrates, and a decrease in diffusion capacity. This problem carries a very high mortality rate.[25] Evidence of preoperative pulmonary toxicity with a decrease in diffusion capacity may contraindicate a cardiac surgical procedure. Avoidance of potential contributing causes, such as a high inspired oxygen fraction, long duration of bypass, and fluid overload, is critical. On rare occasions, this syndrome may occur after a very short course of amiodarone, and it appears to be an idiosyncratic or hypersensitivity reaction.[26] Although baseline PFTs are not necessary in patients on a short-term course of amiodarone for AF prophylaxis, they should be considered when it is anticipated that the amiodarone may be given for more than one month (e.g. after a Maze procedure).

C. A history of heavy **alcohol** abuse identifies potential problems with intraoperative bleeding and postoperative hepatic dysfunction, agitation, and alcohol withdrawal. Prevention of postoperative delirium tremens (DTs) with thiamine, folate, and benzodiazepines should be considered. Bioprosthetic valves should be selected to avoid postoperative anticoagulation.

1. Mildly elevated liver function tests (LFTs) are often of unclear significance and usually do not require further evaluation. However, in a patient with a drinking

history, this does not exclude the possibility of alcoholic hepatitis or cirrhosis, and a gastrointestinal (GI) consultation may be indicated. A common cause of mildly elevated LFTs is use of a statin medication for dyslipidemia. Patients with nonalcoholic steatohepatitis (NASH) can also develop cirrhosis that should be evaluated in a similar fashion.

2. A history of GI bleeding, an elevated prothrombin time (reported as the INR), a low serum albumin indicating impaired synthetic function or malnutrition, an elevated bilirubin, or a low platelet count may suggest the presence of severe cirrhosis with portal hypertension and/or hypersplenism. A liver biopsy may be indicated to evaluate the risk of surgery and the potential for postoperative hepatic failure. If surgery is performed in a patient with esophageal varices, transesophageal echocardiography should probably be avoided.

3. Two risk models that have been used in cirrhotic patients to predict outcomes are the Child-Turcotte-Pugh (CTP) and the Mayo End-Stage Liver Disease (MELD) scores. Patients with CTP class A cirrhosis (Table 3.2) will usually tolerate cardiopulmonary bypass (CPB), but may have a higher risk of postoperative complications, including infections due to immune dysfunction and poor nutritional status, bleeding from impaired coagulation factor synthesis and thrombocytopenia, GI complications, and respiratory, renal, and hepatic failure.[27] Risk factors for mortality in patients with cirrhosis include older age, higher bilirubin levels, high central venous pressures, ascites, emergency surgery, prolonged CPB time, and perioperative thrombocytopenia.[27,28]

4. Patients with advanced alcoholic cirrhosis (class C) or a CTP score ≥8 are generally not candidates for cardiac surgery. The operative mortality rate for patients with cirrhosis in general is very high, with a literature review in 2015 reporting that the average operative mortality after cardiac surgery was 9% for class A, 37.7% for class B, and 52% for class C cirrhosis.[29] Furthermore, the one-year mortality rates were also very high at 27.2, 66.2, and 78.9%, respectively. Nonetheless, there are isolated small series showing better survival rates. One study from Taiwan reported

Table 3.2 • Child-Turcotte-Pugh Classification of Cirrhosis

Total bilirubin (mg/dL)	Albumin (g/dL)	INR
<2: 1 point	>3.5: 1 point	<1.7: 1 point
2–3: 2 points	2.8–3.5: 2 points	1.7–2.2: 2 points
>3: 3 points	<2.8: 3 points	>2.2: 3 points
Ascites	**Encephalopathy**	**CTP Class**
None: 1 point	None: 1 point	Class A: 5–6 points
Controlled: 2 points	Controlled medically: 2 points	Class B: 7–9 points
Poorly controlled: 3 points	Poorly controlled: 3 points	Class C: 10–15 points

an overall operative mortality of 16%, and even though only 9% of the patients were CTP class C, mortality did not correlate with CTP or MELD class.[30]

5. The MELD score includes both hepatic and renal variables and is considered a more sensitive indicator of surgical risk.[28] It is calculated from a summation of multiples of natural logarithms of the INR, serum creatinine, and total bilirubin (see calculator at www.mayoclinic.org/meld). A surgical mortality risk of 50% for a MELD score ≥ 15 was noted in one study,[31] and a mortality risk of 56% for a score exceeding >13.5 was reported in another, which also noted only a 23.8% one-year survival in these patients.[28] An additional ominous sign is an associated platelet count of less than 96,000/μL (reflecting advanced liver fibrosis).[32]

6. With recognition that CPB is a major contributing factor to adverse outcomes, off-pump surgery should be considered in patients with advanced liver disease if their lifestyle and lifespan are compromised primarily by their heart disease.[33]

D. **Diabetes mellitus** is a condition associated with extensive and diffuse atherosclerotic disease due to metabolic derangements and a proinflammatory and prothrombotic state.[34] It may range in severity from mild hyperglycemia controlled with diet or oral medications to more severe diabetes requiring insulin. The more severe and uncontrolled the diabetes, the greater the risk of obesity, congestive HF, PVD, extensive coronary artery disease (CAD), and chronic kidney disease.[35] Nonetheless, the long-term prognosis in diabetics with multivessel disease is improved with surgery.[36,37]

1. Generally, diabetes is associated with an increased postoperative risk of stroke, infection, renal dysfunction, and operative mortality, even after off-pump surgery.[35,38] A decrease in saphenous vein graft patency (hence the desire to use more arterial grafts) and a worse long-term survival have also been noted.[39] Noninsulin-dependent diabetics tend to fare somewhat better, with a lower immediate risk of postoperative complications, including respiratory and renal failure and mediastinitis. Their long-term prognosis is favorable in the absence of significant comorbidities.[34,37]

2. An elevated hemoglobin A1c (HbA1c) >7% is a marker for poorly controlled diabetes in the previous 3–4 months and has been associated with more adverse outcomes, including sternal wound infection, stroke, renal failure, and MI, as well as reduced long-term survival after CABG.[40–43] One study showed that the CABG mortality risk increased fourfold when the HbA1c was >8.6%.[44]

3. To optimize perioperative care, careful attention to potential diabetic-related complications is essential.

a. Any preexisting infections must be treated (urinary infections are particularly common in diabetic women).

b. The STS guidelines recommend that oral hypoglycemics should be withheld for 24 hours prior to surgery and insulin should not be used after an evening meal the night before surgery.[45,46] Monitoring of intraoperative glucose levels and aggressive treatment to maintain blood glucose in the 120–180 mg/dL range is essential to reduce neurologic morbidity and the risk of infection.[46] Interestingly, a literature review suggested that patients with perioperative hyperglycemia, even if not diabetic, had worse outcomes, with twice the mortality at one year compared with normoglycemic patients; however, patients with well-controlled diabetes may have comparable outcomes to those without diabetes with similar glycemic control.[47]

c. In diabetic patients with any element of chronic kidney disease, steps must be taken during cardiac catheterization and surgery to optimize renal function (see Chapter 12).

d. The long-term results of CABG in diabetics are improved with use of bilateral internal thoracic arteries (BITA) or radial artery grafts, since saphenous vein graft patency is compromised in diabetics. Despite multiple reports indicating an association between BITA use and the increased risk of deep sternal wound infections, especially in obese diabetic woman, other reports suggest that this is not the case with meticulous skeletonized ITA harvesting.[48–52] Notably, diabetics may be more prone to phrenic nerve dysfunction after ITA harvesting, so cauterizing near the phrenic nerve must be avoided.[53]

e. Although most patients are currently managed with glargine insulin (Lantus), which has improved efficacy and safety outcomes compared with NPH insulin,[54] the few patients currently taking NPH insulin are at increased risk of experiencing an allergic reaction to protamine.[55]

f. Management of postoperative hyperglycemia with a defined protocol (see Appendix 6) is an essential element of perioperative care and has been shown to reduce operative morbidity and mortality.[45] An endocrine consultation may be helpful in patients with refractory hyperglycemia.

E. **Neurologic symptoms**, whether active (transient ischemic attack [TIA]) or remote (history of a stroke), increase the risk of perioperative stroke and warrant evaluation.[56,57] Approximately 10–15% of patients requiring CABG have significant carotid disease. Selective screening limited to patients >age 65, or those with carotid bruits, TIA, or stroke can identify most patients at high risk.[58] Patients with hypertension, PVD, and particularly women with left main disease or calcified aortas are also at higher risk and should be screened.[59]

1. Generally, a carotid noninvasive study with ultrasound imaging and measurement of flow velocities should be performed in the patient with neurologic symptoms, a history of a carotid endarterectomy (CEA), or asymptomatic carotid bruits to assess for significant stenoses or flow-limiting lesions. A peak systolic velocity (PSV) >230 cm/s in the internal carotid artery (ICA), an ICA/common carotid artery PSV >4.0 cm/s, or an end-diastolic velocity >100 cm/s associated with significant plaque burden by ultrasonic imaging is consistent with significant stenosis. Further evaluation by carotid arteriography (usually magnetic resonance angiography) may be considered if noninvasive studies are inconclusive or a more precise visualization of the carotid vessels is desired.

2. Actively symptomatic carotid disease always warrants CEA either prior to or at the time of cardiac surgery. A combined CABG–CEA should be performed in the patient with unstable angina or significant myocardium at risk if neurologic symptoms are present.

3. The management of asymptomatic carotid lesions in patients requiring cardiac surgery is controversial and is noted in the discussion of carotid bruits (see section III.D, pages 184–185).

F. A history of **saphenous vein stripping and/or ligation or distal vascular reconstructive procedures** using saphenous vein alerts the surgeon to potential problems obtaining satisfactory conduit for bypass grafting.

1. Noninvasive venous mapping of the lower extremities may identify satisfactory greater or lesser saphenous veins for use, but it is not always reliable.[60] Consideration should be given to whether bilateral ITAs can be used to reach the surgical targets or whether their use is contraindicated (morbidly obese and diabetic females in particular).

2. Doppler assessment of the palmar arch or digital plethysmography with radial compression can be performed to assess the feasibility of using the radial artery as a bypass conduit (i.e. confirming that the arm is ulnar-dominant). Contraindications may also include Raynaud's disease, radial dominance, and possibly prior radial artery catheterization. Informing the patient of potential complications of radial artery harvesting, specifically numbness of the dorsum of the thumb and part of the thenar eminence or thumb weakness from trauma to the superficial radial nerve, is essential, as it may occur in 30–35% of patients.[61,62] An increased incidence of forearm neurologic deficits has been noted in smokers, older patients, and those with diabetes, obesity, and PVD.[63,64]

3. Venipunctures and intravenous (IV) catheters should be avoided in the arm from which the radial artery will be harvested. The anesthesiologist should also be alerted to avoid placing a radial artery line or IV catheter in that arm for the surgical procedure.

G. **Urologic symptoms** suggest the presence of an active urinary tract infection (UTI) that must be treated before surgery. In men, a history of prostatic cancer treated by irradiation, a prior transurethral resection, or other urinary symptoms consistent with prostatic hypertrophy identify potential problems with Foley catheter placement in the operating room. Use of a coudé catheter may be necessary. Urologic consultation should be obtained if a catheter cannot be passed. Either a catheter may be placed after dilating the urethra or a suprapubic tube may be inserted. Prolonged postoperative urinary drainage should be anticipated until the patient is fully ambulatory or until further urologic evaluation has been performed.

H. A history of significant **ulcer disease** or **GI bleeding** may necessitate further evaluation by endoscopy, especially if the patient will require postoperative anticoagulation. However, invasive diagnostic tests may need to be deferred in patients with significant coronary disease. Use of postoperative proton pump inhibitors (PPIs) should be considered in these patients, but whether stress prophylaxis should be used routinely or even in ICU patients considered at high risk for GI bleeding remains controversial.[65-67] Gastric acid suppression with PPIs or histamine antagonists may be beneficial in reducing the risk of stress ulceration, but their use is associated with an increased risk of pneumonia. This risk is minimized with the use of sucralfate, which, however, has not been shown to reduce the risk of GI bleeding in critically ill patients.[68] Nonetheless, sucralfate is commonly given routinely, and PPIs should be considered in patients receiving dual antiplatelet therapy or receiving one antiplatelet drug with additional risk factors for bleeding.[66]

I. The risk of **infection** is increased if another infectious source is present in the body (commonly a urinary tract or skin infection). Concurrent infections must be identified and treated before surgery. An upper respiratory infection may increase the risk of pulmonary complications, and bacterial infections may increase the risk of a hematogenous sternal wound infection and can seed a prosthetic heart valve. To reduce the risk of methicillin-resistant *Staphylococcus aureus* (MRSA) infections, prophylaxis with nasal mupirocin can be universally recommended unless a preliminary nasal swab is negative.[69,70]

J. The patient's **medications** should be reviewed to determine which ones to continue up to the time of surgery and which ones to stop in advance or not take the morning of surgery (see section IV, starting on page 186, and section VII, pages 198–199). Patients on chronic steroid therapy should receive a stress dose of hydrocortisone 100 mg IV at the beginning of surgery and should be given a few doses afterwards as well.

K. The patient's **allergies** must be carefully reviewed and listed in the medical record. Commonly, an adverse reaction is considered an allergy to the patient, but it does alert the healthcare team to medications that are best avoided after surgery to minimize side effects. Alternative antibiotic prophylaxis may be required for true antibiotic allergies. Just the mention of a potential latex allergy should be brought to the attention of the operating room to avoid any latex-containing products (including gloves, urinary catheters, Swan-Ganz catheters, and tourniquets used during surgery).

L. Other significant past medical history, such as prior chest irradiation for cancer (usually for mediastinal lymphoma, breast, or lung cancer) or a psychiatric history, should be detailed in the medical record. A thorough review of systems should be able to identify other comorbid conditions likely to affect the outcome of surgery.

III. Physical Examination

A. The patient's general appearance, mental status, and affect should be evaluated and noted in the medical record as a baseline for comparison with the postoperative period. Prior to transcatheter procedures, a mini-mental examination is performed as part of "frailty" testing.

B. An active **skin infection** or **rash** that might be secondarily infected must be treated before surgery to minimize the risk of sternal wound infection.

C. **Dental caries** must be treated before operations during which prosthetic material (valves, grafts) will be placed.[71,72] Dental extractions, however, should be recommended cautiously in patients with severe ischemic heart disease or critical aortic stenosis. Cardiac complications may occur even if dental procedures are performed under local anesthesia. A report from the Mayo Clinic found that 3% of patients died within 30 days of dental work done in anticipation of surgery.[73]

D. **Carotid bruits** are a marker of carotid disease, which is present in about 10–15% of patients with significant coronary disease. Carotid noninvasive studies are warranted in virtually all patients with bruits to assess for high-grade unilateral or bilateral disease because of the association of severe carotid disease with postoperative stroke, which is associated with significant mortality.[74,75]

1. The management of the patient with an asymptomatic carotid lesion requiring open-heart surgery is controversial. A meta-analysis from 1999 suggested that a combined CEA–CABG had a higher death or stroke rate than a staged approach.[76] However, another meta-analysis from 2014 showed equivalent results between the two approaches.[77] Another study showed equivalent results between a staged carotid stenting–CABG approach and a combined CEA–CABG, with both having lower MI rates than a staged CEA–CABG approach.[78] These studies suggest that combined approaches are noninferior to staged approaches, but, for the latter, there must not be too much of a delay before the second procedure (the CABG) to prevent cardiac events in the interim.

2. Because carotid disease is a marker for aortic atherosclerosis, it is not surprising that stroke risk is greater in patients with aortic calcification or atherosclerosis, likely explaining why half of perioperative strokes following combined operations occur contralateral to the operated side.[79]

3. If the patient presents with an acute coronary syndrome or has a large degree of myocardium at risk, most surgeons would consider performing a combined CABG–CEA for a unilateral carotid stenosis >90%. In contrast, preliminary CEA or stenting would be the preferred approach in patients with stable angina and might result in a lower overall risk of stroke, MI, and death. For patients requiring emergency CABG, that procedure alone is indicated, accepting the slightly increased risk of stroke with known carotid disease.

4. The risk of stroke with bilateral disease (>75% bilaterally) is significant during isolated CABG (as high as 10–15% in one report), especially in patients with unilateral stenosis with contralateral occlusion.[74] However, it remains quite significant even with a combined operation. Thus, the operations should be staged with the CEA performed first if cardiac disease permits. If this is not possible because of unstable angina, left main or severe three-vessel disease with a large amount of "myocardium in jeopardy", preliminary carotid stenting or a combined operation should be performed, with the understanding that the risk of stroke is somewhat increased.

E. **Bilateral arm blood pressures** should be measured. A differential systolic blood pressure of >10 mm Hg may identify significant subclavian artery stenosis, which is a relative contraindication to the use of a pedicled ITA graft.[80] This finding is also noted in some patients presenting with a type A aortic dissection.

F. The presence of a **heart murmur** warrants a preoperative echocardiogram if no valvular abnormality had been identified at the time of catheterization. Occasionally, new-onset ischemic mitral regurgitation or unsuspected aortic valve disease will be detected. In terms of valve selection, risk assessment, and informed consent, it is certainly preferable that the need for an additional valve procedure be recognized before surgery, rather than being identified for the first time in the operating room.

G. An **abdominal aortic aneurysm** detected upon palpation should be evaluated by ultrasound. IABP placement through the femoral artery should be avoided to prevent distal atheroembolism. Further evaluation by CT scanning is warranted before considering femoral artery cannulation for a minimally invasive procedure.

H. Severe **peripheral vascular disease** (PVD) must be assessed by a careful pulse examination. It is often associated with cerebrovascular disease and may prompt a preoperative carotid noninvasive study.[59] PVD adversely affects long-term survival after cardiac surgery, but it is not predictive of operative mortality, although it is included in the STS risk calculator.[81–83] Weak femoral pulses may be indicative of "inflow" aortoiliac disease. If the ascending aorta is also significantly diseased and an alternative cannulation site must be utilized for CPB, the axillary artery should be considered.[84]

1. Aortoiliac disease may dictate the unsuitability of the femoral arteries for cannulation, especially for minimally invasive valve surgery, or for placement of an IABP. An abdominal pelvic CT scan to assess the iliofemoral system may dictate whether percutaneous femoral cannulation is feasible or whether it runs the risk of a retrograde dissection or even retrograde embolization of atherosclerotic debris to the brain on CPB.

2. Abdominal-pelvic CT scanning is an essential component of the work-up for transcatheter aortic valve replacements (TAVRs). Vessel tortuosity, calcification, and size need to be assessed to determine whether a transfemoral or alternate access approach is indicated.

3. PVD may contribute to poor leg wound healing after saphenous vein harvesting, although this is generally not a significant problem with endoscopic vein harvesting. If there are plans for future peripheral vascular reconstruction, the vein should be harvested from the opposite leg.

I. The presence of **varicose veins** or a history of **deep venous thrombosis** (DVT) identifies potential problems with conduits for CABG. The distribution of varicosities may indicate whether or not the greater saphenous vein is involved. Noninvasive venous mapping may identify a normal greater saphenous vein despite significant varicosities.[60] The lesser saphenous vein distribution should be inspected to determine whether it might serve as a potential conduit. Assessment of the radial artery, as noted in section II.F, should be considered. BITA grafting may be required, so patients considered at increased risk for a sternal infection should be so informed.

IV. Adjustment of Medications Prior to Cardiac Surgery

Review of the patient's prior and current medications is important. Particular attention should be paid to antiplatelet/anticoagulant medications, which should be either continued or stopped prior to surgery, depending on the clinical situation (Tables 3.3 and 3.4).

A. **Aspirin** (ASA) is commonly taken by patients with known ischemic heart disease and is given routinely to patients presenting with an acute coronary syndrome (ACS). Preoperative use of aspirin is considered beneficial in reducing perioperative

Table 3.3 • Platelet Inhibitors to Be Stopped Prior to Surgery

	Mechanism of Action	Duration of Effect	Discontinue Preoperatively
Aspirin	Inhibits cyclooxygenase	7 days (lifespan of platelets)	3–7 days if at all
Clopidogrel	Inhibits ADP receptor P2Y12 (irreversible)	7 days (lifespan of platelets)	5 days
Prasugrel	Inhibits ADP receptor P2Y12 (irreversible)	7 days (lifespan of platelets)	7 days
Ticagrelor	Inhibits ADP receptor P2Y12 (reversible)	1–2 days ($t_{1/2} = 7$–8 h)	5 days
Tirofiban	Inhibits IIb/IIIa receptor	4–6 hours	4 hours
Eptifibatide	Inhibits IIb/IIIa receptor	4–6 hours	4 hours
Abciximab	Inhibits IIb/IIIa receptor	>24 hours	24 hours

infarction and operative mortality, and improving graft patency and the outcomes of CABG.[85–90] However, although this was documented in several meta-analyses, a trial published by one of the same authors failed to confirm these benefits.[88] Aspirin irreversibly acetylates platelet cyclooxygenase, impairing thromboxane A_2 formation and inhibiting platelet aggregation for the lifespan of the platelet (7–10 days). Thus, aspirin will be superimposing impaired platelet dysfunction on the clotting derangements induced by CPB.

1. Although the preoperative use of aspirin increases perioperative blood loss, this is generally noted in patients taking doses higher than 81 mg daily. Therefore, it is recommended to continue aspirin 81 mg daily up to the day of surgery in most patients undergoing CABG.[87,89,90] In patients undergoing other forms of open-heart surgery, stopping aspirin 3–5 days in advance should be sufficient to allow for significant regeneration of the platelet pool to minimize its antiplatelet effects.

2. Patient response to the antiplatelet effects of aspirin is quite variable. Some patients are somewhat resistant (often from using enteric-coated aspirin), and others have prominent platelet inhibition. A variety of platelet aggregometry tests are available to assess the antiplatelet effect of aspirin, but they do not necessarily correlate with the degree of platelet inhibition, and are rarely indicated before surgery.[91] Patients taking higher doses of aspirin and those with conditions associated with platelet dysfunction, such as uremia and von Willebrand's disease, may also exhibit more bleeding. If these patients are recognized, it may be advisable to stop aspirin a few days before surgery.

3. Studies have shown that there is enhanced platelet aggregation and thromboxane formation in the early postoperative period, even in patients receiving preoperative aspirin.[92] Thus, patients with aspirin resistance will have greater platelet reactivity, which is associated with an increased risk of graft thrombosis.[93] Although various studies provide conflicting data on whether platelet activation is greater following on- or off-pump (OPCAB) surgery,[94,95] routine use of preoperative aspirin and initiation of aspirin within 6–8 hours after surgery should mitigate the extent of platelet activation and aggregation to some degree, most likely accounting for the improved graft patency, lower rate of perioperative MI, and improved operative survival after both types of surgery.[93,96]

B. **The P2Y12 inhibitors** are thienopyridines that inhibit platelet function by irreversibly modifying the platelet adenosine diphosphate (ADP) receptor P2Y12, which then inhibits ADP-mediated activation of the glycoprotein IIb/IIIa receptor. This results in inhibition of platelet activation and aggregation. These medications are given along with aspirin for one month for patients receiving bare-metal stents and for 6–12 months for patients with drug-eluting stents to minimize the risk of stent thrombosis.[97] However, many patients are maintained on them indefinitely after PCI. They are also given to patients presenting with acute coronary syndromes and to those in whom PCI is contemplated, whether elective or not.

1. **Clopidogrel** is biotransformed through a two-step process into an active metabolite which produces its antiplatelet effects. Genetic polymorphisms in the CYP2C19 allele reduce this conversion, resulting in clopidogrel resistance. Prior to PCI, a 300–600 mg load is given, which achieves about 40% platelet inhibition within a few hours, followed by 75 mg daily. Despite a half-life of about seven

hours, the antiplatelet effect lasts for the lifespan of the platelet, so cessation for five days prior to surgery is recommended in elective situations.[89]

2. **Ticagrelor** is a reversible noncompetitive inhibitor of the P2Y12 receptor that has a more rapid onset of action and more pronounced inhibition of platelet function than clopidogrel. Ticagrelor and its metabolite are both pharmacologically active with a peak effect in 1.5 hours after a 180 mg load, which is then followed by 90 mg twice a day. It is more effective than clopidogrel in reducing death in patients with an ACS with a comparable rate (12%) of major bleeding. It has a reversible effect on platelet function with a half-life of 7–8 hours, with 80% recovery of platelet function by 72 hours.[98] This suggests that surgery can be safely performed if ticagrelor has been withheld for 72 hours, although it is still recommended that it be stopped five days prior to surgery.[89]

3. **Prasugrel** is a prodrug that is converted to an active metabolite which produces irreversible antagonism of the P2Y12 receptor. It is approximately 10 times more potent than clopidogrel and produces more rapid onset of action with 50% inhibition within one hour. The maximum platelet inhibition is 80%. Although clinically superior to clopidogrel in ACS patients undergoing PCI, it may be associated with a higher risk of bleeding and it is not recommended in patients >age 75 or patients with a history of TIAs or stroke. Despite a comparable half-life of seven hours, the irreversible effect on platelet function mandates that it be stopped at least seven days before surgery.[89]

4. **Cangrelor** is an intravenous reversible inhibitor of P2Y12 which produces nearly 100% platelet inhibition with a rapid onset of action within minutes since it does not require conversion to an active metabolite. It has a half-life of 3–6 minutes with reversal of effect in 1–2 hours.[99]

5. The risks of perioperative bleeding, need for transfusions, and re-exploration for bleeding are unequivocally increased when patients have received a P2Y12 inhibitor within several days of surgery.[100] This has led to the recommendation that surgery be delayed 5–7 days following cessation of these drugs.[89] However, bleeding is more related to the patient's responsiveness to these medications (primarily clopidogrel) than to the timing of discontinuation.[101] Use of platelet function testing can determine the patient's sensitivity to the P2Y12 inhibitor. If platelet inhibition (platelet reactive units, or PRUs) is <30%, surgery can be safely performed without an increased bleeding risk.[102]

   a. Emergency surgery is indicated for patients with a STEMI or other ACS presentation with refractory ischemia when PCI is not feasible. It is associated with the highest bleeding risk, especially since platelet transfusions given within six hours of a loading dose or four hours after a maintenance dose of a P2Y12 may be less effective because some of the active metabolite may bind exogenous platelets.

   b. Urgent surgery for patients with critical anatomy should usually be performed within a week of catheterization, when antiplatelet effects may not have completely dissipated. Timing of surgery balances the risk of an ischemic event versus the risk of bleeding requiring platelet transfusions. Clearly, surgery should never be delayed if clinically indicated. Use of platelet testing is invaluable in assessing when the risk of bleeding has lessened and surgery can be performed with a lower bleeding risk.

c. Some patients require cardiac surgery despite having received a recent stent. For example, a patient with a STEMI may be found to have multivessel disease, but the culprit lesion may be stented to promptly reperfuse the potential infarct zone, and urgent surgery is then recommended to address the other lesions. Another example is the patient with recurrent chest pain within a few months of receiving a drug-eluting stent. Stopping a P2Y12 inhibitor for one week prior to surgery will increase the risk of stent thrombosis, so two feasible approaches, other than operating without stopping the P2Y12 inhibitor, are to (1) stop the medication for three days, continue aspirin, and operate with mild residual antiplatelet activity or, preferably, (2) stop the P2Y12 inhibitor five days prior to surgery, continue aspirin, and admit the patient for a glycoprotein IIb/IIIa inhibitor for a few days, and stop that four hours prior to surgery. Following the operation, the P2Y12 inhibitor is restarted as soon as possible with a loading dose.[103]

d. It has been suggested that use of an antifibrinolytic medication, such as tranexamic acid, can mitigate some of the bleeding noted in patients in whom a P2Y12 inhibitor was not stopped prior to surgery.[104]

C. **Heparin** is given to patients with an ACS before and after cardiac catheterization if urgent surgery is recommended. It is also used in patients in whom an IABP is placed preoperatively. It may also be used as a bridge to surgery in patients taking preoperative warfarin.

Table 3.4 • Other Anticoagulants to Be Stopped Prior to Surgery

	Mechanism of Action	Duration of Effect	Discontinue Preoperatively
Warfarin	Inhibits clotting factor synthesis	4–5 days	4–5 days
Unfractionated heparin	Binds to antithrombin III, primarily inhibiting thrombin and factor Xa	4 hours	4 hours
LMWH	Inhibits factors Xa and II	12–18 hours ($t_{1/2}$ = 4.5 h)	24 hours
Fondaparinux	Inhibits factor Xa	48 hours ($t_{1/2}$ = 17–21 hours)	60 hours
Bivalirudin	Direct thrombin inhibitor	2 hours ($t_{1/2}$ = 25 min)	1–2 hours
NOACs	Factor IIa (dabigatran) and factor Xa inhibitors (apixaban, rivaroxaban, edoxaban	8–12 hours	48 hours

1. **Unfractionated heparin (UFH)** is given using a weight-based protocol (see Appendix 7) and requires monitoring by a partial thromboplastin time (PTT) to ensure a therapeutic range of approximately 50–60 seconds. Heparin is usually stopped about four hours before surgery. However, in patients with critical CAD, it is best to continue heparin into the operating room. This should not pose a significant risk during the insertion of central lines. When heparin is given for several days, the platelet count should be checked on a daily basis to assess for the development of heparin-induced thrombocytopenia (HIT) (see pages 251–253).

2. **Low-molecular-weight heparin (LMWH)** (enoxaparin) binds to antithrombin, which then accelerates inhibition of activated factor Xa, with minimal inhibition of thrombin (factor IIa). It is commonly used in patients with an ACS (1 mg/kg SC twice a day) due to its efficacy and simplicity of use, with no requirement for blood monitoring. It may also be used as an alternative to UFH during cardiac catheterization procedures. It is commonly used for venous thromboembolism (VTE) prophylaxis in hospitalized patients at a dose of 40 mg SC once daily. Studies have reported an increased risk of perioperative bleeding in patients on LMWH.[105] It has an elimination half-life of 4–5 hours and exhibits 30% of anti-factor Xa activity at 12 hours. It is recommended that the last dose should be given five half-lives or approximately 24 hours prior to surgery to minimize perioperative bleeding. Only 60% of LMWH can be neutralized by protamine, although its effect can be reversed by platelet factor 4.[106]

D. **Warfarin** is given primarily to patients with mechanical prosthetic valves, AF, a history of DVT or pulmonary embolism (PE), or hypercoagulable disorders. Warfarin should be stopped five days prior to surgery and the INR should be rechecked within 24 hours before the procedure. Bridging anticoagulation is not necessary in low-risk patients.[107,108]

1. Patients at high risk for a clinical event should be bridged to surgery with either UFH or LMWH. For outpatients, LMWH (enoxaparin 1 mg/kg SC) is usually given for 2–3 days, starting when the INR is below therapeutic range (usually two days after stopping warfarin) and should be discontinued 24 hours prior to surgery. Since there will still be some residual anticoagulant effect after it is stopped, admission for UFH for a few hours prior to surgery is not necessary. Inpatients may receive UFH, which is then stopped four hours prior to surgery. High-risk patients include those with the following:[108]

   a. Mechanical mitral valve replacement

   b. Mechanical aortic valve replacement with any thromboembolic risk factor (e.g. AF, prior thromboembolism, hypercoagulable condition, non-bileaflet valve, LV systolic dysfunction, or >1 mechanical valve).

   c. AF at high risk for embolic stroke (CHA_2DS_2-VASc score ≥5, stroke or systemic embolism within three months, associated rheumatic mitral stenosis)

   d. VTE within the preceding three months

   e. History of prior thromboembolism during interruption of anticoagulation

2. If the patient requires urgent surgery and has an elevated INR, administration of 5 mg of vitamin K given PO should reduce the INR within 12–24 hours. IV vitamin K given intravenously over 30 minutes is more expeditious in reversing the INR, but it runs the risk of an anaphylactic reaction. Subcutaneous vitamin K has unpredictable and delayed absorption and is not recommended. Fresh frozen plasma

may be necessary if more emergent surgery is indicated and prothrombin complex concentrate (PCC [Kcentra]) in a dose of 500 units of factor IX (usually 25–50 units/kg) may also be considered for rapid reversal.[109]

3. For patients requiring pacemaker or ICD implantation, bleeding risk is increased if the patient is on dual antiplatelet therapy or if a high-risk patient is bridged off of warfarin with heparin. Most studies have not shown an increased bleeding risk if the patient has a therapeutic INR, so for high-risk patients, it is best not to stop the warfarin prior to these procedures; for low-risk patients, stopping the warfarin for four days without a bridge is the safest approach.[110]

E. The **non-vitamin K antagonist oral anticoagulants** (NOACs), also termed direct oral anticoagulants (DOACs), inhibit either factor IIa (dabigatran, a direct thrombin inhibitor) or factor Xa (apixaban, rivaroxaban, and edoxaban) (Table 3.5). They are equivalent, if not superior, to warfarin in reducing the risk of stroke in patients with nonvalvular AF and in the treatment of VTE. They are commonly used in many patients with AF with valvular and structural heart disease, but should **not be used** in higher-risk patients with mechanical valves or rheumatic mitral valve disease.[108,111] Their half-lives average about 12 hours, so they should be stopped 4–5 half-lives or approximately 48 hours prior to surgery. However, clinical studies have shown that this may not be sufficient in patients with renal dysfunction, so a longer interval of cessation is recommended.[108,112] Reversal agents are available when patients require emergency surgery or have significant bleeding (Table 3.5). If these are not available, PCC can be used in a dose of 50–75 units/kg.

F. **Fondaparinux** (Arixtra) is an indirect factor Xa inhibitor that acts by catalyzing factor Xa inhibition by antithrombin. It is given in a daily dose of 2.5 mg SC for VTE prophylaxis and in a higher weight-based protocol for established thrombosis (5 mg if

Table 3.5 • Non-Vitamin K Antagonist Oral Anticoagulants (NOACs)					
	Inhibitor of factor	Half-life[1]	Dose	Excretion	Reversal agent
Dabigatran	IIa	12–17 hours	150 mg bid	80% renal	idarucizumab 5 mg IV × 2
Apixaban	Xa	8–15 hours	5 mg bid	15% hepatic/ 27% renal	Andexanet/PCC*
Rivaroxaban	Xa	5–13 hours	20 mg qd	30% hepatic/ 33% renal	Andexanet/PCC*
Edoxaban	Xa	10–14 hours	60 mg qd	50% renal	PCC*

*Doses: Andexxa (andexanet alfa) = factor Xa (recombinant): 400–800 mg given at 30 mg/min, then 4–8 mg/min × 2 h
Prothrombin complex concentrate: 25–50 units/kg
[1]These are the estimated half-lives with normal renal function; the half-life is influenced by age and GFR.

<50 kg, 7.5 mg if 50–100 kg, 10 mg if >100 kg). Its use has been essentially supplanted by the NOACs for VTE treatment. Its effects cannot be reversed by protamine and, because of its long elimination half-life of 17–21 hours, the dose should be withheld for at least 60 hours prior to surgery.

G. **Bivalirudin** (Angiomax) is a direct thrombin inhibitor that is approved as an alternative to UFH during PCI. Its benefits are a short half-life (25 minutes) and avoidance of exposure to heparin. The usual dose is a 0.7 mg/kg IV bolus followed by an infusion of 1.75 mg/kg/h during the procedure. Due to its short half-life, the potential risk of significant surgical bleeding (other than from a femoral artery puncture) would be increased only if an emergency procedure were required within 1–2 hours of its administration. It is the anticoagulant of choice for CPB in the patient with HIT.

H. **Eptifibatide** (Integrilin) and **tirofiban** (Aggrastat) are short-acting IV reversible antagonists of fibrinogen binding to the glycoprotein IIb/IIIa platelet receptor.[113] They are occasionally used in patients with an ACS and non-ST-elevation myocardial infarctions (non-STEMI) in whom an early invasive strategy is planned. They are usually continued after catheterization along with heparin if CABG is considered the best option for revascularization.

1. Eptifibatide is given as a 180 μg/kg bolus followed by an infusion of 2 μg/kg/min for 72–96 hours. It has a half-life of 2.5 hours and platelet function returns to 50–80% of normal within four hours of its cessation.

2. Tirofiban is given in a dose of 0.4 μg/kg/min for 30 minutes followed by an infusion of 0.1 μg/kg/min for 48–96 hours. It has a half-life of two hours and platelet aggregation returns to 90% of normal within 4–8 hours after it is stopped.

3. It is recommended that either medication be stopped approximately four hours prior to surgery (Table 3.3). It is noteworthy, however, that some studies have not identified an increased risk of postbypass bleeding even if these medications are stopped two hours preoperatively or even as late as the time of skin incision. This may be attributable to their transient "platelet anesthesia" effects, which may offset the adverse influence of CPB on platelet number and function.[114]

4. **Abciximab** (ReoPro) is the Fab fragment of a monoclonal antibody that binds to the IIb/IIIa receptor on the surface of platelets. Platelet aggregation is significantly inhibited by preventing the binding of fibrinogen and von Willebrand's factor to this receptor site on activated platelets. This drug has a half-life of 12 hours, and platelet function may take up to 48 hours to recover. If possible, surgery should be delayed for at least 24 hours after a patient has received abciximab. If emergency surgery is indicated, significant bleeding can be anticipated. Platelet transfusions are effective in producing hemostasis by reducing the overall number of platelet receptors bound to abciximab.[115] A hemoconcentrator can remove some of the residual free abciximab, allowing platelets to function more for hemostasis than for binding free antibodies.[116] Fortunately, this medication has been supplanted in most centers by the shorter-acting reversible IIb/IIIa antagonists.

I. **Thrombolytic therapy** with tissue plasminogen activator (tPA) is rarely used for STEMI patients, except in centers where emergency catheterization and surgery are not available. If emergency surgery is recommended, one can anticipate a significant bleeding problem. Although the half-life of these medications is less than 30 minutes, they cause persistent systemic hemostatic defects that outlive their short half-lives.

These effects include depletion of fibrinogen, reduction in factor II, V, and VIII levels, impairment of platelet aggregation, and the appearance of fibrin split products. Therefore, surgery should be delayed for at least 24 hours, if possible.

J. **Nonsteroidal anti-inflammatory drugs** have a reversible effect on platelet cyclooxygenases (COX-1 and COX-2), and cause platelet dysfunction by inhibiting formation of thromboxane A2. Their antiplatelet effects are primarily determined by their dosing and half-lives. Generally, they only need to be stopped a few days before surgery.[117]

K. **Omega-3 fatty acids (fish oils)** have been shown to reduce the incidence of AF after surgery, but have seen limited use due to concerns that they may produce bleeding by inhibiting platelet adhesion and platelet-stimulated thrombin generation. However, this is apparently evident only when taken with aspirin or factor Xa inhibitors.[118,119] There is also a synergistic effect when taken with warfarin due to its inhibitory effect on thrombin generation. Because of these concerns, it has usually been recommended that fish oil, flaxseed oil, and krill oil should be stopped prior to surgery. However, numerous studies and the OPERA randomized trial published in 2018 reported that use of fish oils did not increase perioperative bleeding after cardiac surgery, but all antiplatelet drugs and anticoagulants were stopped preoperatively in these studies.[118–120]

L. Other products, including vitamin E, ginkgo biloba, garlic, and even flavonoids in purple grape juice, have been shown to inhibit platelet function.[121–124] Whether these have any impact on perioperative bleeding or operative outcomes is not defined, but it is not unreasonable to stop them prior to surgery. It is imperative to specifically ask the patient if these products are being taken, since they are usually not volunteered when a list of medications is reviewed.

M. Inquiry should be made about any known clinical bleeding disorder or hypercoagulable state. This may direct perioperative anticoagulant management or provide direction in the treatment of bleeding problems.

1. **Antiphospholipid syndrome** is an autoimmune disorder in which antiphospholipid (APL) antibodies (anticardiolipin antibodies) and/or lupus anticoagulant are present. It is a rare phenomenon, but has been associated with valvular pathology. These antibodies produce a hypercoagulable state that may cause arterial and venous thrombosis, even though the coagulation profile shows an elevated PTT and commonly thrombocytopenia. The APL antibodies affect the kaolin-activated activated clotting time (ACT), so Celite ACTs have been recommended for intraoperative monitoring. However, because the ACT does not necessarily correlate with heparin levels during surgery, it is suggested that the heparin–protamine titration test be used to ensure adequate anticoagulation, aiming for a heparin level of 3.4 units/mL.[125,126] One report recommended a heparin level of 3 units/mL for a normal-risk APS patient and 5 units/mL for a high-risk patient with a history of APL-antibody-associated thrombocytopenia.[126] Alternatively, bivalirudin might be considered as a substitute anticoagulant during bypass (see Chapter 4).

2. Other hypercoagulable states, such as **factor V Leiden mutation, prothrombin gene mutation, or protein C or S deficiency**, are usually not recognized until the patient sustains a postoperative thrombotic event. However, if these syndromes are known to be present, aggressive anticoagulant measures should be taken to reduce the risk of postoperative thrombosis. Bridging after discontinuation of warfarin

therapy is recommended when the INR is subtherapeutic. If the patient has **antithrombin III deficiency**, which is also a hypercoagulable condition, either fresh frozen plasma or antithrombin III concentrate (Thrombate) may be required to achieve adequate heparinization during CPB.[127]

V. Laboratory Assessment

A. **Complete blood count (CBC), PT, PTT, and platelet count**

1. Patients with moderate anemia (hemoglobin <10 g/dL) have a significantly higher risk of adverse events after surgery as well as a higher operative mortality.[128–130] It is likely that the association of anemia with comorbidities such as congestive HF and chronic kidney disease leaves organ systems less tolerant to impaired oxygen delivery, thus contributing to an increase in noncardiac events, such as stroke, renal failure, and even sternal wound infection. Although both anemia and transfusions have been independently associated with adverse outcomes, including mortality, the stronger association may be with the use of transfusions.[131,132] Studies continue to be published attesting to the adverse effects of transfusions on surgical results, including an increased risk of graft occlusion, mandating careful patient assessment prior to ordering a transfusion.[133–136] Large studies and a meta-analysis of restrictive vs. liberal transfusion strategies show comparable rates of postoperative infection, stroke, cardiac, respiratory, and renal complications, as well as mortality.[137–139]

   a. It is not uncommon for hospitalized patients undergoing cardiac catheterization to have a moderate decrease in hematocrit. This may result from repeat blood draws, hydration prior to and after catheterization, and blood loss during the cath procedure itself, although this is much less extensive using radial rather than femoral access for catheterization.

   b. Although a transfusion trigger of a hemoglobin <8 g/dL is recommended in patients with ischemic heart disease, it must be remembered that very low hematocrits on CPB are associated with adverse neurologic and renal outcomes. Furthermore, patients receiving multiple units of blood intraoperatively often have coagulopathies requiring the use of additional blood components. If the anticipated hematocrit on CPB is calculated to be less than 20%, it is not unreasonable to transfuse a hospitalized patient with a hematocrit <26% prior to surgery. This might be beneficial in reducing potential preoperative cardiac ischemia, but more importantly, it may reduce the extent of hemodilution during surgery and the amount of blood and blood component transfusions required during surgery.

2. An elevated WBC may be associated with an infectious process that should be identified before surgery. However, it may also be a generalized marker of inflammation or could reflect the use of steroids or a myelodysplastic disorder. Studies indicate that preoperative leukocytosis is associated with an increased risk of perioperative myocardial injury, stroke, and operative mortality, as well as decreased one-year survival.[140,141]

3. It is important to check a daily platelet count in patients maintained on heparin to allow for prompt recognition of potential HIT. If this is suspected based on a falling platelet count, further work-up is indicated with testing for heparin-induced platelet aggregation (usually by the serotonin release assay) or serologic testing for

IgG-specific heparin antibodies.[142] If these tests are positive, an alternative means of anticoagulation during bypass may be necessary (see pages 251–253). Routine assessment for heparin antibodies in the absence of thrombocytopenia is not recommended. Preoperative platelet aggregation testing may be beneficial in assessing the residual antiplatelet effects of aspirin and, in particular, the P2Y12 inhibitors, and may influence the appropriate timing of surgery.[102,103]

B. **Basic metabolic panel** (electrolytes, BUN, creatinine, blood glucose) and **hemoglobin A1c**

1. Postoperative acute kidney injury is more common in patients with stage III–IV chronic kidney disease, especially in diabetic patients, and this portends a higher operative mortality and lower long-term survival.[143,144] Adequate hydration during and after cardiac catheterization and delaying on-pump (not off-pump) surgery for at least 24 hours after catheterization may minimize renal toxicity.[145,146] The serum creatinine should be rechecked after catheterization in patients at increased risk of developing renal dysfunction. If the serum creatinine has increased, surgery should be deferred, if clinically feasible, until it has returned to baseline. However, surgery should not be delayed in critically ill patients with hemodynamic compromise and worsening renal function, since delay will often lead to less reversible renal failure and multisystem organ failure. Specific intraoperative measures and postoperative hemodynamic support are critical to minimize the renal insult (see Chapter 12).

2. Hyperglycemia is associated with adverse outcomes, including stroke, wound infection, renal failure, and mortality.[46] Therefore, aggressive perioperative control of blood glucose is essential. An elevated hemoglobin A1c reflects poor diabetic control over the preceding three months and correlates with an increased risk of infection and compromised short- and long-term survival.[40–44]

3. Hyponatremia is often present in patients on diuretic therapy and those with worse LV function and HF. It is associated with a higher risk of coronary events, wound infections, pneumonia, a prolonged hospital stay, and increased operative mortality.[147,148] It can be categorized as hyper-, eu-, or hypovolemic hyponatremia based on the serum osmolarity. Assessment of urine sodium levels will help dictate whether treatment may involve fluid restriction, modification of diuretics, or even IV saline solutions.[149]

4. Hyperkalemia often reflects renal dysfunction and should be treated prior to surgery, since most cardioplegia solutions utilize potassium as the primary arresting agent.

C. **Liver function tests (LFTs)** including bilirubin, alkaline phosphatase (alk phos), alanine aminotransferase (ALT), aspartate aminotransferase (AST), albumin, and serum amylase should be obtained. New York State registry data have shown that an elevated alk phos and AST were significant predictors of CABG mortality and suggested they should be included in risk models.[150] Abnormalities suggestive of hepatitis or cirrhosis may warrant further evaluation. Those associated with chronic passive congestion (tricuspid valve pathology, right heart failure or constriction) may not improve until after surgery has been performed. Occasionally, emergency surgery is indicated in patients with cardiogenic shock and an acute hepatic insult with markedly increased liver enzymes. In this situation, there is a higher risk of severe hepatic dysfunction after surgery. Baseline LFTs are also valuable because all patients should be placed on pre- and postoperative statins, the most common side effect of which is an elevation in LFTs.

D. Other laboratory tests to be considered

1. **Thyroid-stimulating hormone (TSH)** levels should be measured preoperatively in the event that amiodarone will be used either prophylactically or therapeutically after surgery for AF. Amiodarone is an iodine-rich compound that can have a variety of effects on thyroid function, producing either thyrotoxicosis or hypothyroidism in about 15% of patients receiving chronic amiodarone therapy.[151]

2. **BNP and pro-BNP levels** may be drawn to differentiate among the causes of dyspnea. In patients with systolic or diastolic dysfunction, or heart failure resulting from valvular dysfunction, levels are invariably elevated. Elevated BNP levels are associated with postoperative ventricular dysfunction, an increased need for inotropic or IABP support, and a higher mortality rate after CABG and aortic valve surgery.[11-16]

3. **C-reactive protein** levels are often drawn when patients are admitted to the medical service with acute coronary syndromes. Levels are elevated in patients with infections or inflammatory processes. An elevated preoperative level (>10 mg/L) is associated with increased operative mortality, and a level >5 mg/L is associated with reduced long-term survival following CABG.[152] Elevated levels are also associated with an increased incidence of graft occlusion.

E. Urinalysis. If an initial urinalysis suggests contamination, a "clean-catch" specimen with proper cleansing should be obtained. If there is suspicion of a UTI, a culture should be obtained. An appropriate antibiotic should be given for several days prior to elective surgery. If the patient requires urgent bypass surgery, one or two doses of an antibiotic providing gram-negative coverage should suffice, although a few days of treatment might be considered before performing valve surgery.

F. Chest x-ray (PA and lateral). The x-ray is essential to rule out any active pulmonary disease that should be treated prior to surgery. Identification of pulmonary nodules should be further evaluated by a preoperative chest CT scan, since radiographic interpretation can be difficult postoperatively. Evidence of severe aortic calcification should prompt a careful review of the ascending aorta from the catheterization films and often a noncontrast CT scan to identify ascending aortic calcification. If present, this may necessitate modification of the operative approach and, in some elderly patients, a determination of inoperability. A lateral film should always be obtained before reoperations through a median sternotomy incision in patients with prior bypass grafting. This gives an assessment of the proximity of the cardiac structures and the ITA pedicle clips to the posterior sternal table. The PA film allows for optimal planning of minimally invasive incisions. Additional significant information that can be derived from a chest x-ray is noted on pages 123 and 125.

G. Electrocardiogram (ECG). A baseline study should be obtained for comparison with postoperative ECGs. Evidence of an interval infarction or new ischemia since the time of catheterization may warrant reevaluation of ventricular function and, on occasion, a repeat coronary angiogram. Patients being evaluated for elective surgery with active ischemia on ECG should be hospitalized and undergo prompt surgery.

1. If AF is present, it should be rate-controlled and its duration ascertained. The likelihood of conversion to sinus rhythm after surgery is nearly 80% for patients in AF for less than six months, but it is unlikely if the AF has been of longer duration. Thus, the duration of AF would influence the aggressiveness of postoperative treatment and possibly influence the decision to perform a Maze procedure in addition to the planned operation.

2. The presence of a left bundle branch block raises the risk of complete heart block occurring during the insertion of a Swan-Ganz catheter. Advancement of the catheter into the pulmonary artery may be delayed until after the chest is open, unless other provisions for urgent pacing (external pads, transvenous pacing wires) are available. The presence of a bundle branch block also makes it more difficult to detect ischemia. A right bundle branch block with a first-degree block raises the risk of complete heart block following a TAVR procedure.

3. Patients with significant preoperative bradycardia, especially if not taking β-blockers, will often require pacing after surgery. Both atrial and ventricular pacing wires should be placed during surgery. Care must be taken to avoid using prophylactic β-blockers and amiodarone to prevent postoperative AF in these patients since a profound bradycardia might ensue.

H. Most test results are acceptable when performed within one month of surgery. However, it is beneficial to have a CBC, electrolytes, BUN, and creatinine checked within a few days of surgery.

VI. Preoperative Blood Donation and Management of Anemia

A. Preoperative autologous blood donation is a feasible objective in patients with stable angina or valvular heart disease.[153] However, its limited use can be ascribed to several factors: (1) the urgency of surgery in most cases; (2) concerns about precipitating angina in patients with severe coronary disease; (3) lessened concern about the transmission of hepatitis C and human immunodeficiency virus; (4) questions about its cost-effectiveness with the availability of other measures to reduce blood loss, such as antifibrinolytic drugs, cell-saving devices, and off-pump surgery; and (5) logistic blood bank considerations. Thus, it is commonly neither necessary nor encouraged. One unit of blood may be donated every week as long as the hematocrit exceeds 33%, allowing an additional 2–3 weeks before surgery for the hematocrit to return to normal.

B. The use of recombinant erythropoietin with iron supplementation can induce erythropoiesis very rapidly. This is particularly helpful in anemic patients, patients who donate their own blood, and Jehovah Witness patients.[154] Single doses in the range of 500–1000 units/kg SC given 1–2 days prior to surgery have been shown to reduce transfusion requirements.[155,156] An alternative regimen of 14,000 units SC daily for two days prior to surgery and then 8000 units daily for three more days has also been effective.[157]

C. Refinement in testing for hepatitis C (1/250,000–1/1,500,000 units) and human immunodeficiency virus (1/750,000 units) has lowered their risks to extremely low levels. This has allayed the morbid fear of many patients of receiving transfusions. Nonetheless, blood transfusions are not benign: they may still cause febrile, allergic, or transfusion reactions and are associated with an increased risk of infection, stroke, renal dysfunction, respiratory complications, and overall mortality.[135] A conscientious blood conservation program is beneficial in reducing the need for transfusions (see Chapter 9).[136]

D. The percentage of patients requiring perioperative blood transfusions has gradually been decreasing, with less than 40% of patients receiving any blood products. Although transfusions may be necessary to maintain a hematocrit >20% during CPB, a restrictive postoperative transfusion policy (transfusing for a Hb <7.5 g/dL) has evolved with the recognition that clinical outcomes are comparable to those seen with a more liberal strategy (transfusing for a Hb <9 g/dL).[137–139]

VII. Preoperative Medications

A. All **antianginal medications** should be continued up to and including the morning of surgery to prevent recurrence of ischemia. The substitution of a shorter-acting β-blocker or calcium channel blocker for a longer-acting one (metoprolol tartrate for succinate [Toprol XL], diltiazem for Cardizem CD) should be considered. Whether preoperative β-blockers lower the mortality rate of coronary bypass surgery remains controversial, since several studies have shown this to be of benefit only in patients with a recent MI.[158–160] Nonetheless, this is an STS quality measure incorporated into public reporting.

B. **Anti-hypertensive medications** such as β-blockers or calcium channel blockers can be given preoperatively to prevent rebound hypertension and provide for a more stable anesthetic course. However, whether angiotensin-converting enzyme (ACE) inhibitors or angiotensin receptor blockers (ARBs) should be withheld the morning of surgery remains controversial. Their use is associated with reduced systemic resistance and a vasoplegic state during and after CPB, and studies have shown an association with higher mortality rates, an increasing need for inotropic support, and a higher risk of AF.[161,162] However, effects on kidney function are controversial, with various studies showing either an increased and decreased risk of renal dysfunction when given up to the time of surgery.[163,164]

C. Digoxin should be given the morning of surgery if used for rate control.

D. Any medication that can affect renal function during surgery should be withheld. This includes thiazides and loop diuretics, such as furosemide.

E. Anticoagulants and antiplatelet agents should be modified as follows (see section IV on pages 186–193 for more details):

1. Aspirin 81 mg should be continued up to the time of surgery in patients with coronary disease, but may be stopped 3–5 days prior to noncoronary surgery.

2. Clopidogrel and ticagrelor should be stopped five days prior to surgery and prasugrel should be stopped seven days prior to surgery. If the patient has received a bare-metal stent within the past month or a drug-eluting stent within the past 6–12 months, options include (a) continuing the medication, (b) stopping it for only three days before surgery, or (c) considering bridging with a IIb/IIIa inhibitor. The urgency of surgery to prevent an ischemic event always takes precedence over the time interval over which the medication has been stopped.

3. Warfarin should be stopped five days before surgery to allow for normalization of the INR. Bridging with LMWH should be considered in high risk outpatients (see page 190). If the INR remains elevated, 5 mg of oral vitamin K is effective in reducing the INR within 1–2 days. If more urgent reversal is necessary, 5 mg of IV vitamin K, fresh frozen plasma, or prothrombin complex concentrate (25–35 units/kg) may be used.

4. UFH is generally continued up to the time of surgery in patients with critical coronary disease, but when used as a bridge, it can be stopped about four hours before surgery.

5. LMWH: the last dose should be given 24 hours preoperatively.

6. NOACs: the last dose should be given 48 hours preoperatively or stopped even earlier if the patient has renal dysfunction. If the patient requires emergency surgery, expensive antidotes are available but may not be on formulary (idarucizumab for dabigatran, activated factor Xa ([andexanet alfa] for apixaban or rivaroxaban)

7. Fondaparinux should be stopped at least 60–72 hours prior to surgery.

8. Short-acting IIb/IIIa inhibitors should be stopped four hours preoperatively.

9. Surgery should be delayed 12–24 hours in patients receiving abciximab or thrombolytic therapy.

10. If the patient requires truly urgent or emergency surgery, platelets and clotting factors must be available to combat the lingering antihemostatic effects of any of the above drugs.

F. Diabetic patients should refrain from taking insulin or oral hypoglycemic medications after the preceding evening meal. The STS guidelines recommend that oral hypoglycemic medications should be withheld for 24 hours prior to surgery, which should allow for an early-morning dose on the day prior to surgery.[46] Blood glucose should be routinely checked in the operating room and treated with IV insulin to maintain the blood glucose <180 mg/dL.

G. Antiarrhythmic therapy should be continued until the time of surgery. Long-term use of **amiodarone** may be associated with postoperative respiratory failure, and it should be stopped as soon as surgery is being contemplated if there is evidence of any pulmonary complications. Otherwise, there is little benefit in stopping it for a short period of time to reduce perioperative risks because it has a very long half-life. Amiodarone may be used for AF prophylaxis, either starting with a preoperative oral load over several days (10 mg/kg/day) or initiating it IV in the operating room (see pages 623–624).

H. **Statins** should be given to all patients undergoing cardiac surgery, as they have been shown to reduce the risk of AF, delirium, and operative mortality.[165–169] Although several studies have shown a reduced risk of acute kidney injury after surgery in patients on statins,[168,169] one study of rosuvastatin showed that it increased that risk.[170]

I. Stress dose steroids are indicated in patients on chronic steroid therapy, usually for COPD or autoimmune disorders. Administration of perioperative steroids in other patients has marginal benefit.[171]

J. Preoperative prophylactic **antibiotics** must be administered before surgical incision. Vancomycin should be started within two hours of incision, and other antibiotics within one hour of incision.

1. A first-generation cephalosporin, such as cefazolin, is commonly chosen because of its effectiveness against Gram-positive organisms. There is some evidence that overall infection rates may be lower with use of a second-generation cephalosporin, such as cefuroxime.

2. Vancomycin is used if there is a severe allergy to penicillin or the cephalosporins and is often selected in patients undergoing valvular surgery because of its excellent efficacy against Gram-positive organisms. Since vancomycin provides poor Gram-negative coverage, the STS guidelines suggest that the addition of an aminoglycoside be considered to improve prophylaxis, although that is not a common practice.[172] Some centers will use both vancomycin and cefazolin or levofloxacin in penicillin-allergic patients. Vancomycin should not

be used indiscriminately, however, to minimize the emergence of strains of vancomycin-resistant enterococci, a growing concern in intensive care units. If the patient is allergic to vancomycin and it is preferred not to use a cephalosporin, daptomycin is the next best alternative.

K. Preoperative medications are ordered by the anesthesia service. Although some patients may benefit from receiving mild sedation "on-call" to the operating room, most patients are given midazolam and/or fentanyl by the anesthesiologist once the initial IV lines are inserted. The surgical or anesthesia team is responsible for ordering the preoperative antibiotics.

VIII. Preoperative Orders and Checklist

Once the patient has been accepted for surgery, orders should be placed to address general and patient specific concerns (tests, medications) before surgery. Standardized preprinted order sheets that are usually incorporated into computerized order sets are helpful and can be individualized as necessary (Table 3.6 and Appendix 2). The evening before surgery, the covering physician/physician assistant/nurse practitioner should write a brief preoperative note summarizing essential information that should be reviewed before proceeding with the operation. Writing this note prevents important details from being overlooked (Table 3.7 and Appendix 3). For patients undergoing elective surgery, the surgical team must take the responsibility of confirming that all of the requisite information has been reviewed, abnormalities addressed, and the information placed in the patient's office chart the night before admission to be available to the operating room when the patient arrives in the morning. The following should be noted:

A. The planned operative procedure

B. Indication for surgery

C. Brief summary of the cardiac catheterization data

D. Results of the laboratory data obtained

E. Surgical note and **consent** in chart

F. Anesthesia note and consent in chart

G. STS risk score (or EuroSCORE)

H. Confirmation of blood bank cross-match and blood setup

1. Guidelines for blood setup are shown in Table 3.8. One can generally determine the potential need for transfusion based on the patient's blood volume (which correlates with body size and usually with gender), and the preoperative hemoglobin level. More blood transfusions are commonly required during complex procedures requiring long durations of CPB, during which a large amount of crystalloid is usually given. Blood transfusions are indicated to maintain a satisfactory hematocrit (>18–20%) on pump.

2. Other comorbid factors that increase the need for transfusion include older age, urgent or emergent operations, poor ventricular function, reoperations, an elevated INR or use of preoperative antiplatelet drugs, insulin-dependent diabetes, PVD, chronic kidney disease, and an albumin <4 g/dL, consistent with poor nutrition.[173,174]

Table 3.6 • Typical Preoperative Order Sheet

1. Admit to: _____
2. Surgery date: _____
3. Planned procedure: _____
4. Diagnostic studies
   - ☐ CBC with differential
   - ☐ PT/INR ☐ PTT
   - ☐ Electrolytes, BUN, creatinine, blood glucose
   - ☐ Liver function tests (bilirubin, AST, ALT, alkaline phosphatase, albumin)
   - ☐ TSH level
   - ☐ Lipid profile
   - ☐ Hemoglobin A1c level
   - ☐ Urinalysis and urine culture, if indicated
   - ☐ Electrocardiogram
   - ☐ Chest x-ray PA and lateral
   - ☐ Room air oxygen saturation by pulse oximetry; obtain arterial blood gas if <90%
   - ☐ Antibody screen ☐ Crossmatch: ____ units packed red blood cells (PRBCs)
   - ☐ Carotid duplex studies
   - ☐ Bilateral digital radial artery studies
   - ☐ Bilateral venous mapping
   - ☐ Pulmonary function tests
   - ☐ Other: _____
5. Treatments/Assessments
   - ☐ Admission vital signs
   - ☐ Measure height and weight
   - ☐ NPO after midnight except sips of water with meds
   - ☐ Surgical clippers to remove hair at 5:00 AM morning of surgery from chest, legs, and both groins
   - ☐ Hibiclens scrub to chest and legs night before and AM of surgery
   - ☐ Incentive spirometry teaching
   - ☐ Smoking cessation education
6. Medications
   - ☐ Mupirocin 2% (Bactroban ointment): apply Q-tip nasal swabs the evening before and the morning of surgery
   - ☐ Chlorhexidine 0.12% (Peridex) gargle on-call to OR
   - ☐ Ascorbic acid 2 g at 9:00 PM night before surgery
   - ☐ Cefazolin ☐ 1 g IV ☐ 2 g IV – send to OR with patient
   - ☐ Vancomycin 20 mg/kg = _____ g IV – send to OR with patient
   - ☐ Discontinue P2Y12 inhibitor immediately (check with surgeon about PRU testing)
   - ☐ Reduce aspirin to 81 mg daily if patient on a higher dose
   - ☐ Discontinue NOAC after AM/PM dose on ___ (48 hours in advance of surgery)
   - ☐ Discontinue heparin at _____
   - ☐ Continue heparin drip into operating room
   - ☐ Discontinue low-molecular-weight heparin after AM/PM dose on _____
   - ☐ Discontinue IIb/IIIa inhibitor at 4:00 AM prior to surgery
   - ☐ Metoprolol ____ mg PO every 12 hours; hold for SBP <100 or HR <60 (CABG patients)
   - ☐ Discontinue ACE inhibitor or ARB morning of surgery
   - ☐ Discontinue all diabetic medications morning of surgery
   - ☐ Discontinue all diuretics morning of surgery

Table 3.7 • Preoperative Checklist (see also Appendix 3)

1. Planned operation: _____
2. Surgical note and consent obtained
3. Anesthesia consent in chart
4. Indication for surgery: _____
5. Brief summary of cardiac catheterization and echo results
6. STS risk score (or EuroSCORE)
7. Lab results
   a. Electrolytes, BUN, creatinine, blood glucose
   b. PT, PTT, platelet count, CBC
   c. Urinalysis
   d. Chest x-ray
   e. Electrocardiogram
   f. Additional test results: carotid studies, PFTs, vein mapping
8. Confirmation of blood bank setup
9. Preoperative orders written: antibiotics, medication changes
10. Confirmation with patient about cessation of medications

Table 3.8 • Blood Setup Guidelines for Open-Heart Surgery

Procedure	PRBC Setup
Minimally invasive CABG without pump	Type and screen
Weight >70 kg and hematocrit >35%	One unit
Weight <70 kg or hematocrit <35%	Two units
Reoperations	Three units
Ascending aortic surgery	Three units
Descending aortic surgery	Six units
PRBC, packed red blood cells	

I. Preoperative orders are written (in some hospitals, the anesthesia team is responsible for this):

1. Antibiotics: (always check for allergy)

   a. Cefazolin 1–2 g IV to be given in the operating room within one hour of incision. The dose should be weight-based. The STS recommendation is to give 1 g to patients <60 kg and 2 g for patients >60 kg.[172] Most groups routinely give 2 g to patients <120 kg and 3 g if >120 kg. An IV bolus injection achieves a peak plasma concentration within 20 minutes and peak interstitial levels within 60 minutes, so ideally, it should be given 20–30 minutes before surgery starts. Because the half-life of cefazolin is 1.8 hours and serum levels fall up to 50% on pump, an additional 1 g should be given on pump or every 3–4 hours during surgery.

b. Vancomycin 20 mg/kg to be started within two hours of surgery but infused over at least 30 minutes to avoid hypotension and the "red-neck syndrome".[172]

  i. It usually does not need to be redosed on pump.

  ii. The STS guidelines recommend a dose of 15 mg/kg, but most groups use a weight-based strategy of 20 mg/kg.[175] This produces more satisfactory vancomycin levels. A simple method that approximates precise weight-based dosing is to use 1 g for patients <80 kg, 1.5 g if 80–120 kg, and 2 g if >120 kg.

  iii. The STS guidelines provide a level IIb indication to also administer an aminoglycoside, such as gentamicin 4 mg/kg, to provide gram-negative coverage.[172]

2. Specific orders to stop medications listed in section VII, pages 198–199.

3. Antiseptic scrub (chlorhexidine) with which to shower the night before and the morning of surgery. Preferably, this should be applied several times rather than during a single shower.[176]

4. Mupirocin 2% (Bactroban) nasal ointment is effective in reducing nasal carriage of *S. aureus* and can reduce the incidence of surgical-site infections with these organisms. In patients who are not nasal carriers, mupirocin has no benefit and may potentially increase the risk of infection from antibiotic-resistant organisms.[177–180] If polymerase chain reaction (PCR) testing is available, mupirocin administration can be limited to patients who test positive for MRSA carriage. Otherwise, a routine policy of pre-, intra-, and a few days of postoperative nasal mupirocin can be recommended (one swab bid × three days).

5. Chlorhexidine 0.12% (Peridex) mouthwash

6. Skin preparation. This is best performed the morning of surgery, as it has been well documented that the closer the prep to the time of surgery, the lower the wound infection rate. Use of clippers is preferable to shaving with a razor, which increases the risk of infection.[181]

7. NPO after midnight

8. Preoperative medications per anesthesia service

J. For outpatients, it is important that documentation of a very brief updated history and physical exam be written in the medical record the day of surgery, indicating whether there has been any change since the patient's preoperative evaluation.

IX. Risk Assessment and Informed Consent

A. General comments

1. An important element of the preoperative preparation for cardiac surgery is an assessment of the patient's surgical risk. Risk stratification can afford patients and their families insight into the **real** risk of complications and mortality. It can also increase the awareness of the healthcare team to the high-risk patient for whom more aggressive therapy in the perioperative period may be beneficial. Documentation in the chart of an informed-consent discussion is **mandatory** prior to any cardiac surgical procedure. This note should quantify the predicted risk of operative mortality (PROM), preferably using the STS risk calculator (www.STS.org) or the EuroSCORE (www.euroscore.pil-media.com), should list some of the more common complications of the operation being performed, and should address risks that may be unique to the individual patient.

2. Although public reporting of hospitals' and individual surgeons' mortality rates is becoming more commonplace, the correlation of mortality with quality of care is imprecise. Mortality is more commonly related to the underlying cardiac disease and comorbidities and perhaps, most importantly, to patient selection. Nonetheless, the incidence of postoperative complications remains quite substantial, especially in older patient populations, and many of these complications are simply not preventable. Although the ability to predict and hopefully prevent postoperative complications may have some influence on overall mortality rates, it usually has more of an impact of the rapidity of the patient's recovery back to a satisfactory quality of life.

B. **Risk stratification** is based on an assessment of four important interrelated categories of risk factors, many of which are included in the STS and EuroSCORE risk models.

1. **Patient demographics.** These include patient-related factors independent of disease, such as age, gender, and race.

2. **Patient-related comorbidities.** These refer to coexisting diseases that are not necessarily directly related to the cardiac disease, but can have significant impact on the patient's ability to recover from surgery. In fact, in most patients, mortality and morbidity are related to preexisting issues, such as diabetes, renal dysfunction, cerebrovascular disease, and COPD. These render the patient more susceptible to the insults of CPB or to complications from a low cardiac output state. Abnormal lab tests (e.g. anemia, leukocytosis, elevated creatinine or blood sugar) that are linked to increased mortality are usually associated with patient comorbidities.

3. **Cardiac and procedure-related factors.** The clinical presentation (stable ischemic heart disease vs. acute coronary syndrome, recent MI, HF), nature and extent of cardiac disease (isolated CAD, associated valve disease, pulmonary hypertension), and the degree of ventricular dysfunction are important considerations in determining operative risk. Abnormal lab tests that reflect these conditions (elevated BNP, CRP, or troponin levels) are all associated with increased operative mortality.[13,152,182] For the vast majority of patients at low to moderate risk, these clinical factors generally do not raise the operative risk significantly. The extent of the planned operation raises the baseline risk, and reoperations nearly always double or triple the operative risk. Uncommon surgical situations, such as a very recent MI (within 24 hours), profound LV dysfunction (EF <20%), or cardiogenic shock with or without mechanical complications of infarction (ventricular septal rupture or papillary muscle rupture) are powerful risk factors for mortality. Postcardiotomy ventricular dysfunction can exacerbate organ system dysfunction related to preexisting comorbidities, such as chronic kidney disease, and may contribute to operative mortality.

4. **Preoperative status.** The immediate risk of death is greatest in patients requiring emergency surgery. Such patients usually have a "critical preoperative state" with unstable cardiac disease, which may include ongoing ischemia, hemodynamic compromise (such as cardiogenic shock) that requires inotropes or IABP support, or even ongoing cardiopulmonary resuscitation.

C. **Preoperative predictors of operative mortality**

1. Several risk models are available to determine a patient's operative risk. The STS risk model has been continuously upgraded with the incorporation of more data

entry points and is available online at www.sts.org under the "resources" and "risk calculator" links.[183,184] This model provides not just an estimated mortality but a delineation of the risk of re-exploration for bleeding, renal failure, wound infection, respiratory failure, and a length of stay (LOS) analysis. With appropriate data entry for each patient and quarterly submissions of data to the STS database, each cardiac surgical program is provided with risk-adjusted results and a comparison with STS benchmarks. The STS risk calculator has improved to include more lab tests and clinical conditions, but it is not inclusive of all factors that can influence operative risk. The STS risk model and the ASCERT long-term survival probability calculator (both available at www.sts.org) provide comparable information on long-term survival out to seven years.[185,186]

2. Another risk model is the EuroSCORE (see www.euroscore.pil-media.com). The initial additive EuroSCORE model tended to overestimate mortality in low-risk patients and underestimate it in high-risk patients compared with other risk models. A more sophisticated logistic EuroSCORE using a computerized model was then designed that appeared to be more accurate in predicting mortality in high-risk patients. These scoring systems were updated in 2011 to the EuroSCORE II model, which added such fields as LFTs and creatinine clearance and adjusted the weight of some variables. This system was also more applicable to types of surgery not included in the STS risk model.

3. Comparative studies suggest that the STS score and the EuroSCORE II score are comparable in predicting risk and are better than the original EuroSCORE system. However, based on the type of surgery being assessed, the STS model was felt to be most useful for patients having AVR or CABG–valve surgery, whereas the EuroSCORE II was more accurate for isolated CABGs and mitral valve surgery and was also more accurate in patients at high risk.[187]

4. Clinical conditions that are considered the most important risk factors for operative mortality include, in approximate decreasing order of significance:

   a. Emergency surgery, which includes some of the powerful but fairly uncommon risk factors (cardiogenic shock, ongoing CPR)

   b. Renal dysfunction

   c. Reoperations

   d. Older age (>75–80)

   e. Poor ventricular function (EF <30%)

   f. Female gender

   g. Left main disease

   h. Other comorbidities, such as COPD, PVD, diabetes, and cerebrovascular disease

D. Preoperative predictors of operative morbidity and their management

   1. Although the risk factors for morbidity and mortality may differ slightly, complications are more common when any of the problems just listed are present.[188] Although most factors are not modifiable, such as patient age, gender, redo status, urgency status, or the extent of cardiac disease, they do heighten awareness of the increased risk for postoperative complications. Recognizing preexisting organ system dysfunction or risk factors for their development is essential to reduce

postoperative morbidity and mortality. This is especially important in elderly patients, who are more predisposed to renal dysfunction, ventilatory issues, stroke, bleeding, and atrial arrhythmias. The risk ratios and mortality rates for some of the most significant postoperative complications are noted in Table 3.9. Although these data are somewhat dated, and hopefully results have improved since that time, they do delineate the importance of trying to avoid complications at all costs to optimize surgical outcomes. Concern about the following complications should prompt specific measures to prevent their occurrence or minimize their impact if they occur.

2. **Renal failure** that requires dialysis carries a mortality rate of nearly 50%. There are several models to predict the risks of postoperative acute kidney injury and the need for dialysis (see Figures 12.1–12.4, pages 684–686).[189,190] Optimizing renal function before, during, and after surgery is critical in patients with preexisting renal dysfunction. Even if dialysis is not required, chronic kidney disease is associated with increased operative mortality and reduced long-term survival (see Chapter 12).

Table 3.9 • Postoperative Complications of Coronary Bypass Surgery and Their Mortality Risks (STS database)*

Risk Variable	Incidence for First Operations	Risk Ratio	Mortality (%)
Multisystem failure	0.6	28.52	74.4
Cardiac arrest	1.3	29.63	64.1
Renal failure (dialysis)	0.8	17.61	47.6
Septicemia	0.9	13.92	38.6
Renal failure (no dialysis: creatinine >2.0)	2.8	13.53	30.6
Ventilated >5 days	5.5	10.73	21
Permanent stroke	1.5	10.35	28
Tamponade	0.3	8.25	25
Anticoagulation-related bleeding	0.4	8.23	25
Perioperative MI	1.2	6.64	19
GI complication	2.0	6.02	17
Re-exploration for bleeding	2.1	4.53	13
Deep sternal infection	0.6	3.74	11

*Data obtained from STS database website in mid-1990s; data no longer available

3. **Prolonged ventilation.** The STS database definition considers postoperative mechanical ventilation for over 24 hours, measured from the time the patient exits the operating room, to represent a postoperative complication. The operative mortality for patients requiring intubation for over five days is approximately 20%. Several risk models have been evaluated to predict the risk of postoperative prolonged ventilation (see Figure 10.2, page 471).[21,191] In patients with compromised pulmonary function, aggressive preoperative treatment of remediable conditions is essential. This may involve use of antibiotics for pulmonary infiltrates or bronchitis (and delay of surgery), bronchodilators for bronchospasm, diuresis for congestive HF, or even mechanical ventilation for hypoxemia or hypercarbia. Intraoperative management should entail judicious fluid administration, steps to reduce pulmonary artery pressures, steroids and bronchodilators for bronchospasm, and inotropic support if indicated. Postoperatively, aggressive diuresis as tolerated by hemodynamic performance, bronchodilators, early mobilization, and incentive spirometry are a few of the routine measures that can be utilized to minimize pulmonary morbidity (see Chapter 10).

4. Preexisting **cerebrovascular disease**, whether symptomatic or not, increases the risk of stroke. Oftentimes, it is a marker for severe atherosclerosis, and most strokes are related to aortic manipulation rather than to preexisting carotid disease. Although the overall risk of permanent stroke is only 1–2%, this incidence is higher in elderly patients. Development of a permanent perioperative stroke carries about a 25% mortality rate. Identifying carotid disease in patients at higher risk, using epiaortic imaging in the operating room to identify ascending aortic or arch atherosclerosis, using cerebral oximetry, maintaining a higher blood pressure on pump, or performing off-pump surgery are a few examples of measures that should be considered in elderly patients to reduce the risk of stroke and neurocognitive dysfunction.

5. **Mediastinal bleeding** remains a concern after all cardiac operations, whether performed on- or off-pump. It may result from surgical bleeding sites, a coagulopathy, or a combination of both. A higher prevalence is noted following more complex operations, especially valve surgery. Meticulous attention to hemostasis remains imperative, especially in elderly patients with poor tissue quality. Bleeding may produce hemodynamic compromise from a low output state or tamponade, and also increases the requirement for blood and blood component transfusions, which independently increase the risk of infection, respiratory failure, renal dysfunction, and mortality. Reoperation for bleeding and the development of tamponade carry significant mortality rates (about 13% and 25%, respectively).[192] Particular attention to modifying preoperative antiplatelet therapy or anticoagulants, use of antifibrinolytic drugs, and vigilance and patience in the operating room should minimize the risk of bleeding and its adverse consequences.

6. **Anticoagulation-related hemorrhage**, specifically delayed tamponade, is a potential complication of postoperative anticoagulation. Aspirin is routinely started within the first 24 hours after surgery once postoperative bleeding has tapered to a minimal level. Some surgeons use clopidogrel postoperatively, especially after OPCABs or CABG for non-STEMIs. Heparin may be given to patients with AF, for mechanical valve prostheses until warfarin has achieved a therapeutic INR, or for VTE prophylaxis. The risk of delayed bleeding is heightened

in patients receiving multiple antiplatelet or anticoagulant drugs, which may be indicated for several concurrent issues. One must always weigh the risks and benefits of early anticoagulation and maintain constant vigilance for the early clinical signs of delayed tamponade. This is an easily correctable problem if identified. If not, it can be lethal.

7. **Deep sternal wound infections** (DSWIs) occur in less than 1% of patients, but they can be difficult to treat. They occasionally occur in critically ill patients in the ICU and thus are associated with a significant mortality rate (about 10–20%). Treating infections noted preoperatively, using perioperative mupirocin in nasal carriers of S. *aureus*, administering prophylactic antibiotics appropriately in the operating room and continuing for no more than 48 hours, proper invasive line care, and strict control of intraoperative and postoperative hyperglycemia with an insulin protocol are essential in minimizing this problem. Unfortunately, it is highly unlikely that DSWIs can be entirely eliminated, no matter how ideal the care the patient receives.

References

1. Ad N, Henry L, Halpin L, et al. The use of spirometry testing prior to cardiac surgery may impact the Society of Thoracic Surgeons risk prediction score: a prospective study in a cohort of patients at high risk for chronic lung disease. *J Thorac Cardiovasc Surg* 2010;139:686–91.
2. Adabag AS, Wassif HS, Rice K, et al. Preoperative pulmonary function and mortality after cardiac surgery. *Am Heart J* 2010;159:691–7.
3. Angouras DC, Anagnostopoulos CE, Chamogeorgakis TP, et al. Postoperative and long-term outcome of patients with chronic obstructive pulmonary disease undergoing coronary artery bypass grafting. *Ann Thorac Surg* 2010;89:1112–8.
4. Manganas H, Lacasse Y, Bourgeois S, Perron J, Dagenais F, Maltais F. Postoperative outcome after coronary artery bypass grafting in chronic obstructive pulmonary disease. *Can Respir J* 2007;14:19–24.
5. Najafi M, Sheikhvatan M, Mortazavi SH. Do preoperative pulmonary function indices predict morbidity after coronary artery bypass surgery? *Ann Card Anaesth* 2015;18:293–8.
6. Saleh HZ, Mohan K, Shaw M, et al. Impact of chronic obstructive pulmonary disease on surgical outcomes in patients undergoing non-emergent coronary artery bypass grafting. *Eur J Cardiothorac Surg* 2012;42:108–13.
7. Fuster RG, Argudo JA, Albarova OG, et al. Prognostic value of chronic obstructive pulmonary disease in coronary artery bypass grafting. *Eur J Cardiothorac Surg* 2006;29:202–9.
8. Sharif-Kashani B, Shahabi P, Mandegar MH, et al. Smoking and wound complications after coronary artery bypass grafting. *J Surg Res* 2016;200:743–8.
9. Almassi GH, Shroyer AL, Collins JF, et al. Chronic obstructive pulmonary disease impact upon outcomes: the Veteran Affairs Randomized On-Off Bypass Trial. *Ann Thorac Surg* 2013;96:1302–9.
10. McKeon J, Mckeon N, Stevens S, Stewart H. Respiratory function tests prior to cardiac surgery: prediction of post-operative outcomes. *Eur Resp J* 2014;44:1268.
11. Jeong DS, Kim KH, Kim CY, Kim JS. Relationship between plasma B-type natriuretic peptide and ventricular function in adult cardiac surgery patients. *J Int Med Res* 2008;36:31–9.
12. Mueller C, Scholer A, Laule-Kilian K, et al. Use of B-type natriuretic peptide in the evaluation and management of acute dyspnea. *N Engl J Med* 2004;350:647–54.
13. Fox AA, Shernan SK, Collard CD, et al. Preoperative B-type natriuretic peptide is an independent predictor of ventricular dysfunction and mortality after primary coronary artery bypass grafting. *J Thorac Cardiovasc Surg* 2008;136:452–61.
14. Ramkumar N, Jacobs JP, Berman RB, et al. Cardiac biomarkers predict long-term survival after cardiac surgery. *Ann Thorac Surg* 2019;108:1776–82.
15. Eliasdóttir SV, Klemenzson G, Torfason B, Valsson F. Brain natriuretic peptide is a good predictor for outcome in cardiac surgery. *Acta Anaesthesiol Scand* 2008;52:182–7.

16. Murad Junior JA, Nakazone MA, Machado Mde N, Godoy MF. Predictors of mortality in cardiac surgery: brain natriuretic peptide type B. *Rev Bras Cir Cardiovasc.* 2015;30:182–7.

17. Januzzi JL, van Kimmenade R, Lainchbury J, et al. NT-proBNP testing for diagnosis and short-term prognosis in acute destabilized heart failure: an international pooled analysis of 1256 patients: the International Collaborative of NT-proBNP Study. *Eur Heart J* 2006;27:330–7.

18. Hulzebos EH, Van Meeteren NL, De Bie RA, Dagnelie PC, Helders PJ. Prediction of postoperative pulmonary complications on the basis of preoperative risk factors in patients who had undergone coronary artery bypass graft surgery. *Phys Ther* 2003;83:8–16.

19. Rady MY, Ryan T, Starr NJ. Early onset of acute pulmonary dysfunction after cardiovascular surgery: risk factors and clinical outcome. *Crit Care Med* 1997;25:1831–9.

20. Al-Sarraf N, Thalib L, Hughes A, Tolan M, Young V, McGovern E. Effect of smoking on short-term outcome of patients undergoing coronary artery bypass surgery. *Ann Thorac Surg* 2008;86:517–23.

21. Filsoufi F, Rahmanian PB, Castillo JG, Chikwe J, Adams DH. Logistic risk model predicting postoperative respiratory failure in patients undergoing valve surgery. *Eur J Cardiothorac Surg* 2008;34:953–9.

22. Nakagawa M, Tanaka H, Tsukuma H, Kishi Y. Relationship between the duration of the preoperative smoke-free period and the incidence of postoperative pulmonary complications after pulmonary surgery. *Chest* 2001;120:705–10.

23. Buja A, Zampieron A, Cavalet S, et al. An update review on risk factors and scales for prediction of deep sternal wound infections. *Int Wound J* 2012;9:372–86.

24. Hulzebos EHJ, Helders PJ, Favié NJ, De Bie RA, Brutel de la Riviere AB, Van Meeteren NL. Preoperative intensive inspiratory muscle training to prevent postoperative pulmonary complications in high-risk patients undergoing CABG surgery: a randomized clinical trial. *JAMA* 2006;296:1851–7.

25. Mickleborough LL, Maruyama H, Mohamed S, et al. Are patients receiving amiodarone at increased risk for cardiac operations? *Ann Thorac Surg* 1994;58:622–9.

26. Kaushik S, Hussain A, Clarke P, Lazar HL. Acute pulmonary toxicity after low-dose amiodarone therapy. *Ann Thorac Surg* 2001;72:1760–1.

27. Lopez-Delgado JC, Esteve F, Javierre C, et al. Influence of cirrhosis in cardiac surgery outcomes. *World J Hepatol* 2015;7:753–60.

28. Thielmann M, Mechmet A, Neuhäuser M, et al. Risk prediction and outcomes in patients with liver cirrhosis undergoing open-heart surgery. *Eur J Cardiothorac Surg* 2010;38:592–9.

29. Jacob JA, Hjortnaes J, Kranenburg G, de Heer F, Kluin J. Mortality after cardiac surgery in patients with liver cirrhosis classified by the Child-Pugh score. *Interact Cardiovasc Thorac Surg* 2015;20:520–30.

30. Lin CH, Hsu RB. Cardiac surgery in patients with liver cirrhosis: risk factors for predicting mortality. *World J Gastroenterol* 2014;20:12608–14.

31. Morimoto N, Okada K, Okita Y. The model for end-stage liver diseases (MELD) predicts early and late outcomes of cardiovascular operations in patients with liver cirrhosis. *Ann Thorac Surg* 2013;96:1672–8.

32. Morisaki A, Hosono M, Sasaki Y, et al. Risk factor analysis in patients with liver cirrhosis undergoing cardiovascular operations. *Ann Thorac Surg* 2010;89:811–8.

33. Gopaldas RR, Chu D, Cornwell DD, et al. Cirrhosis as a moderator of outcomes in coronary artery bypass grafting and off-pump coronary artery bypass operations: a 12 year population-based study. *Ann Thorac Surg* 2013;96:1310–5.

34. Luciani N, Nasso G, Gaudino M, et al. Coronary artery bypass grafting in type II diabetic patients: a comparison between insulin-dependent and non-insulin-dependent patients at short- and mid-term follow-up. *Ann Thorac Surg* 2003;76:1149–54.

35. Marcheix B, Vanden Eynden F, Demers P, Bouchard D, Cartier R. Influence of diabetes mellitus on long-term survival in systematic off-pump coronary artery bypass surgery. *Ann Thorac Surg* 2008;86:1181–8.

36. Hueb W, Gersh BJ, Costa F, et al. Impact of diabetes on five-year outcomes of patients with multivessel coronary artery disease. *Ann Thorac Surg* 2007;83:93–9.

37. Mohammadi S, Dagenais F, Mathieu P, et al. Long-term impact of diabetes and its comorbidities in patients undergoing isolated primary coronary artery bypass graft surgery. *Circulation* 2007;116(suppl I):I220–5.

38. Kogan A, Ram E, Levin S, et al. Impact of type 2 diabetes mellitus on short- and long-term mortality after coronary artery bypass surgery. *Cardiovascular Diabetology* 2018;17:151.

39. Singh SK, Desai ND, Petroff SD, et al. The impact of diabetic status on coronary artery bypass graft patency: insights from the radial artery patency study. *Circulation* 2008;118(suppl 1):S222–5.

40. Halkos ME, Lattouf OM, Puskas JD, et al. Elevated preoperative hemoglobin A1c is associated with reduced long-term survival after coronary artery bypass surgery. *Ann Thorac Surg* 2008;86:1431–7.

41. Alserius T, Anderson RE, Hammar N, Nordqvist T, Ivert T. Elevated glycosylated haemoglobin (HbA1c) is a risk marker in coronary artery bypass surgery. *Scand Cardiovasc J* 2008;42:392–8.

42. Kim HJ, Shim JK, Youn YN, Song JW, Lee H, Kwak YL. Influence of preoperative hemoglobin A1c on early outcomes in patients with diabetes mellitus undergoing off-pump coronary artery bypass surgery. *J Thorac Cardiovasc Surg* 2020;159:568–76.

43. Tennyson C, Lee R, Attia R. Is there a role for HbA1c in predicting mortality and morbidity outcomes after coronary artery bypass graft surgery? *Interact Cardiovasc Thorac Surg* 2013;17:1000–8.

44. Halkos ME, Puskas JD, Lattouf OM, et al. Elevated preoperative hemoglobin A1c level is predictive of adverse events after coronary artery bypass surgery. *J Thorac Cardiovasc Surg* 2008;136:631–40.

45. Reddy P, Duggar B, Butterworth J. Blood glucose management in the patient undergoing cardiac surgery: a review. *World J Cardiol* 2014;26:1209–17.

46. Lazar HL, McDonnell M, Chipkin SR, et al. The Society of Thoracic Surgeons practice guidelines series: blood glucose management during adult cardiac surgery. *Ann Thorac Surg* 2009;87:663–9.

47. Navaratnarajah M, Rea R, Evans R, et al. Effect of glycaemic control on complications following cardiac surgery: literature review. *J Cardiothorac Surg* 2018;13:10.

48. Savage EB, Grab JD, O'Brien SM, et al. Use of both internal thoracic arteries in diabetic patients increases deep sternal wound infection. *Ann Thorac Surg* 2007;83:1002–7.

49. Nakano J, Okabayashi H, Hanyu M, et al. Risk factors for wound infection after off-pump coronary artery bypass grafting: should bilateral internal thoracic arteries be harvested in patients with diabetes? *J Thorac Cardiovasc Surg* 2008;135:540–5.

50. Crawford TC, Zhou X, Fraser CD III, et al. Bilateral internal mammary artery use in diabetic patients: friend or foe? *Ann Thorac Surg* 2018;106:1088–94.

51. Deo SV, Shah IK, Dunlay SM, et al. Bilateral internal thoracic artery harvest and deep sternal wound infection in diabetic patients. *Ann Thorac Surg* 2013;95:862–9.

52. Iribarne A, Westbrook BM, Malenka DJ, et al. Should diabetes be a contraindication to bilateral internal mammary artery grafting? *Ann Thorac Surg* 2018;105:709–14.

53. Yamazaki K, Kato H, Tsujimoto S, Kitamura R. Diabetes mellitus, internal thoracic artery grafting, and the risk of an elevated hemidiaphragm after coronary artery bypass surgery. *J Cardiothorac Vasc Anesth* 1994;8:437–40.

54. Rys P, Woyciechowski P, Rogoz-Sitek A, et al. Systematic review and meta-analysis of randomized clinical trials comparing efficacy and safety outcomes of insulin glargine with NPH insulin, premixed insulin preparation or insulin detemir in type 2 diabetes mellitus. *Acta Diabetol* 2015;52:649–62.

55. Shokri H, Ali I, El Sayed HM. Protamine adverse reactions in NPH insulin treated diabetics undergoing coronary artery bypass grafting. *Egypt J Cardiothorac Anesth* 2016;10:25–30.

56. Halkos ME, Puskas JD, Lattouf OM, Kilgo P, Guyton RA, Thourani VH. Impact of preoperative neurologic events on outcomes after coronary artery bypass grafting. *Ann Thorac Surg* 2008;86:504–10.

57. Redmond JM, Greene PS, Goldsborough MA, et al. Neurologic injury in cardiac surgical patients with a history of stroke. *Ann Thorac Surg* 1996;61:42–7.

58. Durand DJ, Perler BA, Roseborough GS, et al. Mandatory versus selective preoperative carotid screening: a retrospective analysis. *Ann Thorac Surg* 2004;78:159–66.

59. Salasidis GC, Latter DA, Steinmetz OK, Blair JF, Graham AM. Carotid artery duplex scanning in preoperative assessment for coronary artery revascularization: the association between peripheral vascular disease, carotid artery stenosis, and stroke. *J Vasc Surg* 1995;21:154–80.

60. Manetta F, Yu PJ, Mattia A, Karaptis JC, Hartman AR. Bedside vein mapping for conduit size in coronary artery bypass surgery. *JSLS* 2017;21:pii:e2016.00083. doi: 10.4293/JSLS.2016.00083.

61. Denton TA, Trento L, Cohen M, et al. Radial artery harvesting for coronary bypass operations: neurologic complications and their potential mechanisms. *J Thorac Cardiovasc Surg* 2001;121:951–6.

62. Siminelakis S, Karfis E, Anagnostopolous C, Toumpoulis I, Katsaraki A, Drossos G. Harvesting radial artery and neurologic complications. *J Card Surg* 2004;19:505–10.

63. Shah SA, Chark D, Williams J, et al. Retrospective analysis of local sensorimotor deficits after radial artery harvesting for coronary artery bypass grafting. *J Surg Res* 2007;139:203–8.

64. Allen RH, Szabo RM, Chen JL. Outcome assessment of hand function after radial artery harvesting for coronary artery disease. *J Hand Surg (Am)* 2004;29:628–37.

65. Krag M, Marker S, Perner A, et al. Pantoprazole in patients at risk for gastrointestinal bleeding in the ICU. *N Engl J Med* 2018;379:2199–208.

66. Cook D, Guyatt G. Prophylaxis against upper gastrointestinal bleeding in hospitalized patients. *N Engl J Med* 2018;378:2506–16.

67. Shin JS, Abah U. Is routine stress ulcer prophylaxis of benefit for patients undergoing cardiac surgery? *Interact Cardiovasc Thorac Surg* 2012;14:622–8.

68. Alquraini M, Alshamsi F, Møller MH, et al. Sucralfate versus histamine 2 receptor antagonists for stress ulcer prophylaxis in adult critically ill patients: a meta-analysis and trial sequential analysis of randomized trials. *J Crit Care* 2017;40:21–30.

69. van Rijen MM, Bonten M, Wenzel R, Kluytmans JA. Intranasal mupirocin for reduction of *Staphylococcus aureus* infections in surgical patients with nasal carriage: a systematic review. *Antimicrob Chemother* 2008;61:254–61.

70. Shrestha NK, Banbury MK, Weber M, et al. Safety of targeted perioperative mupirocin treatment for preventing infections after cardiac surgery. *Ann Thorac Surg* 2006;81:2183–8.

71. Terezhallmy GT, Safaddi TJ, Longworth DL, Muercke DD. Oral disease burden in patients undergoing prosthetic heart valve implantation. *Ann Thorac Surg* 1997;63:402–4.

72. Yaony JS, Silvay G. The value of optimizing dentition before cardiac surgery. *J Cardiothorac Vasc Anesth* 2007;21:587–91.

73. Smith MM, Barbara DW, Mauermann WJ, Viozzi CF, Dearani JA, Grim KJ. Morbidity and mortality associated with dental extraction before cardiac operation. *Ann Thorac Surg* 2014;97:838–44.

74. D'Agostino RS, Svensson LG, Neumann DJ, Balkhy HH, Williamson WA, Shahian DM. Screening carotid ultrasonography and risk factors for stroke in coronary artery surgery patients. *Ann Thorac Surg* 1996;62:1714–23.

75. Hirotani T, Kameda T, Kumamoto T, Shirota S, Yamano M. Stroke after coronary artery bypass grafting in patients with cerebrovascular disease. *Ann Thorac Surg* 2000;70:1571–6.

76. Borger MA, Fremes SE, Weisel RD, et al. Coronary bypass and carotid endarterectomy: does a combined approach increase risk? A meta-analysis. *Ann Thorac Surg* 1999;68:14–21.

77. Sharma V, Deo SV, Park SJ, Joyce LD. Meta-analysis of staged versus combined carotid endarterectomy and coronary artery bypass grafting. *Ann Thorac Surg* 2014;97:102–10.

78. Shishehbor MH, Venkatachalam S, Sun Z, et al. A direct comparison of early and late outcomes with three approaches to carotid revascularization and open heart surgery. *J Am Coll Cardiol* 2013;62:1948–56.

79. Akins CW, Hilgenberg AD, Vlahakes GJ, et al. Late results of combined carotid and coronary surgery using actual versus actuarial methodology. *Ann Thorac Surg* 2005;80:2091–7.

80. Clark CE, Gaylor RS, Shore AC, Okoumunne OC, Campbell JL. Association of a difference in systolic blood pressure between arms with vascular disease and mortality: a systematic review and meta-analysis. *Lancet* 2012;379:905–14.

81. van Straten AH, Firanescu C, Soliman Hamad MA, et al. Peripheral vascular disease as a predictor of survival after coronary artery bypass grafting: comparison with a matched general population. *Ann Thorac Surg* 2010;89:414–20.

82. Chu D, Bakaeen FG, Wang XL, et al. The impact of peripheral vascular disease on long-term survival after coronary artery bypass graft surgery. *Ann Thorac Surg* 2008;86:1175–80.

83. Nakamura T, Toda K, Miyagawa S, et al. Symptomatic peripheral artery disease is associated with decreased long-term survival after coronary artery bypass: a contemporary retrospective analysis. *Surg Today* 2016;46:1334–40.

84. Sinclair MC, Singer RL, Manley NJ, Montesano RM. Cannulation of the axillary artery for cardiopulmonary bypass: safeguards and pitfalls. *Ann Thorac Surg* 2003;75:931–4.

85. Aboul-Hassan SS, Stankowski T, Marczak J, et al. The use of preoperative aspirin in cardiac surgery: a systematic review and meta-analysis. *J Card Surg* 2017;32:758–74.

86. Hastings S, Myles P, McIlroy D. Aspirin and coronary artery surgery: a systematic review and meta-analysis. *Br J Anaesth* 2015;115:378–85.

87. Hastings S, Myles PS, McIlroy DR. Aspirin and coronary artery surgery: an updated meta-analysis. *Br J Anaesth* 2016;116:716–7.

88. Myles PS, Smith JA, Forbes A, et al. Stopping vs. continuing aspirin before coronary artery surgery. *N Engl J Med* 2016;374:728–37.

89. Ferraris VA, Saha SP, Oestreich JH, et al. 2012 Update to the Society of Thoracic Surgeons Guideline on use of antiplatelet drugs in patients having cardiac and noncardiac operations. *Ann Thorac Surg* 2012;94:1761–81.

90. Mahla E, Metzler H, Tantry US, Gurbel PA. Controversies in oral antiplatelet therapy in patients undergoing aortocoronary bypass surgery. *Ann Thorac Surg* 2010;90:1040–51.

91. Santilli F, Rocca B, De Cristofaro R, et al. Platelet cyclooxygenase inhibition by low-dose aspirin is not reflected consistently by platelet function assays: implications for aspirin "resistance". *J Am Coll Cardiol* 2009;53:667–77.

92. Suwalski G, Suwalski P, Filipiak KJ, Postula M, Majstrak F, Opolski G. The effect of off-pump coronary artery bypass grafting on platelet activation in patients on aspirin until surgery day. *Eur J Cardiothorac Surg* 2008;34:365–9.

93. Gluckman TJ, McLean RC, Schulman SP, et al. Effects of platelet responsiveness and platelet reactivity on early vein graft thrombosis after coronary artery bypass graft surgery. *J Am Coll Cardiol* 2011;57:1069–77.

94. Bednar F, Osmancik P, Vanek T, et al. Platelet activity and aspirin efficacy after off-pump compared with on-pump coronary artery bypass surgery: results from the prospective randomized trial (PRAGUE 11-Coronary Artery Bypass and REactivity of Thrombocytes CABARET). *J Thorac Cardiovasc Surg* 2008;136:1054–60.

95. Balotta A, Saleh HZ, El Baghdady HW, et al. Comparison of early platelet activation in patients undergoing on-pump versus off-pump coronary artery bypass surgery. *J Thorac Cardiovasc Surg* 2007;134:132–8.

96. Wu H, Wang J, Sun H, et al. Preoperative continuation of aspirin therapy may improve perioperative saphenous venous graft patency after off-pump coronary artery bypass grafting. *Ann Thorac Surg* 2015;99:576–81.

97. Misumida N, Abo-Aly M, Kim SM, Ogunbayo GO, Abdel-Latif A, Ziada KM. Efficacy and safety of short-term dual antiplatelet therapy (≤6 months) after percutaneous coronary intervention for acute coronary syndrome: a systematic review and meta-analysis of randomized controlled trials. *Clin Cardiol* 2018;41:1455–62.

98. Gurbel PA, Bliden KP, Butler K, et al. Randomized double-blind assessment of the ONSET and OFFSET of the antiplatelet effects of ticagrelor versus clopidogrel in patients with stable coronary artery disease: the ONSET/OFFSET study. *Circulation* 2009;120:2577–85.

99. Droppa M, Spahn P, Takhgiriev K, et al. Periprocedural platelet inhibition with cangrelor in P2Y-inhibitor naive patients with acute coronary syndromes: a matched-control pharmacodynamic comparison in real-world patients. *Int J Cardiol* 2016;223:848–51.

100. Herman CR, Buth KJ, Kent BA, Hirsch GM. Clopidogrel increases blood transfusion and hemorrhagic complications in patients undergoing cardiac surgery. *Ann Thorac Surg* 2010;89:397–402.

101. Kwak YL, Kim JC, Choi YS, Yoo KJ, Song Y, Shim JK. Clopidogrel responsiveness regardless of the discontinuation date predicts increased blood loss and transfusion requirement after off-pump coronary artery bypass graft surgery. *J Am Coll Cardiol* 2010;56:1994–2002.

102. Mahla E, Suarez TA, Bliden KP, et al. Platelet function measurement-based strategy to reduce bleeding and waiting time in clopidogrel-treated patients undergoing coronary artery bypass graft surgery: the timing based on platelet function strategy to reduce clopidogrel-associated bleeding related to CABG (TARGET-CABG) Study. *Circ Cardiovasc Interv* 2012;5:261–9.

103. Abualsaud AO, Eisenberg MG. Perioperative management of patients with drug-eluting stents. *J Am Coll Cardiol Intv* 2010;3:131–42.

104. Shi J, Wang G, Lv H, et al. Tranexamic acid in on-pump coronary artery bypass grafting without clopidogrel and aspirin cessation: randomized trial and 1-year follow-up. *Ann Thorac Surg* 2013;95:793–802.

105. McDonald SB, Renna M, Spitznagel EL, et al. Preoperative use of enoxaparin increases the risk of postoperative bleeding and re-exploration in cardiac surgery patients. *J Cardiothorac Vasc Anesth* 2005;19:4–10.

106. Fiore MM, Mackie IM. Mechanism of low-molecular-weight heparin reversal by platelet factor 4. *Throm Res* 2009;124:149–55.

107. Nishimura RA, Otto CM, Bonow RO, et al. 2017 AHA/ACC Focused Update of the 2014 AHA/ACC Guideline for the management of patients with valvular heart disease: A Report of the American College of Cardiology/American Heart Association Task Force on Clinical Practice Guidelines. *Circulation* 2017;1335:e1159–95.

108. Doherty JU, Gluckman TJ, Hucker WJ, et al. 2017 ACC Expert consensus decision pathway for periprocedural management of anticoagulation in patients with nonvalvular atrial fibrillation. *J Am Coll Cardiol* 2017;69:871–92.

109. Yasaka M, Sakata T, Naritomi H, Minematsu K. Optimal dose of prothrombin complex concentrate for acute reversal of oral anticoagulation. *Thromb Res* 2005;115:455–9.

110. Tompkins C, Cheng A, Dalal D, et al. Dual antiplatelet therapy and heparin "bridging" significantly increases the risk of bleeding complications after pacemaker or implantable cardioverter-defibrillator device implantation. *J Am Coll Cardiol* 2010;55:2376–82.

111. Renda G, Ricci F, Giugliano RP, De Caterina R. Non-vitamin K antagonist oral anticoagulants in patients with atrial fibrillation and valvular heart disease. *J Am Coll Cardiol* 2017;69:1363–71.

112. Hassan K, Bayer N, Schlingloff F, et al. Bleeding complications after use of novel oral anticoagulants in patients undergoing cardiac surgery. *Ann Thorac Surg* 2018;105:702–8.

113. Chun R, Orser BA, Madan M. Platelet glycoprotein IIb/IIIa inhibitors: overview and implications for the anesthesiologist. *Anesth Analg* 2002;95:879–88.

114. Bizzari F, Scolletta S, Tucci E, et al. Perioperative use of tirofiban hydrochloride (Aggrastat) does not increase surgical bleeding after emergency or urgent coronary artery bypass grafting. *J Thorac Cardiovasc Surg* 2001;122:1181–5.

115. Silvestry SC, Smith PK. Current status of cardiac surgery in the Abciximab-treated patient. *Ann Thorac Surg* 2000;70:S12–9.

116. Poullis M, Manning R, Haskard D, Taylor K. ReoPro removal during cardiopulmonary bypass using a hemoconcentrator. *J Thorac Cardiovasc Surg* 1999;117:1032–4.

117. Schafer AI. Effects of nonsteroidal anti-inflammatory therapy on platelets. *Am J Med* 1999;106:S25–36.

118. Langlois PL, Hardy G, Manzanares W. Omega-3 polyunsaturated fatty acids in cardiac surgery: an updated systematic review and meta-analysis. *Clin Nutri* 2017;36:737–46.

119. Carr JA. Role of fish oil in post-cardiotomy bleeding: a summary of the basic science and clinical trials. *Ann Thorac Surg* 2018;105:1563–7.

120. Akintoye E, Sethi P, Harris WS, et al. Fish oil and perioperative bleeding: insights from the OPERA randomized trial. *Circulation: Cardiovasc Qual Outcomes* 2018;11:e004584.

121. Celestini A, Pulcinelli FM, Pignatelli P, et al. Vitamin E potentiates the antiplatelet activity of aspirin in collagen-stimulated platelets. *Haematologica* 2002;87:420–6.

122. Antiplatelet effects of herbal products. *Dermatol Nurs* 2002;14:207.

123. Valli G, Giardina EGV. Benefits, adverse effects, and drug interactions of herbal therapies with cardiovascular effects. *J Am Coll Cardiol* 2002;39:1083–95.

124. Freedman JE, Parker C III, Li L, et al. Select flavonoids and whole juice from purple grapes inhibit platelet function and enhance nitric oxide release. *Circulation* 2001;103:2792–8.

125. Seki T, Shingu Y, Sugiki H, et al. Anticoagulation management during cardiopulmonary bypass in patients with antiphospholipid syndrome. *J Artif Organs* 2018;21:363–6.

126. Mishra PK, Khazi RM, Yiu P, Billing JS. Severe antiphospholipid syndrome and cardiac surgery: perioperative management. *Asian Cardiovasc Thorac Ann* 2016;24:473–6.

127. Avidan MS, Levy JH, van Aken H, et al. Recombinant human antithrombin III restores heparin responsiveness and decreases activation of coagulation in heparin-resistant patients during cardiopulmonary bypass. *J Thorac Cardiovasc Surg* 2005;130:107–13.

128. Williams ML, He X, Rankin JS, Slaughter MS, Gammie JS. Preoperative hematocrit is a powerful predictor of adverse outcomes in coronary artery bypass graft surgery: a report from the Society of Thoracic Surgeons adult cardiac surgery database. *Ann Thor Surg* 2013;96:1628–34.

129. Scrascia G, Guida P, Caparrotti SM, et al. Incremental value of anemia in cardiac surgical risk prediction with the European System for Cardiac Operative Risk Evaluation (EuroSCORE) II model. *Ann Thorac Surg* 2014;98:869–76.

130. Padmanabhan H, Siau K, Curtis J, et al. Preoperative anemia and outcomes in cardiovascular surgery: systematic review and meta-analysis. *Ann Thorac Surg* 2019;108:1840–8.

131. LaPar DJ, Hawkins RB, McMurry TL, et al. Preoperative anemia versus blood transfusion: which is the culprit for worse outcomes in cardiac surgery? *J Thorac Cardiovasc Surg* 2018;156:66–74.

132. Engoren M, Schwann TA, Jewell E, et al. Is transfusion associated with graft occlusion after cardiac operations? *Ann Thorac Surg* 2015;99:502–8.

133. Arias-Morales CE, Stoicea N, Gonzalez-Zacarias AA, et al. Revisiting blood transfusion and predictors of outcome in cardiac surgery patients: a concise perspective. *F1000Res* 2017; 6: F1000 Faculty Rev–168.

134. Crawford TC, Magruder JT, Fraser C, et al. Less is more: results of a statewide analysis of the impact of blood transfusion on coronary artery bypass outcomes. *Ann Thorac Surg* 2018;105:129–36.

135. Rawn JD. Blood transfusion in cardiac surgery: a silent epidemic revisited. *Circulation* 2007;116:2523–4.

136. Kilic A, Whitman GJR. Blood transfusions in cardiac surgery: indications, risks, and conservation strategies. *Ann Thorac Surg* 2014;97:726–34.

137. Chen QH, Wang HL, Liu L, Shao J, Yu J, Zheng RQ. Effects of restrictive red blood cell transfusion on the prognoses of adult patients undergoing cardiac surgery: a meta-analysis of randomized controlled trials. *Crit Care* 2018;22:142.

138. Mazer CD, Whitlock RP, Fergusson DA, et al. Six-month outcomes after restrictive or liberal transfusion for cardiac surgery. *N Engl J Med* 2018;379:1224–33.

139. Kheiri B, Abdalla A, Osman M, et al. Restrictive versus liberal red blood cell transfusion for cardiac surgery: a systematic review and meta-analysis of randomized controlled trials. *J Thromb Thrombolysis* 2019;47:179–85.

140. Dacey LJ, DeSimone J, Braxton JH, et al. Preoperative white blood cell count and mortality and morbidity after coronary artery bypass grafting. *Ann Thorac Surg* 2003;76:760–4.

141. Newall N, Grayson AD, Oo AY, et al. Preoperative white blood cell count is independently associated with higher perioperative cardiac enzyme release and increased 1-year mortality after coronary artery bypass grafting. *Ann Thorac Surg* 2006;81:583–90.

142. Salter BS, Weiner MM, Trinh MA, et al. Heparin-induced thrombocytopenia: a comprehensive clinical review. *J Am Coll Cardiol* 2016;67:2519–32.

143 Cooper WA, O'Brien SM, Thourani VH, et al. Impact of renal dysfunction on outcomes of coronary artery bypass surgery: results from the Society of Thoracic Surgeons National Adult Cardiac Database. *Circulation* 2006;113:1063–70.

144. Brown JR, Cochran RP, MacKenzie TA, et al. Long-term survival after cardiac surgery is predicted by estimated glomerular filtration rate. *Ann Thorac Surg* 2008;86:4–11.

145. Hu Y, Zhiping L, Chen J, Shen C, Song Y, Zhong Q. The effect of the time interval between coronary angiography and on-pump cardiac surgery on risk of postoperative acute kidney injury: a meta-analysis. *J Cardiothorac Surg* 2013;8:178.

146. Lee EH, Chin JH, Joung KW, et al. Impact of the time of coronary angiography on acute kidney injury after elective off-pump coronary artery bypass surgery. *Ann Thorac Surg* 2013;96:1635–42.

147. Crestellano JA, Phillips G, Firstenberg MS, et al. Preoperative hyponatremia predicts outcomes after cardiac surgery. *J Surg Res* 2013;181:60–6.

148. Leung AA, McAlister FA, Rogers SO Jr, Pazo V, Wright A, Bates DW. Preoperative hyponatremia and perioperative complications. *Arch Intern Med* 2012;172:1474–81.

149. Braun MM, Barstow CH, Pyzocha NJ. Diagnosis and management of sodium disorders: hyponatremia and hypernatremia. *Am Fam Physician* 2015;91:299–307.

150. Hannan EL, Qian F, Pine M, Fry DE, Whitman K, Dennison BA. The value of adding laboratory data to coronary artery bypass grafting registry data to improve models for risk-adjusting provider mortality rates. *Ann Thorac Surg* 2015;99:495–501.

151. Burch HB. Drug effects on the thyroid. *N Engl J Med* 2019;381:749–61.

152. van Straten AHM, Soliman Hamad M, van Zundert AJ, et al. Preoperative C-reactive protein levels to predict early and late mortalities after coronary artery bypass surgery: eight years of follow-up. *J Thorac Cardiovasc Surg* 2009;138:954–8.

153. Karkouti K, McCluskey S. Pro: preoperative autologous blood donation has a role in cardiac surgery. *J Cardiothorac Vasc Anesth* 2003;17:121–5.

154. Alghamdi AA, Albanna MJ, Guru V, Brister SJ. Does the use of erythropoietin reduce the risk of exposure to allogeneic blood transfusion in cardiac surgery? A systematic review and meta-analysis. *J Card Surg* 2008;21:320–6.

155. Weltert L, Rondinelli B, Bello R, et al. A single dose of erythropoietin reduces perioperative transfusions in cardiac surgery: results of a prospective single-blind randomized controlled trial. *Transfusion* 2015;55:1644–54.

156. Yoo YC, Shim JK, Kim JC, Jo YY, Lee JH, Kwak YL. Effect of single recombinant human erythropoietin injection on transfusion requirements in preoperatively anemic patients undergoing valvular heart surgery. *Anesthesiology* 2011;115:929–37.

157. Weltert L, D'Alessandro S, Nardella S, et al. Preoperative very short-term, high-dose erythropoietin administration diminishes blood transfusion rate in off-pump coronary artery bypass: a randomized blind controlled study. *J Thorac Cardiovasc Surg* 2010;139:621–6.

158. Thaper A, Kulik A. Rationale for administering beta-blocker therapy to patients undergoing coronary artery bypass surgery: a systematic review. *Expert Opin Drug Saf* 2018;17:805–13.

159. Brinkman W, Herbert MA, O'Brien S, et al. Preoperative β-blocker use in coronary artery bypass surgery: national database analysis. *JAMA Intern Med* 2014;174:1320–7.

160. Bleessberger H, Lewis SR, Pritchard MW, et al. Perioperative beta-blockers for preventing surgery-related mortality and morbidity in adults undergoing cardiac surgery. *Cochrane Database Syst Rev* 2019;9:CD013435. doi: 10.1002/14651858.

161. Miceli A, Capoun R, Fino C, et al. Effects of angiotensin-converting enzyme inhibitor therapy on clinical outcome in patients undergoing coronary artery bypass grafting. *J Am Coll Cardiol* 2009;54:1778–84.

162. Disque A, Neelankavil J. Con: ACE inhibitors should be stopped prior to cardiovascular surgery. *J Cardiothorac Vasc Anesth* 2016;30:820–2.

163. Arora P, Rajagopalam S, Ranjan R, et al. Preoperative use of angiotensin-converting enzyme inhibitors/angiotensin receptor blockers is associated with increased risk for acute kidney injury after cardiovascular surgery. *Clin J Am Soc Nephrol* 2008;3:1266–73.

164. Benedetto U, Sciarretta S, Roscitano A, et al. Preoperative angiotensin-converting enzyme inhibitors and acute kidney injury after coronary artery bypass grafting. *Ann Thorac Surg* 2008;86:1160–5.

165. Liakopoulos OJ, Choi YH, Haldenwang PL, et al. Impact of preoperative statin therapy on adverse postoperative outcomes in patients undergoing cardiac surgery: a meta-analysis of over 30,000 patients. *Eur Heart J* 2008;29:1548–59.

166. Curtis M, Deng Y, Lee VV, et al. Effect of dose and timing of preoperative statins on mortality after coronary artery bypass surgery. *Ann Thorac Surg* 2017;104:782–9.

167. Katznelson R, Djaiani GN, Borger MA, et al. Preoperative use of statins is associated with reduced early delirium rates after cardiac surgery. *Anesthesiology* 2009;110:67–73.

168. Wang J, Gu C, Gao M, Yu W, Yu Y. Preoperative statin therapy and renal outcomes after cardiac surgery: a meta-analysis and meta-regression of 59,771 patients. *Can J Cardiol* 2015;31:1051–60.

169. Singh I, Rajagopalan S, Srinivasan A, et al. Preoperative statin therapy is associated with lower requirement of renal replacement therapy in patients undergoing cardiac surgery: a meta-analysis of observational studies. *Interact Cardiovasc Thorac Surg* 2013;17:342–52.

170. Zheng Z, Jayaram R, Jiang L, et al. Perioperative rosuvastatin in cardiac surgery. *N Engl J Med* 2016;374:1744–53.

171. Whitlock RP, Chan S, Devereaux PJ, et al. Clinical benefit of steroid use in patients undergoing cardiopulmonary bypass: a meta-analysis of randomized trials. *Eur Heart J* 2008;29:2592–600.

172. Engelman R, Shahian D, Shemin R, et al. The Society of Thoracic Surgeons practice guideline series: antibiotic prophylaxis in cardiac surgery: part II: antibiotic choice. *Ann Thorac Surg* 2007;83:1569–76.

173. The Society of Thoracic Surgeons Blood Conservation Guideline Taskforce. Perioperative transfusion and blood conservation in cardiac surgery: the Society of Thoracic Surgeons and the Society of Cardiovascular Anesthesiologists clinical practice guidelines. *Ann Thorac Surg* 2007;83(5 Suppl):S27–86.

174. Arora RC, Légaré JF, Buth KJ, Sullivan JA, Hirsch GM. Identifying patients at risk of intraoperative and postoperative transfusion in isolated CABG: toward selective conservation strategies. *Ann Thorac Surg* 2004;78:1547–55.

175. Hafermann MJ, Kiser TH, Lyda C, et al. Weight-based versus set dosing of vancomycin for coronary artery bypass grafting or aortic valve surgery. *J Thorac Cardiovasc Surg* 2014;147:1925–30.

176. Kaiser AB, Kernodle DS, Barg NL, Petracek MR. Influence of preoperative showers on staphylococcal skin colonization: a comparative trial of antiseptic skin cleansers. *Ann Thorac Surg* 1988;45:35–8.

177. Muñoz P, Hortal J, Giannella M, et al. Nasal carriage of *S. aureus* increases the risk of surgical site infection after major heart surgery. *J Hosp Infect* 2008;68:25–31.

178. Tom TSM, Kruse MW, Reichman RT. Update: methicillin-resistant *Staphylococcus aureus* screening and decolonization in cardiac surgery. *Ann Thorac Surg* 2009;88:695–702.

179. Kallen AJ, Wilson CT, Larson RJ. Perioperative intranasal mupirocin for the prevention of surgical-site infections: systematic review of the literature and meta-analysis. *Infect Control Hosp Epidemiol* 2005;26:916–22.

180. Jog S, Cunningham R, Cooper S, et al. Impact of preoperative screening for methicillin-resistant *Staphylococcus aureus* by real-time polymerase chain reaction in patients undergoing cardiac surgery. *J Hosp Infect* 2008;69:124–30.

181. Ko W, Lazenby D, Zelano JA, Isom OW, Krieger KH. Effects of shaving methods and intraoperative irrigation on suppurative mediastinitis after bypass operations. *Ann Thorac Surg* 1992;53:301–5.

182. Beller JP, Hawkins RB, Mehaffey JH, et al. Does preoperative troponin level impact outcomes after coronary artery bypass grafting? *Ann Thorac Surg* 2018;1056:46–51.

183. Shahian DM, Jacobs JP, Badhwar V, et al. The Society of Thoracic Surgeons 2018 adult cardiac surgery risk models: part 1: background, design considerations, and model development. *Ann Thorac Surg* 2018;105:1411–8.

184. O'Brien SM, Feng L, He X, et al. The Society of Thoracic Surgeons 2018 adult cardiac surgery risk models: part 2: statistical methods and results. *Ann Thorac Surg* 2018;105:1419–28.

185. Shahian DM, O'Brien SM, Shen S, et al. Predictors of long-term survival following coronary artery bypass grafting surgery: results from The Society of Thoracic Surgeons adult cardiac surgery database (The ASCERT Study). *Circulation* 2012;125:1491–500.

186. Lancaster TS, Schill MR, Greenberg JW, et al. Long-term survival prediction for coronary artery bypass grafting: validation of the ASCERT model compared with the Society of Thoracic Surgeons predicted risk of mortality. *Ann Thorac Surg* 2018;1065:1336–43.

187. Ad N, Holmes SD, Patel J, Pritchard G, Shuman DJ, Halpin L. Comparison of EuroSCORE II, original EuroSCORE, and the Society of Thoracic Surgeons risk score in cardiac surgery patients. *Ann Thorac Surg* 2016;102:573–9.

188. Ferraris VA, Ferraris SP. Risk factors for postoperative morbidity. *J Thorac Cardiovasc Surg* 1996;111:731–41.

189. Mehta RH, Grab JD, O'Brien SM, et al. Bedside tool for predicting the risk of postoperative dialysis in patients undergoing cardiac surgery. *Circulation* 2006;114:2208–16.

190. Thakar CV, Arrigain S, Worley S, Yared JP, Paganin EP. A clinical score to predict acute renal failure after cardiac surgery. *Am J Soc Nephrol* 2005;16:162–8.

191. Reddy SLC, Grayson AD, Griffiths EM, Pullan DM, Rashid A. Logistic risk model for prolonged ventilation after adult cardiac surgery. *Ann Thorac Surg* 2007;84:528–36.

192. Ranucci M, Bozzetti G, Ditta A, Cotza M, Carboni G, Ballotta A. Surgical reexploration after cardiac operations: why a worse outcome? *Ann Thorac Surg* 2008;86:1557–62.

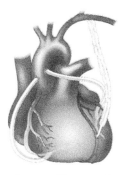

CHAPTER 4

Cardiac Anesthesia

4 Cardiac Anesthesia

Although excellence in pre- and postoperative care can often make the difference between an uneventful and a complicated recovery, the care provided in the operating room (OR) usually has the most significant impact on patient outcome. Performing a technically proficient, complete, and expeditious operation is only one component of this phase. Refinements in anesthetic techniques and monitoring, cardiopulmonary bypass (CPB), and myocardial protection have enabled surgeons to operate successfully on extremely ill patients with far advanced cardiac disease and multiple comorbidities. Use of off-pump modalities to avoid CPB is particularly useful in patients at high risk because of associated comorbidities. Minimally invasive surgery and percutaneous approaches to address valve pathology may lessen the trauma of a procedure and expedite recovery. This chapter describes intraoperative monitoring, transesophageal echocardiography (TEE), concepts of anesthetic management unique to different types of cardiac surgical procedures, and various considerations in the management of patients undergoing procedures in the OR, hybrid OR, or hybrid cath lab with or without use of CPB.

I. Preoperative Visit

A. A preoperative visit by the cardiac anesthesiologist is essential before all operations. This provides an opportunity to review the patient's history, perform a relevant examination, and explain the techniques of monitoring and postoperative ventilatory support. This evaluation should identify any potential problems that might require further work-up or could influence intraoperative management.

   1. History: cardiac symptoms, significant comorbidities, previous anesthetic experiences, surgical procedures, allergies, medications, and recent use of steroids.

   2. Examination: heart, lungs, loose teeth, intubation concerns based on oral anatomy (the Mallampati score), the thyromental distance, which is measured from the thyroid notch to the jaw with the head extended, >7 cm suggesting possible difficult intubation, range of motion of the neck, and jaw laxity.

B. The anesthesiologist should confirm with the patient the surgeon's instructions on which medications to continue up to the time of surgery, which ones to stop, and which ones to take in modified doses. Specifically, they should tell the patient to:

   1. Continue all antihypertensive and antianginal medications up to and including the morning of surgery. Exceptions may include angiotensin-converting enzyme (ACE) inhibitors and angiotensin receptor blockers (ARBs), which arguably should be withheld the morning of surgery to reduce the risk of low systemic resistance in the perioperative period.[1-4]

Manual of Perioperative Care in Adult Cardiac Surgery, Sixth Edition. Robert M. Bojar.
© 2021 John Wiley & Sons Ltd. Published 2021 by John Wiley & Sons Ltd.

2. Withhold long-acting insulin the night before and not take any insulin or oral hypoglycemic medications the morning of the surgery. Blood glucose should be obtained on arrival in the OR and checked frequently during surgery with coverage provided by intravenous (IV) insulin.

3. Follow the surgeon's recommendations for cessation of anticoagulants and antiplatelet agents.[5,6]

   a. Warfarin should be stopped at least four days preoperatively so that the INR will normalize before surgery. The INR can be reversed for more urgent surgery with vitamin K, fresh frozen plasma, or prothrombin complex concentrate (Kcentra).[7]

   b. Aspirin can be stopped 3–5 days before valvular surgery in patients without coronary disease. However, aspirin 81 mg daily should be continued in most coronary patients and should have little impact on perioperative bleeding. The benefits of its preoperative use on improving graft patency remain controversial.[8–11]

   c. The P2Y12 inhibitors should be stopped five days (clopidogrel and ticagrelor) and seven days (prasugrel) before elective surgery. If surgery is indicated within 6–12 months after a drug-eluting stent (DES) has been placed, stopping these medications prior to surgery may increase the risk of stent thrombosis. Therefore, in this situation, as well as when the patient needs urgent surgery after DES placement, the surgeon may adopt a bridging plan, such as stopping the P2Y12 for a few days and then initiating a glycoprotein IIb/IIIa inhibitor for a few days, which is then stopped four hours prior to surgery.[12,13]

   d. Unfractionated heparin (UFH) may be continued into the OR for patients with critical coronary disease, but otherwise it can be stopped about four hours before surgery.

   e. Dissipation of the full effect of other anticoagulants takes 4–5 half-lives. Therefore, low-molecular-weight heparin (LMWH), which has a half-life of 4–5 hours, should be held for 24 hours. The non-vitamin K antagonist oral anticoagulants (NOACs), including dabigatran, apixaban, and rivaroxaban have half-lives of about 12 hours in older patients with normal renal function, so the last dose should be given 48 hours prior to surgery.[6]

C. Informed consent should be obtained for anesthesia management, including the insertion of monitoring lines, with a discussion of potential complications.

II. Preoperative Medications

These are usually not given before the patient is brought into the holding area or the OR for line insertion. Once the initial IV lines are inserted, low doses of midazolam (1–5 mg IV) with fentanyl (0.2–2 µg/kg or about 50–200 µg) can be given to reduce the patient's anxiety and produce amnesia and allow for the safe insertion of additional monitoring lines without producing hemodynamic stress. Prophylactic antibiotics should be given within one hour of skin incision (starting two hours beforehand for vancomycin).[14]

III. Intraoperative Monitoring and Transesophageal Echocardiography

A. Patients undergoing cardiac surgical procedures are extensively monitored. Hemodynamic alterations and myocardial ischemia that occur during the induction of anesthesia, in the prebypass period, during CPB, and following resumption of cardiac activity can have significant adverse effects on myocardial function and recovery. It should be noted that, even though both hypertension and tachycardia can increase myocardial oxygen demand, an increase in heart rate results in more myocardial ischemia at an equivalent increase in oxygen demand.[15]

B. Standard monitoring in the OR consists of a five-lead ECG system, a radial (and occasionally femoral) arterial line, noninvasive blood pressure cuff, pressure monitoring from a central venous pressure (CVP) line or Swan-Ganz pulmonary artery (PA) catheter, pulse oximetry, and an end-tidal CO_2 measurement (Figure 4.1). In addition, cerebral oximetry, core body temperature (usually from a "temp probe" Foley catheter) and urine output through the Foley catheter are monitored.

1. For uncomplicated coronary artery bypass surgery in patients with normal or mildly depressed ventricular function, the use of a CVP monitoring line instead of a PA catheter can provide an adequate assessment of filling pressures.[16]

2. Specially designed Swan-Ganz catheters can be used to obtain continuous cardiac outputs and mixed venous oxygen saturations.

3. TEE is routine and is cost-effective in providing useful information that may alter the operative approach.[17–19] There should be provisions available to perform epiaortic scanning to assess for ascending aortic atherosclerosis, which may also influence the conduct of the operation.[20,21]

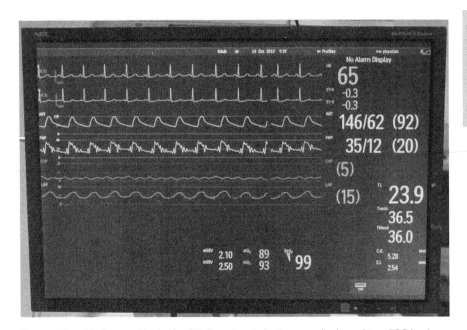

Figure 4.1 • Display monitor in the OR. From top to bottom are displays of two ECG leads, the arterial pressure, pulmonary artery and central venous pressures from the Swan-Ganz catheter, a third pressure tracing (initially the retrograde cardioplegia pressure and later a second arterial tracing, usually from the femoral artery), and pulse oximetry. The right side displays the digital values of the heart rate and pressures (phasic and mean pressures), three temperature readings, reflecting the myocardial, systemic (Tblood from the pulmonary artery), and core (Tvesic) temperatures and cardiac output and index values. At the bottom are the doses of inhalational gases being administered, the inspired (FiO_2) and end-tidal O_2 saturations, and the arterial oxygen saturation.

C. **Swan-Ganz pulmonary artery catheters** are usually placed after induction and intubation to minimize patient discomfort. However, they may be placed before the induction of anesthesia in patients with severe left ventricular (LV) dysfunction. Flow-directed catheters are used to measure right- (CVP) and left-sided filling pressures (pulmonary artery diastolic [PAD] and pulmonary capillary wedge [PCW] pressures), and obtain thermodilution cardiac outputs. Despite the nearly universal use of these catheters to carefully monitor patients and provide objective data on cardiac performance in the pre- and postbypass periods, it has not been demonstrated that they influence the outcome of cardiac surgery.

   1. The catheter is usually inserted through an 8.5 Fr introducer placed into the internal jugular (IJ) vein or, less commonly, the subclavian vein. Ultrasound-guided access, using an echo probe on the neck to identify the IJ vein, is very helpful in facilitating line placement (Figure 4.2). The introducer sheath contains one side port that provides central venous access for the infusion of vasoactive medications and potassium. Multilumen introducers, such as the 8.5 Fr and 9 Fr high-flow advanced venous access (AVA) device (Edwards Lifesciences) or the Teleflex

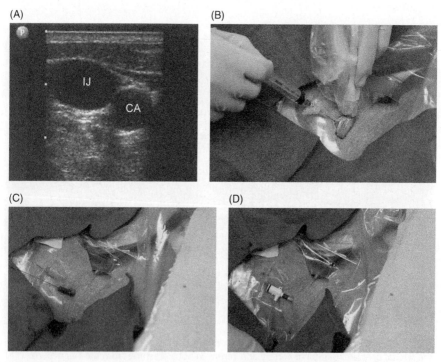

(A)   (B)

(C)   (D)

Figure 4.2 • (A) An echo probe is used to identify the location of the internal jugular (IJ) vein and its relationship to the carotid artery. (B) Using the echo probe, a small caliber finder needle is used to locate the IJ vein. (C) A larger needle then accesses the vein through which a wire and a dilator are placed into the IJ vein. (D) The introducer sheath is then advanced over the wire into the IJ through which the Swan-Ganz catheter is then placed.

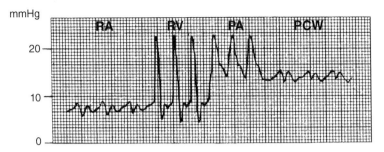

Figure 4.3 • Swan-Ganz catheter pressures. Intracardiac pressures are recorded from the distal (PA) port as the catheter is passed through the right atrium (RA), right ventricle (RV), and pulmonary artery (PA), into the pulmonary capillary wedge (PCW) position.

multilumen access catheter (MAC) with a 12-gauge proximal lumen and a 9 Fr distal lumen, can provide additional venous access in patients with poor arm veins and limited peripheral access. A manifold with multiple stopcocks is attached to the side port of the introducer or to one of the additional ports of the AVA/MAC through which all medications are administered.

2. The catheter is passed into the right atrium, and the balloon at the catheter tip is inflated. The catheter is advanced through the right ventricle (RV) and PA into the PCW position, as confirmed by pressure tracings (Figure 4.3). The PA tracing should reappear when the balloon is deflated. **Note:** caution is essential in passing the catheter through the RV in patients with a left bundle branch block (LBBB), in whom complete heart block might occur. In this situation, unless provisions for urgent pacing are available, such as external pacing/defibrillator pads, it is best to wait until the chest is open before advancing the catheter, so that the surgeon can directly pace the heart if necessary.[22]

3. The proximal port of the Swan-Ganz catheter (30 cm from the tip) is used for CVP measurements from the right atrium and for fluid injections to determine the cardiac output. Care must be exercised when injecting sterile fluid for cardiac outputs to prevent bolusing of vasoactive medications that might be running through the CVP port. **Note:** one must **never** infuse anything through this port if the catheter has been pulled back so that the tip lies in the right atrium and the CVP port lies outside the patient! This might not be noticed, because the catheter is usually placed through a sterile sheath that allows for advancement or withdrawal of the catheter. This concept must always be kept in mind when critical medications, such as heparin prior to cannulation, are being administered.

4. The distal port should always be transduced and displayed on a monitor to allow for the detection of catheter advancement into the permanent wedge position, which could result in PA injury. Balloon inflation ("wedging" of the catheter) is rarely necessary during surgery. Medication should never be given through the distal PA port.

5. A variety of advanced technology Swan-Ganz catheters are available that provide additional functions.

a. Swan-Ganz Paceport catheters have additional ports for the placement of right atrial and ventricular pacing probes, which is helpful during minimally invasive surgery when access to the heart is limited.

b. Catheters have been designed for assessment of continuous cardiac outputs (CCO) or mixed venous oxygen saturations (SvO$_2$) by fiberoptic oximetry (Figure 4.4). These are helpful during off-pump surgery to evaluate the patient's hemodynamic status and may contribute to a therapeutic maneuver in many patients. The Vigileo/FloTrac (Edwards Lifesciences) cardiac output monitoring system is also useful during off-pump surgery,[23,24] and may be considered when there is difficulty placing a Swan-Ganz catheter or when thermodilution cardiac outputs are unreliable (moderate–severe tricuspid regurgitation).[25]

c. Swan-Ganz catheters for CCO and SvO$_2$ monitoring may also include the technology to provide measurements of RV ejection fraction and RV end-diastolic volume. They are particularly valuable in patients with pulmonary hypertension and compromised RV function.[26]

6. The primary concerns during the insertion of a PA catheter are arterial puncture, arrhythmias during passage through the RV, and potential heart block in patients with preexisting LBBB. Other complications of Swan-Ganz catheters are noted on pages 354–355.

7. **Pulmonary artery perforation** is a very serious complication.[27-29] It may occur during insertion of the catheter or during the surgical procedure when hypothermia causes the catheter to become rigid. Since a cold, stiff catheter may advance into the lung when the heart is manipulated, it is advisable to pull it back slightly during CPB to prevent perforation and then to re-advance it after CPB. Migration of the catheter into the wedge position may be evident by a loss of pulse pressure in the PA waveform before or after bypass or by a very high PA pressure measurement on bypass when the heart is decompressed.

a. If perforation occurs, blood will appear in the endotracheal tube. The goals of management are to maintain gas exchange and arrest the hemorrhage. Positive end-expiratory pressure (PEEP) should be applied to the ventilator circuit. If the degree of hemoptysis is not severe, it may abate once CPB is terminated and protamine is administered.

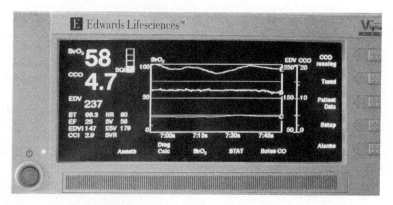

Figure 4.4 • Continuous cardiac output monitor display.

b. If the airway is compromised by bleeding, CPB should be resumed with venting of the PA. Bronchoscopy is then performed with placement of a bronchial blocker or a double-lumen endotracheal tube to provide differential lung ventilation. The pleural space should be entered to evaluate the problem. If significant bleeding does not abate after application of PEEP or occlusion of the hilar vessels, pulmonary resection may be required. Use of femoral artery–femoral venous extracorporeal membrane oxygenation (ECMO) has been described to control bleeding by lowering the PA pressures, but it is risky because it requires persistent heparinization.[30] Because of the risk of recurrence, pulmonary angiography and embolization may be considered once the bleeding is controlled.

D. **Intraoperative TEE** has become routine in most cardiac surgical centers, being beneficial in coronary artery bypass grafting (CABG) operations and essential during valvular surgery.[17–19,31] The probe is placed after the patient is anesthetized and before heparinization. TEE provides an analysis of regional and global RV and LV function, is very sensitive in detecting ischemia,[32] and identifies the presence of valvular pathology or intracardiac masses (Table 4.1 and see Figures 2.21–2.28, pages 148–153). Color flow, continuous wave, and pulsed wave Doppler are used to analyze valvular function or suspected shunts. Although TEE may image the aorta for atheromatous disease, epiaortic imaging provides better visualization of the ascending aorta and arch when there are significant concerns about atheromatous disease.[20,21] Having an individual trained in performing and reading TEEs, be they a cardiac anesthesiologist or a cardiologist, is essential to optimize its usefulness.

Table 4.1 • Specific Uses of Intraoperative Echocardiography

Prebypass	Identify or confirm preoperative pathology (see Table 2.3, page 154) Epiaortic imaging for aortic atherosclerosis in ascending aorta and arch Intracardiac thrombus (LA appendage, LV apex)
During Off-pump Surgery	Regional wall motion abnormalities
Postbypass Coronary disease Valve surgery	Regional dysfunction (incomplete/inadequate revascularization) Presence of intracardiac air on weaning from CPB RV and LV function (circumflex artery entrapment after MVR, coronary ostial obstruction after AVR) Valve regurgitation from paravalvular leak or inadequate repair Outflow tract obstruction after mitral valve repair or replacement Obstruction to prosthetic leaflet opening or closing Residual stenosis after commissurotomy
VSD closure	Residual VSD
IABP	Location of device relative to aortic arch
All patients	Evaluation of iatrogenic aortic dissection

1. Before the probe is placed, consideration must be given to contraindications to TEE placement that could produce catastrophic complications, such as hypopharyngeal, or proximal or distal esophageal perforation or bleeding, which are noted in less than 0.1% of patients.[33-36] TEE must be used cautiously or avoided in patients with prior esophageal surgery or with known esophageal pathology, such as strictures, Schatzki's ring, or esophageal varices.

2. TEE allows for advancement/withdrawal, rotation, and "multiplaning" of the probe through 180 degrees, thus affording excellent images of the heart in multiple views. The probe is advanced up and down the esophagus and then into the stomach for transgastric views. The American Society of Echocardiography (ASE) and the Society of Cardiovascular Anesthesiologists defined 20 standard views for a routine examination in their report from 1999[37] and expanded the recommendations to 28 standard views in their 2013 update.[31] These include 15 mid-esophageal (ME) views, nine transgastric (TG) views, and four aortic views, which can be obtained in a sequential fashion. These images provide multiple long-axis (LAX) and short-axis (SAX) views of all four cardiac valves, the four cardiac chambers, and the great vessels. The 2013 update can be accessed online at www.onlinejase.org and provides links to videos of each of the views. The most important views during cardiac surgery (Figures 4.5–4.7) include the following:

   a. Multiplaning of the probe in the mid-esophagus allows for acquisition of four- and five-chamber views (0–10°), the mitral commissural view (50–70°), and the two-chamber view (80–100°) (Figure 4.5). These views are helpful in assessing which mitral valve scallops are involved in patients with degenerative mitral regurgitation (MR). The bicaval view (Figure 4.5E) and SAX view at the base of the aortic valve are used to optimize the site for transseptal puncture during percutaneous mitral valve procedures. The ME SAX view (Figure 4.6A) is used to visualize the three aortic valve leaflets, and the ME LAX LVOT view (Figure 4.6B) is an excellent image for evaluation of aortic and mitral valve pathology, LV function, intracardiac air when weaning from CPB, and for positioning of MitraClip devices.

   b. With the probe anteflexed in the TG position (Figure 4.7), the most helpful views include the following:

      i. The LV SAX views (0–20°) extending from the apex toward the base to assess global and regional LV function and LV wall thickness.

      ii. The TG two-chamber view (90–110°) to identify the mitral valve, submitral apparatus, and the anterior and inferior walls of the LV.

Figure 4.5 • Best TEE views for mitral valve procedures. For mitral valve repairs, the probe is rotated in the mid-esophagus (ME) to identify which scallops are involved. These views include the (A) five-chamber, (B) four-chamber, (C) mitral commissural, and (D) two-chamber views. The ME LAX view (Figure 4.6B) shows A2-P2 as well as the LVOT and aortic valve. The best TEE views for a MitraClip include (E) the bicaval view and the SAX at the base view for transseptal puncture, the mitral commissural view to determine lateral–medial orientation of the clip and the ME LAX (LVOT) view for proper anterior–posterior orientation of the clip.

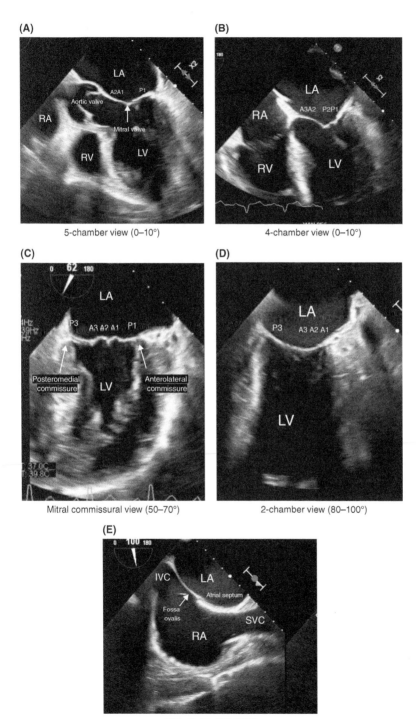

(A) 5-chamber view (0–10°)

(B) 4-chamber view (0–10°)

(C) Mitral commissural view (50–70°)

(D) 2-chamber view (80–100°)

(E) Bicaval view (90–110°)

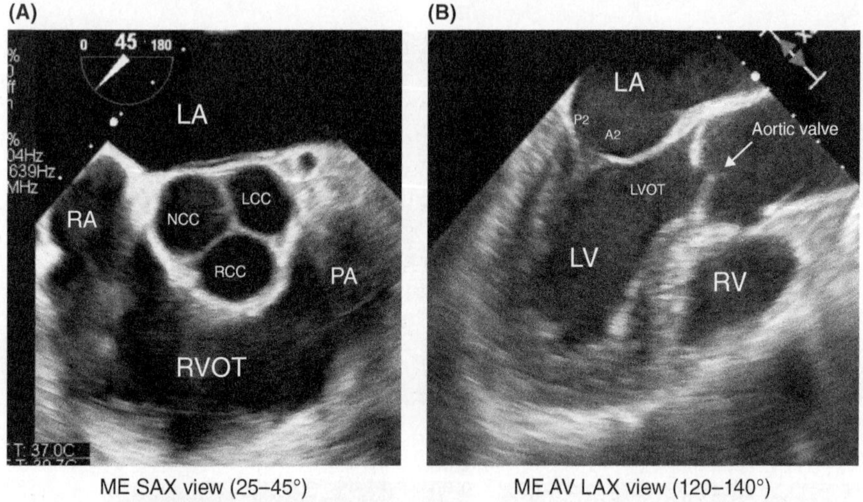

(A)

(B)

ME SAX view (25–45°)   ME AV LAX view (120–140°)

Figure 4.6 • Best TEE views of the aortic valve are the (A) ME aortic valve SAX and (B) ME aortic valve LAX views. These views are also useful during MitraClip procedures, with the ME SAX at the base view used to determine the anterior–posterior location for transseptal puncture, and the ME LAX or LVOT view used to determine positioning of the clip below the anterior and posterior mitral valve leaflets. The ME LAX view is most helpful in assessing mitral valve function, LV function, and detecting air when weaning from bypass after both aortic and mitral valve surgery.

> iii. The TG RV two-chamber (inflow) view (with clockwise rotation of the probe at 90–110°) to show the tricuspid valve and right heart chambers.
>
> iv. The TG LAX view (120–140°) to measure aortic valve gradients.
>
> v. The deep TG five-chamber view to assess LV function, but primarily to measure the aortic valve gradient.
>
> c. Imaging of the aorta is usually performed after obtaining the TG views and is obtained in both SAX and LAX views as the probe is pulled back into the esophagus. This allows for imaging of the ascending and descending aorta and the aortic arch.

Figure 4.7 • Transgastric (TG) views. With the probe anteflexed in the TG position, the most helpful views are the (A) SAX views of the LV extending upwards from the apex to assess LV function, (B) the longitudinal TG two-chamber LV view to image the mitral valve apparatus and anterior and inferior wall function, and (C) the TG two-chamber RV (inflow) view to assess tricuspid valve pathology. (D) The TG LAX and (E) deep TG five-chamber views are used to obtain aortic valve gradients.

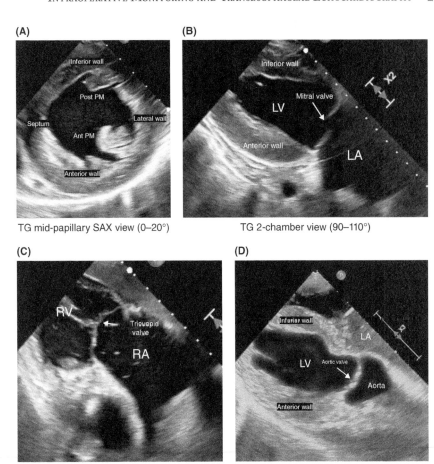

TG mid-papillary SAX view (0–20°)

TG 2-chamber view (90–110°)

TG 2-chamber RV view (90–110°)

TG LAX view (120–140°)

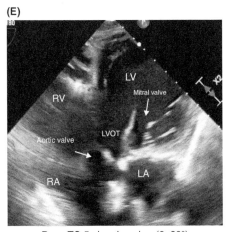

Deep TG 5-chamber view (0–20°)

3. During **on-pump coronary artery surgery**, a prebypass TEE will provide a baseline analysis of regional and global ventricular function. The TG mid-papillary SAX view and most ME LAX views of the LV can be used to assess regional wall motion (RWM). The ability of the heart muscle to thicken is consistent with viability, whereas areas of thinned-out muscle represent infarcted areas. Following bypass, slight improvement in previously ischemic zones may be noted, especially with inotropic stimulation. Areas of hypokinesis may represent stunned or hibernating myocardium that have contractile reserve and may gradually recover function after revascularization. The new onset of hypokinesis raises the specter of hypoperfusion from an anastomotic or graft problem, incomplete revascularization, or inadequate myocardial protection. The new onset of MR may reflect loading conditions but is also consistent with ischemic dysfunction.

4. During **off-pump surgery**, the ME windows are best for assessing RV and LV function and the presence of MR. Baseline views are obtained. During vessel occlusion, TEE should assess for the acute development of regional LV dysfunction or acute MR during construction of left-sided grafts and for RV dysfunction during right coronary grafting. The TG views are not helpful when the heart is elevated out of the chest.[38,39] The development and persistence of a new RWM abnormality after a graft anastomosis is completed suggest a flow problem, usually at the anastomosis. However, the latter may be present even in the absence of a RWM abnormality.

5. In **minimally invasive** access procedures (usually aortic or mitral valve surgery), TEE can confirm the location of the retrograde coronary sinus catheter since it cannot be palpated by the surgeon. It can also visualize the intracardiac location of a femoral venous catheter and identify the location of an aortic endoballoon. Upon weaning from bypass, TEE is essential to identify intracardiac air and assess valve competence.

6. **Aortic valve surgery.** The best TEE views of the aortic valve are obtained in the ME SAX and LAX views, with use of the TG views to obtain aortic valve gradients. These images are important for the surgeon to:

   a. Quantify the degree of aortic stenosis (AS) by planimetry and by continuous wave and pulsed wave Doppler flow analysis. This provides peak and mean transvalvular pressure gradients and calculates the aortic area using the continuity equation.

   b. Quantify the degree of aortic regurgitation (AR) using color flow and continuous wave Doppler analysis. If moderate to severe, this will render delivery of antegrade cardioplegia into the aortic root ineffective.

   c. Assess the degree of LV hypertrophy and its nature (concentric, septal).

   d. Assess annular and aortic root size and identify an annular abscess in patients with endocarditis.

   e. Identify the presence of systolic and/or diastolic dysfunction (by looking at transmitral flow), which may influence filling pressures and pharmacologic management coming off-pump.

f. After bypass, intracardiac air is best assessed in the ME LAX view, and ventricular function is best determined in the ME LAX, TG LAX, and SAX views. Imaging to assess opening and closing of valve leaflets, identify transvalvular and paravalvular leaks, and calculate aortic valve gradients is then performed. Transvalvular regurgitation should be minor and located centrally after a bioprosthetic AVR, but may be eccentric if a leaflet has been distorted by the aortic closure sutures. Multiple trace jets are anticipated after St. Jude (Abbott) bileaflet valve replacements. Paravalvular leaks may need to be reevaluated by direct visualization. Competence of homografts, autografts (Ross procedure), and the native aortic valve in a valve-sparing root procedure should be confirmed. Rarely, an unusual finding may be demonstrated, such as a ventricular septal defect or an aorto-left atrial fistula. Flow into the left main coronary artery can be visualized in the ME SAX view.

g. Following transcatheter aortic valve replacement (TAVR), TEE is used if the procedure is performed under general anesthesia. If the procedure is performed under sedation, transthoracic imaging is adequate to identify paravalvular leaks in the parasternal LAX and SAX views, and to calculate a transvalvular gradient in the apical four-chamber view.

7 **Mitral valve surgery.** TEE is essential to identify the anatomic abnormality responsible for the MR, quantitate its severity, and evaluate the surgical result. The best visualization of the mitral valve is from the mid-lower esophagus and includes the ME two- and four-chamber views, the ME mitral commissural view, and the ME LAX views. These, along with the three-dimensional (3D) en face views, allow for the visualization of all of the mitral valve scallops to help identify the precise location of the pathology causing the MR.[40]

a. Prebypass assessment should confirm the valvular pathology and identify the mechanism of MR. For example, degenerative MR with a flail leaflet will produce an eccentric jet, whereas functional MR with depressed LV function may produce a central jet from remodeling with papillary muscle displacement or an eccentric jet from leaflet tethering (see Figures 2.22–2.24, pages 148–150). Rotation of the probe to sequentially provide the four-chamber, mitral commissural, and two-chamber views should allow for localization of the prolapsed scallop.[41] In some patients with MR, it is not uncommon to note a discrepancy in the degree of MR between preoperative echoes and intraoperative TEE due to alteration in loading conditions. The left atrial appendage should be evaluated for the presence of thrombus.

b. In anticipation of a mitral valve repair, markers for systolic anterior motion should be analyzed. These include an end-diastolic diameter (EDD) <45 mm. aorto-mitral angle <120°, coaptation–septum distance <25 mm, posterior leaflet height >15 mm, and basal septal diameter ≥15 mm.[42]

c. Assessment of RV function is also important during mitral valve surgery. Markers of RV dysfunction include an RV fractional area change (FAC) <35%

or a tricuspid annular plane systolic excursion (TAPSE, the distance traveled between end-diastole and end-systole at the lateral corner of the tricuspid annulus) <16 mm.[43]

d. During weaning from bypass, TEE is essential to identify intracardiac air. After termination of bypass, it should be used to assess the competence of valve repairs, identify paravalvular leaks after mitral valve replacement (MVR) (Figure 4.8), and assess LV and RV function. Occasionally, the TEE will reveal an unsuspected finding such as:

i. Systolic anterior motion (SAM) of the anterior mitral valve leaflet obstructing the LV outflow tract (after valve repairs or MVR with retention of the anterior leaflet)

ii. Evidence of valve dysfunction with a trapped or obstructed leaflet

iii. Aortic valve regurgitation after a difficult mitral valve operation (due to suture entrapment of an aortic valve cusp or distortion of the aortic annulus from placement of too small a mitral valve)

iv. Marked lateral wall hypokinesis from circumflex artery entrapment by valve sutures

e. Percutaneous mitral valve repair with the MitraClip device is performed under general anesthesia with TEE guidance. Specific views are utilized to perform the septal puncture (bicaval, SAX at the base, four-chamber) and then for

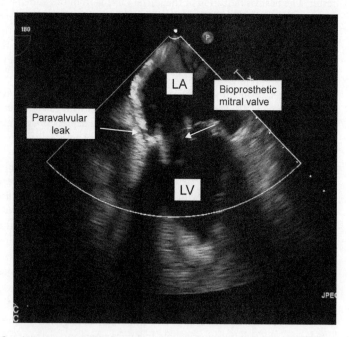

Figure 4.8 • Intraoperative TEE showing a paravalvular leak following tissue mitral valve replacement.

maneuvering the system down to the mitral valve to avoid passage into the pulmonary veins or left atrial appendage. The mitral commissural and LVOT views are used to place the clip in the proper position with the aid of the 3D en face view to ensure correct clip orientation. Clip stability should be assessed prior to and after the clip has been deployed.

8. The diagnosis of an **aortic dissection** can be confirmed by TEE once the patient is anesthetized (see Figure 2.27, page 152). It may not only identify the intimal flap but can also determine whether AR is present, mandating aortic valve resuspension or replacement. If a large pericardial effusion is present, axillary or groin cannulation may be necessary for the emergent institution of CPB before opening the pericardium. TEE can also identify flaps in cases of iatrogenic dissections at the cannulation or clamp sites.[44]

9. In **thoracic aortic surgery**, TEE is useful in assessing cardiac performance and intracardiac volume status during the period of clamping and after unclamping, when PA pressures tend to be elevated out of proportion to preload. This may influence fluid and pharmacologic management.[45] Positioning of an endograft for thoracic aortic repairs, including traumatic aortic tears, type B dissections, and thoracic aortic aneurysms, is usually confirmed by fluoroscopy, and the TEE probe should be pulled back to avoid interference with the x-ray beam.

IV. Anesthetic Considerations for Various Types of Heart Surgery

A. Anesthetic management must be individualized, taking into consideration the patient's age, comorbidities, the nature and extent of coronary or valvular disease, the degree of LV dysfunction, and plans for early extubation. These factors will determine which medications should be selected to avoid myocardial depression, tachycardia or bradycardia, or to counteract changes in vasomotor tone. Generally, a balanced anesthetic technique using a combination of narcotics and potent inhalational agents is used for all open-heart surgery to minimize myocardial depression. Specific anesthetic concerns for various disease processes are presented in this section.

B. **Coronary artery bypass surgery**

1. Factors that increase myocardial oxygen demand, such as tachycardia and hypertension, must be prevented in the prebypass period, especially during the induction of anesthesia. Hypotension, often resulting from the vasodilating effects of narcotics, anxiolytics (midazolam), and sedatives (propofol), should be counteracted with fluids and α-agents, since hypotension is more likely to produce ischemia than hypertension.

2. Detection and treatment of ischemia is critical in the prebypass period. TEE is the most sensitive means of detecting ischemic RWM abnormalities and can be recommended for all cardiac cases. Ischemia may also be manifested by an elevation in the PA pressures or by ST segment changes in the ECG leads. Aggressive management with nitroglycerin, β-blockers (esmolol), and narcotics can usually control prebypass ischemia.[46] Placement of an intra-aortic balloon

pump (IABP) may be considered for ischemia, but if the patient is truly unstable, prompt initiation of CPB may be necessary.

3. Narcotic/sedative regimens are the standard for coronary surgery, especially in patients with LV dysfunction. Use of low-dose fentanyl or sufentanil with inhalational anesthetics during the surgery, and use of propofol or dexmedetomidine at the conclusion of surgery allow for early postoperative extubation. Use of the short-acting narcotic remifentanil along with a volatile inhalational anesthetic with rapid onset and offset of effect, such as sevoflurane or desflurane, allows for "ultra-fast tracking" with extubation in the OR or upon arrival in the ICU.[47] Remifentanil has been shown to minimize the systemic inflammatory response and shorten ventilation time, but it is associated with chest wall rigidity and the occurrence of chronic pain syndromes for up to one year.[48,49]

4. Monitoring techniques for **off-pump surgery** (OPCAB) commonly involve a continuous cardiac output Swan-Ganz catheter with in-line mixed venous oxygen saturation monitoring. Tilting of the OR table (Trendelenburg position and to the right) to augment cardiac filling, judicious fluid administration, antiarrhythmic therapy (lidocaine/magnesium), α-agents (phenylephrine) and inotropes (epinephrine/milrinone), and, on occasion, insertion of an IABP may be used to produce hemodynamic stability when the heart is rotated for exposure of the coronary arteries. ß-blockers to reduce the heart rate may be helpful to reduce cardiac motion during the distal anastomoses. The blood pressure may be lowered to the 80–90s during construction of the proximal anastomoses to reduce the risk of aortic injury when a sideclamp is placed on the aorta. Use of a warming system, especially the Kimberly-Clark warming system (formerly the Arctic Sun temperature management system), is helpful in preventing hypothermia during OPCAB surgery.[50] The essential elements of a successful off-pump operation include a patient surgeon who uses good judgment in deciding when off-pump surgery is feasible and when conversion to CPB or right-heart assist is necessary, an anesthesiologist who is experienced and comfortable with off-pump surgery, and a qualified, actively involved first assistant. See section IX (pages 262–264) for a more detailed discussion of anesthesia for off-pump surgery.

5. **MIDCAB** procedures involve internal thoracic artery (ITA) takedown either under direct vision or with endoscopic or robotic assistance. The anastomosis to the left anterior descending (LAD) artery is then performed through a small thoracotomy incision, but it can also be performed robotically. One-lung anesthesia is generally used. Even with use of stabilization platforms, slowing the heart down pharmacologically may be helpful. Robotic coronary surgery can be performed off-pump or on-pump with groin cannulation.

C. **Left ventricular aneurysms (LVAs).** Anesthetic drugs that cause myocardial depression must be avoided because of the association of LVAs with significant LV dysfunction. Swan-Ganz monitoring is important in optimizing preload and contractility before and after bypass. TEE is the most sensitive means of detecting the presence of LV thrombus and provides an excellent assessment of ventricular wall thickness and motion (akinesia, hypokinesia, and dyskinesia noted with aneurysms). Aneurysm repairs may be performed with an unclamped aorta, allowing the surgeon to palpate the margin between viable and scarred myocardium. Proper deairing during closure is essential and can be monitored by TEE.

D. **Ventricular septal defects** are usually operated upon on an emergent basis when the patient is in cardiogenic shock, usually on inotropic support and an IABP. Thus, myocardial depression must be avoided. Systemic hypertension may increase the shunt and should be prevented. TEE is invaluable in identifying the persistence of a left-to-right shunt.

E. **Aortic valve surgery**

1. **Aortic stenosis (AS).** The induction of anesthesia is a critical period for patients with AS. The LV is generally hypertrophied and stiff with evidence of diastolic dysfunction. Avoidance of hypovolemia, myocardial depression, vasodilation, tachycardia, or dysrhythmias is important, as all of these can lower the cardiac output precipitously.

   a. **Blood pressure issues.** Hypotension, usually as a result of vasodilation, can produce myocardial ischemia. Volume should be given to maintain intravascular volume, with the understanding that PA pressures may rise quickly with small infusions of volume in noncompliant ventricles and can adversely affect pulmonary function. Systemic resistance should be supported with a small bolus or infusion of an α-agent, such as phenylephrine or norepinephrine. Hypertension can make aortic cannulation for CPB dangerous. It should be addressed by increasing the depth of anesthesia, use of propofol, or use of ß-blockers. Post-CPB, strict adherence to blood pressure control is essential to minimize bleeding from the aortotomy site and avoid the risk of dissection.

   b. **Heart rate.** Loss of "atrial kick" can substantially compromise the cardiac output in patients with LV hypertrophy. Thus, atrial fibrillation (AF) developing before the initiation of bypass is often associated with profound hypotension for which cardioversion may be necessary. Tachyarrhythmias will compromise LV filling and can also precipitate ischemia. A short-acting ß-blocker, such as esmolol or IV metoprolol, may be helpful to control a sinus tachycardia. A reentrant supraventricular or junctional tachycardia may require cardioversion. Sinus bradycardia or a slow junctional rhythm may cause hypotension and can be treated by attaching "alligator" leads to the right atrium to restore a supraventricular mechanism once the pericardium has been opened. Prior to that time, very slow rhythms can be treated by a bolus dose of 5–15 mg of ephedrine, 5–10 μg of epinephrine, or 0.2–0.4 mg of glycopyrrolate.

   c. The best TEE views of the aortic valve are obtained in the ME SAX and LAX views (Figure 4.6). The important information prior to initiating CPB includes confirmation of the degree of AS and regurgitation and the estimated aortic annular diameter. During weaning from bypass, assessment for intracardiac air is essential and is best seen in the ME LVOT LAX view. Postbypass, valve competence, valve gradient, and LV function are important and should be evaluated by the anesthesiologist and surgeon. Significant abnormalities in valve function (primarily paravalvular or transvalvular regurgitation), and especially a significant RWM abnormality possibly related to coronary ostial obstruction by the valve sewing ring, need to be addressed.

d. Most procedures are performed through a median sternotomy incision. "Minimally invasive" approaches include an upper sternotomy and right upper thoracotomy approach. Both central and peripheral cannulation for CPB may be used and the anesthesiologist may on occasion be asked to place venous drainage catheters, a PA vent, or a cardioplegia catheter. Anesthetic management of minimally invasive AVR is discussed in section XI on page 268.

e. Transient AV block necessitating AV pacing upon termination of CPB is not uncommon in aortic valve surgery, and about 5% of patients may require a permanent pacemaker if this persists. It is critical that the pacing threshold be adequate prior to chest closure if the patient has third-degree heart block.

f. Comments on anesthetic management during TAVRs are noted in section VII on pages 268–269.

2. **Aortic regurgitation (AR).** Chronic AR produces volume overload and progressive LV dilatation and compromise of ventricular function. It is associated with a low diastolic pressure that can compromise coronary perfusion.

a. Hypotension will worsen coronary ischemia while hypertension and bradycardia will increase regurgitation. Thus, a delicate balance must be sought to optimize hemodynamics by maintaining satisfactory preload, treating bradycardia, and avoiding hyper- or hypotension before going on CPB. Volatile anesthetics that depress contractility should be avoided. These patients tend to be vasodilated on pump and afterwards as well, often requiring vasopressor support.

b. The ME aortic valve LAX and SAX and TG LAX views with color Doppler are best for assessing AR, and allow for the measurement of the pressure half-time (P1/2t). Careful examination of the valve in the ME SAX view is best to determine whether it is repairable or not.

c. Myocardial protection, especially of the RV, may be compromised in patients with severe AR, since antegrade cardioplegia cannot be administered into the aortic root. Retrograde cardioplegia and use of ostial antegrade perfusion are usually used. Patients with occluded right coronary arteries are at higher risk for RV dysfunction. Post-CPB, inotropic support may be necessary in patients with pre-existing LV dysfunction, and many patients are vasodilated and hypotensive despite good cardiac function, requiring an α-agent or vasopressin for blood pressure support.

d. The LV is usually dilated and compliant and significant volume infusions may be necessary to maintain preload and cardiac output coming off-pump.

F. **Hypertrophic obstructive cardiomyopathy.** Measures that produce hypovolemia or vasodilation must be avoided because they increase the outflow tract gradient. Volume infusions should be used to maintain preload, with the use of α-agents to maintain systemic resistance. Use of β-blockers and calcium channel blockers to reduce the heart rate and contractility are beneficial in the immediate preoperative and prebypass periods. Inotropic drugs with predominantly β-adrenergic effects could provoke the gradient and must be avoided. TEE assessment of subvalvular pathology is essential so that the surgeon can address issues with papillary muscle pathology in addition to performing a septal myectomy. Assessment of the degree of MR prior to and after surgical repair is essential.[51]

G. **Mitral valve surgery**

1. **Mitral stenosis (MS).** Severe MS is associated with impairment to LV filling resulting in an elevation of left atrial and PA pressures to maintain cardiac output. This may result in RV dilatation and functional TR as well. The LV is usually small. Severe MS is often associated with AF with dilated atrial chambers, for which patients should be on preoperative anticoagulation to reduce the risk of formation of thrombus in the left atrial appendage. Attention should be paid to maintaining preload, reducing heart rate, and preventing an increase in pulmonary vascular resistance (PVR) in the prebypass period.

   a. Preload must be adjusted judiciously to ensure adequate LV filling across the stenotic valve while simultaneously avoiding excessive fluid administration that could lead to pulmonary edema.

   b. In patients with severe pulmonary hypertension and RV dysfunction, a volumetric (RVEF) Swan-Ganz catheter is valuable in the assessment of RV volume and the RV ejection fraction. The PA diastolic pressure may be inconsistent with the left atrial pressure, and placement of a left atrial line for monitoring postbypass may be considered. Balloon inflation ("wedging") of a PA catheter should be avoided or performed with a minimal amount of balloon inflation in patients with pulmonary hypertension because of the increased risk of PA rupture. If the patient remains hypotensive despite adequate preload, an α-agent is preferable to restore the blood pressure. Inotropic agents are usually not of much value, since LV function is usually normal, but they may be beneficial if there is evidence of RV dysfunction (usually epinephrine +/- milrinone).

   c. Prebypass TEE is helpful in identifying left atrial thrombus. It should also be used to assess RV function, which can be compromised due to pulmonary hypertension.

   d. The heart rate should be reduced to <80/min to prolong the diastolic filling period. For patients in AF, small doses of esmolol or diltiazem can be used to control a rapid ventricular response. If the AF is of short duration, cardioversion can be performed for an uncontrolled rate with hypotension as long as the TEE confirms absence of thrombus in the left atrial appendage. Cardiac output is usually marginal in patients with MS and can be further compromised if the ventricular rate is excessively slow.

   e. Factors that can increase the PVR must be avoided. Preoperative sedation can induce hypercarbia and should be minimized. Hypoxemia, hypercarbia, acidosis, and nitrous (not nitric) oxide should be avoided in the OR. The PVR can be reduced with systemic vasodilators (propofol) or nonspecific pulmonary vasodilators (usually nitroglycerin) before bypass. Following bypass, RV support is best achieved using inotropic agents that can produce pulmonary vasodilation (usually milrinone). In patients with severe pulmonary hypertension and RV dysfunction, inhaled nitric oxide, epoprostenol (Flolan), or iloprost (Ventavis) can be used. Further discussion of the postoperative management of mitral valve surgery and the management of RV dysfunction is noted on pages 396–397 and 530–534.

f. TEE should be used during weaning from bypass to identify intracardiac air. Once off bypass, TEE should assess the mean gradient if a commissurotomy is performed, and check for paravalvular or transvalvular leaks of a mitral prosthesis. For mechanical valves, proper opening and closing of the leaflets must be confirmed.

g. Although the INR should be corrected prior to surgery, levels of clotting factors are rarely normal despite a lowering of the INR into the normal range, so one should anticipate a potential coagulopathy and the potential need for clotting factors (fresh frozen plasma and/or cryoprecipitate). Rarely, AV groove disruption may occur, especially in patients with mitral annular calcification, which will cause catastrophic hemorrhage.

2. **Mitral regurgitation (MR)**

a. MR results in volume overload of the left atrium and ventricle, which subsequently dilate and develop increased compliance. Eventually, the PA pressure rises, causing RV dysfunction and TR, and then the LV, despite the low pressure unloading, begins to fail. Poor LV function with severe MR is an ominous prognostic sign since restoration of mitral valve competence will "unmask" LV dysfunction that was not appreciated due to LV unloading through the regurgitant valve.

b. Measures that can increase PA pressure, such as hypoxemia, hypercarbia, acidosis, and nitrous oxide, should be avoided. Preoperative sedation should be light or avoided altogether.

c. In the prebypass period, adequate preload must be maintained to ensure forward output. Some patients come to the OR "dry" because of chronic diuretic usage, while others may be in heart failure from severe MR. Systemic hypertension should be avoided, because the increased resistance to outflow will usually worsen MR. If the patient has ischemic MR or a borderline cardiac output, use of systemic vasodilators or an IABP will improve forward flow. Inotropes with vasodilator properties (i.e. milrinone or dobutamine) should be considered in patients with markedly compromised LV function. Heart rate should be optimized; a slightly faster heart rate in the 80–90s will reduce the degree of MR, and a slow heart rate may cause hypotension.

d. TEE is invaluable in identifying the precise anatomic cause for MR, assessing the risk of SAM[42] (see section D.7.b, page 231), and in evaluating the surgical result. TEE is performed once the patient is anesthetized. The critical views include the ME two- and four-chamber views, the ME mitral commissural view, and the ME LAX views. These, along with the 3D en face views, allow for the visualization of all of the mitral valve scallops to help identify the precise location of the pathology causing the MR. Occasionally, there is a discrepancy between preoperative and intraoperative studies, due to alterations in systemic resistance and loading conditions. Elevating the blood pressure with an α-agent may increase the amount of regurgitation in patients with moderate ischemic MR and aid in the decision to repair the valve during coronary bypass surgery. TEE is evaluated for intracardiac air when weaning from bypass and for evaluating mitral valve competence after a repair, regurgitant leaks after a mitral valve replacement, and RV and LV function.

e. Measures noted above to decrease PA pressures may be used before or after bypass to optimize RV function. Both RV and LV function may be compromised after mitral valve surgery, requiring judicious hemodynamic support. This is discussed in detail on pages 385–396 and 530–534.

f. **Percutaneous mitral valve repairs** (MitraClip) are performed under general anesthesia with the use of TEE monitoring. A Swan-Ganz catheter may be placed for documentation of right heart pressures, but it is not essential. Left atrial pressures (assessment of the "v" wave) before and after clip placement are obtained by direct measurement through the guide catheter. Familiarity with all of the requisite TEE images and with 3D echo imaging is critical to the success of the procedure. Reduction in the degree of MR is anticipated but is generally not as successful as a surgical repair. Further comments on anesthesia for these repairs is noted in section XIII on pages 269–271.

H. **Maze procedure for atrial fibrillation**

1. The cut-and-sew Cox-Maze procedure to eliminate AF has been generally replaced by devices that produce comparable transmural ablation lines using either radiofrequency or cryoablation. A left atrial Maze procedure is most commonly performed as a concomitant procedure with mitral valve surgery, although a biatrial Maze may be more successful in eliminating AF (see Figures 1.28 and 1.29). Anesthesia management is directed toward the primary pathology for which surgery is being performed if the Maze procedure is performed as an adjunct. Medications may be used for rate control pre-CPB.

2. Bilateral pulmonary vein isolation (PVI) with resection and oversewing of the left atrial appendage is an appropriate procedure for patients with paroxysmal AF. This operation can be performed as an adjunct to any cardiac procedure or as an isolated operation. Surgery for lone AF may be performed through a sternotomy incision or through bilateral thoracoscopic ports. This requires repositioning of the patient with the operated side elevated about 30 degrees and the use of one-lung anesthesia to allow the surgeon better exposure to isolate the pulmonary veins. The "convergent" procedure entails a subcostal incision to place epicardial ablation lines followed by an endocardial approach by the electrophysiologist (see Chapter 1).

3. Most surgeons will use amiodarone for early AF prophylaxis, and this is usually given IV during the procedure (unless previously given) and then continued orally for several months.

I. **Tricuspid valve disease**

1. Maintenance of an elevated CVP is essential to achieve satisfactory forward flow in tricuspid stenosis. A Swan-Ganz catheter can be placed for monitoring PA pressures, although cardiac output determinations are of little value if TR is present. If placed at the beginning of surgery, it is withdrawn into the superior vena cava (SVC) when the tricuspid valve is being addressed and then is readvanced through a repaired valve or a bioprosthetic valve replacement. If not done under direct vision by the surgeon, advancement may need to be deferred until the SVC cannula has been removed. The Vigileo/FloTrac monitor can provide adequate cardiac output measurements based on the arterial line pulse wave, but it will be inaccurate with AF.

2. Normal sinus rhythm provides better hemodynamics than AF, although the latter is frequently present. Slower heart rates are preferable for tricuspid stenosis and faster heart rates for TR.

3. Tricuspid valve surgery requires entry into the right atrium. Therefore, tourniquets are placed around the SVC and inferior vena cava (IVC) cannulas to avoid air entry into the venous lines. With the SVC tourniquet tightened, the patient's head should be observed for congestion, which indicates inadequate drainage by the SVC cannula. An elevated CVP may be noted, depending on the location of the measurement.

4. Functional TR usually results from RV dilatation and dysfunction due to increased RV afterload from pulmonary hypertension. TEE assessment of tricuspid annular diameter may be helpful to the surgeon in determining whether a tricuspid valve repair is indicated for functional TR even when mild–moderate in severity.[52] A dilated annulus ≥40 or ≥21 mm^2 is a Class IIa indication for tricuspid repair during left-sided repairs.[53]

5. RV dysfunction is not uncommon once valve competence has been restored and may be exacerbated by suboptimal RV protection during cardioplegic arrest. Tricuspid valve repair for severe TR in patients with preexisting RV dysfunction is very high risk, and use of inotropes that can also lower the PVR (milrinone, dobutamine, and rarely isoproterenol), selective pulmonary vasodilators, or right ventricular assist device (RVAD) support may be required.

6. Patients with hepatic congestion often have abnormal liver function that can impair the synthesis of clotting factors. A coagulopathy may develop after CPB, necessitating use of multiple blood component transfusions (especially fresh frozen plasma and cryoprecipitate) to control bleeding.

J. Endocarditis

1. Anesthetic management is dictated by the hemodynamic derangements associated with the particular valve involved. TEE is invaluable in identifying valve pathology, vegetations, and perivalvular abscesses, and may occasionally demonstrate involvement of other valves not appreciated on preoperative studies.

2. Surgery may be required urgently for HF or cardiogenic shock when there are acute regurgitant lesions, or for persistent sepsis. These patients tend to be quite ill, often with significant respiratory, cardiac, renal, and hematologic problems. Those operated upon for large vegetations or peripheral embolization tend to be more stable. Patients with aortic valve endocarditis may develop heart block from involvement of the conduction system by periannular infection. This may require preoperative placement of a transvenous pacing wire.

3. Ongoing sepsis may produce refractory hypotension on pump despite the use of α-agents. Vasopressin may be necessary to maintain blood pressure.

K. Aortic dissections

1. Maintenance of hemodynamic stability and especially avoidance of hypertension are critical to prevent aortic rupture, especially during the induction of anesthesia and line insertion. Use of a Swan-Ganz catheter is helpful in optimizing perioperative hemodynamics. Its insertion should be delayed until after intubation to minimize the stress response or can be performed later for postoperative management.

2. Most patients require emergency surgery and should be considered to have a full stomach. A modified rapid-sequence induction should be performed to minimize the risk of aspiration while ensuring hemodynamic stability.

3. TEE is useful in localizing the site of the intimal tear and the proximal (and occasionally the distal) extent of the dissection, the degree of AR, and the presence of a

hemopericardium. Because the diagnosis of an aortic dissection is usually obtained by a contrast CT scan, TEE is best performed once the patient has been anesthetized. If the diagnosis is in doubt, a TEE may be performed in an awake patient. In this situation, TEE must be performed **very cautiously** with light sedation for fear of precipitating hypertension, rupture, and then tamponade.

4. Repair of a type A dissection is usually performed during a period of deep hypothermic circulatory arrest (DHCA). The head is packed in ice, and medications may be given to potentially provide additional cerebral protection (see section L.1). To document reaching 18–20 °C for DHCA, tympanic temperatures correlate better with arterial blood temperatures than do bladder and rectal measurements, which are considered to represent the core temperature.[54] Use of a temperature management system is important to prevent temperature afterdrop during the rewarming phase. Uncommonly, the repair does not require DHCA and these measures are not necessary.[55] Coagulopathies should be anticipated with this procedure, and blood clotting factors should be requested early and should be available immediately after protamine administration, if needed.

5. Repair of type B dissections should be accomplished by an endovascular approach if at all possible. An open surgical approach requires a period of descending aortic cross-clamping. Because less collateral flow is present in patients with dissections than with atherosclerotic aneurysms, the risk of paraplegia is greater. Left-heart bypass may reduce the risk of paraplegia.[56] A cerebrospinal fluid (CSF) drainage catheter should be placed before the patient is anesthetized. Proximal hypertension must be controlled during application of the cross-clamp, but it should not be so low as to compromise spinal cord perfusion. A CSF drain is also useful if an endovascular stent procedure is performed for a complicated type B dissection.[57]

L. **Ascending aortic and arch aneurysms**

1. Aneurysms limited to the ascending aorta are repaired on CPB with application of an aortic cross-clamp. If they extend more distally or the arch is extensively involved, a period of DHCA at 18–20 °C core temperature is used. This usually ensures a lower nasopharyngeal or tympanic temperature, which correlates best with brain temperature. At this point, it is inferred that there is EEG silence with a bispectral index (BIS) analysis reading of 0. This should provide about 45 minutes of safe arrest time and minimize the risk of neurologic insult.

2. Adjuncts to improve cerebral protection include selective antegrade (ACP) or retrograde cerebral perfusion (RCP), and packing the head in ice.[58–60] Administration of methylprednisolone 30 mg/kg may be considered, but evidence of any benefit is unclear.[61,62] Some groups prefer to use cold cerebral perfusion techniques to protect the brain while maintaining the body at only moderate hypothermia (21–28 °C).[62–64] One study found no difference in neurologic outcome between the use of DHCA + RCP and moderate HCA with ACP, but twice as many new diffusion-weighted MRI lesions were noted in the latter group.[64]

3. Profound hypothermia and warming are associated with a coagulopathy. Platelets, fresh frozen plasma, and cryoprecipitate are helpful in achieving hemostasis. Supplemental use of warming devices is beneficial in warming the patient and preventing temperature afterdrop.

M. **Descending aortic and thoracoabdominal aneurysms (TAAs)**

1. Arterial monitoring lines are inserted in the right radial and femoral arteries to monitor proximal and distal pressures during the period of aortic cross-clamping. The femoral line is valuable when left-heart bypass techniques are used.

2. A Swan-Ganz catheter is important to monitor filling pressures during the period of cross-clamping. TEE is helpful in evaluating myocardial function and often demonstrates a hypovolemic LV chamber despite elevated PA pressures when the cross-clamp is removed. Ensuring adequate intravascular volume will reduce the risk of "declamping shock" upon release of the aortic cross-clamp.

3. One-lung anesthesia using a double-lumen or Univent tube with a bronchial blocker improves operative exposure.

4. Control of proximal hypertension is essential during the cross-clamp period to minimize the adverse effects of increased afterload on LV function. However, lowering the pressure too much can reduce renal and spinal cord perfusion and increase the CSF pressure, so maintaining a pressure >130 mm Hg is recommended. Additional steps should be taken to optimize distal perfusion pressure to minimize the risk of distal ischemic injury during aortic cross-clamping. This includes use of CSF drainage, distal perfusion to maintain collateral network perfusion pressure, and reattachment of segmental arteries T8–12.[65] Cold renal perfusion, epidural cooling, or use of DHCA may also be considered.[66–68]

5. Endovascular stent placement is performed under conscious sedation or general anesthesia. Devices may be placed percutaneously or via a surgical groin incision with placement either directly into the femoral artery or through a side graft in patients with extensive aortoiliac disease. The landing zones are located by fluoroscopy. Spinal cord ischemia remains a concern with extensive endovascular repairs, and CSF drainage is recommended.[69]

N. **Implantable cardioverter-defibrillator (ICD) placement**

1. Transvenous ICD implantation is usually performed in an electrophysiology laboratory under moderate sedation with propofol or dexmedetomidine, allowing the patient to breathe spontaneously. When ventricular fibrillation is induced, deepening the level of sedation and assisted ventilation usually suffices. This requires close nursing or anesthesia attendance and careful monitoring. Most patients have markedly depressed ventricular function, and provisions for cardiac resuscitation (personnel and equipment) should be immediately available. External defibrillator pads should be placed for rescue defibrillation.

2. Medications that could be potentially arrhythmogenic, such as the catecholamines, must be avoided. Antiarrhythmic medications are continued unless there are plans for an electrophysiology study, which is usually performed with the patient off medications.

3. Subcutaneous ICD implants may require a higher level of sedation than transvenous implants, but generally it can be accomplished without the use of general anesthesia.[70]

O. **Cardioversion**

1. Awake patients requiring emergency cardioversion in the ICU are generally hemodynamically unstable and should be given extremely light sedation prior to being cardioverted (1–2.5 mg of midazolam or 2–5 mg morphine). If the patient

is still anesthetized and sedated, an increase in the infusion rate of propofol may be considered.

2. Patients requiring less urgent cardioversion for hemodynamic compromise or undergoing elective cardioversion (usually after TEE confirmation of absence of left atrial appendage thrombus) should receive a small dose of propofol (0.5–1 mg/kg or approximately 50–100 mg). Alternatively, etomidate (0.3 mg/kg or a 10–20 mg bolus) can be used, especially in patients with compromised ventricular function. Etomidate may produce myoclonus in up to 50% of patients, often causing ECG interference, which makes synchronized cardioversion very difficult.[71] Anesthesia stand-by is recommended to provide airway support during the short period of sedation.

P. **Surgery for pericardial disease**

1. Pericardial drainage of a large pericardial effusion or for tamponade is often performed urgently or emergently. In the immediate postoperative period, emergent exploration through a full sternotomy incision may be carried out in the ICU if tamponade is associated with severe hypotension or cardiac arrest. Otherwise, emergency exploration is carried out in the OR. Most patients are still intubated and sedated, and most still have a Swan-Ganz catheter and satisfactory venous access in place, and there is little time for insertion of additional lines. Patients are generally in a low cardiac output state, and blood pressure is dependent on adequate preload, increased heart rate, and increased sympathetic tone. Volume infusions and less commonly, β-agonists are beneficial in trying to maintain hemodynamic stability. Any medications that slow the heart rate must be avoided, and sedatives and anesthetic drugs that produce vasodilation must be given judiciously to avoid profound hypotension and cardiac arrest. Since loss of sympathetic tone can be catastrophic in a patient with tamponade physiology, prepping and draping of the patient should be considered before the administration of additional anesthetic agents. There is generally striking hemodynamic improvement once the pericardial blood is evacuated.

2. In less emergent situations, drainage is usually indicated for hemodynamically significant effusions. This may be accomplished by a pericardiocentesis performed in the cath lab with local anesthesia, depending on the size and location of the effusion. If this cannot be accomplished, the procedure is performed in the OR. A large-bore central venous line should be inserted. A subxiphoid incision can be made under local anesthesia with moderate sedation, but more commonly it is done under general anesthesia. Again, if there is evidence of tamponade, blood pressure is dependent on adequate preload, heart rate, and increased sympathetic tone, so agents that produce vasodilation, bradycardia, or myocardial depression must be avoided. The patient may need to be prepped and draped before the induction of anesthesia, to prevent cardiovascular collapse.

3. TEE is invaluable in identifying the size and hemodynamic effects of an effusion. With limited surgical approaches, such as a subxiphoid window or thoracoscopy, TEE can identify whether the effusion has been adequately drained.

4. After resolution of tamponade, filling pressures generally fall, blood pressure increases, and a brisk diuresis occurs. Depending on the duration of tamponade, some patients may require transient inotropic support after the fluid is removed.

5. Patients with chronic constrictive pericarditis are usually in a chronic, compensated low cardiac output state. It is similarly essential to avoid hypovolemia, vasodilation, bradycardia, or myocardial depression. After the constricted heart is decorticated, filling pressures may transiently fall, but many patients develop a low output state associated with RV dilatation and will require inotropic support. Inadequate decortication may be evident when a fluid challenge that restores the preoperative filling pressures fails to increase cardiac output. Pulmonary edema may develop if the surgeon decorticates the RV while the LV remains constricted.

V. Induction and Maintenance of Anesthesia

A. Cardiac anesthesia is provided by a combination of medications, including induction agents, anxiolytics, amnestics, analgesics, muscle relaxants, and inhalational anesthetics.[72] Although most centers used a "balanced anesthesia" technique, studies have reported comparable results with regimens of volatile inhalational anesthetics vs. total IV anesthesia for cardiac surgery.[73]

B. Induction agents may include propofol, etomidate, ketamine, or a benzodiazepine. Most commonly, anesthesia is induced with a combination of propofol, a narcotic, and a neuromuscular blocker to provide muscle relaxation and prevent chest wall rigidity that is associated with high-dose narcotic inductions. The most common doses for induction are propofol 1–2 mg/kg (50–100 mg), fentanyl 2.5–5 µg/kg (250–500 µg), and vecuronium 0.1 mg/kg IV followed by 0.01–0.03 mg/kg every 30 minutes. Alternative narcotics, such as sufentanil and remifentanil, are rarely used. Low-dose fentanyl has a duration of action of 1–4 hours, which allows the patient to awaken within hours of completion of the operation. Remifentanil is a very short-acting narcotic with a duration of action of only 10 minutes. It is beneficial in shorter operations and allows for very early awakening and extubation.

   1. Succinylcholine is a depolarizing agent with rapid onset that can be used during rapid-sequence inductions or in patients with difficult airways.

   2. Although rarely used, ketamine given with a benzodiazepine is very useful in patients with compromised hemodynamics or tamponade. Ketamine does not produce myocardial depression, and its dissociative effects and sympathetic stimulant properties that produce hypertension and tachycardia are attenuated by use of a benzodiazepine.[74]

C. Subsequently, anesthesia is maintained by additional dosing of narcotics and muscle relaxants in combination with an anxiolytic, such as propofol, and an inhalational agent (Tables 4.2 and 4.3). Bispectral electroencephalographic monitoring (BIS) can be used during on- and off-pump surgery to titrate and minimize the amount of medication required to maintain adequate anesthesia (a level around 55–60) while minimizing hemodynamic alterations and preventing awareness.[75,76] This is useful during off-pump surgery and during bypass, when hemodilution increases the effective volume of distribution of anesthetic medications and may necessitate redosing. The dose and selection of anesthetic agents must provide adequate anesthesia and analgesia during surgery, but it may be modified to allow for extubation in the OR or, more frequently, several hours after arrival in the ICU.

Table 4.2 • Hemodynamic Effects of Commonly Used Anesthetic Agents

	HR	Contractility	SVR	Net Effect on BP
Induction Agents				
Propofol (bolus)	↓	↓	↓↓	↓↓
Etomidate	↔	↔	↔	↔
Anxiolytics				
Midazolam	↑	↔	↓	↓
Propofol (drip)	↓	↓	↓	↓
Narcotics				
Fentanyl	↓	↔	↓	↓
Sufentanil	↓	↔	↓	↓
Alfentanil	↓	↔	↓	↓
Remifentanil	↓	↔	↓	↓
Muscle Relaxants				
Vecuronium	↔	↔	↔	↔
Atracurium	↔	↔	↓	↓
Cisatracurium	↔	↔	↔	↔
Rocuronium	↔	↔	↔	↔
Succinylcholine	↑↓	↓	↔	↑↓

HR, heart rate; SVR, systemic vascular resistance; BP, blood pressure

D. Midazolam has an elimination half-life of over 10 hours in patients undergoing cardiac surgery. Therefore, its use is best limited to the prebypass period.

E. Propofol is used for induction, may be given during bypass at doses of 20–30 μg/kg/min, and is usually given at the termination of CPB and continued in the ICU at a dose of 25–75 μg/kg/min.[77] Propofol can be used to control postbypass hypertension because of its strong vasodilator properties. When the patient is stable, the propofol is turned off and the patient is allowed to awaken.

F. Inhalational agents provide muscle relaxation and unconsciousness, with variable effects on myocardial depression. Agents commonly used include sevoflurane, desflurane, and isoflurane, with relatively comparable influence on outcomes.[78-81] They are generally given during CPB to maintain anesthesia and reduce blood pressure, and allow for use of lower doses of IV medications, although they provide

Table 4.3 • Doses of Commonly Used Drugs for Cardiac Anesthesia		
	Usual Dosage	**Duration of Action**
Induction Agents		
Propofol	1–2 mg/kg	2–8 min
Etomidate	0.2–0.4 mg/kg	3–8 min
Anxiolytics		
Propofol	25–30 µg/kg/min	up to 20 min
Midazolam	2.5–5 mg IV q2h or 1–4 mg/h	up to 10 h
Narcotics		
Fentanyl	5–10 µg/kg → 1–5 µg/kg	1–4 h
Remifentanil	1 µg/kg → 0.05–2 µg/kg/min	10 min
Muscle Relaxants		
Vecuronium	0.1 mg/kg → 0.01–0.03 mg/kg q30 min	45–90 min[a]/25–40 min[b]
Cisatracurium	0.15 mg/kg → 0.03 mg/kg q45–60 min	60 min
Rocuronium	0.6–1.2 mg/kg IV → 0.1–0.2 mg/kg q45 min	30–60 min
Succinylcholine	1 mg/kg	5–10 min

[a]After initial intubating dose; [b]after repeat dose in OR (continuous infusions used in ICU)

no analgesia. Desflurane and sevoflurane have been found to be cardioprotective. They have less lipid solubility with a rapid onset of action and are quickly reversible, allowing for early extubation. Nitrous oxide is contraindicated in that it reduces the amount of oxygen that can be delivered and it also may increase PA pressures.

G. Muscle relaxants are given throughout the operation to minimize patient movement and suppress shivering during hypothermia. Adequate muscle relaxation might reduce some of the paraspinal muscle soreness often noted after surgery due to sternal retraction. Most neuromuscular blockers have minimal effect on myocardial function or blood pressure other than atracurium, which tends to lower the blood pressure (Tables 4.2 and 4.3).

1. **Vecuronium** (Norcuron) does not undergo renal elimination and may be selected in patients with renal insufficiency. It does not have vagolytic properties, so the heart rate is generally fairly slow when used with fentanyl. **Rocuronium** (Zemuron) and **cisatracurium** (Nimbex) are short-acting neuromuscular blockers with rapid onset of action that can be used if very early

extubation is planned. **Pancuronium** is an excellent neuromuscular blocker that is beneficial in offsetting the bradycardia often noted with administration of narcotics. It has been in short supply since 2016 and is now used infrequently.

2. Although some centers reverse muscle relaxants at the end of the operation to expedite extubation, this may prove detrimental if the patient becomes agitated and develops hemodynamic alterations. A conservative approach is to observe the patient in the ICU for several hours, during which time most of the neuromuscular blockade dissipates, and extubation can then be achieved. **Adequate sedation must be maintained in the ICU while a patient remains pharmacologically paralyzed.**

H. **Dexmedetomidine** (Precedex) is an α_2-adrenergic agonist with numerous properties, including sedation, analgesia, anxiolysis, and sympatholysis. However, it lacks an amnesic effect. During surgery, it can be used to reduce the dosage of other medications, allowing for early, comfortable extubation. It may also reduce shivering and myocardial ischemia and may improve hemodynamic performance. It can be used alone to provide sedation during a TAVR. Another benefit of this drug is that it aids in weaning the patient from the ventilator when they develop agitation or patient–ventilator dyssynchrony as the propofol dose is decreased. In comparison with propofol, dexmedetomidine appears to shorten the duration of ventilation and is associated with a lower incidence of delirium, especially in older patients.[82,83] It is, however, associated with more bradycardia than propofol due to its sympatholytic effects. It is given as a loading dose of 1 µg/kg over 10 minutes followed by a continuous infusion of 0.2–1.5 µg/kg/h (most commonly in the 0.5–0.75 µg/kg/h range).

VI. General Prebypass Considerations

A. Prior to the commencement of surgery, the anesthesiologist is responsible for the safe insertion of monitoring lines, avoidance or treatment of hemodynamic or ischemic changes during the induction of anesthesia and intubation, and the placement and initial interpretation of the TEE (Table 4.4). In addition, the anesthesiologist is responsible for:

1. The administration of prophylactic antibiotics starting within one hour (cephalosporins) or two hours (vancomycin) of the initiation of surgery[14]

2. Placing external defibrillator pads (over the midaxillary line and back) for reoperations or TAVRs

3. Ensuring that positioning of the head and arms is safe (with nursing)

4. Ensuring adequate functioning of the cerebral oximetry pads (with perfusion)

B. Avoidance of ischemia prior to initiating bypass is critical for all types of heart surgery. Identification of ischemic ECG changes, elevation in filling pressures, or RWM abnormalities on TEE requires prompt attention. Manipulation of the heart by the surgeon for cannula placement, blood loss during redo dissections, ongoing blood loss from leg incisions, and AF during atrial cannulation are a few of the potential insults that must be addressed. Judicious use of fluids and α-agents to counteract vasodilation and hypotension, β-blockers or additional anesthetic agents to treat hypertension or tachycardia, and nitroglycerin to treat ischemia must be selected

Table 4.4 • Anesthetic Considerations Prior to Cardiopulmonary Bypass
1. Line insertion and monitoring
2. Antibiotics prior to skin incision
3. External defibrillator pads for reoperations
4. Selection of medications for "balanced anesthesia" and plans for early extubation
5. Endotracheal intubation
6. Transesophageal echocardiography
7. Antifibrinolytic drug administration
8. Insertion of coronary sinus catheter or vents in minimally invasive surgery
9. Maintaining hemodynamics and avoiding or treating ischemia
10. Monitoring and treatment of abnormal cerebral oximetry
11. Heparinization for CPB

appropriately to maintain stable hemodynamics. In the prebypass period, fluids are usually administered in the form of crystalloid, but excessive infusions in vasodilated patients and those with significant preoperative anemia should be avoided. During minimally invasive surgery, the limited exposure may prevent the surgeon from directly visualizing most of the heart, reinforcing the importance of the anesthesiologist in using appropriate monitoring to identify and address abnormalities to ensure a stable perioperative course.

C. **Transesophageal echocardiography** should be performed after intubation and line placement to provide a baseline assessment of RWM abnormalities and to identify known or overlooked valvular pathology. A comprehensive TEE examination should be performed according to ASE guidelines.[31] In minimally invasive valve cases, it is used to identify the placement of the coronary sinus catheter and PA vent and the positioning of the femoral venous line in the right atrium. For off-pump bypass surgery, it is utilized to assess RWM abnormalities during bypass grafting.

D. **Autologous blood withdrawal** before the institution of bypass protects platelets from the damaging effects of CPB. The quality of this blood is excellent, with only slight activation of platelets, and it has been demonstrated to preserve red cell mass and reduce transfusion requirements.[84,85] It can be considered in patients for whom the calculated hematocrit on pump will remain adequate after withdrawal of 1–2 units of blood with nonheme fluid replacement.

E. **Steroids** might be considered to mitigate the systemic inflammatory response to CPB, although evidence of significant clinical benefit is weak. Use of high doses of methylprednisolone (30 mg/kg) or dexamethasone (1 mg/kg) may reduce emetic symptoms and improve appetite after surgery, but they have been associated with hyperglycemia, metabolic acidosis, an increased risk of delayed tamponade, transient subclinical organ system damage, as well as more pronounced pulmonary dysfunction.[86–93]

F. **Antifibrinolytic drugs** have been demonstrated to reduce perioperative blood loss in cardiac operations.[94,95] They should be used for all on-pump procedures and may be of benefit in off-pump cases as well. Most protocols include giving the first dose at the time of skin incision, giving a dose in the pump prime, and administering a constant infusion throughout the operation. One report suggests that the initial dose should be given after heparinization, since thrombus was noted on a PA catheter when given earlier.[96]

1. **ε-aminocaproic acid** (Amicar) is an inexpensive medication that has antifibrinolytic properties, and it may also preserve platelet function by inhibiting the conversion of plasminogen to plasmin. It is primarily effective in reducing bleeding when given prophylactically, with questionable benefit if given only for postoperative bleeding with suspected fibrinolysis.[97] There are not that many reports on its efficacy, but it is the most commonly used antifibrinolytic medication in the US. Studies suggest equal benefit to that of tranexamic acid.[98]

   a. One common regimen is to give 5 g after the induction of anesthesia, 5 g on pump, and 1 g/h during the procedure. Twice this dose is commonly used in patients weighing over 100 kg.

   b. A pharmacokinetic study showed that the clearance of ε-aminocaproic acid decreases and the volume of distribution increases during CPB. To maintain a plasma level of 260 mg/mL, an alternative weight-based protocol of a 50 mg/kg load over 20 minutes followed by a maintenance infusion of 25 mg/kg/h has been described.[99]

   c. Few adverse clinical effects have been noted with use of ε-aminocaproic acid. There is no increased risk of stroke.[100] Although a subtle degree of renal tubular dysfunction may occur, as demonstrated by an increase in urine β_2-microglobulin levels, a 10 g dose was not shown to alter creatinine clearance.[101]

2. **Tranexamic acid** (TXA) has similar properties to ε-aminocaproic acid, inhibiting fibrinolysis at a serum concentration of 10 μg/mL, and reducing plasmin-induced platelet activation at a level of 16 μg/mL.[102] It has been shown to reduce perioperative blood loss in on- and off-pump surgery.[103,104] Two studies showed that it significantly reduced blood loss in patients in whom aspirin and clopidogrel were given within seven days of surgery, possibly implying that surgery need not be delayed for a patient on clopidogrel. However, in those studies, the last dose was actually given on average five days prior to surgery, and there was most likely good recovery of platelet function within that time.[105,106] There are a variety of dosing protocols that have been recommended with slightly better efficacy at higher doses.[107] However, TXA has been associated with dose-related convulsive seizures in about 1% of patients. The commonly utilized protocols are the following:[94]

   a. Modified low dose: 5 mg/kg load followed by 5 mg/kg/h

   b. Low dose: 10 mg/kg over 20 minutes with 1–2 mg/kg in the pump prime, followed by a 1 mg/kg/h infusion – probably preferable in patients at low risk for bleeding

   c. High dose: 30 mg/kg loading dose, 2 mg/kg in the pump prime, and 16 mg/kg/h continuous infusion – probably preferable in patients at high risk for bleeding[108]

3. **Aprotinin** is a serine protease inhibitor that was found to be extremely effective in reducing perioperative bleeding in most cardiac procedures. It exhibited antifibrinolytic effects, preserved platelet function, and inhibited kallikrein, producing an anti-inflammatory effect. Although it was withdrawn from the US market in 2007, it is still available in other countries under select circumstances.

G. Anticoagulation for cardiopulmonary bypass

1. Anticoagulation is essential during CPB to minimize the generation of thrombin and fibrin monomers caused by the interaction of blood with a synthetic interface. UFH is universally used because it is an effective anticoagulant and is reversible with protamine. In contrast, other anticoagulants that can be used for CPB, such as the direct thrombin inhibitors, are not reversible.[109]

2. **Heparin dosing.** Heparin inhibits the coagulation system by binding to antithrombin (AT, previously called antithrombin III), inactivating primarily thrombin and factor Xa. Inactivation of thrombin prevents fibrin formation and also inhibits thrombin-induced activation of platelets and factors V, VIII, and XI. A baseline activated clotting time (ACT) should be drawn after the operation has commenced and before systemic heparinization. One study recommended that the initial ACT should be drawn through the introducer sheath prior to placing a heparin-coated PA catheter which may artificially elevate the baseline ACT.[110] A small dose of heparin (5000 units = 50 mg) is given before division of the ITA or radial artery. The level IIa recommendation from joint societies is to administer an empiric total dose of 3 mg/kg of heparin prior to cannulation for CPB. Porcine heparin is associated with a lower risk of heparin antibody formation than bovine heparin and is therefore recommended.[111]

3. **Heparin monitoring** is performed using a number of systems that measure the ACT.[112]

   a. The ACT qualitatively assesses the anticoagulant effect of heparin, but does not measure nor necessarily correlate with heparin concentrations.[113] There is great variability in patient response to heparin, and the ACT can be affected by hypothermia, hemodilution, and to a lesser degree by thrombocytopenia. Nonetheless, due to its simplicity and overall safety, achieving and maintaining a satisfactory ACT (>480 seconds for routine circuits and >400 seconds in biocompatible circuits) throughout the pump run is acceptable and universally utilized. ACTs should be monitored every 20–30 minutes during bypass (or prior to bypass if there is a significant delay before initiating bypass after initial heparinization), and additional heparin should be given as necessary. The Hepcon (Medtronic), Hemochron (Accriva Diagnostics), and i-STAT (Abbott Point of Care) devices are commonly used to measure ACTs with this approach.

   b. Because of individual patient variability in response to heparin, anticoagulation can also be assessed by calculating dose-response curves using the Medtronic Hemostasis Management Systems (HMS or HMS Plus) or the Hemochron Response RxDx heparin and protamine dosing system. These systems measure circulating levels of heparin (desired level is >2–2.5 units/mL), determine the appropriate amount of heparin to achieve a desired ACT, and calculate the dose of protamine required to neutralize the heparin. Whole blood heparin concentrations correlate better with plasma anti-Xa levels than the ACT. Achieving patient-specific heparin levels more effectively suppresses hemostatic system activation than standard dosing based on an ACT alone, with less thrombin generation, less fibrinolysis, and less platelet activation. Although more heparin is often given with this system, less protamine is required for reversal, and less bleeding is noted after protamine neutralization.[112,114] Despite these advantages, use of these systems has only a level IIb indication for use because they have not been shown to influence clinical outcomes.[112] During cases involving DHCA, maintenance of blood heparin concentrations, rather than ACTs, has been shown to preserve the coagulation system better.[115]

c. Use of heparin-bonded circuits to reduce the inflammatory response has reduced the requisite level of heparinization necessary to minimize activation of the coagulation system. However, underanticoagulation results in thrombin generation, which then triggers platelet activation, resulting in clotting within the bypass circuit. An ACT exceeding 400 seconds is generally recommended with use of these circuits.

d. During off-pump surgery, the optimal ACT is most likely >250 seconds and can be achieved with 2.5 mg/kg of heparin in most cases. This should minimize thrombin formation, reduce activation of the coagulation system, and minimize fibrinolysis. This ACT level is not associated with an increased risk of thrombotic complications.[116,117]

4. **Heparin resistance** is present when a heparin dose of 5 mg/kg fails to raise the ACT to an adequate level (>480 seconds). This is usually caused by AT deficiency, which can lead to a hypercoagulable state.

a. This is more likely to occur in patients on preoperative heparin, IV nitroglycerin, or an IABP, with elevated platelet counts >300,000/mm³, and with infective endocarditis.[118] Other risk factors associated with heparin resistance include high fibrinogen levels, which reduce the capacity of heparin to bind to AT, and smoking and COPD, which activate platelets and increase inflammatory markers and fibrinogen levels.[119] Interestingly, it has been noted that heparin resistance can occur despite normal AT levels assessed by lab testing. Conversely, heparin resistance does not necessarily occur when AT levels are low. One study suggested that prophylactic AT administration in high-risk patients might be considered despite a normal AT level to achieve optimal heparinization for CPB.[119]

b. If additional heparin does not elevate the ACT, fresh frozen plasma is usually given first to achieve an adequate ACT.[120] However, this may not be effective and is associated with potential transfusion-related side effects.[121] Human AT is commercially available from a number of companies, the most common product being Thrombate III (Grifols) which contains 500 units per vial.[122] Precise dosing of this product is difficult because baseline levels of AT are unknown in most cases and are most likely higher than levels noted in the rare patient with a hereditary AT deficiency. The amount needed is calculated as (desired – baseline AT level) × weight (kg) divided by 1.4. For example, to reach 120% of normal levels (which is recommended) in a 70 kg man with a baseline level 80% of normal would require $[(120 - 80)/1.4] \times 70 = 2000$ units or 28 units/kg. If the baseline level is 50% of normal, 3500 units (50 units/kg) should be given. Another alternative is to use bivalirudin as the anticoagulant during bypass.[123]

5. **Heparin-induced thrombocytopenia (HIT)** is a condition associated with the development of heparin-platelet factor 4 (PF4) complex antibodies that bind to platelets, triggering arterial and venous thrombosis.[124,125] A fall of >50% in platelet count following administration of heparin is noted in most patients with HIT, but

other potential etiologies for thrombocytopenia must be considered (especially the use of glycoprotein IIb/IIIa inhibitors). If HIT is not identified and appropriately dealt with by using alternative anticoagulation regimens during surgery, it may be associated with life-threatening postoperative complications.

a. Most patients have been exposed to heparin for catheterization, and heparin-PF4 antibodies are detected by ELISA testing prior to surgery in 5–19% of patients in various studies.[125–129] However, ELISA serologic testing for IgG-specific heparin-dependent platelet antibodies has replaced prior testing that also detected non-HIT causing IgM antibodies. Such testing was positive in about 20% of preoperative cardiac surgical patients, but only a minority of these patients actually have HIT-causing antibodies and are susceptible to thrombotic complications that can be avoided by using alternative anticoagulation.[130]

b. The benefit of assessing for the presence of preoperative heparin PF4 antibodies is not defined, and testing for preoperative antibodies in the absence of thrombocytopenia, thrombosis, or a known history of HIT is not indicated. The presence of antibodies alone is arguably not associated with an increased thrombotic risk, but it may be associated with other adverse outcomes, independent of the occurrence of HIT. However, if IgG platelet antibodies are present along with thrombocytopenia or thrombosis, it is beneficial to perform functional washed platelet activation assays, including the serotonin release assay, to confirm the diagnosis of HIT.

c. If HIT is present and the surgery is not urgent, it is best to wait three months before performing surgery. Antibodies usually clear in less than three months, at which time UFH can be used safely during surgery if the washed platelet activation assay is negative.

d. When surgery is necessary on a more urgent basis and either acute HIT or subacute HIT (recovery from thrombocytopenia but a positive washed platelet activation assay) is present, use of UFH alone increases the risk of rapid-onset HIT. Therefore, an alternate anticoagulation regimen is indicated.

   i. **Bivalirudin**, a direct thrombin inhibitor, is the best alternative for anticoagulation for CPB when HIT is present. It has a rapid onset of action and a half-life of 25 minutes. It is primarily metabolized by proteolytic cleavage with only 20% renal elimination, so slight modification is necessary in patients with renal dysfunction. It cannot be reversed, but it can be eliminated by hemofiltration and plasmapheresis. Studies comparing bivalirudin with UFH for cardiac surgery (on- and off-pump) in patients with and without HIT have shown comparable outcomes.[131–133] Attention must be paid to avoiding blood stagnation, which will cause nonenzymatic degradation of bivalirudin and allow for clotting to occur within the pump system, and to limiting the use of cardiotomy suction, so as to minimize the activation of the coagulation cascade.

   - Dosing for on-pump surgery: 1.25 mg/kg load over five minutes, 50 mg in the pump prime, then a 2.5 mg/kg/h infusion. The infusion rate may be increased in increments of 0.1–0.5 mg/kg/h to maintain the ACT >2.5 times baseline or >500 seconds. The drug should be stopped 10–15 minutes before coming off CPB. If more than 20 minutes is anticipated before terminating bypass, the bivalirudin should be redosed with 0.5

mg/kg and a 2.5 mg/kg/h infusion should be restarted. Ultrafiltration can remove 70% of the bivalirudin after coming off CPB.

- Dosing for off-pump surgery: 0.75 mg/kg bolus, then 1.75 mg/kg/h to maintain an ACT >300 seconds.

   ii. If it is elected not to use bivalirudin for anticoagulation, other protocols include the use of UFH in the usual dose along with drugs that inhibit platelet activation, such as the prostacyclin analogs and IIb/IIIa inhibitors.

- **Epoprostenol** is given in a dose of 5 ng/kg/min and increased by 5 ng/kg/min increments every five minutes (observing for systemic hypotension) up to 25 ng/kg/min, following which a heparin bolus is given. After protamine administration, the dose is weaned in 5 ng/kg decrements.[134]

- **Iloprost** can be given starting at a dose of 3 ng/kg/min with a doubling of the dose every five minutes to a dose determined by preoperative *in vitro* testing. The usual dose required is 6–24 ng/kg/min.[135]

- **Tirofiban**, a short-acting glycoprotein IIb/IIIa inhibitor, can be given as a 10 mg/kg bolus 10 minutes prior to administration of standard-dose heparin, followed by 0.15 μg/kg/min. It should be stopped one hour before the anticipated conclusion of CPB. Generally, 80% of the antiplatelet effect dissipates within four hours. Thus, bleeding may persist for a period of time after CPB has terminated, for which recombinant factor VIIa has been found beneficial.[136]

VII. Considerations During Cardiopulmonary Bypass

  A. Virtually all valve surgery and most coronary bypass surgery is performed using CPB (Table 4.5). The essential components of the CPB circuit are discussed in Chapter 5. Basically, the blood drains by gravity or with vacuum assist from the right atrium into a reservoir, is oxygenated, cooled or warmed, and then returned to the patient through an arterial cannula, which is usually placed in the ascending aorta. The same principles apply during minimally invasive surgery, although the cannulation sites may vary. Desired hemodynamic and laboratory values during bypass are noted in Table 5.2 (page 299).

  B. The lungs are not ventilated during bypass, as oxygenation occurs within the oxygenator and carbon dioxide is eliminated by the gas flow into the oxygenator (the

---

Table 4.5 • Anesthetic Considerations During Bypass (with Perfusionist)

1. Use of vasopressor drugs to support systemic blood pressure
2. Administration of adjunctive drugs to optimize renal perfusion
3. Maintain adequate level of anesthesia with inhalational anesthetics or IV medications
4. Monitor cerebral oximetry
5. Sample blood for ACTs
6. Re-administer antibiotics (cephalosporin) either when going on pump or at four-hour intervals
7. Maintain blood glucose <180 mg/dL with IV insulin infusion

sweep rate). Although some studies have suggested that the efficacy of gas exchange post-pump is improved if the lungs remain inflated with continuous positive airway pressure (CPAP) during CPB, this is not common practice.[137] Arterial blood gases are measured to ensure that the oxygenator is providing adequate oxygenation and that CO_2 extraction is sufficient. Venous oxygen saturation is measured to determine if the systemic flow rate is adequate, and should be >65%. If in-line monitoring is not available, studies should be repeated every 15–20 minutes by the perfusionist.

C. Systemic hypothermia is utilized to varying degrees during on-pump surgery as a means of organ system protection while the heart–lung machine provides nonphysiologic, nonpulsatile flow at low mean pressures. Cooling is initiated soon after CPB is started, and warming is commenced based on the amount of additional surgery anticipated so as to achieve near-normothermia when CPB is terminated. Temperature is usually measured in the bladder using a Foley catheter with a temperature sensor, which is considered to represent core temperature. It is also measured in the venous return line and from the PA catheter. The STS guidelines recommend avoiding overwarming the patient to a core temperature greater than 37 °C to reduce the risk of neurologic damage, since the recorded bladder temperature will underestimate brain temperature and the brain receives the initial warmer flow from the aortic cannula.[138] Temperature afterdrop is uncommon when mild–moderate hypothermia (>30 °C) is used, and warming devices are not necessary. In contrast, these devices are very helpful in preserving body temperature upon warming from deeper hypothermia. A warming device should be considered for blood and blood-product transfusions, which may be given at a rapid rate.

D. The serum level of antibiotics falls approximately 30–50% at the time of initiation of CPB, and an additional dose of a cephalosporin should be considered at that time. Alternatively, a second dose can be given 3–4 hours after the initial dose.[14] An additional dose of vancomycin is not necessary.

E. The optimal mean blood pressure during CPB to maintain adequate organ system perfusion is controversial. It has been shown that cerebral blood flow is more dependent on blood pressure than on flow rate.[139,140] The brain is able to maintain cerebral blood flow by autoregulation until the pressure falls below 40 mm Hg, but this response is inadequate in diabetic and hypertensive patients, in whom a higher pressure must be maintained. Systemic pressures are subject to a number of variables.

1. Hypotension occurring on bypass is usually multifactorial. It may be related to hemodilution, use of preoperative vasodilators (ACE inhibitors, ARBs, calcium channel blockers, and amiodarone), vasodilators used during bypass (inhalational anesthetics and propofol), vasodilation during rewarming, and autonomic dysfunction. It may also result from inadequate systemic flow rates, impairment of venous drainage, aortic regurgitation, the administration of cardioplegia, and the return of large amounts of cardiotomy-suctioned blood into the circulation.

2. Hypertension may be related to vasoconstriction with hypothermia, inadequate levels of anesthesia and analgesia, elevation in endogenous catecholamine levels, and alterations in acid–base balance and blood gas exchange.

3. Standard management is to maintain a mean blood pressure around 65 mm Hg on CPB using vasodilators (narcotics, propofol, or inhalational anesthetics) or vasopressors (phenylephrine, norepinephrine, or vasopressin) as long as flow rates are

adequate. A venous oxygen saturation exceeding 65%, which is measured on-line by the perfusionist, generally indicates that the systemic flow rate is satisfactory, although there are usually differences in regional flow (i.e. less to the kidneys and splanchnic circulation). The venous saturation will be higher during systemic hypothermia, due to lower oxygen extraction, and may decrease significantly during rewarming, necessitating an increase in flow rates.

F. Cerebral oximetry to assess the adequacy of cerebral oxygenation during CPB is an essential element of intraoperative care. Three commonly used systems are the INVOS (Medtronic), Equanox (NONIN Medical), and Foresight (Edward Lifesciences) devices.[141] They use near-infrared technology to assess regional cerebral oxygen saturations (rSO_2) from bifrontal sensing pads placed on the patient's forehead (Figure 4.9).

1. The rSO_2 tends to fall during initiation of bypass and during rewarming, even with an increase in systemic flow. The rSO_2 promptly detects problems with arterial desaturation even before it is evident by pulse oximetry.[142] A reduction in rSO_2 greater than 20% may be associated with adverse neurologic outcomes and should be treated. Prior to bypass, steps to increase the systemic pressure or the PCO_2 will improve cerebral blood flow. Once on pump, modifications of flow rate, blood pressure, PCO_2, or the hematocrit may be beneficial.

2. Although a reduction in the monitored rSO_2 often reflects a poorly adherent sensor, a legitimate decrease in cerebral saturation may not only reflect moderate hypotension from vasodilatation or low pump flow rates, but could indicate cannula malplacement, aortic dissection, oxygenator or other pump-related failures, air embolism, or anaphylactic reactions to drugs, such as protamine. Although interventions to improve rSO_2 should intuitively reduce the adverse effects of desaturation, few studies have documented improvements in clinical outcome.[143,144]

3. Cerebral oximetry may be a surrogate measure of cerebral autoregulation. Although most patients can autoregulate down to a pressure of 40–50 mm Hg, studies suggest that this level may vary quite considerably in different patients (between 40 and 90 mm Hg) and is unpredictable based on patient demographics. Because of a documented association between the duration and extent of time below the

(A)

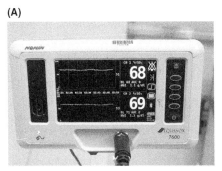

(B)

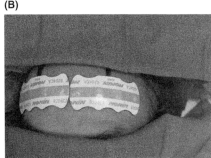

Figure 4.9 • (A) The NONIN Equanox cerebral oximeter. This device uses near-infrared spectroscopy to measure the regional saturation of predominantly venous blood directly in the brain through optical sensors placed on the right and left sides of the forehead (B).

limits of autoregulation and major morbidity after cardiac surgery, it has been recommended that maintaining an adequate mean pressure within the autoregulatory range for the brain, as calculated from the cerebral oximetry readings, may ensure adequate perfusion to other organs such as the kidney, where blood flow is also autoregulated.[145,146]

G. Blood glucose tends to be elevated due to the hormonal stress response to surgery and CPB with insulin resistance. An infusion of insulin to maintain blood glucose <180–200 mg/dL during surgery has not been shown to reduce inotropic requirements or the occurrence of arrhythmias, but it may reduce the incidence of neurocognitive dysfunction and other adverse outcomes, including death.[147–150] Overly aggressive protocols to maintain blood glucose <100 mg/dL during surgery may increase the risk of stroke and death.[151]

H. Measures to optimize renal function to reduce the risk of acute kidney injury (AKI) should be considered in patients with preoperative renal dysfunction (stage III–IV chronic kidney disease), especially in diabetic, hypertensive patients. The primary considerations should be maintaining a higher mean perfusion pressure (around 80 mm Hg) or, at the minimum, above the cerebral autoregulatory threshold,[145,146] keeping the pump run as short as possible, or avoiding it entirely with off-pump techniques. Profound anemia (hematocrit <20%) should be avoided, as it may increase the risk of AKI.[152,153] Pharmacologic means to optimize renal perfusion have been studied, with variable results.[154–157] Fenoldopam (0.03–0.1 μg/kg/min) may reduce the risk of AKI without any reduction in the need for renal replacement therapy or mortality.[158,159] Sodium bicarbonate or statins cannot be recommended, and nesiritide, which did show some promise, has not been manufactured since 2018. Although both renal-dose dopamine (3 μg/kg/min) and furosemide may increase urine output during CPB, neither has been found to be renoprotective.[160] In fact, furosemide has actually been shown to increase the incidence of postoperative renal dysfunction. However, the major cause of postoperative renal dysfunction is a low output state, so maintenance of satisfactory hemodynamics at the termination of CPB is essential so that any intraoperative renal insults are transient.

I. When the cross-clamp is removed, lidocaine (100 mg) and magnesium (1–2 g) may be given to reduce the incidence of atrial and ventricular arrhythmias.[161] Ventricular fibrillation tends to occur when the heart is maintained at cold temperatures during the period of cardioplegic arrest and usually requires defibrillation, although spontaneous conversion to a sinus mechanism may occur. Del Nido cardioplegia uses lidocaine as a major ingredient, so the heart is less likely to fibrillate with removal of the aortic cross-clamp.

J. Administration of perioperative amiodarone reduces the incidence of postoperative AF.[162] Based on the classic PAPABEAR trial published in 2005, amiodarone given for six days prior to and after surgery nearly halved the incidence of postoperative AF.[163] Since this is rarely feasible or cost-effective, a common protocol is to give a 150 mg bolus intraoperatively, followed by a 24-hour IV infusion and then conversion to oral therapy. Postoperative initiation of IV and then PO amiodarone is also effective in reducing AF, so it is surprising that one study suggested that intraoperative initiation of amiodarone was not effective.[164]

VIII. Termination of Bypass and Reversal of Anticoagulation

A. Once the cardiac portion of the operation has been completed, the lungs are ventilated, and pacing is initiated, if necessary. Just prior to weaning from CPB, calcium chloride 1 g may be given to increase systemic vascular resistance (SVR) and provide some initial inotropic support (Table 4.6).

B. Inotropic medications should be started before terminating bypass if it is anticipated that hemodynamic support may be necessary. This should be considered in patients with preexisting LV dysfunction, prebypass ischemia, recent infarction, suboptimal or incomplete revascularization, LV hypertrophy, and long cross-clamp times. If an α-agent (phenylephrine, norepinephrine) or vasopressin was necessary to support systemic pressure on pump, it will usually be required for a brief period of time after CPB is terminated.

C. Bypass is weaned by gradually reducing the venous return to the CPB circuit, increasing intravascular volume in the patient and reducing the arterial flow rate.

D. **Arterial blood pressure** monitoring in the radial artery is commonly inconsistent with the central aortic pressure, due to the presence of peripheral vasodilation. Measurement of the central aortic pressure using a stopcock on the aortic line is very helpful in sorting out discrepancies. If this problem persists for a short period of time, it is helpful to insert a femoral arterial monitoring line.

E. **TEE** is utilized as the patient is being weaned from bypass and after bypass is terminated (Table 4.1). Significant benefits include:

  1. Identifying intracardiac air. This is essential in valvular heart procedures or any procedure in which the left side of the heart has been entered (including venting). It is particularly valuable during minimally invasive procedures, in which exposure to the heart for deairing is limited.

Table 4.6 • Anesthetic Considerations at the Conclusion of CPB

When Terminating Bypass

1. Establish pacing as indicated
2. Resume mechanical ventilation
3. TEE to identify intracardiac air and assess ventricular function
4. Initiate pharmacologic therapy to support cardiac function and blood pressure as identified by TEE and Swan-Ganz catheter assessments

After Terminating Bypass

1. TEE to assess ventricular function and valve issues (native valves, repairs, replacements); identify residual air
2. Adjustment of pharmacologic support based on systemic blood pressure, TEE, and Swan-Ganz catheter measurements
3. Protamine administration
4. Use of blood and/or blood-component therapy as indicated (point-of-care testing)

2. Assessing regional and global ventricular function and correlating the cardiac output with loading conditions. TEE is the only means of assessing intravascular volume (preload) directly. The volume–pressure relationship is altered by decreased ventricular compliance after cardioplegic arrest, so higher filling pressures measured with the Swan-Ganz catheter are usually necessary to achieve adequate intravascular volume, especially with hypertrophied hearts. The TEE assessment of ventricular volume should be correlated with pressure measurements to determine optimal filling pressures for subsequent management. TEE is invaluable in determining whether hypotension should be treated by volume infusions, inotropic medications, or α-agents.

3. After valve surgery, detecting paravalvular leaks, obstructed valve leaflets, or the competence of a valve repair.

F. In most patients with satisfactory cardiac function, fluid administration to optimize preload is usually sufficient to obtain adequate hemodynamic parameters. Initially, filling pressures are increased by transfusing volume from the pump. After protamine administration, the blood remaining in the pump circuit is processed through the cell-saving device into bags and reinfused by the anesthesiologist into the patient. If this is not immediately available, a colloid is often chosen to maintain intravascular volume. Albumin is preferable to hetastarch compounds, which have been shown to increase bleeding and transfusion requirements.[165,166] Even the rapidly degradable low-molecular-weight hetastarch compounds have been shown to impair fibrin formation and clot strength and should be avoided.

G. If hemodynamic performance is not ideal, the anesthesiologist must work with the surgeon in assessing myocardial function and the need for inotropes. Visual inspection of the heart, assessment of serial cardiac outputs and filling pressures with a Swan-Ganz catheter, and TEE imaging can be used to assess ventricular function and identify potential problems.

1. Inotropic support is usually initiated with a catecholamine, such as epinephrine (1–2 μg/min) or dobutamine (5–10 μg/kg/min). If cardiac performance remains unsatisfactory, milrinone is extremely helpful in unloading the heart and providing inotropic support. Its preemptive use just prior to terminating bypass has been suggested as a means of ameliorating postoperative deterioration in cardiac performance and oxygen transport, and for reducing the need for catecholamine support.[167]

2. If the patient has a satisfactory cardiac output and good ventricular function on TEE, but has persistent hypotension ("vasoplegic" state), increasing doses of norepinephrine or phenylephrine are indicated. If the patient remains refractory to these medications, a bolus of 1 unit of vasopressin may be sufficient to "turn the corner". It may be necessary to continue vasopressin as an infusion of 0.01–0.1 units/min to maintain vascular tone. If the patient remains hypotensive, methylene blue 1.5–2 mg/kg is recommended.[168,169]

3. If the patient has persistent hypotension or a low cardiac output state for more than a minute or so, reinstitution of CPB to reperfuse the heart at a low workload will frequently result in improved ventricular function. This will also allow time to sort out the nature of the problem. In most situations, time and patience are all that is required to allow the heart to recover on bypass as additional

inotropic support is initiated. Remediable problems that might be encountered include:

    a. Air embolism down the right coronary artery, which may cause RV dysfunction and hypotension, necessitating a brief period of resumption of bypass to resolve. This is not an uncommon phenomenon after mitral valve surgery.

    b. A new RWM abnormality, which may suggest a technical problem with graft flow (kinking, twisting, anastomotic problem) that can be remedied. In mitral valve surgery, it might suggest circumflex artery entrapment if associated with lateral ECG changes. After aortic valve surgery or aortic root procedures, it might suggest impairment of coronary ostial flow by the valve prosthesis or kinking of the proximal coronary artery after coronary button reimplantation, respectively.

    c. A paravalvular leak, unexplained transvalvular leak, or impairment in mechanical valve leaflet motion that may require additional surgery.

4. If the heart still does not function well after being rested on bypass or after use of multiple pharmacologic agents, insertion of an IABP is usually necessary. When all of the above fail, consideration should be given to the use of ECMO or a circulatory assist device in appropriate candidates (see pages 555–574).

H. Reversal of anticoagulation. Protamine is a polycationic peptide administered to counteract the effects of heparin and is usually given in a 0.5-1 to 1:1 mg/mg ratio to the dose of heparin to return the ACT to baseline. The ACT may remain elevated from residual heparin effect, for which small additional doses of protamine may be given. This is helpful if the patient is transfused with several bags of cell-saver blood, which does contain a small amount of heparin. However, the ACT may also be elevated in patients with significant thrombocytopenia or a coagulopathy despite complete neutralization of heparin. Thus, additional protamine administered for an elevated ACT may not return it to baseline. Although moderate thrombocytopenia has not been shown to increase the ACT in patients with normally functioning platelets, it may increase it when associated with platelet dysfunction after bypass.[170]

1. The systems that perform heparin–protamine titration tests measure heparin levels in the bloodstream and determine the appropriate dose of protamine necessary to neutralize the remaining heparin. This usually results in less protamine being administered than empiric dosing based on the heparin dose. This may restore platelet responsiveness to thrombin and attenuate platelet α-granule secretion, resulting in less bleeding.[171] Thus, these systems should prevent the unnecessary administration of protamine to correct an abnormal ACT that is not attributable to excessive heparin. In fact, additional protamine, even just exceeding a 1:1 reversal ratio, may activate platelets and elevate the ACT, thus serving as an anticoagulant that may cause more bleeding![172,173]

2. "Heparin rebound" may occur when heparin reappears in the bloodstream after protamine neutralization. This is more likely to occur in patients who have received large doses of heparin during bypass and is more common in obese patients. This may occur because the half-life of protamine is only about 5 minutes and it has nearly completely disappeared from the bloodstream within 20 minutes.[174] A normal ACT may be noted despite residual heparin

activity, although the Medtronic HMS system and thromboelastography can assess whether there is still some circulating heparin.[175] If there is residual heparin or a heparin "rebound", it can be reversed with additional doses of protamine.[176]

3. IV administration of protamine may cause histamine release from the lungs, contributing to a decrease in systemic resistance and blood pressure, an effect not seen with intra-arterial injection. Nonetheless, evidence supporting any hemodynamic advantage to intra-arterial vs IV administration is controversial.[177,178]

I. **Protamine reactions** are unusual and often unpredictable, although they have been noted with greater frequency in patients taking NPH insulin, those with fish (not shellfish) or medication allergies, those with prior protamine exposure, and men who have had vasectomies. Awareness of the possibility of a protamine reaction, with a prompt therapeutic response if it occurs, is essential because protamine reactions are associated with increased perioperative mortality.[179–182]

1. **Type I.** Systemic hypotension from rapid administration (entire neutralizing dose after CPB given within three minutes). This is caused by a histamine-related reduction in systemic and pulmonary vascular resistance. It can be avoided by infusing the protamine over a 10- to 15-minute period and should be reversible with α-agent support.

2. **Type II.** Anaphylactic or anaphylactoid reaction resulting in hypotension, tachycardia, bronchospasm, flushing, and pulmonary edema.

   a. IIA. Idiosyncratic IgE- or IgG-mediated anaphylactic reaction. Release of histamine, leukotrienes, and kinins produces a systemic capillary leak causing hypotension and pulmonary edema. This tends to occur within the first 10 minutes of administration.

   b. IIB. Immediate nonimmunologic anaphylactoid reaction

   c. IIC. Delayed reactions, usually occurring 20 minutes or more after the protamine infusion has been started, probably related to complement activation and leukotriene release, producing wheezing, hypovolemia, and noncardiogenic pulmonary edema from a pulmonary capillary leak.

3. **Type III.** Catastrophic pulmonary vasoconstriction (CPV) manifested by elevated PA pressures, systemic hypotension from peripheral vasodilation, decreased left atrial pressures, RV dilatation, and myocardial depression. This reaction tends to occur about 10–20 minutes after the protamine infusion has started. One proposed mechanism involves activation of complement by the heparin-protamine complex that triggers leukocyte aggregation and release of liposomal enzymes that damage pulmonary tissue leading to pulmonary edema. Activation of the arachidonic acid pathway produces thromboxane, which constricts the pulmonary vessels. Pulmonary vasoconstriction usually abates after about 10 minutes.[182]

4. Prevention of protamine reactions is usually not possible. Skin testing has not proved of any value. In patients considered at high risk, type II reactions might be attenuated by the prophylactic use of histamine blockers (ranitidine 150 mg IV, diphenhydramine 50 mg IV) and steroids (hydrocortisone 100 mg IV). This common practice has not been shown clinically to be of much benefit.

5. Treatment of protamine reactions involves correction of any hemodynamic abnormalities that are identified. They must be differentiated from other conditions that can cause hemodynamic deterioration, such as hypoperfusion, air embolism, poor myocardial protection, or valve dysfunction. Measures must be taken to support the systemic blood pressure while reversing pulmonary vasoconstriction if also present. Preparations to reinstitute CPB are frequently necessary. The following options may be effective:

    a. Calcium chloride 500 mg IV to increase systemic resistance and provide some inotropic support

    b. α-agents (phenylephrine, norepinephrine, vasopressin) to support systemic resistance

    c. β-agents for inotropic support that can also reduce pulmonary resistance (low-dose epinephrine, dobutamine, milrinone)

    d. Readily available drugs to reduce preload and pulmonary pressures (nitroglycerin)

    e. Aminophylline for wheezing

    f. Re-administration of heparin to reverse the protamine reaction by reducing heparin–protamine complex size

    g. Steroids (hydrocortisone 100 mg IV)

    h. Methylene blue might be beneficial because of the possible involvement of nitric oxide in the pathogenesis of CPV.[182]

J. **Alternatives to reverse anticoagulation.** Although simply not reversing heparin and administering clotting factors may suffice in ameliorating the bleeding caused by residual heparin when protamine cannot be used, other measures have been evaluated to reverse heparin effect. These include use of heparinase I, recombinant PF4, and heparin removal devices.[183-186] Interestingly, PF4 has been shown to reverse the effects of LMWH, which is incompletely accomplished by protamine.[187]

K. **Treatment of coagulopathy.** Cessation of antiplatelet medications (except low-dose aspirin) and other anticoagulants, performing a meticulous operation, and the routine use of antifibrinolytic drugs should result in minimal postoperative bleeding in most patients undergoing cardiac surgery. However, a coagulopathy of varying degrees is probably present in all patients after CPB. Generally, the longer the duration of CPB, the more profound the degree of systemic hypothermia, and the more blood transfusions required on pump, the greater the coagulopathy.

1. Most groups treat coagulopathies in the OR by the "shotgun approach". This entails the empiric administration of small additional doses of protamine for an elevated ACT, and the transfusion of platelets, fresh frozen plasma, and/or cryoprecipitate for suspected coagulopathic bleeding. It is best to prioritize these products based on suspicion of the hemostatic defect while awaiting the results of coagulation studies. For example, platelet transfusions should be given first to patients on aspirin or with recent use of P2Y12 inhibitors (clopidogrel, ticagrelor, or prasugrel) or with uremia; fresh frozen plasma should be considered first for patients on preoperative warfarin, with hepatic dysfunction, or when multiple transfusions are given on pump; and uremic patients might benefit from desmopressin (see page 439). Cryoprecipitate is helpful in improving platelet

function, especially when the fibrinogen level is low. Alternative products include prothrombin complex concentrate and fibrinogen concentrates (see pages 444–445). Recombinant factor VIIa is particularly effective in achieving hemostasis when the coagulopathy is severe, although it may be associated with thrombotic complications.[188,189]

2. Although this particular approach will usually stem the "coagulopathic tide", it is more scientific and cost-effective to use point-of-care testing to assess the specific hemostatic defect and direct care accordingly.[113] Systems are available to measure the PT, PTT, and platelet count, and several are capable of measuring platelet function as well. Rotational thromboelastometry and thromboelastography are valuable tests that evaluate the entire clotting process and are very effective in identifying the exact hemostatic defect in the bleeding patient that needs to be addressed (see Figure 9.1).[190–192] However, their routine use in cardiac surgery may not be justifiable.

3. Further comments on the prevention, assessment, and management of mediastinal bleeding can be found in Chapter 9.

IX. Anesthetic Considerations During Off-pump Coronary Surgery[193]

A. Monitoring considerations

1. In contrast to on-pump surgery, off-pump surgery via a median sternotomy requires that the heart provide adequate systemic perfusion at all times. Hemodynamics may be compromised by positioning of the heart, myocardial ischemia, ventricular arrhythmias, bleeding, and valvular regurgitation (Table 4.7).

2. To assess for myocardial ischemia and dysfunction when the heart is positioned at unorthodox angles, more intensive monitoring is required than for on-pump surgery. Swan-Ganz catheters that provide in-line continuous cardiac outputs and mixed venous oxygen saturations are very beneficial. These will dictate whether volume infusion or pharmacologic management is indicated. Pulse contour analysis using the Vigileo/FloTrac or other available systems attached to the radial

---

Table 4.7 • Key Elements of Anesthetic Management of Off-Pump Surgery

1. Continuous cardiac output and mixed venous oxygen monitoring
2. Transesophageal echocardiography
3. Antifibrinolytic drugs
4. Low-level heparinization with ACT >250 seconds
5. Short-acting anesthetic agents
6. Maintenance of systemic normothermia with use of warming devices
7. Arrhythmia prophylaxis with lidocaine and magnesium
8. Availability of pacing capability
9. Maintenance of hemodynamics with fluid, α-agents, and inotropes
10. Patience and emotional support for the surgeon!

artery catheter can also provide accurate cardiac output measurements during heart displacement when TEE imaging may be suboptimal.[194] Simply maintaining an adequate blood pressure and heart rate pharmacologically may not suffice and often will provide no premonitory indication that the heart is becoming ischemic and subject to precipitous deterioration into ventricular fibrillation.

3. TEE is helpful in assessing for the development of RWM abnormalities during construction of an anastomosis that may be indicative of acute ischemia.[39] The anesthesiologist should be well trained in TEE and must immediately communicate any problem to the surgeon. Steps can then be taken to resolve the problem, often with the placement of a shunt to improve flow.[195] During vessel occlusion, TEE should assess for the acute development of regional LV dysfunction or acute MR during construction of left-sided grafts and for RV or inferior wall dysfunction during right-sided grafting. If RWM abnormalities persist after the graft is completed, a technical problem with the anastomosis should be suspected. The ME windows are best for assessing RV and LV function. The TG views are not helpful when the heart is elevated out of the chest. TEE will lead to modifications of the surgical strategy in a significant number of patients.[196]

B. **Anesthetic agents** are similar to those used for on-pump surgery, although shorter-acting medications may be selected, depending on plans for extubation. Although patients can be extubated in the OR, a more common practice is to use propofol for sedation at the end of surgery and for several hours in the ICU before considering extubation.

C. **Heparinization** is essential during off-pump surgery during vessel occlusion, and the extrinsic coagulation system is still activated by release of tissue factor. Usually about 2–2.5 mg/kg of heparin suffices to raise the ACT to >250 seconds, with some patient variability. There have been concerns about the prothrombotic tendency noted after OPCAB, since the hemodilution, platelet dysfunction, and fibrinolysis associated with CPB may not be seen.[197,198] This prothrombotic tendency may be related to the procoagulant activity of platelets or to the activation of fibrinogen and other acute-phase reactants that result from the surgery. However, this recommended dose of heparin is not associated with significant thrombin generation, activation of the coagulation system, or fibrinolysis, and it has not been associated with graft closure problems.[116,117]

D. **Antifibrinolytic therapy** with TXA has been to shown to minimize bleeding in OPCAB surgery.[103] Although the blood is not subject to contact activation in an extracorporeal circuit, heparinization does induce fibrinolysis, and antifibrinolytic agents may be beneficial without causing a hypercoagulable state. ε-aminocaproic acid (Amicar) can also be used with the same anticipated benefit.

E. **Patient temperature** tends to drift during open-chest procedures, but it should be maintained as close to normothermia as possible to prevent arrhythmias, bleeding, and subsequent shivering in the ICU. The ambient room temperature must be raised into the low-70s Fahrenheit and some form of warming blanket should be considered. These include a sterile Bair Hugger (3M Company) and heat-emitting devices, such as the Kimberly-Clark temperature management system.[199] The endovascular Thermogard system (Zoll Medical Corporation) has also been used effectively in optimizing intraoperative temperature control during OPCAB.[200] All fluids must be warmed as they are being administered.[201]

F. **Maintenance of hemodynamics.** During cardiac positioning, the patient is placed in the Trendelenburg position and the OR table is rotated to the right. Deep pericardial sutures are placed to aid with retraction. Apical suction devices can also be used to rotate the heart cephalad and to the right. Central venous and PA pressures increase in the head-down position, and care must be taken not to administer too much fluid and increase these pressures even further. Transducer location may need to be adjusted to ensure accuracy. The possibility of producing cerebral edema should be kept in mind.

1. Magnesium and lidocaine should be given to increase the arrhythmic threshold.

2. Blood pressure should be maintained in the 120–140 mm Hg systolic range to optimize coronary perfusion, especially via collateral flow. This can be done with some fluid administration, but usually with liberal administration of α-agents.

3. Atrial pacing wires may be placed if there is a concern about bradycardia developing with heart positioning. Transesophageal pacing may be utilized. Induced bradycardia is not essential when using current stabilizing devices. However, tachycardia should be controlled. Ventricular pacing cables should be immediately available in case heart block develops. Coronary shunting may be helpful during bypass of the right coronary artery, during which there may be compromise of flow to the AV node, producing heart block.

4. Detection of ischemia can be difficult, since the ECG and TEE can be difficult to interpret in the translocated heart. A reduction in the SvO_2 is one of the first signs of the struggling heart. Intracoronary shunting or aortocoronary shunting during construction of an anastomosis ameliorates distal ischemia. Upon the first suspicion of ventricular dysfunction, the surgeon should be informed immediately so that a shunt may be placed, if not done so prophylactically, to try to minimize ischemia.

5. If inotropic support is required, low-dose epinephrine is given first, and then milrinone may be given if more support is needed. In high-risk cases, such as severe left main disease, a prophylactic IABP may be helpful. Unless there is a strong indication for OPCAB, such as severe comorbidities, immediate conversion to an on-pump procedure may be a wise decision if instability persists.

G. **Blood loss** can be insidious during OPCAB if proximal and distal vessel control is suboptimal, especially if the proximal vessel does not have a critical stenosis. Blood should be scavenged into a cell saver and retransfused to the patient. Not infrequently, a significant amount of blood drains into the left pleural space that can be aspirated, processed with the cell saver, and transfused.

H. **Proximal anastomoses** are usually performed last. During construction of proximal anastomoses with a sideclamp, the systolic blood pressure should be reduced to 90–100 mm Hg systolic to reduce the risk of aortic injury and atheroembolism. However, induced hypotension may increase the risk of renal dysfunction, and distal coronary perfusion through vein grafts is compromised until all grafts are sewn to the aorta and the clamp is removed. Thus, the patient may become unstable at this time. Induced hypotension is not necessary if an aortic sealing device, such as the Heartstring proximal seal system (MAQUET Cardiovascular), is used during the construction of proximal anastomoses.

I. Protamine is given in a 1:1 ratio to heparin. Bleeding should be minimal if the anastomoses are hemostatic. Pacing wires may be placed on the atrium and ventricle, chest tubes are placed, and the chest is closed.

X. Anesthetic Considerations During Minimally Invasive or Robotic CABG and Mitral Valve Surgery[202,203]

A. General comments

1. Appropriate draping is essential in case an emergency conversion to a median sternotomy incision is required. Positioning of anesthesia and TEE equipment must be well planned in order to optimize access to the patient in robotic cases. Body warmers are useful in off-pump procedures. External defibrillator pads must be placed in appropriate positions to avoid being near the operative field.

2. Intubation for one-lung anesthesia is required to improve surgical exposure with small thoracotomy incisions or multiple robotic ports, but it can compromise pulmonary function in patients with advanced lung disease. Hypoxemia may induce hypoxic pulmonary vasoconstriction. One-lung anesthesia is accomplished with either a double-lumen endotracheal tube or a single-lumen endotracheal tube with a bronchial blocker. Prior to going on CPB, hypoxemia can be managed by the addition of PEEP to the ventilated lung, although this may shunt blood to the nonventilated lung and worsen oxygenation. Applying CPAP to the nonventilated lung can also improve oxygenation, but this may be bothersome to the surgeon. A few moments of two-lung ventilation can usually deal with these issues. It has been noted that oxygenation tends to be worse after CPB than it was before in these cases.[203]

3. For robotic cases, CO_2 is inflated into the chest to improve exposure and will reduce the amount of intracardiac air at the conclusion of CPB. As long as the intrapleural pressure remains <10 mm Hg with an insufflation rate of 2–3 L/min, a tension capnothorax should not occur. If it does, it can produce hypotension due to mediastinal shift, decreased venous return, and RV compression.

4. Because these operations are less invasive, anesthetic agents should be selected to allow for early extubation, with the use of lower doses of narcotics. This requires the provision of additional analgesia because of the pain associated with lateral chest incisions. For thoracotomy approaches, intercostal blocks at the conclusion of surgery are beneficial. For robotic procedures, paravertebral nerve blocks are helpful in reducing postoperative pain. If the patient is not extubated in the OR and it is anticipated that mechanical ventilatory support will be necessary for more than an hour or so in the ICU, the endotracheal tube will need to be exchanged for a single-lumen tube prior to transfer to the ICU.

5. On-pump procedures require femoral arterial and venous cannulation for CPB. TEE is essential to assist in the positioning of catheters, since limited exposure prevents the surgeon from palpating their location. Although antegrade cardioplegia can be administered with thoracotomy and robotic approaches, the anesthesiologist may be asked to place a retrograde cardioplegia catheter into the coronary sinus, a 15–18 Fr venous drainage catheter into the IJ vein, and/or a pulmonary "endovent" via the IJ vein. Their positions are monitored by TEE. Although direct clamping of the aorta is feasible in most cases, an "endoballoon" may be used for aortic occlusion. This requires placement of bilateral radial artery catheters (or contralateral radial and femoral lines if axillary cannulation is used) to monitor pressures during balloon inflation to identify distal migration. In addition, TEE can identify the distal and proximal locations of the inflated endoballoon, to avoid

obstruction of the innominate artery distally and the coronary arteries proximally. TEE can identify aortic dissections and SVC injury from cannula placement.

6. Cerebral oximetry should be used to assess cerebral perfusion, since perfusion from the heart–lung machine is retrograde from the femoral arteries. It is also helpful during endoballoon inflation, because a reduction in regional oxygen saturation (rSO_2) on either side of the forehead may reflect compromise of flow into the ipsilateral brachiocephalic vessel. In the unusual case of an aberrant right subclavian artery, cerebral oximetry may show a reduction in cerebral oxygenation despite a normal right radial pressure.[204]

7. If femoral arterial cannulation is used for a prolonged period of time, ischemia/reperfusion injury to the leg may result, potentially causing a compartment syndrome of the lower extremity. The risk of leg ischemia is greater in larger patients, with use of large cannulas, and with longer operating times.[205] The anesthesiologist should remind the surgeon to evaluate the patient's calves at the conclusion of surgery for tenseness. Although edema is common after a long case, there should be a low threshold for measuring compartment pressures if the leg has been ischemic for over 4–6 hours. If significantly elevated, a fasciotomy should be considered to prevent muscle necrosis.

B. **Endoscopic or robotic CABG** through limited thoracotomy incisions are less extensive procedures than those performed through sternotomy incisions and do not result in much cardiac manipulation. Robotic surgery performed through small ports can be used for ITA takedown as well as for construction of coronary anastomoses, which may be performed with clips or distal anastomotic connector devices. However, despite endoscopic/robotic ITA takedown, many surgeons will hand-sew anastomoses through small thoracotomy incisions. Procedures may be done on- or off-pump.

1. The patient is positioned with the left side slightly elevated. The left arm may be abducted to improve exposure, but excessive abduction can cause brachial plexus stretch. The limited exposure to the heart and avoidance of CPB for off-pump procedures mandate adequate monitoring for ischemia, comparable to that noted for OPCABs.

2. For robotic cases, the lateral ECG leads must be placed posteriorly and laterally to avoid the port access sites. Defibrillator pads must be placed out of the way of the ports as well, which may produce a suboptimal axis for defibrillation in the event of ventricular fibrillation.

3. For off-pump procedures, a single radial arterial line is placed for monitoring. If the procedure will be done on CPB using cardioplegic arrest, two arterial lines should be placed if an endoballoon is used for aortic cross-clamping. TEE is helpful in off-pump procedures by identifying RWM abnormalities during construction of anastomoses or afterwards.

4. Pacing capabilities using Swan-Ganz pacing catheters may be beneficial.

C. **Minimally invasive mitral valve procedures** may be performed through lower sternotomy incisions, but are usually performed under direct vision through a limited right thoracotomy incision or robotically using small ports.[203]

1. The patient is positioned with the right side elevated about 15°. Defibrillator pads are placed with one pad on the patient's back to the left of the spine and the other

near the apex of the heart in the anterior axillary line. A left radial artery line is placed with consideration of another radial line (or femoral line in case of axillary cannulation) if a balloon endoclamp will be used. For most cases, antegrade cardioplegia administration and direct aortic clamping with a "Chitwood" clamp are feasible. This is usually placed through a separate stab wound on the chest wall. A supplemental retrograde cardioplegia catheter may be placed by the anesthesiologist via the right IJ vein. An additional 15–18 Fr catheter placed in the right IJ is beneficial to augment venous return, and drainage may be vacuum-assisted. It is critical to pay attention to clamping and unclamping of the IJ catheter to prevent inadvertent (and potentially exsanguinating) drainage when the patient is not on bypass. A pulmonary endovent is rarely necessary.

2. One-lung anesthesia, femoral cannulation, and possible use of a Swan-Ganz Paceport catheter are as described in section X.A. TEE is essential in identifying mitral valve pathology, the location of guidewires (arterial and venous) prior to cannulation, and the positions of the femoral venous cannula (which should be about 5 cm into the SVC to prevent dislodgment), the IJ venous cannula, the aortic endoballoon (which should be about 2 cm above the aortic root), and the coronary sinus catheter. It may also detect other previously unsuspected pathology that could impact the operative procedure (more than mild AR, atrial septal defect). During aortic clamping, TEE can visualize flow of antegrade cardioplegia into the coronary arteries, potential AR, and LV distention that the surgeon is unable to see. It may also visualize retrograde cardioplegia flow into the coronary sinus.

3. During weaning from bypass, the antegrade cardioplegia catheter is attached to suction and used for venting of air. TEE is **essential** in identifying air during weaning from CPB, as the amount of air in the LV can be quite striking in these cases. If the mitral valve repair is satisfactory, bypass is briefly resumed to allow for the removal of the vent line under lower pressure, and then the patient is weaned off bypass.

4. Special considerations in robotic mitral valve surgery

   a. Robotic procedures are not pain-free. Use of standard opiate-based anesthesia may be considered, but the narcotic requirement may be lessened using alternative methods to provide analgesia and expedite extubation. Paravertebral nerve blocks at three sites are very useful in accomplishing this. Other approaches include intrathecal or thoracic epidural opiates, intercostal nerve blocks, or pectoral blocks. Local infiltration of long-acting, liposomal bupivacaine has also been described.[203]

   b. The endotracheal tube must be well secured because access to the patient's airway can be difficult with use of the robot.

   c. Muscle relaxation is essential to prevent patient movement during use of the robotic arms that could damage the heart.

   d. Defibrillation may be impaired by the presence of a capnothorax. Establishing two-lung ventilation to reduce electrical impedance and using biphasic defibrillation at 150–200 joules will usually suffice to ensure defibrillation.

   e. The importance of TEE in these procedures cannot be overemphasized.

XI. Anesthetic Considerations During Minimally Invasive Aortic Valve Surgery[206]

A. Minimally invasive AVR through an upper sternotomy incision leaves the lower sternum intact and may improve postoperative pulmonary function after surgery. This approach allows for the direct cannulation of the aorta with venous drainage either from the right atrium or from the right femoral vein, guided by TEE visualization of the cannula. It is usually possible for the surgeon to place a vent through the right superior pulmonary vein and a cardioplegia catheter into the coronary sinus, although its position will need to be confirmed by TEE. Deairing is more problematic than with a full exposure sternotomy, so use of CO_2 insufflation is helpful, and TEE monitoring for evacuation of air prior to terminating bypass is essential. Otherwise, the anesthesia for this procedure is similar to that of a full sternotomy.

B. The upper thoracotomy approach through the right second or third intercostal space limits access to the heart. Some surgeons prefer femoral arterial and venous cannulation, but others have used central aortic and right atrial cannulation successfully. The surgeon can place the vent through the right superior pulmonary vein and often the retrograde cardioplegia catheter as well, but it may be necessary for the anesthesiologist to insert that through the IJ vein. The surgeon can place an antegrade catheter and will directly clamp the aorta. Because of limited access to the LV, deairing is an issue requiring careful TEE monitoring during weaning from bypass. This procedure is more technically challenging with less exposure and usually has a longer pump run than a standard approach.

XII. Anesthetic Considerations During Transcatheter Aortic Valve Replacement (TAVR)

A. TAVR for calcific AS is preferentially performed through a percutaneous transfemoral approach using sedation. General anesthesia is only indicated if the patient has ventilatory issues lying flat, whether from advanced heart failure, COPD, or sleep apnea. Sedation with dexmedetomidine (1 µg/kg over 10 minutes followed by 0.2–1 µg/kg/h) with supplemental 2% lidocaine in the groins allows the patient to tolerate the procedure well. Occasionally at the time of rapid ventricular pacing and valve deployment (for Edwards valves), a small dose of propofol (10–20 mg) or fentanyl (25–50 µg) may be given.

B. **Monitoring.** With use of sedation rather than general anesthesia, no monitoring lines need to be placed by the anesthesiologist, unless the patient has markedly impaired LV function or is in profound heart failure. Rarely is it necessary to place a Swan-Ganz catheter. Arterial monitoring can be done through a femoral access site (usually using the side port of a 7 Fr sheath through which the pigtail catheter is placed), obviating the need for a radial artery line. One of the femoral venous sheaths (through which a transvenous pacing wire is placed) can be used for additional venous access. Proper placement of defibrillator pads is essential in the event of ventricular fibrillation. These need to be far enough to the right on the anterior chest wall to avoid interference with a potential sternotomy incision and far enough away from the LV apex to allow for transthoracic apical echo imaging to assess the gradient post deployment. On rare occasions, assessment of annular size is inadequate from preoperative studies and a TEE may need to be performed, but this can be accomplished without general anesthesia.

C. **Hemodynamic stability.** Hypertension is common in these patients and is best controlled with clevidipine. For balloon-deployed valves (Edwards SAPIEN series), hemodynamic instability most commonly occurs following a period of rapid ventricular pacing, whether for balloon valvuloplasty or valve deployment. Obstruction of the native valve by the undeployed transcatheter heart valve or production of significant AR can cause hypotension. Refractory hemodynamic instability at any point in the procedure may occur in patients with markedly impaired LV function, and can be managed by an IABP and rarely by the establishment of CPB via the femoral vessels. The blood pressure should be maintained above 100 mm Hg prior to valve deployment. Rapid ventricular pacing is initiated, and ventilation is held if performed under general anesthesia. The blood pressure should not be allowed to overshoot too much after valve deployment, although that is a fairly common phenomenon if phenylephrine or norepinephrine was given for hypotension prior to valve deployment.

D. For self-expanding valves (the Medtronic CoreValve/Evolut series), ventricular pacing at a rate of around 100–110/min is usually used as the valve is being unsheathed, and the valve is repeatedly checked for its position relative to the native annulus. There is a brief period of compromised blood pressure during mid-deployment which then recovers just prior to reaching the "point of no return" at 80% unsheathing. If the valve remains in a good position, it is completely unsheathed.

E. **Echocardiography.** Following valve deployment, a transthoracic echo is performed to assess for paravalvular leaks in the LAX and SAX views, and the transvalvular gradient is measured in the apical four-chamber view. Persistent hemodynamic instability may indicate coronary ostial obstruction, ischemia with significant coronary disease, cardiac tamponade, aortic annular disruption, aortic dissection, or valve malposition. Virtually all of these can be identified by a root angiogram and echocardiogram.

F. Following the procedure, the dexmedetomidine is stopped and the patient can be transferred to a routine recovery area. Occasionally, especially in patients with an underlying right bundle branch block and first degree block, complete heart block will develop and persist, and the transvenous pacing wire placed during the procedure will need to be retained. The wire should also be left in for marked bradycardia and for some patients with a new LBBB (see pages 390 and 615).

G. In patients with extensive iliofemoral disease that precludes transfemoral access, alternatives include transcaval, transaxillary, transcarotid, upper sternotomy, and transapical approaches, all of which are usually performed under general anesthesia.[207-209]

H. In patients undergoing a valve-in-valve procedure, the preliminary CT scan is critical in assessing whether displacement of the prosthetic valve leaflet may obstruct the coronary ostia. If that is the case, a BASILICA procedure (Bioprosthetic Aortic Scallop Intentional Laceration to prevent Iatrogenic Coronary Artery obstruction) can be performed.[210]

XIII. Anesthetic Considerations During Transcatheter Mitral Valve Procedures[211]

A. The mitral valve apparatus is a complex structure which has made percutaneous approaches more challenging. Devices producing leaflet repairs, such as the MitraClip system, are performed through a transseptal approach, whereas chordal repairs are performed through a transapical approach. Annuloplasty devices are also being investigated. A transcatheter MVR (TMVR) using a transcatheter aortic valve has primarily been used as a "valve-in-valve" and sometimes a "valve-in-ring" procedure to address bioprosthetic valve stenosis/regurgitation or a failed repair. "Valve-in-MAC" (mitral annular calcification) procedures have also been performed, with suboptimal results.[212] Several other valves are being evaluated for MVRs in high-risk patients.

B. **Percutaneous mitral valve repair with the MitraClip system** can be considered in very high-risk surgical patients with degenerative and functional MR. It reapproximates the anterior and posterior leaflets in the same plane, and is effective in reducing, but rarely eliminating MR.

1. The procedure is done under general anesthesia with TEE guidance. Femoral venous access with transseptal puncture is used. A Swan-Ganz catheter may be helpful in assessing right-heart pressures, but it is not essential. A radial arterial line is helpful.

2. Standard TEE images used for transseptal puncture include the bicaval and SAX at the base views for anterior–posterior positioning and the four-chamber view for the height of the puncture site relative to the mitral valve coaption plane. After this has been accomplished, the patient is systemically heparinized to reach an ACT >300 seconds. Positioning of a ProTrack stiff pigtail wire (Baylis Medical) in the left atrium is confirmed by TEE. Once the steerable guide catheter has been positioned in the left atrium and the wire is removed, the left atrial "v" wave may be measured directly (see Figure 2.5, page 137).

3. The clip delivery system is then advanced into the left atrium. TEE imaging is critical to make sure the device clears the pulmonary veins and left atrial appendage as it is manipulated down to the mitral valve. Initial clip orientation is confirmed in the 3D en face view, then the clip arms are closed to 60° and the system is advanced into the LV. Using the mitral commissural view for medial–lateral orientation, the LVOT view for anterior–posterior orientation, and the 3D en face view, the clip is placed in the desired position. After the clip is closed, the quality of leaflet grasp, the degree of residual MR, and the degree of MS are assessed. If the mean gradient is <5 mm Hg, it is feasible to apply a second clip to improve the degree of regurgitation. A subsequent measurement of the left atrial "v" wave after removal of the clip delivery system gives an appreciation of the hemodynamic improvement from the clip application.

4. When the guide catheter is pulled back into the right atrium, the size of the residual atrial septal defect and the degree of shunting are evaluated by TEE. If the latter appears to be significant or there is evidence of hypoxemia from right-to-left shunting, a septal occluder may be placed. The pericardium should be checked for the presence of an effusion.

5. Complications are uncommon with careful technique in wire and catheter placement and continuous visualization on TEE. This should prevent left atrial perforation and hemopericardium. The clip can get trapped in the subvalvular apparatus and can cause chordal rupture, worsening the MR. There appears to be less compromise of LV function with the reestablishment of valve competence than noted with surgical mitral valve repairs, so use of inotropic support is

unusual, even with markedly impaired LV function. Patients can usually be extubated at the conclusion of the procedure.

C. **Percutaneous mitral "valve-in-valve" and "valve-in-ring" procedures**

   1. These procedures require careful planning to select the proper size valve and to ensure that valve placement will not produce LV outflow tract obstruction. A radial arterial line should be placed, but a Swan-Ganz catheter is not necessary. Defibrillators pads are essential.

   2. A transseptal or transapical approach via a small thoracotomy incision has been used for these procedures. General anesthesia with TEE and fluoroscopic guidance is utilized. The transseptal approach is similar to the MitraClip approach, using femoral venous access. However, these procedures usually require a balloon septostomy with a 12–14 Fr balloon to position an 8.5 Fr sheath across the septum through which a Safari (Boston Scientific) or Confida (Medtronic) extra stiff wire is passed into the LV. A transvenous pacing wire is passed from the contralateral femoral vein up to the RV apex for pacing during valve deployment. The transcatheter valve is then advanced over the wire and positioned in an appropriate position relative to each type of tissue valve using fluoroscopy. The valve is then deployed during a period of rapid ventricular pacing.

   3. Potential complications of these procedures include arrhythmias, hemopericardium, cardiac tamponade, and device embolization. With a TMVR, a paravalvular leak or LVOT obstruction may occur. The latter may result from displacement of the anterior mitral leaflet of a native valve or tissue prosthetic valve leaflet into the outflow tract. Preoperative assessment of the "neo-LVOT" may dictate whether this may occur, and a LAMPOON procedure (intentional Laceration of the Anterior Mitral leaflet to Prevent left ventricular Outflow tract ObstructioN) may need to be performed in patients at risk.[213,214]

D. The **transapical approach** is used for chordal procedures and has been used for TMVR in the native annulus and with severe mitral annular calcification.[215] The Neochord device anchors a suture in the papillary muscle and then anchors the suture to the edge of the prolapsed leaflet segment. This is done primarily under TEE guidance.[216]

   1. Large-bore IV access is essential because there is a greater likelihood of bleeding from the apical puncture site. A central venous line is also helpful for volume infusions, but a Swan-Ganz catheter may only be useful in patients with significant LV dysfunction. Defibrillator pads must be well positioned because arrhythmias may be triggered by cardiac manipulation, and the limited thoracotomy incision does not allow for internal defibrillation. One-lung anesthesia is not necessary. The blood pressure should be kept around 100 during apical access and decannulation. Lidocaine may be given to reduce ventricular irritability. Heparin is administered just prior to apical access.

   2. The most significant complications of any transapical procedure are malignant ventricular arrhythmias and hemorrhage from the cannulation site. Adequate pursestring or mattress suture placement prior to apical access and tying down of the sutures with the blood pressure lowered are important. Thoracotomy incisions are painful, so use of thoracic epidural analgesia or paravertebral blockade may reduce the intraoperative and postoperative opioid requirement.

References

1. Disque A, Neelankavil J. Con: ACE inhibitors should be stopped prior to cardiovascular surgery. *J Cardiothorac Vasc Anesth* 2016;30:820–2.

2. Bhatia M, Arora H, Kumar PA. Pro: ACE inhibitors should be continued perioperatively and prior to cardiovascular operations. *J Cardiothorac Vasc Anesth* 2016;30:816–9.

3. Ouzounian M, Buth KJ, Valeeva L, Morton CC, Hassan A, Ali IS. Impact of preoperative angiotensin-converting enzyme inhibitor use on clinical outcomes after cardiac surgery. *Ann Thorac Surg* 2012;93:559–64.

4. Miceli A, Capoun R, Fino C, et al. Effects of angiotensin-converting enzyme inhibitor therapy on clinical outcome in patients undergoing coronary artery bypass grafting. *J Am Coll Cardiol* 2009;54:1778–84.

5. Ferraris VA, Saha SP, Oestreich JH, et al. 2012 update to the Society of Thoracic Surgeons guideline on use of antiplatelet drugs in patients having cardiac and noncardiac operations. *Ann Thorac Surg* 2012;94:1761–81.

6. Hornor MA, Duane TM, Ehlers AP, et al. American College of Surgeons' guidelines for the perioperative management of antithrombotic medications. *J Am Coll Surg* 2018;227:521–36.

7. Franchini M, Lippi G. Prothrombin complex concentrates: an update. *Blood Transfus* 2010;8:149–54.

8. Sun JC, Whitlock R, Cheng J, et al. The effect of pre-operative aspirin on bleeding, transfusion, myocardial infarction, and mortality in coronary artery bypass surgery: a systematic review of randomized and observational studies. *Eur Heart J* 2008;29:1057–71.

9. Chello M, Nenna A. Continuing aspirin before coronary artery bypass grafting surgery: old fears challenged by new evidences. *Ann Transl Med* 2016;4(Suppl 1):S34.

10. Hastings S, Myles PA, McIlroy DM. Aspirin and coronary artery surgery: an updated meta-analysis. *Br J Anaesth* 2016;116:716–7.

11. Myles PS, Smith JA, Forbes A, et al. Stopping vs. continuing aspirin before coronary artery surgery. *N Engl J Med* 2016;374:728–37.

12. Misumida N, Abo-Aly M, Kim SM, Ogunbayo GO, Abdel-Latif A, Ziada KM. Efficacy and safety of short-term dual antiplatelet therapy (≤6 months) after percutaneous coronary intervention for acute coronary syndrome: a systematic review and meta-analysis of randomized controlled trials. *Clin Cardiol* 2018;41:1455–62.

13. Chun R, Orser BA, Madan M. Platelet glycoprotein IIb/IIIa inhibitors: overview and implications for the anesthesiologist. *Anesth Analg* 2002;95:879–88.

14. Engelman R, Shahian D, Shemin R, et al. The Society of Thoracic Surgeons practice guideline series: antibiotic prophylaxis in cardiac surgery: part II: antibiotic choice. *Ann Thorac Surg* 2007;83:1569–76.

15. Loeb HS, Saudye A, Croke RP, Talano JV, Klodnycky ML, Gunnar RM. Effects of pharmacologically-induced hypertension on myocardial ischemia and coronary hemodynamics in patients with fixed coronary obstruction. *Circulation* 1978;57:41–6.

16. Djaini G, Karski J, Yudin M, et al. Clinical outcomes in patients undergoing elective coronary artery bypass graft surgery with and without utilization of pulmonary artery-generated data. *J Cardiothorac Vasc Anesth* 2006;20:307–10.

17. Eltzschig HK, Rosenberger P, Löffler M, Fox JA, Aranki SF, Shernan SK. Impact of intraoperative transesophageal echocardiography on surgical decisions in 12,566 patients undergoing cardiac surgery. *Ann Thorac Surg* 2008;85:845–52.

18. Minhaj M, Patel K, Muzic D, et al. The effect of routine intraoperative transesophageal echocardiography on surgical management. *J Cardiothorac Vasc Anesth* 2007;21:800–4.

19. Desjardins G, Cahalan M. The impact of routine trans-oesophageal echocardiography (TOE) in cardiac surgery. *Anaesthesiology* 2009;23:263–71.

20. Rosenberger P, Shernan SK, Löffler M, et al. The influence of epiaortic ultrasonography on intraoperative management in 6051 cardiac surgical patients. *Ann Thorac Surg* 2008;85:548–53.

21. Ikram A, Mohiuddin H, Zia A, et al. Does epiaortic ultrasound screening reduce perioperative stroke in patients undergoing coronary surgery? A topical review. *J Clin Neurosci* 2018;50:30–4.

22. Wadsworth R, Littler C. Cardiac standstill, pulmonary artery catheterisation and left bundle branch block. *Anaesthesia* 1996;51:97.

23. Zimmermann A, Kufner C, Hofbauer S, et al. The accuracy of the Vigileo/FloTrac continuous cardiac output monitor. *J Cardiothorac Vasc Anesth* 2008;22:388–93.

24. Mehta Y, Chand RK, Sawhney R, Bhise M, Singh A, Trehan N. Cardiac output monitoring: comparison of a new arterial pressure waveform analysis to the bolus thermodilution technique in patients undergoing off-pump coronary artery bypass surgery. *J Cardiothorac Vasc Anesth* 2008;22:394–9.

25. Balik M, Pachl J, Hendl J. Effect of the degree of tricuspid regurgitation on cardiac output measurements by thermodilution. *Intensive Care Med* 2002;28:1117–21.

26. Edwards.com (2020). The Swan-Ganz catheter. https://www.edwards.com/devices/hemodynamic-monitoring/swan-ganz-catheters (accessed 24 April 2020).

27. Mullerworth MH, Angelopoulos P, Couyant MA, et al. Recognition and management of catheter-induced pulmonary artery rupture. *Ann Thorac Surg* 1998;66:1242–5.

28. Bossert T, Gummert JF, Bittner HB, et al. Swan-Ganz catheter-induced severe complications in cardiac surgery: right ventricular perforation, knotting, and rupture of the pulmonary artery. *J Card Surg* 2006;21:292–5.

29. Abreu AR, Campos MA, Krieger BP. Pulmonary artery rupture induced by a pulmonary artery catheter: a case report and review of the literature. *J Intensive Care Med* 2004;19:291–6.

30. Bianchini R, Melina G, Benedetto U, et al. Extracorporeal membrane oxygenation for Swan-Ganz induced intraoperative hemorrhage. *Ann Thorac Surg* 2007;83:2213–4.

31. Hahn RT, Abraham T, Adams MS, et al. Guidelines for performing a comprehensive transesophageal echocardiographic examination: recommendations from the American Society of Echocardiography and the Society of Cardiovascular Anesthesiologists. *J Am Soc Echocardiogr* 2013;26:921 64.

32. Koide Y, Keehn L, Nomura T, Long T, Oka Y. Relationship of regional wall motion abnormalities detected by biplane transesophageal echocardiography and electrocardiographic changes in patients undergoing coronary artery bypass graft surgery. *J Cardiothorac Vasc Anesth* 1996;10:719–27.

33. Kallmeyer IJ, Collard CD, Fox JA, Body SC, Shernan SK. The safety of intraoperative transesophageal echocardiography: a case series of 7200 cardiac surgical patients. *Anesth Analg* 2001;92:1126–30.

34 Lennon MJ, Gibbs NM, Weightman WM, Leber J, Ee HC, Yusoff IF. Transesophageal echocardiography-related gastrointestinal complications in cardiac surgical patients. *J Cardiothorac Vasc Anesth* 2005;19:141–5.

35. Piercy M, McNicol L, Dinh DT, Story DA, Smith JA. Major complications related to the use of transesophageal echocardiography in cardiac surgery. *J Cardiothorac Vasc Anesth* 2009;23:62–5.

36. Min JK, Spencer KT, Furlong KT, et al. Clinical features of complications from transesophageal echocardiography: a single-center case series of 10,000 consecutive examinations. *J Am Soc Echocardiogr* 2005;18:925–9.

37. Shanewise JS, Cheung AT, Aronson S, et al. ASE/SCA guidelines for performing a comprehensive intraoperative multiplane transesophageal echocardiography examination: recommendations of the American Society of Echocardiography Council for Intraoperative Echocardiography and the Society of Cardiovascular Anesthesiologists Task Force for certification in perioperative transesophageal echocardiography. *Anesth Analg* 1999;89:870–84.

38. Shanewise JS, Zaffer R, Martin RP. Intraoperative echocardiography and minimally invasive cardiac surgery. *Echocardiography* 2002;19:579–82.

39. Wang J, Filipovic M, Rudzitis A, et al. Transesophageal echocardiography for monitoring segmental wall motion during off-pump coronary artery bypass surgery. *Anesth Analg* 2004;99:965–73.

40. Quader N, Rigolin VH. Two and three dimensional echocardiography for pre-operative assessment of mitral valve regurgitation. *Cardiovasc Ultrasound* 2014;12:42.

41. Foster GP, Isselbacher EM, Rose GA, Torchiana D, Akins CW, Picard MH. Accurate localization of mitral regurgitant defects using multiplane transesophageal echocardiography. *Ann Thorac Surg* 1998;65:1025–31.

42. Varghese R, Itagaki S, Anyanwu AC, Trigo P, Fischer G, Adams DH. Predicting systolic anterior motion after mitral valve reconstruction: using intraoperative transoesophageal echocardiography to identify those at greatest risk. *Eur J Cardiothoracic Surg* 2014;45:132–7.

43. Wu VCC, Takeuchi M. Echocardiographic assessment of right ventricular systolic function. *Cardiovasc Diag Ther* 2018;8:70–9.

44. Jansen Klomp WW, Peelan LM, Brandon Bravo Bruinsma GJ, Van't Hof AW, Grandjean JG, Nierich AP. Modified transesophageal echocardiography of the dissected thoracic aorta: a novel diagnostic approach. *Cardiovasc Ultrasound* 2016;14:28.

45. Iafrati MD, Gordon G, Staples MH, et al. Transesophageal echocardiography for hemodynamic management of thoracoabdominal aneurysm repair. *Am J Surg* 1993;166:179–85.

46. Zangrillo A, Turi S, Crescenzi G, et al. Esmolol reduces perioperative ischemia in cardiac surgery: a meta-analysis of randomized controlled studies. *J Cardiothorac Vasc Anesth* 2009;23:625–32.

47. Greco M, Landoni G, Biondi-Zoccai G, et al. Remifentanil in cardiac surgery: a meta-analysis of randomized controlled trials. *J Cardiothorac Vasc Anesth* 2012;26:110–6.

48. Lee HJ, Tin TD, Kim JY, Chung SS, Kwak SH. Remifentanil attenuates systemic inflammatory response in patients undergoing cardiac surgery with cardiopulmonary bypass. *Arch Med* 2017;9:5.

49. de Hoogd S, Ahlers SJGM, van Dongen EPA, et al. Randomized controlled trial on the influence of intraoperative remifentanil versus fentanyl on acute and chronic pain after cardiac surgery. *Pain Pract* 2018;18:443–51.

50. Calcaterra D, Ricci M, Lombardi P, Katariya K, Panos A, Salerno TA. Reduction of postoperative hypothermia with a new warming device: a prospective randomized study in off-pump coronary artery surgery. *J Cardiovasc Surg (Torino)* 2009;50:813–7.

51. Sherrid MV, Balaram S, Kim B, Axel L, Swistel DG. The mitral valve in obstructive hypertrophic cardiomyopathy: a test in context. *J Am Coll Cardiol* 2016;67:1846–58.

52. Mangieri A, Montalto C, Pagnesi M, et al. Mechanism and implications of the tricuspid regurgitation: from the pathophysiology to the current and future therapeutic options. *Circ Cardiovasc Interv* 2017;10:pii:e005043.

53. Benedetto U, Melina G, Angeloni E, et al. Prophylactic tricuspid annuloplasty in patients with dilated tricuspid annulus undergoing mitral valve surgery. *J Thorac Cardiovasc Surg* 2012;143:632–8.

54. Gobolos L, Phillip A, Ugocsai P, et al. Reliability of different body temperature measurement sites during aortic surgery. *Perfusion* 2014;29:75–81.

55. Geirsson A, Shioda K, Olsson C, et al. Differential outcomes of open and clamp-on distal anastomotic techniques in acute type A aortic dissection. *J Thorac Cardiovasc Surg* 2019;157:1750–8.

56. Shimokawa T, Horiuchi K, Ozawa N, et al. Outcome of surgical treatment in patients with acute type B aortic dissection. *Ann Thorac Surg* 2008;86:103–7.

57. Hnath JC, Mehta M, Taggert JB, et al. Strategies to improve spinal cord ischemia in endovascular thoracic aortic repair: outcomes of a prospective cerebrospinal fluid drainage protocol. *J Vasc Surg* 2008;48:836–40.

58. Tian DH, Weller J, Hasmat S, et al. Adjunct retrograde cerebral perfusion provides superior outcomes compared with hypothermic circulatory arrest alone: a meta-analysis. *J Thorac Cardiovasc Surg* 2018;156:1339–48.

59. Apostolakis E, Shuhaiber JH. Antegrade or retrograde cerebral perfusion as an adjunct during hypothermic circulatory arrest for aortic arch surgery. *Expert Rev Cardiovasc Ther* 2007;5:1147–61.

60. Dewhurst AT, Moore SJ, Liban JB. Pharmacologic agents as cerebral protectants during deep hypothermic circulatory arrest in adult thoracic aortic surgery. *Anaesthesia* 2002;57:1016–21.

61. Schubert S, Stoltenburg-Didinger G, Wehsack A, et al. Large-dose pretreatment with methylprednisolone fails to attenuate neuronal injury after deep hypothermic circulatory arrest in a neonatal piglet model. *Anesth Analg* 2005;101:1311–8.

62. Minatoya K, Ogino H, Matsuda H, et al. Evolving selective cerebral perfusion for aortic arch replacement: high flow rate with moderate hypothermic circulatory arrest. *Ann Thorac Surg* 2008;86:1827–31.

63. Keeling WB, Leshnower BG, Hunting JC, Binongo J, Chen EP. Hypothermia and selective antegrade cerebral perfusion is safe for arch repair in type A dissection. *Ann Thorac Surg* 2017;104:767–72.

64. Leshnower BG, Rangaraju S, Allen JW, Stringer AY, Gleason TG, Chen EP. Deep hypothermia + retrograde cerebral perfusion vs. moderate hypothermia + antegrade cerebral perfusion for arch surgery. *Ann Thorac Surg* 2019;107:1104–10.

65. Tanaka A, Safi HJ, Estrera AL. Current strategies of spinal cord protection during thoracoabdominal aortic surgery. *Gen Thorac Cardiovasc Surg* 2018;66:307–14.

66. Black JH, Davison JK, Cambria RP. Regional hypothermia with epidural cooling for prevention of spinal cord ischemic complications after thoracoabdominal aortic surgery. *Semin Thorac Cardiovasc Surg* 2003;15:345–52.

67. Lemaire SA, Jones MM, Conklin LD, et al. Randomized comparison of cold blood and cold crystalloid renal perfusion for renal protection during thoracoabdominal aortic aneurysm repair. *J Vasc Surg* 2009;49:11–9.

68. Fehrenbacher JW, Hart DW, Huddleston E, Siderys H, Rice C. Optimal end-organ protection for thoracic and thoracoabdominal aneurysm repair using deep hypothermic circulatory arrest. *Ann Thorac Surg* 2007;83:1041–6.

69. Spanos K, Kölbel T, Kubitz JC, et al. Risk of spinal cord ischemia after fenestrated or branched endovascular repair of complex aortic aneurysms. *J Vasc Surg* 2019;69:357–66.

70. Essandoh MK, Mark GE, Aasbo, JD, et al. Anesthesia for subcutaneous implantable cardioverter-defibrillator implantation: perspectives from the clinical experience of a U.S. panel of physicians. *Pacing Clin Electrophysiol* 2018;41:807–16.

71. Hullander RM, Leivers D, Wingler K. A comparison of propofol and etomidate for cardioversion. *Anesth Analg* 1993;77:690–4.

72. Barry AE, Chaney MA, London MJ. Anesthetic management during cardiopulmonary bypass: a systematic review. *Anesth Analg* 2015;120:749–69.

73. Landoni G, Lomivorotov VV, Nigro Neto C, et al. Volatile anesthetics versus total intravenous anesthesia for cardiac surgery. *N Engl J Med* 2019;380:1121–25.

74. Dhadphale PR, Jackson AP, Alseri S. Comparison of anesthesia with diazepam and ketamine vs. morphine in patients undergoing heart-valve replacement. *Anesthesiology* 1979;51:200–3.

75. Puri GD, Murthy SS. Bispectral index monitoring in patients undergoing cardiac surgery under cardiopulmonary bypass. *Eur J Anaesthesiol* 2003;20:451–6.

76. Muralidhar K, Banakal S, Murthy K, Garg R, Rani GR, Dinesh R. Bispectral index-guided anaesthesia for off-pump coronary artery bypass grafting. *Ann Card Anaesth* 2008;11:105–10.

77. Landoni G, Biondi-Zoccai GG, Zangrillo A, et al. Desflurane and sevoflurane in cardiac surgery: a meta-analysis of randomized clinical trials. *J Cardiothorac Vasc Anesth* 2007;21:502–11.

78 Delphin E, Jackson D, Gubenko Y, et al. Sevoflurane provides earlier tracheal extubation and assessment of cognitive recovery than isoflurane in patients undergoing off-pump coronary artery bypass surgery. *J Cardiothorac Vasc Anesth* 2007;21:690–5.

79. Jones PM, Bainbridge D, Chu MW, et al. Comparison of isoflurane and sevoflurane in cardiac surgery: a randomized non-inferiority comparative effectiveness trial. *Can J Anaesth* 2016;63:1128–39.

80. Zorrilla-Vaca A, Núñez-Patiño RA, Torres V, Salazar Gomez Y. The impact of volatile anesthetic choice on postoperative outcomes of cardiac surgery: a meta-analysis. *BioMed Res Int* 2017;7073401.

81. Jakobsen CJ, Berg H, Hindsholm KB, Faddy N, Sloth E. The influence of propofol versus sevoflurane anesthesia on outcome in 10,535 cardiac surgical procedures. *J Cardiothorac Vasc Anesth* 2007;21:664–71.

82. Liu X, Zie G, Zhang K, et al. Dexmedetomidine vs propofol sedation reduces delirium in patients after cardiac surgery: a meta-analysis with trial sequential analysis of randomized clinical trials. *J Crit Care* 2017;38:190–6.

83. Wang G, Niu J, Li Z, Lv H, Cai H. The efficacy and safety of dexmedetomidine in cardiac surgery patients: a systematic review and meta-analysis. *PLoS One* 2018;13:e0202620.

84. Society of Thoracic Surgeons Blood Conservation Guidelines Taskforce. 2011 update to the Society of Thoracic Surgeons and the Society of Cardiovascular Anesthesiologists blood conservation clinical practice guidelines. *Ann Thorac Surg* 2011;91:944–82.

85. Flom-Halvorsen HI, Øvrum E, Øystese R, Brosstad F. Quality of intraoperative autologous blood withdrawal for retransfusion after cardiopulmonary bypass. *Ann Thorac Surg* 2003;76:744–8.

86. Whitlock RP, Chan S, Devereaux PJ, et al. Clinical benefit of steroid use in patients undergoing cardiopulmonary bypass: a meta-analysis of randomized trials. *Eur Heart J* 2008;29:2592–600.

87. Kristeller JL, Jankowski A, Reinaker T. Role of corticosteroids during cardiopulmonary bypass. *Hosp Pharm* 2014;49:232–6.

88. Augoustides JG. The inflammatory response to cardiac surgery with cardiopulmonary bypass: should steroid prophylaxis be routine? *J Cardiothorac Vasc Anesth* 2012;26:952–8.
89. Bourbon A, Vionnet M, Leprince P, et al. The effect of methylprednisolone treatment on the cardiopulmonary bypass-induced systemic inflammatory response. *Eur J Cardiothorac Surg* 2004;26:932–8.
90. Morariu AM, Loef BG, Aarts LP, et al. Dexamethasone: benefit and prejudice for patients undergoing on-pump coronary artery bypass grafting: a study on myocardial, pulmonary, renal, intestinal, and hepatic injury. *Chest* 2005;128:2677–87.
91. Sobieski MA 2nd, Graham JD, Pappas PS, Tatooles AJ, Slaughter MS. Reducing the effects of the systemic inflammatory response to cardiopulmonary bypass: can single dose steroids blunt systemic inflammatory response syndrome? *ASAIO J* 2008;54:203–6.
92. Halvorsen P, Raeder J, White PF, et al. The effect of dexamethasone on side effects after coronary revascularization procedures. *Anesth Analg* 2003;96:1578–83.
93. van Osch D, Dieleman JM, Nathoe HM, et al. Intraoperative high-dose dexamethasone in cardiac surgery and the risk of rethoracotomy. *Ann Thorac Surg* 2015;100:2237–42.
94. Koster A, Faraoni D, Levy JH. Antifibrinolytic therapy for cardiac surgery: an update. *Anesthesiology* 2015;123:214–21.
95. Pustavoitau A, Faraday N. Pro: antifibrinolytics should be used in routine cardiac cases using cardiopulmonary bypass (unless contraindicated). *J Cardiothorac Vasc Anesth* 2016;30:245–7.
96. Dentz ME, Slaughter TF, Mark JB. Early thrombus formation on heparin-bonded pulmonary artery catheters in patients receiving epsilon aminocaproic acid. *Anesthesiology* 1995;82:583–6.
97. Ray MJ, Hales MM, Brown L, O'Brien MF, Stafford EG. Postoperatively administered aprotinin or epsilon aminocaproic acid after cardiopulmonary bypass has limited benefit. *Ann Thorac Surg* 2001;72:521–6.
98. Chauhan S, Gharde P, Bisoi A, Kale S, Kiran U. A comparison of aminocaproic acid and tranexamic acid in adult cardiac surgery. *Ann Card Anaesth* 2004;7:40–3.
99. Butterworth J, James RL, Lin Y, Prielipp RC, Hudspeth AS. Pharmacokinetics of epsilon-aminocaproic acid in patients undergoing aortocoronary bypass surgery. *Anesthesiology* 1999;90:1624–35.
100. Bennett-Guerrero E, Spillane WF, White WD, et al. Epsilon-aminocaproic acid administration and stroke following coronary artery bypass graft surgery. *Ann Thorac Surg* 1999;67:1283–7.
101. Stafford-Smith M, Phillips-Bute B, Reddan DN, Black J, Newman MF. The association of epsilon-aminocaproic acid with postoperative decrease in creatinine clearance in 1502 coronary bypass patients. *Anesth Analg* 2000;91:1085–90.
102. Fiechtner BK, Nuttall GA, Johnson ME, et al. Plasma tranexamic acid concentrations during cardiopulmonary bypass. *Anesth Analg* 2001;92:1131–6.
103. Murphy GJ, Mango E, Lucchetti V, et al. A randomized trial of tranexamic acid in combination with cell salvage plus a meta-analysis of randomized trials evaluating tranexamic acid in off-pump coronary artery bypass grafting. *J Thorac Cardiovasc Surg* 2006;132:475–80.
104. Myles PS, Smith JA, Forbes A, et al. Tranexamic acid in patients undergoing coronary-artery surgery. *N Engl J Med* 2017;376:136–48.
105. Shi J, Wang G, Lv H, et al. Tranexamic acid in on-pump coronary artery bypass grafting without clopidogrel and aspirin cessation: randomized trial and 1-year follow-up. *Ann Thorac Surg* 2013;95:793–802.
106. Shi J, Ji H, Ren F, et al. Protective effects of tranexamic acid on clopidogrel before coronary artery bypass grafting: a multicenter randomized trial. *JAMA Surg* 2013;148:538–47.
107. Sigaut S, Tremey B, Ouattara A, et al. Comparison of two doses of tranexamic acid in adults undergoing cardiac surgery with cardiopulmonary bypass. *Anesthesiology* 2014;120:590–600.
108. Hodgson S, Larvin JT, Dearman C. What dose of tranexamic acid is most effective and safe for adult patients undergoing cardiac surgery? *Interact Cardiovasc Thorac Surg* 2015;21:384–8.
109. Warkentin TE. Anticoagulation for cardiopulmonary bypass: is a replacement for heparin on the horizon? *J Thorac Cardiovasc Surg* 2006;131:515–6.

110. Haering JH, Maslow AD, Parker RA, Lowenstein E, Comunale ME. The effect of heparin-coated pulmonary artery catheters on activated coagulation time in cardiac surgical patients. *J Cardiothorac Vasc Anesth* 2000;14:260–3.

111. Francis JL, Palmer GJ 3rd, Moroose R, Drexler A. Comparison of bovine and porcine heparin in heparin antibody formation after cardiac surgery. *Ann Thorac Surg* 2003;75:17–22.

112. Shore-Lesserson L, Baker RA, Ferraris V, et al. STS/SCA/AmSECT clinical practice guidelines: anticoagulation during cardiopulmonary bypass. *Ann Thorac Surg* 2018;105:650–62.

113. Shore-Lesserson L. Point-of-care coagulation monitoring for cardiovascular patients: past and present. *J Cardiothorac Vasc Anesth* 2002;16:99–106.

114. Despotis GJ, Joist JH, Hogue CW Jr, et al. More effective suppression of hemostatic system activation in patients undergoing cardiac surgery by heparin dosing based on heparin blood concentrations rather than ACT. *Thromb Haemost* 1996;76:902–8.

115. Shirota K, Watanabe T, Takagi Y, Ohara Y, Usui A, Yasuura K. Maintenance of blood heparin concentration rather than activated clotting time better preserves the coagulation system in hypothermic cardiopulmonary bypass. *Artif Organs* 2000;24:49–56.

116. Cartier R, Robitaille D. Thrombotic complications in beating heart operations. *J Thorac Cardiovasc Surg* 2001;121:920–2.

117. Englberger L, Immer FF, Eckstein FS, Berdat PA, Haeberli A, Carrel TP. Off-pump coronary artery bypass operation does not increase procoagulant and fibrinolytic activity: preliminary results. *Ann Thorac Surg* 2004;77:1560–6.

118. Ranucci M, Isgrò G, Cazzaniga A, Soro G, Menicanti L, Frigiola A. Predictors for heparin resistance in patients undergoing coronary artery bypass grafting. *Perfusion* 1999;14:437–42.

119. Kawatsu S, Sasaki K, Sakatsume K, et al. Predictors of heparin resistance before cardiovascular operations in adults. *Ann Thorac Surg* 2018;105.1316–21.

120. Finley A, Greenberg C. Review article: heparin sensitivity and resistance: management during cardiopulmonary bypass. *Anesth Analg* 2013;116:1210–22.

121. Beattie GW, Jeffrey RR. Is there evidence that fresh frozen plasma is superior to antithrombin administration to treat heparin resistance in cardiac surgery? *Interact Cardiovasc Thorac Surg* 2014;18:117–20.

122. Avidan MS, Levy JH, van Aken H, et al. Recombinant human antithrombin III restores heparin responsiveness and decreases activation of coagulation in heparin-resistant patients during cardiopulmonary bypass. *J Thorac Cardiovasc Surg* 2005;130:107–13.

123. McNair E, Marcoux JA, Bally C, Gamble J, Thomson D. Bivalirudin as an adjunctive anticoagulant to heparin in the treatment of heparin resistance during cardiopulmonary-bypass assisted cardiac surgery. *Perfusion* 2016;31:189–99.

124. Salter BS, Weiner MM, Trinh MA, et al. Heparin-induced thrombocytopenia: a comprehensive clinical review. *J Am Coll Cardiol* 2016;67:2519–32.

125. Selleng S, Selleng K. Heparin-induced thrombocytopenia in cardiac surgery and critically ill patients. *Thromb Haemost* 2016;116:843–51.

126. Bennett-Guerrero E, Slaughter TF, White WD, et al. Preoperative anti-PF4/heparin antibody level predicts adverse outcome after cardiac surgery. *J Thorac Cardiovasc Surg* 2005;130:1567–72.

127. Kress DC, Aronson S, McDonald ML, et al. Positive heparin-platelet factor 4 antibody complex and cardiac surgical outcomes. *Ann Thorac Surg* 2007;83:1737–43.

128. Everett BM, Yeh R, Foo SY, et al. Prevalence of heparin/platelet factor 4 antibodies before and after cardiac surgery. *Ann Thorac Surg* 2007;83:592–7.

129. Bauer TL, Arepally G, Konkle BA, et al. Prevalence of heparin-associated antibodies without thrombosis in patients undergoing cardiopulmonary bypass surgery. *Circulation* 1997;95:1242–6.

130. Greinacher A, Levy JH. HIT happens: diagnosing and evaluating the patient with heparin-induced thrombocytopenia. *Anesth Analg* 2008;107:356–8.

131. Dyke CM, Smedira NG, Koster A, et al. A comparison of bivalirudin to heparin with protamine reversal in patients undergoing cardiac surgery with cardiopulmonary bypass: the EVOLUTION-ON study. *J Thorac Cardiovasc Surg* 2006;131:533–9.

278   CARDIAC ANESTHESIA

132. Koster A, Dyke CM, Aldea G, et al. Bivalirudin during cardiopulmonary bypass in patients with previous or acute heparin-induced thrombocytopenia and heparin antibodies: results of the CHOOSE-ON trial. *Ann Thorac Surg* 2007;83:572–7.
133. Dyke CM, Aldea G, Koster A, et al. Off-pump coronary artery bypass with bivalirudin for patients with heparin-induced thrombocytopenia or antiplatelet factor four/heparin antibodies. *Ann Thorac Surg* 2007;84:836–9.
134. Mertzlufft F, Kuppe H, Koster A. Management of urgent high-risk cardiopulmonary bypass with heparin-induced thrombocytopenia type II and coexisting disorders of renal function: use of heparin and epoprostenol combined with on-line monitoring of platelet function. *J Cardiothorac Vasc Anesth* 2000;14:304–8.
135. Palatianos G, Michalis A, Alivizatos P, et al. Perioperative use of iloprost in cardiac surgery patients diagnosed with heparin-induced thrombocytopenia-reactive antibodies or with true HIT (HIT-reactive antibodies plus thrombocytopenia): an 11-year experience. *Am J Hematol* 2015;90:608–17.
136. Durand M, Lecompte T, Hacquard M, Carteaux JP. Heparin-induced thrombocytopenia and cardiopulmonary bypass: anticoagulation with unfractionated heparin and the glycoprotein IIb/IIIa inhibitor tirofiban and successful use of rFVIIa for post-protamine bleeding due to persistent platelet blockade. *Eur J Cardiothorac Surg* 2008;34:687–9.
137. Wang YC, Huang CH, Tu YK. Effects of positive airway pressure and mechanical ventilation of the lungs during cardiopulmonary bypass on pulmonary adverse events after cardiac surgery: a systematic review and meta-analysis. *J Cardiothorac Vasc Anesth* 2018;32:748–59.
138. Engelman R, Baker RA, Likosky DS, et al. The Society of Thoracic Surgeons, the Society of Cardiovascular Anesthesiologists, and the American Society of ExtraCorporeal Technology: clinical practice guidelines for cardiopulmonary bypass–temperature management during cardiopulmonary bypass. *Ann Thorac Surg* 2015;100:748–57.
139. Schwartz AE, Sandhu AA, Kaplon RJ, et al. Cerebral blood flow is determined by arterial pressure and not cardiopulmonary bypass flow rate. *Ann Thorac Surg* 1995;60:165–70.
140. Schwartz AE. Regulation of cerebral blood flow during hypothermic cardiopulmonary bypass: review of experimental results and recommendations for clinical practice. *CVE* 1997;2:133–7.
141. Fischer GW, Silvay G. Cerebral oximetry in cardiac and major vascular surgery. *HSR Proc Intensive Care Cardiovasc Anesth* 2010;2:249–56.
142. Tobias JD. Cerebral oximetry monitoring with near infrared spectroscopy detects alterations in oxygenation before pulse oximetry. *J Intensive Care Med* 2008;23:384–8.
143. Murkin JM, Adams SJ, Novick RJ, et al. Monitoring brain oxygen saturation during coronary bypass surgery: a randomized, prospective study. *Anesth Analg* 2007;104:51–8.
144. Slater JP, Guarino T, Stack J, et al. Cerebral oxygen desaturation predicts cognitive decline and longer hospital stay after cardiac surgery. *Ann Thorac Surg* 2009;87:36–45.
145. Ono M, Arnaoutakis GJ, Fine DM, et al. Blood pressure excursions below the cerebral autoregulation threshold during cardiac surgery are associated with acute kidney injury. *Crit Care Med* 2013;41:464–71.
146. Ono M, Brady K, Easley RB, et al. Duration and magnitude of blood pressure below cerebral autoregulation threshold during cardiopulmonary bypass is associated with major morbidity and operative mortality. *J Thorac Cardiovasc Surg* 2014;147:483–9.
147. Lazar HL, McDonnell M, Chipkin SR, et al. The Society of Thoracic Surgeons practice guideline series: blood glucose management during adult cardiac surgery. *Ann Thorac Surg* 2009;87:663–9.
148. Gandhi GY, Nuttall GA, Abel MD, et al. Intraoperative hyperglycemia and perioperative outcomes in cardiac surgical patients. *Mayo Clin Proc* 2005;80:862–6.
149. Puskas F, Grocott HP, White WD, Mathew JP, Newman MF, Bar-Yosef S. Intraoperative hyperglycemia and cognitive decline after CABG. *Ann Thorac Surg* 2007;84:1467–73.
150. Butterworth J, Wagenknecht LE, Legault C, et al. Attempted control of hyperglycemia during cardiopulmonary bypass fails to improve neurologic or neurobehavioral outcomes in patients without diabetes mellitus undergoing coronary artery bypass grafting. *J Thorac Cardiovasc Surg* 2005;130:1319–25.
151. Gandhi GY, Nuttall GA, Abel MD, et al. Intensive intraoperative insulin therapy versus conventional glucose management during cardiac surgery: a randomized trial. *Ann Intern Med* 2007;146:233–43.

152. Karkouti K, Wijeysundera DN, Yau TM, et al. Acute kidney injury after cardiac surgery: focus on modifiable risk factors. *Circulation* 2009;119:495–502.

153. Karkouti K, Wijeysundera DN, Yau TM, McCluskey SA, van Rensburg A, Beattie WS. The influence of baseline hemoglobin concentration on tolerance of anemia in cardiac surgery. *Transfusion* 2008;48:666–72.

154. Vives M, Wijeysundera D, Marczin N, Mondedero P, Rao V. Cardiac surgery-associated acute kidney injury. *Interact Cardiovasc Thorac Surg* 2014;18:637–45.

155. Di Tomasso N, Monaco F, Landoni G. Renal protection in cardiovascular surgery. *F1000Res* 2016;5:F1000 Faculty Rev-331.

156. Chen X, Huang T, Cao X, Xu G. Comparative efficacy of drugs for preventing acute kidney injury after cardiac surgery: a network meta-analysis. *Am J Cardiovasc Drugs* 2018;18:49–58.

157. Mao H, Katz N, Ariyanon W, et al. Cardiac-surgery associated acute kidney injury. *Blood Purif* 2014;37(Suppl 2):34–50.

158. Zangrillo A, Biondi-Zocci GG, Frati E, et al. Fenoldopam and acute renal failure in cardiac surgery: a meta-analysis of randomized placebo-controlled trials. *J Cardiothorac Vasc Anesth* 2012;26:407–13.

159. Sun H, Xie Q, Peng Z. Does fenoldopam protect kidney in cardiac surgery? A systemic review and meta-analysis with trial sequential analysis. *Shock* 2019;52:326–33.

160. Lassnigg A, Donner E, Grubhofer G, Presterl E, Druml W, Hiesmayr M. Lack of renoprotective effects of dopamine and furosemide during cardiac surgery. *J Am Soc Nephrol* 2000;11:97–104.

161. Wilkes NJ, Mallett SV, Peachey T, Di Salvo C, Walesby R. Correction of ionized magnesium during cardiopulmonary bypass reduces the risk of postoperative cardiac arrhythmia. *Anesth Analg* 2002;95:828–34.

162. Yagdi T, Nalbantgil S, Ayik F, et al. Amiodarone reduces the incidence of atrial fibrillation after coronary artery bypass grafting. *J Thorac Cardiovasc Surg* 2003;125:1420–5.

163. Mitchell LB, Exner DV, Wyse DG, et al. Prophylactic oral amiodarone for the prevention of arrhythmias that begin early after revascularization, valve replacement, or repair: PAPABEAR: a randomized controlled trial. *JAMA* 2005;294:3093–100.

164. Dörge H, Schoendube FA, Schoberer M, Stellbrink C, Voss M, Messmer BJ. Intraoperative amiodarone as prophylaxis against atrial fibrillation after coronary operations. *Ann Thorac Surg* 2000;69:1358–62.

165. Knutson JE, Deering JA, Hall FW, et al. Does intraoperative hetastarch administration increase blood loss and transfusion requirements after cardiac surgery? *Anesth Analg* 2000;90:801–7.

166. Schramko AA, Suojaranta-Ylinen T, Kuitunen AH, Kukkonen SI, Niemi TT. Rapidly degradable hydroxyethyl starch solutions impair blood coagulation after cardiac surgery: a prospective randomized trial. *Anesth Analg* 2009;108:30–6.

167. Kikura M, Sato S. The efficacy of preemptive milrinone or amrinone therapy in patients undergoing coronary artery bypass grafting. *Anesth Analg* 2002;94.22–30.

168. Shaefi S, Mittel A, Klick J, et al. Vasoplegia after cardiovascular procedures: pathophysiology and targeted therapy. *J Cardiothorac Vasc Anesth* 2018;32:1013–22.

169. McCartney SL, Duce L, Ghadimi K. Intraoperative vasoplegia: methylene blue to the rescue! *Curr Opin Anaesthesiol* 2018;31:43–9.

170. Ammar T, Fisher CF, Sarier K, Coller BS. The effects of thrombocytopenia on the activated coagulation time. *Anesth Analg* 1996;83:1185–8.

171. Shigeta O, Kojima H, Hiramatsu Y, et al. Low-dose protamine based on heparin-protamine titration method reduces platelet dysfunction after cardiopulmonary bypass. *J Thorac Cardiovasc Surg* 1999;118:354–60.

172. Boer C, Meesters MI, Veerhoek D, Vonk ABA. Anticoagulant and side-effects of protamine in cardiac surgery: a narrative review. *Br J Anaesth* 2018;120:914–27.

173. Meesters MI, Verrhoek D, de Lange F, et al. Effect of high or low protamine dosing on postoperative bleeding following heparin anticoagulation in cardiac surgery: a randomized controlled trial. *Thromb Haemost* 2016;116:251–61.

174. Butterworth J, Lin YA, Prielipp RC, Bennett J, Hammon JW, James RL. Rapid disappearance of protamine in adults undergoing cardiac operation with cardiopulmonary bypass. *Ann Thorac Surg* 2002;74:1589–95.

175. Galeone A, Rotunno C, Guida P, et al. Monitoring incomplete heparin reversal and heparin rebound after cardiac surgery. *J Cardiothorac Vasc Anesth* 2013;127:853–8.

176. Teoh KH, Young E, Blackall MH, Roberts RS, Hirsh J. Can extra protamine eliminate heparin rebound following cardiopulmonary bypass surgery? *J Thorac Cardiovasc Surg* 2014;128:211–9.

177. Milne B, Rogers K, Cervenko F, Salerno T. The haemodynamic effects of intraaortic versus intravenous administration of protamine for reversal of heparin in man. *Can Anaesth Soc J* 1983;30:347–51.

178. Chaney MA, Devin Roberts J, Wroblewski K, Shahul S, Gaudet R, Jeevanandam V. Protamine administration via the ascending aorta may prevent cardiopulmonary instability. *J Cardiothorac Vasc Anesth* 2016;30:647–55.

179. Nybo M, Madsen JS. Serious anaphylactic reactions due to protamine sulfate: a systematic literature review. *Basic Clin Pharmacol Toxicol* 2008;103:192–6.

180. Kimmel SE, Sekeres MA, Berlin JA, Ellison N, DiSesa VJ, Strom BL. Risk factors for clinically important adverse events after protamine administration following cardiopulmonary bypass. *J Am Coll Cardiol* 1998;32:1916–22.

181. Hiong YT, Tang YK, Chui WH, Das SR. A case of catastrophic pulmonary vasoconstriction after protamine administration in cardiac surgery: role of intraoperative transesophageal echocardiography. *J Cardiothorac Vasc Anesth* 2008;22:727–31.

182. Viaro F, Dalio MB, Evora PR. Catastrophic cardiovascular adverse reactions to protamine are nitric oxide/cyclic guanosine monophosphate dependent and endothelium mediated: should methylene blue be the treatment of choice? *Chest* 2002;122:1061–6.

183. Stafford-Smith M, Lefrak EA, Qazi AG, et al. Efficacy and safety of heparinase I versus protamine in patients undergoing coronary artery bypass grafting with and without cardiopulmonary bypass. *Anesthesiology* 2005;103:229–40.

184. Mixon TA, Dehmer GJ. Recombinant platelet factor 4 for heparin neutralization. *Semin Thromb Hemost* 2004;30:369–77.

185. Demma L, Levy JH. A case series of recombinant platelet factor 4 for heparin reversal after cardiopulmonary bypass. *Anesth Analg* 2012;115:1273–8.

186. Zwischenberger JB, Tao W, Deyo DJ, Vertrees RA, Alpard SK, Shulman G. Safety and efficacy of a heparin removal device: a prospective randomized preclinical outcomes study. *Ann Thorac Surg* 2001;71:270–7.

187. Fiore MM, Mackie IM. Mechanism of low-molecular-weight heparin reversal by platelet factor 4. *Throm Res* 2009;124:149–55.

188. Elizalde M, Slobodskoy L, Diodato M, Chang J, Chedrawy EG. Use of recombinant factor VII in cardiac surgery. *Recent Pat Cardiovasc Drug Discov* 2012;7:216–20.

189. Habib AM, Calafiore AM, Cargoni M, Foschi M, Di Mauro M. Recombinant activated factor VII is associated with postoperative thromboembolic adverse events in bleeding after coronary surgery. *Interact Cardiovasc Thorac Surg* 2018;27:350–6.

190. Sharma S, Kumar S, Tewari P, Pande S, Murari M. Utility of thromboelastography versus routine coagulation tests for assessment of hypocoagulable state in patients undergoing cardiac bypass surgery. *Ann Card Anaesth* 2018;21:151–7.

191. Sharp G, Young CJ. Point-of-care-viscoelastic assay devices (rotational thromboelastometry and thromboelastography): a primer for surgeons. *ANZ J Surg* 2019;89:291–5.

192. Lodewyks C, Heinrichs J, Grocott HP, et al. Point-of-care viscoelastic hemostatic testing in cardiac surgery patients: a systematic review and meta-analysis. *Can J Anaesth* 2018;65:1333–47.

193. Michelsen LG, Horswell S. Anesthesia for off-pump coronary artery bypass grafting. *Semin Thorac Cardiovasc Surg* 2003;15:71–82.

194. Missant C, Rex S, Wouters PF. Accuracy of cardiac output measurements with pulse contour analysis (PulseCO) and Doppler echocardiography during off-pump coronary artery bypass grafting. *Eur J Anaesthesiol* 2008;25:243–8.

195. Bergsland J, Lingaas PS, Skulstad H, et al. Intracoronary shunt prevents ischemia in off-pump coronary artery bypass surgery. *Ann Thorac Surg* 2009;87:54–60.

196. Gurbuz AT, Hecht ML, Arslan AH. Intraoperative transesophageal echocardiography modifies strategy in off-pump coronary artery bypass grafting. *Ann Thorac Surg* 2007;83:1035–40.

197. Tanaka KA, Thourani VH, Williams WH, et al. Heparin anticoagulation in patients undergoing off-pump and on-pump bypass surgery. *J Anesth* 2007;21:297–303.

198. Englberger L, Streich M, Tevaearai H, Carrel TP. Different anticoagulation strategies in off-pump coronary artery bypass operations: a European survey. *Interact Cardiovasc Thorac Surg* 2008;7:378–82.

199. Zangrillo A, Pappalardo F, Talò G, et al. Temperature management during off-pump coronary artery bypass graft surgery: a randomized clinical trial on the efficacy of a circulating water system versus a forced-air system. *J Cardiothorac Vasc Anesth* 2006;20:788–92.

200. Allen GS. Intraoperative temperature control using the Thermogard system during off-pump coronary artery bypass grafting. *Ann Thorac Surg* 2009;87:284–8.

201. Jeong SM, Hahm KD, Jeong YB, Yang HS, Choi IC. Warming of intravenous fluids prevents hypothermia during off-pump coronary artery bypass graft surgery. *J Cardiothorac Vasc Anesth* 2008;22:67–70.

202. Bernstein WK, Walker A. Anesthetic issues in robotic cardiac surgery. *Ann Card Anaesth* 2015;18:58–68.

203. Rehfeldt KH, Andre JV, Ritter MJ. Anesthetic considerations in robotic mitral valve surgery. *Ann Cardiothorac Surg* 2017;6:47–53.

204. Scohy TV, Bentala M, van der Meer NJM, Gerritse BM. Minimally invasive mitral valve surgery with endoaortic balloon requires cerebral monitoring. *Ann Thorac Surg* 2018;106:e295–6.

205. Tarui T, Miyata K, Shigematsu S, Watanabe G. Risk factors to predict leg ischemia in patients undergoing single femoral artery cannulation in minimally invasive cardiac surgery. *Perfusion* 2018;33:533–7.

206. Mikus E, Turci S, Calvi S, Ricci M, Dozza L, Del Giglio M. Aortic valve replacement through right minithoracotomy: is it really biologically minimally invasive? *Ann Thorac Surg* 2015;99:826–30.

207. Young MN, Singh V, Sakhuja R. A review of alternative access for transcatheter aortic valve replacement. *Curr Treat Options Cardiovasc Med* 2018;20:62.

208. Greenbaum AB, Babaliaros VC, Chen MY, et al. Transcaval access and closure for transcatheter aortic valve replacement: a prospective investigation. *J Am Coll Cardiol* 2017;69:511–21.

209. Mathur M, Krishnan SK, Levin D, Aldea G, Reisman M, McCabe JM. A step-by-step guide to fully percutaneous transaxillary transcatheter aortic valve replacement. *Structural Heart* 2017;1:209–15.

210. Lederman R, Babaliaros VC, Rogers T, et al. Preventing coronary obstruction during transcatheter aortic valve replacement: from computed tomography to BASILICA. *JACC Cardiovasc Interv* 2019;12:1197–1216.

211. Gregory SH, Sodhi N, Zoller JK, et al. Anesthetic considerations for the transcatheter management of mitral valve disease. *J Cardiothorac Vasc Anesth* 2019;33:796–807.

212. Long A, Mahoney P. Transcatheter mitral valve-in-valve and valve-in-ring replacement in high-risk surgical patients: feasibility, safety, and longitudinal outcomes in a single-center experience. *J Invasive Cardiol* 2018;30:324–8.

213. Blanke P, Naoum C, Dvir D, et al. Predicting LVOT obstruction in transcatheter mitral valve implantation: concept of the neo-LVOT. *JACC Cardiovasc Imaging* 2017;10:482–5.

214. Greenbaum AB, Condado JF, Eng M, et al. Long or redundant leaflet complicating transcatheter mitral valve replacement: case vignettes that advocate for removal or reduction of the anterior mitral leaflet. *Catheter Cardiovasc Interv* 2018;92:627–32.

215. Sorajja P, Gössi M, Babaliaros V, et al. Novel transcatheter mitral valve prosthesis for patients with severe mitral annular calcification. *J Am Coll Cardiol* 2019;74:1431–40.

216. Samalavicius RS, Norkiene I, Drasutiene A, et al. Anesthetic management and procedure outcome of patients undergoing off-pump transapical implantation of artificial chordae to correct mitral regurgitation: case series of 76 patients. *Anesth Analg* 2018;126:776–84.

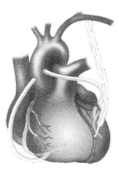

CHAPTER 5

Cardiopulmonary Bypass

5 Cardiopulmonary Bypass

Cardiopulmonary bypass (CPB) is a form of extracorporeal circulation provided by a heart–lung machine that provides systemic perfusion of oxygenated blood during open-heart surgery. It is utilized for "on-pump" coronary bypass surgery and is required for all types of "surgical" valve and aortic procedures. Vascular access for the CPB circuit may vary, depending on the operative approach, but the technology and physiologic concepts remain virtually the same. Although there has been a significant trend toward "minimally invasive" approaches for many types of cardiac surgery, including transcatheter valve procedures, off-pump bypass surgery, and endovascular procedures, CPB remains an essential element of cardiac surgical practice. Additional applications of CPB, such as extracorporeal membrane oxygenation (ECMO), have been invaluable in improving outcomes in patients with cardiogenic shock after surgery and other clinical situations requiring cardiac or respiratory support.

I. General Comments

A. CPB (the "pump") involves an extracorporeal circuit that drains blood from the venous system and returns oxygenated blood to the systemic circulation when the heart and lungs are not functional. CPB is accompanied by normovolemic hemodilution and nonpulsatile flow.[1]

B. The contact of blood with the extracorporeal circuit generates a systemic inflammatory response that is related to a multitude of pathophysiologic factors. CPB results in the activation of numerous cascades, including the kallikrein, coagulation, and complement systems.[2,3] These may cause thrombin generation, the release of proinflammatory cytokines, and a systemic inflammatory response. Endothelial-based reactions, including platelet adhesion, aggregation, and activation, as well as leukocyte adhesion and activation, have been implicated in myocardial reperfusion damage, pulmonary and renal dysfunction, neurocognitive changes, and a generalized capillary leak.

C. Use of membrane oxygenators, biocompatible circuits and centrifugal pumps, adopting a restrictive transfusion threshold, avoiding cardiotomy suction, and equivocally use of leukocyte filters and steroids may reduce some of these inflammatory responses to CPB.[4-9] Most patients will experience few adverse effects from the systemic inflammatory response, but those with long pump runs or with significant hemodynamic issues following surgery may experience significant tissue edema and organ system dysfunction that may persist for days.

Manual of Perioperative Care in Adult Cardiac Surgery, Sixth Edition. Robert M. Bojar.
© 2021 John Wiley & Sons Ltd. Published 2021 by John Wiley & Sons Ltd.

II. The Cardiopulmonary Bypass Circuit

A. The extracorporeal circuit consists of polyvinylchloride tubing and polycarbonate connectors. Circuits with biocompatible coatings (most commonly the Medtronic Cortiva BioActive Surface and Trillium Biosurface polymer coating circuits) have been shown to improve biocompatibility, which reduces complement, leukocyte, and platelet activation, and lessens the release of proinflammatory mediators.[8,9] Although biocompatible circuits may reduce bleeding, atrial fibrillation, tissue edema, and the degree of pulmonary dysfunction, other clinical benefits of their anti-inflammatory properties are modest. Studies have not shown that these circuits decrease thrombin generation, which is a marker of coagulation system activation and a trigger of endothelial cell dysfunction.

B. The bypass circuit is a potent activator of the coagulation system with generation of factor Xa and thrombin, which may contribute to a systemic inflammatory response and ischemia/reperfusion injury.[10] Anticoagulation, generally with heparin, is essential during CPB to minimize activation of the coagulation system, thrombus formation, and fibrinolysis.[11] Use of heparin-coated circuits allows for the safe use of lower doses of heparin, which might be associated with less bleeding.[12,13] A number of factors associated with the use of CPB, including hemodilution of clotting factors and platelets, platelet dysfunction, and fibrinolysis, may contribute to a coagulopathy.

C. The pump is primed with a balanced electrolyte solution, such as Lactated Ringer's, Normosol, or Plasmalyte, although normal saline may be used in patients with chronic kidney disease to reduce the potassium load associated with the use of cardioplegia solutions. The average priming volume is about 1000–1500 mL. A colloid, usually albumin, is usually not added to the pump prime, but it may be given during the pump run to increase oncotic pressure and reduce fluid requirements, thus decreasing extravascular lung water. It may also ameliorate bleeding by delaying fibrinogen absorption and reducing platelet activation.[14] The use of acute normovolemic hemodilution reduces blood loss and the number of blood transfusions required.[15]

D. Miniaturized circuits with lower priming volumes (500–800 mL) minimize hemodilution and reduce the blood–artificial surface interface, possibly minimizing the inflammatory response. These systems also allow for centrifugation of shed blood for retransfusion to reduce blood activation and lipid embolism. Studies using these circuits have demonstrated improved clinical outcomes, with decreased transfusion rates, lower troponin release, a reduced incidence of neurologic damage and atrial fibrillation, and a shorter duration of ventilation. The decrease in the inflammatory response may be equivalent to that seen during off-pump surgery.[16,17] However, these circuits do lower the safety margins for volume loss and air emboli, and make weaning and termination of bypass more difficult because of low volume reserve in the system.

E. The establishment of CPB involves the drainage of venous blood from the right atrium or venae cavae into a hardshell cardiotomy reservoir or bag. This usually occurs by gravity, but it may also occur by vacuum-assisted drainage. The blood then passes through an antifoam and sock filter into the oxygenator attached to a heater/cooler unit, and is returned to the arterial system through a filter using either a roller or, preferably, a centrifugal pump.

1. In a closed reservoir system, which contains a collapsible bag, air passing through the venous lines can be vented through ports at the top of the bag. In a hardshell open system, air can potentially get entrained into the oxygenator if the cardiotomy

volume is too low, so low-volume alarms must be utilized and keen attention paid to reservoir volumes.

2. Active venous drainage using vacuum assist or kinetic assist (with a centrifugal pump) can be used to augment venous drainage.[18,19] This is valuable during minimally invasive procedures or when small venous catheters are utilized. The least amount of negative pressure necessary to augment drainage should be used, although a pressure up to -60 mm Hg is acceptable. Vacuum assist causes an insignificant degree of hemolysis and may reduce hemodilution and transfusion requirements. However, one must always consider the possibility of venous air entrainment and undetected air microembolism when this technique is utilized. Excessive vacuum may pull air retrograde through the oxygenator membrane, causing depriming of a centrifugal pump. Monitoring for gaseous emboli on both the venous and arterial side should be utilized to minimize these risks.

F. Centrifugal pumps have replaced roller pumps to provide systemic flow in most current systems. Both provide nonpulsatile flow, unless additional technology is utilized to provide pulsatile flow. Roller pumps are pressure-insensitive and can pressurize the arterial line in the face of outflow obstruction. Centrifugal pumps are afterload-sensitive, such that they will reduce flow if outflow is obstructed. Centrifugal pumps cause less blood trauma than roller pumps, but the inflammatory response and effects on perioperative bleeding are fairly similar with both types of pumps.[20,21] Roller pumps are used, however, for suction lines and cardioplegia delivery (Figure 5.1).

G. Oxygenators have integral heater–cooler coils which are located proximal to the oxygenator to minimize gas embolization. A separate heater–cooler unit is utilized to control the temperature of the arterial inflow to provide systemic warming and cooling. In 2015, the FDA published an alert that contamination occurring during manufacturing of the Sorin 3T heater–cooler units caused delayed sternal wound infections with *Mycoplasma chimaera*, leading to recommendations for strict adherence to instructions about the maintenance and cleaning of these units.

H. Suction lines return extravasated blood from the surgical field to the cardiotomy reservoir to conserve blood and blood elements and to maintain pump volume.

1. Despite the nearly universal use of these suction lines, the benefits of blood salvage into the pump may be offset by the adverse effects of the aspirated blood. Studies have shown that blood in contact with tissue factor in the pericardium is replete with fat and procoagulant and proinflammatory mediators, such as complement and cytokines.[22-25] Thus, aspirated blood is a significant activator of coagulation, causing increased generation of thrombin and complement that promote inflammation, and is a major cause of hemolysis. Cytokines may contribute to increased perioperative bleeding and neurologic sequelae. Elimination of cardiotomy suction may reduce thrombin generation, platelet activation, and the systemic inflammatory response.[25] Notably, return of cardiotomy suction into the circuit usually causes systemic hypotension, most likely because of the high levels of inflammatory mediators present.

2. The routine use of cell-saving devices to aspirate and wash shed blood can preserve red cells while eliminating many of these inflammatory mediators while also removing fat from the blood. However, centrifugation of shed blood does remove coagulation factors and platelets from the blood. Most surgeons continue to use cardiotomy suction while still using cell-saving devices.[26]

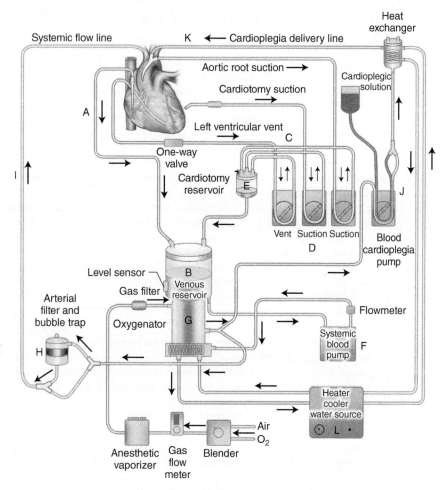

Figure 5.1 • The basics of a "closed" extracorporeal circuit. Blood drains through the venous line (A) into a venous reservoir bag (B), while blood from vent lines and the cardiotomy sucker (C) are actively suctioned using a roller pump (D) into a cardiotomy reservoir (E), which drains into the venous reservoir. The blood is then pumped by a centrifugal pump (F) through an integrated oxygenator–heat exchanger unit (G) and returned through an arterial filter (H) to the arterial circulation (I). For blood cardioplegia setups, a mixture of blood from the oxygenator and a stock cardioplegia solution is pumped through a roller pump head (J) using different size tubing (depending on the mixture ratio) and returned to the ascending aorta for antegrade cardioplegia delivery (K) and the coronary sinus for retrograde cardioplegia. The heater–cooler system is used for systemic and cardioplegia temperature management (L).

I. An additional suction line can be connected to an intracardiac vent, draining blood from the left ventricle (LV) or other cardiac chamber into the reservoir by active suctioning by a roller pump head. These lines are useful in providing ventricular decompression and/or improving surgical exposure. Active root venting should be used in all valve cases upon weaning from CPB to evacuate ejected air.

J. Oxygen and compressed air pass into the oxygenator from a blender which regulates oxygen concentration by adjusting the FiO_2 and determines the gas flow by adjusting a "sweep rate". The sweep rate is generally maintained at slightly less than the systemic flow rate to eliminate CO_2 from the blood to achieve a desired value (generally around 40–50 mm Hg). To minimize blood activation, the oxygenator may be coated with heparin or Trillium to improve biocompatibility.[27]

K. The pump setup includes a separate heat exchanger for cardioplegia delivery. Tubes of differing diameters are passed through the same roller pump head, delivering a preselected ratio of pump volume to cardioplegia solution (such as 4:1). The final mixture then passes through this heat exchanger for the delivery of cold or warm cardioplegia. Monitoring of infusion pressure is essential, especially for retrograde delivery, which generally provides about 200 mL/min of flow at a pressure that should not exceed 40 mm Hg to prevent coronary sinus rupture. Very high line pressures indicate obstruction to flow, either because the line is clamped or kinked or because the cardioplegia catheter is obstructed. A low line pressure generally indicates misplacement of the catheter, either back into the right atrium or from perforation of the coronary sinus. Microplegia systems (such as the Quest MPS system) minimize the volume of crystalloid vehicle required during cardioplegia delivery. They mix the essential cardioplegia contents (primarily potassium and magnesium) with the blood in a specified ratio that is then delivered to the heart. This allows for a large amount of cardioplegia to be delivered with minimal hemodilution.

L. Additional features of the CPB circuit usually include the following:

1. In-line monitoring of arterial and venous blood gases, electrolytes, hematocrit, and temperatures at multiple sites simultaneously. The last of these is useful during deep hypothermia cases.

2. An arterial line filter (usually 40 μm), which is essential to remove microemboli before blood is returned to the patient. Microemboli may consist of air, blood, or platelet microaggregates, or other particulate matter. Fat microemboli are found in abundance in cardiotomy suction and can be removed by 20 μm filters. Large emboli may become fractionated before reaching the arterial line filter, and then may not be completely removed.

3. Recirculation lines to allow for venting of air and to prevent stagnation of blood. This is essential during circulatory arrest cases and when direct thrombin inhibitors are used for anticoagulation in patients with heparin-induced thrombocytopenia.

4. Hemofilters or hemoconcentrators, which can be placed in the circuit to remove excessive volume in patients with preexisting fluid overload or renal dysfunction. Modified ultrafiltration (MUF) at the end of the pump run can hemoconcentrate the pump contents by pumping blood from the arterial cannula through the concentrator for retransfusion through the venous cannula into the right atrium.[28]

5. A cell-saving device into which blood is scavenged from the operative field to be centrifuged, washed, and collected in a bag. This can then be drained into the cardiotomy device for transfusion during CPB or after CPB is terminated, or placed in a transfer bag and given to the anesthesiologist for infusion. This has been shown to decrease blood transfusion requirements during cardiac surgical procedures.[26]

M. A detailed checklist must be utilized by the perfusionist before every case to make sure that no detail is overlooked. The patient's life depends on the perfusionist and proper function of the heart–lung machine. Accurate record keeping during bypass is essential (Figure 5.2 and 5.3).

Saint Vincent Hospital at Worcester Medical Center
DEPARTMENT OF SURGERY

Perfusion Record

- ☐ Patient chart reviewed and assessed
- ☐ Heart-Lung machine properly plugged in; all batteries checked and operational
- ☐ Centrifugal pump in correct position and properly mounted
- ☐ Hand cranks available
- ☐ All pump tubing connections correct and tightened
- ☐ MPS machine properly set up and primed, correct ratio, KCL, MgSO4 and temps
- ☐ Cardioplegia tubing placement in correct direction in pump head raceway and occlusions checked and set
- ☐ Adequate tubing clamps available
- ☐ Sweep gas line attached to oxygenator / FIO2 and gas flow selected
- ☐ Fluotec checked and filled with Isoflourane
- ☐ Scavenger line prepared
- ☐ Venous sat. monitor, battery checked
- ☐ Venous sat. probe attached and checked for proper functioning and positioning
- ☐ Pump cart available with adequate supply of drugs, solutions, syringes, needles, filters, etc.
- ☐ Centrifugal pump flow probe attched properly
- ☐ Oxygen analyzer calibrated and battery checked
- ☐ Connections to table lines properly made and checked, A-V Loop primed
- ☐ Heater/Cooler connected and primed and properly set
- ☐ Ice in room and added to appropriate heater/cooler
- ☐ Cardioplegia solution prepared and correct for surgeon
- ☐ Hepcon machine set up, with adequate supplies and patient data entered
- ☐ Baseline ACT performed and heparin dose calculated/reported to anesthesiologist
- ☐ Heparin given by anesthesiologist
- ☐ Adequate post-heparin ACT achieved
- ☐ Arterial and venous lines properly clamped
- ☐ Cardiotomy reservoir set up and vented
- ☐ Pump suction and vent line placed correctly in pump head
- ☐ Occlusions properly checked and set
- ☐ Blood gas analyzer shift Q.C. completed

Signature: _____ Date: _____

DISPOSABLES	MANUFACTURER	LOT #
Oxygenator:		
Cardioplegia:		
Tubing Pack:		
Cell Saver:		
Hemoconcentrator:		

Figure 5.2 • Example of a pre-bypass checklist.

Saint Vincent Hospital
DEPARTMENT OF SURGERY
Perfusion Record

				Date	OR #	Case #	
				Preop Diagnosis		Procedure	
Surgeon		Anesthesiologist		Perfusionist		Assistant	
BSA	Ht.	Wt.	☐ M ☐ F	Age	Bld. Type	Preop Heparin: ☐ Yes ☐ No	
Labs	BUN/Creat	K	Glucose	WBC	HGB	Hct	Plts
PMH and Meds			On Pump	Xclamp On	IABP ☐ Preop ☐ Intraop	Art. Can.	Prime
			Off Pump	Xclamp Off	Inotropes ☐ Yes ☐ No	Ven. Can.	Blood ID #
			ECP Total	Xclamp Time	Defibx	Retro. Can	Cell Saver Vol.

Map X Flows •	Time		Grafts	Flows
	MAP/(L) Flows			
	100	5		
	90			
	80	4		
	70			
	60	3		
	50			
	40	2		
	30			
	20	1		
	10			

			Comments:
In-Line	SVO_2%		
Temp			
Gas	FiO_2%		
	Flow L/m		
Labs	pH	A	
Prehyness	pCO_2	A	
	pO_2	A	
	HCO3	A	
	BE		
	Sat	A	
	%		
	K+		
	Hct/Hgb		
	Glucose		
	iCa/Na+		
	ACT		
Fluid	Crystalloid		
	Colloid		Cardioplegia: ☐ MPS ☐ 4:1
ccs	Blood		Time / Temp / Ant cc / Ret cc
	FFP		
	Urine		
	Hemoconc		
Drugs	HCO3		
	Heparin		
	Mannitol		
	Forane		
	CaCl		
	Lidocaine		
	Pressor (NEO)		
	Dilator (TNG)		
			Total Blood:
			Cryst:

FORM #11132 (Rev. 3/06))

8

Figure 5.3 Typical perfusion record.

III. Anticoagulation and Cannulation for Bypass

A. **Anticoagulation.** Prior to cannulation, achievement of adequate anticoagulation is essential to minimize thrombus formation on the cannulas and within the extracorporeal circuit (see also pages 250–251).[1]

1. Unfractionated heparin may be administered in a dose of 3–4 mg/kg for uncoated circuits with monitoring of its anticoagulant effect by the activated clotting time (ACT).[11] A blood sample is drawn 3–5 minutes after heparin administration and

should achieve an ACT >480 seconds in non-heparin-coated circuits and an ACT >400 seconds in heparin-coated circuits. Patients with heparin resistance may require more heparin or administration of other blood products (2–4 units of fresh frozen plasma, antithrombin (AT) 500–1000 units) or even bivalirudin to achieve adequate anticoagulation (see page 251).[29-32] Common systems to measure ACTs include the Hepcon (Medtronic), Hemochron (Accriva Diagnostics), and i-STAT (Abbott) devices.

2. Because of patient variability in response to heparin and the effects of hypothermia and hemodilution on the ACT, the correlation between ACTs and the level of thrombin markers is imprecise. Using the Medtronic Heparin Hemostasis Management System (HMS), an individual dose–response curve can be generated which calculates the precise amount of heparin necessary to achieve a specified ACT. Monitoring of heparin concentrations is important during CPB as this may reduce heparin over- or underdosing and has been shown to reduce thrombin generation, fibrinolysis, and neutrophil activation.[33] A level of ≥2.0 units/mL is recommended. During off-pump surgery, the ACT should reach 250 seconds because the coronary artery being bypassed is occluded during the procedure.

B. In a patient with documented **heparin-induced thrombocytopenia (HIT)**, an alternative means of anticoagulation must be sought. Although one can give an antiplatelet medication (glycoprotein IIb/IIIa inhibitor or a prostaglandin analog) with heparin during bypass, the preferred approach is to use bivalirudin, a short-acting direct thrombin inhibitor, to avoid heparin entirely.[34,35] This issue is discussed in more detail on pages 251–253.

C. **Antifibrinolytic drugs.** CPB is associated with a variety of abnormalities in coagulation, among which is fibrinolysis. ε-aminocaproic acid (Amicar) and tranexamic acid decrease fibrinolysis by inhibiting plasminogen activation and through antiplasmin activity. When given prior to going on bypass and during the pump run, they have both been demonstrated to reduce perioperative bleeding. Although a variety of different dosing regimens are used, ε-aminocaproic acid is usually given in a dose of 10 g intravenously (IV) with 5–10 g in the pump prime. A common dose of tranexamic acid is 10 mg/kg with 1 mg/kg/h infusion during surgery (see page 249).[36,37] Although many groups give the initial dose of antifibrinolytic medication prior to skin incision, it may be best to defer the bolus dose until after heparinization, to avoid a transient procoagulant state.[38]

D. **Arterial cannulation** is usually accomplished by placement of a cannula in the ascending aorta just proximal to the innominate artery (Figure 5.4). Cannula size is determined by the anticipated flow rate for the patient based on body surface area, so as to minimize line pressure and shear forces (Table 5.1).

1. Cannula designs have been modified in a variety of ways to minimize shear forces and jet effects on the aortic wall (Figure 5.5). Most commonly used are those with end holes and/or multiple side holes through which blood exits at lower velocity (the Medtronic EOPA and Soft-flow cannulas).[39]

2. Steps to prevent systemic embolization, primarily to the brain, are imperative when CPB is used during surgery. Although gaseous microembolization can be addressed by improvements in CPB technology, cannulation and clamping are the primary causes of atheroembolism and stroke. Although most surgeons palpate the proposed

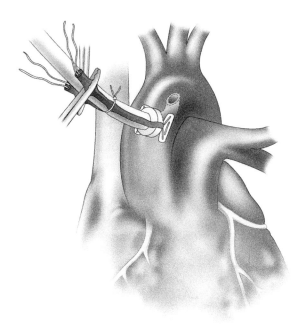

Figure 5.4 • Arterial cannulation. The arterial cannula is placed amidst two pursestrings in the ascending aorta just proximal to the innominate artery. The outflow should be directed into the arch, not into the innominate artery.

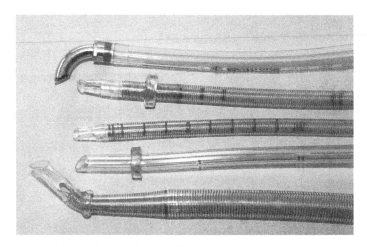

Figure 5.5 • Arterial cannulas include (top to bottom): Medtronic DLP 20 Fr curved metal cannula, Sarns Terumo 7 Fr Soft-Flow cannula with multiple side holes, Medtronic 20 Fr EOPA cannula with end and side holes, Medtronic DLP 22 Fr straight arch cannula, and Medtronic 22 mm three-dimensional select cannula.

Table 5.1 • Flow Rates and Desired Cannula Sizes

BSA	Venous		Arterial		Flow L/min
	Bicaval (Fr)	2 or 3 Stage (Fr)	French	Metric	
1.3	26 & 28		18 Fr	6.5 mm (curved)	3.1
1.4		29/37 29/29/29			3.4
1.5	28 & 30				3.6
1.6					3.8
1.7	30 & 32		20 Fr (EOPA)		4.1
1.8		32/40 29/37/37			4.3
1.9	32 & 34				4.6
2.0					4.8
2.1				7–8 mm (Soft-flow)	5.0
2.2					5.3
2.3	34 & 36		22/24 Fr (Select 3D)		5.5
2.4		36/46 29/46/37			5.8
2.5					6.0
2.6					6.2

Note that smaller venous cannulas can be used when vacuum-assisted drainage is employed
BSA, body surface area (m^2)

cannulation site in the ascending aorta to assess for the presence of atherosclerotic plaque and calcification, this is a very insensitive means of detecting plaque. Transesophageal echocardiography (TEE) may identify protruding atheromas, but epiaortic imaging is the gold standard for identifying plaque and may lead to modification of the surgical approach.[40–42] Cannulas with attached intra-aortic filtration devices (Embol-X catheter) and suction-based extraction devices have been devised to trap embolic material upon unclamping with equivocal benefits.[43–45]

3. If ascending aortic cannulation is not feasible, an alternative cannulation site must be sought. Femoral artery cannulation, either percutaneously or via cutdown, is feasible if aortoiliac atherosclerosis is not severe and the TEE does not demonstrate significant descending aortic atherosclerosis which could produce retrograde cerebral embolization and stroke. In fact, one study of reoperative mitral valve surgery demonstrated a greater than fourfold incidence of stroke comparing retrograde arterial perfusion to central cannulation.[46] Femoral cannulation also

runs the risk of a retrograde dissection. Satisfactory flow into the cannula must be assured before connecting the cannula to the CPB circuit. After decannulation, distal flow must be confirmed after the femoral access site has been repaired.

4. Although central aortic cannulation can be accomplished in many types of minimally invasive surgery, femoral arterial cannulation is commonly used. In these patients, it is important to assess the patient's iliofemoral system prior to surgery to identify whether femoral artery cannulation will be feasible. Furthermore, when a long duration of CPB is anticipated (complex minimally invasive or robotic surgery), there is an increased risk of a lower-extremity compartment syndrome from ischemia/reperfusion injury.[47-50] In these situations, options include placing the cannula percutaneously, placing it using the Seldinger technique to allow some distal flow, placing it through a sidearm graft sewn to the femoral artery to ensure distal flow, or placing an additional small cannula to provide distal perfusion.

5. If femoral cannulation is not feasible, or for surgery of the ascending aorta and arch, cannulation of the distal subclavian/axillary artery is an excellent alternative (Figure 5.6).[51] This may be performed directly through an arteriotomy or preferably through an 8 mm sidearm graft anastomosed to the vessel, which provides distal arm circulation during bypass. With snaring of the proximal innominate artery, axillary cannulation allows for selective antegrade brain perfusion during deep hypothermic circulatory arrest (DHCA). In these cases, additional cannulation of the left carotid artery may also be considered.[52-54]

6. Either femoral or axillary arterial cannulation should be immediately available when there is concern about potential cardiac, aortic, or graft damage during resternotomy or for patients with ruptured ascending aortic aneurysms or aortic dissections with hemopericardium. The artery should be exposed and occasionally may need to be cannulated, either for immediate initiation of bypass if problems are encountered after sternotomy or, on occasion, to initiate bypass and systemic cooling before the sternotomy is performed, depending on the patient's clinical condition.

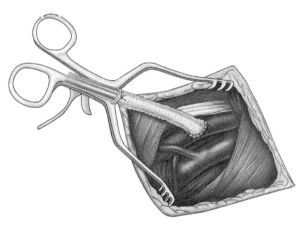

Figure 5.6 • Axillary artery cannulation. An 8 mm side graft is sewn to the distal subclavian/axillary artery, into which the cannula is placed and secured in position.

7. In patients developing hemodynamic instability during transcatheter aortic valve replacement (TAVR) despite pharmacologic management, an intra-aortic balloon pump is usually placed first for additional support. If the patient remains unstable, develops refractory arrhythmias, or has a cardiac arrest or life-threatening tamponade, institution of CPB may be life-saving. Use of 15 Fr arterial and 17 Fr venous cannulas placed through a percutaneous transfemoral approach can allow for systemic flow rates of up to 2.5 L/min while problems are rectified.

E. **Venous drainage** for most open-heart surgery is accomplished with a double- or triple-stage cavoatrial cannula (Figure 5.7). This is placed through the right atrial appendage or right atrial free wall with the distal end situated in the inferior vena cava (IVC) (Figure 5.8A). Blood drains from the IVC through several apertures near the end and from the right atrium through additional side holes. These catheters are used for most procedures that do not require opening of the right heart. The triple-stage cannula provides excellent flow and allows for use of a smaller outer-diameter cannula, especially with vacuum-assisted drainage.

1. Mitral valve surgery may be accomplished using a double- or triple-staged cannula or with bicaval cannulation, the latter being required if a biatrial transseptal approach is planned. Tricuspid valve surgery through a sternotomy incision is performed using bicaval cannulation with placement of caval snares around the cannulas to prevent air entry into the venous lines. A cannula may be placed directly into the superior vena cava (SVC) or passed through the right atrial appendage into the SVC. The IVC cannula is placed through a pursestring suture low in the right atrial free wall (Figure 5.8B).

2. Femoral venous cannulation is used in robotic and minimally invasive cases and may be supplemented by a 15 or 17 Fr venous line placed into the internal jugular vein. The femoral catheter is 50 cm long and is passed through the femoral vein

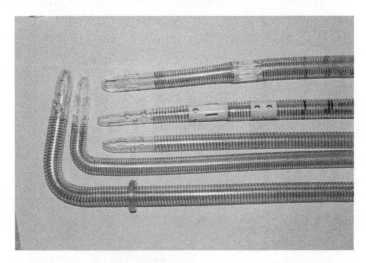

Figure 5.7 • Venous cannulas include (top to bottom): Medtronic 32/40 double-stage cavoatrial cannula, RMI 29/37/37 triple-stage cannula, RMI 30 Fr straight "lighthouse" tipped cannula, and short DLP 32 Fr and long RMI 36 Fr right-angle cannulas.

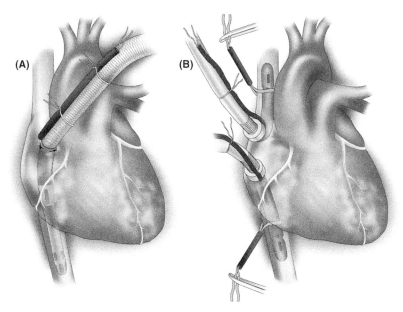

Figure 5.8 • Venous cannulation. (A) The cavoatrial catheter is placed through a pursestring in the right atrial appendage. The tip consists of multiple side holes and is placed into the IVC. The "basket" lies in the mid-atrium and drains blood from the SVC and coronary sinus through multiple holes 9 cm back from the tip for dual-stage cannulas and 6 and 11 cm from the tip for triple-stage cannulas. (B) Bicaval cannulation. The SVC cannula may be placed into the SVC directly or via the right atrial appendage. The IVC cannula is placed through a pursestring low on the right atrial free wall.

to lie within the right atrium to ensure adequate venous drainage. Shorter venous catheters can be used, if necessary. Exposure of the femoral vein or even cannulation and establishment of CPB may also be used in high-risk situations of hemodynamic instability or redo surgery. Minimally invasive tricuspid valve surgery can also be performed using femoral venous drainage. The transfemoral catheter is withdrawn into the IVC and the IVC is snared. An additional drainage catheter is placed in the SVC either directly or through the right atrium and the SVC is snared to eliminate air entry into the venous line. This is usually supplemented with vacuum-assisted drainage. In redo cases, the cannula may be left in the SVC and snares are not necessary.[55]

3. Femoral arterial and venous cannulation have been used to systemically warm patients presenting with profound accidental hypothermia and can be used in emergency situations, such as cardiac arrest, to establish an ECMO circuit (see pages 312–315 and 563–565).

F. **Cannulation for cardioplegia administration.** Antegrade cardioplegia is delivered through a catheter placed in the aortic root just proximal to the position of the aortic cross-clamp. This should provide the best myocardial protection in the absence of coronary disease. A retrograde catheter is routinely used to augment protection and ease the flow of an operation. It is very useful in patients with coronary disease and those with severe aortic regurgitation in whom antegrade cardioplegia cannot be delivered into the root (it can subsequently be given directly into the coronary ostia). The catheter is placed through a pursestring suture in the right atrial free wall, although some surgeons open the right atrium to place the catheter under direct vision, and place a suture around the coronary sinus ostium to optimize flow. Cannulas are held in position within the sinus with a balloon which may be self-inflating or manually inflated which allows for pressure measurements near the tip of the catheter to prevent overpressurization and potential coronary sinus rupture.[56]

G. Figure 5.9 provides an illustration of cannulation and clamping for a routine on-pump coronary bypass operation.

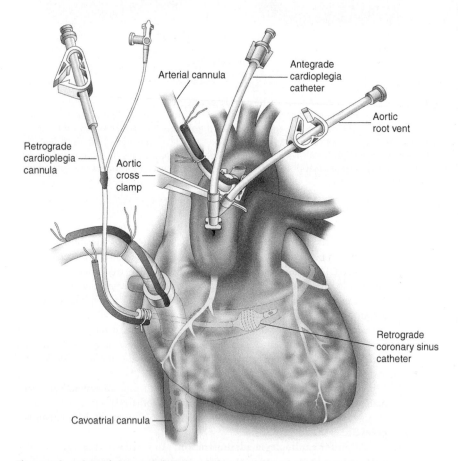

Figure 5.9 • Cannulation and clamping during a routine on-pump coronary bypass operation. Note aortic and venous cannulation, antegrade and retrograde cardioplegia catheters, and the aortic cross-clamp just proximal to the aortic cannulation site.

IV. Initiation and Conduct of Cardiopulmonary Bypass (Table 5.2)

A. **Retrograde autologous priming (RAP)** along with venous antegrade priming (VAP) can be used to reduce the hemodilutional effects of the priming solution and maintain a higher hematocrit on pump. The process involves back-draining the arterial line, then the venous reservoir and oxygenator, and then the venous line to remove about 1100 mL of crystalloid from the pump setup prior to initiating bypass. Simultaneously, an α-agent may be given to maintain systemic pressure. RAP does maintain a higher oncotic pressure during the pump run and has been shown to minimize the accumulation of extravascular lung water and postoperative weight gain. It may also improve tissue perfusion on pump leading to lower lactate levels. It is probably most beneficial in small patients with low blood volumes and low hematocrits, and might be considered in patients who refuse transfusions (Jehovah Witnesses). Although the impact of RAP on clinical outcomes is not significant, it may reduce the overall number of transfusions required.[57–61]

B. **Systemic pressures and flows.** When pump flow is initiated, the patient's pulsatile perfusion is replaced by nonpulsatile flow. The blood pressure initially decreases from hemodilution with a reduction in blood viscosity. The mean arterial pressure should then be maintained between 50 and 70 mm Hg during the pump run. It may transiently decrease during cardioplegia delivery (probably from potassium delivery into the systemic circulation), from return of large volumes of cardiotomy suction (from inflammatory mediators), and during rewarming (from vasodilation). Blood pressure may rise due to vasoconstriction from hypothermia, and from dilution of narcotics by the pump prime.

Table 5.2 • Desired Values on Pump	
1. ACT	>480 seconds >400 seconds for biocompatible circuits
2. Systemic flow rates	2–2.5 L/min/m² at 37 °C 1.7–2.0 (low flow) or 2.0–2.5 L/min/m² (high flow) at 30 °C
3. Systemic blood pressure	50–70 mm Hg

4. Arterial blood gases	PO_2 >250 torr, PCO_2 40–50 torr with pH 7.40
	Deep hypothermia:
	  α–stat pH 7.40 measured at 37 °C
	  pH–stat pH 7.40 at systemic temperature

5. SVO_2	>65%
6. Hematocrit	>18% or higher depending on patient age and comorbidities
7. Blood glucose	100–180 mg/dL

1. The systemic flow rate is calculated based on the patient's body surface area and is modified by the degree of hypothermia and the venous oxygen saturation (SvO_2). It should also take into account the degree of anemia, which can influence whole-body oxygen delivery. The flow rate should exceed 2 L/min/m² at normothermia and can be reduced to 1.5–1.7 L/min/m² at 30 °C with "low flow" bypass. Flow needs to be increased during rewarming, when increased metabolism usually decreases the SvO_2. Low-flow bypass during moderate hypothermia has been shown to improve myocardial protection, reduce collateral flow improving exposure, reduce hemolysis, and reduce fluid requirements without any compromise in tissue perfusion.[62]

2. The optimal flow rate should be based on an assessment of adequate oxygen delivery. Means of assessing this include the SvO_2, blood lactate levels, and in-line monitoring of CO_2 production.[63] The latter two together may be the best way of predicting anaerobic metabolism, which is not assessed by the SvO_2. Nonetheless, in most practices, as long as the SvO_2 exceeds 65%, the flow rate is considered adequate, although this may not reflect regional flow.[64,65]

   a. For example, at normothermia, the brain and kidney autoregulate to maintain perfusion as the flow rate is reduced at the expense of skeletal muscle and splanchnic flow. Due to concerns that the combination of hemodilution and a lower flow rate may reduce the mean arterial pressure below the autoregulatory threshold and compromise organ system function, there are proponents of using "high flow" (2–2.4 L/min/m²) rather than "low flow" bypass during hypothermia. Hypothermia may cause more regional variation in flow.[65]

   b. CPB has significant adverse effects on renal perfusion, filtration, and oxygenation.[66–68] Renal blood flow is determined primarily by the systemic flow rate, but hypothermia impairs renal autoregulation and induces renal vasoconstriction. This results in blood being shunted away from the kidneys while the glomerular filtrate rate and renal oxygen consumption remain unchanged. Thus, renal oxygen extraction increases significantly as there is a significant mismatch between oxygen supply and demand that is exacerbated by the anemia of hemodilution. One study demonstrated that renal function was not affected by using lower target blood pressures on CPB (<60 mm Hg vs. 60–69 mm Hg vs. >70 mm Hg), although urine output was less at the lower pressures.[69] It does appear, however, that lower systemic flow rates and low hematocrits do adversely affect renal function, so in older patients, those with known chronic kidney disease, and with longer pump runs, maintenance of higher flow rates and a hematocrit above 21% may minimize the risk of acute kidney injury.[67–73]

3. One of the primary concerns with CPB is maintenance of adequate cerebral oxygenation, which is determined by the blood pressure, the systemic flow rate, and the pCO_2. Cerebral autoregulation allows for maintenance of cerebral blood flow down to a mean arterial pressure as low as 40–50 mm Hg, but autoregulation may be inadequate in hypertensive or diabetic patients, in whom it may be desirable to maintain a higher pressure.[74] In fact, some studies have shown that cerebral oxygenation is impaired at this level even if the flow rate is satisfactory, so the blood pressure must be maintained at an adequate level regardless of the flow rate, usually using vasopressors, such as phenylephrine, norepinephrine, or vasopressin.[75] This may improve cerebral oxygenation but reduce flow to other regions, specifically the kidneys and splanchnic viscera.

4. The adequacy of cerebral oxygenation during CPB is usually assessed by cerebral oximetry using bifrontal sensors with near-infrared spectroscopy. Numerous products are available, including the INVOS (Medtronic), Equanox (NONIN Medical), and ForeSight (Edwards) cerebral oximeters (see Figure 4.9, page 255). The regional cerebral oxygen saturation (rSO_2) tends to fall during initiation of bypass and during rewarming, even with an increase in systemic flow. The rSO_2 promptly detects problems with arterial desaturation even before it is evident by pulse oximetry.[76] Studies have demonstrated that oxygen desaturation is associated with an increased incidence of neurocognitive changes.[77] If the oxygen saturation falls more than 20% below baseline or below 40%, an intervention is recommended to restore cerebral blood flow. Before initiating bypass, an increase in blood pressure or an elevation in PCO_2 will be effective in increasing cerebral blood flow. Once on bypass, modifications of flow rate, blood pressure, PCO_2, or the hematocrit are beneficial. This technology may also alert the cardiac surgical team to potential catastrophes associated with brain malperfusion from cannula malplacement, dissections, oxygenator or other pump-related failures, air embolism, anaphylactic reactions (such as from protamine), and monitoring problems. Although interventions to improve rSO_2 should intuitively reduce the adverse effects of cerebral oxygen desaturation, few studies have documented improvements in clinical outcome.[78]

C. Both the **hematocrit (HCT)** on pump and the systemic flow rate determine the amount of oxygen delivery to the body. Hemodilution from the pump prime commonly reduces oxygen delivery by 25% as estimated from the following equation:

$$\text{Predicted HCT on pump} = \frac{\left(70 \times \text{kg} \times \text{preop HCT}/100\right)}{\left(70 \times \text{kg}\right) + \text{prime volume} + \text{IV fluids pre-CPB}}$$

where 70 × kg equals the blood volume and 70 × kg × preoperative HCT is the RBC volume.

1. Hemodilution reduces blood viscosity and improves microcirculatory flow, but at the extremes of hemodilution, there is a significant reduction in oncotic pressure that increases fluid requirements. This can exacerbate the systemic inflammatory response and capillary leak, causing substantial tissue edema. This may contribute to cerebral edema, papilledema, and ischemic optic neuropathy,[79] and can lead to respiratory compromise, among other adverse effects.

2. Very low hematocrits on pump have been associated with increased mortality and an increase in the incidence of renal dysfunction, stroke, and prolonged mechanical ventilation.[71,72,80] Profound anemia will compromise oxygen delivery despite adequate systemic flow rates and may lead to ischemic organ system damage that at its extreme can produce life-threatening complications, such as mesenteric ischemia. Although the acceptable lower limit for a hematocrit on pump has been considered 18% according to the STS guidelines,[81] numerous studies have shown that the risk of renal dysfunction increases below a hematocrit of 21%, and if that is considered a surrogate for organ system malperfusion, it is feasible to recommend that 21% should be the limit below which transfusion is indicated.[69–72] However, transfusions are not benign: administering blood to raise the hematocrit

to over 24% offers little advantage during bypass and may prove deleterious because of immunomodulatory effects and other potential adverse organ system sequelae of transfusions.

D. **Temperature management.** The systemic temperature may be maintained at normothermia or at varying degrees of hypothermia, depending on the surgeon's preference and the operative procedure. Most surgeons use moderate hypothermia to 34–35 °C to provide some organ system protection during nonpulsatile perfusion and also in the event that a temporary problem arises with surgery (need to reduce flow to place sutures) or with perfusion (impaired drainage, low blood pressure, air embolism, pump head failure, oxygenator failure, etc.). No conclusive advantage of using either normothermic or hypothermic bypass has been established in terms of inflammatory activation, perioperative hemostasis, or neurocognitive outcome.[82] However, the rate of rewarming and its extent may affect neurocognitive outcome.[83,84] The STS guidelines suggest that the oxygenator arterial outlet temperature is a surrogate for cerebral temperature measurements even though it underestimates the cerebral perfusate temperature. It is recommended the outlet temperature be kept at less than 37 °C during rewarming. When the patient's arterial temperature is ≥ 30 °C, the difference between the arterial outlet and venous inflow temperatures should be ≤ 4 °C; when the patient's temperature is < 30 °C, the gradient should be no more than 10° to minimize generation of gaseous emboli (during cooling) or "outgassing" when blood is returned to the patient upon warming.[84]

E. **Gas exchange.** Oxygenation and elimination of CO_2 are determined by the sweep rate, which is adjusted on the blender. Most oxygenators are not stressed until the flow rate exceeds 7 L/min, which should be adequate for even a 175 kg patient. The PO_2 should be maintained above 250 torr in the event of a temporary reduction in flow or pump malfunction, and can be monitored in-line or by intermittent blood gases every 30 minutes. Inhalational anesthetics, such as sevoflurane, desflurane, or isoflurane, are administered through the blender and must be scavenged via the oxygenator.

F. **Ventilation.** Upon initiation of full flow on bypass, ventilation is stopped. Although ventilation or use of continuous positive airway pressure (CPAP) during bypass may improve pulmonary function and gas exchange with less release of inflammatory mediators, this is not a common practice.[85,86]

G. **pH management.** With progressive hypothermia, CO_2 production decreases and pH normally rises. With mild or moderate hypothermia, pH is generally maintained between 7.40 and 7.50 by adjusting the sweep rate and maintaining the PCO_2 around 40–50 torr. Evidence of metabolic acidosis on pump may be a sign of inadequate tissue oxygenation despite normal blood gases. Regional hypoperfusion, especially of the splanchnic bed, may be contributory to this problem. In fact, lactate release with levels greater than 4 mmol/L during reperfusion is predictive of an increased risk of complications and death.[87,88] During deep hypothermia, two pH management strategies can be used. With pH-stat, the pH is temperature-corrected and maintained at 7.40 by adding a mixture of O_2 and CO_2 ("carbogen") to the circuit. With this strategy, there is an increase in cerebral blood flow with a potentially increased risk of cerebral microembolism. This strategy is associated with improved tissue oxygenation during hypothermia.[89] In contrast, with α-stat, the pH is maintained at 7.40 measured at 37 °C (i.e. not temperature-corrected). Cerebral blood flow is autoregulated and coupled to cerebral oxygen demand. The latter strategy is preferred during DHCA cases.[90,91]

(A)   (B)

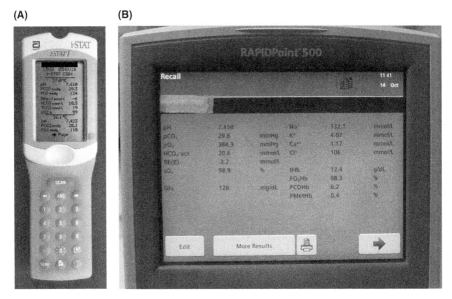

Figure 5.10 • Point-of-care testing devices available to the perfusionist to obtain arterial blood gases, electrolytes, glucose levels, oxygen saturations, and hematocrit levels. (A) The i-STAT handheld device and (B) the Siemens RAPIDpoint system.

H. **Medications** to maintain anesthesia or to control blood pressure are given into a sampling manifold that flows into the venous reservoir. Medications that may be given by the perfusionist into the circuit during bypass include mannitol, insulin, sodium bicarbonate, calcium chloride, magnesium sulfate, antibiotics, vasopressors, and inotropes.

I. Intermittent measurements of serum potassium, glucose, and hematocrit should be performed in addition to arterial and venous blood gases and ACTs. This should be performed using point-of-care machines in the operating room. Commonly used systems include the Siemens RAPIDpoint and the i-STAT handheld system (Figure 5.10). An elevated potassium may necessitate a change in the composition or frequency of cardioplegia delivery and may require administration of diuretics or insulin for control. An elevated glucose is related to increased levels of endogenous epinephrine and insulin resistance and may be associated with an increased risk of neurologic injury.[3] Blood glucose should generally be maintained at a level below 180 mg/dL, but excessively stringent control (glucose <100 mg/dL) may be more harmful than beneficial.[92–94]

V. Terminating Bypass

A. Before terminating bypass, the patient should be warmed toward normothermia (to at least 36 °C). As noted above, the rate of rewarming should be appropriate and cerebral hyperthermia should be avoided, as both may affect neurocognitive outcome.[84]

B. The lungs are ventilated, taking care to identify the course of the internal thoracic artery (ITA) to avoid tension on the ITA pedicle. Pacing is initiated, if necessary.

Calcium chloride 1 g may be given prior to coming off bypass to provide an increase in systemic vascular resistance and some inotropic support. The heart is filled by restricting venous return as bypass flow is reduced and turned off by the perfusionist. Active root venting is used in cases of intracardiac entry (primarily valve operations) to evacuate any ejected air with the patient in the Trendelenburg position.

C. Cardiac performance is assessed by incorporating visual assessment with echocardiographic imaging, filling pressures, and cardiac output measurements. Inotropic support should be considered for marginal cardiac performance. Low systemic resistance is common and α-agents or vasopressin may be necessary to improve the blood pressure. In primarily valve cases, right ventricular (RV) dysfunction from coronary air embolism is not uncommon, and bypass occasionally must be resumed for a short period of time until myocardial function improves. Insertion of an intra-aortic balloon may be necessary if cardiac performance is suboptimal on multiple inotropic medications. Attention should be paid to the ECG monitor to identify ischemic changes that may require revision of the procedure.

D. When the patient is stable, protamine is administered to reverse any heparin effect and should return the ACT to normal. The dosage is commonly based on a 1:1 mg:mg ratio to the administered heparin, although with use of the HMS system, which measures heparin levels, a heparin–protamine titration test can be used to determine the actual heparin concentration in the blood and the precise dose of protamine needed to reverse its effects. A protamine reaction is uncommon, but can be life-threatening (see pages 260–261). It requires immediate attention and occasionally the reinstitution of CPB after the re-administration of heparin. Ongoing bleeding may be surgical in etiology, but the availability of routine coagulation studies and particularly thromboelastography may be helpful in ascertaining the exact nature of a hemostatic problem.[95]

E. The suction lines are turned off once the protamine administration has started. The venous line is removed first and drained into the cardiotomy reservoir. Blood may then be transfused through the arterial cannula as needed to maintain filling pressures. Once the aorta is decannulated and the patient is stable, the pump contents are drained into a cell-saving device, centrifuged and washed, and made available in transfer bags for the anesthesiologist to transfuse as necessary.

F. The cannulation sites are secured. Hemostasis is then achieved and the chest is closed. Issues related to perioperative bleeding are discussed in detail in Chapter 9.

VI. Potential Problems Encountered During Cardiopulmonary Bypass and upon Weaning from Bypass (Table 5.3)

A. **Inadequate ACT** from standard doses of heparin usually results from antithrombin (AT) deficiency. AT is a major inhibitor of thrombin and factors Xa and IXa, and its deficiency leads to a hypercoagulable state. The basis for anticoagulation with heparin is the rapid activation of AT inhibitory activity. AT deficiency results in resistance to treatment with heparin and is noted most frequently in patients maintained preoperatively on heparin therapy or intravenous nitroglycerin or those with high platelet counts.[96] Additional administration of 1–2 mg/kg of heparin will usually achieve an adequate ACT. If not, AT can be provided by transfusion of fresh frozen plasma or,

Table 5.3 • Potential Problems on Pump and on Weaning from Bypass
A. Inadequate heparinization (low ACT)
B. Inadequate venous drainage
C. Distention of the heart (right and left)
D. Air entry into the venous lines
E. Inadequate systemic pressures
F. Vasoplegia post-pump
G. Inadequate systemic oxygenation
H. High arterial line pressure
I. Inadequate retrograde cardioplegia delivery
J. Inadequate antegrade cardioplegia delivery
K. Cannulation/decannulation problems
L. Systemic or coronary air embolism
M. Clotting within the extracorporeal circuit from cold agglutinins

if available, by a commercial AT product (Thrombate III), which provides 500 units per vial.[29-31] Because preoperative AT levels are rarely known, the exact dose required to reach 120% of normal, which is recommended, can only be estimated. Studies have shown successful elevation of the ACT using a wide dosage range of AT doses to as high as 75 units/kg. The calculation of the amount needed equals the (desired − baseline AT level) × weight (kg) divided by 1.4. For example, to reach 120% of normal levels in a 70 kg man with a baseline level that is 80% of normal would require ([120 − 80]/1.4) × 70 = 2000 units (or 28 units/kg); if the baseline level is 50% of normal, 3500 units (50 units/kg) should be given.

B. **Inadequate venous drainage** will be detected by the surgeon as a distended right heart and by the perfusionist as a drop in the blood level in the venous reservoir (which should trigger a low-volume alarm with use of a hardshell reservoir), with an inability to maintain systemic flow rates. It may result from an airlock in the venous line, kinking of the line on the field or close to the reservoir, inadvertent clamping of the venous line, retraction of the heart impeding flow into the venous cannula, or malposition of the venous cannula (either being too far in or not in enough). Inadequate venous drainage not only warms the heart during systemic hypothermia, potentially compromising myocardial protection, but may adversely affect the organs that are not drained well. A high central venous pressure (CVP) may indicate impaired SVC drainage and can produce cerebral edema. More commonly, drainage from the IVC is impaired, which could result in renal impairment or hepatic or splanchnic congestion with significant fluid sequestration in the bowel. Simply readjusting the depth of the cannula in the IVC usually resolves this issue. Rarely, when the SVC or IVC is snared with a tourniquet and the catheter has inadvertently pulled back into the atrium, there will be compromise of virtually all flow into the cannula and the right atrium.

C. **Distention of the heart** on bypass is indicative of poor venous drainage, aortic valve insufficiency, or significant collateral flow. It may stretch the ventricular fibers producing myocardial injury, increase pulmonary artery pressures producing pulmonary barotrauma, or contribute to ventricular warming, impairing myocardial protection.

The cause of distention should be remedied, either by readjusting the venous lines and/or by placing a vent, either in the LV or in the pulmonary artery. Occasionally, a distended heart during aortic cross-clamping is related to incomplete occlusion of the aorta, with creation of aortic regurgitation when the heart is retracted.

D. **Air entry into the venous lines** usually arises from the venous cannulation site or the retrograde cardioplegia site, and can be controlled by an additional suture around the catheter. Rarely, it may result from inadvertent damage to the IVC or coronary sinus, or from an atrial septal defect. Air entrapment with use of vacuum assist can result in arterial gaseous embolization.[18]

E. **Inadequate systemic pressures** on pump have been incriminated as the cause of multisystem organ dysfunction, including neurocognitive changes, renal failure, and splanchnic hypoperfusion. Whether low-flow or high-flow CPB is optimal for organ system protection is controversial, but a minimum pressure of 50–70 mm Hg should be maintained unless it is desired to intentionally maintain a higher pressure (e.g. the patient with significant uncorrected carotid disease or the hypertensive, diabetic patient with preexisting renal dysfunction). Phenylephrine or norepinephrine is commonly used on pump to maintain systemic pressures, accepting the transient dips that occur with cardioplegia infusion or reinfusion of shed blood aspirated through the cardiotomy suckers. However, adequate flow rates must be maintained, because α-agents will shunt blood away from the muscles and splanchnic circulation.

F. **Vasodilatory shock post-pump ("vasoplegia").** Not infrequently, a patient may be hypotensive from profound peripheral vasodilation despite an adequate cardiac output when terminating bypass. These patients often require a substantial amount of pressor support on pump as well. This phenomenon of "vasoplegia" appears to be mediated by high levels of nitric oxide due to activation of nitric acid synthase, activation of vascular smooth muscle ATP-sensitive potassium channels, and relative vasopressin deficiency.[97] Risk factors include older age, recent myocardial infarction, dialysis-dependent renal failure, and valve operations.[98] It may also occur more frequently in patients on preoperative ACE inhibitors or ARBs, as well as those on amiodarone.[99] Although norepinephrine or phenylephrine are initially used to offset hypotension, vasopressin may be given in doses of 0.01–0.1 units/min and is usually successful in restoring the blood pressure and has been shown to improve clinical outcomes.[100] If vasopressin is not successful, methylene blue (1.5 mg/kg) has been recommended.[101,102] Hydroxocobalamin has also been used successfully to treat vasoplegia on pump by its effect on nitric oxide metabolism.[103]

G. **Inadequate systemic oxygenation** can result in tissue ischemia and acidosis, potentially resulting in multisystem organ dysfunction. Despite regional variations in flow, it is presumed that a SvO_2 exceeding 65% is indicative of satisfactory oxygenation. If the saturation is low, as is often noted during rewarming, this problem can be mitigated by improving the systemic flow rates and/or increasing the hematocrit. Evidence of cerebral oxygen desaturation is first evident by cerebral oximetry, then by pulse oximetry, and eventually by systemic venous oxygen desaturation. Mild systemic hypothermia can provide some element of organ system protection. However, significant arterial desaturation may also result from a catastrophic problem requiring immediate attention. This may include failure of the oxygenator or oxygen blender, or disconnection from an oxygen source. It might also result from an aortic dissection or malperfusion syndrome. Pump issues should be immediately recognizable by a change in the color of the blood in the arterial return line. On rare occasions, when the patient is no longer on pump, inadequate systemic oxygenation may result from the anesthesiologist failing to provide adequate ventilation to the patient (usually after the surgeon has asked that the lungs not be ventilated to improve exposure and then forgetting that request!).

H. **High arterial line pressure** measured by the perfusionist is a potentially alarming situation. With pressurized roller pumps, this could result in a catastrophic line disconnection. With centrifugal pumps, which are afterload-sensitive, unsafe high line pressures should not occur, because the flow is automatically reduced. A high line pressure caused by a high flow rate through a small cannula should not occur if the appropriately sized cannula is selected. For example, a 20 Fr curved-tip cannula may provide up to 5 L/min flow at acceptable line pressures, but excessive shear force with higher line pressures may be noted at higher flow rates. In contrast, a 7 or 8 mm Medtronic Soft-flow or EOPA cannula can flow more than 6 L/min without producing high line pressures. Malposition of the tip of the aortic cannula, kinking or clamping of the line, or an aortic dissection can also account for a high line pressure. When a dissection occurs, the high line pressure is accompanied by very low systemic pressures, and mandates immediate cessation of pump flow and relocation of the arterial inflow cannula.

I. **Inadequate retrograde cardioplegia delivery** may produce inadequate myocardial protection. Low retrograde cardioplegia line pressures may be associated with rupture of the coronary sinus, a left SVC, or catheter displacement back into the right atrium.[56,104] High line pressures may be noted in patients with a small coronary sinus, impingement of the end of the catheter on the sinus wall, inadvertent clamping of the catheter, or kinking of the cardioplegia line or catheter. Placement too far into the sinus may reduce flow to the RV and impair its protection. Filling of the posterior descending vein suggests that the RV is being adequately protected, but this may not always be the case.

J. **Inadequate antegrade cardioplegia delivery** is usually associated with the presence of aortic regurgitation, thus mandating the use of retrograde cardioplegia for myocardial protection unless direct coronary ostial cannulation is used after performing an aortotomy. The efficacy of antegrade delivery can also be in doubt in patients with very severe coronary disease, so monitoring of myocardial pH or temperature may provide the surgeon with some assurance that adequate protection is being achieved. If the antegrade catheter is not completely within the aortic lumen, it is possible to infuse cardioplegia into the aortic wall, creating a dissection. Note that there are very small side holes a few millimeters away from the tip of the cannula and flow exiting those holes within the aortic wall could also cause a dissection.

K. **Cannulation/decannulation problems** in the ascending aorta can cause catastrophic bleeding or stroke and can be quite problematic. Always respect the ascending aorta! Femoral cannulation also can cause significant life-threatening problems when complications develop.

   1. The surgeon must carefully assess the ascending aorta prior to cannulation to avoid areas of plaque and calcification which could dislodge during cannulation (or clamping/unclamping) causing an embolic stroke.

   2. Suture placement in dilated aortas, especially those with bicuspid valves, can produce significant bleeding even with superficial passage of the needle through the

aortic wall. Cannulating these sites must be done carefully to avoid tearing of the wall, which can result in significant bleeding around the cannula and potentially can cause an iatrogenic dissection. The latter may on occasion be repaired by additional suturing but, in most cases, requires repair during circulatory arrest and carries a high mortality rate. Cannula malposition should be rare with ascending aortic cannulation, especially if multiple side hole cannulas are used. The cannula must be securely positioned with tourniquets to prevent dislodgement.

3. Adequate imaging of the iliofemoral vessels is essential prior to femoral cannulation in patients undergoing minimally invasive surgery to determine if femoral cannulation can be safely performed. Nonetheless, retrograde aortic dissections can occur with femoral cannulation if not careful. Upstream malperfusion can occur in patients with aortic dissections despite true lumen femoral cannulation. All femoral cannulas must be securely sewn to the skin, because malposition may impair pump flow and dislodgement can cause catastrophic bleeding, often not initially noted when the cannula is covered by a towel.

4. Right atrial cannulation is usually done through the atrial appendage, but free wall cannulation is used during bicaval cannulation and for placement of the retrograde cardioplegia catheter, except in some minimally invasive cases. The atrial wall can be inordinately fragile and can tear, requiring additional sutures for control upon decannulation. Care must be taken to properly place all venous cannulas to optimize venous return. Improper positioning of a cavoatrial or IVC cannula can impair venous drainage from the splanchnic bed causing organ system dysfunction, and poor positioning of an SVC cannula can cause cerebral edema. This will be extreme if a tourniquet is tightened around the SVC or IVC when the cannula has pulled back into the right atrium. Poor right-sided drainage will cause RV and often LV distention and will compromise myocardial protection.

L. **Systemic or coronary air embolism** is always a possibility upon termination of bypass when there has been intracardiac entry, but its occurrence during CPB is a catastrophic problem.

1. Careful attention to deairing of the left-heart chambers is important when there has been intracardiac entry (valve surgery) or active intracardiac or root venting. Various maneuvers, including ventilating the lungs, restricting venous return, stopping LV vent return, and gently massaging the heart with the patient in the Trendelenburg position should be considered prior to removing the aortic cross-clamp in these cases. Needle aspiration of the LV apex should be considered after aortic valve surgery. Carbon dioxide flooding of the field may minimize the amount of air retained during intracardiac procedures.[105] Active root venting with gentle cardiac massage and sideways "shaking" of the patient on the OR table upon weaning from bypass are important maneuvers to evacuate any ejected air. It is not uncommon for some air to pass down the right coronary artery or an aorto-coronary venous bypass graft and cause RV dysfunction upon weaning from bypass. This problem usually resolves quickly, but CPB should be reinstituted if hemodynamics are compromised. TEE monitoring is the best means of identifying retained air as the heart is weaned from bypass.

2. Systemic air embolism occurring during CPB is usually related to inattention to the venous reservoir level in open circuits with delivery of air through a roller pump head. It may also occur with use of vacuum-assisted drainage. Air embolism may also occur on bypass when the aorta is not clamped and air trapped in the left

heart is ejected when the pressure generated by the LV exceeds that in the aorta. Significant air embolism requires cessation of bypass with immediate venting of air from the aorta with a needle or through a stopcock on the aortic line and then removal of air from the bypass circuit. Ventilation with 100% oxygen, steep Trendelenburg position, and retrograde SVC perfusion should be used to try to eliminate air from the cerebral circulation. Steroids, barbiturates, and reinstitution of bypass with deep hypothermia may also reduce the degree of cerebral injury.[106]

3. Systemic air embolism may occur if there is air entry into the inflow drainage lines of an assist device, because there is no reservoir or means available for venting or filtration of the air. The air will fragment and be pumped back into the arterial system.

M. Cold-reactive autoimmune diseases are rarely detected preoperatively, but may result in red cell agglutination and hemolysis on bypass at cold temperatures. This may be noted in the bypass or cardioplegia circuit.[107–109]

1. Cold hemagglutinin disease is caused by an IgM autoimmune antibody that causes red cell agglutination and hemolysis at cold temperatures. This may cause microvascular thrombosis that may contribute to myocardial infarction, renal failure, or other organ system failure. Since less than 1% of patients have cold agglutinins, screening is not routinely performed, and it rarely poses a problem during bypass, because hemodilution lowers antibody titers. However, should antibody titers be measured and be in high concentration (> 1.1000), agglutination will occur at warmer temperatures.

2. If high-titer agglutinins are present, systemic hypothermia and cold blood cardioplegia must be avoided. Either warm cardioplegia or cold crystalloid cardioplegia after an initial normothermic flush can be used.[108,109] Even better would be performance of off-pump coronary bypass surgery or on-pump beating- or fibrillating-heart surgery.

3. De novo discovery of cold agglutinins may occur on-pump by detecting agglutination and sedimentation in the blood cardioplegia heat exchanger or any stagnant line containing blood. It has also been identified when the retrograde cardioplegia line develops high pressure due to obstruction from agglutination. In these circumstances, the patient should be warmed back to normothermia, and crystalloid cardioplegia used to flush out the coronary arteries.

4. Paroxysmal cold hemoglobinuria (PCH) is an autoimmune disease in which a nonagglutinating IgG antibody binds to red cells in the cold, causing hemolysis. It should be managed in a similar fashion.[110]

VII. Modifications of Extracorporeal Circulation

A. **Deep hypothermic circulatory arrest (DHCA)** is used primarily in situations when the aorta cannot be clamped to perform an aortic anastomosis.

1. Indications for DHCA include:

a. Severe aortic atherosclerosis or calcification (porcelain aorta for aortic valve replacement) (see Figure 2.10, page 139)

b. Acute type A aortic dissections to avoid aortic wall damage and perform the distal anastomosis

c. Clamp placement too close to a planned suture line – ascending aortic or hemiarch repairs, arch repair, proximal descending thoracic aneurysms

    d. Complex descending thoracic aortic surgery to improve anastomotic exposure while providing neuroprotection for the brain and/or spinal cord

    e. Resection of IVC tumors

2. With traditional DHCA, the patient is cooled systemically to 18 °C to achieve electroencephalographic (EEG) silence. The temperature is measured at multiple sites, including the tympanic membrane, nasopharynx, bladder, and/or rectum, with the presumption that this will ensure uniform cooling of the cerebral cortex. Since an EEG is usually not performed, surgeons rely on clinical studies that have shown that about 45 minutes of DHCA at 18 °C is safe in minimizing cerebral damage.[111] The head is packed in ice, and methylprednisolone 20 mg/kg is also given. The arterial line is clamped and blood is drained from the circulation, taking care not to allow air entry into the lines.

3. Near-infrared spectroscopy usually shows an increase in rSO_2 as the patient is cooled systemically, but it usually falls during the first five minutes of DHCA. If the rSO_2 has not reached a steady state >90% of baseline despite reaching the desired temperature, a few additional minutes of cooling may be beneficial.[112]

4. Measures that may extend the acceptable period of DHCA to minimize the risk of CNS injury include antegrade or retrograde cerebral perfusion.

    a. **Antegrade cerebral perfusion (ACP)** provides flow into the arch vessels during the period of circulatory arrest and provides cold oxygenated blood to the brain at temperatures between 20–28 °C. Although core cooling to 18 °C is commonly used, moderate hypothermia to 30 °C can also be used with ACP without an added risk of cerebral damage.[113–116]

        i. Axillary artery cannulation with occlusion of the proximal innominate artery can provide flow to the right side of the brain, and, through the circle of Willis, to the left side. It may be augmented by a catheter placed into the left common carotid artery (LCCA), which may be beneficial for circulatory arrest times greater than 40 minutes.[117] Generally, infusing arterial blood at a rate of 6–10 mL/kg at a pressure of 40–60 mm Hg appears to give the best protection.[113,118]

        ii. If the patient is undergoing aortic arch reconstruction, use of a trifurcation graft sewn to the arch vessels can minimize the time during which there is no cerebral perfusion and can potentially shorten the duration of DHCA. The brain can then be perfused and the patient warmed while the distal aortic anastomosis is performed. The proximal end of the trifurcation graft is then sewn off the proximal aortic graft (Figure 1.26, page 81).[119]

    b. **Retrograde cerebral perfusion (RCP)** provides oxygenated, cold blood into the SVC at a flow rate up to 500 mL/min and at a pressure of up to 20 mm Hg. Studies suggest that this is not effective in providing nutrients to the brain, but it can maintain cerebral hypothermia. Although this is an effective technique for neuroprotection, it is probably most effective when the duration of DHCA will not be prolonged much beyond 45 minutes. RCP is beneficial in flushing air and debris out of the cerebral vessels.[120]

5. Extensive cooling and rewarming are often associated with a coagulopathy that may require blood-product transfusions. Warming generally takes twice as long as cooling, and the gradient between the arterial inflow and the patient's

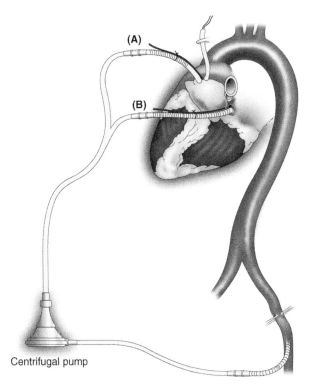

Figure 5.11 • Left-heart bypass setup. Inflow to the pump comes from either the left atrial appendage (A) or the left inferior pulmonary vein (B). Blood is then returned by a centrifugal pump to the femoral artery or to the distal aorta in cases of limited disease, such as traumatic tears of the aorta.

temperature should be no more than 10–12 °C to prevent generation of gaseous emboli.[84]

6. When hypaco flow is reinstituted, care must be taken to eliminate any air or atherosclerotic debris from the arterial tree.

B. **Left-heart bypass for thoracic aortic surgery**

1. Impairment of blood supply to the lower body is inherent to any aortic procedure involving descending aortic cross-clamping. The greatest risks are those of paraplegia and renal dysfunction. Even though thoracic endovascular aortic repair (TEVAR) is the procedure of choice for most descending thoracic aneurysms, an open surgical approach may be indicated in some patients.[121] To minimize the risk of ischemic complications during cross-clamping, techniques such as circulatory arrest or left-heart bypass can be used. The latter entails drainage of oxygenated blood from the left side of the heart and returning it more distally in the arterial tree (Figure 5.11).[122]

2. Inflow to a centrifugal pump may come from the left atrium or preferentially from the inferior pulmonary vein, which may be associated with fewer complications.[123] The blood is returned either to the femoral artery or to the distal aorta

below the lowest clamp in patients with limited disease (such as traumatic tears or Crawford type I aneurysms; see Figure 1.25, page 79). The blood does not pass through an oxygenator, although one can be placed in the circuit to improve oxygenation during one-lung anesthesia.[124]

3. Minimal heparinization is necessary for this setup (about 5000 units to achieve an ACT of 250 seconds), which is beneficial in trauma cases or cases requiring extensive dissection. Flow rates of up to 3 L/min can be used, with monitoring of lower-extremity mean pressures in the femoral artery that should approximate 50 mm Hg. Drainage should not be so excessive as to compromise antegrade flow from the heart to the brain.

C. **Assisted right-heart bypass for off-pump surgery.** During manipulation of the heart for off-pump surgery, especially with hypertrophied hearts, there may be compromise of RV filling. Several devices have been designed that provide right-heart assist by draining blood from the right atrium and pumping it into the pulmonary artery during these procedures.[125]

D. **Perfusion-assisted direct coronary artery bypass (PADCAB).** During off-pump surgery, there is compromise of distal flow during temporary vessel occlusion required for the construction of an anastomosis. This may lead to a subtle or severe degree of ischemia and potential myocardial necrosis. Intracoronary or aortocoronary shunts can be used to provide distal perfusion when constructing the anastomosis, either routinely or if there is evidence of ischemia.[126] PADCAB provides perfusion-assisted flow at a designated pressure (usually 120 mm Hg) that is independent of the systemic blood pressure. Additionally, medications such as nitroglycerin can be administered in the perfusate to provide coronary vasodilation. Placing a small catheter directly into the coronary artery allows for distal perfusion as the anastomosis is being constructed. Subsequently, flow can be directed through 2–3 mm cannulas placed into the conduits until the proximal anastomoses are performed. A comparative study of no shunting, passive shunting, and active perfusion showed that myocardial protection (measured by troponin levels) and performance were superior with active perfusion.[127,128]

VIII. Extracorporeal Membrane Oxygenation (ECMO)

A. **Indications and circuit setup.** ECMO is a means of providing a prolonged period of either pulmonary or cardiac support or both, depending on the nature of the circuit. It can be used in anticipation of recovery of organ system function or as a bridge to an assist device or transplantation.[129,130]

1. Veno-arterial (VA) ECMO can provide oxygenation and circulatory support in cases of LV and RV failure. Such conditions include refractory cardiogenic shock (postinfarction, postcardiotomy, myocarditis), cardiac arrest, or progressively worsening heart failure. After cardiac surgery, the right atrial and aortic cannulas can be utilized and connected to the ECMO circuit. Otherwise, a venous drainage cannula is placed in the femoral vein with return of oxygenated blood to the femoral, axillary, or carotid artery (see Figure 11.7, page 564). To avoid distal ischemia with femoral arterial cannulation, a cannula placed into a sidearm graft will ensure distal perfusion of the leg. Alternatively, a small distal cannula (such as a 6 or 7 Fr Pinnacle sheath) can be directed distal to the cannula, with distal perfusion directed through a stopcock in the arterial line tubing.

2. Veno-venous (VV) ECMO is only useful for patients with advanced respiratory failure, as it does not provide any cardiac support (Figure 5.12). This can be considered in patients with hypoxemic respiratory failure with a PaO_2/FiO_2 <100, hypercapneic respiratory failure with a pH <7.20 and as a potential bridge to lung transplantation. Dual-site cannulation involves drainage from the femoral vein with return of oxygenated blood to either the contralateral femoral vein or the internal jugular vein. A single-stage setup involves placing a dual-lumen single-stage cannula through the internal jugular vein which is positioned in the right atrium. The return port directs oxygenated blood flow toward the tricuspid valve to minimize recirculation. Oxygenation is not as good with VV ECMO as it is with VA ECMO.

3. The ECMO circuit resembles that used for standard CPB with a gas exchange device (oxygenator), centrifugal pump, and heat exchanger. Advanced membrane oxygenators are constructed of a polymethylpentene membrane (e.g. the MAQUET Quadrox and Terumo CAPIOX membrane oxygenators) which can function efficiently for weeks, providing improved gas exchange and reducing blood and blood product transfusion requirements. Cumbersome makeshift systems have been replaced by compact devices, such as the MAQUET Cardiohelp system, that incorporates a Rotaflow centrifugal pump and allows for easy transportability.

4. A modified circuit that can be used for pulmonary support and RV failure is called RVAD ECMO. One example is the Tandem Heart Protek Duo system, which uses a dual lumen cannula and a Tandem Heart pump. Blood is drained through a 29 Fr cannula from the right atrium with return of oxygenated blood through the inner 16 Fr cannula into the pulmonary artery (see Figure 11.6, page 561).

B. **Management concerns during ECMO and prognosis**

1. Satisfactory oxygenation can be achieved using a target SaO_2 >90% for patients on VA ECMO and >75% for VV ECMO. Reduction in FiO_2 and PEEP will reduce barotrauma until pulmonary function recovers. Patients with ARDS often take weeks to recover, but the 30-day survival is 50–70%.

2. Mediastinal bleeding is common when ECMO is used for postcardiotomy support due to an ongoing coagulopathy, the use of heparin to maintain an ACT >180 seconds, and platelet activation and consumption. Although heparin is required to minimize thrombus formation within the circuit and reduce the possibility of a stroke, heparinization is usually withheld immediately after surgery to minimize mediastinal bleeding. This is well tolerated with commonly used systems, such as the CentriMag circulatory support system with magnetically levitated pump heads, even as a coagulopathy is corrected with clotting factors. Once bleeding is under control, heparin in then started. Bivalirudin may be considered when the duration of ECMO is anticipated to be prolonged to reduce the risk of developing HIT.

3. Renal failure requiring dialysis occurs in nearly 50% of patients on ECMO and compromises survival.

4. Cardiac issues
   a. Ventricular thrombus may form if LV output is very poor. Therefore, it is advisable to maintain the patient on inotropic support during ECMO to promote ventricular contraction.

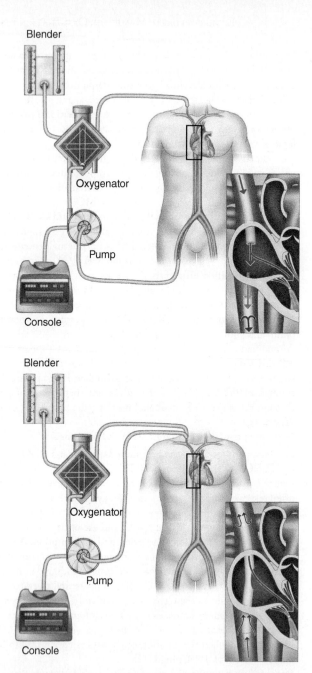

Figure 5.12 • Veno-venous ECMO can be used to provide respiratory support but not cardiac support after cardiac surgery. (A) **Dual site VV ECMO** Blood is withdrawn from the femoral vein, pumped through an oxygenator and reinfused into a central vein to provide oxygenation. (B) **Single site VV ECMO** Bicaval dual lumen cannula withdraws blood, pumps it through an oxygenator and the reinfused blood is directed toward the tricuspid valve to minimize recirculation.

b. In patients with severe LV dysfunction, left-heart distention may occur, causing pulmonary edema and a reduction in subendocardial blood flow, and may reduce the potential for myocardial recovery. Decompression with a transseptal catheter or placement of an Impella device may be helpful.

c. In patients on VA ECMO through femoral arterial and venous cannulation, coronary and cerebral hypoxia may occur, since femoral arterial return of oxygenated blood preferentially perfuses the lower extremities and the splanchnic viscera, while poorly oxygenated blood ejected from the heart perfuses the heart and brain and upper extremities. This so-called Harlequin or North South syndrome can be assessed by monitoring oxygen saturations in the arms and legs as well as the brain. Placement of an additional return cannula in the right atrium neutralizes this problem.

d. Return of pulsatility in the arterial waveform is an early sign of ventricular recovery. Failure to recover within 2–5 days of support is an ominous prognostic sign. However, if organ system function has stabilized, the patient may then be transitioned to an assist device if further support is required. The 30-day survival is 20–30% for patients receiving ECMO after a cardiac arrest and about 35% for patients with cardiogenic shock or failure to wean from bypass.

e. Further comments on the use of ECMO are found on pages 563–565 in Chapter 11.

References

1. Sarkar M, Prabhu BV. Basics of cardiopulmonary bypass. *Indian J Anaesth* 2017;61:760–7.

2. Levy JH, Tanaka KA. Inflammatory response to cardiopulmonary bypass. *Ann Thorac Surg* 2003;75:S715–20.

3. Shann KG, Likosky DS, Murkin JM, et al. An evidence-based review of the practice of cardiopulmonary bypass in adults: a focus on neurologic injury, glycemic control, hemodilution, and the inflammatory response. *J Thorac Cardiovasc Surg* 2006;132:283–90.

4. Kristeller JL, Jankowski A, Reinaker T. Role of corticosteroids during cardiopulmonary bypass. *Hosp Pharm* 2014;49:232–6.

5. de Amorim CG, Malbouisson LMS, da Silva Jr FC, Fiorelli AI, Murakami CKF, Carmona MJC. Leukocyte depletion during CPB: effects on inflammation and lung function. *Inflammation* 2014;37:196–204.

6. Boodhain S, Evans E. Use of leukocyte-depleting filters during cardiac surgery with cardiopulmonary bypass: a review. *J Extra Corpor Technol* 2008;40:27–42.

7. Leal-Noval SR, Amaya R, Herruzo A, et al. Effects of a leukocyte depleting arterial line filter on perioperative morbidity in patients undergoing cardiac surgery: a controlled randomized trial. *Ann Thorac Surg* 2005;80:1394–1400.

8. Ranucci M, Balduini A, Ditta A, Boncilli A, Brozzi S. A systematic review of biocompatible cardiopulmonary bypass circuits and clinical outcome. *Ann Thorac Surg* 2009;87:1311–9.

9. Dickinson T, Mahoney CB, Simmons M, Marison A, Polanski P. Trillium™-coated oxygenators in adult open-heart surgery: a prospective randomized trial. *J Extra Corpor Technol* 2002;34:248–53.

10. Raivio P, Lassila R, Petäjä J. Thrombin in myocardial ischemia-reperfusion during cardiac surgery. *Ann Thorac Surg* 2009;88:318–25.

11. Shore-Lesserson L, Baker RA, Ferraris V, et al. STS/SCA/AmSECT clinical practice guidelines: anticoagulation during cardiopulmonary bypass. *J Extra Corpor Technol* 2018;50:1–14 and *Ann Thorac Surg* 2018;105:650–62.

12. Mirow N, Zittermann A, Koertke H, et al. Heparin-coated extracorporeal circulation in combination with low dose systemic heparinization reduces early postoperative blood loss in cardiac surgery. *J Cardiovasc Surg (Torino)* 2008;49:277–84.

13. Kumano H, Suehiro S, Hattori K, et al. Coagulofibrinolysis during heparin-coated cardiopulmonary bypass with reduced heparinization. *Ann Thorac Surg* 1999;68:1252–6.

14. Kaplan M, Cimen S, Demirtas MM. Effects of different pump prime solutions on postoperative fluid balance and hemostasis. *Chest* 2001;120:172S.

15. Barile L, Fominskiy E, Di Tomasso N, et al. Acute normovolemic hemodilution reduces allogeneic red blood cell transfusion in cardiac surgery: a systematic review and meta-analysis of randomized trials. *Anesth Analg* 2017;124:743–52.

16. Anastasiadis K, Antonitsis P, Haidich AB, Argiriadou H, Deliopoulos A, Papakonstantinou C. Use of minimal extracorporeal circulation improves outcome after heart surgery: a systematic review and meta-analysis of randomized controlled trials. *Int J Cardiol* 2013;164:158–69.

17. Nollert G, Schwabenland I, Maktav D, et al. Miniaturized cardiopulmonary bypass in coronary artery bypass surgery: marginal impact on inflammation and coagulation but loss of safety margins. *Ann Thorac Surg* 2005;80:2326–32.

18. Filho EB, Marson FA, de Costa LN, Antunes N. Vacuum-assisted drainage in cardiopulmonary bypass: advantages and disadvantages. *Rev Bras Cir Cardiovasc* 2014;29:266–71.

19. Wang S, Undar A. Vacuum-assisted venous drainage and gaseous microemboli in cardiopulmonary bypass. *J Extra Corpor Technol* 2008;40:249–56.

20. Baufreton C, Intrator L, Jansen PGM, et al. Inflammatory response to cardiopulmonary bypass using roller or centrifugal pumps. *Ann Thorac Surg* 1999;67:972–7.

21. Scott DA, Silbert BS, Blyth C, O'Brien J, Santamaria J. Blood loss in elective coronary artery surgery: a comparison of centrifugal versus roller pump heads during cardiopulmonary bypass. *J Cardiothorac Vasc Anesth* 2001;15:322–5.

22. Westerberg M, Gäbel J, Bengtsson A, Sellgren J, Eidem O, Jeppsson A. Hemodynamic effects of cardiotomy suction blood. *J Thorac Cardiovasc Surg* 2006;131:1352–7.

23. Westerberg M, Bengstsson A, Jeppsson A. Coronary surgery without cardiotomy suction and autotransfusion reduces the postoperative systemic inflammatory response. *Ann Thorac Surg* 2004;78:54–9.

24. De Somer F, Van Belleghem Y, Caes F, et al. Tissue factor as the main activator of the coagulation system during cardiopulmonary bypass. *J Thorac Cardiovasc Surg* 2002;123:951–8.

25. Aldea GS, Soltow LO, Chandler WL, et al. Limitation of thrombin generation, platelet activation, and inflammation by elimination of cardiotomy suction in patients undergoing coronary artery bypass grafting treated with heparin-coated circuits. *J Thorac Cardiovasc Surg* 2002;123:742–55.

26. Côté CL, Yip AM, MacLeod JB, et al. Efficacy of intraoperative cell salvage in decreasing perioperative blood transfusion rates in first-time cardiac surgery patients: a retrospective study. *Can J Surg* 2016;59:330–6.

27. Vanden Eynden F, Carrier M, Ouellet S, et al. Avecor Trillium oxygenator versus noncoated Monolyth oxygenator: a prospective randomized controlled study. *J Card Surg* 2008;23:288–93.

28. Boodhwani M, Hamilton A, de Varennes B, et al. A multicenter randomized controlled trial to assess the feasibility of testing modified ultrafiltration as a blood conservation technology in cardiac surgery. *J Thorac Cardiovasc Surg* 2010;139:701–6.

29. Finley A, Greenberg C. Review article: heparin sensitivity and resistance: management during cardiopulmonary bypass. *Anesth Analg* 2013;116:1210–22.

30. Avidan MS, Levy JH, van Aken H, et al. Recombinant human antithrombin III restores heparin responsiveness and decreases activation of coagulation in heparin-resistant patients during cardiopulmonary bypass. *J Thorac Cardiovasc Surg* 2005;130:107–13.

31. Beattie GW, Jeffrey RR. Is there evidence that fresh frozen plasma is superior to antithrombin administration to treat heparin resistance in cardiac surgery? *Interact Cardiovasc Thorac Surg* 2014;18:117–20.

32. McNair E, Marcoux JA, Bally C, Gamble J, Thomson D. Bivalirudin as an adjunctive anticoagulant to heparin in the treatment of heparin resistance during cardiopulmonary-bypass assisted cardiac surgery. *Perfusion* 2016;31:189–99.

33. Koster A, Fischer T, Praus M, et al. Hemostatic activation and inflammatory response during cardiopulmonary bypass: impact of heparin management. *Anesthesiology* 2002;97:837–41.

34. Palatianos G, Michalis A, Alivizatos P, et al. Perioperative use of iloprost in cardiac surgery patients diagnosed with heparin-induced thrombocytopenia-reactive antibodies or with true HIT (HIT-reactive antibodies plus thrombocytopenia): an 11-year experience. *Am J Hematol* 2015;90:608–17.

35. Koster A, Dyke CM, Aldea G, et al. Bivalirudin during cardiopulmonary bypass in patients with previous or acute heparin-induced thrombocytopenia and heparin antibodies: results of the CHOOSE-ON trial. *Ann Thorac Surg* 2007;83:572–7.

36. Falana O, Patel G. Efficacy and safety of tranexamic acid versus ε-aminocaproic acid in cardiovascular surgery. *Ann Pharmacother* 2014;48:1563–9.

37. Pustavoitau A, Faraday N. Pro: antifibrinolytics should be used in routine cardiac cases using cardiopulmonary bypass (unless contraindicated). *J Cardiothorac Vasc Anesth* 2016;30:245–7.

38. Dentz ME, Slaughter TF, Mark JB. Early thrombus formation on heparin-bonded pulmonary artery catheters in patients receiving epsilon aminocaproic acid. *Anesthesiology* 1995;82:583–6.

39. Grooters RK, Ver Steeg DA, Stewart MJ, Thieman KC, Schneider RF. Echocardiographic comparison of the standard end-hole cannula, the soft-flow cannula, and the dispersion cannula during perfusion into the aortic arch. *Ann Thorac Surg* 2003;75:1919–23.

40. Ikram A, Mohiuddin H, Zia A, et al. Does epiaortic ultrasound screening reduce perioperative stroke in patients undergoing coronary surgery? A topical review. *J Clin Neurosci* 2018;50:30–4.

41. Gold JP, Torres KE, Maldarelli W, Zhuravlev I, Condit D, Wasnick J. Improving outcomes in coronary surgery: the impact of echo-directed aortic cannulation and perioperative hemodynamic management in 500 patients. *Ann Thorac Surg* 2004;78:1579–85.

42. Suvarna S, Smith A, Kolvecar SJ, Walesby R, Harrison M, Newman S. An intraoperative assessment of the ascending aorta: a comparison of digital palpation, transesophageal echocardiography, and epiaortic ultrasonography. *J Cardiothorac Vasc Anesth* 2007;21:805–9.

43. Sobielski MA 2nd, Pappas PS, Tatooles AJ, Slaughter MS. Embol-X intra-aortic filtration system: capturing particulate emboli in the cardiac surgery patient. *J Extra Corpor Technol* 2005;37:222–6.

44. Mack MJ, Acker MA, Gelijns AC, et al. Effect of cerebral embolic protection devices on CNS infarction in surgical aortic valve replacement: a randomized clinical trial. *JAMA* 2017;318:536–47.

45. Gerriets T, Schwarz N, Sammer G, et al. Protecting the brain from gaseous and solid micro-emboli during coronary artery bypass grafting: a randomized controlled trial. *Eur Heart J* 2010;31:360–8.

46. Crooke GA, Schwartz CF, Ribakove GH, et al. Retrograde arterial perfusion, not incision location, significantly increases the risk of stroke in reoperative mitral valve procedures. *Ann Thorac Surg* 2010;89:723–9.

47. Ramchandani M, Jabbari OA, Saleh WKA, Ramlawi B. Cannulation strategies and pitfalls in minimally invasive cardiac surgery. *Methodist DeBakey Cardiovasc J* 2016;12:10–3.

48. Lamelas J, Williams RF, Mawad M, LaPietra A. Complications associated with femoral cannulation during minimally invasive cardiac surgery. *Ann Thorac Surg* 2017;103:1927–32.

49. James T, Friedman SG, Scher L, Hall M. Lower extremity compartment syndrome after coronary artery bypass. *J Vasc Surg* 2002;36:1069–70.

50. Rudersdorf PD, Wheaton MD, Abolhoda A. Lower limb compartment syndrome after femoral artery cannulation for cardiopulmonary bypass. *Am Surg* 2013;79:E175–6.

51. Sinclair MC, Singer RL, Manley NJ, Montesano RM. Cannulation of the axillary artery for cardiopulmonary bypass: safeguards and pitfalls. *Ann Thorac Surg* 2003;75:931–4.

52. Etz CD, Plestis KA, Kari FA, et al. Axillary cannulation significantly improves survival and neurologic outcome after atherosclerotic aneurysm repair of the aortic root and ascending aorta. *Ann Thorac Surg* 2008;86:441–7.

53. Ogino H, Sasaki H, Minatoya K, et al. Evolving arch surgery using integrated antegrade selective cerebral perfusion: impact of axillary artery perfusion. *J Thorac Cardiovasc Surg* 2008;136:641–8.

54. Malvindi PG, Scrascia G, Vitale N. Is unilateral antegrade cerebral perfusion equivalent to bilateral cerebral perfusion for patients undergoing aortic arch surgery? *Interact Cardiovasc Thorac Surg* 2008;7:891–7.

55. Lamelas J. Minimal access tricuspid valve surgery. *Ann Cardiothorac Surg* 2017;6:283–6.

56. Langenberg CJ, Pietersen HG, Geskes G, Wagenmakers AJM, Soeters PB, Durieux M. Coronary sinus catheter placement: assessment of placement criteria and cardiac complications. *Chest* 2003;124:1259–65.

57. Rosengart TK, Krieger KH. Retrograde autologous priming for cardiopulmonary bypass: a safe and effective means of decreasing hemodilution and transfusion requirements. *J Thorac Cardiovasc Surg* 1998;115:426–39.

58. Cheng M, Li JQ, Wu TC, Tian WC. Short-term effects and safety analysis of retrograde autologous priming for cardiopulmonary bypass in patients with cardiac valve replacement surgery. *Cell Biochem Biophys* 2015;73:441–6.

59. Trapp C, Schiller W, Mellert F, et al. Retrograde autologous priming as a safe and easy method to reduce hemodilution and transfusion requirements during cardiac surgery. *Thorac Cardiovasc Surg* 2015;63:628–34.

60. Nanjappa A, Gill J, Sadat U, Colah S, Abu-Omar Y, Nair S. The effect of retrograde autologous priming on intraoperative blood product transfusion in coronary artery bypass grafting. *Perfusion* 2013;28:530–5.

61. Sun P, Ji B, Sun Y, et al. Effects of retrograde autologous priming on blood transfusion and clinical outcomes in adults: a meta-analysis. *Perfusion* 2013;28:238–43.

62. DiNardo JA, Wegner JA. Pro: low-flow cardiopulmonary bypass is the preferred technique for patients undergoing cardiac surgical procedures. *J Cardiothorac Vasc Anesth* 2001;15:649–51.

63. De Somer F. What is optimal flow and how to validate this. *J Extra Corpor Technol* 2007;39:278–80.

64. Boston US, Slater JM, Orszulak TA, Cook DJ. Hierarchy of regional oxygen delivery during cardiopulmonary bypass. *Ann Thorac Surg* 2001;71:260–4.

65. Schmid FX, Philipp A, Foltan M, Jueckstock H, Wiesenack C, Birnbaum, D. Adequacy of perfusion during hypothermia: regional distribution of cardiopulmonary bypass flow, mixed venous and regional venous oxygen saturation: hypothermia and distribution of flow and oxygen. *Thorac Cardiovasc Surg* 2003;51:306–11.

66. Lannemyr L, Bragadottir G, Krumbholz V, Redfors B, Sellgren J, Ricksten SE. Effects of cardiopulmonary bypass on renal perfusion, filtration and oxygenation in patients undergoing cardiac surgery. *Anesthesiology* 2017;126:205–13.

67. Lanneemyr L, Bragadottir G, Hjärpe A, Redfors B, Ricksten SE. Impact of cardiopulmonary bypass flow on renal oxygenation in patients undergoing cardiac surgery. *Ann Thorac Surg* 2019;107:506–11.

68. Andersson LG, Bratteby LE, Ekroth R, et al. Renal function during cardiopulmonary bypass: influence of pump flow and systemic blood pressure. *Eur J Cardiothorac Surg* 1994;8:597–602.

69. Sirvinskas E, Andrejaitiene J, Raliene L, et al. Cardiopulmonary bypass management and acute renal failure: risk factors and prognosis. *Perfusion* 2008;23:323–7.

70. Ghatanatti R, Teli A, Narayan P, et al. Ideal hematocrit to minimize renal injury on cardiopulmonary bypass. *Innovations (Phila)* 2015;10:420–4.

71. Karkouti K, Beattie WS, Wijeysundera DN, et al. Hemodilution during cardiopulmonary bypass is an independent risk factor for acute renal failure in adult cardiac surgery. *J Thorac Cardiovasc Surg* 2005;129:391–400.

72. Habib RH, Zacharias A, Schwann TA, Riordan DJ, Durham SJ, Shah A. Adverse effects of low hematocrit during cardiopulmonary bypass in the adult: should current practice be changed? *J Thorac Cardiovasc Surg* 2003;125:1438–50.

73. Ranucci M, Romitti F, Isgrò G, et al. Oxygen delivery during cardiopulmonary bypass and acute renal failure after coronary operations. *Ann Thorac Surg* 2005;80:2213–20.

74. Croughwell N, Lyth M, Quill TJ, et al. Diabetic patients have abnormal cerebral autoregulation during cardiopulmonary bypass. *Circulation* 1990;82(5 Suppl):IV-407–12.

75. Schwartz AE, Sandhu AA, Kaplon RJ, et al. Cerebral blood flow is determined by arterial pressure and not cardiopulmonary bypass flow rate. *Ann Thorac Surg* 1995;60:165–70.

76. Tobias JD. Cerebral oximetry monitoring with near infrared spectroscopy detects alterations in oxygenation before pulse oximetry. *J Intensive Care Med* 2008;23:384–8.

77. Slater JP, Guarino T, Stack J, et al. Cerebral oxygen desaturation predicts cognitive decline and longer hospital stay after cardiac surgery. *Ann Thorac Surg* 2009;87:36–45.

78. Zheng F, Sheinberg R, Yee MS, Ono M, Zheng Y, Hogue CW. Cerebral near-infrared spectroscopy monitoring and neurologic outcomes in adult cardiac surgery patients: a systematic review. *Anesth Analg* 2013;116:664–76.

79. Kalyani SD, Miller NR, Dong LM, Baumgartner WA, Alejo DE, Gilbert TB. Incidence of and risk factors for perioperative optic neuropathy after cardiac surgery. *Ann Thorac Surg* 2004;78:34–7.

80. Ranucci M, Conti D, Castelvecchio S, et al. Hematocrit on cardiopulmonary bypass and outcome after coronary surgery in nontransfused patients. *Ann Thorac Surg* 2010;89:11–18.

81. Society of Thoracic Surgeons Blood Conservation Guideline Task Force, Ferraris VA, Brown JR, Desposits GJ, et al. 2011 update to the Society of Thoracic Surgeons and the Society of Cardiovascular Anesthesiologists blood conservation clinical practice guidelines. *Ann Thorac Surg* 2011;91:944–82.

82. Engelman RM, Pleet AB, Rousou JA, et al. Influence of cardiopulmonary bypass perfusion temperature on neurologic and hematologic function after coronary artery bypass grafting. *Ann Thorac Surg* 1999;67:1547–56.

83. Grigore AM, Grocott HP, Mathew JP, et al. The rewarming rate and increased peak temperature alter neurocognitive outcome after cardiac surgery. *Anesth Analg* 2002;94:4–10.

84. Engelman R, Baker RA, Likosky DS, et al. The Society of Thoracic Surgeons, the Society of Cardiovascular Anesthesiologists, and the American Society of ExtraCorporeal Technology: clinical practice guidelines for cardiopulmonary bypass: temperature management during cardiopulmonary bypass. *Ann Thorac Surg* 2015;100:748–57.

85. Gabriel EA, Fagionato Locali R, Katsumi Matsuoka P, et al. Lung perfusion during cardiac surgery with cardiopulmonary bypass: is it necessary? *Interact Cardiovasc Thorac Surg* 2008;7:1089–95.

86. Wang YC, Huang CH, Tu YK. Effects of positive airway pressure and mechanical ventilation of the lungs during cardiopulmonary bypass on pulmonary adverse events after cardiac surgery: a systematic review and meta-analysis. *J Cardiothorac Vasc Anesth* 2018;748–59.

87. Demers P, Elkouri S, Martineau R, Couturier A, Cartier R. Outcome with high blood lactate levels during cardiopulmonary bypass in adult cardiac operation. *Ann Thorac Surg* 2000;70:2082–6.

88. Ranucci M, De Toffol B, Isgrò G, Romitti F, Conti D, Vicentini M. Hyperlactatemia during cardiopulmonary bypass: determinants and impact on postoperative outcome. *Crit Care* 2006;10:R167.

89. Duebner LF, Hagino I, Sakamoto T, et al. Effects of pH management during deep hypothermic bypass on cerebral microcirculation: alpha-stat versus pH-stat. *Circulation* 2002;106:1103–8.

90. Patel RL, Turtle MR, Chambers DJ, James DN, Newman S, Venn GE. Alpha-stat acid–base regulation during cardiopulmonary bypass improves neuropsychological outcome in patients undergoing coronary artery bypass grafting. *J Thorac Cardiovasc Surg* 1996;111:1267–79.

91. Dahlbacka S, Alaoja H, Mäkelä J, et al. Effects of pH management during selective antegrade cerebral perfusion on cerebral microcirculation and metabolism: alpha-stat versus pH-stat. *Ann Thorac Surg* 2007;84:847–56.

92. Lazar HL, McDonnell M, Chipkin SR, et al. The Society of Thoracic Surgeons practice guideline series: blood glucose management during adult cardiac surgery. *Ann Thorac Surg* 2009;87:663–9.

93. Gandhi GY, Nuttall GA, Abel MD, et al. Intensive intraoperative insulin therapy versus conventional glucose management during cardiac surgery: a randomized trial. *Ann Intern Med* 2007;146:233–43.

94. Doenst T, Wijeysundera D, Karkouti K, et al. Hyperglycemia during cardiopulmonary bypass is an independent risk factor for mortality in patients undergoing cardiac surgery. *J Thorac Cardiovasc Surg* 2005;130:1144–50.

95. Deppe AC, Weber C, Zimmermann J, et al. Point-of-care thromboelastography/thromboelastometry-based coagulation management in cardiac surgery: a meta-analysis of 8332 patients. *J Surg Res* 2016;203:424–33.

96. Ranucci M, Ingrò G, Cazzaniga A, Soro G, Menicanti L, Frigiola A. Predictors for heparin resistance in patients undergoing coronary artery bypass grafting. *Perfusion* 1999;14:437–42.

97. Shaefi S, Mittel A, Klick J, et al. Vasoplegia after cardiovascular procedures: pathophysiology and targeted therapy. *J Cardiothorac Vasc Anesth* 2018;32:1013–22.

98. Tsiouris A, Wilson L, Haddadin AS, Yun JJ, Mangi AA. Risk assessment and outcomes of vasoplegia after cardiac surgery. *Gen Thorac Cardiovasc Surg* 2017;65:557–65.

99. Liu H, Yu L, Yang L, Green MS. Vasoplegic syndrome: an update on perioperative considerations. *J Clin Anesth* 2017;40:63–71.

100. Hajjar LA, Vincent JL, Barbposa Gomes Galas FR, et al. Vasopressin versus norepinephrine in patients with vasoplegic shock after cardiac surgery: the VANCS randomized controlled trial. *Anesthesiology* 2017;126:85–93.

101. Leyh RG, Kofidis T, Struber M, et al. Methylene blue: the drug of choice for catecholamine-refractory vasoplegia after cardiopulmonary bypass? *J Thorac Cardiovasc Surg* 2003;125:1426–31.

102. Shanmugam G. Vasoplegic syndrome: the role of methylene blue. *Eur J Cardiothorac Surg* 2005;28:705–10.

103. Shah PR, Reynolds PS, Pal N, Tang D, McCarthy H, Spiess BD. Hydroxocobalamin for the treatment of cardiac surgery-associated vasoplegia: a case series. *Can J Anaesth* 2018;65:560–8.

104. Economopoulos GC, Michalis A, Palatianos GM, Sarris GE. Management of catheter-related injuries to the coronary sinus. *Ann Thorac Surg* 2003;76:112–6.

105. Webb WR, Harrison LH Jr, Helmcke FR, et al. Carbon dioxide field flooding minimizes residual intracardiac air after open heart operations. *Ann Thorac Surg* 1997;64:1489–91.

106. Mills NL, Ochsner JL. Massive air embolism during cardiopulmonary bypass. *J Thorac Cardiovasc Surg* 1980;80:708–17.

107. Barbara DW, Mauermann WJ, Neal JR, Abel MD, Schaff HV, Winters JL. Cold agglutinins in patients undergoing cardiac surgery requiring cardiopulmonary bypass. *J Thorac Cardiovasc Surg* 2013;146:668–80.

108. Atkinson VP, Soeding P, Horne G, Tatoulis J. Cold agglutinins in cardiac surgery: management of myocardial protection and cardiopulmonary bypass. *Ann Thorac Surg* 2008;85:310–1.

109. Patel PA, Ghadimi K, Coetzee E, et al. Incidental cold agglutinins in cardiac surgery: intraoperative surprises and team-based problem-solving strategies during cardiopulmonary bypass. *J Cardiothorac Vasc Anesth* 2017;31:1109–18.

110. Kypson AP, Warner JJ, Telen MJ, Milano CA. Paroxysmal cold hemoglobinuria and cardiopulmonary bypass. *Ann Thorac Surg* 2003;75:579–81.

111. Svensson LG, Crawford ES, Hess KR, et al. Deep hypothermia with circulatory arrest: determinants of stroke and early mortality in 656 patients. *J Thorac Cardiovasc Surg* 1993;106:19–28.

112. Tobias JD, Russo P, Russo J. Changes in near infrared spectroscopy during deep hypothermic circulatory arrest. *Ann Card Anaesth* 2009;12:17.

113. Spielvogel D, Tang GHL. Selective cerebral perfusion for cerebral protection: what we do know. *Ann Cardiothorac Surg* 2013;2:326–30.

114. Keeling WB, Leshnower BG, Hunting JC, Binongo J, Chen EP. Hypothermia and selective antegrade cerebral perfusion is safe for arch repair in type A dissection. *Ann Thorac Surg* 2017;104:767–72.

115. Misfeld M, Mohr RW, Etz CD. Best strategy for cerebral protection in arch surgery: antegrade selective cerebral perfusion and adequate hypothermia. *Ann Cardiothorac Surg* 2013;2:331–8.

116. Spielvogel D, Kai M, Tang GHL, Malekan R, Lansman SL. Selective cerebral perfusion: a review of the evidence. *J Thorac Cardiovasc Surg* 2013;145:(suppl):S59–62.

117. Malvindi PG, Scrascia G, Vitale N. Is unilateral antegrade cerebral perfusion equivalent to bilateral cerebral perfusion for patients undergoing aortic arch surgery? *Interact Cardiovasc Thorac Surg* 2008;7:891–7.

118. Halstead JC, Meier M, Wurm M, et al. Optimizing selective cerebral perfusion: deleterious effects of high perfusion pressures. *J Thorac Cardiovasc Surg* 2008;135:784–91.

119. Spielvogel D, Etz CD, Silovitz D, Lansman SL, Griepp RB. Aortic arch replacement with a trifurcated graft. *Ann Thorac Surg* 2007;83:S791–5.

120. Tian DH, Weller J, Hasmat S, et al. Adjunct retrograde cerebral perfusion provides superior outcomes compared with hypothermic circulatory arrest alone: a meta-analysis. *J Thorac Cardiovasc Surg* 2018;156:1339–48.

121. Chiu P, Goldstone AB, Schaffer JM, et al. Endovascular versus open repair of intact descending thoracic aortic aneurysms. *J Am Coll Cardiol* 2019;73:643–5.

122. Coselli JS, LeMaire SA. Left heart bypass reduces paraplegia rates after thoracoabdominal aortic aneurysm repair. *Ann Thorac Surg* 1999;67:484–90.

123. Szwerc MF, Benckhart DH, Lin JC, et al. Recent clinical experience with left heart bypass using a centrifugal pump for repair of traumatic aortic transection. *Ann Surg* 1999;230:484–90.

124. Karmy-Jones R, Carter Y, Meissner M, Mulligan MS. Choice of venous cannulation for bypass during repair of traumatic rupture of the aorta. *Ann Thorac Surg* 2001;71:39–41.

125.. Leach WR, Sundt TM 3rd, Moon MP. Oxygenator support for partial left-heart bypass. *Ann Thorac Surg* 2001;72:1770–1.

126. Mathison M, Buffolo E, Jatene AD, et al. Right heart circulatory support facilitates coronary artery bypass without cardiopulmonary bypass. *Ann Thorac Surg* 2000;70:1083–5.

127. Bergsland J, Lingaas PS, Skulstad H, et al. Intracoronary shunt prevents ischemia in off-pump coronary artery bypass surgery. *Ann Thorac Surg* 2009;87:54–60.

128. Vassiliades TA Jr, Nielsen JL, Lonquist JL. Coronary perfusion methods during off-pump coronary artery bypass: results of a randomized clinical trial. *Ann Thorac Surg* 2002;74:S1383–9.

129. Makdisi G, Wang IW. Extra corporeal membrane oxygenation (ECMO) review of a lifesaving technology. *J Thorac Disease* 2015;7:E166–76.

130. Squiers JJ, Lima B, DiMaio JM. Contemporary extracorporeal membrane oxygenation therapy in adults: fundamental principles and systematic review of the evidence. *J Thorac Cardiovasc Surg* 2016;152:20–32.

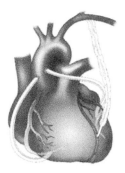

CHAPTER 6

Myocardial Protection

6 Myocardial Protection

Optimizing clinical outcomes in cardiac surgery depends upon the performance of a technically proficient operation without incurring myocardial damage during the procedure. Adherence to this principle is imperative, whether a minimally invasive, robotic, off-pump, or conventional surgical approach through a median sternotomy is performed. With the widespread application of percutaneous coronary interventions, patients requiring surgical revascularization tend to have severe coronary disease and more impaired ventricular function, requiring optimal myocardial preservation. The same holds true for patients undergoing surgery for complex valve problems that may not be amenable to percutaneous approaches. In most of these cases, the surgeon must conscientiously apply the well-developed principles of cardioplegic arrest to minimize ischemia/reperfusion injury, which contributes to postischemic myocardial dysfunction. Excellent myocardial protection is essential to optimize the short- and long-term results of surgery. In some situations, modifications of traditional approaches to myocardial protection with cardioplegia may prove beneficial.

I. Techniques to Minimize Myocardial Injury During Cardiac Surgical Procedures (Table 6.1)

A. **The problem of ischemic arrest.** Aortic cross-clamping interrupts the coronary circulation and will result in conversion to anaerobic metabolism with lactate accumulation, myocardial acidosis, depletion of myocardial energy stores, and cellular swelling. There is an accelerated accumulation of intracellular calcium during ischemia as the ATP-dependent active transport mechanism to extract sodium and calcium is impaired. Upon reperfusion, the high intracellular calcium levels cause severe myocardial dysfunction. Thus, without a reduction in myocardial metabolism, either by hypothermia or chemical cardiac arrest, aortic occlusion producing ischemic arrest for more than 15–20 minutes results in severe myocardial dysfunction.

B. **Cardioplegic arrest** with aortic cross-clamping is used during most types of cardiac surgery to allow the surgeon to operate upon an arrested heart with a relatively bloodless field. This produces diastolic arrest, preserves energy stores, and minimizes calcium entry into myocardial cells. With appropriate replenishment, this allows the surgeon to arrest the heart for several hours without experiencing ischemic myocardial damage.[1-3]

C. **Off-pump coronary artery bypass surgery (OPCAB)** is performed without cardiopulmonary bypass (CPB) and thus on a beating heart. The need to provide myocardial protection is limited, because only the region subtended by the artery which is transiently occluded while being bypassed should be in ischemic jeopardy. Careful positioning of the heart for anastomoses to the inferior and lateral walls is essential to

Manual of Perioperative Care in Adult Cardiac Surgery, Sixth Edition. Robert M. Bojar.
© 2021 John Wiley & Sons Ltd. Published 2021 by John Wiley & Sons Ltd.

Table 6.1 • Options for Myocardial Protection

1. Off-pump surgery
   a. Intraluminal shunting
   b. Aortocoronary shunting
   c. Perfusion-assisted shunting
   d. Ischemic preconditioning
2. On-pump surgery
   a. Cardioplegic arrest (antegrade/retrograde)
   b. On-pump beating heart
   c. Hypothermic fibrillatory arrest
   d. Intermittent ischemic arrest
   e. Redo AVR with patent ITA – cold retrograde blood or blood cardioplegia

AVR, aortic valve replacement; ITA, internal thoracic artery

minimize systemic hypotension, which can also induce ischemia. If ischemia develops during vessel occlusion, as evidenced by ECG changes or ventricular dysfunction, intracoronary shunting or aortocoronary shunting can be used to provide distal flow until the anastomosis is completed.[4,5] Additional support using miniaturized CPB systems or right ventricular (RV) assist can be used in high-risk off-pump cases.[6–8] Despite fairly comparable morbidity and mortality to standard on-pump/cardioplegic arrest techniques, off-pump surgery may have some advantages in patients with severe left ventricular (LV) dysfunction.[9]

D. **On-pump beating-heart surgery** for coronary bypass grafting can be performed without aortic cross-clamping, using stabilizing OPCAB platforms to allow for the construction of distal anastomoses on a beating heart while the pump provides systemic flow. Despite the lower oxygen demand of the empty beating heart, ischemia in the distribution of severely diseased nonbypassed arteries is often noted due to the lower perfusion pressures on pump. Although ischemia should be better tolerated than during a standard OPCAB, shunting techniques can still be used to optimize protection. Applications of this technique include:

1. When safe aortic clamping cannot be performed (usually with a calcified or severely atherosclerotic aorta), when off-pump surgery is not technically feasible, or when the risk of arresting the heart is considered very high due to a recent myocardial infarction, ongoing ischemia, marked LV hypertrophy, or severe ventricular dysfunction.[10] In these high-risk cases, studies have shown equivalent if not better results with this technique than with OPCABs and conventional CABGs.[11–13]

2. Intracardiac operations, such as resection of a LV aneurysm or surgical ventricular restoration, allowing the surgeon to palpate the border zone between viable muscle and scar tissue better than if the heart were arrested.

3. Minimally invasive mitral valve surgery when access to the aorta for clamping may be difficult (although a balloon "endoclamp" can be used). This is tolerated as long

as there is no aortic valve regurgitation, either at baseline or with retraction of the left atrial wall during valve exposure.[14–18] The latter problem can be avoided using a transseptal approach.

4. Reoperative aortic valve surgery with a patent internal thoracic artery (ITA) graft that cannot be dissected free and controlled during cardioplegic arrest. Use of continuous retrograde cold blood or blood cardioplegia with at least moderate systemic hypothermia can be used for myocardial protection.[19–21] Performing reoperative aortic valve surgery using normothermic noncardioplegic retrograde blood perfusion has been used successfully as well.[14,15]

E. **Hypothermic fibrillatory arrest** is a variant of the "empty beating heart" approach. It can be used for coronary surgery, with the aorta remaining unclamped and the distal anastomoses performed on a cold vented fibrillating heart with high perfusion pressures. Stabilizing platforms can be used if necessary to optimize exposure. This technique provides less than ideal protection, especially in the hypertrophied heart. Although it confirmed the concept that coronary surgery could be performed safely without aortic cross-clamping, this technique is rarely used anymore.[22]

F. **Intermittent ischemic arrest** involves multiple short periods of cross-clamping during mild systemic hypothermia to perform each distal anastomosis. Conceptually, this is a violation of the principle of preserving the heart by inducing diastolic arrest during the period of aortic cross-clamping. However, the heart is able to tolerate these brief periods of ischemia without adverse sequelae.[23,24]

G. **Ischemic preconditioning** refers to a phenomenon in which a transient reduction in blood flow to myocardial tissue enables it to tolerate a subsequent longer period of ischemia. The ideal application of this concept is in off-pump surgery, because, in the absence of collateral flow, there is obligatory transient ischemia with occlusion of a target vessel that might be lessened by ischemic preconditioning. Although some studies suggest that this technique reduces troponin leakage, myocardial dysfunction, and arrhythmias compared with surgery using cardioplegic arrest, others have not.[25–28]

H. **Ischemic postconditioning** involves the administration of medications at the time of initial reperfusion when the aortic cross-clamp is removed to modify ischemia/reperfusion damage. Use of adenosine 1.5 mg/kg has been shown to reduce troponin leakage.[29]

II. Principles of Cardioplegia[1–3] (Table 6.2)

A. Prompt **diastolic arrest** of the heart is achieved using a delivery solution containing about 20–25 mEq/L of potassium chloride (KCl). The potassium may be added to a crystalloid solution which is administered undiluted ("crystalloid cardioplegia"), or it may be concentrated in a smaller bag of crystalloid solution and administered in a mixture with blood in varying ratios (most commonly 4:1 or 8:1 blood:cardioplegia solution) ("blood cardioplegia"). Systems are available that add the potassium directly to blood to minimize hemodilution (so-called miniplegia or microplegia). In these systems, the lack of hemodilution provides superior oxygen-carrying capacity to diluted blood cardioplegia along with natural osmotic properties. They have been shown to reduce postoperative myocardial edema, increase buffering, and permit more rapid recovery of LV function compared with 8:1 blood cardioplegia.[30–32]

Table 6.2 • Principles and Composition of Modified Buckberg Cardioplegia

Principle	Composition
1. Prompt diastolic arrest	KCl 20–25 mEq/L
2. Buffering	THAM, bicarbonate
3. Reduction of calcium levels	Citrate-phosphate-dextrose (CPD) or double-dextrose (CP2D)
4. Adequate delivery	Antegrade ± retrograde administration
5. Temperature	Cold vs. tepid vs. warm
6. Substrate additives to optimize myocardial metabolism or prevent cell damage	Aspartate–glutamate Na^+/H^+ exchange inhibitors Insulin Magnesium L-arginine Calcium-channel blockers

THAM, tromethamine; CPD, citrate-phosphate-dextrose; CP2D, double-dextrose

1. **Crystalloid cardioplegia (CCP)** provides little substrate and no oxygen to the heart during the period of ischemic arrest. It functions primarily by arresting the heart at cold temperatures. It can be oxygenated by bubbling oxygen through the solution, but this is not a common practice.

   a. **St. Thomas** and **Plegisol** are extracellular solutions with high potassium levels that produce arrest by depolarization. They require replenishment every 20 minutes or so to optimize protection. St. Thomas solution also contains procaine, and high doses can trigger postoperative seizures. A comparison of these two solutions showed less ventricular fibrillation after unclamping with use of St. Thomas solution.[33]

   b. **Bretschneider solution (Custodiol)** is an intracellular hyperpolarizing solution with low sodium and potassium that contains histidine–tryptophan–ketoglutarate.[34] The histidine provides a buffer and is a free-radical scavenger, and this reduces the risk of ischemia-reperfusion injury. This solution can provide myocardial protection for up to 2–3 hours with just one dose.[35–37] Studies comparing cold antegrade blood cardioplegia with Custodiol showed similar or better protection with Custodiol for mitral valve surgery and equivalent results in aortic valve surgery, although better results were noted with blood cardioplegia in patients with reduced ejection fractions.[36–38]

2. **Blood cardioplegia (BCP)** solutions provide oxygen, natural buffering agents, antioxidants, and free-radical scavengers. Standard supplemental additives to these solutions include other buffers to achieve an alkaline pH (THAM), citrate-phosphate-dextrose (CPD) or double-dextrose (CP2D) to lower the level of calcium, and occasionally drugs to maintain slight hyperosmolarity (mannitol).

a. **Buckberg solution** and its modifications contain the ingredients listed above in a variety of different concentrations. It produces potassium-induced cellular depolarization and requires replenishment every 20–30 minutes. The cardioplegia mixture passes through a separate heater/cooler system in the extracorporeal circuit with a 4:1 or 8:1 mixture of blood:cardioplegia stock solution. The infusion rate, temperature, and pressure are controlled by the perfusionist. Various additives can be used to optimize protection in various clinical situations by replenishing ATP stores (see sections II.D and E).

b. **del Nido (DN) cardioplegia** is a hyperkalemic, low calcium solution that contains lidocaine and magnesium (polarizing agents), bicarbonate (to maintain an intracellular pH), and mannitol (a free-radical scavenger that also reduces myocardial edema). Myocardial protection is optimized by low diastolic intracellular calcium levels attributable to lidocaine blockade of Na+ channels and the presence of magnesium. The solution is given in a ratio of 1:4 blood to cardioplegia stock solution.[39,40] Although it has been administered primarily antegrade in most studies, there is no specific reason why it could not be given retrograde as well.

   i. DN cardioplegia was initially developed for congenital heart surgery and has now seen more widespread application in adult cardiac surgery. Earlier studies evaluated its benefits in valvular surgery, with subsequent studies reporting its use in adult congenital cases, complex valve and combined operations, reoperations, and coronary surgery.[41-47] When used with mild hypothermic CPB, it provides equivalent protection in patients with and without LVH and with cross-clamp times of up to about 90 minutes.[48]

   ii. A dose of 20 mL/kg to a maximum of one liter is given antegrade, with half that dose given if the anticipated cross-clamp time will be less than 30 minutes (except a full dose should be given if LVH is present).[39] One dose usually suffices for cross-clamp times less than 90 minutes, and not having to re-administer cardioplegia generally shortens the cross-clamp and bypass times. The heart usually does not fibrillate after unclamping of the aorta.

   iii. If a longer cross-clamp time is anticipated or has occurred, redosing with about 10 mL/kg after 45–90 minutes is suggested.[42,43] However, the heart is often sluggish for a short period of time after unclamping the aorta, especially after redosing or when an additional dose is given close to unclamping.[49,50] Furthermore, very few reports include patients requiring very prolonged cross-clamp times (>2 hours). Thus, it is still not clear when redosing should take place in such patients.

   iv. Clinical results are comparable to those with Buckberg-type solutions and probably better than with St. Thomas solution.[40,41,43-47,51,52]

3. The oxygen demand of the heart is reduced nearly 90% by simply arresting the heart at normothermia, so maintenance of arrest during the cross-clamp period is essential (Figure 6.1). For Buckberg-type solutions, this is accomplished by re-administering the solution every 15–20 minutes to deliver potassium and wash out metabolic byproducts. A low-potassium solution (12–15 mEq/L) is used to maintain the arrest to avoid an excess potassium load. The high-potassium solution should be re-administered if the heart resumes any activity. For DN cardioplegia,

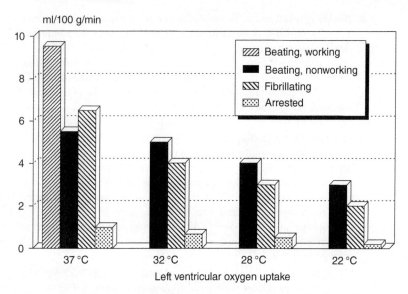

Figure 6.1 • Myocardial oxygen demand (mvO₂). Notice that the most significant decrease in mvO₂ occurs with the induction of the arrested state, and secondarily by the production of hypothermia. (Reproduced with permission from Buckberg et al., *J Thorac Cardiovasc Surg*, 73;87–94. © 1977 Elsevier. Reprinted with permission of Elsevier.)

re-administration may be given empirically every 45–90 minutes or when the heart resumes activity. Cold blood alone can be given retrograde into the coronary sinus as an alternative to subsequent doses of cardioplegia to optimize tissue oxygenation and metabolism while minimizing the potassium load. This is adequate as long as the heart remains arrested. It is especially beneficial in patients with renal dysfunction, who are predisposed to the development of hyperkalemia.

4. Clinical studies generally suggest that both cold and warm BCP provide superior myocardial protection to cold CCP, with less troponin release and better hemodynamic performance post-pump. However, the rate of myocardial infarction and operative mortality has not been shown to differ.[53–57] The advantage of BCP is probably most evident in patients with acute ischemia and more advanced LV dysfunction, especially when given both antegrade and retrograde. However, myocardial protection remains suboptimal even with BCP in hypertrophied hearts.[58]

B. **Temperature.** Before the development of cardioplegia solutions, myocardial protection was provided entirely by systemic and topical hypothermia. It was found that myocardial oxygen consumption did decrease about 50% for every 10 °C decrease in myocardial temperature. It only seemed logical that administering cardioplegia at a cold temperature would be a significant factor in decreasing myocardial metabolism. However, the reduction in myocardial metabolism attributable to hypothermia is actually quite insignificant compared with that achieved by diastolic arrest (Figure 6.1). Nonetheless, systemic hypothermia and topical cold (not iced) saline are routinely used in patients receiving cold cardioplegia, with occasional use of a topical cooling insulation device to surround the LV and protect the phrenic nerve from cold injury.

1. Some surgeons monitor myocardial temperatures with the presumption that adequate hypothermia (<15 °C) of the myocardium is providing satisfactory myocardial protection. However, in clinical practice, only one site is usually selected for monitoring (usually the LV apex or septum), and there is commonly a significant discrepancy between the temperatures of different areas of the LV, and especially between the left and right ventricles. It should be understood that temperature monitoring provides only a relative assessment of the degree of myocardial protection. A more scientific means of doing so can be accomplished using a pH probe. The development of significant acidosis caused by a derangement in myocardial metabolism is indicative of poor protection.[59] Studies have shown little correlation between pH and temperature, suggesting that temperature is actually not a good indicator of the state of myocardial metabolism.[60]

2. Use of intermittent "tepid" BCP (whether at 32 °C or 20 °C) allows the heart to utilize more oxygen and glucose than a colder heart.[61] It may provide better metabolic and functional recovery than cold cardioplegia, with improved long-term results.[62] Optimizing its benefits may require administration through both antegrade and retrograde routes, especially in hypertrophied hearts.[63,64]

3. Since enzymatic and cellular reparative processes function better at normothermia, some surgeons use "warm cardioplegia" for myocardial protection, with excellent results.[56,57,63–68] Compared to cold cardioplegia, there may be a reduction in enzyme release and better ventricular function with comparable clinical events. However, because of the tendency for the heart to resume electrical activity at normothermia, this must be given continuously or with only short periods of interruption to protect the heart. An ischemic time of 15 minutes between repeat administrations is considered safe, and one study showed that supplementing cardioplegia with magnesium could safely extend this time to 25 minutes.[69] When given continuously, it can obscure the operative field. To minimize hemodilution from excessive cardioplegia administration, the "miniplegia" system that simply adds potassium or other substances (magnesium) to the blood is useful. Warm cardioplegia can also be used as an adjunct to cold cardioplegia when given just after aortic cross-clamping (warm induction) or just prior to removing the cross-clamp ("hot shot").

   a. **Warm induction** involves administering approximately 500 mL of warm cardioplegia immediately after aortic cross-clamping. Studies suggest that this may be beneficial in actively ischemic hearts with energy depletion by providing a brief period of time during which oxygen can be used to repair cell damage and replace energy stores.[70]

   b. Terminal warm BCP ("**hot shot**") is commonly given just before removal of the aortic cross-clamp, because it has been shown to improve myocardial metabolism.[71,72] The heart tends to remain asystolic for several minutes after removal of the aortic cross-clamp, during which time it is able to "repair" cellular processes or replenish energy stores while the oxygen demand is low. A combination of warm induction and "hot shot" has been shown to reduce troponin leak in patients undergoing CABG.[73,74] However, a study of patients with LV hypertrophy undergoing AVR did not show any clinical benefit of using "hot shot",[75] and another study comparing standard "hot shot" with a modified reperfusion solution including aspartate and glutamate found no difference in clinical outcome.[76]

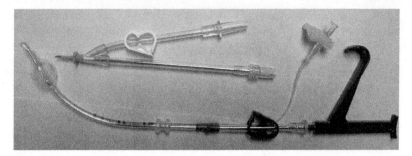

Figure 6.2 • (Top) Antegrade cardioplegia catheter with a side port for venting. (Bottom) A 14 Fr retrograde catheter with self-inflating balloon that allows for measurement of coronary sinus pressures.

C. **Route of delivery.** Cardioplegia is initially administered antegrade into the aortic root, and then may be given retrograde through a catheter placed into the coronary sinus (see Figure 5.9, page 298, and Figure 6.2).

1. The efficacy of **antegrade cardioplegia (ACP)** delivery may be compromised by severe coronary artery stenosis and is often dependent on collateral flow.[77] In addition, in patients with more than mild aortic regurgitation, sufficient root distention may not be achieved, such that ACP delivery will be ineffective. In that situation, the initial dose should be given retrograde, and, if an AVR is being performed, it may be supplemented by an infusion of ACP directly into the coronary ostia once the aortotomy incision has been performed. ACP can be cumbersome and time-consuming to re-administer during aortic valve operations. During mitral valve procedures, left atrial retraction usually distorts the aortic annulus, preventing adequate re-administration of ACP. However, this can be accomplished by readjusting the position of the atrial wall retractor and making sure to eliminate air from the aortic root when ACP is re-administered.

2. **Retrograde cardioplegia (RCP)** is easy to administer, either intermittently or continuously, and does not interrupt the flow of an operation. It is helpful in reducing the risk of atheroembolism from patent yet diseased saphenous vein grafts at reoperation. It generally provides excellent myocardial protection, although protection of the RV and the posterior LV is always of concern.[78-80] Careful monitoring of coronary sinus pressure during the administration of RCP is essential: if it is too high (>50 mm Hg), coronary sinus rupture can occur; if it is too low (<20 mm Hg), there is usually a problem with catheter malposition or coronary sinus rupture.[81] The desired flow rate for warm RCP has been determined to be about 200 mL/min.[82] A variety of catheters, both self-inflating and manual-inflating, have been designed to maintain the catheter within the sinus, prevent retrograde flow of cardioplegia into the right atrium, and allow for pressure monitoring during cardioplegia administration. Transesophageal echocardiography is helpful in locating the position of the coronary sinus catheter, especially in minimally invasive cases or reoperative procedures, during which the surgeon cannot feel the coronary sinus or when the catheter has been placed by the anesthesiologist through the internal jugular vein.

3. Studies that have analyzed the distribution of cardioplegia solutions suggest that the routes of delivery should be complementary, not exclusive. Contrast echo studies have shown that perfusion of the LV is better with warm antegrade delivery than retrograde delivery, and that delivery to the RV is poor with either approach, especially if there is right coronary artery occlusion.[79,83] However, the latter may be improved by constructing the right coronary graft first and infusing cardioplegia down that graft.[79] Use of combined ACP/RCP appears to provide the best protection and can be recommended for all cases.[84–86] Cold RCP is generally given intermittently, although continuous cold RCP may improve ventricular performance with less myocardial ischemia compared with intermittent administration.[87] Tepid or warm cardioplegia should be given as continuously as possible.

4. Administration of simultaneous ACP/RCP usually involves administration down completed vein grafts at the same time as coronary sinus delivery. Despite concerns that this can be disruptive to myocardial cell homeostasis, with increased water accumulation in extracellular and intracellular compartments, this has not been demonstrated to jeopardize myocardial energy metabolism, especially when given for brief periods of time.[88]

D. **Modified reperfusion.** Just prior to removal of the aortic cross-clamp, the administration of a modified cardioplegia solution given under specific conditions has been shown to improve myocardial function.[1–3] Such controlled reperfusion, with or without substrate enhancement, such as aspartate and glutamate, should provide a low potassium load (8–10 mEq/L), CPD or CP2D to limit calcium influx, provide hyperosmolarity, and should be given at a low pressure (<50 mm Hg) over several minutes. Such a regimen is a component of "integrated cardioplegia" but may be beneficial only in high-risk cases.[89] While one study suggested that a substrate-enriched solution given during induction and reperfusion produced a transient improvement in LV function,[72] another found no difference in clinical outcome compared to an unenriched "hot shot".[76] Use of the Buckberg "integrated" cardioplegia approach (antegrade/retrograde with terminal warm substrate-enriched reperfusion) has been shown to improve myocardial protection, especially of the septum.[2,89]

E. **Other cardioplegia additives.** Studies have evaluated the potential myocardial protective benefits of a variety of additives to cardioplegia solutions, with variable results. Krebs cycle intermediates (aspartate and glutamate) appear to have the most benefit in energy-depleted hearts. Studies evaluating use of esmolol and glucose–insulin–potassium given prior to cardioplegic arrest have also shown modest benefit in lowering troponin levels and improving systolic function in high-risk patients.[90,91]

III. Cardioplegia Strategy

Numerous comparative studies have been done to elucidate the best cardioplegia strategy. These have evaluated the distribution of cardioplegia solutions, examined troponin levels and rates of infarction, and assessed hemodynamic performance, the requirement for inotropes, and mortality. There are so many variables that can influence outcomes that it is very difficult to conclude which method of myocardial protection is truly superior in influencing surgical results. In fact, excellent myocardial protection can be obtained with numerous strategies that adhere to the generally accepted principles of cardioplegia delivery.

A. Most studies suggest that, in low-risk cases, multidose cold crystalloid, cold, tepid, or warm BCP, whether given antegrade and/or retrograde, all produce relatively comparable clinical results. In general, protection of the RV is suboptimal with all strategies, especially in patients with right coronary artery disease. A combined ACP/RCP cold, tepid, or warm BCP approach seems to be best for high-risk patients, and can be recommended for all operations. Del Nido cardioplegia appears to provide excellent protection, but the timing of redelivery to optimize protection in cases requiring prolonged periods of cardioplegic arrest has not been clarified.

B. A proposal for BCP strategy (except DN cardioplegia) is as follows:

1. Use warm induction for severely ischemic hearts only.

2. Induce cardioplegic arrest with about one liter of cardioplegia, giving about 750 mL of antegrade infusion (warm, cold, or tepid) initially, followed by 250 mL of RCP. The latter is especially important in patients with severe coronary artery disease. If temperature monitoring is used for cold cardioplegia, it should be maintained at less than 20 °C. The amounts of both ACP and RCP delivered may need to be modified depending on how effective they appear to be, based on the nature of coronary disease, temperature, or pH monitoring.

3. For valve surgery, after the initial antegrade dose, use either continuous warm RCP or intermittent cold retrograde BCP with a low-potassium solution every 20 minutes. If aortic insufficiency is present, administer cardioplegia retrograde, and if there is a large right coronary artery, consider direct antegrade administration into the right coronary ostium.

4. For redo aortic valve surgery in patients with a patent ITA, the ITA pedicle may be left unclamped. Systemic hypothermia to at least 28 °C with use of continuous cold retrograde blood or BCP should provide adequate myocardial protection.

5. For coronary surgery, perform the right coronary graft first and administer low-potassium cardioplegia down that graft simultaneously with RCP for all subsequent administrations. Antegrade delivery, of course, cannot be delivered down pedicled ITA grafts and is best avoided in free grafts (ITA or radial artery) to avoid the potential adverse impact of graft manipulation and hyperkalemia on endothelial function.

   a. Administer cardioplegia down each saphenous vein bypass graft as it is completed along with additional RCP. Concomitant administration down all completed grafts along with RCP might be helpful (Figure 6.3). If it is elected not to use RCP, alternating distal and proximal anastomoses will allow for antegrade delivery down the completed grafts.

   b. The duration of aortic cross-clamping is lengthened when both proximal and distal anastomoses are performed during a single aortic cross-clamp (SAC) period rather than performing the proximal anastomoses with partial aortic clamping (PAC). Although some literature supported the tradeoff of a longer period of cardioplegic arrest for the lower risk of stroke with SAC, other studies have not found any difference in stroke risk comparing SAC with PAC.[92–94] However, the risk is least when the aorta is not clamped at all, using ITA inflow or proximal aortic seal devices, such as the Heartstring device (MAQUET), for the proximal anastomoses.[95]

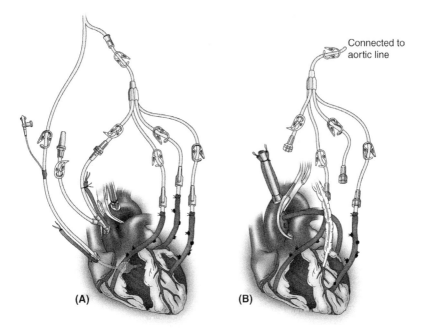

Connected to
aortic line

(A)   (B)

Figure 6.3 • (A) Technique of administering cardioplegia simultaneously down the completed vein grafts and the retrograde cannula. If proximal anastomoses are done during the cross-clamp period, cardioplegia is usually given retrograde, but it can be delivered into the aortic root and down the completed grafts after deairing the root. (B) Blood can be delivered off the aortic line during construction of the proximal anastomoses if they are performed with a sideclamp on the aorta.

6. If warm RCP is used, it should be run as continuously as possible as long as it does not interfere with exposure. A high-potassium solution should be used if there is return of cardiac activity.

7. Administer approximately 500 mL of "hot shot" retrograde just prior to removal of the cross-clamp. If RCP is not used, give this into the aortic root at a pressure that does not exceed 50–80 mm Hg after ensuring that there is no air in the aortic root. This is probably only beneficial in hearts that were actively ischemic or after long cross-clamp times. The addition of aspartate–glutamate to the reperfusion solution may have benefit in actively ischemic hearts.

8. In circulatory arrest cases for aortic root and arch surgery, cardioplegia should be either administered directly into the coronary ostia or given retrograde just prior to or at the time that circulatory arrest is initiated.

9. Careful adherence to the basic principles of cardioplegia, including maintenance of arrest, antegrade and retrograde delivery, and multidosing, in particular for Buckberg-type solutions, should allow surgeons to patiently yet expeditiously perform even the most complex, time-consuming operations without worrying about poor myocardial protection.

References

1. Buckberg GD, Beyersdorf F, Allen BS, Robertson JM. Integrated myocardial management: background and initial application. *J Card Surg* 1995;10:68–89.

2. Buckberg GD, Athanasuleas CL. Cardioplegia: solutions or strategies? *Eur J Cardiothorac Surg* 2016;50:787–91.

3. Buckberg GD, Cohen G, Borger MA, Weisel RD, Rao V. Intraoperative myocardial protection: current trends and future perspectives. *Ann Thorac Surg* 1999;68:1995–2001.

4. Bergsland J, Lingaas PS, Skulstad H, et al. Intracoronary shunt prevents ischemia in off-pump coronary artery bypass surgery. *Ann Thorac Surg* 2009;87:54–60.

5. Vassiliades TA Jr, Nielsen JL, Lonquist JL. Coronary perfusion methods during off-pump coronary artery bypass: results of a randomized clinical trial. *Ann Thorac Surg* 2002;74:S1383–9.

6. Reber D, Fritz M, Tossios P, et al. Beating-heart coronary artery bypass grafting using a miniaturized extracorporeal circulation system. *Heart Surg Forum* 2008;11:E276–80.

7. Lundell DC, Crouch JD. A miniature right heart support system improves cardiac output and stroke volume during beating heart posterior/lateral coronary artery bypass grafting. *Heart Surg Forum* 2003;6:302–6.

8. Lima LE, Jatene F, Buffolo E, et al. A multicenter initial clinical experience with right heart support and beating heart coronary surgery. *Heart Surg Forum* 2001;4:60–4.

9. Ueki C, Miyata H, Motonura N, Sakaguchi G, Akimoto T, Takamoto S. Off-pump versus on-pump coronary artery bypass grafting in patients with left ventricular dysfunction. *J Thorac Cardiovasc Surg* 2016;15:1092–8.

10. Wang J, Liu H, Xiang B, et al. Keeping the heart empty and beating improves preservation of hypertrophied hearts for valve surgery. *J Thorac Cardiovasc Surg* 2006;132:1314–20.

11. Ueki C, Sakaguchi G, Akimoto T, Ohashi Y, Sato H. On-pump beating-heart technique is associated with lower morbidity and mortality following coronary artery bypass grafting: a meta-analysis. *Eur J Cardiothorac Surg* 2016;50:813–21.

12. Xia L, Ji Q, Song K, et al. Early clinical outcomes of on-pump beating-heart versus off-pump technique for surgical revascularization in patients with severe left ventricular dysfunction: the experience of a single center. *J Cardiothoracic Surg* 2017;12:11.

13. Ferrari E, Stalder N, von Segesser LK. On-pump beating heart coronary surgery for high risk patients requiring emergency multiple coronary artery bypass grafting. *J Cardiothorac Surg* 2008;3:38–43.

14. Cicekcioglu F, Tutun U, Babaroglu S, et al. Redo valve surgery with on-pump beating heart technique. *J Cardiovasc Surg (Torino)* 2007;48:513–8.

15. Gersak B, Sutlic Z. Aortic and mitral valve surgery on the beating heart is lowering cardiopulmonary bypass and aortic cross clamp time. *Heart Surg Forum* 2002;5:182–6.

16. Salerno TA, Panos AL, Tian G, Deslauriers R, Calcaterra D, Ricci M. Surgery for cardiac valves and aortic root without cardioplegic arrest ("beating heart"): experience with a new method of myocardial perfusion. *J Card Surg* 2007;22:459–64.

17. Loulmet DF, Patel NC, Jennings JM, Subramanian VA. Less invasive intracardiac surgery performed without aortic clamping. *Ann Thorac Surg* 2008;85:1551–5.

18. Umakanthan R, Leacche M, Petracek MR, et al. Safety of minimally invasive mitral valve surgery without aortic cross-clamp. *Ann Thorac Surg* 2008;85:1544–9.

19. Battellini R, Rastan AJ, Fabricius A, Moscoso-Luduena M, Lachmann N, Mohr FW. Beating heart aortic valve replacement after previous coronary artery bypass surgery with a patent internal mammary artery graft. *Ann Thorac Surg* 2007;83:1206–9.

20. Reber D, Fritz M, Bojara W, Marks P, Laczkovics A, Tossios P. Aortic valve replacement after previous coronary artery bypass grafting: experience with a simplified approach. *J Cardiovasc Surg* 2007;48:73–7.

21. Bar-El Y, Kophit A, Cohen O, Kertzman V, Milo S. Minimal dissection and continuous retrograde cardioplegia for aortic valve replacement in patients with a patent left internal mammary artery bypass graft. *J Heart Valve Dis* 2003;12:454–7.

22. Akins CW. Noncardioplegic myocardial preservation for coronary revascularization. *J Thorac Cardiovasc Surg* 1984;88:174–81.

23. Raco L, Mills E, Millner RJ. Isolated myocardial revascularization with intermittent aortic cross-clamping: experience with 800 cases. *Ann Thorac Surg* 2002;73:1436–40.

24. Alex J, Ansari J, Guerrero R, et al. Comparison of the immediate post-operative outcome of two different myocardial protection strategies: antegrade–retrograde cold St. Thomas blood cardioplegia versus intermittent cross-clamp fibrillation. *Interact Cardiovasc Thorac Surg* 2003;2:584–8.

25. Walsh SR, Tang TY, Kullar P, Jenkins DP, Dutka DP, Gaunt ME. Ischaemic preconditioning during cardiac surgery: systematic review and meta-analysis of perioperative outcomes in randomised clinical trials. *Eur J Cardiothorac Surg* 2008;34:985–94.

26. Ji B, Liu M, Liu J, et al. Evaluation by cardiac troponin I: the effect of ischemic preconditioning as an adjunct to intermittent blood cardioplegia on coronary artery bypass grafting. *J Card Surg* 2007;22:394–400.

27. Codispoti M, Sundaramoorthi T, Saad RA, Reid A, Sinclair C, Mankad P. Optimal myocardial protection strategy for coronary artery bypass grafting without cardioplegia: prospective randomised trial. *Interact Cardiovasc Thorac Surg* 2006;5:217–21.

28. Perrault LP, Menasché P, Bel A, et al. Ischemic preconditioning in cardiac surgery: a word of caution. *J Thorac Cardiovasc Surg* 1996;112:1378–86.

29. Jin ZX, Zhou JJ, Xin M, et al. Postconditioning the human heart with adenosine in heart valve replacement surgery. *Ann Thorac Surg* 2007;83:2066–72.

30. Algarni KD, Weisel RD, Caldarone CA, Maganti M, Tsang K, Yau TM. Microplegia during coronary artery bypass grafting was associated with less low cardiac output syndrome: a propensity-matched analysis. *Ann Thorac Surg* 2013;95:1532–8.

31. McCann UG 2nd, Lutz CJ, Picone AI, et al. Whole blood cardioplegia (miniplegia) reduces myocardial edema after ischemic injury and cardiopulmonary bypass. *J Extra Corpor Technol* 2006;38:11 21.

32. Vinten-Johansen J. Whole blood cardioplegia. do we still need to dilute? *J Extra Corpor Technol* 2016;48:P9–14.

33. Aldemir M, Karatepe C, Baki ED, Çarşanba G, Tecer E. Comparison of Plegisol and modified St. Thomas Hospital cardioplegic solution in the development of ventricular fibrillation after declamping of the aorta. *World J Cardiovasc Surg* 2014;4:159–66.

34. Edelman JJ, Seco M, Dunne B, et al. Custodiol for myocardial protection and preservation: a systematic review. *Ann Cardiothorac Surg* 2013;2:717–28.

35. Preusse CJ. Custodiol cardioplegia: a single-dose hyperpolarizing solution. *J Extra Corpor Technol* 2016;48:P15–20.

36. Hoyer A, Lehmann S, Mende M, et al. Custodiol versus cold Calafiore for elective cardiac arrest in isolated aortic valve replacement: a propensity-matched analysis of 7263 patients. *Eur J Cardiothorac Surg* 2017;52:303–9.

37. Braathen B, Jeppsson A, Scherstén H, et al. One single dose of histidine–tryptophan–ketoglutarate solution gives equally good myocardial protection in elective mitral valve surgery as repetitive doses of blood cardioplegia: a prospective randomized trial. *J Thorac Cardiovasc Surg* 2011;141:995–1001.

38. Sakata J, Morishita K, Ito T, Koshino T, Kazui T, Abe T. Comparison of clinical outcome between histidine–tritophan–ketoglutalate solution and cold blood cardioplegic solution in mitral valve replacement. *J Card Surg* 1998;13:343–7.

39. Kim K, Ball C, Grady P, Mick S. Use of del Nido cardioplegia for adult cardiac surgery at the Cleveland Clinic: perfusion implications. *J Extra Corpor Technol* 2014;46:317–23.

40. Li Y, Lin H, Zhao Y, et al. Del Nido cardioplegia for myocardial protection in adult cardiac surgery: a systematic review and meta-analysis. *ASAIO J* 2018;64:360–7.

41. Mick SL, Robich MP, Houghtaling PL, et al. del Nido versus Buckberg cardioplegia in adult isolated valve surgery. *J Thorac Cardiovasc Surg* 2015;149:626–34.

42. Smigla G. Jaquiss R, Walczak R, et al. Assessing the safety of del Nido cardioplegia solutions in adult congenital cases. *Perfusion* 2014;29:554–8.

43. Kim WK, Kim HR, Kim JB, et al. del Nido cardioplegia in adult cardiac surgery: beyond single-valve surgery. *Interact Cardiovasc Thorac Surg* 2018;27:81–7.

44. Hamad R, Nguyen A, Laliberté E, et al. Comparison of del Nido cardioplegia with blood cardioplegia in adult combined surgery. *Innovations (Phila)* 2017;12:356–62.

45. Sorabella RA, Akashi H, Yerebakan H, et al. Myocardial protection using del Nido cardioplegia solution in adult reoperative aortic valve surgery. *J Card Surg* 2014;29:445–9.

46. Yerebakan H, Sorabella RA, Najjar M, et al. Del Nido cardioplegia can be safely administered in high-risk coronary artery bypass grafting surgery after acute myocardial infarction: a propensity matched comparison. *J Cardiothorac Surg* 2014;9:141.

47. Ad N, Holmes SD, Massimiano PS, Rongione AJ, Fornaresio LM, Fitzgerald D. The use of del Nido cardioplegia in adult cardiac surgery: a prospective randomized trial. *J Thorac Cardiovasc Surg* 2018;155:1011–8.

48. Kim JS, Jeong JH, Moon SJ, Ahn H, Hwang HY. Sufficient myocardial protection of del Nido cardioplegia regardless of ventricular mass and myocardial ischemic time in adult cardiac surgical patients. *J Thorac Dis* 2016;8:2004–10.

49. Mongero LB. Del Nido cardioplegia: not just kids stuff. *J Extra Corpor Technol* 2016;48:P25–8.

50. Valooran GJ, Nair SK, Chandrasekharan K, Simon R, Dominic C. Del Nido cardioplegia in adult cardiac surgery: scopes and concerns. *Perfusion* 2016;31:6–14.

51. Mishra P, Jadhav RB, Mohapatra CKR, et al. Comparison of del Nido cardioplegia and St. Thomas Hospital solution: two types of cardioplegia in adult cardiac surgery. *Kardiochir Torakochirurgia Pol* 2016;13:295–9.

52. Sanetra K, Geber W, Shrestha R, et al. The del Nido versus cold blood cardioplegia in aortic valve replacement: a randomized trial. *J Thorac Cardiovasc Surg* 2020;159:2275–83.

53. Jacob S, Kallikourdis A, Sellke F, Dunning J. Is blood cardioplegia superior to crystalloid cardioplegia? *Interact Cardiovasc Thorac Surg* 2008;7:491–8.

54. Guru V, Omura J, Alghamdi A, Weisel R, Fremes SE. Is blood superior to crystalloid cardioplegia? A meta-analysis of randomized clinical trials. *Circulation* 2006;114(1 Suppl):I-331–8.

55. Zeng J, He W, Qu Z, Tang Y, Zhou Q, Zhang B. Cold blood versus crystalloid cardioplegia for myocardial protection in adult cardiac surgery: a meta-analysis of randomized controlled studies. *J Cardiothorac Vasc Anesth* 2014;38:674–81.

56. Nardi P, Pisano C, Bertoldo F, et al. Warm blood cardioplegia versus cold crystalloid cardioplegia for myocardial protection during coronary artery bypass grafting surgery. *Cell Death Discovery* 2018;4:23.

57. Dar MI. Cold crystalloid versus warm blood cardioplegia for coronary bypass surgery. *Ann Thorac Cardiovasc Surg* 2005;11:382–5.

58. Ascione R, Caputo M, Gomes WJ, et al. Myocardial injury in hypertrophic hearts of patients undergoing aortic valve surgery using cold or warm blood cardioplegia. *Eur J Cardiothorac Surg* 2002;21:440–6.

59. Khabbaz KR, Feng J, Boodhwani M, Clements RT, Bianchi C, Sellke FW. Nonischemic myocardial acidosis adversely affects microvascular and myocardial function and triggers apoptosis during cardioplegia. *J Thorac Cardiovasc Surg* 2008;135:139–46.

60. Dearani JA, Axford TC, Patel MA, Healey NA, Lavin PT, Khuri SF. Role of myocardial temperature measurement in monitoring the adequacy of myocardial protection during cardiac surgery. *Ann Thorac Surg* 2001;72:S2235–43.

61. Badak MI, Gurcun U, Discigil B, Boga M, Ozkisacik EA, Alayunt EA. Myocardium utilizes more oxygen and glucose during tepid cardioplegic infusion in arrested heart. *Int Heart J* 2005;46:219–29.

62. Mallidi HR, Sever J, Tamariz M, et al. The short-term and long-term effects of warm or tepid cardioplegia. *J Thorac Cardiovasc Surg* 2003;125:711–20.

63. Sirvinskas E, Nasvytis L, Raliene L, Vaskelyte J, Toleikis A, Trumbeckaite S. Myocardial protective effect of warm blood, tepid blood, and cold crystalloid cardioplegia in coronary artery bypass grafting surgery. *Croat Med J* 2005;46:879–88.

64. Bezon E, Choplain JN, Khalifa AA, Numa H, Salley N, Barra JA. Continuous retrograde blood cardioplegia ensures prolonged aortic cross-clamping without increasing the operative risk. *Interact Cardiovasc Thorac Surg* 2006;5:403–7.

65. Salerno TA. Warm heart surgery: reflections on the history of its development. *J Card Surg* 2007;22:257–9.

66. Fan Y, Zhang AM, Xiao YB, Weng YG, Hetzer R. Warm versus cold cardioplegia for heart surgery: a meta-analysis. *Eur J Cardiothorac Surg* 2010;37:912–9.

67. Abah U, Roberts PG, Ishaq M, De Silva R. Is cold or warm blood cardioplegia superior for myocardial protection? *Interact Cardiovasc Thorac Surg* 2012;14:848–55.

68. Nardi P, Vacirca SR, Russo M, et al. Cold crystalloid versus warm blood cardioplegia in patients undergoing aortic valve replacement. *J Thorac Dis* 2018;10:1490–9.

69. Casalino S, Tesler UF, Novelli E, et al. The efficacy and safety of extending the ischemic time with a modified cardioplegic technique for coronary artery surgery. *J Card Surg* 2008;23:444–9.

70. Rosenkranz ER, Vinten-Johansen J, Buckberg GD, Okamoto F, Edwards H, Bugyi H. Benefits of normothermic induction of blood cardioplegia in energy-depleted hearts with maintenance of arrest by multidose cold blood cardioplegic solution. *J Thorac Cardiovac Surg* 1982;84:667–77.

71. Teoh KH, Christakis GT, Weisel RD, et al. Accelerated myocardial metabolic recovery with terminal warm blood cardioplegia. *J Thorac Cardiovasc Surg* 1986;91:888–95.

72. Caputo M, Dihmis WC, Bryan AJ, Suleiman MS, Angelini GD. Warm blood hyperkalaemic reperfusion ("hot shot") prevents myocardial substrate derangement in patients undergoing coronary artery bypass surgery. *Eur J Cardiothorac Surg* 1998;13:559–64.

73. Ji B, Liu M, Lu F, et al. Warm induction cardioplegia and reperfusion dose influence the occurrence of post CABG TnI level. *Interact Cardiovasc Thorac Surg* 2006;5:67–70.

74. Wallace AW, Ratcliffe MB, Nosé PS, et al. Effect of induction and reperfusion with warm substrate-enriched cardioplegia on ventricular function. *Ann Thorac Surg* 2000;70:1301–7.

75. Ascione R, Suleiman SM, Angelini GD. Retrograde hot-shot cardioplegia in patients with left ventricular hypertrophy undergoing aortic valve replacement. *Ann Thorac Surg* 2008;85:454–8.

76. Edwards R, Treasure T, Hossein-Nia M, Murday A, Kantidakis GH, Holt DW. A controlled trial of substrate-enhanced, warm reperfusion ("hot shot") versus simple reperfusion. *Ann Thorac Surg* 2000;69:551–5.

77. Aronson S, Jacobsohn E, Savage R, Albertucci M. The influence of collateral flow on the antegrade and retrograde distribution of cardioplegia in patients with an occluded right coronary artery. *Anesthesiology* 1998;89:1099–107.

78. Honkonen EL, Kaukinen L, Pehkonen EJ, Kaukinen S. Myocardial cooling and right ventricular function in patients with right coronary artery disease: antegrade vs. retrograde cardioplegia. *Acta Anaesthesiol Scand* 1997;41:287–96.

79. Borger MA, Wei KS, Weisel RD, et al. Myocardial perfusion during warm antegrade and retrograde cardioplegia: a contrast echo study. *Ann Thorac Surg* 1999;68:955–61.

80. Allen BS, Winkelmann JW, Hanafy H, et al. Retrograde cardioplegia does not adequately perfuse the right ventricle. *J Thorac Cardiovasc Surg* 1995;109:1116–26.

81. Langenberg CJ, Pietersen HG, Geskes G, Wagenmakers AJ, Soeters PB, Durieux M. Coronary sinus catheter placement: assessment of placement criteria and cardiac complications. *Chest* 2003;124:1259–65.

82. Ikonomidis JS, Yau TM, Weisel RD, et al. Optimal flow rates for retrograde warm cardioplegia. *J Thorac Cardiovasc Surg* 1994;107:510–9.

83. Bhaya M, Sudhakar S, Sadat K, et al. Effects of antegrade versus integrated blood cardioplegia on left ventricular function evaluated by echocardiographic real-time 3-dimensional speckle tracking. *J Thorac Cardiovasc Surg* 2015;149:877–84.

84. Buckberg GD. Antegrade cardioplegia, retrograde cardioplegia, or both? *Ann Thorac Surg* 1988;45:589–90.

85. Sanjay OP, Srikrishna SV, Prashanth P, Kajrekar P, Vincent V. Antegrade versus antegrade with retrograde delivery of cardioplegia solution in myocardial revascularisation: a clinical study in patients with triple vessel coronary artery disease. *Ann Card Anaesth* 2003;6:143–8.

86. Radmehr H, Soleimani A, Tatari H, Salehi M. Does combined antegrade–retrograde cardioplegia have any superiority over antegrade cardioplegia? *Heart Lung Circ* 2008;17:475–7.

87. Louagie YA, Jamart J, Gonzalez M, et al. Continuous cold blood cardioplegia improves myocardial protection: a prospective randomized study. *Ann Thorac Surg* 2004;77:664–71.

88. Li G, Tian W, Wang J, et al. The effects of simultaneous antegrade/retrograde cardioplegia on cellular volumes and energy metabolism. *J Card Surg* 2008;23:437–43.

89. Buckberg GD. Controlled reperfusion after ischemia may be the unifying recovery denominator. *J Thorac Cardiovasc Surg* 2010;140:12–8.

90. Fannelop T, Dahle GO, Matre K, et al. Esmolol before 80 min of cardiac arrest with oxygenated cold blood cardioplegia alleviates systolic dysfunction: an experimental study in pigs. *Eur J Cardiothorac Surg* 2008;33:9–17.

91. Ellenberger C, Sologashvili T, Kreienbühl L, Cikirikcioglu M, Diaper J, Licker M. Myocardial protection by glucose–insulin–potassium in moderate- to high-risk patients undergoing elective on-pump cardiac surgery: a randomized controlled trial. *Anesth Analg* 2018;126:1133–41.

92. Aranki SF, Sullivan TE, Cohn LH. The effect of the single aortic cross-clamp technique on cardiac and cerebral complications during coronary bypass surgery. *J Card Surg* 1995;10(4 Suppl): 498–502.

93. Kim RW, Mariconda DC, Tellides G, et al. Single-clamp techniques do not protect against cerebrovascular accident in coronary artery bypass grafting. *Eur J Cardiothorac Surg* 2001;20:127–32.

94. Chen L, Hua X, Song J, Wang L. Which aortic clamp strategy is better to reduce postoperative stroke and death: single center report and a meta-analysis. *Medicine (Baltimore)* 2018;97:e0221.

95. Moss E, Puskas JD, Thourani V, et al. Avoiding aortic clamping during CABG reduces postoperative stroke. *J Thorac Cardiovasc Surg* 2015;149:175–80.

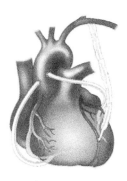

CHAPTER 7

Admission to the ICU and Monitoring Techniques

♡ 7 Admission to the ICU and Monitoring Techniques

I. Admission to the ICU

A. The first critical phase of postoperative care begins at the completion of the surgical procedure. During transfer from the operating room table to an intensive care unit (ICU) bed, from one monitoring system to another, and from the operating room to the ICU, the potential exists for airway and ventilation problems, sudden hypotension or hypertension, arrhythmias, increased mediastinal bleeding, inadvertent medication changes, and problems with invasive catheters and monitoring.

   1. The electrocardiogram (ECG), arterial pressure tracing, and arterial oxygen saturation (SaO_2) are transduced on the transport monitor, after which the patient is transferred to the ICU bed. During this transfer, the anesthesia team should coordinate all movements, paying particular attention to the airway, with hand ventilation provided by an Ambu bag connected to a portable oxygen tank. The entire team should also pay attention to invasive lines, the pacing wires, urinary catheter, and chest tubes to make sure nothing becomes dislodged during transfer.

   2. Drug infusions should be placed on battery-powered infusion pumps to ensure accurate infusion rates. These pumps should be plugged in during the surgical procedure so that battery function is fully charged when ready for transport. A selection of cardiac medications should always be available in the event of an emergency during transport.

B. A standard handoff routine from the anesthesiology team and accompanying providers to the ICU team (nurses, mid-level providers and/or physicians, respiratory therapists) is essential to ensure an expeditious and safe arrival in the ICU.[1]

C. Upon arrival in the ICU, the endotracheal tube is connected to a mechanical ventilator, and the ECG, pressure monitoring lines, and pulse oximetry are transduced on a bedside monitor. Some hospitals have transport modules that plug directly into the ICU monitoring systems. Medication drip rates are confirmed or readjusted on controlled infusion pumps, preferably using the same pumps that were used in the operating room to avoid temporary disconnection from the patient. The thoracic drainage system is connected to suction.[2]

D. During this transition phase, much attention is directed to getting the patient connected to the monitors and attached to the ventilator. To ensure that the patient remains stable while getting settled in, it is critical that the accompanying anesthesia and/or surgical personnel as well as the accepting nurses and respiratory therapists make sure that:

Manual of Perioperative Care in Adult Cardiac Surgery, Sixth Edition. Robert M. Bojar.
© 2021 John Wiley & Sons Ltd. Published 2021 by John Wiley & Sons Ltd.

1. The patient is being well ventilated by observing chest movement, auscultating bilateral breath sounds, and confirming that the oxygen saturation by pulse oximetry is acceptable (>90%).

2. The ECG tracing demonstrates satisfactory rate and rhythm on the transport and then the bedside monitor.

3. The blood pressure is adequate on the portable monitor and remains so after the arterial line is transduced and calibrated on the bedside monitor.

E. Immediate assessment and response to any abnormalities suspected to be present at the time of admission to the ICU, whether real or spurious, is imperative. The two most common problems encountered are a low blood pressure and an indecipherable ECG.

F. **Low blood pressure** (systolic BP <90 mm Hg or mean BP <60 mm Hg) is caused most commonly by hypovolemia or sudden termination of a drug infusion. However, the possibility of a more critical problem, such as acute blood loss, myocardial ischemia, severe myocardial dysfunction, arrhythmias, or ventilatory problems, should always be kept in mind. Low blood pressure may also result from inadequate zeroing of the transducer, or kinking or transient occlusion of the arterial line, producing a dampened tracing. If the transduced blood pressure is low, do the following:

1. Resume manual ventilation and listen for bilateral breath sounds.

2. Palpate the brachial or femoral artery to confirm a pulse and a satisfactory blood pressure. Attach the blood pressure cuff above the radial arterial line site and take an auscultatory or occlusion blood pressure. The latter is done by inflating the cuff until the arterial tracing on the monitor is obliterated; when the pressure tracing reappears, the systolic pressure can be read from the sphygmomanometer. **Never assume that a low blood pressure recording is caused by dampening of the arterial line unless a higher pressure can be confirmed by another method.** Insertion of an additional arterial monitoring line (usually in the femoral artery) may be indicated.

3. Make sure that all medication bottles are appropriately labeled and are connected to the patient and infusing at the designated rate through patent intravenous (IV) lines. **Note:** If hypotension is present, quickly ascertain whether the patient is receiving nitroglycerin or nitroprusside (in the silver wrapper), because both can lower the blood pressure precipitously. Unless you know how to change the drip rate on the particular drug infusion pump, let someone else who is familiar with it take care of it!

4. Quickly examine the chest tubes for massive mediastinal bleeding. Exsanguinating hemorrhage may require emergency sternotomy.

5. Evaluate the cardiac filling pressures on the ICU monitor. Confirm that the transducers are at the appropriate levels relative to the patient's position in the bed and that the monitors are calibrated. Not uncommonly, during the very early stages of admission to the ICU, the observed filling pressures will not be accurate and this may confound an assessment of the patient's volume status. The anesthesiologist should be aware of the filling pressures just prior to transport and can assist in assessing whether a significant change has occurred, with low filling pressures indicating hypovolemia and very high filling pressures consistent with myocardial dysfunction, excessive fluid administration, or tamponade.

6. The initial **treatment** of hypotension should include volume infusion, and, if there is no immediate response, administration of calcium chloride 500 mg IV. Vasoactive medications may be started or the rate of medications already being used can be

adjusted. **If there is no response to these measures, and the ECG is abnormal, assume the worst and prepare to treat the patient as an imminent cardiac arrest until the problem is sorted out. If the patient cannot be immediately resuscitated, call for help and prepare for an emergency sternotomy.**

G. An **indeterminate or undecipherable ECG** is usually caused by artifact with jostling or detachment of the ECG leads. If the arterial waveform and pulse oximetry readings are acceptable, this is usually the case. However, if the arterial pressure is low or not transduced, the pulse is irregular or slow, or the monitor is difficult to interpret, palpate for a pulse and take the steps mentioned above. **If the blood pressure is undetectable and an ECG reading is not available, assume the worst and treat the patient as a cardiac arrest.** Readjust the ECG leads on the patient and monitor. If interpretation remains difficult, attach a standard ECG machine to limb leads to ascertain the rhythm.

1. If ventricular fibrillation or tachycardia is present, immediate defibrillation and a cardiac arrest protocol are indicated (see pages 591–599).

2. If a pacemaker is being used, examine the connections and settings and confirm capture on the bedside monitor or an ECG. Make sure that the pacemaker is appropriately sensing the patient's rhythm, since inappropriate sensing may trigger malignant ventricular arrhythmias.

3. Attach a pacemaker and initiate pacing if bradycardia or heart block is present. The initial default setting on most external pacemakers is the VVI mode, which should produce a ventricular contraction. One should then attempt to pace the atrium (AOO) or initiate AV pacing (DDD or DVI) if atrial pacing wires are present and heart block is present. If there is no response to atrial pacing, ventricular pacing (VVI) should be used. If the patient has a rhythm, but the ventricle fails to pace, reverse the leads in the cable connector, and if that fails, consider placing a skin wire as a ground in case one of the wires has been dislodged from the heart. One of the atrial leads can also be used as the grounding wire (the anode or positive lead, which is the red connector on the pacing cables).

4. Look for the undetected development of atrial fibrillation that can develop during AV pacing. This may account for a fall in cardiac output and blood pressure, despite an adequate ventricular pacing rate.

5. Obtain a 12-lead ECG, looking for evidence of arrhythmias or ischemia that may require treatment.

H. Once the patient's heart rate, rhythm, and blood pressure are found to be satisfactory and adequate oxygenation and ventilation from the ventilator are confirmed, a full report should be given to the ICU staff by the accompanying anesthesiologist/CRNA and/or surgical house staff/PA/NP. This should include the patient's cardiac disease and comorbidities, the operative procedure and any technical issues, the aortic cross-clamp time and duration of cardiopulmonary bypass, medications used to come off bypass and those currently being administered, use of pacing, and special instructions for postoperative care.[1] Further assessment as delineated in Table 7.1 can then be carried out to address the subtleties of patient care. A standardized set of preprinted orders that can be adapted to each patient is invaluable in ensuring that no essential elements of the early postoperative care are overlooked (Table 7.2 and Appendix 4). In most hospitals, this is incorporated into a set of electronic orders which must be individualized for each patient.

Table 7.1 • Initial Evaluation of the Patient in the Intensive Care Unit
1. The patient should be examined thoroughly (heart, lungs, peripheral perfusion).
2. Obtain hemodynamic measurements, including the central venous pressure (CVP) and PA pressures; obtain a cardiac output and calculate the systemic vascular resistance (SVR) (see Table 11.1, page 517).
3. A portable supine chest x-ray should be obtained either in the operating room or soon after arrival in the ICU. Specific attention should be paid to the position of the endotracheal tube and Swan-Ganz catheter, the width of the mediastinum, and the presence of a pneumothorax, fluid overload, atelectasis, or pleural effusion (hemothorax).
4. A 12-lead ECG should be reviewed for ischemic changes or arrhythmias.
5. Laboratory tests should be drawn (see Table 7.2 for sample admission order sheet).

I. It is very important to review the immediate postoperative chest x-ray to assess the position of the endotracheal tube and make sure that a pneumothorax is not missed. If present, an additional chest tube may need to be placed. Obtaining a chest x-ray prior to departure from the operating room is beneficial. However, even if the initial chest x-ray does not show a pneumothorax, one may develop subsequently, usually due to positive pressure ventilation, and is often manifested by unexplained hypoxemia or unstable hemodynamics without evident cause. In addition, review of an ECG obtained soon after arrival in the ICU is essential to identify any ischemic changes that might require urgent attention.

II. Monitoring in the ICU: Techniques and Problems

Careful monitoring is required in the early postoperative period to optimize patient management and outcome.[2] A continuous display of the ECG is provided, and pressures derived from invasive catheters, including arterial and Swan-Ganz catheters placed in the operating room, are transduced on bedside monitors (Figure 7.1). The endotracheal tube is securely connected to the mechanical ventilator and appropriate ventilator settings are selected. A continuous readout of the arterial oxygen saturation (SaO_2) determined by pulse oximetry should be displayed. The drainage outputs of chest tubes and the Foley catheter are measured and recorded. Conscientious data collection on computerized flowsheets is essential. Each invasive technique is used to provide an essential function or obtain special information about the patient's postoperative course, but each has potential complications. Each should be used only as long as necessary to maximize benefit while minimizing morbidity.

A. **ECG display** on a bedside monitor is critical to allow for rapid interpretation of rhythm changes. Most bedside monitors have a memory, and abnormal rhythms will activate a printout. This is helpful in detecting the mechanism of arrhythmia development (such as an R-on-T phenomenon leading to ventricular tachycardia or fibrillation). ST segment analysis is provided by most monitoring systems, but abnormalities must be thoroughly analyzed from a 12-lead ECG.

B. Mechanical ventilation via an endotracheal tube is used for all patients, except those who are extubated in the operating room. The initial settings are determined by the anesthesiologist and respiratory therapist and generally provide a tidal volume around 6–8 mL/kg at a rate of 12–14/min with the initial FiO_2 set at 1.0. Confirmation of bilateral breath sounds and chest movement, intermittent rechecking of ventilator settings, and assessment of the adequacy of gas exchange are essential.

Table 7.2 • Typical Orders for Admission to the ICU

1. Admit to ICU on _____ MD service
2. Procedure: _____
3. Vital signs q15 min until stable, then q30 min or per protocol
4. Continuous ECG, arterial, PA tracings, SaO_2 on bedside monitor
5. Cardiac output q15 min × 1 hour, then q1h × 4 hours, then q2–4h when stable
6. IABP 1:1; check distal pulses manually or with Doppler q1h
7. Chest tubes to chest drainage system with −20 cm H_2O suction; record q15 min until <60 mL/h, then q1h until <30 mL/h, then every 2 hours
8. Bair Hugger warming system if core temperature <35 °C
9. Urinary catheter to gravity drainage and record hourly
10. Elevate head of bed 30°
11. Hourly I & O
12. Daily weights
13. Advance activity after extubation (dangle, OOB to chair)
14. VTE prophylaxis
    - ☐ T.E.D. elastic stockings (apply on POD #1)
    - ☐ Sequential or pneumatic compression devices while in bed
    - ☐ Heparin 5000 units SC bid starting on POD # _____
    - ☐ Low-molecular-weight heparin (Lovenox) 40 mg SC daily starting on POD #_____
15. GI/Nutrition:
    - ☐ NPO while intubated
    - ☐ Nasogastric tube to low suction
    - ☐ Clear liquids as tolerated 1 h after extubation and removal of NG tube
16. Ventilator settings
    FiO_2: _____ in SIMV mode
    IMV rate: _____ breaths/min
    Tidal volume: _____ mL
    PEEP: _____ cm H_2O
17. Respiratory care
    - ☐ Endotracheal suction q4h, then prn
    - ☐ Wean ventilator to extubate per protocol (see Tables 10.3–10.5, pages 475–476)
    - ☐ O_2 via face mask with FiO_2 0.6–1.0 per protocol
    - ☐ O_2 via nasal prongs @ 2–6 L/min to keep SaO_2 >95%
    - ☐ Incentive spirometer q1h when awake
    - ☐ Cough pillow at bedside
    - ☐ Albuterol 0.5 mL of 0.5% solution (2.5 mg) in 3 mL normal saline q6h via nebulizer or metered dose inhaler 6 puffs via endotracheal tube (90 µg/inhalation)
18. Laboratory tests
    - ☐ On arrival: STAT ABGs, CBC, electrolytes, glucose
      STAT PT, PTT, platelet count if chest tube output >100/h (thromboelastogram if available)
      STAT chest x-ray (if not done in operating room)
      STAT ECG
    - ☐ Four and eight hours after arrival and prn: potassium, hematocrit, ABGs (respiratory distress)
    - ☐ ABGs per protocol (prior to weaning and prior to extubation)
    - ☐ 3:00 AM on POD #1: CBC, lytes, BUN, creatinine, blood glucose, ECG, CXR, INR (if patient to receive warfarin after valve procedure)

(continued)

Table 7.2 • (Continued)

19. Pacemaker settings
    Mode: □ Atrial □ VVI □ DVI □ DDD
    Atrial output: _____ mA   Ventricular output: _____ mA
    Rate: _____/min   AV interval: _____ msec
    Sensitivity: □ Asynchronous   □ Demand
    □ Pacer off but attached
20. Cardiac rehab consult
21. Notify MD/PA/NP for:
    a. Systolic blood pressure <90 or >140 mm Hg
    b. Cardiac index <2.0 L/min/m²
    c. Urine output <30 mL/h for two hours
    d. Chest tube drainage >100 mL/h
    e. Temperature >38.5 °C
22. IV Drips/Medications (with suggested ranges)
    a. Allergies_____
       □ IV drips:
       □ Dextrose 5% in 0.45% NS 250 mL via Cordis/triple lumen to KVO
       □ Arterial line and distal Swan-Ganz port: NS flushes at 3 mL/h
       □ Epinephrine 1 mg/250 mL D5W: _____ µg/min to maintain cardiac index >2.0
         (0.01–0.06 µg/kg/min or 1–4 µg/min)
       □ Milrinone 20 mg/100 mL D5W: _____ µg/kg/min (0.25–0.75 µg/kg/min)
       □ Dobutamine 250 mg/250 mL D5W: _____ µg/kg/min (5–20 µg/kg/min)
       □ Norepinephrine 4–8 mg/250 mL D5W: _____ µg/min to keep systolic BP >100
         (0.01–1.0 µg/kg/min)
       □ Phenylephrine 20 mg/250 mL NS: _____ µg/min to keep systolic BP >100
         (0.1–3.0 µg/kg/min)
       □ Vasopressin 100 units/250 mL D5W: _____ units/min (0.01–0.1 units/min)
       □ Nitroprusside 50 mg/250 mL D5W: _____ µg/kg/min to keep systolic BP <130
         (0.1–8 µg/kg/min)
       □ Clevidipine 50 mg/100 mL D5W: _____ mg/h to keep systolic BP <130 (2–21 mg/h)
       □ Nicardipine 25 mg/250 mL D5W: _____ mg/h to keep BP <130 (5–15 mg/h)
       □ Nitroglycerin 50 mg/250 mL D5W: _____ µg/kg/min (0.1–5 µg/kg/min)
       □ Diltiazem: 100 mg/100 mL D5W: _____ mg/h (for radial artery prophylaxis)
       □ Esmolol 2.5 g/250 mL NS: _____ µg/kg/min (25–100 µg/kg/min)
       □ Amiodarone: after initial IV load in OR, 900 mg/500 mL D5W: 1 mg/min × 6
         hours, then decrease to 0.5 mg/min × 18 hours
       □ Lidocaine 2 g/250 mL D5W: _____ mg/min IV; wean off at 6:00 AM POD #1
    b. Antibiotics
       □ Cefazolin 1 g IV q8h for 6 doses
       □ Vancomycin 1 g IV q12h for 4 doses
    c. Sedatives/analgesics
       □ Propofol infusion 10 mg/mL: 25–75 µg/kg/min; wean off per protocol
       □ Dexmedetomidine: 400 µg (2 vials of 2 mL of 100 µg/mL solution)/100 mL NS:
         bolus dose of _____ (1 µg/kg) over 10 minutes, then maintenance infusion of
         _____ µg/kg/h (0.2–1.5 µg/kg/h)
       □ Midazolam 2 mg IV q2h prn agitation; stop after extubation
       □ Morphine sulfate _____ mg IV q2h prn for pain (while intubated)
       □ Meperidine 25–50 mg IV prn shivering
       □ Ketorolac 30–60 mg IV q6h prn for moderate–severe pain (4–10 on pain scale);
         stop after 72 hours

Table 7.2 • (Continued)

- ☐ Acetaminophen 650 mg PO/IV q4h prn pain (maximum 4 g/day)
- ☐ Oxycodone with acetaminophen (Percocet) 5/325 mg 1–2 tabs PO q4h prn for pain after extubation; start with 1 tab for mild pain (1–3 on pain scale); give additional tab 60 minutes later if no change in pain. Give 2 tabs for moderate-severe pain (4–10 on pain scale)

d. Other medications
  - ☐ β-blocker starting at 8:00 AM on POD #1, then q12h; hold for HR <60 or SBP <100
    - ☐ Metoprolol _____ mg PO/per NG tube bid (12.5–100 mg bid)
    - ☐ Carvedilol _____ mg PO/per NG tube bid (3.125–25 mg bid)
  - ☐ Amiodarone 400 mg PO bid to start after amiodarone infusion discontinued
  - ☐ Magnesium sulfate 2 g in 50 mL NS IV over 2 hours on POD #1 in AM
  - ☐ Sucralfate 1 g per NG tube q6h until NG tube removed
  - ☐ Pantoprazole (Protonix) 40 mg IV/PO qd
  - ☐ Aspirin   ☐ 81 mg   ☐ 325 mg PO qd (starting 8 hours after arrival); hold for platelet count <60,000 or chest tube drainage >50 mL/h
  - ☐ Warfarin _____ mg starting _____; check with HO for daily dose (use warfarin protocol) (see Appendix 8)
  - ☐ Ascorbic acid 1 g PO qd × 5 days
  - ☐ Nitroglycerin 50 mg/250 mL D5W at 10–15 µg/min until taking PO (radial artery prophylaxis); then convert to:
    - ☐ Amlodipine 5 mg PO qd   ☐ Amlodipine 10 mg PO qd
    - ☐ Isosorbide mononitrate sustained release (Imdur) 20 mg PO qd
  - ☐ Simvastatin _____ mg qd hs (no more than 20 mg if on amiodarone)
  - ☐ Mupirocin 2% (Bactroban ointment) via Q-tip nasal swab the evening after surgery and bid × 3 days
  - ☐ Chlorhexidine 0.12% oral wash (Peridex) 15 mL soft swab and rub oral cavity while intubated q12h

e. Prn medications
  - ☐ Acetaminophen 650 mg PO/PR q4h prn temp >38.5 °C
  - ☐ Metoclopramide 10 mg IV/PO q6h prn nausea
  - ☐ Ondansetron 4–8 mg IV q4h prn nausea
  - ☐ KCl 20 mEq/50 mL D5W via central line to keep K+ >4.5 mEq/L:
    - ☐ KCl 10 mEq over 30 min for K+ 4.0–4.5
    - ☐ KCl 20 mEq over 60 min for K+ 3.5–3.9
    - ☐ KCl 40 mEq over 90 min for K+ <3.5
  - ☐ Initiate hyperglycemia protocol if blood glucose >150 mg/dL on admission or any time within the first 48 hours (see Appendix 6)
  - ☐ Other

1. Pulse oximetry is routinely used to continuously assess the status of peripheral perfusion and arterial oxygen saturation (SaO_2).[3] It can draw attention to major problems with oxygenation during the period of intubation and following extubation. If the patient is severely vasoconstricted, the recordings from the patient's fingers may be inadequate and a better signal may be derived from the earlobe. Use of pulse oximetry obviates the need to draw arterial blood gases (ABGs) more than a few times during the period of intubation.[4] Nonetheless, it should be kept in mind that pulse oximetry only provides a measurement of SaO_2 (and heart rate), but it does not provide the same information as an ABG, which measures the PCO_2 and pH. These values may be important in assessing the patient's respiratory drive during

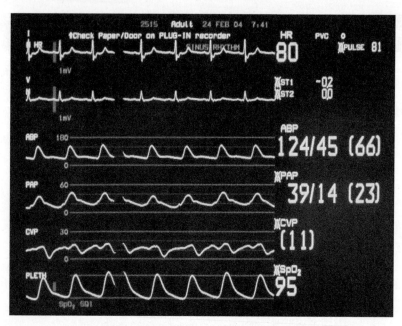

Figure 7.1 • Monitoring in the ICU. From top to bottom: two ECG leads, arterial blood pressure (ABP), pulmonary artery systolic/diastolic waveforms (PAP), central venous pressure (CVP), and pulse oximetry (SpO₂). The digital display of the pressures with the mean pressure in parentheses is noted on the right.

the weaning process and can identify whether the patient has a metabolic or respiratory acidosis/alkalosis. This is particularly valuable in identifying a metabolic acidosis that may reflect borderline hemodynamic function that requires further pharmacologic intervention. A profound metabolic acidosis often suggests the presence of a catastrophic problem, such as mesenteric ischemia.

2. Suctioning should be performed gently every few hours or as necessary to maintain a tube free of secretions but not so frequently as to induce endobronchial trauma or bronchospasm.[5] The endotracheal tube bypasses the protective mechanism of the upper airway and predisposes the patient to pulmonary infection. It should be removed as soon as the patient can maintain satisfactory ventilation and oxygenation and is able to protect their airway. This is generally accomplished within 4–6 hours of surgery. A standard protocol for weaning and extubation is essential in any cardiac surgical ICU (see Tables 10.3–10.5, pages 475–476).

C. **Arterial lines** are placed in either the radial or femoral artery during surgery and are transduced on the bedside monitor.[6] Occasionally, a brachial arterial line may be necessary when a radial line cannot be placed and there are anatomic problems that preclude placement of a femoral arterial line. These may include extensive iliofemoral disease, vascular reconstructive grafts in the groin, or limited availability of the femoral vessels because of the use of an intra-aortic balloon pump (IABP) or femoral cannulation for cardiopulmonary bypass. Accurate pressure recording depends on proper calibration and elimination of air from the transducer.

1. Radial arterial pressure measurements do not correspond to the central aortic pressure immediately after bypass in about one-third of patients, and femoral lines are often placed for more accurate measurements. One study suggested that this phenomenon is more common in patients with short stature, hypertension, or after long complex procedures.[7] This problem usually abates by the time the patient reaches the ICU. Generally, the mean pressures at these two sites do correlate, and systolic overshoot from the femoral lines can be eliminated by using resonance overshoot filters.

2. There is often a discrepancy noted between the auscultatory or occlusion blood pressure and that recorded digitally on the bedside monitor. This may be ascribed to the dynamic response characteristics of catheter–transducer systems.[8] The overdampening of signals usually results from gas bubbles within the fluid-filled system. Underdampening of signals is related to excessive compliance, length, or diameter of the tubing connecting the arterial line to the transducer. If the intra-arterial pressure appears to be dampened or exhibits overshoot, the analog display of the mean pressure is most reliable. The occlusion pressure is probably the most accurate measurement of the systolic pressure.

3. Arterial lines should be connected to continuous saline flushes to improve patency rates and minimize thrombus formation. Heparin flushes do not provide any advantage in maintaining line patency and may potentially increase the risk of developing heparin-induced thrombocytopenia, although this association has not been documented in studies of cardiac surgical ICU patients.[9,10]

4. The incidence of complications associated with radial arterial lines, such as digital ischemia or infection, is extremely low, and empiric changing of arterial lines is not mandatory. However, attention must always be directed to perfusion of the hand when a radial arterial line is present, so that prompt therapy can be initiated if problems develop. Digital ischemia can occur within a few days and usually is associated with low output states and use of vasoconstrictive medications. This may then cause thrombosis at the insertion site with distal embolization.[11] This is a serious problem that mandates immediate removal of the arterial line. It usually does not respond to radial revascularization but can be treated with vasodilators to minimize tissue loss. Infections usually respond to removal of the catheter and antibiotics. An infected pseudoaneurysm usually requires surgery.[12]

5. Arterial lines are invaluable for sampling ABG specimens and obtaining blood for other laboratory tests, but they are often retained when invasive pressure monitoring is no longer essential but IV access for blood sampling is limited. Arterial lines should generally be removed when there is no longer a requirement for pharmacologic support and when satisfactory post-extubation ABGs have been achieved. A room-air blood gas before removal may give a baseline assessment of the patient's oxygenation. However, as long as the PaO_2 and oxygen saturation obtained from an ABG are consistent with the SaO_2 measured by pulse oximetry, the latter may then be used to follow the patient's oxygenation. After removal of a femoral arterial catheter, adequate manual pressure should be maintained to produce adequate hemostasis. A falling hematocrit of unclear etiology could result from bleeding into the groin or retroperitoneum from the femoral access site.

D. **Central venous pressure (CVP)** monitoring may provide adequate information about filling pressures in patients with preserved ventricular function undergoing coronary surgery.[13,14] Whereas a low CVP is invariably associated with hypovolemia, a high CVP is consistent with fluid overload, right ventricular (RV) dysfunction (that may be exacerbated by positive-pressure ventilation), severe tricuspid regurgitation, or cardiac tamponade. It is less precise in estimating left-heart filling pressures, especially in patients with left ventricular (LV) hypertrophy or LV dysfunction. Although both elevated CVP and PA pressures measured by a Swan-Ganz catheter are somewhat insensitive to the status of circulatory blood volume and are imprecise in predicting fluid responsiveness, PA catheter monitoring is still widely used to direct management in patients with compromised cardiac function, especially those undergoing valve procedures. An understanding of the patient's underlying heart disease and correlation of filling pressures with intraoperative echocardiographic findings allows for appropriate therapeutic decisions to be made.[15-21] Patients with PA catheters tend to receive more volume than those managed with only CVP lines, with a tendency towards delayed extubation.[15]

E. **Venous oxygen saturation** reflects the balance between oxygen delivery and consumption by the tissues.[22] The mixed venous oxygen saturation (SvO_2) obtained from the distal PA port of a Swan-Ganz catheter has been considered the best means of assessing this balance, and, although subject to many variables, it is generally reflective of the cardiac output.[23] An improvement in SvO_2 with fluid administration generally correlates with increased oxygen delivery to tissues as noted with an improved cardiac output.[24]

1. An inexpensive alternative to the SvO_2 is the central venous oxygen saturation ($ScvO_2$) obtained from a CVP line, which in some studies has been demonstrated to correlate fairly well with SvO_2.[25] However, there is often a significant discrepancy between these two values which reflects variation in regional blood flow, and it is most marked when the SaO_2, hemoglobin, or cardiac index is low.[26,27] Although the SvO_2 is helpful in assessing the cardiac output, the lack of correlation with the $ScvO_2$ demonstrated in several studies suggests that the latter should only be used as a relative means of detecting trends in oxygen extraction.

2. One study of goal-directed therapy (GDT) in moderate- to high-risk patients evaluated whether use of the Vigileo/FloTrac device (see pages 355–356) to measure cardiac outputs along with continuous $ScvO_2$ measurements provided any clinical benefits compared with standard monitoring including a CVP line. GDT resulted in increased volume infusions, more adjustment of inotropic medications, and a decrease in the duration of ventilation, but otherwise, there were few clinical benefits over standard CVP monitoring.[28]

F. **Swan-Ganz pulmonary artery catheters** are commonly placed in patients undergoing open-heart surgery to assist with intraoperative and postoperative hemodynamic management. In some centers, they are used selectively; in others, they are used uniformly to aid with postoperative care. As noted, PA pressure measurements do not have a precise correlation with volume status, but an integration of filling pressures and cardiac output measurements usually can be used to make evidence-based, scientific decisions about fluid, inotropic, or vasopressor support, although their impact on clinical outcome may only be evident in high-risk patients. They are generally placed either prior to or more commonly after the induction of anesthesia and intubation.

1. The basic flow-directed monitoring catheters measure the CVP, the pulmonary artery (PA), and pulmonary capillary wedge (PCW) pressures indicative of left-sided

filling, and allow for the determination of thermodilution cardiac outputs. Blood sampled from the PA port allows for measurement of the SvO_2. Although the correlation of SvO_2 and cardiac output is subject to many variables (see pages 519–520), the SvO_2 is helpful in several clinical situations:

a. To follow trends in oxygen delivery with fluid administration or inotrope use.

b. To corroborate that the thermodilution output is or is not consistent with the patient's clinical course.

c. To obtain a general estimate of cardiac output in patients with tricuspid regurgitation, in whom the thermodilution cardiac output is inaccurate and tends to underestimate the cardiac output.[29,30] This is a situation when a FloTrac is invaluable, unless the patient is in atrial fibrillation.

2. The introducer sheath for a PA catheter (the Cordis) is an 8.5 Fr catheter with a sidearm for volume infusions. In patients with limited access, a Teleflex multilumen access catheter (MAC) with a 12-gauge proximal lumen and a 9 Fr distal lumen is quite helpful.

3. The proximal port of the Swan-Ganz catheter (30 cm from the tip) is used for CVP measurements from the right atrium and for fluid injections to determine the cardiac output. Care must be exercised when injecting sterile fluid for cardiac outputs to prevent bolusing of vasoactive medications that might be running through the CVP port. **Note:** one must **never** infuse anything through this port if the catheter has been pulled back, such that the tip of the catheter lies in the right atrium and the CVP port is not within the bloodstream!

4. The distal port should always be transduced and displayed on the bedside monitor to allow for detection of catheter advancement into the permanent wedge position, which could result in pulmonary artery injury. This will be detected by loss of the phasic PA trace on the monitor and is suggested by the position of the catheter on a chest x-ray. Because the pulmonary artery diastolic (PAD) pressure and pulmonary capillary wedge pressure (PCWP) are fairly similar (the PAD being slightly higher, in the absence of mitral valve pathology, because of the pulmonary vascular resistance) and tend to move in tandem, the PAD can be used as a surrogate for the PCWP for an assessment of LV volumes. Thus, balloon inflation ("wedging" of the catheter) does not need to be performed routinely, if at all. If it is desired to obtain a PCWP measurement, the balloon should not be inflated for more than two respiratory cycles to prevent PA injury. Balloon inflation should be performed cautiously with minimal inflation volume or should be avoided entirely in patients with pulmonary hypertension. Medications should never be given through the distal PA port.

5. The interpretation of hemodynamic parameters derived from the PA catheter requires an understanding of the patient's underlying disease process, filling pressures and cardiac output at baseline and upon weaning from bypass, the nature and extent of the operative procedure, and the effects of surgery on ventricular compliance. Interpretation of these values can be optimized by integrating intraoperative echocardiographic assessments of ventricular volumes and function. The PA catheter provides pressure measurements and the correlation with the left ventricular end-diastolic volume depends on ventricular compliance (i.e. the less compliant the ventricle, the higher the pressure at equal preload).[18] With an understanding that

"normal" hemodynamic measurements vary from patient to patient, a Swan-Ganz catheter can provide invaluable information for patient management by assessing volume status and response to volume infusions, providing an indirect assessment of systolic function and response to vasoactive drug support, and identifying early evidence of ischemia (rising filling pressures).[31]

6. Advanced technology Swan-Ganz catheters available from Edwards Lifesciences (https://www.edwards.com/devices/hemodynamic-monitoring/swan-ganz-catheters) include those that provide continuous cardiac output measurements and those that provide in-line oximetry (SvO$_2$) assessments. These are invaluable during off-pump bypass surgery. The most sophisticated catheters in the CCOmbo series used with the Vigilance II monitor can measure preload (right atrial pressure, PA diastolic and wedge pressures, and right-ventricular end-diastolic volume), calculate afterload (SVR), and assess contractility by assessing the stroke volume index and RVEF. There are also thermodilution Swan-Ganz Paceport catheters available.

7. Although there is a significant incidence of minor complications associated with the insertion and use of the Swan-Ganz catheter, serious life-threatening complications are very uncommon. The catheter is more commonly placed through the internal jugular vein than the subclavian vein for cardiac surgery, as the catheter may become displaced during sternal retraction with the latter approach.[32] Using ultrasound imaging with an echo probe to identify the location of the internal jugular vein is helpful in avoiding arterial puncture (Figure 4.2, page 222).

   a. Complications associated with insertion include:
      • Arrhythmias and heart block (especially in patients with a left bundle branch block)

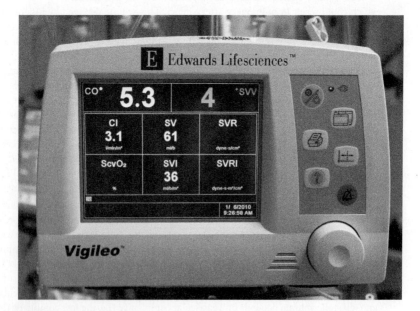

Figure 7.2 • The Edwards Vigileo FloTrac continuous cardiac output monitor, which is connected to the arterial line.

- Arterial puncture
- Pneumothorax
- Air embolism
- Perforation of the right atrium or ventricle
- Catheter knotting

b. Complications of indwelling PA catheters include:

- Arrhythmias and heart block
- Heparin-induced thrombocytopenia (from heparin-coated catheters)
- Infection
- Pulmonary artery rupture and hemorrhage; pulmonary pseudoaneurysms
- Endocardial and valvular damage
- Pulmonary infarction
- Pulmonary infiltrates
- Venous thrombosis

8. Pulmonary artery perforation is a very serious complication that may occur during insertion of the catheter, during surgery, or at any time in the ICU.[33–35] The position of the catheter should always be inspected on an immediate postoperative or any postinsertion chest x-ray. Migration of the catheter into the wedge position should be evident by dampening of the PA tracing on the bedside monitor, and the catheter should be pulled back immediately. Perforation may lead to hemoptysis, bleeding into the endotracheal tube, or intrapleural hemorrhage. The chest x-ray may demonstrate a hematoma surrounding the tip of the catheter. If perforation is suspected, the catheter should be withdrawn and positive end-expiratory pressure (PEEP) added to the ventilator circuit. If bleeding persists, bronchoscopy can be performed with placement of a bronchial blocker to isolate the lung. Use of a double-lumen endotracheal tube or even a thoracotomy with pulmonary resection may be indicated for ongoing pulmonary hemorrhage. Rarely, a false aneurysm of the pulmonary artery branches may develop. This has been treated by transcatheter embolization.[36] The management of pulmonary artery perforation occurring during surgery is discussed on pages 224–225.

G. **Cardiac output monitoring.** Although the flow-directed Swan-Ganz catheter is the gold standard for measuring cardiac outputs intra- and postoperatively, it is an invasive catheter associated with a number of potential complications. Similarly, the Edwards CCO and CCOmbo series are helpful during and after off-pump surgery and can provide additional information. Alternative, less-invasive means of determining the cardiac output may also be useful, and their correlation with thermodilution cardiac outputs is fairly good.[37–42]

1. Of particular value in cardiac surgery is the Edwards Vigileo/FloTrac device, which performs an analysis of the pressure wave signal from the arterial line, correlates the standard deviation of the pulse pressure with the stroke volume using patient demographic data, adjusts for vascular compliance, and then provides continuous cardiac output calculations (Figure 7.2). This is very valuable when a Swan-Ganz catheter has not been placed, is not functioning well, provides cardiac output values that appear inconsistent with the patient's clinical picture, or when moderate-severe tricuspid regurgitation is present. Readings are inaccurate during

conditions of hemodynamic instability or arrhythmias, such as atrial fibrillation or frequent ventricular ectopy. During off-pump surgery, it is extremely helpful in assessing cardiac function when the heart is displaced for posterior anastomoses or when significant ischemia occurs.[40] The correlation with thermodilution cardiac outputs is reasonably accurate.[41–46]

2. A number of other systems using pulse contour or pulse wave velocity analysis, bioimpedance, and esophageal Doppler have been developed to determine cardiac output less invasively. Their role in cardiac surgery patients has been somewhat limited.[37,38,47,48]

H. **Left atrial (LA) lines** can be used in special circumstances to give the most accurate assessment of left-sided filling pressures. They are placed through the right superior pulmonary vein and passed into the left atrium during surgery.

1. LA lines are particularly helpful in patients with high transpulmonary gradients, in whom the PAD pressure is significantly greater than true left-sided filling pressures. They may be used in patients with severe LV dysfunction, severe pulmonary hypertension secondary to mitral valve disease, during use of circulatory assist devices, or following heart transplantation.

2. Although LA lines may provide important hemodynamic information, they are associated with rare but potentially significant complications.[49,50] An LA line should always be considered dangerous because of the risk of air embolism. It must always be aspirated before being flushed to make sure there is no air or thrombus present within the system. It is then connected to a constant infusion flush line that includes an air filter to reduce the risk of systemic air embolism. The line should be removed when the chest tubes are still in place in the event of bleeding from the insertion site.

I. **Chest tubes** are placed in the mediastinum and into the pleural spaces if they are entered during surgery. Straight and right-angled 32 Fr PVC or silicone-coated chest tubes are placed in the mediastinum, either two anteriorly or one anteriorly and one below the heart. The latter should be tacked by the surgeon away from inferior wall grafts, as compression could lead to inferior ischemia, which should be evident on a postoperative ECG. Pleural tubes can be placed subcostally or through the lateral chest wall. The latter may produce more chest wall pain with more impairment of pulmonary function, but theoretically are less likely to contribute to mediastinal infection if left in place for a prolonged period of time.[51–53] Use of silicone fluted Blake drains (J & J Medical Devices) or even Jackson-Pratt silicone or PVC drains (CardinalHealth) has been reported to have equal if not better effectiveness in reducing residual pericardial effusions and the risk of atrial fibrillation, and are more comfortable for the patient.[54–56]

1. Drainage should be recorded every 15 minutes and then less frequently once mediastinal bleeding tapers to minimal levels. The chest tubes are connected to a drainage system to which –20 cm of H_2O suction is applied. The tubes should be gently milked or stripped to prevent blood from clotting within them. There is no particular advantage of any of the common practices (milking, stripping, fanfolding, or tapping) in maintaining chest tube patency.[57–59] Aggressive stripping creates a negative pressure of up to –300 cm H_2O in the mediastinum. This may actually increase bleeding and is quite painful to a patient who has regained consciousness and is not adequately sedated. Suctioning of clotted chest tubes with endotracheal suction catheters is discouraged in the ICU because of the risk of introducing infection.

This has led to the development of a silicone chest tube system with a clearance apparatus that allows for advancement of a loop over a guidewire into the chest tube to break up and extract clot (Pleuraflow ACT, ClearFlow Inc.).[60]

2. Bloody drainage through chest tubes can be best observed if the tubes are not completely covered with tape. Plastic connectors must be tightly and securely attached to both the chest tubes and the drainage tubing to maintain sterility and prevent air leaks within the system. Although an air leak should always raise the possibility of a pulmonary parenchymal leak, the connections should be checked first since a loose connection or disconnection is an easily remediable problem. The development of subcutaneous emphysema may reflect an active air leak with clotted chest tubes, but more frequently is the result of kinking of the tubes.

3. Excessive mediastinal bleeding requires immediate attention because it often leads to hemodynamic instability, metabolic acidosis, the requirement for multiple blood products, and the potential for cardiac tamponade (see Chapter 9).

4. Autotransfusion of shed mediastinal blood can be used as a component of a blood conservation strategy, but its benefits are controversial. It provides volume expansion with the potential for reducing transfusion requirements. However, shed blood also has a low level of platelets, fibrinogen, and factor VIII and a high level of fibrin split products.[61] Although reinfusion in moderate amounts (less than 1 L) does not significantly alter coagulation parameters, larger amounts may.[62] If the patient has bled that much, re-exploration is probably indicated. Autotransfusion can be accomplished either from soft plastic collection bags or directly from the plastic shell via a pump through a 20–40 μm filter.

J. The **urinary Foley catheter** is attached to gravity drainage and the urine output is recorded hourly. Urine output is subject to many variables, but in a patient with normal renal function, it generally reflects the level of renal perfusion, which may be compromised in a low cardiac output state.

1. Foley catheters incorporating temperature probes are commonly used during surgery and can be used in the ICU to record the patient's core temperature.

2. The Foley catheter is usually removed at midnight entering the second postoperative day.[63] It may be left in place if the patient is undergoing a significant diuresis or has a history of prostatic hypertrophy or urinary retention and has not been mobilized. Although earlier removal is associated with a higher risk of voiding problems, it does reduce the risk of developing a urinary tract infection, which is related to the duration of indwelling catheter time. Thus, early removal should be considered in patients with prosthetic valves and grafts when its use is no longer essential.

3. Suprapubic tubes should be left in place and clamped after several days to see if the patient can void per urethra.

K. **Nasogastric tubes** or orogastric tubes may be inserted in the operating room or after the patient's arrival in the ICU to aid with gastric decompression. Insertion may cause hypertension, bradycardia, tachycardia, or arrhythmias if the patient is not well sedated. Insertion may also cause nasopharyngeal bleeding if the patient is still heparinized (during surgery) or has a coagulopathy. Instillation of a medication to reduce stress ulceration, such as sucralfate, should be considered for all patients during the first 12–24 hours. Proton-pump inhibitors are preferred for patients at high risk for stress-ulcer-related bleeding, and may provide some benefit to any patient taking aspirin, a P2Y12 inhibitor, warfarin, or non-vitamin K antagonist oral anticoagulant (NOAC) soon after surgery, which basically includes all patients undergoing cardiac surgery.[64,65]

L. **Pacing wires.** Most surgeons place two atrial and two ventricular temporary epicardial pacing wire electrodes at the conclusion of open-heart surgery. If the pacing wires are being used, they must be securely attached to the patient and to the cable connector, and the cable must be securely attached to the pacing box. The pacemaker box itself should be easily accessible. **Everyone caring for the patient should understand how the particular pacemaker generator works and what the current pacemaker settings are.** Pacing wires that are not being used should be placed in insulating needle caps to isolate them from stray electrical currents that could potentially trigger arrhythmias. Particular issues of concern are pacing thresholds in patients with complete heart block and no escape mechanism, and inappropriate sensing and pacing that could trigger malignant arrhythmias. Issues regarding pacing wire removal are discussed on pages 609 and 758.

III. Summary of Guidelines for Removal of Lines and Tubes in the ICU

A. The Swan-Ganz catheter should be removed when inotropic support and vasodilators are no longer necessary. If central venous access is required after several days but hemodynamic monitoring is no longer essential, the Swan-Ganz catheter can be replaced by a double- or triple-lumen catheter. Alternatively, a peripherally inserted central catheter (PICC) line can be placed. If the Swan-Ganz catheter is removed but the introducer sheath is left in place for fluid or medication administration, the port must be covered with a small adhesive drape to minimize the risk of infection. A one-way valve present on most introducer sheaths eliminates the possibility of air embolism. The introducer should be removed as soon as possible because of its size to minimize the risk of infection and venous thrombosis (let alone patient discomfort).

B. Any central line should be removed when no longer necessary, to reduce the risk of infection. If central access is indicated but the patient has a fever of unknown origin or suspected bacteremia, the catheter should be removed and cultured, and another catheter inserted in a different site. If neither of these indications is present, the catheter can be changed over a guidewire to reduce the risk of mechanical complications associated with a new insertion. The catheter tip should still be cultured, and if this returns positive, the catheter should be changed to a new site.[66,67] If the patient has very poor peripheral access but needs continued IV access, a PICC line through an upper arm vein is useful.

C. An additional ABG obtained on room air is frequently worthwhile because it provides a relative indication of the patient's baseline postoperative oxygenation and it can be correlated with the SaO_2 measured by pulse oximetry. Subsequently, the latter may be used to follow the patient's oxygenation. The arterial line should not be left in place as a convenience for blood sampling. Adequate pressure should be maintained over the groin upon removal of a femoral arterial catheter. Early removal of femoral artery catheters enables the patient to be mobilized out of bed.

D. LA lines must be removed in the ICU with the chest tubes remaining in place in the event that intrapericardial bleeding occurs.

E. The urinary catheter can be left in place if the patient is undergoing a vigorous diuresis or has an increased risk of urinary retention. It should otherwise be removed once the patient is mobilized out of bed, usually at midnight entering the second postoperative day.

F. Chest tubes should be removed when the total drainage is less than 100 mL for eight hours.

1. Serous drainage related to fluid overload will usually taper with additional diuresis. One study found that prolonging the duration of drainage may increase total chest-tube output without any effect on the incidence of postoperative pericardial effusions.[68] Another showed that there was no difference in the incidence of pericardial effusions if tubes were withdrawn when drainage was less than 50 mL over five hours or when the fluid became serosanguineous (either upon visual inspection or when the drain:blood hematocrit ratio was <0.3).[69] However, another study did find that leaving chest tubes in at least until the second postoperative day and removing them only after the drainage was <50 mL/4 h more than halved the incidence of delayed tamponade.[70]

2. Generally, there is a potential advantage and little downside to leaving mediastinal chest tubes in for a few additional days if there is evidence of persistent serosanguineous drainage. Additionally, leaving a supplemental drain in the pleural space for 3–5 days is useful in reducing the incidence of symptomatic pleural effusions. If this is contemplated at the time of surgery, this tube should preferably be placed through the lateral chest wall, although it may cause the patient more discomfort and adversely affect pulmonary function.[51–53,71]

3. Mediastinal tubes should **always be removed off suction**, because graft avulsion might theoretically occur if suction is maintained. A chest x-ray is not essential after mediastinal tube removal, but it should be performed after removal of pleural chest tubes to check for the development of a pneumothorax.

References

1. Dixon JL, Staff HW, Wehbe-Janek H, Jo C, Culp WC Jr, Shake JG. A standard handoff improves cardiac surgical patient transfer: operating room to intensive care unit. *J Healthc Qual* 2015;37:22–32.

2. Stephens RS, Whitman GJR. Postoperative critical care of the adult cardiac surgical patient: part I: routine postoperative care. *Crit Care Med* 2015;43:1477–97.

3. Bierman MI, Stein KL, Snyder JV. Pulse oximetry in the postoperative care of cardiac surgical patients: a randomized controlled trial. *Chest* 1992;102:1367–70.

4. Durbin CG Jr, Rostow SK. More reliable oximetry reduces the frequency of arterial blood gas analyses and hastens oxygen weaning after cardiac surgery: a prospective randomized trial of the clinical impact of a new technology. *Crit Care Med* 2002;30:1735–40.

5. Guglielminotti J, Desmonts JM, Dureuil B. Effects of tracheal suctioning on respiratory resistances in mechanically ventilated patients. *Chest* 1999;113:1135–8.

6. Haddad F, Zeeni C, El Rassi I, et al. Can femoral artery pressure monitoring be used routinely in cardiac surgery? *J Cardiothorac Vasc Anesth* 2008;22:418–22.

7. Bouchard-Dechêne V, Couture P, Su A, et al. Risk factors for radial-to-femoral artery pressure gradient in patients undergoing cardiac surgery with cardiopulmonary bypass. *J Cardiothorac Vasc Anesth* 2018;32:692–8.

8. Gibbs NC, Gardner RM. Dynamics of invasive pressure monitoring systems: clinical and laboratory evaluation. *Heart Lung* 1988;17:43–51.

9. Whitta RK, Hall KF, Bennetts TM, Welman L, Rawlins P. Comparison of normal or heparinised saline flushing on function of arterial lines. *Crit Care Resusc* 2006;8:205–8.

10. Hall KF, Bennetts TM, Whitta RK, Welman L, Rawlins P. Effect of heparin in arterial line flushing solutions on platelet count: a randomised double-blind study. *Crit Care Resusc* 2006;8:294–6.

11. Valentine RJ, Modrall JG, Clagett GP. Hand ischemia after radial artery cannulation. *J Am Coll Surg* 2005;201:18–22.

12. El-Hamamsy I, Dürrleman N, Stevens LM, et al. Incidence and outcome of radial artery infections following cardiac surgery. *Ann Thorac Surg* 2003;76:801–4.

13. Stewart RD, Psyhojos T, Lahey SJ, Levitsky S, Campos CT. Central venous catheter use in low-risk coronary artery bypass grafting. *Ann Thorac Surg* 1998;66:1306–11.

14. Schwann TA, Zacharias A, Riordan CJ, Durham SJ, Engoren M, Habib RH. Safe, highly selective use of pulmonary artery catheters in coronary artery bypass grafting: an objective patient selection method. *Ann Thorac Surg* 2002;73:1394–401.

15. Yamauchi H, Biuk-Aghai EN, Yu M, et al. Circulating blood volume measurements correlate poorly with pulmonary artery catheter measurements. *Hawaii Med J* 2008;67:8–11.

16. Breukers RM, Trof RJ, de Wilde RB, et al. Relative value of pressures and volumes in assessing fluid responsiveness after valvular and coronary artery surgery. *Eur J Cardiothorac Surg* 2009;35:62–8.

17. Buhre W, Weyland A, Schorn B, et al. Changes in central venous pressure and pulmonary capillary wedge pressure do not indicate changes in right and left heart volume in patients undergoing coronary artery bypass surgery. *Eur J Anesthesiol* 1999;16:11–7.

18. Reddy YN, El-Sabbagh A, Nishimura RA. Comparing pulmonary arterial wedge pressure and left ventricular end diastolic pressure for assessment of left-sided filling pressures. *JAMA Cardiol* 2018;3:453–4.

19. Hoeft AM, Schorn B, Weyland A, et al. Bedside assessment of intravascular volume status in patients undergoing coronary bypass surgery. *Anesthesiology* 1994;81:76–86.

20. St. André AC, DelRossi A. Hemodynamic management of patients in the first 24 hours after cardiac surgery. *Crit Care Med* 2005;33:2082–93.

21 Li P, Qu LP, Qi D, et al. Significance of perioperative goal-directed hemodynamic approach in preventing postoperative complications in patients after cardiac surgery: a meta-analysis and systematic review. *Ann Med* 2017;49:342–51.

22. Shepherd SJ, Pearse RM. Role of central and mixed venous oxygen saturation measurement in perioperative care. *Anesthesiology* 2009;111:649–56.

23. Sommers MS, Stevenson JS, Hamlin RL, Ivey TD, Russell AC. Mixed venous oxygen saturation and oxygen partial pressure as predictors of cardiac index after coronary artery bypass grafting. *Heart Lung* 1993;22:112–20.

24. Kuiper AN, Troff RJ, Groeneveld ABJ. Mixed venous O_2 saturation and fluid responsiveness after cardiac or major vascular surgery. *J Cardiothorac Surg* 2013;8:189.

25. Ramakrisha MN, Hegde DP, Kumaraswamy GN, Gupta R, Girish TN. Correlation of mixed venous and central venous oxygen saturation and its relation to cardiac index. *Indian J Crit Care Med* 2006;10:230–4.

26. Yazigi A, El Khoury C, Jebara S, Haddad F, Hayeck G, Sleilaty G. Comparison of central venous to mixed venous oxygen saturation in patients with low cardiac index and filling pressures after coronary artery surgery. *J Cardiothorac Vasc Anesth* 2008;22:77–83.

27. Lorentzen AG, Lindskov C, Sloth E, Jakobsen CJ. Central venous oxygen saturation cannot replace mixed venous saturation in patients undergoing cardiac surgery. *J Cardiothorac Vasc Anesth* 2008;22:853–7.

28. Kapoor PM, Kakani M, Chowdhury U, Choudhury M, Lakshmy R, Kiran U. Early goal-directed therapy in moderate to high-risk cardiac surgery patients. *Ann Card Anaesth* 2008;11:27–34.

29. Balik M, Pachl J, Hendl J. Effect of the degree of tricuspid regurgitation on cardiac output measurements by thermodilution. *Intensive Care Med* 2002;28:1117–21.

30. Heerdt PM, Blessios GA, Beach ML, Hogue CW. Flow dependency of error in thermodilution measurement of cardiac output during acute tricuspid regurgitation. *J Cardiothorac Vasc Anesth* 2001;15:183–7.

31. Mark JB. Multimodal detection of perioperative myocardial ischemia. *Tex Heart Inst J* 2005;32: 461–6.
32. Ruesch S, Walder B, Tramèr MR. Complications of central venous catheters: internal jugular versus subclavian access: a systematic review. *Crit Care Med* 2002;30:454–60.
33. Mullerworth MH, Angelopoulos P, Couyant MA, et al. Recognition and management of catheter-induced pulmonary artery rupture. *Ann Thorac Surg* 1998;66:1242–5.
34. Bossert T, Gummert JF, Bittner HB, et al. Swan-Ganz catheter-induced severe complications in cardiac surgery: right ventricular perforation, knotting, and rupture of the pulmonary artery. *J Card Surg* 2006;21:292–5.
35. Abreu AR, Campos MA, Krieger BP. Pulmonary artery rupture induced by a pulmonary artery catheter: a case report and review of the literature. *J Intensive Care Med* 2004;19:291–6.
36. Karak P, Dimick R, Hamrick KM, Schwartzberg M, Saddekni S. Immediate transcatheter embolization of Swan-Ganz catheter-induced pulmonary artery pseudoaneurysm. *Chest* 1997;111:1450–2.
37. Arora D, Mehta Y. Recent trends on hemodynamic monitoring in cardiac surgery. *Ann Card Anaesth* 2016;19:580–3.
38. Thiele RH, Bartels K, Gan TJ. Cardiac output monitoring; a contemporary assessment and review. *Crit Care Med* 2015;43:177–85.
39. Imakiire N, Omae T, Matsunaga A, Sakata R, Kanmura Y. Can a NICO monitor substitute for thermodilution to measure cardiac output in patients with coexisting tricuspid regurgitation? *J Anesth* 2010;24:511–7.
40. Mehta YM, Chand RK, Sawhney R, Bhise M, Singh A, Trehan N. Cardiac output monitoring: comparison of a new arterial pressure waveform analysis to the bolus thermodilution technique in patients undergoing off-pump coronary artery bypass surgery. *J Cardiothorac Vasc Anesth* 2008;22:394–9.
41. Breukers RM, Sepehrkhouy S, Speigelenberg SR, Groeneveld ABJ. Cardiac output measured by a new arterial pressure waveform analysis method without calibration compared with thermodilution after cardiac surgery. *J Cardiothorac Vasc Anesth* 2007;21:632–5.
42. Maus TM, Lee DE. Arterial pressure-based cardiac output assessment. *J Cardiothorac Vasc Anesth* 2008;22:468–73.
43. Senn A, Button D, Zollinger A, Hofer CK. Assessment of cardiac output changes using a modified FloTrac/Vigileo algorithm in cardiac surgery patients. *Crit Care* 2009;13:R32.
44. Peyton PJ, Chong SW. Minimally invasive measurement of cardiac output during surgery and critical care: a meta-analysis of accuracy and precision. *Anesthesiology* 2010;113:1220–35.
45. Ham JB, Nguyen BV, Kiss G, et al. Assessment of a cardiac output device using arterial pulse waveform analysis, Vigileo, in cardiac surgery compared to pulmonary artery thermodilution. *Anaesth Intensive Care* 2010;38:295–301.
46. Zimmermann A, Kufner C, Hofbauer S, et al. The accuracy of the Vigileo/FloTrac continuous cardiac output monitor. *J Cardiothorac Vasc Anesth* 2002;22:388–93.
47. DiCorte CJ, Latham P, Greilich PE, Cooley MV, Grayburn PA, Jessen ME. Esophageal Doppler monitor determinations of cardiac output and preload during cardiac operations. *Ann Thorac Surg* 2000;69:1782–6.
48. Bein B, Worthmann F, Tonner PH, et al. Comparison of esophageal Doppler, pulse contour analysis, and real-time pulmonary artery thermodilution for the continuous measurement of cardiac output. *J Cardiothorac Vasc Anesth* 2004;18:185–9.
49. Santini F, Gatti G, Borghetti V, Oppido G, Mazzucco A. Routine left atrial catheterization for the post-operative management of cardiac surgical patients: is the risk justified? *Eur J Cardiothorac Surg* 1999;16:218–21.
50. Feerick AE, Church JA, Zwischenberger J, Conti V, Johnston WE. Systemic gaseous microembolism during left atrial catheterization: a common occurrence? *J Cardiothorac Vasc Anesth* 1995;9:395–8.
51. Guden M, Korkmaz AA, Onan B, Onan IS, Tarakci SI, Fidan F. Subxiphoid versus intercostal chest tubes: comparison of postoperative pain and pulmonary morbidities after coronary artery bypass grafting. *Tex Heart Inst J* 2012;39:507–12.
52. Hagl C, Harringer W, Gohrbandt B, Haverich A. Site of pleural drain insertion and early postoperative pulmonary function following coronary artery bypass grafting with the internal mammary artery. *Chest* 1999;115:757–61.

53. Guizilini S, Viceconte M, Esperanca GT, et al. Pleural subxyphoid drain confers better pulmonary function and clinical outcomes in chronic obstructive pulmonary disease after off-pump coronary artery bypass grafting: a randomized controlled trial. *Rev Bras Cir Cardiovasc* 2014;29:588–92.

54. Sakopoulous AG, Hurwitz AS, Suda RW, Goodwin JN. Efficacy of Blake drains for mediastinal and pleural drainage following cardiac operations. *J Card Surg* 2005;20:574–7.

55. Ege T, Tatli E, Canbaz S, et al. The importance of intrapericardial drain selection in cardiac surgery. *Chest* 2004;126:1559–62.

56. Mirmohammad-Sadeghi M, Pourazari P, Akbari M. Comparison consequences of Jackson-Pratt drain versus chest tube after coronary artery bypass grafting: a randomized controlled clinical trial. *J Res Med Sci* 2017;22:134.

57. Wallen M, Morrison A, Gillies D, O'Riordan E, Bridge C, Stoddart F. Mediastinal chest drain clearance for cardiac surgery. *Cochrane Database Syst Rev* 2004;4:CD003042. https://doi.org/10.1002/14651858.CD003042.pub2.

58. Day TG, Perring RR, Gofton K. Is manipulation of mediastinal chest drains useful or harmful after cardiac surgery? *Interact Cardiovasc Thorac Surg* 2008;7:888–90.

59. Charnock Y, Evans D. Nursing management of chest drains: a systematic review. *Aust Crit Care* 2001;14:156–60.

60. Vistarini N, Gabrysz-Forget F, Beaulieu Y, Perrault LP. Tamponade relief by active clearance of chest tubes. *Ann Thorac Surg* 2016;101:1159–63.

61. Hartz RS, Smith JA, Green D. Autotransfusion after cardiac operation: assessment of hemostatic factors. *J Thorac Cardiovasc Surg* 1988;96:178–82.

62. Marberg H, Jeppsson A, Brandrup-Wognsen G. Postoperative autotransfusion of mediastinal shed blood does not influence haemostasis after elective coronary artery bypass grafting. *Eur J Cardiothorac Surg* 2010;38:767–72.

63. Griffiths R, Fernandez R. Strategies for the removal of short-term indwelling urethral catheters in adults. *Cochrane Database Syst Rev* 2007;2:CD004011. https://doi.org/10.1002/14651858.CD004011.pub3.

64. Shin JS, Abah U. Is routine stress ulcer prophylaxis of benefit for patients undergoing cardiac surgery? *Interact Cardiovasc Thorac Surg* 2012;14:622–8.

65. Patel AJ, Som R. What is the optimum prophylaxis against gastrointestinal haemorrhage for patients undergoing adult cardiac surgery: histamine receptor antagonists, or proton-pump inhibitors? *Interact Cardiovasc Thorac Surg* 2013;16:356–60.

66. Cobb DK, High KP, Sawyer RG, et al. A controlled trial of scheduled replacement of central venous and pulmonary-artery catheters. *N Engl J Med* 1992;327:1062–8.

67. Hagley MT, Martin B, Gast P, Traeger SM. Infectious and mechanical complications of central venous catheters placed by percutaneous venipuncture and over guidewires. *Crit Care Med* 1992;20:1426–30.

68. Smulders YM, Wiepking ME, Moulijn AC, Koolen JJ, van Wezel HB, Visser CA. How soon should drainage tubes be removed after cardiac operations? *Ann Thorac Surg* 1989;48:540–3.

69. Gercekoglu H, Aydin NB, Dagdeviren B, et al. Effect of timing of chest tube removal on development of pericardial effusion following cardiac surgery. *J Card Surg* 2003;18:217–24.

70. Khan J, Khan N, Mannander A. Lower incidence of late tamponade after cardiac surgery by extended chest tube drainage. *Scand Cardiovasc J* 2019;53:104–9.

71. Payne M, Magovern GJ Jr, Benckart DH, et al. Left pleural effusion after coronary artery bypass decreases with a supplemental pleural drain. *Ann Thorac Surg* 2002;73:149–52.

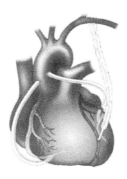

CHAPTER 8

Early Postoperative Care

♡ 8 Early Postoperative Care

The early postoperative course for most patients undergoing cardiac surgery with use of cardiopulmonary bypass (CPB) is characterized by a typical pattern of pathophysiologic derangements that benefits from standardized management.[1] CPB is associated with a systemic inflammatory response that causes systemic vasodilatation and a capillary leak, which, along with hemodilution from a crystalloid prime, leads to total body volume overload. Use of CPB causes a dilutional and functional coagulopathy, and cardioplegic arrest may cause transient myocardial depression. Intraoperative monitoring to assess filling pressures and transesophageal echocardiography (TEE) are used to direct hemodynamic management and fluid administration upon termination of CPB. Anesthetic techniques and early extubation protocols should be designed to achieve "fast-track" recovery of most patients (Table 8.1).[2] The pathophysiology noted after off-pump surgery is slightly different in that patients are not subjected to the insults of CPB and cardioplegic arrest. This chapter will summarize the basic clinical features of the post-CPB patient and will then present scenarios commonly seen in the early postoperative period. It will then discuss aspects of postoperative care unique to various types of cardiac surgery, including off-pump and catheter-based procedures. The subsequent chapters will describe in greater detail the assessment and management of the major concerns of the postoperative period: mediastinal bleeding and respiratory, cardiovascular, renal, and metabolic problems.

I. Basic Features of the Early Postoperative Period

A. Overview

1. Following most cardiac procedures, patients arrive in the intensive care unit (ICU) fully anesthetized and sedated, requiring mechanical ventilation for several hours. Considerations during transfer to the ICU and a discussion of ICU monitoring techniques are presented in Chapter 7.[3] Adequate pharmacologic sedation and pain control are essential at this time and during the weaning process from the ventilator, which generally should be started once standard criteria are met (Table 10.3, page 475). Early extubation is usually defined as withdrawal of mechanical ventilation within six hours of surgery, and many protocols are designed to achieve "ultra-fast" extubation within a few hours.

2. Extubation can be accomplished at the conclusion of surgery following both on- and off-pump surgery.[4,5] After extubation, the blood pressure may be higher due to increased sympathetic tone and less vasodilation from sedatives (i.e. propofol, dexmedetomidine, and morphine). Right ventricular (RV) function may be improved when positive-pressure ventilation is not required. However, it is important to provide adequate analgesia at this time without producing respiratory depression,

Manual of Perioperative Care in Adult Cardiac Surgery, Sixth Edition. Robert M. Bojar.
© 2021 John Wiley & Sons Ltd. Published 2021 by John Wiley & Sons Ltd.

Table 8.1 • Options for a Fast-track Protocol

Operating Room

Anesthetic agents	Fentanyl 5–10 µg/kg, then 0.3–5 µg/kg/h Inhalational agents + low-dose opiates, then propofol or dexmedetomidine Remifentanil 1 µg/kg for induction, then 0.05–2 µg/kg/min
Sedatives	Midazolam 2.5–5 mg before bypass Propofol 25–75 µg/kg/min (2–10 mg/kg/h) after bypass Dexmedetomidine 1 mg/kg over 10 minutes followed by a continuous infusion of 0.2–1.5 µg/kg/h
Cardiopulmonary bypass	Withdrawal of autologous blood before starting bypass Consider retrograde autologous priming to maintain higher hematocrit Echo imaging for aortic atherosclerosis Maintain blood glucose <180 mg/dL Warm to slightly less than 37 °C before terminating bypass
Myocardial protection	Antegrade/retrograde blood cardioplegia with terminal "hot shot"
Antifibrinolytic agents	ε-aminocaproic acid 5 g at skin incision and in pump prime, and 1 g/h infusion Tranexamic acid 10 mg/kg, then 1 mg/kg/h
Fluids	Minimize fluid administration
Other medications	Amiodarone 150 mg IV over 30 minutes, then continue as an infusion in the ICU for 24 hours Methylprednisolone 1 g before bypass, then dexamethasone 4 mg q6h × 4 doses

Intensive Care Unit

Analgesia	Morphine as small boluses or an infusion of 0.01–0.02 mg/kg/h depending on age Ketorolac 15–30 mg IV after extubation × 72 hours Acetaminophen 650 mg IV
Anxiolysis	Propofol 25 µg/kg/min Dexmedetomidine 1 mg/kg over 10 minutes followed by a continuous infusion of 0.2–1.5 µg/kg/h (if not started in the OR)
Shivering	Meperidine 25–50 mg IV
Hypertension	Sodium nitroprusside/clevidipine/esmolol (avoid sedatives)
Anemia	Tolerate hematocrit of 22% if stable
Other medications	Metoprolol by POD #1 (AF prophylaxis) Magnesium sulfate 2 g on POD #1 (AF prophylaxis) Consider amiodarone for AF prophylaxis

generally using nonsteroidal anti-inflammatory drugs (NSAIDs), intravenous (IV) acetaminophen, or low doses of narcotics.

3. Ventricular function is commonly compromised for several hours following operations on CPB with cardioplegic arrest.[6] Inotropic medications may be required for postcardiotomy hemodynamic support during this time as the heart recovers from the insult imposed by ischemia and reperfusion. Furthermore, diastolic function is impaired with reduced compliance. Therefore, volume administration to achieve satisfactory preload will require higher filling pressures than noted preoperatively.

4. Urine output may be copious because of hemodilution during surgery. However, even though the patient is total body fluid overloaded, fluid administration is usually necessary to maintain intravascular volume to optimize hemodynamic status. Hypokalemia associated with excellent urine output must be monitored and treated. Renal function is generally a good marker of hemodynamic function, although it is subject to numerous variables. Consequently, an initial good urine output may be noted despite poor cardiac function, but a low urine output is of more concern.

5. Hyperglycemia is commonly noted, even in nondiabetic patients, and the blood sugar should be maintained at <180 mg/dL using intravenous insulin protocols (see Appendix 6).

6. Patients may have mediastinal bleeding as a result of surgical issues or a coagulopathy, and careful monitoring of chest tube drainage is essential. Blood or blood product transfusions may be indicated for profound anemia or ongoing bleeding.

7. Postoperative care requires an integration of a myriad of hemodynamic measurements and laboratory tests to ensure a swift and uneventful recovery from surgery. Use of a comprehensive handwritten or computerized flowsheet is essential in evaluating the patient's course in the ICU.

B. **Warming from hypothermia to 37 °C**

1. Hypothermia (<36 °C) upon admission to the ICU has been associated with adverse outcomes.[7] Therefore, it is imperative that adequate rewarming be performed prior to termination of CPB, since the temperature at that time correlates best with core temperature at the time of arrival in the ICU.[8] Hypothermia upon arrival to the ICU must be actively treated since it may:

   a. Predispose to atrial and ventricular arrhythmias and lower the ventricular fibrillation threshold

   b. Produce peripheral vasoconstriction, increasing the systemic vascular resistance (SVR). This will elevate filling pressures, masking hypovolemia, increase afterload, raising myocardial oxygen demand, and often cause hypertension, potentially increasing mediastinal bleeding.

   c. Precipitate shivering, which increases peripheral O_2 consumption and CO_2 production

   d. Produce platelet dysfunction and a generalized impairment of the coagulation cascade

   e. Prolong the duration of action of anesthetic drugs and prolong the time to extubation[9]

   f. Increase the risk of wound infection, possibly related to immunosuppression

2. CPB for most nonaortic surgery is usually accompanied by mild systemic hypothermia to 33–35 °C and is terminated after the patient has been rewarmed to a core

body temperature of at least 36.5 °C. Although it is common practice to warm patients to 37 °C before terminating bypass, this may require higher arterial inflow temperatures and may be associated with impairment in neurocognitive function.[10] The brain temperature is several degrees warmer than the nasopharyngeal temperature during rewarming, suggesting that temperatures measured at other sites may underestimate the degree of cerebral hyperthermia. Even the rectum and bladder, two commonly monitored sites considered to represent the core temperature, are in an "intermediate compartment" where the temperature is close, but not identical, to core temperature. Thus, although hypothermia has potential adverse effects, aggressive "overwarming" during CPB may also prove detrimental.

3. Despite adequate core rewarming on pump, progressive hypothermia may ensue in the post-pump period when the chest is still open and hemostasis is being achieved (so-called temperature afterdrop). This results from insufficient rewarming of peripheral tissues that leaves a significant temperature gradient between the core temperature and the periphery. Thus, heat is subsequently redistributed to the periphery, resulting in a gradual reduction in core temperature. Heat loss is further exacerbated by continued intraoperative heat loss from exposure to cool ambient temperatures in the operating room, poor peripheral perfusion, administration of cold blood products or room-temperature fluids, and anesthetic-induced inhibition of normal thermoregulatory control.

4. Prevention of temperature afterdrop can be achieved by prolonging the warming phase on CPB, warming the periphery, warming blood products before administration, or using pharmacologic vasodilation. Increasing the ambient air temperature to a tolerable level for the surgeon is helpful, especially in patients undergoing off-pump surgery. In these patients, the use of the Kimberly-Clark temperature-management system[11] or a cutaneous forced-air warming device, such as the Bair Hugger (3M), is helpful in avoiding hypothermia (Figure 8.1). These devices are also very helpful in preventing temperature afterdrop when deep hypothermic circulatory arrest (DHCA) is used, but they cannot actively warm the patient or reduce redistribution of heat.[12] Sodium nitroprusside has been successful in reducing postbypass afterdrop because it produces peripheral vasodilation and improves peripheral perfusion. However, this benefit is usually noticed only in patients cooled to less than 32 °C.[12,13]

5. In the ICU, most patients are peripherally vasoconstricted as a compensatory mechanism to provide core warming. Pharmacologic vasodilation with medications such as nitroprusside, clevidipine, or propofol may facilitate the redistribution of core heat to peripheral tissues and improve tissue perfusion, but at the same time they may delay central warming because peripheral vasodilation augments heat loss. Forced-air warming systems, radiant warming systems, and resistive heating blankets all appear to be effective in treating postoperative hypothermia, although forced-air systems appear to be most comfortable for the patient.[14] Other measures, such as heating intravenous fluids or using heated humidifiers in the ventilator circuit, are of some benefit in preventing progressive hypothermia, but generally they do not contribute to warming.

6. Shivering is associated with hypothermia and increases oxygen consumption and patient discomfort. Control of shivering is important in the postoperative period and is best controlled with meperidine (25 mg IV), which has specific antishivering

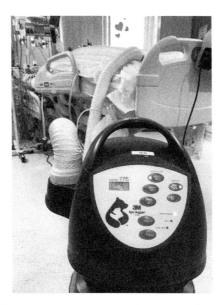

Figure 8.1 • The Bair Hugger warming system, used to warm patients arriving in the ICU at temperatures <36 °C.

properties related to several possible mechanisms.[15] Dexmedetomidine is also effective in controlling shivering.[16]

7. Occasionally a patient will rapidly rewarm to 37 °C and then "overwarm" to higher temperatures due to resetting of the central thermoregulating system. Narcotics tend to increase the core temperature required for sweating and may contribute to this problem.[17] Since warming may lead to profound peripheral vasodilation and hypotension, gradual vasodilation with nitroprusside or clevidipine and concomitant volume infusion can minimize this problem (see postoperative scenarios II.A and II.B, pages 376–380).

C. **Control of mediastinal bleeding** (see Chapter 9)

1. Numerous factors may predispose to mediastinal bleeding following CPB. These include residual heparin effect, thrombocytopenia and platelet dysfunction, clotting factor depletion, fibrinolysis, technical issues during surgery, hypothermia, and postoperative hypertension.[18,19]

2. Antifibrinolytic medications, including ε-aminocaproic acid and tranexamic acid, are recommended for all cardiac surgical procedures to reduce intraoperative bleeding. These medications not only inhibit fibrinolysis but, to varying degrees, also preserve platelet function.[20]

3. A universal definition of perioperative bleeding was proposed by an expert panel in 2014.[21] This took into consideration the amount of bleeding over 12 hours, the administration of transfusions, and the need for exploration, but did not define a specific amount of bleeding for which interventions were indicated. As anticipated, the more significant the degree of bleeding, the greater the risk of low cardiac output syndrome, inotrope use, acute kidney injury, and mortality.[22]

Generally, an arbitrary bleeding rate of >200 mL/h is of concern, since it may contribute to hemodynamic problems and trigger blood and blood product transfusions.[23]

4. Careful monitoring of the extent of postoperative bleeding dictates the aggressiveness with which bleeding should be treated. Many patients with "nonsurgical" causes will drain about 100–200 mL/h for several hours before bleeding eventually tapers. Unless that produces anemia with a hematocrit <22–24% or there is evidence of hemodynamic compromise or end-organ dysfunction, transfusion should not be necessary. A faster rate of bleeding without evidence of diminution requires systematic evaluation and treatment, often prompting re-exploration, as described in Chapter 9.

5. Thromboelastography is helpful in delineating the specific coagulation defect that needs to be addressed and may improve clinical outcomes.[24] Routine coagulation studies (INR, PTT, fibrinogen, platelet count) should also be analyzed. Even though they tend to be abnormal in patients with coagulopathic bleeding, they may also be abnormal in patients with ongoing surgical bleeding. Thus, abnormal coagulation studies should not delay exploration for significant bleeding. Persistent bleeding with normal coagulation studies tends to be more surgical in nature.

6. Recognition of the early signs of cardiac tamponade and the importance of prompt mediastinal exploration for severe bleeding or tamponade are critical to improving patient outcomes.[25]

D. **Ventilatory support, emergence from anesthesia, weaning, and extubation** (see Chapter 10)

1. Following off-pump or uneventful on-pump surgery, some groups prefer to extubate patients in the OR or upon arrival in the ICU.[4,5] This can be accomplished using short-acting narcotics, such as remifentanil, low doses of another narcotics, such as sufentanil 0.15 μg/kg/h, or primarily inhalational agents.[26] Sevoflurane rather than isoflurane may be used as an inhalational agent to allow for early awakening and extubation in the OR or soon after arrival in the ICU.[27] Alternative approaches to achieve early extubation include high thoracic epidural analgesia or spinal (intrathecal) analgesia with bupivacaine, fentanyl, or morphine with clonidine, often combined with remifentanil.[28–31] Neuromuscular blockers that have a short duration of action and do not require renal or hepatic elimination, such as cisatracurium or rocuronium, are best in this regard.

2. Careful monitoring of the patient's mental status and respiratory drive is imperative after extubation as the patient is still in an early phase of recovery from anesthesia. Just prior to and after extubation, analgesia should be provided to minimize splinting and improve inspiratory effort, but narcotics must be used with caution as they depress the respiratory drive. NSAIDs are usually helpful and might reduce narcotic requirements.[32,33] Ketorolac is a COX-1 inhibitor that inhibits platelet aggregation, so in addition to providing analgesia, it also been shown to improve graft patency and reduce mortality after CABG.[34,35] Ibuprofen given with a proton-pump inhibitor has also been effective and devoid of major side effects.[36] However, NSAIDs must be used with caution in patients with ongoing bleeding or chronic kidney disease. Intravenous acetaminophen might also be beneficial, although a randomized trial failed to show a reduction in opioid use.[37] Acetaminophen combined with propofol or dexmedetomidine has been shown to reduce the incidence of delirium.[38]

3. Most groups select anesthetic agents to allow for early extubation within 6–8 hours of arrival in the ICU. Thus, fentanyl or sufentanil are used for narcotic-based balanced anesthesia. Patients will remain anesthetized and sedated upon arrival in the ICU and will require mechanical ventilation for a short period of time. Propofol or dexmedetomidine will provide sedation as the narcotic effects dissipate, the latter generally being associated with shorter intubation times.[39] The initial fraction of inspired oxygen (FiO_2) of 1.0 is gradually weaned to below 0.5 as long as the PaO_2 remains above 80 torr or the arterial oxygen saturation (SaO_2) exceeds 95%. The respiratory rate or tidal volume of the mechanical ventilator is adjusted to accommodate the increased CO_2 production that occurs with warming, awakening, and shivering. Use of a low tidal volume (6 mL/kg rather than 10 mL/kg) has been shown to be beneficial in patients with ARDS, and a study in cardiac surgery patients found a trend towards earlier extubation, with fewer patients requiring reintubation with this ventilatory strategy.[40]

4. Early extubation is feasible in most patients, conditional upon their mental status, gas exchange, and hemodynamic performance.

    a. Virtually all patients have some compromise of pulmonary function after surgery related to a median sternotomy, entrance into the pleural cavity, and noncardiogenic pulmonary edema from the capillary leak caused by a systemic inflammatory response and fluid overload from crystalloid hemodilution. These issues are more prominent in patients undergoing prolonged complex operations with long bypass runs, who often receive multiple blood products as well. Superimposing these insults on preexisting heart failure or underlying lung disease, such as COPD, will predictably result in suboptimal oxygenation and ventilatory issues after surgery that might require a longer period of intubation.

    b. Even so, as long as certain criteria are met, there is no reason to exclude a patient based upon age, comorbidities, cardiac disease, or the extent of surgery from a protocol of early extubation. Even if it takes a few hours longer to extubate a patient, the benefits of an early extubation strategy usually translate into a quicker recovery from surgery.[41–43] The longer the patient remains intubated receiving sedation, the greater the risk of delirium.[44]

    c. Once criteria for weaning are satisfied (see Table 10.3, page 475), propofol is weaned off, neuromuscular blocking agents are allowed to wear off, low-dose narcotics or nonopioids may be given for analgesia (note that propofol is not an analgesic), and hypertension is controlled with nonsedating antihypertensive medications. If extubation criteria are met, the patient is extubated. Propofol-based regimens allow for earlier extubation than fentanyl-based regimens,[45] but as noted, dexmedetomidine allows for earlier extubation than propofol because it has less sedative and respiratory depressant effects, and can "take the edge off" because of its anxiolytic properties.[39] As such, it is also extremely useful when a patient exhibits agitation and dyssynchronous breathing while still on the ventilator.

5. Despite the desirability of early extubation, there are patients in whom it is ill-advised to "rush to extubate" (Table 10.2, page 472).[41–43,46,47]

    a. **Preoperative** factors predictive of prolonged postoperative ventilation are often cardiac in origin, including poor left ventricular (LV) function with congestive heart failure, cardiogenic shock, or pulmonary edema, especially if an intra-aortic balloon pump (IABP) is required for hemodynamic support. Other risk factors include need for urgent or emergent surgery, reoperations, and the presence of significant comorbidities, including severe COPD, marked obesity, peripheral vascular disease, and chronic kidney disease. In these cases, use of sufentanil or fentanyl is advisable, rather than shorter-acting medications. It is reasonable to use narcotics for the control of hypertension.

b. **Postoperative** clinical issues that may necessitate prolonged ventilation include hemodynamic instability requiring multiple inotropes and/or IABP dependence, low cardiac output syndrome, depressed level of consciousness or a stroke, ongoing mediastinal bleeding, oliguria from renal failure, and especially poor oxygenation or poor respiratory mechanics. In these patients, propofol can provide adequate sedation for several days and may be converted to other sedatives, such as fentanyl, if prolonged intubation is required. Careful review of the patient's chest x-ray, ECG, arterial blood gases, hemodynamic parameters, and renal function should allow for identification of problems that need to be addressed. Issues related to the management of hypoxia and acute respiratory failure are discussed in detail in Chapter 10.

E. **Analgesia and sedation**

1. An essential element of postoperative care is the provision of adequate analgesia without inducing too much sedation that may contribute to delirium or respiratory depression.[48,49] Pain control reduces the sympathetic response, reducing the risk of myocardial ischemia and arrhythmias, and improves the patient's respiratory efforts, overall mental status, mobilization, and physical rehabilitation after surgery. Pain is especially prominent with coughing and deep breathing as well as with movement. "Cough pillows" to brace the chest wall are very helpful in reducing splinting. Pain often improves following removal of chest tubes.

a. Parasternal intercostal blocks or subcutaneous local anesthetic infusions of bupivacaine 0.5% 4 mL/h (ON-Q Pain Relief System, Avanos) initiated at the time of surgery can ameliorate chest wall pain and decrease opioid requirements.[50,51] This is especially beneficial when patients are extubated in the operating room.

b. While the patient remains intubated, there may be some residual analgesic effects of the intraoperative narcotics, but propofol is not an analgesic, and additional analgesic medications may be required around the time of extubation. Dexmedetomidine is beneficial in this regard since it has both sedative and analgesic properties. Use of narcotics is appropriate in patients in whom prolonged ventilation is anticipated. However, if extubation is considered imminent, a variety of analgesic regimens may be able to reduce or eliminate opioid requirements around the time of extubation. These include use of an NSAID, such as ketorolac 30 mg IV, and IV acetaminophen. A multimodal approach using a combination of dexamethasone, gabapentin, ibuprofen, and acetaminophen has been shown to provide superior analgesia to opiates with less nausea after surgery through a median sternotomy incision.[52]

c. After extubation, adequate analgesia can be provided by a variety of medications and via different routes.

i. Use of nonopioid analgesia is always preferable and may provide adequate pain relief in most patients. IV ketorolac (15–30 mg) for 72 hours or IV acetaminophen can often bridge the patient to oral analgesics within a few days. Gabapentin 300 mg up to three times a day is usually recommended to treat nerve pain, but it is often helpful in providing analgesia early after surgery. Tramadol 50–100 mg every 4–6 hours may also be considered.

ii. Patient-controlled analgesia (PCA) IV pumps using a variety of opioids provide excellent analgesia.[53,54] One study found that use of morphine (1 mg bolus and 0.3 mg/h infusion), fentanyl (10 μg bolus and 1 μg/kg/h infusion), or remifentanil (0.5 mg/kg bolus and 0.05 μg/kg/min infusion) started after the completion of surgery for 24 hours provided comparable analgesia, but fewer side effects were noted with use of remifentanil.[54]

iii. Thoracic epidural or intrathecal analgesia with narcotics and bupivacaine are beneficial in reducing pain, expediting extubation, and improving pulmonary function, especially in patients with COPD and obesity.[28–30,55,56]

iv. Small bolus doses of IV narcotics or a continuous infusion of narcotics (such as morphine sulfate 0.02 mg/kg/h for patients under age 65 and 0.01 mg/kg/h for patients over age 65) may be considered to provide analgesia while minimizing respiratory depression.

v. On occasion, persistent pain refractory to the above regimens, especially in opioid tolerant patients, may require use of IV hydromorphone (Dilaudid) 1–2 mg q2–3h, which runs the risk of respiratory depression, or a fentanyl patch (25–50 μg/h patch every 72 hours).

2. **Sedation**

a. If the patient does not tolerate the weaning process, often becoming agitated with the weaning of propofol, substitution of dexmedetomidine can provide anxiolysis, analgesia, sympatholysis, and mild sedation to expedite a more tolerable weaning process from the ventilator.[57] It can be continued after the patient is extubated.

b. If delayed extubation is anticipated, propofol remains an excellent choice for several days and may be converted to IV fentanyl for longer-term sedation.[58] It should be noted that the offset of action of propofol depends on the duration of use, the depth of sedation, and body habitus. One study showed that, with light sedation for up to 24 hours, emergence occurs in only 13 minutes, but in heavily sedated patients it may take up to 25 hours![59] Although use of dexmedetomidine has only been recommended for 24 hours, several studies have found it to be comparable to or better than propofol or midazolam for long-term sedation.[60,61]

F. **Hemodynamic support** during a period of transient myocardial depression (see Chapter 11)[1,6,62]

1. Myocardial function following a period of cardioplegic arrest may be transiently depressed from ischemia/reperfusion injury and will often benefit from low-dose inotropic support for several hours. Systolic dysfunction may also be accompanied by diastolic dysfunction due to impaired ventricular compliance from cardioplegic arrest and myocardial edema. The reduction in ejection fraction (EF) is about 10–15% in patients with relatively normal LV function, but it may be even greater in those with preexisting LV dysfunction. Additionally, hypothermia and elevated levels of catecholamines lead to an increase in SVR and systemic hypertension, which increase afterload and can further depress myocardial performance. Factors influencing the need for inotropic support include the extent of preoperative LV

dysfunction, a recent infarction or ongoing ischemia at the time of surgery, and the duration of aortic cross-clamping. In patients sustaining a perioperative infarction, the period of myocardial depression tends to last somewhat longer, and may require more prolonged support.

2. Serial assessments of filling pressures, cardiac output and cardiac index (CI), and SVR allow for the appropriate selection of fluids, inotropes, and/or vasodilators to optimize preload, afterload, and contractility to provide hemodynamic support during this period of temporary myocardial depression. The objective is to maintain a cardiac index above 2.2 L/min/m^2 with a stable blood pressure (systolic 100–130 mm Hg or a mean pressure of 70–80 mm Hg). Adequate tissue oxygenation is the primary goal of hemodynamic management and can be assessed by measuring the mixed venous O_2 saturation (SvO$_2$) from the pulmonary artery port of the Swan-Ganz catheter (normal >65%).

3. Traditionally, the Swan-Ganz catheter has been used to monitor filling pressures, assess the cardiac output, and measure the SvO$_2$. Numerous studies have documented an imprecise correlation of measured filling pressures with intravascular volume and fluid responsiveness and have questioned the benefits of this catheter.[63] In most low-risk patients, not using a Swan-Ganz catheter has not influenced outcomes; in fact, some have found its use prolongs the duration of ventilation with no impact on outcomes even in high-risk patients.[64] One study found not only poor correlation between echocardiography and a Swan-Ganz catheter or FloTrac device in the assessment of hemodynamics, but also little correlation between the latter two devices![65] Nonetheless, numerous studies have suggested that a "goal-directed" hemodynamic approach to optimize fluid status and cardiac output may reduce complications, facilitate recovery, and shorten the hospital length of stay, although a mortality benefit may not be evident.[66,67] A survey reported that most centers are still using a Swan-Ganz catheter as a matter of routine because of a perceived benefit in postoperative management.[68]

4. The initial intervention to augment cardiac output is fluid administration. The filling pressures do tend to underestimate volume status, because of impaired ventricular compliance. Furthermore, the response to volume may differ, depending on whether the heart is hypertrophied with a "pressure overload" condition, as noted with hypertension or aortic stenosis (AS), or is somewhat dilated from a "volume overload" condition, as noted with long-standing aortic or mitral regurgitation. Observation of trends in filling pressures is essential when making clinical decisions about fluid administration.

5. Atrial or atrioventricular (AV) pacing at a rate of 80–90 beats/min is commonly required at the conclusion of surgery to achieve optimal hemodynamics, especially in hypertrophied hearts. Pacing is frequently required in patients taking β-blockers before surgery. A slow heart rate may reduce myocardial oxygen demand but will compromise cardiac output. In a well-revascularized heart, raising the heart rate to augment cardiac output is indicated and generally well tolerated. Ventricular pacing to increase heart rate will always produce inferior hemodynamic performance to atrial pacing, so atrial pacing wires should be placed in virtually all patients with preoperative sinus rhythm.

6. Inotropes should be selected based on an understanding of their hemodynamic benefits and potential complications (see pages 535–548). If a marginal cardiac output

is present after adequate fluid status has been achieved, inotropic support is initiated and should improve the cardiac output to acceptable levels. When the thermodilution cardiac output appears inconsistent with the patient's clinical course, a mixed venous oxygen saturation reflects the adequacy of tissue oxygenation. This indirectly correlates with cardiac output, since it is also influenced by arterial oxygen saturation. If a satisfactory cardiac output still cannot be achieved or begins to deteriorate, additional inotropes, an IABP, or rarely an assist device may be necessary. However, in most patients, cardiac function improves to baseline within a few hours and inotropes can be usually weaned off within 12 hours of surgery. In patients with preexisting severe ventricular dysfunction or acute perioperative cardiac insults (ischemia, infarction, prolonged cross-clamp time), it may take somewhat longer.

7. Monitoring of serial hematocrits is important to ensure the adequacy of tissue oxygen delivery. The hematocrit may be influenced by hemodilution or mediastinal bleeding and should generally be maintained at a level greater than 22%. In elderly or critically ill patients, especially those with a low cardiac output state, hypotension, tachycardia, low mixed venous oxygen saturation, evidence of ischemia, metabolic acidosis, or hypoxemia, transfusion to a higher level should be considered, weighing the potential risks and benefits of transfusion.[69]

G. **Fluid administration** to maintain filling pressures in the presence of a capillary leak and vasodilation (see Chapter 12)

  1. Following CPB, the patient will be total body salt and water overloaded and should theoretically be diuresed. However, numerous factors may contribute to inadequate preload that may compromise hemodynamic performance.

    a. Mediastinal bleeding or bleeding from leg incisions from vein harvesting.

    b. A capillary leak from the CPB-induced systemic inflammatory response which contributes to interstitial edema.

    c. Peripheral vasodilatation from medications (propofol, narcotics, antihypertensive medications), and rewarming. Note that peripheral vasoconstriction that is present when the patient is hypothermic or in a low flow state will mask intravascular hypovolemia despite adequate left-heart filling pressures.

    d. Decreased ventricular compliance producing higher filling pressures at lower intravascular volumes.

    e. Impaired systolic function due to transient myocardial depression that requires increased preload to maintain stroke volume.

  2. Fluid administration is necessary in most patients to maintain adequate preload and cardiac output. Crystalloid and colloid infusions are used to maintain intravascular volume, although this usually occurs at the expense of expansion of the interstitial space. After the capillary leak has ceased and hemodynamics have stabilized, the patient may be aggressively diuresed to eliminate the excessive salt and water administered during surgery and the early postoperative period. Scenario B in the next few pages addresses issues related to fluid resuscitation in the vasodilated patient.

H. **Electrolytes and acid–base balance**

  1. Monitoring of serum **potassium (KCl)** is essential in the early postoperative period. Potassium levels may be elevated from cardioplegia solutions delivered for myocardial protection, but most patients with normal renal function and preserved myocardial function will make large quantities of urine during the first few hours after CPB, often

resulting in hypokalemia. To minimize the risk of developing arrhythmias, potassium levels should be checked every four hours and KCL replaced as necessary.

2. Magnesium levels are usually lower due to hemodilution on CPB and should be replenished because of potential benefits in reducing postoperative arrhythmias.[70]

3. Metabolic acidosis may result from the use of epinephrine, but may be an ominous sign of inadequate tissue perfusion, especially in the vasoconstricted patient. In several studies that evaluated central venous oxygen saturations (ScvO2), an elevated lactate level was found to be a sensitive sign of inadequate perfusion, with levels >4 mmol/L that cleared slowly, even with a normal ScvO2, correlating with a higher rate of complications.[71,72] In fact, complications were also found to be common in patients with lactate levels of 2–4 mmol/L and a $ScvO_2$ <70%, despite normal mean arterial pressures, CVP, and urine output, and may be a marker of global tissue hypoxia from "occult hypoperfusion".[73] Metabolic acidosis generally resolves with improvement in hemodynamic parameters. Use of sodium bicarbonate may be considered for profound acidosis because of its adverse effects on cardiac function, but it only acts as a "bandaid" until the cause of the acidosis is corrected (see pages 715–716 in Chapter 12).

I. Strict management of **hyperglycemia** has been shown to reduce the incidence of sternal wound infection and surgical mortality.[74,75] Factors that contribute to hyperglycemia are insulin resistance, endogenous catecholamine release on pump, and use of epinephrine post-pump for hemodynamic support. A hyperglycemia protocol should be utilized to determine the appropriate amount of insulin to be given to maintain blood glucose <180 mg/dL (see Appendix 6).

II. Management of Common Postoperative Scenarios

There are several typical hemodynamic scenarios that are noted during the early phase of recovery from open-heart surgery. An understanding of these patterns allows for therapeutic maneuvers to be undertaken in anticipation of hemodynamic changes, rather than as reactions to problems once they have occurred.

A. **Vasoconstriction from hypothermia with hypertension and borderline cardiac output**

1. The patient arriving in the ICU with a temperature below 35–36 °C will vasoconstrict in an attempt to increase core body temperature. The elevation in SVR may produce hypertension at a time when cardiac function is still somewhat depressed from surgery. These patients should be managed by a combination of fluid replacement to reach a pulmonary artery diastolic (PAD) pressure or pulmonary capillary wedge pressure (PCWP) around 15–20 mm Hg, pharmacologic vasodilation to maintain a systolic pressure of 100–120 mm Hg (mean pressure 70–80 mm Hg), and inotropic support if the cardiac index remains <2.0 L/min/m². Warming methods noted above should also be employed. Among the commonly used vasodilators, clevidipine is a short-acting calcium channel blocker that reduces SVR and is usually the drug of first choice.[76] Nitroprusside is preferable to intravenous nitroglycerin (IV NTG) in reducing SVR, but it is a very powerful drug which requires careful monitoring. IV NTG is useful in patients with potential ischemia, but it tends to lower preload and reduce cardiac output to a greater degree while producing less systemic vasodilation than the other drugs. Nicardipine is a longer-acting calcium channel blocker that can also be considered.

2. The use of arterial vasodilators is beneficial in the vasoconstricted patient in that they:

   a. Reduce afterload, improving myocardial metabolism and LV function

   b. Improve peripheral tissue perfusion and redistribute heat to the periphery

   c. Facilitate gentle and adequate fluid administration

3. Vasodilators will reduce the SVR and blood pressure, and left-sided filling pressures will fall modestly, requiring the simultaneous infusion of fluids to maintain cardiac output. The optimal left-sided filling pressures depend on the state of myocardial contractility and compliance. Preload (generally the PA diastolic pressure) should generally not be raised above 20 mm Hg, because of the deleterious effects of elevated wall tension on myocardial metabolism and function. However, if preload is allowed to fall too low, the patient may become hypovolemic and hypotensive when normothermia is achieved. The general principle is to "optimize preload → reduce afterload → restore preload".

4. If the patient has a marginal cardiac index (<2.0 L/min/m²), has adequate filling pressures, yet is somewhat hypertensive, a low dose of a vasodilator can be initiated. If the patient is already on inotropic support, it is imperative to assess the cardiac index before modifying the therapeutic approach. Despite the temptation to do so, **stopping an inotropic medication in a hypertensive patient without first ensuring that a satisfactory cardiac output is present can be very dangerous.** Some patients with very marginal cardiac function maintain a satisfactory blood pressure by intense vasoconstriction from enhanced sympathetic tone. Loss of this compensatory mechanism may result in rapid deterioration from loss of perfusion pressure.

B. **Vasodilation and hypotension during the rewarming phase**

   1. Vasodilation reduces filling pressures and, in the hypovolemic patient, may produce hypotension and often a decrease in cardiac output despite good cardiac function. There are several reasons why a patient may vasodilate during the early postoperative period.

      a. Medications used for analgesia and anxiolysis are vasodilators (narcotics, propofol, midazolam). Recent use of ACE inhibitors or angiotensin receptor blockers (ARBs) tends to cause hypotension during and after bypass.

      b. Intravenous NTG used in the OR or in the ICU to control blood pressure, minimize ischemia, or prevent radial artery spasm will lower preload and cardiac output as well as blood pressure. To counteract these problems, significant fluid administration is frequently required. Unless active ischemia is present, IV NTG is best avoided during the rewarming phase to reduce fluid requirements.

      c. Resolution of hypothermia leads to peripheral vasodilation, which is accentuated in patients who warm to higher than 37 °C.

      d. Improvement in cardiac output often leads to relaxation of peripheral vasoconstriction.

      e. A vasoplegic state of refractory hypotension may develop despite the presence of an adequate cardiac output. This may be a consequence of a systemic inflammatory response (although it has been noted after off-pump surgery as well) and may be related to vasodilation induced by nitric oxide.

    f. Transfusion reactions or anaphylactic reactions to medications will cause vasodilation.

    g. Sepsis is very uncommon immediately after surgery but should be considered in the differential diagnosis.

2. To avoid hypotension, fluids must be given to maintain filling pressures. The quandary is whether crystalloid or colloid should be selected and how much should be given. If the basic reason for hypovolemia is a capillary leak syndrome, the use of colloid could be detrimental, because its oncotic elements may pass into the interstitial tissues, exacerbating tissue edema and compromising organ function. However, if vasodilation of the peripheral and splanchnic beds is the major problem, then colloids should be preferable, because they will augment the intravascular volume to a greater extent than crystalloids. Generally, if filling pressures are not elevated, the amount of extravascular lung water will not be influenced significantly whether colloid or crystalloid is infused.[77] Volume resuscitation is usually required during the initial six hours after arrival in the ICU, following which most mechanisms for vasodilation are no longer present and the capillary leak begins to abate.

3. It is generally best to start with a 500 mL bolus of lactated Ringer's, rather than normal saline. The latter may contribute to a hyperchloremic acidosis and worsen acute kidney injury.[78,79] If there is a minimal increase in filling pressures, a colloid such as 5% albumin may be chosen because more volume is retained in the intravascular space. Hetastarch compounds increase the intravascular volume more effectively than crystalloid and for longer than 5% albumin, but they have fallen out of favor as they may contribute to a coagulopathy or renal dysfunction. If given, tetrastarches should be used and the total infusion volume limited to 1500–1750 mL (20 mL/kg) per 24 hours.[80] If the patient's hematocrit is low (<22%), a packed red cell transfusion is the most appropriate means of increasing intravascular volume. If the patient is bleeding, use of blood component transfusions may be indicated as well. It must always be remembered that any volume, but more so colloids and blood products than crystalloids, will also lower the hematocrit from hemodilution.

4. There is often a tendency to administer a tremendous amount of fluid during the period of vasodilation in order to maintain filling pressures and systemic blood pressure. Although most patients with satisfactory cardiac function will simultaneously produce a copious amount of urine, many patients will not. One should resist the temptation to "flood" the patient with fluid, because excessive fluid administration (>2 L within six hours) will exacerbate interstitial pulmonary edema and delay extubation, and may contribute to cerebral or bowel edema. It will also produce significant hemodilution, often necessitating blood transfusions for anemia, and will reduce the levels of clotting factors, possibly increasing mediastinal bleeding and necessitating plasma or platelet administration. **Preload should be increased only as necessary to maintain satisfactory cardiac output and tissue perfusion.**

5. The response to fluid administration is not always predictable and depends on the compliance of the left atrium and ventricle, the degree of "capillary leak", and the intensity of peripheral vasoconstriction.

    a. An increase in preload with repeated fluid challenges will generally raise the cardiac output and blood pressure to satisfactory levels. Less volume is required in noncompliant hearts, usually those with LV hypertrophy. Peripheral vasoconstriction tends to relax as the cardiac output improves and the patient warms. As this occurs, filling pressures tend to fall and some additional volume may be necessary. If cardiac function and filling pressures are adequate, yet the blood pressure remains marginal, use of an α-agent (phenylephrine or norepinephrine) to support the blood pressure can limit the amount of fluid that needs to be given. If these drugs cannot maintain a satisfactory blood pressure with adequate filling pressures, yet the cardiac output is satisfactory, a "vasoplegic syndrome" may be present. This generally responds to vasopressin 0.01–0.1 units/min.[81] This syndrome may be attributable to leukocyte activation and release of proinflammatory mediators caused by the systemic inflammatory response to CPB, although it has been described after off-pump surgery as well. If vasoplegia persists, methylene blue 2 mg/kg IV followed by 0.5–1 mg/kg/h may be beneficial.[82]

b. Failure of filling pressures to rise with volume infusions may be noted in patients with highly compliant, volume-overloaded hearts (such as mitral regurgitation), in whom the cardiac output improves before the filling pressures are noted to increase. Thus, further fluid therapy can be guided by the cardiac output. Consideration must always be given to possible sources of blood loss, including accumulation in the chest cavity not drained by chest tubes.

c. In other patients, filling pressures may not rise due to persistent vasodilation and the capillary leak of fluid into the interstitial space rather than retention in the intravascular space. This is particularly common in very sick patients with a long duration of CPB. Sometimes it seems virtually impossible to maintain filling pressures and cardiac output despite a tremendous amount of fluid administration, yet, on occasion, this may be necessary. One often has to accept the adverse consequences of excessive total body water to improve hemodynamics. Use of drugs to provide inotropic support and produce an increase in systemic resistance may reduce the amount of fluid administered.

d. If filling pressures do rise with fluid administration, but the blood pressure and cardiac output remain marginal, RV and LV distention may ensue, increasing myocardial oxygen demand and decreasing coronary blood flow. At this point, further fluid administration is contraindicated, and inotropic support must be initiated. An echocardiographic assessment may be necessary to rule out tamponade or assess for unsuspected additional pathology (ventricular septal defect, valvular pathology). A chest x-ray may demonstrate a tension pneumothorax.

6. The following is a general guideline to hemodynamic management during the rewarming phase.

a. If the blood pressure is marginal, push the PAD pressure or PCWP to 18–20 mm Hg (often up to 25 mm Hg in hypertrophied hearts) using crystalloid and then colloid. Once this level is reached and the patient remains hypotensive, if the urine volume begins to match the infused volume, or if more than 2000 mL of fluid has been administered and filling pressures are not rising, consider the following:

i. If CI >2.2 L/min/m^2, use phenylephrine (pure α), or if unsuccessful, vasopressin for a potential "vasoplegic" state

ii. If CI is 1.8–2.2 L/min/m^2, use norepinephrine (α and β)

iii. If CI <1.8 L/min/m^2, use an inotrope, then norepinephrine to support the blood pressure

b. **Note:** use of an α-agent may not be able to minimize a capillary leak, but it does counteract vasodilation. This may decrease the volume requirement and improve SVR and blood pressure with little effect on myocardial function.

C. **Copious urine output and falling filling pressures.** Some patients will make large quantities of urine, resulting in a reduction in filling pressures, blood pressure, and cardiac output. Several factors should be considered when determining why this might be occurring.

1. Did the patient receive mannitol or furosemide in the OR because of a low urine output or hyperkalemia? Urine output is no longer a direct reflection of myocardial function when a diuretic has been administered. Excessive urine output often necessitates a significant amount of fluid administration to maintain filling pressures and confounds the selection of the appropriate fluid to administer (crystalloid vs. colloid).

2. Is the patient hyperglycemic and developing an osmotic diuresis? A hyperglycemia protocol should be used routinely to maintain blood glucose below 180 mg/dL (see Appendix 6).

3. Does the patient have normal LV function and the kidneys are simply mobilizing excessive interstitial fluid from hemodilution on pump? This beneficial effect is often seen in healthy patients with a short CPB run and reflects excellent cardiac output and renal function that should lead to a rapid postoperative recovery. However, copious urine output can be problematic when it lowers filling pressures, blood pressure, and cardiac output.

   a. Any contributing factors or medications causing the diuresis should be addressed.

   b. Crystalloid and colloid should be administered to keep the fluid balance modestly negative during this phase of spontaneous diuresis. The temptation should be resisted to administer too much colloid, because this can produce hemodilution and progressive anemia despite the negative fluid balance and can dilute clotting factors, potentially contributing to mediastinal bleeding. Use of an α-agent or vasopressin may maintain filling pressures and decrease the volume requirement in some of these patients.

D. **Low cardiac output syndrome with impaired left ventricular function**

1. Isolated LV dysfunction requiring postcardiotomy inotropic support may be noted in patients with active ischemia at the time of surgery, preexisting LV dysfunction, a remote or recent myocardial infarction, or advanced valvular heart disease. It may also result from intraoperative problems, such as a prolonged period of cardioplegic arrest, inadequate myocardial protection, incomplete revascularization, or compromised graft flow. Poor RV or LV function often reflects reversible myocardial stunning rather than perioperative ischemia and infarction. Both are managed in similar fashion, but the suspicion of ongoing ischemia by ECG may require reevaluation and potential treatment in the cardiac cath lab.[83–86]

2. Appropriate measures should be taken at the conclusion of surgery to assess and optimize a patient's hemodynamic status before arrival in the ICU, including pacing, optimal preload, inotropic support, and use of an IABP, if indicated. It is critical that the surgeon, along with the anesthesiologist, establish a "game plan" for how the patient should be managed in the ICU. Assessment of cardiac function by

direct visualization and TEE allows for correlation with hemodynamic parameters obtained with the Swan-Ganz catheter to establish an individualized therapeutic approach. Decisions on desired filling pressures, inotropic selection, plans for maintaining or weaning inotropes, and ventilatory requirements must be communicated to those caring for the patient in the ICU on a minute-by-minute basis. Careful monitoring and continuous reevaluation in the ICU are essential to identify whether the patient is recovering as desired or requires further evaluation and intervention.

3. In addition to careful examination and standard monitoring of critically ill patients, **echocardiography** in the ICU is very beneficial in clarifying potential problems. A typical scenario that may benefit from echo evaluation is the patient with a low cardiac output on substantial doses of inotropes, borderline and labile blood pressure, elevated filling pressures (often ascribed to volume infusions), worsening oxygenation, and bleeding that is ongoing or has tapered. In such a situation, an echo is indicated to assess whether there are factors other than LV dysfunction that may be causing the low cardiac output syndrome. Conditions such as circumferential or regional cardiac tamponade, severe diastolic dysfunction, RV dysfunction, regurgitant valvular lesions, or septal shunting may be identified. The most likely alternative cause of the scenario noted is cardiac tamponade, which, fortunately, is the most remediable. If a transthoracic echo does not provide adequate acoustic windows, a transesophageal study can easily be performed, especially in the intubated patient.[87]

4. A comprehensive discussion of the management of the low cardiac output syndrome is provided starting on page 521 in Chapter 11.

E. Normal left ventricular function but low cardiac output: diastolic dysfunction

1. A disturbing postoperative scenario is that of a low cardiac output syndrome associated with normal or elevated left-heart filling pressures yet preserved LV function. This scenario is noted most commonly in small women with systemic hypertension who have small, hypertrophied LVs. A variant of this problem is seen in patients with AS and hyperdynamic hearts that manifest near cavity obliteration.[88]

2. The problem of severe diastolic dysfunction is characterized by reduced ventricular compliance exacerbated by myocardial edema from ischemia/reperfusion injury. Contributing factors to the low cardiac output are lack of AV synchrony with impaired ventricular filling, occasionally impaired RV function, and perhaps excessive use of inotropic agents.

3. The hemodynamic data derived from the Swan-Ganz catheter typically show elevated filling pressures and a low cardiac output, suggestive of LV dysfunction. Thus, a typical therapeutic response would be to ensure AV conduction, administer some volume, and initiate inotropic support. However, this may lead to little improvement in cardiac output, even higher filling pressures leading to pulmonary congestion, a reduction in renal blood flow (often exacerbated by systemic venous hypertension), and progressive oliguria. The use of inotropes may also produce a significant sinus tachycardia that is detrimental to myocardial metabolism and recovery.

4. Transesophageal echocardiography (TEE) has been invaluable in the assessment and management of this problem. TEE will usually confirm a hypertrophic, stiff

LV with hyperdynamic systolic function and signs of diastolic dysfunction. Fluid should be administered to raise the PAD pressure to about 20–25 mm Hg. This will increase the LV end-diastolic volume, which tends to be lower than would be suggested by pressure measurements because of poor LV compliance. Lusitropic drugs that relax the LV should be substituted for catecholamines that have strong β-adrenergic inotropic and chronotropic properties. Dobutamine or milrinone may be beneficial in this regard and can support RV function as well.

5. Other considerations include use of low-dose calcium channel blockers or β-blockers to improve diastolic relaxation, although it is conceptually difficult to start these when the cardiac output is compromised. Aggressive diuresis to reduce interstitial edema while providing colloid (salt-poor albumin) to maintain intravascular volume may also improve diastolic relaxation. If the patient can survive the first few days of low output syndrome without end-organ dysfunction, a gradual improvement in cardiac output generally results.

F. **Low cardiac output states from right ventricular dysfunction**

1. The problem of a marginal cardiac output and blood pressure with preserved LV function may also be noted in patients with markedly impaired RV function. This may result from RV infarction and prior RV dysfunction from pulmonary hypertension (PH) of any cause, most commonly mitral valve disease. Intraoperative issues include surgical correction of severe TR with preexisting RV dysfunction, poor intraoperative protection of the RV, especially with RV hypertrophy in patients with PH, and use of multiple blood products. Inadequate pulmonary blood flow compromises oxygenation, and RV dilatation and distention can then cause septal shift, compromising LV filling.

2. RV function can be improved by moderate volume infusions, maintenance of a satisfactory systemic perfusion pressure, and measures to improve RV contractility and reduce RV afterload. These include normalizing arterial blood gases with correction of acidosis, use of appropriate inotropes (usually milrinone or dobutamine), and initiation of a pulmonary vasodilator (inhaled nitric oxide, epoprostenol [Flolan], iloprost or milrinone).[89-91] If these steps are insufficient, consideration should be given to use of an RV assist device or extracorporeal membrane oxygenation (ECMO).

3. The management of RV dysfunction is discussed in more detail on pages 530–534.

III. Postoperative Considerations Following Commonly Performed Procedures[92]

A. On-pump coronary artery bypass grafting (CABG)

1. Even with relatively normal preoperative LV function, most centers use a low-dose inotrope to support myocardial function at the termination of bypass and for several hours in the ICU during the early phase of transient myocardial dysfunction. The initial first-line drug is usually epinephrine or dobutamine. Epinephrine (1–2 μg/min) is the preferred inotrope and usually produces less tachycardia than the other drugs. If there is an inadequate response to one of these catecholamines, milrinone is of great benefit in improving cardiac output. It is a positive inotrope that produces systemic vasodilation that frequently requires the addition of norepinephrine to support systemic resistance. When hemodynamic performance

remains very marginal, placement of an IABP should be considered. In contrast to the catecholamines, the IABP can reduce myocardial oxygen demand and improve coronary perfusion. Inotropic support beyond 6–12 hours may be necessary if the patient has sustained a perioperative infarction or has a severely "stunned" myocardium that exhibits a prolonged period of dysfunction in the absence of infarction. A persistent low output state despite optimal pharmacologic therapy and an IABP may require placement of an assist device.

2. While the patient is intubated, propofol is an effective vasodilator to mitigate hypertension, but the blood pressure tends to creep upwards as the level of sedation is weaned. At this point, if the patient is otherwise hemodynamically stable, it is advisable to start a vasodilator which reduces SVR, such as clevidipine or nitroprusside, rather than give additional sedation or narcotics to control hypertension, in order to minimize respiratory depression. IV NTG may be used, especially if there is evidence of ischemia, but it will lower preload and cardiac output. Short-acting antihypertensives are preferable, because, as the patient warms, hypertension will start to resolve as peripheral vasoconstriction abates.

3. Although patients who are β-blocked preoperatively frequently require pacing at the conclusion of bypass, tachycardia may be present in those who are not well β-blocked, especially in young, anxious patients. Although the potential causes of a tachycardia always need to be assessed, the combination of hypertension and tachycardia with a supranormal cardiac output can be managed by β-blockers (esmolol or intermittent doses of IV metoprolol). Patients with a **hyperdynamic left ventricle** may develop progressive tachycardia when vasodilators are used to control hypertension. This should be managed by allowing the blood pressure to drift up to 140 mm Hg systolic and then using a β-blocker to control both the tachycardia and the hypertension.

4. Atrial and ventricular pacing wires should be placed in all patients undergoing CABG. If the patient has sinus bradycardia or a junctional rhythm, atrial pacing at 90 beats/min should be used to ensure optimal LV filling and improve the cardiac output. If there is normal AV conduction, it is always preferable to use atrial pacing rather than AV sequential pacing, since the latter involves pacing of the right atrium (RA) and right ventricle (RV), which will produce ventricular dyssynchrony. If second- or third-degree heart block is present, pacing in the DVI or DDD mode is appropriate. In patients with moderate–severe LV dysfunction, biventricular pacing (RA–BiV) using an extra set of leads will provide a superior cardiac output to standard RA–RV pacing.[93,94] If the patient has a slow ventricular response to atrial fibrillation (AF), VVI pacing should be initiated. Atrial pacing wires are probably not necessary in patients with long-standing AF, but many of these patients will be in sinus rhythm at the conclusion of surgery and for a few days afterwards, and, if bradycardic, they might benefit from atrial pacing.

5. A common practice is to initiate antiarrhythmic therapy with lidocaine in the OR to suppress ventricular arrhythmias, although there is little documented evidence of benefit.[95] It is given at the time of removal of the aortic cross-clamp and then continued on a prophylactic basis until the following morning. Alternatively, prophylactic amiodarone may be used to reduce the incidence of postoperative AF, especially in elderly patients, and it can also provide benefits in controlling ventricular ectopy. A common approach is to give the initial load intravenously during

surgery, although protocols of preoperative oral loading or a postoperative IV load may be just as effective in reducing the incidence of postoperative AF.[96]

6. **Atrial fibrillation** is noted in about 25% of patients following CABG. It may be related to poor atrial preservation during surgery or to withdrawal of β-blockers. Most centers initiate a β-blocker by the first postoperative morning (usually metoprolol 25–50 mg bid) because of the overwhelming evidence that β-blockers reduce the incidence of AF.[97] Magnesium sulfate has been shown in several studies to reduce the incidence of AF as well as the occurrence of ventricular arrhythmias.[70,98] Administration of 2 g at the termination of CPB and on the first postoperative morning can be recommended. Amiodarone may be used alone or in addition to β-blockers for AF prophylaxis, the latter being perhaps the best approach.[97,99] A detailed discussion of the prevention and management of AF is presented on pages 620–632.

7. Close attention must be paid to the postoperative **ECG**. Evidence of ischemia may represent incomplete revascularization, poor myocardial protection, or impaired myocardial perfusion due to anastomotic stenosis, acute graft occlusion, or coronary spasm (Figure 8.2).[100] Regardless of the etiology, IV NTG (starting at 0.25 µg/kg/min) is usually indicated. Calcium channel blockers (nifedipine 30 mg SL or diltiazem 0.25 mg/kg IV over two minutes, then 5–15 mg/h IV) are useful if coronary spasm is suspected. These medications may resolve ischemic changes or minimize infarct size if necrosis is already under way. Placement of an IABP should also be considered. If a problem with a bypass graft is suspected as the cause of the ischemia, emergency angiography followed by percutaneous coronary intervention or re-exploration may be indicated.[83–86] Coronary spasm can be so refractory as to cause cardiogenic shock that can only be treated by emergency ECMO.[101]

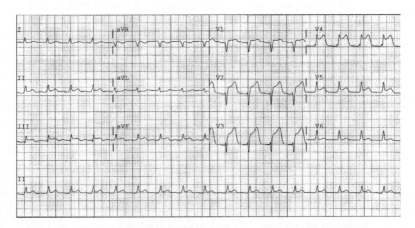

Figure 8.2 • An ECG obtained from a patient following a coronary bypass operation that required an endarterectomy of a diffusely diseased LAD. Note the profound ST elevations in precordial leads consistent with a current of injury. The patient was returned to the cath lab and found to have an obstruction distal to the anastomosis from an elevated plaque, and a stent was satisfactorily placed.

8. ST elevation noted in multiple ECG leads is often consistent with acute pericarditis, although computerized interpretation of these ECGs often indicates "acute infarction" (Figure 8.3). The ECG must be interpreted carefully, taking into consideration the heart's hemodynamic performance and an accurate perception by the surgeon of the quality of revascularization. An echocardiogram should be considered to assess for regional wall motion abnormalities.

9. The development of new postoperative ventricular arrhythmias should always raise the specter of ischemia and may prompt consideration of postoperative coronary angiography. A full 12-lead ECG should be reviewed. Reentrant ventricular tachycardias are usually related to prior heart damage. Nonsustained ventricular tachycardia (VT) in patients with an EF >35% is best managed with β-blockers and/or amiodarone. In patients with a low EF, amiodarone should be given, and if VT recurs, an electrophysiologic study may be indicated and placement of an implantable cardioverter-defibrillator (ICD) may be considered. The timing of placement may depend on the frequency and severity of VT, since randomized studies have suggested waiting three months after revascularization, during which time improvement in LV function may occur. A LifeVest (ZOLL Medical Corporation) might be considered in the interim.

10. Virtually all open-heart surgery on pump is associated with some degree of perioperative myocardial injury with elevation in cardiac biomarkers. For that reason, some surgeons do not routinely obtain troponin or CK-MB values postoperatively. Therefore, the diagnosis of a **perioperative myocardial infarction (PMI)** can be difficult to make, but may be suspected when there are persistent ECG changes and new regional wall motion abnormalities on echocardiography.[102,103] Biomarkers are very sensitive to myocardial injury, and higher levels do reflect more myocardial necrosis and correlate with adverse outcomes. Management of a PMI consists primarily of hemodynamic support. A common finding in the patient sustaining a small PMI is a low SVR that requires a vasopressor for several days to support blood pressure. A more extensive infarction may require pharmacologic support or an IABP for longer periods of time. The diagnosis and management of a PMI are discussed in more detail on pages 586–589.

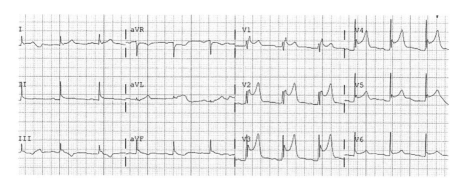

Figure 8.3 • An ECG obtained several hours after an uneventful valve operation. Note the diffuse elevation in ST segments with PR depression, which is consistent with acute pericarditis.

11. For patients receiving **radial artery grafts**, a vasodilator is used to prevent graft spasm. A variety of "cocktails" including IV NTG with verapamil or nicardipine may be used during preparation of the conduit, and IV diltiazem 10 mg/h or IV NTG 10–15 μg/min (0.1–0.2 μg/kg/min) is given intraoperatively and continued for 18–24 hours postoperatively. These intravenous medications are then converted to amlodipine 5 mg qd, long-acting diltiazem 120–180 mg PO qd, or isosorbide mononitrate (Imdur) 20 mg PO qd, and arbitrarily continued for six months.[100]

12. **Antiplatelet therapy** has been shown to inhibit platelet deposition on vein grafts and may delay or attenuate the development of fibrointimal hyperplasia and atherosclerosis. This may translate into reduced perioperative mortality and long-term improvement in graft patency rates.

   a. The immediate postoperative period is a time of increased platelet reactivity, and aspirin should be started within 6–24 hours after surgery.[104] There are concerns that platelet aggregation may not be sufficiently inhibited at doses of 75–100 mg, suggesting that 325 mg daily may be more beneficial.[105,106] Aspirin can be recommended for one year to improve graft patency and indefinitely for secondary prevention of coronary disease. Thus, it should also be given to patients receiving all arterial grafts as well. If a patient is unable to take aspirin, a 300 mg clopidogrel load followed by 75 mg daily is recommended, since failure to give a load will cause inadequate platelet inhibition for several days.

   b. Most studies suggest that dual antiplatelet therapy (DAPT) with ASA and a P2Y12 inhibitor does not provide any additional benefit in patients with stable ischemic heart disease undergoing CABG, including diabetics, as shown in the FREEDOM trial.[107–109] However, the AHA guidelines give a level IIb indication to consider DAPT for one year in such patients,[104] whereas the European guidelines give a level IIb indication to consider DAPT only for patients who had coronary endarterectomies during on-pump CABG (but for all off-pump CABGs).[109]

   c. For patients undergoing CABG for an acute coronary syndrome, the AHA guidelines give a level IIa indication for DAPT, with the recommendation to use aspirin with ticagrelor or prasugrel rather than clopidogrel.[104] A meta-analysis showed the former two P2Y12 inhibitors were effective in reducing mortality and graft occlusion rates.[110] The ESC guidelines recommend DAPT only if the patient had received DAPT preoperatively, which is often the case in most patients presenting with a non-STEMI undergoing surgery.[109]

   d. Statins should be given following surgery to improve vein graft patency.[111] Better efficacy may be achieved by giving a loading dose rather than regular dosing immediately after surgery.[112] The 2015 AHA recommendations were to give a high-dose statin (atorvastatin 40–80 mg or rosuvastatin 20–40 mg) after surgery to patients <age 75 and a lower dose to patients >age 75.[104]

B. **Off-pump coronary artery bypass grafting (OPCAB)** is performed through a sternotomy incision and avoids use of CPB. Numerous studies have documented that OPCAB is associated with reduced blood loss, reduced transfusion requirements, less renal dysfunction, and arguably less AF, less neurocognitive decline, and a lower risk of stroke.[113,114] However, most studies indicate that it is associated with less complete revascularization, more repeat revascularization, and compromised long-term surivval.[115–120] Patients are intensively monitored during OPCAB using continuous cardiac output measurements, in-line mixed venous oxygen saturations, and TEE to ensure stability during the procedure. Aspects of this operation which can impact postoperative care include temperature regulation, the influence of intraoperative ischemia on cardiac performance, potential anastomotic problems or incomplete revascularization causing perioperative ischemia or infarction, fluid administration to maintain hemodynamics during cardiac positioning, and bleeding due to use of heparin or transfusion of scavenged blood.

1. Patient temperature tends to drift during surgery and must be maintained by having a higher temperature in the OR, warming all intravenous fluids,[121] and using a topical warming device, such as the Bair Hugger or Kimberly-Clark temperature-controlling system. The Thermogard XP endovascular heating system (ZOLL Medical Corporation), which is placed within the inferior vena cava, has also been found to be very effective in maintaining normothermia.[122] If the patient arrives in the unit hypothermic, the standard measures noted in section I.B, pages 367–369 should be utilized.

2. Hemodynamic performance is generally stable after arrival in the ICU, although ischemia occurring during construction of anastomoses may lead to transient diminution in cardiac performance. Generally, the initial deterioration in cardiac output noted in CPB patients does not occur. However, low doses of inotropes are commonly used during surgery, especially in patients with impaired ventricular function, and should be continued until a satisfactory output can be maintained.

3. The immediate postoperative ECG must be evaluated. Intraoperative assessment of graft patency by Doppler flow analysis should be considered. The likelihood of an anastomotic problem is greater during OPCAB than an on-pump CABG due to suboptimal visualization from bleeding or cardiac motion. This may be evidenced by ECG changes or regional wall motion abnormalities on TEE, but this is not always the case. Occasionally, an abnormal ECG reflects incomplete revascularization when arteries have not been bypassed, either due to exposure issues, hemodynamic instability, or small size. There should be a low threshold for postoperative coronary angiography if there is any question about graft flow and patency.

4. Pacing wires should be placed on all patients, because patients well managed preoperatively on β-blockers will have slower heart rates that will persist into the postoperative period. Although heart rates of 60–70 bpm are acceptable, cardiac output can be optimized by achieving a heart rate of at least 80 bpm in the early postoperative period.

5. The benefits of OPCAB in reducing the incidence of AF are controversial, with benefits most likely seen in elderly patients.[114,123] Thus, the early initiation of β-blockers remains essential. Magnesium is usually given in the OR to raise the arrhythmia threshold during construction of anastomoses, and may also be given on the first postoperative day to reduce the risk of AF. Use of amiodarone in high-risk patients may be considered.

6. Although the hemodilution of CPB has been avoided, there is a tendency for anesthesiologists to administer a significant amount of fluid during surgery to maintain preload and offset the adverse effects of cardiac manipulation and positioning on hemodynamic performance, especially during grafting of the

posterolateral wall. Thus, patients tend to be somewhat fluid overloaded and need to be diuresed once hemodynamic stability has been achieved. Although the incidence of renal dysfunction may arguably be less with OPCAB, there is an obligatory period of relative hypotension during the construction of proximal anastomoses with an aortic sideclamp that can adversely affect kidney function in patients with preexisting renal dysfunction. This is less of a problem when proximal anastomoses are constructed using devices such as the HEARTSTRING proximal seal system (MAQUET Cardiovascular).

7. Many centers extubate OPCAB patients in the OR or soon after arrival in the ICU. Standard criteria for weaning and extubation should be used. These include the achievement of normothermia, hemodynamic stability, absence of bleeding, an adequate level of alertness without significant pain, and satisfactory gas exchange. Use of short-acting anesthetic agents and propofol or dexmedetomidine should allow for the safe early extubation of most patients once these criteria are met.[124] Because of the increased fluid administration to maintain hemodynamic stability, pulmonary compliance is reduced.[125] Although one comparative study of OPCAB and routine CABG showed better gas exchange and earlier extubation after OPCABs, another showed no difference, and both studies showed comparable deterioration in pulmonary function tests after either type of operation.[125,126]

8. Anemia is less common after OPCAB than on-pump surgery because hemodilution and other adverse effects of CPB on the coagulation system are avoided. Thus, significant mediastinal bleeding should be extremely uncommon in the absence of a surgical bleeding site. However, the potential for a coagulopathy may still exist.

   a. Heparinization is necessary during the procedure, and some degree of fibrinolysis is also probably present. Antifibrinolytic drugs have been shown to be beneficial in reducing bleeding in OPCAB, and thus should be utilized.[127]

   b. Insidious blood loss occurring during the construction of distal anastomoses is scavenged into a cell-saving device. Centrifugation and washing eliminate clotting factors and platelets from reinfused blood.

   c. Both pleural spaces are entered during OPCAB, and failure to place a chest tube in a pleural cavity (or poor drainage through a pleural tube that is placed) may result in the undetected collection of blood that spills over from the mediastinum. Vigilance remains necessary in assessing and managing significant mediastinal bleeding, with a high level of suspicion that it might be occurring if the patient is hemodynamically unstable.

9. Following OPCAB, a hypercoagulable state may exist, in part related to enhanced platelet reactivity and less platelet dysfunction than noted with use of CPB.[128] Early institution of aspirin plus clopidogrel has been shown to reduce postoperative cardiac events without an increased risk of bleeding. A meta-analysis showed a reduction in early vein graft occlusion and perioperative infarction (yet an increased risk of bleeding) with DAPT after OPCAB.[129] Thus, the American Heart Association (AHA) recommendation is to use DAPT for one year after surgery,[104] although one study showed no additional benefit of giving clopidogrel for more than one month after surgery.[130]

C. Minimally invasive direct coronary artery bypass grafting (MIDCAB) entails performance of an anastomosis of the left internal thoracic artery (LITA) to the left anterior descending artery (LAD). This is performed through a left thoracotomy incision using one-lung anesthesia. The LITA may be taken down with direct vision, thoracoscopically or robotically.

1. Patients are generally extubated in the OR or soon after arrival in the ICU. Epidural or intrathecal morphine analgesia (Duramorph) is helpful in reducing splinting and improving respiratory efforts in patients who might otherwise have significant chest wall pain from rib retraction, resection, or fracture.[131] A local infusion of bupivacaine into the wound is also helpful and may provide superior pain relief to the use of PCA alone.[132]

2. No pacing wires are placed, so a heart rate in the 60–70 bpm range is acceptable. Ventricular pacing wires placed through a Swan-Ganz Paceport catheter can be used for bradycardia, but generally they do not provide optimal hemodynamics. External pacing may be used, if necessary.

3. A postoperative ECG must be obtained and carefully reviewed for any evidence of ischemia, because anastomotic problems are more common when surgery is performed on a beating, rather than an arrested, heart.

4. Intrapericardial or intrapleural bleeding may originate from the chest wall, the anastomotic site, or side branches of the ITA. Blood will more readily accumulate in the pleural space during spontaneous ventilation. The possibility of bleeding should be monitored by observing chest tube drainage and a postoperative chest x-ray.

D. Aortic valve surgery and TAVRs (surgical and transcatheter)

1. **Aortic stenosis (surgical aortic valve replacement [SAVR])**

   a. Aortic stenosis (AS) leads to the development of a hypertrophied, noncompliant LV that depends on synchronized atrial and ventricular contractions for nearly 30% of its stroke volume. Postoperatively, it is imperative that sinus rhythm be present or that atrial or AV pacing be used. The optimal heart rate early after surgery is probably around 80–90 bpm for patients with LVH. There should be a low threshold for cardioversion of AF, because profound hemodynamic deterioration may occur, especially during the first 24 hours after surgery.

   b. Adequate **preload** must be maintained (PCWP often >20 mm Hg) to ensure adequate LV filling. Filling pressures may rise rapidly with minimal volume infusion because of the noncompliant hypertrophied LV.

   c. Although the LV pressure is often very high in patients with high transvalvular gradients, significant **systolic hypertension** is usually not seen at the conclusion of surgery, despite elimination of most of the gradient by valve replacement. However, hypertension tends to develop after several hours in the ICU and must be controlled to reduce myocardial oxygen demand and protect the aortic suture line. Use of vasodilators for a hyperdynamic heart may reduce diastolic perfusion pressure and produce a tachycardia. A β-blocker, such as esmolol or IV metoprolol, is beneficial in this situation. Subsequently, if the patient remains hypertensive, an oral β-blocker should be used. ARBs have been shown to improve diastolic function and should be considered as well.[133]

d. The patient with a hypertrophied, hyperdynamic LV may demonstrate mid-cavity obliteration and intracavitary flow acceleration, a problem associated with increased perioperative risk.[88] The LV demonstrates diastolic dysfunction with increased stiffness after surgery and is unable to fill well. This results in elevated filling pressures, low stroke volumes, and a low cardiac output. This problem may be exacerbated by patient/prosthesis mismatch. TEE in the OR can define the nature of the pathophysiology and direct management appropriately. Volume infusions to improve LV filling are beneficial despite the high filling pressures, but initiation of inotropic support with catecholamines for a low cardiac output state is counterproductive. Milrinone or dobutamine might be beneficial because of their lusitropic effects that promote ventricular relaxation. β-blockers can be used cautiously. ARBs, as noted, may also promote diastolic relaxation.

2. **Aortic stenosis (transcatheter aortic valve replacement [TAVR])**

a. TAVR has become the procedure of choice for most patients with AS. Even in elderly patients in whom this initially had been performed, recovery is expeditious and most patients are discharged from the hospital the day after the procedure.

b. **Hemodynamics.** Most patients following TAVR are somewhat hypertensive and may require intravenous antihypertensive medications (preferably clevidipine) until their oral medications can be started. Instability and hypotension during the procedure may be related to tamponade from wire perforation or annular disruption, or to ischemia from coronary ostial occlusion or significant coronary stenoses that were left unaddressed. Hypotension and bradycardia commonly result from the use of dexmedetomidine for sedation and improve once it is weaned off. In the absence of myocardial ischemia or bleeding, most patients respond to phenylephrine.

c. **Conduction abnormalities.** A pre-procedural ECG is helpful in determining whether the patient is at risk for advanced heart block, but telemetry is recommended overnight for all patients following a TAVR procedure.

i. A temporary pacemaker wire may be left at the conclusion of the procedure if the heart rate is very slow or there is evidence or predictors of advanced heart block. An ACC expert consensus panel recommended leaving the temporary pacing wire in overnight for patients with a pre-existing right bundle branch block (RBBB), who are at the highest risk for developing advanced or complete heart block, or with a pre-existing QRS >120 ms or first-degree AV block if there is an increase in the PR or QRS duration >20 ms.[134] If there is no progression in these parameters, the wire can be removed the following morning.

ii. A post-procedure ECG should be reviewed to ascertain the likelihood of needing a permanent pacemaker (PPM).[135] Generally, PPM implantation is indicated for patients with complete heart block, and further monitoring and possibly an electrophysiologic evaluation should be considered to evaluate the need for a PPM if there are pre-existing conduction abnormalities (QRS >120 ms or first-degree AVR block) with an increase >20 ms in the PR or QRS intervals, or a RBBB or LBBB with a QRS >150 ms or PR interval >240 ms.

    iii. Some patients may develop advanced heart block after 48 hours, and this may develop after hospital discharge. Independent predictors of the development of late (>48h) advanced heart block are a baseline RBBB and the amount of increase in the PR length.[136]

    iv. The development of a new LBBB or the requirement for a PPM has adverse effects on LV function, and both may impact survival, although the latter has not been noted in all studies.[137,138]

    v. A follow-up study reported that only 40% of patients receiving a PPM within 10 days after TAVR were pacer-dependent at one year, and this was more likely to occur in patients receiving self-expanding valves.[139]

d. **Renal function.** Contrast used during the procedure can contribute to acute kidney injury, especially in elderly patients with compromised renal function. A similar fluid protocol to that used during cardiac catheterization, which may be based on the patient's LVEDP that is measured when the valve is crossed, should be used (see page 688).

e. **Mental status** can be influenced by the use of anesthesia or sedatives, including dexmedetomidine, which is commonly used for deep sedation. Elderly patients may be very sensitive to medications and have delayed clearance. Depressed mental status may lead to hypoxemia and hypercarbia during recovery from sedation or after extubation, so careful monitoring of pulse oximetry and respiratory effort is mandatory until the patient is more alert. Delirium is noted more commonly in patients with AF, NYHA class III/IV, dementia, and nonfemoral TAVRs (usually done under general anesthesia), with delirium noted in 7% with a femoral approach vs. 21% with a nonfemoral approach in one study.[140] Although postprocedure delirium may be associated with increased mortality, after adjusting for other postoperative events, it was not found to be an independent predictor of mortality.[141]

f. **Neurologic deficits** have decreased in incidence to about 2% with improvements in transcatheter valve design and delivery systems.[142] However, MRI studies have demonstrated new ischemic lesions in more than 75% of patients,[143] although they are generally not associated with immediate neurocognitive decline. Use of cerebral embolic protection devices may reduce the volume and size of embolic material, but these devices have not reduced the incidence of new lesions or improved neurologic outcome.[143,144]

g. **Anticoagulation** is recommended following TAVR to reduce the risk of thromboembolism. A 300–600 mg load of clopidogrel is given along with aspirin 81 mg a few hours after the procedure, followed by clopidogrel 75 mg daily for six months and aspirin 81 mg daily indefinitely. However, a few studies have found that DAPT increases the risk of bleeding without any impact on the risk of stroke and may therefore be unnecessary.[145,146] In patients with AF, warfarin or a non-vitamin K antagonist oral anticoagulant (NOAC) is recommended without an antiplatelet medication. The GALILEO study comparing rivaroxaban + aspirin with clopidogrel + aspirin in patients without AF showed that rivaroxaban reduced the incidence of subclinical leaflet thrombosis, but increased the risk of bleeding, thromboembolism, and death. Thus, this study indicated that use of a NOAC plus aspirin cannot be recommended in the absence of AF, but it did not address whether a NOAC alone was noninferior to aspirin plus clopidogrel in these patients.[147]

h. **Bleeding.** Most TAVR procedures are performed transfemorally, and assessment for femoral arterial or venous bleeding causing a hematoma or thigh ecchymosis is important. Distal pulses should also be assessed, because closure devices (Perclose ProGlide [Abbott] and Angio-Seal [Terumo]) may produce moderate compromise of the femoral access site. Elderly TAVR patients often have poor-quality, calcified vessels that are more prone to bleeding, especially with the early institution of antiplatelet therapy or anticoagulants. Hemodynamic instability may lead to suspicion of a retroperitoneal hematoma with transfemoral or transcaval access, prompting evaluation by a CT scan (see Figure 2.38, page 163). A chest wall hematoma from percutaneous transaxillary access or intrapleural bleeding with a transapical approach should be considered in the unstable patient.

3. **Aortic regurgitation**

   a. Aortic regurgitation (AR) produces both volume and pressure overload of the LV, resulting in a dilated and frequently hypertrophied chamber. Maintenance of a supraventricular rhythm is important. Filling pressures often rise minimally despite large fluid challenges because of the enlarged, compliant LV, although the cardiac output will usually improve.

   b. Despite the placement of a competent aortic valvular prosthesis, most patients with AR remain vasodilated after surgery and require the use of an α-agent, such as phenylephrine or norepinephrine, to maintain a satisfactory blood pressure. Systolic hypertension is often better controlled with β-blockers than with vasodilators.

4. **Heart block** may complicate a SAVR because of edema, hemorrhage, suturing, or debridement near the conduction system, which lies adjacent to the base of the right coronary cusp near the commissure with the noncoronary cusp.

   a. Preoperative conduction system disease (first-degree block, left anterior hemiblock, RBBB, or LBBB) has been shown to be a risk factor for heart block in most studies.[148,149] Other risk factors for heart block requiring a PPM include procedures that require more manipulation in the region of the conduction system (endocarditis, reoperations, bicuspid valves, annular calcification) and the presence of AR, septal hypertrophy, larger end-systolic diameters, longer pump times, and preexisting hypertension.[148–150] The incidence of bundle branch blocks and complete heart block is much higher following implantation of rapid-deployment valves (23% for the Sorin Perceval and 14% for Edwards Intuity in separate studies).[151–153]

   b. Both the presence of a bundle branch block and the necessity for a PPM early after surgical AVR (noted in about 5% of patients) have adverse prognostic significance, with a compromise in long-term survival.[154–156]

5. On rare occasions, the sewing ring of the valve may compromise flow into the left or right coronary ostium. This should be identified by the surgeon prior to closing the aorta, but if not, there is usually evidence of severe RV or LV dysfunction or ventricular arrhythmias upon termination of bypass. This problem must be addressed at the time of surgery. If not, a postoperative ECG may show significant ischemia, although this may be obscured by the presence of LVH or a bundle branch block pattern. Coronary embolization of residual calcium fragments or

even small amounts of thrombus forming on sutures or the sewing ring may also produce evidence of ischemia.

6. **Anticoagulation (ACC and European 2017 guidelines)**[157,158]

    a. **Tissue aortic valves:** most surgeons implanting tissue aortic valves do so to avoid the use of anticoagulant therapy since the evidence supporting the superiority of a vitamin K antagonist (VKA) such as warfarin over aspirin is weak.[159] Hence antiplatelet therapy with aspirin 75–100 mg once daily is commonly used and is a level IIa recommendation in the European guidelines.[158] However, because of some evidence that the risk of stroke and subclinical leaflet thrombosis is greater during the initial 3–6 postoperative months, the 2017 ACC updated guidelines give a level IIa recommendation ("is reasonable") to use a VKA with a target INR of 2.5 for "at least three months and for as long as six months" if the patient is at low risk for bleeding.[157] Aspirin also received a level IIa recommendation, and it was not specified whether the recommendation was to use either aspirin or a VKA or both together. These guidelines did give a level IIa recommendation to use aspirin indefinitely. The European guidelines give a level IIb indication for a VKA and recommend it for three months.[158] These guidelines reflect the uncertainty of the preferable medication in patients at low risk for thromboembolism. Previous recommendations were to use warfarin for patients at high risk, including AF, a prior thromboembolic event, EF <35% or a hypercoagulable state. It may be feasible to use a NOAC for patients receiving tissue valves as an alternative to warfarin, but preferably after three months if the patient is in AF.[160]

    b. **Mechanical aortic valves:** all patients with current-generation single tilting-disc or bileaflet aortic valves should receive warfarin indefinitely to achieve a target INR of 2.5 (1.5–2.0 for On-X valves). The ACC guidelines also recommend aspirin 75–100 mg, but the European guidelines only recommend aspirin if there has been a thromboembolic event at a therapeutic INR or there is concomitant atherosclerotic disease. The 2017 ACC guidelines recommend a target INR of 3.0 if any of the above-mentioned additional risk factors for thromboembolism are present.[157]

    c. In patients receiving mechanical valves, there is a potential increased risk of thromboembolism in the early postoperative period when the patient is not therapeutically anticoagulated. Therefore, use of heparin is recommended until the INR becomes therapeutic. However, the timing of initiation of heparin as a bridge is not well defined. Early postoperative use of either unfractionated heparin (UFH) or low-molecular-weight heparin (LMWH) 1 mg/kg bid is effective, but both increase the risk of cardiac tamponade.[161,162] Since patients are generally hypocoagulable and often thrombocytopenic for several days after surgery, a safe approach would be to give aspirin as soon as mediastinal bleeding is minimal, give warfarin the night of surgery, and then start either heparin product on the 3rd–5th postoperative day if the INR is less than 1.8. The heparin is continued until the INR is >2.0 for two consecutive days. A bridge is important after hospital discharge if the INR is still <2.0 in a patient with a mechanical valve, AF, or a hypercoagulable disorder. Use of a NOAC is contraindicated as the anticoagulant for patients receiving a mechanical valve.[163]

E. Mitral valve surgery

1. **Mitral stenosis (MS).** Most patients with MS have a small LV cavity with preserved function. They are prone to a low cardiac output syndrome following surgery because of small LV end-diastolic and end-systolic volumes. Maintenance of adequate filling pressures is essential to ensure a satisfactory stroke volume, especially in patients with permanent AF. The "ideal" filling pressure varies for each patient, depending on the level of preexisting PH and the degree of its reversibility. Generally, there is a substantial reduction in PA pressures postoperatively, even in patients with severe preoperative PH, and this may translate into a greater reduction in associated tricuspid regurgitation.[164] One study found that, for patients with severe PH, the use of IV NTG, induced hypocarbia, and longer ventilation times were associated with a significant reduction in PA pressures, improved cardiac outputs and improved oxygenation, with comparable results to patients without severe PH.[165]

   a. Hemodynamic support may be required for RV dysfunction. Use of dobutamine and milrinone are most effective, but the use of pulmonary vasodilators, such as inhaled epoprostenol (Flolan) or nitric oxide, may also be beneficial.

   b. Postoperative ventilatory failure is not uncommon in patients with chronic MS as a result of PH, fluid overload, and chronic cachexia with poor ventilatory reserve. Aggressive diuresis, nutritional support, and a plan for ventilatory support and weaning are essential.

   c. Most patients with MS are diuretic-dependent. Despite correction of their valvular abnormality, they often require substantial doses of diuretics during the hospital stay to achieve their preoperative weight. They should be maintained on diuretics for several months after discharge.

   d. A Maze procedure should be considered in any patient undergoing mitral valve surgery with AF. However, this procedure may not be effective in patients with long-standing permanent AF or a markedly enlarged left atrium, and atrial inactivity may remain even if successful. A rapid ventricular response to AF will reduce LV filling and lower cardiac outputs, and should usually be managed by a calcium channel blocker or low-dose ß-blocker. Additional comments on the Maze procedure are provided in section III.E.7, pages 397–399.

   e. Anticoagulation following mitral surgery is noted in section III.E.9, pages 399–400.

2. **Mitral regurgitation (MR)** reduces LV wall stress by systolic unloading through the regurgitant valve. An EF in the normal range may represent early LV dysfunction, supporting the concept of early mitral valve repair for asymptomatic patients with severe MR.[166] When mitral valve competence has been restored, eliminating low pressure unloading, there may be unmasking of LV dysfunction because of the greater systolic wall stress required to achieve forward ejection. Although wall stress may be attenuated to some degree by a reduction in preload, this newly created "afterload mismatch" may result in LV failure, requiring inotropic support and systemic unloading with vasodilators.

   a. A reduction in LVEF should be anticipated after surgery, whether MR is addressed by mitral valve repair or mitral valve replacement (MVR) with preservation of the subchordal apparatus. This decline is more prominent in patients with large left ventricular end-diastolic dimensions (LVEDD), lower EFs, more advanced NYHA class, large left atria, and AF. It was found that, after surgery, the LVEDD decreased due to reduced volume overload, but the left ventricular end-systolic diameter (LVESD) remained the same, resulting in a reduction in EF.[167]

b. Postoperative LV dysfunction is common when there is evidence of preoperative LV dysfunction (EF <40%), LV dilatation (LVESD >19 mm/m²), an RV systolic pressure >45 mm Hg, or an ischemic etiology of the MR.[168,169] One study reported that the postoperative EF recovered to preoperative levels in only two-thirds of patients with a preoperative EF >50% and in only one-third of patients with a preoperative EF <50%.[166] Thus, one can anticipate hemodynamic issues after surgery in any patient with a dilated, dysfunctional LV preoperatively, and even in those with documented "normal" LV function as well.[166] Use of TEE with speckle tracking to determine LV strain measurements may be useful in identifying LV dysfunction despite preserved preoperative EF.[170] One study found that EF normalized after surgery only in patients with an EF >65% and an LVESD <36 mm.[171]

c. Current guidelines for surgery reflect these concerns that long-term results will be compromised by delaying surgery until symptoms or LV dysfunction develop. Nonetheless, LV dysfunction remains a significant issue after mitral valve surgery. Notably, patients requiring valve replacement for mitral valve endocarditis often require excision of the entire subvalvular apparatus, leading to even worse LV function.

d. On rare occasions, LV dysfunction may be attributable to inadvertent circumferential entrapment of the circumflex coronary artery during suture placement, either for valve repair or replacement (usually in left-dominant circulations) or during a left atrial reduction procedure.[172] This should be identifiable by significant regional wall motion abnormalities on TEE and by ECG changes in the distribution of the artery.

3. Management of **left ventricular dysfunction** after MV surgery for MR entails optimizing preload, providing inotropic support, and reducing afterload.

a. To optimize the systemic output, the LV volume status usually has to be maintained at fairly high levels. Administering a large quantity of fluid is frequently required because of increased left atrial and ventricular chamber size and compliance. In the presence of concomitant RV dysfunction, this can be problematic, because attempts to achieve adequate left-sided filling may lead to progressive RV dilatation and failure, with subsequent impairment in LV filling. Careful monitoring of CVP and RV end-diastolic volumes with volumetric Swan-Ganz catheters may indicate when fluid challenges are detrimental rather than beneficial.

b. Assessment of LV end-diastolic volumes requires echocardiographic evaluation because of the imprecise correlation with Swan-Ganz catheter pressure measurements. It is generally best to correlate the PAD pressure with direct observation of LV volumes by TEE at the conclusion of surgery. This can establish a baseline from which trends can be identified in the ICU.

c. The extent of reversibility of preexisting PH is unpredictable, and PAD pressures may not correlate well with the volume status of the LV. The PCWP is more accurate than PAD pressures, especially in patients with a high transpulmonary gradient (PA mean pressure minus PCWP), but "wedging" of the balloon is ill advised in patients with PH. Left atrial pressures measured through a left atrial line provide the most accurate assessment of LV volume status, but these are rarely used.

d. Inotropic support is usually selected to support both RV and LV function, since most patients with mitral valve disease have some degree of PH causing RV dilatation and dysfunction. Use of epinephrine or dobutamine and the addition of milrinone, as necessary, is the best approach. Milrinone is effective as an "inodilator" that can also reduce afterload to improve forward flow with a competent mitral valve. If the blood pressure is elevated, use of clevidipine or nitroprusside is helpful in reducing systemic resistance. If the patient still has a low output state, unloading with an IABP is helpful.

4. **Right ventricular dysfunction** is not uncommon following mitral valve surgery, especially in patients with preexisting PH.[173] RV failure may be precipitated by poor myocardial protection or factors that increase RV afterload. These include positive-pressure ventilation, increased extravascular lung water, blood and blood component transfusions, blood gas and acid–base abnormalities, and reversible pulmonary vascular spasm associated with perfusion-related phenomena and the systemic inflammatory response. In the OR, various TEE measurements can be used to identify RV dysfunction, which include RV fractional area change (FAC) <35% or a tricuspid annular plane systolic excursion (TAPSE) <16 mm.[174] However, once the patient is transferred to the ICU, assessment of RV function is more difficult. Volumetric Swan-Ganz catheters that measure RVEF and end-diastolic volumes may be helpful.

a. Isolated RV dysfunction may be present at times and is manifested by a high CVP, variable PA pressures, a hypovolemic LV, and a low cardiac output. However, these hemodynamic parameters may be influenced by the presence of LV dysfunction or preexisting PH (causing an elevated PA pressure), inability to calculate a thermodilution cardiac output (due to the presence of residual TR), inaccuracy of the FloTrac system (if in AF), and lack of continuous echo monitoring.

b. The initial management of RV dysfunction is fluid administration to optimize preload. However, if the CVP rises above 20 mm Hg without achieving a satisfactory cardiac output, further volume should not be given. This may cause further deterioration of RV function and also impair LV filling by producing a septal shift.

c. Inotropic drugs should be given to support both RV and LV performance. Preferably, those that can also reduce the PVR, such as milrinone, should be chosen. Low-dose epinephrine or dobutamine may be helpful. Probably the strongest drug to improve RV performance is isoproterenol, which is commonly used following heart transplantation, but its utility may be limited by a significant tachycardia.

d. In patients with severe RV dysfunction, selective pulmonary vasodilators may improve RV function by lowering RV afterload. IV NTG is effective in reducing preload, although it also produces systemic vasodilation at higher doses. Selective pulmonary vasodilators include inhaled nitric oxide (20–40 ppm through the ventilator), inhaled epoprostenol (Flolan) (up to 50 ng/kg/min), inhaled iloprost (Ventavis) (25 µg of a 20 µg/mL mixture via nebulizer), inhaled milrinone (5 mg bolus in the endotracheal tube), or oral sildenafil.[175–181] Additional comments on the management of RV failure are noted on pages 530–534.

5. Left ventricular outflow tract obstruction (LVOTO) has been described following MVR due to strut malposition in the outflow tract, especially in patients with small LV cavities or septal hypertrophy. It may also occur when there has been retention of the anterior mitral leaflet.[182] In many patients, the obstruction requires an additional procedure, but in some, it can be minimized by volume infusions and avoidance of β-agonists. Systolic anterior motion (SAM) producing LVOTO is most commonly noted following mitral valve repair when there is excess posterior leaflet height. If this does not respond to volume, stopping catecholamines and increasing systemic resistance, it may require revision of the repair with a "sliding plasty" technique to lower posterior leaflet height.[183] SAM is commonly noted preoperatively in patients with hypertrophic obstructive cardiomyopathy due to mitral–septal apposition with a hypertrophied basal septum. This produces not only outflow tract obstruction but also MR from incomplete leaflet apposition as the leaflet is displaced anteriorly and pulled into the outflow tract. With an adequate extended septal myectomy, SAM and MR should be eliminated, but, if persistent, additional subvalvular surgery may be indicated. If organic MR is present, an MVR may be necessary.[184]

6. Maintenance of **sinus rhythm** is beneficial to optimize cardiac output after mitral valve surgery, although it is not as critical as in hypertrophied hearts. Faster heart rates are preferable in volume-overloaded hearts to reduce diastolic filling, which, by reducing wall stress, may improve systolic emptying.

   a. It is controversial whether exposure to the mitral valve through the dome of the left atrium (superior approach), the superior transseptal approach which divides the sinus node artery, or a biatrial transseptal approach with or without connecting the atrial incisions ("minitransseptal" approach) is associated with more junctional rhythms or an increased need for pacemakers than the standard posterior left atriotomy approach.[185–187] Nonetheless, it is not uncommon to have some difficulty with atrial pacing despite preoperative sinus rhythm with transseptal approaches.

   b. In patients with long-standing persistent AF, it is frequently possible to atrially or AV pace the heart for several hours or days after surgery, but most patients will revert back to AF. Maintenance of sinus rhythm beyond the early postoperative period is highly unlikely when AF has been present for more than one year or the left atrial dimension exceeds 50 mm. β-blockers or calcium channel blockers may be used for rate control, but medications to maintain sinus rhythm, such as amiodarone, are generally not indicated in patients with long-standing persistent AF.

7. Because the presence of AF with degenerative MR compromises long-term survival with or without mitral valve reparative surgery,[188] the Cox-Maze IV (CMIV) procedure using radiofrequency and cryoablation technologies (see Figures 1.28 and 1.29, pages 85 and 86) can be used to treat paroxysmal or persistent AF. Although widely adopted as a simpler procedure than the "cut-and-sew"

Cox-Maze III (CMIII), freedom from recurrent AF does appear to be superior with the latter. These procedures are most commonly performed as an adjunct to mitral valve surgery. Bilateral pulmonary vein isolation (PVI) with resection and oversewing of the left atrial appendage is an acceptable operation for paroxysmal AF, but additional ablation lines within the left atrium are essential for persistent AF. Biatrial Maze procedures may produce greater freedom from recurrent AF, but this has not been uniformly demonstrated.[189,190]

a. Sinus node (SN) dysfunction or high-grade AV block may be present after the Cox-Maze procedures, so it is essential that epicardial atrial and ventricular pacing wires are functional at the conclusion of surgery. Subsequently, careful follow-up for recurrence of AF or the development of SN dysfunction or AV block is important to optimize long-term outcomes.

    i. A study from an experienced arrhythmia center found that PPMs were implanted in 5 and 11% of patients undergoing lone and concomitant CMIV procedures, respectively, mostly due to SN dysfunction which appeared unlikely to recover.[191] Their data contrasted with previously reported PPM rates of 8 and 23% for lone and concomitant CMIII procedures. Thus, there is a tradeoff of a lower need for PPM vs. a higher AF recurrence rate with the CMIV procedure.

    ii. However, other studies have reported an even higher rate of PPM after Maze procedures, which in fact increased one-year mortality.[192] A study from the Cardiothoracic Surgery Network of patients undergoing mitral valve surgery with preoperative AF reported that, at one year, pacemakers were required in 7.8% of patients after isolated mitral valve surgery alone, but in 16% after mitral valve surgery with PVI and in 25% after mitral valve surgery with a biatrial Maze. The primary risk factors were advanced NYHA class, multivalve surgery, and performing a biatrial Maze. Nearly 83% of patients who required a PPM received it during their initial hospitalization, the indications being equally divided between SN dysfunction and high-grade AV block. These data also reiterate the importance of placing and utilizing pacemaker wires immediately after surgery to optimize hemodynamics.

b. Recurrence of atrial tachyarrhythmias (ATAs) during the early postoperative period is quite common after a Maze procedure, especially in older patients, but it does not appear to correlate with the late recurrence of AF, since the mechanism triggering the AF differs.

    i. One report of patients undergoing "cut-and-sew" Maze procedures found a 43% incidence of postoperative ATA, with equal incidence in those with persistent and paroxysmal AF. AF was present in 59% of patients, atrial flutter in 14%, and both in 27%. With initiation of antiarrhythmic drugs once ATA developed, ATAs persisted for more than five days in 21% of patients, but lasted over two weeks in less than 3% of patients.[193]

    ii. Since this study found a correlation of ATA with the duration of aortic cross-clamping and CPB, it might be inferred that expediting the procedure with a CMIV approach might reduce the incidence of postop AF. There was also no protocol to initiate amiodarone prior to the development of ATAs, which might have reduced their occurrence. Generally, amiodarone is recommended prophylactically and continued for about 3–6 months. If the patient reverts to AF, a cardioversion should be attempted after three months. Generally, if a patient had been in AF for more than five years prior to a CMIV, the three-year freedom from AF is only about 55%.[194]

   iii. Both right and left atrial flutter have been noted to occur after Maze procedures and may require an endocardial ablation.[195]

  c. After a Maze procedure, anticoagulation with warfarin or a NOAC is given for about six months and can be safely stopped at that time if synchronous atrial contractions are noted on echocardiogram. However, ongoing monitoring is required because AF has about a 15% recurrence rate at five years and may be greater in older patients and those with longer durations of AF.[196] The decision to stop anticoagulation must be individualized, taking into account the patient's bleeding risk and echo findings, not just their $CHADS_2$ score.[197] If the patient desires to be off of, or has a contraindication to, anticoagulation with evidence of AF recurrence, a Watchman device should be offered. However, some form of anticoagulation or antiplatelet therapy is recommended for a short course after implantation.[198]

8. The acute onset of exsanguinating bleeding through the chest tubes or the development of tamponade soon after a MVR suggests the possibility of **left ventricular rupture.** This may occur at the AV groove, at the base of the papillary muscles, or in between. This problem can be avoided by meticulous surgical technique (especially if there is mitral annular calcification), chordal preservation during MVR, and avoiding tissue valves in patients with very small LV chambers (usually in elderly women with MS). LV rupture may be precipitated by LV distention or excessive afterload after bypass. Once identified, emergency surgical intervention on bypass is required and carries a significant mortality rate.[199]

9. **Anticoagulation**

  a. **Mitral annuloplasty rings.** There are insufficient data to determine whether aspirin is an acceptable alternative to a VKA following ring annuloplasties for patients in sinus rhythm. Some studies have shown that aspirin alone is sufficient,[200] yet both the ESC and ACC/AHA guidelines recommend three months of warfarin, albeit based on very limited evidence.[157,158] One rationale for using warfarin is that many of these patients will develop AF during the early postoperative period for which they should be on a VKA. If the patient has AF beyond three months, warfarin is recommended, but NOACs may be a reasonable alternative despite lack of confirmatory data.

  b. **Tissue mitral valves.** Guidelines on anticoagulation are essentially identical for tissue valves in the aortic and mitral position.[157] Thus, 3–6 months of a VKA given with aspirin is recommended per the ACC guidelines[157] and three months of a VKA is recommended per the European guidelines.[158] Similar to aortic tissue valves, one might consider initiating heparin before the INR becomes therapeutic, usually starting heparin on the 4th–5th postoperative day and continuing it until the INR exceeds 1.8 if the patient is in sinus rhythm. After three months, aspirin may be substituted if the patient remains in sinus rhythm. A VKA is recommended if the patient remains in AF after three months, with limited evidence supporting use of a NOAC.[160]

   c. **Mechanical mitral valves.** Aspirin is given on the first postoperative day along with warfarin to achieve a target INR of 3.0. The warfarin is continued indefinitely with aspirin 75–100 mg per the ACC guidelines to further reduce the thromboembolic risk.[157] The European guidelines only recommend the addition of aspirin if there has been a thromboembolic event at a therapeutic INR or there is concomitant atherosclerotic disease.[158] Heparin should be started around the fourth postoperative day if the INR is <2.0 and should be given until the INR is >2.0 for two consecutive days, and this can easily be accomplished using LMWH in the hospital and as an outpatient. It should be reemphasized that early postoperative initiation of either UFH or LMWH may increase the risk of tamponade, although some surgical groups do recommend very early initiation of anticoagulation in these patients.

F. Minimally invasive/robotic surgery

1. Procedures performed through small incisions limit surgical exposure to the heart. Since all minimally invasive valve procedures and some totally endoscopic/robotic coronary bypass grafting are performed on-pump, CPB-related problems, whether pulmonary, cardiac, or renal in nature, are similar to those noted above for specific valve pathology. However, there are a few specific issues that may arise in these patients.

2. Pain control is essential following ministernotomy and rib-spreading procedures. Similar to MIDCABs, use of epidural analgesia or intercostal blocks can optimize patient comfort and pulmonary status.

3. Access to the RV is limited, making placement of pacemaker wires somewhat difficult. The ability to pace the heart using pacing pads (which are fairly uncomfortable) or using a ventricular pacing wire placed through a Swan-Ganz Paceport catheter is useful.

4. Placement of chest tubes may not be ideal, because of exposure limitations. Usually one pleural and one anterior mediastinal tube are placed, but they may not provide ideal drainage. It is essential to be alert to the potential for undetected accumulation of blood in the pleural space or for the development of tamponade when the patient is hemodynamically unstable.

5. Although some minimally invasive incisions allow for central aortic and venous cannulation, all robotic cases and other minimally invasive cases with limited exposure require alternative cannulation sites – usually the femoral artery and/or vein. The presence of aortoiliac disease, tortuosity with calcification, very small femoral arteries, or thoracic or abdominal aneurysmal disease generally contraindicates femoral cannulation, so axillary or central cannulation must be used. Insertion of a femoral cannula is accomplished by direct cutdown or percutaneous placement. Following decannulation, the artery is repaired under direct vision unless placed percutaneously. The potential for hemorrhage, femoral artery injury, development of an AV fistula or false aneurysm, focal thrombosis, or distal atheroembolism exists. It is absolutely essential that distal perfusion be assessed at the conclusion of surgery by pulse or Doppler examination.

6. Because these operations can be tedious, especially in the early part of the learning curve, the bypass run may be quite long, often over four hours. This could potentially lead to a lower-extremity compartment syndrome. Since the anesthetized patient cannot complain of pain or sensory changes or exhibit motor function,

assessment of calf size and tenseness at the conclusion of surgery and in the ICU on a frequent basis is essential to recognize the very early stages of a compartment syndrome. Early fasciotomy can salvage muscle and limb function; delayed fasciotomy may be the first step towards an amputation.

G. Aortic dissections

1. Virtually all patients with dissections that involve the ascending aorta (type A dissections) undergo surgical repair (see Figure 1.23, page 75). The reestablishment of vascular continuity involves suturing of a Dacron graft to very fragile tissues, often supplemented with PTFE felt, and suture-line bleeding is commonly noted. In addition, surgical repair is predicated on stabilization of the entry site of the dissection, but this does not completely eliminate the distal false channel or a distal exit site, which may then be converted to an entry site. Thus surgery is palliative and leaves the patient predisposed to distal aneurysm formation in the future.

2. Aggressive management of hypertension following surgery is just as important as preoperative control, although the primary indication after surgery is to protect suture lines and minimize bleeding. Similar antihypertensive medications should be used to reduce systolic blood pressure and the force of cardiac contraction (dp/dt). The most common regimens are a β-blocker (IV esmolol, metoprolol, or labetalol) alone or in combination with clevidipine or nitroprusside. The patient is then converted to oral metoprolol or labetalol with use of additional antihypertensives, such as calcium channel blockers, ACE inhibitors, or ARBs as necessary. The risk of subsequent aneurysmal disease in the descending aorta is reduced with the use of β-blockers, reinforcing that heart rate control is an important component of postoperative long-term care.[201] This is also true for patients with type B dissections (not involving the ascending aorta), in whom control of both blood pressure and heart rate reduces the frequency of aortic events, including distal ischemia, recurrent dissection, expansion, and aortic rupture.[202]

3. The repair of a type A dissection usually involves a period of deep hypothermic circulatory arrest (DHCA) while the distal anastomosis is performed. The extensive period of profound cooling and rewarming may be associated with a significant coagulopathy, but bleeding can be minimized by use of felt reinforcement at the suture lines and use of tissue adhesives, such as BioGlue. Early and aggressive use of blood products is indicated if a coagulopathy is suspected to be the cause of significant bleeding, but early re-exploration is indicated for suspected surgical bleeding.

4. Careful preoperative and postoperative neurologic assessments are important to distinguish a preoperative neurologic deficit from a new stroke. Although antegrade and retrograde cerebral perfusion can be used to provide neuroprotection during the period of DHCA, the occurrence of a stroke may be related to the use of circulatory arrest, cerebral malperfusion on CPB, or air or atheroembolism.[203] Although femoral cannulation would seemingly increase the risk of retrograde malperfusion, and axillary cannulation can provide unilateral cerebral perfusion during a period of DHCA, outcomes are fairly similar with either cannulation site.[204] Distal perfusion in the cannulated limb (leg or arm) must be assessed following the procedure.

5. For type B dissections, medical therapy is associated with a 95% hospital survival rate, and interventions are usually reserved for patients with "complicated" dissections,

defined as those with refractory pain or hypertension, evidence of expansion, leaking or rupture, or malperfusion.[205–207] Surgical repairs have high mortality and substantial potential morbidity, including respiratory failure and problems related to aortic cross-clamping or malperfusion (renal failure and paraplegia). Therefore, thoracic endovascular aortic repair (TEVAR) is the preferred approach to promote thrombosis of the false lumen, although it may still be associated with paraplegia. Patients with uncomplicated type B dissections who are considered at high risk for potential expansion may also be considered for early TEVAR.[208] Careful preoperative assessment of branch artery flow is essential, and fenestration or branch artery stenting/grafting may be necessary if there is mesenteric or renal ischemia. A careful preoperative and postoperative neurologic examination of the lower extremities, and measures to support renal function in the perioperative period, are important. Other comments on management after descending thoracic aortic surgery are noted in section I.

H. Ascending aortic and arch aneurysms

1. Ascending aortic aneurysms may be associated with normal or dysfunctional bicuspid or trileaflet valves, and may involve or spare the sinuses of Valsalva. The extent of involvement dictates the type of operative procedure.

   a. When there is an indication for AVR due to AS or AR, the procedure may be a root replacement using a valved conduit, which incorporates either a mechanical or tissue valve at the proximal end of the graft, or a stentless miniroot or homograft. If the sinuses are not involved, an AVR and supracoronary graft will be placed, sparing the proximal aortic segment from which the coronary arteries arise. If the sinuses are dilated but valve function is relatively preserved, a valve-sparing root procedure can be performed.

   b. In addition to postoperative concerns noted following AVR for AS or AR, the two concerns after ascending aortic surgery are bleeding and issues related to coronary button implantation, which is performed during root replacements or valve-sparing root procedures. Strict control of hypertension is essential to minimize bleeding, and aggressive steps to control a coagulopathy should be taken starting intraoperatively to minimize bleeding from the suture lines. If there is compromise of coronary blood flow due to kinking of the proximal coronary arteries, ECG changes or ventricular dysfunction should be evident in the OR, but it may also occur later. A careful review of the postoperative ECG is essential to identify this problem.

2. For aneurysms limited to the ascending aorta, cannulation sites for CPB include the proximal arch, the femoral artery (in the absence of significant distal atherosclerosis), or the axillary artery. It is important to confirm satisfactory distal flow in the limb beyond the cannulation site after decannulation. The risk of stroke is low, but it may occur if there is atherosclerotic disease at the level of the aortic cross-clamp or in the thoracic or abdominal aorta that could embolize retrograde during femoral perfusion.

3. For aneurysms extending to the proximal arch that require DHCA, the ascending aorta is cannulated. During these procedures, ACP, either directly or through the axillary artery, or RCP through the superior vena cava, can be utilized to optimize neuroprotection during the period of circulatory arrest.[209] Although some surgeons use cold ACP with moderate (25 °C) systemic perfusion to eliminate some

of the issues related to deep hypothermia, this may not be safe in older patients with long DHCA times and multiple comorbidities.[210] An alternative approach in aortic arch surgery is a "debranching" operation, which restores cerebral flow to individual arch vessels before the distal aortic anastomosis is sewn. This may limit the duration of DHCA and optimize cerebral protection.[211]

4. Following operations using DHCA, neurologic recovery can be expedited using short-acting medications, but this may take up to 24 hours in some patients. The anesthetic agents and postoperative protocols for sedation and control of hypertension should acknowledge plans for a slightly prolonged duration of ventilation. It is enticing to promptly awaken the patient to assess a response to verbal commands and motor function of all extremities, but this could result in a period of inadequate analgesia and hypertension that is best avoided. The maintenance of adequate cerebral oximetry during the early rewarming phase from DHCA has been shown to reduce the incidence of delayed awakening.[212]

5. Use of DHCA to 18 °C requires a substantial time to rewarm to normothermia, because it is important to maintain a perfusion temperature gradient of <10 °C between venous return and arterial inflow. Despite active rewarming to 37 °C on bypass, significant temperature afterdrop is common, and a temperature-controlling device during surgery (Bair Hugger or Kimberly-Clark) and a forced-air system in the ICU (Bair Hugger) should be used. Coagulopathies are commonly present and require aggressive management to minimize mediastinal bleeding. The duration of DHCA correlates with perioperative bleeding and the need for transfusions, and both are risk factors for postoperative ARDS.[213,214]

I. **Descending thoracic and thoracoabdominal aneurysms**

1. Surgical repairs of descending thoracic and thoracoabdominal aneurysms are complex operations fraught with a significant incidence of postoperative complications involving numerous organ systems.

2. Surgery involves a thoracotomy incision and often takedown of the diaphragm. Extensive blood loss requiring massive transfusions of blood is not uncommon and usually produces a coagulopathy requiring multiple blood components and often a re-exploration. Prolonged ventilation should be anticipated and medications selected accordingly. The extensive incisions required for these operations can produce significant pain that requires adequate analgesia. More than 10% of patients undergoing these repairs may require a postoperative tracheostomy for prolonged ventilatory support.

3. Cross-clamping of the descending aorta can result in paraplegia or renal failure, even if distal perfusion is provided during the cross-clamp period. Because hypoperfusion due to reduced collateral flow and ischemic intolerance is considered the mechanism producing spinal cord ischemia, intraoperative blood pressure management (avoidance of hypotension) and cerebrospinal fluid (CSF) drainage initiated before surgery are important to improve spinal cord perfusion pressure.[215–218] The drain is left in place for up to three days after surgery to keep the CSF pressure less than 10 mm Hg. A mean arterial pressure of at least 90 mm Hg should be maintained with an understanding that this could worsen bleeding. Particular attention to a pre- and postoperative neurologic evaluation on a daily basis is essential.

4. **Delayed onset of paraplegia** occurring in the ICU may develop after several days and is actually more common than immediate postoperative paraplegia even when protective steps, including distal perfusion, CSF drainage, or circulatory arrest, are used.[219–221] It is usually, but not always, triggered by an episode of hypotension. If recognized immediately, it is usually reversible with elevation of the systemic blood pressure to a mean pressure of 95 mm Hg, and reinsertion of the CSF drain if it has been removed, to reduce the CSF pressure to 10 mm Hg. High-dose steroids might prove beneficial.

5. Cross-clamping of the aorta impairs renal perfusion and can produce acute kidney injury in 10–15% of patients. When it occurs, it is associated with a 40% mortality rate and compromises long-term survival as well. Numerous strategies to reduce the risk of acute kidney injury have been tried with minimal success, but the most useful technique may be cold crystalloid renal perfusion with the addition of mannitol.[222–225]

6. TEVAR has proven very beneficial in the management of descending thoracic aneurysms, with a substantially lower mortality rate. However, significant complications may still occur, related to access issues, thromboembolism, and ischemia due to branch artery coverage by the endograft.

   a. The risk of spinal cord ischemia is reported to be as high as 13%, comparable to that of open repairs. Thus, repeated assessment of neurologic function is essential during the few days following surgery. Delayed paraplegia should be treated as noted in section I.4. Spinal cord ischemia is more common in patients with prior TEVAR or open aneurysm repairs, extensive coverage of the aorta, internal iliac occlusions, with lengthy procedures, and with perioperative hypotension.[226–229] Intraoperative measures to reduce the risk of paraplegia include use of somatosensory evoked potentials,[230] CSF drainage to maintain a pressure <10 mm Hg, moderate hypothermia to 34 °C, maintaining a mean arterial pressure >90 mm Hg, and use of naloxone (1 µg/kg/h), methylprednisolone (30 mg/kg), and mannitol 12.5 g.[231]

   b. Acute kidney injury is noted in 10–15% of patients, increases operative mortality, and compromises survival, just as after open surgery. It is more common in those with preexisting chronic kidney disease, extensive thoracoabdominal surgery, use of multiple stents, intraoperative hypotension, and extensive blood loss requiring transfusions.[232,233] The best management is proactive, using intravascular ultrasound and less contrast, optimizing hemodynamics, and minimizing blood loss.

   c. Stroke has been noted in 4–8% of patients and usually results from embolization of mobile arch or descending aortic atheroma during stent positioning and deployment, especially with a very proximal landing zone. Treatment is supportive.[228]

   d. Upper extremity ischemia may occur if the proximal landing zone occludes the left subclavian artery. This should be avoidable if a preliminary carotid–subclavian graft is performed.

J. **Left ventricular aneurysms and ventricular arrhythmia surgery**

   1. Patients undergoing resection of a LV aneurysm usually have markedly depressed LV function. Although ventricular size and geometry are better preserved using

the endoaneurysmorrhaphy or endoventricular circular patch plasty techniques than with a linear closure, the LV chamber size is reduced, and the stroke volume is usually lower after surgery. Achieving adequate filling pressures (usually a PCWP around 20–25 mm Hg) is essential to optimize stroke volume. Filling pressures may rise precipitously with minimal volume infusion because of the small noncompliant LV chamber. Many patients generate a satisfactory cardiac output by virtue of a faster heart rate, which should not be reduced pharmacologically unless the stroke volume is satisfactory. Hemodynamic support and an IABP are frequently necessary to allow weaning from CPB.

2. Surgery for VT is relatively uncommon and usually involves blind endocardial resection with cryoablation. To minimize the risk of postoperative ventricular arrhythmias, lidocaine may be used prophylactically for 24 hours. Most of these patients will be candidates for postoperative ICD placement with or without electrophysiologic testing. Recurrent VT may be managed by an ablation procedure in an attempt to reduce the use of antiarrhythmic drugs.

3. Transvenous or subcutaneous ICDs are usually placed in the electrophysiology lab in patients with sustained VT, other suspected life-threatening arrhythmias, or prophylactically in patients with poor LV function.[234] If the patient has had heart surgery and had a preoperative indication for the device (other than poor LV function), it is placed several days after surgery. Similarly, if the patient has poor ventricular function and develops nonsustained or sustained VT after surgery, an ICD may be considered before hospital discharge. Otherwise, guidelines recommend that ICD placement should be delayed 90 days after surgery with reassessment of LV function, which may have improved. However, because the risk of sudden death remains elevated in patients with impaired LV function, it is not unreasonable to recommend a LifeVest (ZOLL Medical Corporation) in the interim.[235,236]

4. An ICD device is tested and usually left in the active mode. There should be a card posted above the head of the patient's bed indicating the status of the ICD so that anyone who responds to an emergency knows whether the device is activated or not. Generally, patients are placed on either β-blockers or amiodarone if they have malignant ventricular arrhythmias, but long-term use of the latter is not recommended due to numerous adverse effects.

References

1. Stephens RS, Whitman GJR. Postoperative critical care of the adult cardiac surgical patient: part I: routine postoperative care. *Crit Care Med* 2015;43:1477–97.

2. Wong WT, Lai VK, Chee YE, Lee A. Fast-track cardiac care for adult cardiac surgical patients. *Cochrane Database Syst Rev* 2016;9:CD003587. https://doi.org/10.1002/14651858.CD003587.pub3.

3. Dixon JL, Staff HW, Wehbe-Janek H, Jo C, Culp WC Jr, Shake JG. A standard handoff improves cardiac surgical patient transfer: operating room to intensive care unit. *J Health Qual* 2015;37:22–32.

4. Totonchi Z, Azarfarin R, Jafari L, et al. Feasibility of on-table extubation after cardiac surgery with cardiopulmonary bypass: a randomized clinical trial. *Anesth Pain Med* 2018;8:e380158.

5. Nagre AS, Jambures NP. Comparison of immediate extubation versus ultrafast tracking strategy in the management of off-pump coronary artery bypass surgery. *Ann Card Anaesth* 2018;21:129–33.

6. St. André AC, DelRossi A. Hemodynamic management of patients in the first 24 hours after cardiac surgery. *Crit Care Med* 2005;33:2082–93.

7. Reynolds L, Beckmann J, Kurz A. Perioperative complications of hypothermia. *Best Pract Res Clin Anaesthesiol* 2008;22:645–57.

8. El-Rahmany HK, Frank SM, Vannier CA, Schneider G, Okasha AS, Bulcao CF. Determinants of core temperature at the time of admission to intensive care following cardiac surgery. *Clin Anesth* 2000;12:177–83.

9. Pezewas T, Rajek A, Plöchel W. Core and skin surface temperature course after normothermic and hypothermic cardiopulmonary bypass and its impact on extubation time. *Eur J Anaesthesiol* 2007;24:20–5.

10. Engelman R, Baker RA, Likosky DS, et al. The Society of Thoracic Surgeons, The Society of Cardiovascular Anesthesiologists, and The American Society of ExtraCorporeal Technology: clinical practice guidelines for cardiopulmonary bypass-temperature management during cardiopulmonary bypass. *J Cardiothorac Vasc Anesth* 2015;29:1104–13.

11. Grocott HP, Mathew JP, Carver EH, et al. A randomized controlled trial of the Arctic Sun Temperature Management System versus conventional methods for preventing hypothermia during off-pump cardiac surgery. *Anesth Analg* 2004;98:298–302.

12. Rajek A, Lenhardt R, Sessler DI, et al. Efficacy of two methods for reducing postbypass afterdrop. *Anesthesiology* 2000;92:447–56.

13. Noback CR, Tinker JH. Hypothermia after cardiopulmonary bypass in man: amelioration by nitro-prusside-induced vasodilation during rewarming. *Anesthesiology* 1980;53:277–80.

14. Nieh HC, Su SF. Meta-analysis: effectiveness of forced-air warming for prevention of perioperative hypothermia in surgical patients. *J Adv Nurs* 2016;72:2294–314.

15. De Witte J, Sessler DI. Perioperative shivering: physiology and pharmacology. *Anesthesiology* 2002;96:467–84.

16. Bicer C, Esmaoglu A, Akin A, Boyaci A. Dexmedetomidine and meperidine prevent postanaesthetic shivering. *Eur J Anaesthesiol* 2006;23:149–53.

17. Kurz A, Go JC, Sessler DI, Kaer K, Larson MD, Bjorksten AR. Alfentanil slightly increases the sweating threshold and markedly reduces the vasoconstriction and shivering thresholds. *Anesthesiology* 1995;83:293–9.

18. Despotis GJ, Hogue CW Jr. Pathophysiology, prevention, and treatment of bleeding after cardiac surgery: a primer for cardiologists and an update for the cardiothoracic team. *Am J Cardiol* 1999;83:15B–30B.

19. Despotis GJ, Avidan MS, Hogue CW Jr. Mechanisms and attenuation of hemostatic activation during extracorporeal circulation. *Ann Thorac Surg* 2001;72:S1821–31.

20. Pustavoitau A, Faraday N. Pro: antifibrinolytics should be used in routine cardiac cases using cardiopulmonary bypass (unless contraindicated). *J Cardiothorac Vasc Anesth* 2016;30:245–7.

21. Dyke C, Aronson S, Dietrich W, et al. Universal definition of perioperative bleeding in adult cardiac surgery. *J Thorac Cardiovasc Surg* 2014;147:1458–63.

22. Kinnunen EM, Juvonen T, Airaksinen KE, et al. Clinical significance and determinants of the universal definition of perioperative bleeding classification in patients undergoing coronary artery bypass surgery. *J Thorac Cardiovasc Surg* 2014;148:1640–6.

23. Kilic A, Whitman GJ. Blood transfusions in cardiac surgery: indications, risks, and conservation strategies. *Ann Thorac Surg* 2014;97:726–34.

24. Redfern RE, Fleming K, March RL, et al. Thromboelastography-directed transfusion in cardiac surgery: impact on postoperative outcomes. *Ann Thorac Surg* 2019;107:1313–8.

25. Karthik S, Grayson AD, McCarron EE, Pullan DM, Desmond MJ. Reexploration for bleeding after coronary artery bypass surgery: risk factors, outcomes, and effect of time delay. *Ann Thorac Surg* 2004;78:527–34.

26. Zakhary WZA, Turton EW, Flo Forner A, von Aspern K, Borger MA, Ender JK. A comparison of sufentanil vs. remifentanil in fast-track cardiac surgery patients. *Anaesthesia* 2019;74:602–8.

27. Delphin E, Jackson D, Gubenko Y, et al. Sevoflurane provides earlier tracheal extubation and assessment of cognitive recovery than isoflurane in patients undergoing off-pump coronary artery bypass surgery. *J Cardiothorac Vasc Anesth* 2007;21:690–5.

28. Hemmerling TM, Lê N, Olivier JF, Choinière JL, Basile F, Prieto I. Immediate extubation after aortic valve surgery using high thoracic epidural analgesia or opioid-based analgesia. *J Cardiothorac Vasc Anesth* 2005;19:176–81.

29. Turker G, Goren S, Sahin S, Korfali G, Sayan E. Combination of intrathecal morphine and remifentanil infusion for fast-track anesthesia in off-pump coronary artery bypass surgery. *J Cardiothorac Vasc Anesth* 2005;19:708–13.

30. Parlow JL, Steele RG, O'Reilly D. Low dose intrathecal morphine facilitates early extubation after cardiac surgery: results of a retrospective continuous quality improvement audit. *Can J Anaesth* 2005;52:94–9.

31. Lena P, Balarac N, Lena D, et al. Fast-track anesthesia with remifentanil and spinal analgesia for cardiac surgery: the effect on pain control and quality of recovery. *J Cardiothorac Vasc Anesth* 2008;22:536–42.

32. Ralley FE, Day FJ, Cheng DCH. Pro: nonsteroidal anti-inflammatory drugs should be routinely administered for postoperative analgesia after cardiac surgery. *J Cardiothorac Vasc Anesth* 2000;14:731–4.

33. Hynninen MS, Cheng DC, Hossain I, et al. Non-steroidal anti-inflammatory drugs in treatment of postoperative pain after cardiac surgery. *Can J Anaesth* 2000;47:1182–7.

34. Engoren MC, Habib RH, Zacharias A, et al. Postoperative analgesia with ketorolac is associated with decreased mortality after isolated coronary artery bypass graft surgery in patients already receiving aspirin: a propensity-matched study. *J Cardiothorac Vasc Anesth* 2007;21:820–6.

35. Engoren M, Haday J, Schwann TA, Habib RH. Ketorolac improves graft patency after coronary artery bypass grafting: a propensity-matched analysis. *Ann Thorac Surg* 2011;92:603–9

36. Qazi SM, Sindby EJ, Nørgaard MA. Ibuprofen: a safe analgesic during recovery? A randomized controlled trial. *J Cardiovasc Thor Res* 2015;7:141–8.

37. Mamoun NF, Lin P, Zimmerman NM, et al. Intravenous acetaminophen analgesia after cardiac surgery: a randomized, blinded, controlled superiority trial. *J Thorac Cardiovasc Surg* 2016;152:881–8.

38. Subramaniam B, Shankar P, Shaefi S, et al. Effect of intravenous acetaminophen vs placebo combined with propofol or dexmedetomidine on postoperative delirium among older patients following cardiac surgery: the DEXACET randomized clinical trial. *JAMA* 2019;321:686–96.

39. Curtis JA, Hollinger MK, Jain HB. Propofol-based versus dexmedetomidine-based sedation in cardiac surgery patients. *J Cardiothorac Vasc Anesth* 2013;27:1289–94.

40. Sundar S, Novack V, Jervis K, et al. Influence of low tidal volume ventilation on time to extubation in cardiac surgical patients. *Anesthesiology* 2011;114:1102–10.

41. Kogan A, Ghosh P, Preisman S, et al. Risk factors for failed "fast-tracking" after cardiac surgery in patients older than 70 years. *J Cardiothorac Vasc Anesth* 2008;22:530–5.

42. Parlow JL, Ahn R, Milne B. Obesity is a risk factor for failure of "fast track" extubation following coronary artery bypass surgery. *Can J Anaesth* 2006;53:288–94.

43. Kiessling AH, Huneke P, Reyher C, Bingold T, Zierer A, Moritz A. Risk factor analysis for fast track protocol failure. *J Cardiothorac Surg* 2013;8:47.

44. Barr J, Fraser FL, Puntillo K, et al. Clinical practice guidelines for the management of pain, agitation, and delirium in adult patients in the intensive care unit. *Crit Care Med* 2013;41:263–306.

45. Oliver WC Jr, Nuttall GA, Murari T, et al. A prospective, randomized double-blind trial of 3 regimens for sedation and analgesia after cardiac surgery. *J Cardiothorac Vasc Anesth* 2011;25:110–19.

46. Constantinides VA, Tekkis PP, Fazil A, et al. Fast-track failure after cardiac surgery: development of a prediction model. *Crit Care Med* 2006;34:2875–82.

47. Yende S, Wunderlink R. Causes of prolonged mechanical ventilation after coronary artery bypass surgery. *Chest* 2002;122:245–52.

48. Mazzeffi M, Khaleminsky Y. Poststernotomy pain: a clinical review. *J Cardiothorac Vasc Anesth* 2011;25:1163–78.

49. Huang APS, Sakata RK. Pain after sternotomy: review. *Rev Bras Anestesiol* 2016;66:395–401.

50. Barr AM, Tutungi E, Almeida AA. Parasternal intercostal block with ropivacaine for pain management after cardiac surgery: a double-blind, randomized controlled trial. *J Cardiothorac Vasc Anesth* 2007;21:547–53.

51. White PF, Rawal S, Latham P, et al. Use of a continuous local anesthetic infusion for pain management after median sternotomy. *Anesthesiology* 2003;99:918–23.

52. Rafiq S, Steinbrüchel DA, Wanscher MJ, et al. Multimodal analgesia versus traditional opiate based analgesia after cardiac surgery: a randomized controlled trial. *J Cardiothorac Surg* 2014;9:52.

53. Gurbet A, Goren S, Sahin S, Uckunkaya N, Korfali G. Comparison of analgesic effects of morphine, fentanyl, and remifentanil with intravenous patient-controlled analgesia after cardiac surgery. *J Cardiothorac Vasc Anesth* 2004;18:755–8.

54. Baltali S, Turkoz A, Bozdogan N, et al. The efficacy of intravenous patient-controlled remifentanil versus morphine anesthesia after coronary artery surgery. *J Cardiothorac Vasc Anesth* 2009;23:170–4.

55. Sharma M, Mehta Y, Sawhney R, Vats M, Trehan N. Thoracic epidural analgesia in obese patients with body mass index of more than 30 kg/m² for off pump coronary artery bypass surgery. *Ann Card Anaesth* 2010;13:28–33.

56. Mehta Y, Vats M, Sharma M, Arora R, Trehan N. Thoracic epidural analgesia for off-pump coronary artery bypass surgery in patients with chronic obstructive lung disease. *Ann Card Anaesth* 2010;13:224–30.

57. Herr DL, Sum-Ping ST, England M. ICU sedation after coronary artery bypass graft surgery: dexmedetomidine-based versus propofol-based sedation regimens. *J Cardiothorac Vasc Anesth* 2003;17:576–84.

58. Ho KM, Ng JY. The use of propofol for medium and long-term sedation in critically ill adult patients: a meta-analysis. *Intensive Care Med* 2008;34:1969–79.

59. Barr J, Egan TD, Sandoval NF, et al. Propofol dosing regimens for ICU sedation based upon an integrated pharmacokinetic–pharmacodynamic model. *Anesthesiology* 2001;95:324–33.

60. Ruokonen E, Parviainen I, Jakob SM, et al. Dexmedetomidine versus propofol/midazolam for long-term sedation during mechanical ventilation. *Intensive Care Med* 2009;35:282–90.

61. Riker RR, Shehabi Y, Bokesch PM, et al. Dexmedetomidine vs midazolam for sedation of critically ill patients: a randomized trial. *JAMA* 2009;301:489–99.

62. Lomivorotov VV, Efremov SM, Kirov MY, Fominskiy EEV, Karaskov AM. Low-cardiac-output after cardiac surgery. *J Cardiothorac Vasc Anesth* 2017;31:291–308.

63. Buhre W, Weyland A, Schorn B, et al. Changes in central venous pressure and pulmonary capillary wedge pressure do not indicate changes in right and left heart volume in patients undergoing coronary artery bypass surgery. *Eur J Anesthesiol* 1999;16:11–7.

64. Chiang Y, Hosseinian L, Rhee A, Itagaki S, Cavallaro P, Chikwe J. Questionable benefit of the pulmonary artery catheter after cardiac surgery in high-risk patients. *J Cardiothorac Vasc Anesth* 2015;29:76–81.

65. Power P, Bone A, Simpson N, Yap CH, Gower S, Bailey M. Comparison of pulmonary artery catheter, echocardiography, and arterial waveform analysis monitoring in predicting the hemodynamic state during and after cardiac surgery. *Int J Crit Illn Inj Sci* 2017;7:156–62.

66. Li P, Qu LP, Qi D, et al. Significance of perioperative goal-directed hemodynamic approach in preventing postoperative complications in patients after cardiac surgery: a meta-analysis and systematic review. *Ann Med* 2017;49:343–51.

67. Osawa EA, Rhodes A, Landoni G, et al. Effect of perioperative goal-directed hemodynamic resuscitation therapy on outcomes following cardiac surgery: a randomized clinical trial and systematic review. *Crit Care Med* 2016;44:724–33.

68. Judge O, Ji F, Fleming N, Liu H. Current use of the pulmonary artery catheter in cardiac surgery: a survey study. *J Cardiothorac Vasc Anesth* 2015;29:69–75.

69. Arias-Morales CE, Stoicea N, Gonzalez-Zacarias AA, et al. Revisiting blood transfusion and outcome in cardiac surgery patients: a concise perspective. *F1000Res* 2017;6:pii: F1000 Faculty Rev-168.

70. Fairley JL, Zhang L, Glassford NJ, Bellomo R. Magnesium status and magnesium therapy in cardiac surgery: a systematic review and meta-analysis focusing on arrhythmia prevention. *J Crit Care* 2017;42:69–77.

71. Laine GA, Hu BY, Wang S, Thomas Solis R, Reul GJ Jr. Isolated high lactate or low central venous oxygen saturation after cardiac surgery and association with outcome. *J Cardiothorac Vasc Anesth* 2013;27:1271–6.

72. Lindsay AJ, Xu M, Sessler DI, Blackstone EH, Bashour CA. Lactate clearance time and concentration linked to morbidity and death in cardiac surgical patients. *Ann Thorac Surg* 2013;95:486–92.

73. Hu BW, Laine GA, Wang S, Solis RT. Combined central venous oxygen saturation and lactate as markers of occult hypoperfusion and outcome following cardiac surgery. *J Cardiothorac Vasc Anesth* 2012;26:52–7.

74. Jones KW, Cain AS, Mitchell JH, et al. Hyperglycemia predicts mortality after CABG: postoperative hyperglycemia predicts dramatic increases in mortality after coronary artery bypass graft surgery. *J Diabetes Complications* 2008;22:365–70.

75. Lazar HL, McDonnell M, Chipkin SR, et al. The Society of Thoracic Surgeons practice guidelines series: blood glucose management during adult cardiac surgery. *Ann Thorac Surg* 2009;87:663–9.

76. Espinosa A, Ripollés-Melchor J, Casans-Francés R, et al. Perioperative use of clevidipine: a systematic review and meta-analysis. *PLoS One* 2016;11:e0150625.

77. Gallagher JD, Moore RA, Kerns D, et al. Effects of colloid or crystalloid administration on pulmonary extravascular water in the postoperative period after coronary artery bypass grafting. *Anesth Analg* 1985;64:753–8.

78. Yunos NM, Bellomo R, Hegarty C, Story D, Ho L, Bailey M. Association between a chloride-liberal and chloride-restrictive intravenous fluid administration strategy and kidney injury in critically ill adults. *JAMA* 2012;308:1566–72.

79. Raghunathan K, Murray PT, Beattie WS, et al. Choice of fluid in acute illness: what should be given? An international consensus. *Br J Anaesth* 2014;113:772–83.

80. Jacob M, Fellahi JL, Chappell D, Kurz A. The impact of hydroxyethyl starches in cardiac surgery: a meta-analysis. *Crit Care* 2014;18:656.

81. Shaefi S, Mittel A, Klick J, et al. Vasoplegia after cardiovascular procedures: pathophysiology and targeted therapy. *J Cardiothorac Vasc Anesth* 2018;32:1013–22.

82. Habib AM, Elsherbeny AG, Almehizia RA. Methylene blue for vasoplegic syndrome postcardiac surgery. *Indian J Crit Care Med* 2018;22:168–73.

83. Hultgen K, Andreasson A, Axelsson TA, Albertsson P, Lepore V, Jeppsson A. Acute coronary angiography after coronary artery bypass grafting. *Scand Cardiovasc J* 2016;50:123–7.

84. Fleißner F, Issam I, Martens A, Cebotari S, Haverich A, Shrestha ML. The unplanned postoperative coronary angiogram after CABG: identifying the patients at risk. *Thorac Cardiovasc Surg* 2017;65:292–5.

85. Gaudino M, Nesta M, Burzotta F, et al. Results of emergency postoperative re-angiography after cardiac surgery procedures. *Ann Thorac Surg* 2015;99:1576–82.

86. Alqahtani F, Ziada KM, Badhwar V, Sandhu G, Rihal CS, Alkhouli M. Incidence, predictors, and outcomes of in-hospital percutaneous coronary intervention following coronary artery bypass grafting. *J Am Coll Cardiol* 2019;73:415–23.

87. Imren Y, Tasoglu I, Oktar GL, et al. The importance of transesophageal echocardiography in diagnosis of pericardial tamponade after cardiac surgery. *J Card Surg* 2008;23:450–3.

88. Bartunek J, Sys SU, Rodrigues AC, van Schuerbeeck E, Mortier L, de Bruyne B. Abnormal systolic intracavity flow velocities after valve replacement for aortic stenosis: mechanisms, predictive factors, and prognostic significance. *Circulation* 1996;93:712–9.

89. McGinn K, Reichert M. A comparison of inhaled nitric oxide versus inhaled epoprostenol for acute pulmonary hypertension following cardiac surgery. *Ann Pharmacother* 2016;50:22–6.

90. Winterhalter M, Simon A, Fischer S, et al. Comparison of inhaled iloprost and nitric oxide in patients with pulmonary hypertension during weaning from cardiopulmonary bypass in cardiac surgery: a prospective randomized trial. *J Cardiothorac Vasc Anesth* 2008;22:406–13.

91. Theodoraki K, Thanopoulos A, Rellia P, et al. A retrospective comparison of inhaled milrinone and iloprost in post-bypass pulmonary hypertension. *Heart Vessels* 2017;32:1488–97.

92. Stephens RS, Whitman GJR. Postoperative critical care of the adult cardiac surgical patient: part II: procedure-specific considerations, management of complications, and quality improvement. *Crit Care Med* 2015;43:1995–2014.

93. Cannesson M, Farhat F, Scarlata M, Cassar E, Lehot JJ. The impact of atrio-biventricular pacing on hemodynamics and left ventricular dyssynchrony compared with atrio-right ventricular pacing alone in the postoperative period after cardiac surgery. *J Cardiothorac Vasc Anesth* 2009;23:306–11.

94. Gielgends RCW, Herold IHF, van Straten AHM, et al. The hemodynamic effects of different pacing modalities after cardiopulmonary bypass in patients with reduced left ventricular function. *J Cardiothorac Vasc Anesth* 2018;32:259–66.

95. Johnson RG, Goldberger AL, Thurer RL, Schwartz M, Sirois S, Weintraub RM. Lidocaine prophylaxis in coronary revascularization patients: a randomized, prospective trial. *Ann Thorac Surg* 1993;55:1180–4.

96. Zebis LR, Christensen TD, Thomsen HF, et al. Practical regimen for amiodarone use in preventing postoperative atrial fibrillation. *Ann Thorac Surg* 2007;83:1326–31.

97. Osmanovic E, Ostojic M, Avdic S, et al. Pharmacological prophylaxis of atrial fibrillation after surgical myocardial revascularization. *Med Arch* 2019;73:19–22.

98. Henyan NN, Gillespie EL, White CM, Kluger J, Coleman CI. Impact of intravenous magnesium on post-cardiothoracic surgery atrial fibrillation and length of hospital stay: a meta-analysis. *Ann Thorac Surg* 2005;80:2402–6.

99. van der Does WFB, de Broot NMS. Prophylaxis with amiodarone for postoperative atrial fibrillation: when and who? *J Thorac Dis* 2018;10(Suppl 33):S3831–3.

100. He GW, Taggart DP. Antispastic management in arterial grafts in coronary artery bypass grafting surgery. *Ann Thorac Surg* 2016;102:659–68.

101. Lorusso R, Crudeli E, Lucà F, et al. Refractory spasm of coronary arteries and grafted conduits after isolated coronary artery bypass surgery. *Ann Thorac Surg* 2012;93:545–51.

102. Thygesen K, Alpert JS, Jaffe AS, et al. Fourth universal definition of myocardial infarction (2018). *J Am Coll Cardiol* 2018;72:2231–64.

103. Thielmann M, Sharma V, Al-Attar N, et al. ESC Joint Working Groups on cardiovascular surgery and the cellular biology of the heart position paper: peri-operative myocardial injury and infarction in patients undergoing coronary artery bypass graft surgery. *Eur Heart J* 2017;38:2392–407.

104. Kulik A, Ruel M, Jneid H, et al. Secondary prevention after coronary artery bypass graft surgery: a scientific statement from the American Heart Association. *Circulation* 2015;131:927–64.

105. Bednar F, Osmancik P, Hlavicka J, Jedlickova V, Paluch Z, Vanek T. Aspirin is insufficient in inhibition of platelet aggregation and thromboxane formation early after coronary artery bypass surgery. *J Thromb Thrombolysis* 2009;27:394–9.

106. Bednar F, Tencer T, Plasil P, et al. Evaluation of aspirin's effect on platelet function early after coronary artery bypass grafting. *J Cardiothorac Vasc Anesth* 2012;26:575–86.

107 van Diepen S, Fuster V, Verma S, et al. Dual antiplatelet therapy versus aspirin monotherapy in diabetics with multivessel disease undergoing CABG: FREEDOM insights. *J Am Coll Cardiol* 2017;69:119–27.

108. Mori M, Shioda K, Bin Mahmood K, Mangi AA, Yun JJ, Giersson A. Dual antiplatelet therapy versus aspirin monotherapy in diabetics with stable ischemic heart disease undergoing coronary artery bypass grafting. *Ann Cardiothorac Surg* 2018;7:628–35.

109. Sousa-Uva M, Head SJ, Milojevic M, et al. 2017 EACTS guidelines on perioperative medication in adult cardiac surgery. *Eur J Cardiothorac Surg* 2018;53:5–33.

110. Verma S, Goodman SG, Mehta SR, et al. Should dual antiplatelet therapy be used in patients following coronary artery bypass surgery? A meta-analysis of randomized controlled trials. *BMC Surg* 2015;15:112.

111. Kulik A, Voisine P, Mathieu P, et al. Statin therapy and saphenous vein graft disease after coronary bypass surgery: analysis from the CASCADE randomized trial. *Ann Thorac Surg* 2011;92:1284–90.

112. Bin C, Junsheng M, Jianqun Z, Ping B. Meta-analysis of medium and long-term efficacy of loading statins after coronary artery bypass grafting. *Ann Thorac Surg* 2016;101:990–5.

113. Cavallaro P, Itagaki S, Seigerman M, Chikwe J. Operative mortality and stroke after on-pump vs off-pump surgery in high-risk patients: an analysis of 83,914 coronary bypass operations. *Eur J Cardiothorac Surg* 2014;45:159–64.

114. Lewicki L, Siebert J, Rogowski J. Atrial fibrillation following off-pump versus on-pump coronary artery bypass grafting: incidence and risk factors. *Cardiol J* 2016;23:518–23.

115. Neumann A, Vöhringer L, Fischer J, et al. Off-pump coronary artery bypass grafting in acute coronary syndrome: focus on safety and completeness of revascularization. *Thorac Cardiovasc Surg* 2019. doi:10.1055/s-0039-1677834. [Epub ahead of print]

116. Thakur U, Nerlekar N, Muthalaly RG, et al. Off- vs. on-pump coronary artery bypass grafting long-term survival is driven by incompleteness of revascularisation. *Heart Lung Circ* 2020;29:149–55.

117. Chikwe J, Lee T, Itagaki S, Adams DH, Egorova NN. Long-term outcomes after off-pump versus on-pump coronary artery bypass grafting by experienced surgeons. *J Am Coll Cardiol* 2018;72:1478–86.

118. Filardo G, Hamman BL, de Graca B, et al. Efficacy and effectiveness of on- versus off-pump coronary artery bypass grafting: a meta-analysis of mortality and survival. *J Thorac Cardiovasc Surg* 2018;155:172–9.

119. Takagi H, Mizuno Y, Niwa M, et al, A meta-analysis of randomized trials for repeat revascularization following off-pump versus on-pump coronary artery bypass grafting. *Interact Cardiovasc Thorac Surg* 2013;17:878–80.

120. Gaudino M, Angelini GD, Antoniades C, et al. Off-pump coronary artery bypass grafting: 30 years of debate. *J Am Heart Assoc* 2018;7:e009934.

121. Jeong SM, Hahm KD, Jeong YB, Yang HS, Choi IC. Warming of intravenous fluids prevents hypothermia during off-pump coronary artery bypass graft surgery. *J Cardiothorac Vasc Anesth* 2008;22:67–70.

122. Allen GS. Intraoperative temperature control using the Thermogard system during off-pump coronary artery bypass grafting. *Ann Thorac Surg* 2009;87:284–8.

123. Athanasiou T, Aziz O, Mangoush O, et al. Do off-pump techniques reduce the incidence of postoperative atrial fibrillation in elderly patients undergoing coronary artery bypass grafting? *Ann Thorac Surg* 2004;77:1567–74.

124. Zientara AM, Mariotti S, Matter-Ensner S, et al. Fast-track management in off-pump coronary artery bypass grafting: dexmedetomidine provides rapid extubation and effective pain modulation. *Thorac Cardiovasc Surg* 2019;67:450–7.

125. Staton GW, Williams WH, Mahoney EM, et al. Pulmonary outcomes of off-pump vs on-pump coronary artery bypass surgery in a randomized trial. *Chest* 2005;127:892–901.

126. Cimen S, Ozkul V, Ketenci B, et al. Daily comparison of respiratory functions between on-pump and off-pump patients undergoing CABG. *Eur J Cardiothorac Surg* 2003;23:589–94.

127. Dai Z, Chu H, Wang S, Liang Y. The effect of tranexamic acid to reduce blood loss and transfusion on off-pump coronary artery bypass surgery: a systematic review and cumulative meta-analysis. *J Clin Anesth* 2018;44:23–31.

128. Bednar F, Osmancik P, Vanek T, et al. Platelet activity and aspirin efficacy after off-pump compared with on-pump coronary artery bypass surgery: results from the prospective randomized PRAGUE 11-Coronary Artery Bypass and REactivity of Thrombocytes (CABARET). *J Thorac Cardiovasc Surg* 2008;136:1054–60.

129. Deo SV, Dunlay SM, Shah IK, et al. Dual anti-platelet therapy after coronary artery bypass grafting: is there any benefit? A systematic review and meta-analysis. *J Card Surg* 2013;28:109–16.

130. Gurbuz AT, Zia AA, Vuran AC, Cui H, Aytac A. Postoperative clopidogrel improves mid-term outcome after off-pump coronary artery bypass graft surgery: a prospective study. *Eur J Cardiothorac Surg* 2006;29:190–5.

131. Zisman E, Shenderey A, Ammar R, Eden A, Pizov R. The effects of intrathecal morphine on patients undergoing minimally invasive direct coronary artery bypass surgery. *J Cardiothorac Vasc Anesth* 2005;19:40–3.

132. Chiu KM, Wu CC, Wang MJ, et al. Local infusion of bupivacaine combined with intravenous patient-controlled analgesia provides better pain relief than intravenous patient-controlled analgesia alone in patients undergoing minimally invasive cardiac surgery. *J Thorac Cardiovasc Surg* 2008;135:1348–52.

133. Zaid RR, Barker CM, Little SH, Nagueh SF. Pre- and post-operative diastolic dysfunction in patients with valvular heart disease: diagnosis and therapeutic implications. *J Am Coll Cardiol* 2013;62:1922–30.

134. Rodés-Abau J, Ellenbogen KA, Krahn AD, et al. Management of conduction disturbances associated with transcatheter aortic valve replacement: JACC Scientific Expert Panel. *J Am Coll Cardiol* 2019;74:1086–106.

135. Jergensen TH, De Backer O, Gerds TA, Bieliauskas G, Svendsen JH, Sondergaard L. Immediate post-procedure 12-lead electrocardiography as predictor of late conduction defects after transcatheter aortic valve replacement. *JACC Cardiovasc Interv* 2018;11:1509–18.

136. Mangieri A, Lanzillo G, Bertoldi L, et al. Predictors of advanced conduction disturbances requiring a late (≥48 H) permanent pacemaker following transcatheter aortic valve replacement. *JACC Cardiovasc Interv* 2018;11:1519–26.

137. Urena M, Webb JG, Tamburino C, et al. Permanent pacemaker implantation after transcatheter aortic valve implantation: impact on late clinical outcomes and left ventricular function. *Circulation* 2014;129:1233–43.

138. Nazif TM, Chen S, George I, et al. New-onset left bundle branch block after transcatheter aortic valve replacement is associated with adverse long-term clinical outcomes in intermediate-risk patients: an analysis from the Partner II trial. *Eur Heart J* 2019;40:2218–27.

139. Kaplan RM, Yadlapati A, Cantey EP, et al. Conduction recovery following pacemaker implantation after transcatheter aortic valve replacement. *Pacing Clin Electrophysiol* 2019;42:146–52.

140. Abawi M, Pagnesi M, Agostoni P, et al. Postoperative delirium in individuals undergoing transcatheter aortic valve replacement: a systematic review and meta-analysis. *J Am Geriatr Soc* 2018;66:2417–24.

141. Stachon P, Kaier K, Zirlik A, et al. Risk factors and outcome of postoperative delirium after transcatheter aortic valve replacement. *Clin Res Cardiol* 2018;107:756–62.

142. Patel PA, Patel S, Feinman JW, et al. Stroke after transcatheter aortic valve replacement: incidence, definitions, etiologies, and management options. *J Cardiothorac Vasc Anesth* 2018;32:968–81.

143. Pagnesi M, Martino EA, Chiarito M, et al. Silent cerebral injury after transcatheter aortic valve implantation and the preventive role of embolic protection devices: a systematic review and meta-analysis. *Int J Cardiol* 2016;221:97–106.

144. Gallo M, Putzu A, Conti M, Pedrazzini G, Demertzis S, Ferrari E. Embolic protection devices for transcatheter aortic valve replacement. *Eur J Cardiothorac Surg* 2018;53:1118–26.

145. Zuo W, Yang M, He Y, Hao C, Chen L, Ma G. Single or dual antiplatelet therapy after transcatheter aortic valve replacement: an updated systemic review and meta-analysis. *J Thorac Dis* 2019;11:959–68.

146. Brouwer J, Nijenhuis VJ, Delewi R, et al. Aspirin with or without clopidogrel after transcatheter aortic-valve implantation. *N Engl J Med* 2020;383:1447–57.

147. Dangas GD, Tijssen JG, Wöhrle J, et al., on behalf of the GALILEO Investigators. A controlled trial of rivaroxaban after transcatheter aortic-valve replacement. *N Engl J Med* 2020;382:120–9.

148. Mathews IG, Fazal IA, Bates MG, Turley AJ. In patients undergoing aortic valve replacement, what factors predict the requirement for permanent pacemaker implantation? *Interact Cardiovasc Thorac Surg* 2011;12:475–9.

149. Nardi P, Pellegrino A, Scafuri A, et al. Permanent pacemaker implantation after isolated aortic valve replacement: incidence, risk factors and surgical technical aspects. *J Cardiovasc Med (Hagerstown)* 2010;11:14–9.

150. Erdogan HB, Kayalar N, Ardal H, et al. Risk factors for requirement of permanent pacemaker implantation after aortic valve replacement. *J Card Surg* 2006;21:211–5.

151. Romano MA, Koeckert M, Mumtaz MA, et al. Permanent pacemaker implantation after rapid deployment aortic valve replacement. *Ann Thorac Surg* 2018;106:685–90.

152. Ensminger S, Fujita B, Bauer T, et al. Rapid deployment versus conventional bioprosthetic valve replacement for aortic stenosis. *J Am Coll Cardiol* 2018;71:1417–28.

153. Bouhout I, Mazine A, Rivard L, et al. Conduction disorders after sutureless aortic valve replacement. *Ann Thorac Surg* 2017;103:1254–60.

154. Thomas JL, Dickstein RA, Parker FB Jr, et al. Prognostic significance of the development of left bundle conduction defects following aortic valve replacement. *J Thorac Cardiovasc Surg* 1982;84:382–6.

155. Greason KL, Lahr BD, Stulak JM, et al. Long-term mortality effect of early pacemaker implantation after surgical aortic valve replacement. *Ann Thorac Surg* 2017;104:1259–64.

156. Mehaffey JH, Haywood NS, Hawkins RB, et al. Need for permanent pacemaker after surgical aortic valve replacement reduces long-term survival. *Ann Thorac Surg* 2018;108:460–5.

157. Nishimura RA, Otto CM, Bonow RO, et al. 2017 AHA/ACC focused update of the 2014 AHA/ACC guideline for the management of patients with valvular heart disease. *Circulation* 2017;135:e1159–95.

158. Baumgartner H, Falk V, Bax JJ, et al. 2017 ESC/EACTS Guidelines for the management of valvular heart disease. *Eur Heart J* 2017;38:2739–91.

159. Papak JN, Chiovaro JC, Noelck N, et al. Antithrombotic strategies after bioprosthetic aortic valve replacement: a systematic review. *Ann Thorac Surg* 2019;107:1571–81.

160. Guimarães PO, Pokorney SD, Lopes RD, et al. Efficacy and safety of apixaban vs warfarin in patients with atrial fibrillation and prior bioprosthetic valve replacement or valve repair: insights from the ARISTOTLE trial. *Clin Cardiol* 2019;42:568–71.

161. Jones HU, Mulestein JB, Jones KW, et al. Early postoperative use of unfractionated heparin or enoxaparin is associated with increased surgical re-exploration for bleeding. *Ann Thorac Surg* 2005;80:519–22.

162. Kindo M, Gerelli S, Hoanag Minh T, et al. Exclusive low-molecular-weight heparin as bridging anticoagulant after mechanical valve replacement. *Ann Thorac Surg* 2014;97:789–95.

163. Eikelboom JW, Connolly SJ, Brueckmann M, et al. Dabigatran versus warfarin in patients with mechanical heart valves. *N Engl J Med* 2013;369:1206–14.

164. Kim DJ, Lee S, Joo HC, et al. Effect of pulmonary hypertension on clinical outcomes in patients with rheumatic mitral stenosis. *Ann Thorac Surg* 2020;109:496–508.

165. Tempe DK, Hasija S, Datt V, et al. Evaluation and comparison of early hemodynamic changes after elective mitral valve replacement in patients with severe and mild pulmonary arterial hypertension. *J Cardiothorac Vasc Anesth* 2009;23:298–305.

166. Quintana E, Suri RM, Thalji NM, et al. Left ventricular dysfunction after mitral valve repair: the fallacy of "normal" preoperative myocardial function. *J Thorac Cardiovasc Surg* 2014;148:2752–60.

167. Suri RM, Schaff HV, Dearani JA, et al. Determinants of early decline in ejection fraction after surgical correction of mitral regurgitation. *J Thorac Cardiovasc Surg* 2008;136:442–7.

168. Maganti M, Badiwala M, Sheikh A, et al. Predictors of low cardiac output syndrome after isolated mitral valve surgery. *J Thorac Cardiovasc Surg* 2010;140:790–6.

169. Chan V, Ruel M, Elmistekawy E, Mesana TG. Determinants of left ventricular dysfunction after repair of chronic asymptomatic mitral regurgitation. *Ann Thorac Surg* 2015;99:38–42.

170. Kislitsina ON, Thomas JD, Crawford E, et al. Predictors of left ventricular dysfunction after surgery for degenerative mitral regurgitation. *Ann Thorac Surg* 2020;19:669–77.

171. Suri RM, Schaff HV, Dearani JA, et al. Recovery of left ventricular function after surgical correction of mitral regurgitation caused by leaflet prolapse. *J Cardiovasc Thorac Surg* 2009;137:1071–6.

172. Hiltrop N, Bennett J, Desmet W. Circumflex coronary artery injury after mitral valve surgery: a report of four cases and comprehensive review of the literature. *Catheter Cardiovasc Interv* 2017;89:78–92.

173. Hyllén S, Nozohoor S, Ingvarsson A, Meurling C, Wierup P, Sjögren J. Right ventricular performance after valve repair for chronic degenerative mitral regurgitation. *Ann Thorac Surg* 2014;98:2023–31.

174. Wu VCC, Takeuchi M. Echocardiographic assessment of right ventricular systolic function. *Cardiovasc Diag Ther* 2018;8:789–9.

175. Elmi-Sarabi M, Descamps A, Delisle S, et al. Aerosolized vasodilators for the treatment of pulmonary hypertension in cardiac surgical patients: a systematic review and meta-analysis. *Anesth Analg* 2017;125:393–402.

176. Rex S, Schaelte G, Metzelder S, et al. Inhaled iloprost to control pulmonary artery hypertension in patients undergoing mitral valve surgery: a prospective, randomized-controlled trial. *Acta Anaethesiol Scand* 2008;52:65–72.

177. Wang H, Gong M, Zhou B, Dai A. Comparison of inhaled and intravenous milrinone in patients with pulmonary hypertension undergoing mitral valve surgery. *Adv Ther* 2009;26:462–8.

178. Laflamme M, Perrault LP, Carrier M, Elmi-Sarabi M, Fortier A, Denault AY. Preliminary experience with combined inhaled milrinone and prostacyclin in cardiac surgical patients with pulmonary hypertension. *J Cardiothorac Vasc Anesth* 2015;29:38–45.

179. Gebhard CE, Rochon A, Cogan J, et al. Acute right ventricular failure in cardiac surgery during cardiopulmonary bypass separation: a retrospective case series of 12 years' experience with intratracheal milrinone administration. *J Cardiothorac Vasc Anesth* 2019;33:651–60.

180. Shim JK, Choi YS, Oh YJ, Kim DH, Hong YW, Kwak YL. Effect of oral sildenafil citrate on intraoperative hemodynamics in patients with pulmonary hypertension undergoing valvular heart surgery. *J Thorac Cardiovasc Surg* 2006;132:1420–5.

181. Ram E, Sternik L, Klempfner R, et al. Sildenafil for pulmonary hypertension in the early postoperative period after mitral valve surgery. *J Cardiothorac Vasc Anesth* 2019;33:1648–56.

182. Okamoto K, Kiso I, Inoue Y, Matayoshi H, Takahashi R, Umezu Y. Left ventricular outflow obstruction after mitral valve replacement preserving native anterior leaflet. *Ann Thorac Surg* 2006;82:735–7.

183. Crescenzi G, Landoni G, Zangrillo A, et al. Management and decision-making strategy for systolic anterior motion after mitral valve repair. *J Thorac Cardiovasc Surg* 2009;137:320–5.

184. Sherrid MV, Balaram S, Kim B, Axel L, Swistel DG. The mitral valve in obstructive hypertrophic cardiomyopathy: a test in context. *J Am Coll Cardiol* 2016;67:1846–58.

185. Tambuer L, Meyns B, Flameng W, Daenen W. Rhythm disturbances after mitral valve surgery: comparison between left atrial and extended transseptal approach. *Cardiovasc Surg* 1996;4:820–4.

186. Little S, Flynn M, Pettersson GB, Gillinov AM, Blackstone EH. Revisiting the dome approach to partial sternotomy/minimally invasive mitral valve surgery. *Ann Thorac Surg* 2009;87:694–7.

187. Nienaber JJ, Glower DD. Minitransseptal versus left atrial approach to the mitral valve: a comparison of outcomes. *Ann Thorac Surg* 2006;82:834–9.

188. Grigioni F, Benfari G, Vanoverschelde JL, et al. Long-term implications of atrial fibrillation in patients with degenerative mitral regurgitation. *J Am Coll Cardiol* 2019;73:264–74.

189. Zheng S, Zhang H, Li Y, Han J, Jia Y, Meng X. Comparison of left atrial and biatrial maze procedure in the treatment of atrial fibrillation: a meta-analysis of clinical studies. *Thorac Cardiovasc Surg* 2016;64:661–71.

190. Li H, Lin X, Ma X, et al. Biatrial versus isolated left atrial ablation in atrial fibrillation: a systematic review and meta-analysis. *Biomed Res Int* 2018;2018:3651212. https://doi.org/10.1155/2018/3651212.

191. Robertson JO, Cuculich PS, Saint LL, et al. Predictors and risk of pacemaker implantation after the Cox-Maze IV procedure. *Ann Thorac Surg* 2013;95:2015–20.

192. DeRose JJ, Mancini DM, Chang HL, et al. Pacemaker implantation after mitral valve surgery with atrial fibrillation ablation. *J Am Coll Cardiol* 2019;73:2427–35.

193. Ishii Y, Gleva MJ, Gamache C, et al. Atrial tachyarrhythmias after the Maze procedure: incidence and prognosis. *Circulation* 2004;110:II-164–8.

194. Takagi M, Yamaguchi H, Ikeda N, et al. Risk factors for atrial fibrillation recurrence after Cox Maze IV performed without pre-exclusion. *Ann Thorac Surg* 2020;109:771–9.

195. Dresen W, Mason PK. Atrial flutter after surgical maze: incidence, diagnosis, and management. *Cur Opin Cardiol* 2016;31:57–63.

196. Hwang SK, Yoo JS, Kim JB, et al. Long-term outcomes of the maze procedure combined with mitral valve repair: risk of thromboembolism without anticoagulation therapy. *Ann Thorac Surg* 2015;100:840–4.

197. Ad N, Henry L, Shuman DJ, Holmes SD. A more specific anticoagulation regimen is required for patients after the Cox-Maze procedure. *Ann Thorac Surg* 2014;98:1331–8.

198. Pacha HM, Hritani R, Alraeis MC. Antithrombotic therapy after percutaneous left atrial appendage occlusion using the WATCHMAN device. *Ochsner J* 2018;18:193–4.

199. Karlson KH, Ashraf MM, Berger RL. Rupture of the left ventricle following mitral valve replacement. *Ann Thorac Surg* 1988;46:590–7.

200. van der Wall SJ, Olsthoorn JR, Huets S, et al. Antithrombotic therapy after mitral valve repair: VKA or aspirin? *J Thoromb Thrombolysis* 2018;46:473–81.

201. Suzuki T, Asai T, Kinoshita T. Predictors for late reoperation after surgical repair of acute type A aortic dissection. *Ann Thorac Surg* 2018;106:63–9.

202. Kodama K, Nishigami K, Sakamoto T, et al. Tight heart rate control reduces secondary adverse events in patients with type B aortic dissection. *Circulation* 2008;118(14 Suppl):S167–70.

203. Stamou SC, Rausch LA, Kouchoukos NT, et al. Comparison between antegrade and retrograde cerebral perfusion or profound hypothermia as brain protection strategies during repair of type A aortic dissection. *Ann Cardiothorac Surg* 2016;5:328–35.

204. Stamou SC, Gartner D, Louchoukos NT, et al. Axillary versus femoral artery cannulation during repair of type A aortic dissection? An old problem seeking new solutions. *Aorta (Stamford)* 2016;4:115–23.

205. Nauta AJH, Trimarchi S, Kamman AV, et al. Update in the management of type B aortic dissection. *Vasc Med* 2016;21:251–63.

206. Moulakakis KG, Mylonas SN, Daleinas I, Kakisis J, Kotsis T, Liapis CD. Management of complicated and uncomplicated acute type B dissection: a systematic review and meta-analysis. *Ann Cardiothorac Surg* 2014;3:234–46.

207. Tadros ROI, Tang GHL, Barnes JH, et al. Optimal treatment of uncomplicated type B aortic dissection. *J Am Coll Cardiol* 2019;74:1494–504.

208. Krol E, Panneton JM. Uncomplicated acute type B aortic dissection: selection guidelines for TEVAR. *Ann Vasc Dis* 2017;10:pii:ra.17-00061.

209. Perreas K, Samanidis G, Thanopoulos A, et al. Antegrade or retrograde cerebral perfusion in ascending aorta and hemiarch surgery? A propensity-matched analysis. *Ann Thor Surg* 2016;101:146–52.

210. Khaladj N, Shrestha M, Meck S, et al. Hypothermic circulatory arrest with selective antegrade cerebral perfusion in ascending aortic and aortic arch surgery: a risk factor analysis for adverse outcome in 501 patients. *J Thorac Cardiovasc Surg* 2008;135:908–14.

211. Spielvogel D, Etz CD, Silovitz D, Lansman SL, Griepp RB. Aortic arch replacement with a trifurcated graft. *Ann Thorac Surg* 2007;83:S791–5.

212. Shirasaka T, Okada K, Kano H, Matsumori M, Inoue T, Okita Y. New indicator of postoperative delayed awakening after total aortic arch replacement. *Eur J Cardiothorac Surg* 2015;47:101–5.

213. Mazzeffi M, Marotta M, Lin HM, Fischer G. Duration of deep hypothermia during aortic surgery and the risk of perioperative blood transfusion. *Ann Card Anaesth* 2012;15:266–73.

214. Chen MF, Chen LW, Cao H, Lin Y. Analysis of risk factors for and the prognosis of postoperative acute respiratory distress syndrome in patients with Stanford type A aortic dissection. *J Thorac Dis* 2016;8:2862–71.

215. Estrera AL, Sheinbaum R, Miller CC, et al. Cerebrospinal fluid drainage during thoracic aortic repair: safety and current management. *Ann Thorac Surg* 2009;88:9–15.

216. Tanaka A, Safi HJ, Estrera AL. Current strategies of spinal cord protection during thoracoabdominal aortic surgery. *Gen Thorac Cardiovasc Surg* 2018;66:307–14.

217. Bilal H, O'Neill B, Mahmood S, Waterworth P. Is cerebrospinal fluid drainage of benefit to neuroprotection in patients undergoing surgery on the descending thoracic aorta or thoracoabdominal aorta? *Interact Cardiovasc Thorac Surg* 2012;15:702–8.

218. Archer C, Wynn M. Paraplegia after thoracoabdominal aortic surgery: not just assisted circulation, hypothermic arrest, clamp and sew, or TEVAR. *Ann Cardiothorac Surg* 2012;1:365–72.

219. Maniar HS, Sundt TM III, Prasad SM, et al. Delayed paraplegia after thoracic and thoracoabdominal aneurysm repair: a continuing risk. *Ann Thorac Surg* 2003;75:113–20.

220. Hunt I, Deshpande RP, Aps C, Young CP. Delayed paraplegia after thoracic and thoracoabdominal aneurysm repair: timing of reinsertion of spinal drain. *Ann Thorac Surg* 2004;78:2213

221. Cheung AT, Weiss SJ, McGarvey ML, et al. Interventions for reversing delayed-onset postoperative paraplegia after thoracic aortic reconstruction. *Ann Thorac Surg* 2002;74:413–9.

222. Coselli JS, Amarasekara HS, Zhang Q, et al. The impact of preoperative chronic kidney disease on outcomes after Crawford extent II thoracoabdominal aneurysm repairs. *J Thorac Cardiovasc Surg* 2018;156:2053–64.

223. Girardi LN. Perioperative renal function and thoracoabdominal aneurysm repair: where do we go from here? *J Thorac Cardiovasc Surg* 2018;50:2049–50.

224. Wynn MM, Acher C, Marks E, Engelbert T, Acher CW. Postoperative renal failure in thoracoabdominal aortic aneurysm, repair with simple cross-clamp technique and 4 °C renal perfusion. *J Vasc Surg* 2015;61:611–22.

225. Aftab M, Coselli JS. Reprint of: renal and visceral protection in thoracoabdominal aortic surgery. *J Thorac Cardiovasc Surg* 2015;149(2 Suppl):S130–3.

226. Gravereax EC, Faries PL, Burks JA, et al. Risk of spinal cord ischemia after endograft repair of thoracic aortic aneurysm. *J Vasc Surg* 2001;34:997–1003.

227. Von Aspern K, Luehr M, Mohr FW, Etz CD. Spinal cord protection in open- and endovascular thoracoabdominal aortic aneurysm repair: critical review of current concepts and future perspectives. *J Cardiovasc Surg (Torino)* 2015;56:745–9.

228. Khoynezhad A, Donayre CE, Bui H, Kopchok GE, Walot I, White RA. Risk factors of neurologic deficit after thoracic aortic endografting. *Ann Thorac Surg* 2007;83:S882–9.

229. Miranda V, Sousa J, Mansilha A. Spinal cord injury in endovascular thoracoabdominal aortic aneurysm repair: prevalence, risk factors and preventive strategies. *Int Angiol* 2018;37:112–26.

230. Liu LY, Callahan B, Peterss S, et al. Neuromonitoring using motor and somatosensory evoked potentials in aortic surgery. *J Card Surg* 2016;31:383–9.

231. Acher C, Acher CW, Marks E, Wynn M. Intraoperative neuroprotective interventions prevent spinal cord ischemia and injury in thoracic endovascular aortic repair. *J Vasc Surg* 2016;63:1458–65.

232. Piffaretti G, Mariscalco G, Bonardelli S, et al. Predictors and outcomes of acute kidney injury after thoracic aortic endograft repair. *J Vasc Surg* 2012;56:1527–34.

233. Pisimisis GT, Khoynezhad A, Bashir K, Kruse MJ, Donayre CE, White RA. Incidence and risk factors of renal dysfunction after thoracic endovascular aortic repair. *J Thorac Cardiovasc Surg* 2010;140(6 Suppl): S161–7.

234. De Maria E, Olaaru A, Cappelli S. The entirely subcutaneous defibrillator (s-icd): state of the art and selection of the ideal candidate. *Curr Cardiol Rev* 2015;11:180–6.

235. Olgin JE, Pletcher MJ, Vitinghoff E, et al. Wearable cardioverter-defibrillator after myocardial infarction. *N Engl J Med* 2018;379:1205–15.

236. Kutyifa V, Moss AJ, Klein H, et al. Use of the wearable cardioverter defibrillator in high-risk cardiac patients: data from the Prospective Registry of Patients Using the Wearable Cardioverter Defibrillator (WEARIT-II Registry). *Circulation* 2015;132:1613–9.

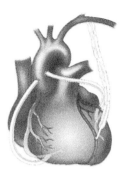

CHAPTER 9

Mediastinal Bleeding

♡ 9 Mediastinal Bleeding

I. Overview

A. The use of cardiopulmonary bypass (CPB) during cardiac surgical procedures causes a significant disruption of the coagulation system that may contribute to a coagulopathy of varying degrees.[1] In addition to hemodilution from a crystalloid prime, which reduces levels of clotting factors and platelets, contact of blood with the extracorporeal circuit activates platelets and the extrinsic and intrinsic coagulation systems and triggers fibrinolysis. In fact, systemic heparinization alone causes platelet dysfunction and induces fibrinolysis.[2] In addition, cell-saving devices that are routinely used for red cell salvage eliminate platelets and coagulation factors from the blood.

B. Off-pump coronary artery bypass surgery (OPCAB) avoids hemodilution, minimizes platelet activation, and reduces usage of blood products.[3] The ability of the antifibrinolytic agents to reduce bleeding during these procedures suggests that low-grade fibrinolysis is still present.[4] Although a coagulopathy after OPCAB is very unusual, it may occur in patients who have sustained substantial blood loss with blood scavenged in and returned from the cell-saving device. This will result in depletion of coagulation factors and platelets. The occurrence of substantial bleeding after an OPCAB procedure generally indicates a surgical source.

C. Either 28–32 Fr PVC or silicone malleable chest tubes or 24 Fr silicone fluted (Blake) drains are placed in the mediastinum and opened pleural cavities at the conclusion of surgery. They are connected to a drainage system and placed to –20 cm of H_2O suction. They are gently milked or stripped to maintain patency after surgery. Both are equally effective in evacuating blood, although the Blake drains may be more comfortable for the patient.[5,6]

1. Some surgeons do not obligatorily place chest tubes into widely opened pleural spaces, especially after off-pump surgery. However, any bleeding that occurs in the pleural space will tend to accumulate and not be drained by the mediastinal tubes. This can produce a deceptive picture with insidious bleeding that can only be detected by chest x-ray.

2. Following minimally invasive surgery, the number and location of tubes may vary. After MIDCABs, only one pleural chest tube is placed, so blood could potentially accumulate around the heart and not be drained through the pericardial opening. Following ministernotomy incisions, one mediastinal tube is placed unless the pleural cavity is entered. With right thoracotomy approaches to the aortic or mitral valve, one mediastinal and one pleural tube are placed. Chest tube positioning is difficult and not ideal after these procedures, so the potential for undetected blood

Manual of Perioperative Care in Adult Cardiac Surgery, Sixth Edition. Robert M. Bojar.
© 2021 John Wiley & Sons Ltd. Published 2021 by John Wiley & Sons Ltd.

accumulation around the heart or in the pleural spaces is enhanced. Thus, extra vigilance for undrained blood in the unstable patient is imperative.

D. Postoperative bleeding gradually tapers over the course of several hours in the majority of patients, but about 1–3% of patients will require re-exploration for persistent mediastinal bleeding. Prompt assessment and aggressive treatment in the intensive care unit (ICU) may frequently arrest "medical bleeding", but evidence of persistent or increasing amounts of bleeding should prompt early exploration (see section VIII, pages 446–449).

E. Persistent mediastinal bleeding invariably requires the use of various blood products to maintain normovolemia and adequate hemodynamic parameters, correct anemia to ensure adequate tissue oxygen delivery, and correct a coagulopathy to help arrest the bleeding. Understandably, increased chest tube drainage in the early postoperative period is associated with adverse outcomes. One study showed that drainage of >200 mL/h in one hour or >2 mg/kg for two consecutive hours was associated with an increased risk of stroke, re-exploration, prolonged ventilation, and mortality.[7] The need for transfusions and re-exploration are both independent risk factors for morbidity and mortality.[8]

F. Transfused blood is not benign, contributing to increased postoperative morbidity, including graft occlusion, pulmonary, infectious, neurologic, renal, and gastrointestinal complications, as well as increased short-term and long-term mortality.[9-13] Although a "restrictive" transfusion strategy (transfusion threshold of a hemoglobin of 7–8 g/dL or a hematocrit [HCT] of 21–24%) might be safe in stable patients,[14-16] hemodynamic considerations and potential impairment of tissue oxygen delivery with ongoing bleeding mandate transfusions to maintain a safe HCT, which is probably at least 24%. Blood component therapy ideally should be selected based upon identification of specific coagulation abnormalities by point-of-care testing and treatment algorithms, although clinical judgment remains essential in making prompt and appropriate therapeutic decisions.[17,18]

G. Mediastinal bleeding can be a highly morbid and lethal problem. Although hypovolemia can be corrected by volume infusions, the bleeding patient tends to be hemodynamically unstable out of proportion to the degree of bleeding and fluid replacement. Most importantly in the immediate postoperative period is the potential for blood to accumulate around the heart, causing cardiac tamponade. The restriction to cardiac filling may produce severe hemodynamic compromise that can precipitously cause cardiac arrest. Constant attention to the degree of bleeding and to trends in hemodynamic parameters should allow for steps to be taken to avert this problem. If profound hypotension or a cardiac arrest develops, emergency sternotomy in the ICU is indicated.

II. Etiology of Mediastinal Bleeding

Mediastinal bleeding is somewhat arbitrarily categorized as "surgical" or "medical" in nature (Table 9.1). Significant bleeding after uneventful surgery is usually "surgical", especially when initial coagulation studies are fairly normal. However, persistent bleeding depletes coagulation factors and platelets, causing a coagulopathy that is self-perpetuating. Bleeding that is noted after complex operations with long durations of CPB is frequently associated with abnormal coagulation studies and is considered "medical". However, even after correction of coagulation abnormalities, discrete bleeding sites may be present that will not stop without re-exploration.

Table 9.1 • Etiology of Mediastinal Bleeding

1. Surgical bleeding sites
2. Residual anticoagulant/antiplatelet effects from medications
3. Platelet dysfunction
4. Thrombocytopenia
5. Heparin effect – residual or rebound
6. Excessive protamine administration
7. Clotting factor deficiency
8. Fibrinolysis

Table 9.2 • Patients at Increased Risk for Mediastinal Bleeding

Patient-related Variables

1. Older patients
2. Females or smaller body surface area
3. Preoperative anemia
4. Advanced cardiac disease (shock, poor left ventricular function)
5. Comorbidities (renal or hepatic dysfunction, diabetes, peripheral vascular disease)
6. Known coagulopathies (von Willebrand's disease, uremia)

Preoperative Medications

1. High-dose aspirin
2. P2Y12 inhibitors (clopidogrel, ticagrelor, prasugrel)
3. Low-molecular-weight heparin (LMWH) within 18 hours
4. Nonvitamin K antagonist oral anticoagulants (NOACs), including dabigatran, apixaban, rivaroxaban, and edoxaban, within 48 hours
5. Incomplete reversal of INR off warfarin
6. Emergency surgery after IIb/IIIa inhibitors or thrombolytic therapy

Procedure-related Variables

1. Complex operations (valve-CABG, thoracic aortic surgery, aortic dissections, especially requiring deep hypothermic circulatory arrest)
2. Urgent/emergent operations
3. Reoperations
4. Use of bilateral ITA grafting

Most studies suggest that a surgical source is identified in about two-thirds of patients who are re-explored.[19] Thus, the initial approach to bleeding is to try to identify any contributing factors that might account for the degree of bleeding and then take the appropriate steps to correct them.

A. A number of risk factors have been identified that increase perioperative bleeding and/or the requirement for transfusions (Table 9.2).[14,20-22] One risk stratification model found an excellent correlation of only five factors with the risk of significant bleeding, which included nonelective surgery, more than a CABG or isolated valve operation, presence of aortic valve disease, a body mass index (BMI) >25, and age >75.[23] Aside from stopping antiplatelet or anticoagulant medications preoperatively, most risk factors cannot be modified. However, they should alert the healthcare team to the increased risk of a coagulopathy, the necessity of utilizing blood conservation measures, and the importance of early aggressive treatment of bleeding to minimize or prevent hemodynamic compromise and organ system dysfunction.

B. Surgical bleeding is usually related to:
   1. Anastomotic sites (suture lines)
   2. Side branches of arterial or venous conduits
   3. Substernal soft tissues, sternal suture sites, bone marrow, periosteum
   4. Raw surfaces caused by previous surgery, pericarditis, or radiation therapy

C. Residual anticoagulant effects of medications taken preoperatively, which include:
   1. Unfractionated heparin that is continued into the operating room
   2. Low-molecular-weight heparin (LMWH) given within 18 hours
   3. Nonvitamin K antagonist oral anticoagulants (NOACs), including dabigatran, apixaban, rivaroxaban, and edoxaban when given within 48 hours or even longer in patients with chronic kidney disease
   4. Intravenous direct thrombin inhibitors (bivalirudin)
   5. Indirect factor Xa inhibitors (fondaparinux)

D. Qualitative platelet defects – a major concern with the liberal use of antiplatelet agents in patients with acute coronary syndromes and recently placed stents.[14,24,25]
   1. Preoperative platelet dysfunction may result from antiplatelet medications (aspirin and P2Y12 inhibitors [clopidogrel, ticagrelor, prasugrel]), glycoprotein IIb/IIIa inhibitors (tirofiban, eptifibatide, abciximab), herbal medications and vitamins (fish oils, ginkgo products, vitamin E), or uremia.
   2. Exposure of platelets to the CPB circuit with alpha-granule release and alteration of platelet membrane receptors impairs platelet function. The degree of platelet dysfunction correlates with the duration of CPB and the degree of hypothermia after bypass.
   3. Inadequate heparinization is a potent trigger for thrombin release, which activates platelets.

E. Quantitative platelet defects
   1. Preoperative thrombocytopenia may result from use of heparin, drug reactions (P2Y12 inhibitors including clopidogrel and prasugrel, but not ticagrelor, antibiotics and IIb/IIIa inhibitors), infection, hypersplenism in patients with liver disease, and other chronic conditions (idiopathic thrombocytopenic purpura [ITP]). If a patient developing thrombocytopenia has recently been given heparin, it is essential to rule out heparin-induced thrombocytopenia (HIT).
   2. Hemodilution on CPB and consumption in the extracorporeal circuit reduce the platelet count by about 30–50%, and thrombocytopenia will be progressive as the duration of CPB lengthens.
   3. Protamine administration transiently reduces the platelet count by about 30%.

F. Intraoperative heparin and protamine usage
   1. Residual heparin effect may result from inadequate neutralization with protamine at the conclusion of CPB. Administering fully heparinized "pump" blood towards the end of the protamine infusion will reintroduce unneutralized heparin into the

blood. Blood washed in cell-saving devices is usually given after protamine administration, but it has been shown to contain insignificant amounts of heparin.[26]

2. Heparin rebound may occur when heparin reappears from tissue stores after protamine administration. This is more common in patients receiving large amounts of heparin, especially obese patients.

3. Excessive protamine may cause a coagulopathy.[14,27,28]

G. Depletion of coagulation factors

1. Preoperative hepatic dysfunction, residual warfarin effect with vitamin K-dependent clotting factor deficiencies, and thrombolytic therapy reduce the level of clotting factors. Increased bleeding may specifically be related to a low fibrinogen level.[29]

2. von Willebrand's disease caused by a deficiency in von Willebrand's factor, a clotting protein that binds to factor VIII and platelets to form a platelet plug. An acquired form is associated with aortic stenosis.[30]

3. Hemodilution on CPB reduces most factors by 50%, including fibrinogen. This is most pronounced in patients with a small blood volume.

4. Loss of clotting factors results from use of intraoperative cell-saving devices.

H. Fibrinolysis results in clotting factor degradation and platelet dysfunction.

1. Preoperative use of thrombolytic agents causes fibrinolysis.

2. Use of CPB causes plasminogen activation.

3. Heparinization itself induces a fibrinolytic state.

III. Prevention of Perioperative Blood Loss: Blood Conservation Measures (Table 9.3)[14,22]

A. Preoperative assessment of the patient's coagulation system should entail measurement of a prothrombin time, as measured by the international normalized ratio (INR), partial thromboplastin time (PTT), and platelet count. Any abnormality should be investigated and corrected, if possible, prior to surgery. Platelet function testing to assess platelet responsiveness to P2Y12 inhibitors is helpful in determining when the bleeding risk is low enough to proceed with urgent, but not emergent, surgery.[31]

B. Considerations in patients with preoperative anemia

1. Preoperative anemia is associated with increased morbidity and mortality after cardiac surgery, being most likely a surrogate for clinical disease and increasing the requirement for transfusions.[32] Preoperative iron supplementation and use of erythropoietin should be considered in anemic patients undergoing elective surgery, especially Jehovah Witness patients, who refuse any blood transfusions (see doses on page 197 in Chapter 3).

2. Hemodilution during CPB can produce a profound anemia in patients with a low preoperative HCT. This may increase the risk of renal dysfunction if the HCT on CPB is much less than 21%,[33,34] and can contribute to neurologic events, such as ischemic optic neuropathy.[35,36] Although preoperative transfusion for a HCT <26% will reduce the need for intraoperative transfusions, it is controversial as to whether there is any clinical benefit to this approach. However, patients who require multiple blood transfusions during surgery tend to be more coagulopathic and require additional blood component therapy, providing some justification for a preoperative transfusion strategy.

Table 9.3 • Methods of Minimizing Operative Blood Loss and Transfusion Requirements

1. Stop all anticoagulant and antiplatelet medications preoperatively if feasible (except low-dose ASA for CABG patients)
2. Consider erythropoietin with iron for anemic patients prior to elective surgery
3. Identify preoperative hematologic abnormalities (HIT, antiphospholipid syndrome)
4. Transfuse patients requiring urgent surgery to a HCT >26% preoperatively
5. Use antifibrinolytic therapy (ε-aminocaproic acid or tranexamic acid)
6. Consider off-pump coronary bypass grafting, if feasible
7. Perfusion considerations
   a. Autologous blood withdrawal prior to CPB if HCT >30% with plateletpheresis
   b. Use heparin-coated (biocompatible) circuit, if available
   c. Use miniaturized CPB circuit, if available
   d. Use heparin–protamine titration test to optimize anticoagulation and heparin reversal
   e. Consider retrograde autologous priming of the bypass circuit
   f. Avoid more than mild systemic hypothermia
   g. Avoid use of cardiotomy suction
   h. Salvage pump blood via either hemofiltration or cell saver
8. Employ meticulous surgical technique with careful inspection of anastomotic sites and all artery and vein side branches before coming off bypass
9. Complete neutralization of heparin with protamine based on heparin levels to return ACT to baseline
10. Administer appropriate blood component therapy based upon suspicion of the hemostatic defect (especially platelet dysfunction) or use point-of-care testing to direct blood component therapy
11. Use recombinant factor VIIa for intractable coagulopathic bleeding
12. Exercise patience

C. Heparin-induced thrombocytopenia (HIT) may develop in patients receiving intravenous heparin for several days before surgery. Thus, it is very important to recheck the platelet count on a daily basis in these patients. If the patient develops thrombocytopenia, with documented heparin antibodies by ELISA testing and a positive functional assay (serotonin release assay or heparin-induced platelet aggregation test), an alternative means of anticoagulation will be necessary during surgery (see pages 251–253).

D. Cessation of medications with antiplatelet or anticoagulant effects is essential to allow their effects to dissipate to minimize blood loss.[14,22] A more detailed discussion of these medications is presented in Chapter 3 (pages 186–193). Specific recommendations are as follows:

   1. **Warfarin** should be stopped 4–5 days before surgery to allow for the resynthesis of vitamin-K-dependent clotting factors and normalization of the INR. Bridging anticoagulation with either LMWH or unfractionated heparin is indicated in patients at high thromboembolic risk, including those with a mechanical valve, recent pulmonary embolism (<4 weeks), and atrial fibrillation

with rheumatic mitral stenosis or a CHA$_2$DS$_2$-VASc Score >4.[14] Otherwise, bridging is not indicated.

    a. If the patient requires urgent surgery, vitamin K should be given to normalize the INR. A slow IV infusion of 5 mg over 30 minutes is effective in promptly correcting the INR, but it is preferable to give 5 mg of oral vitamin K if surgery can be delayed a day or two to avoid the risk of anaphylaxis.

    b. If emergency surgery is indicated, fresh frozen plasma (FFP) or prothrombin complex concentrate (PCC) may be given. PCC is more effective and expeditious in reducing the INR and is the preferred product.[37,38] The recommended doses are 25 units/kg for an elevated INR <4, 35 units/kg for an INR of 4–6, and 50 units/kg for an INR >6.

    c. Factor eight inhibitor bypassing activity (FEIBA) is an activated four-factor PCC. It is an anti-inhibitor coagulant complex that contains nonactivated factors II, IX, X, activated factor VII and factor VIII inhibitor bypassing activity, and some factor VIII coagulant antigen. It has been used to control warfarin-related coagulopathic bleeding and thus could be used to achieve rapid reversal of warfarin prior to emergency surgery. It can normalize the INR within an hour, but may be associated with thrombotic events.[39]

2. **Unfractionated heparin (UFH)** is used for patients with acute coronary syndromes, during catheterization, for critical coronary disease, or during use of an intra-aortic balloon pump (IABP). It can be continued up to the time of surgery without increasing morbidity during line placement or increasing the risk of perioperative bleeding. A common practice is to stop it four hours in advance of surgery for patients at low risk for instability.

3. **Low-molecular-weight heparin (LMWH)** is given in a dose of 1 mg/kg SC q12h for acute coronary syndromes or as a bridge to surgery once warfarin has been stopped. LMWH has a half-life of approximately four hours, so the last dose should be given 24 hours prior to surgery to minimize the perioperative bleeding risk, since only 60–80% of LMWH is reversible with protamine.

4. **Aspirin (ASA)** should be continued up to the time of surgery in patients undergoing bypass surgery, but it may be stopped 3–5 days prior to noncoronary surgery. Because an 81 mg dose is usually not associated with an increased risk of bleeding and has arguably lowered the risk of infarction and mortality, it can be recommended before all coronary bypass operations.[40–42] Antifibrinolytic drugs, which should be routinely used, may reduce bleeding associated with preoperative use of aspirin and possibly P2Y12 inhibitors.[43–45]

5. **The P2Y12 inhibitors** are commonly given to patients presenting with an acute coronary syndrome and are generally recommended for at least a year in patients undergoing percutaneous coronary intervention (PCI) with drug-eluting stents to avoid stent thrombosis. They exhibit antiplatelet effects that last for the lifespan of the platelet, which is 5–7 days, and an increased risk of bleeding is noted when they are stopped for shorter periods of time prior to surgery.[46] It is generally recommended that ticagrelor be stopped 3–5 days, clopidogrel 5 days, and prasugrel 7 days before surgery.[14,22,47] Use of PRU testing, which is an abbreviation for both platelet reactivity units and P2Y12 reaction units, may reveal patient resistance to P2Y12 inhibitors, allowing for safer earlier surgery than the recommended five-day interval.[31,48] If surgery is required on an emergent or urgent

basis, significant bleeding may be encountered, and exogenously administered platelets may be ineffective if given within several hours of a dose of a P2Y12 inhibitor, because the active metabolite may still be present in the bloodstream. Nonetheless, the urgency of surgery to prevent an ischemic event always takes precedence over the time interval from cessation of a P2Y12 inhibitor. If a patient requires urgent but not emergent surgery after receiving one of these drugs or is taking them for recent stent placement, feasible options are to:

a. Continue the P2Y12 inhibitor and accept the potential for more bleeding.

b. Stop it for three days to restore some platelet function while maintaining a lesser degree of platelet inhibition.

c. Stop it for 5 days and use a short-acting glycoprotein IIb/IIIa inhibitor for a few days as a bridge to surgery.

6. **Nonvitamin K antagonist (or novel) oral anticoagulants (NOACs)**, also referred to as direct oral anticoagulants (DOACs), are generally recommended for nonvalvular atrial fibrillation or deep venous thrombosis. However, they are commonly used off-label for patients with AF and structural heart disease exclusive of rheumatic mitral stenosis, although some studies do suggest an excellent safety profile and clinical benefit even in patients with mitral stenosis.[49] NOACs should not be used for patients with mechanical heart valves.[50] Since the dissipation of anticoagulant effects generally takes 4–5 half-lives and NOACs have half-lives averaging around 12 hours, the last dose of these medications should be taken 48 hours prior to surgery and stopped even earlier if the patient has renal dysfunction.[51] If the patient requires more urgent surgery, other products can be used to offset their anticoagulant effects.[52]

a. Idarucizumab (Praxbind) 5 g IV can reverse dabigatran

b. Andexanet alfa (recombinant factor Xa) can be used to reverse the effects of apixaban and rivaroxaban.[53] A recommended low-dose protocol is 400 mg IV given at a target infusion rate of 30 mg/min, to be followed by 4 mg/min for 120 minutes. This is recommended if the patient had been taking apixaban ≤5 mg or rivaroxaban ≤10 mg. The high-dose protocol is twice that dose at the same infusion rates if the patient had been taking >5 mg of apixaban or >10 mg of rivaroxaban. This product prevents factor Xa inhibition for about one hour after the infusion has been stopped.

c. Antibody-based targeted therapy for these medications is on the horizon.[54]

d. FEIBA can be used to minimize bleeding associated with NOACs if emergency surgery is required. It is usually given in a dose of 20–30 units/kg.[55]

e. In the absence of availability of the above products, PCC can be given in a dose of 25–50 units/kg.

7. **Fondaparinux**, a factor Xa inhibitor, has a half-life of nearly 20 hours and should be stopped at least 60 hours before surgery, although there are reports that 24 hours should suffice.[14]

8. **Tirofiban** (Aggrastat) and **eptifibatide** (Integrilin) are short-acting IIb/IIIa inhibitors that allow for recovery of 80% of platelet function within 4–6 hours of being discontinued. They should be stopped about four hours prior to surgery. Some studies have shown that continuing these medications up to the time of surgery may preserve platelet function on pump, leading to increased platelet number and function after CPB with no adverse effects on bleeding.[56]

9. **Abciximab** (ReoPro) is a long-acting IIb/IIIa inhibitor used for high-risk PCI that has a half-life of 12 hours. If surgery needs to be performed on an emergency basis, platelets are effective in producing hemostasis, since there is very little circulating unbound drug. Ideally, surgery should be delayed for at least 12 hours and preferably 24 hours. Although platelet function remains abnormal for up to 48 hours, there is little hemostatic compromise at receptor blockade levels less than 50%.

10. **Intravenous direct thrombin inhibitors** are primarily used in patients with HIT, but bivalirudin has been used as an alternative to UFH in patients undergoing PCI. It has a short half-life of 25 minutes and should not pose a significant issue if emergency surgery is required. Its use as an alternative to heparin during surgery in patients with HIT has been associated with comparable outcomes, although bleeding tends to be more problematic.[57]

11. **Thrombolytic therapy** is an alternative to primary PCI for patients presenting with ST-elevation myocardial infarctions (STEMIs) in centers without PCI capability. Although most agents have short half-lives measured in minutes, the systemic hemostatic defects persist much longer. These effects include depletion of fibrinogen, reduction in factors II, V, and VIII, impairment of platelet aggregation, and the appearance of fibrin split products. If surgery is required for persistent ischemia after failed thrombolytic therapy, it should be delayed for at least 12–24 hours. If it is required emergently, blood component therapy with FFP, PCC, and/or cryoprecipitate will probably be necessary to correct the anticipated coagulopathy.

E. **Antifibrinolytic therapy** with lysine analogues should be used to reduce intraoperative blood loss in all on- and off-pump surgical cases (see doses on page 249).[14,43–45]

1. **ε-aminocaproic acid** (Amicar) is an antifibrinolytic agent that preserves platelet function by inhibiting the conversion of plasminogen to plasmin. It is effective in reducing blood loss and the amount of transfusions, although it has not been shown to reduce the rate of re-exploration for bleeding. Because of its low cost, it is usually the drug of choice for most cardiac surgical procedures.

2. **Tranexamic acid** (Cyklokapron) has similar properties and benefits to ε-aminocaproic acid, with more clinical evidence of benefit in reducing perioperative blood loss in both on- and off-pump surgery. One study found that topical tranexamic acid (2 g/500 mL NS) poured into the pericardial cavity just prior to closure significantly reduced blood loss and the need for transfusions.[58]

F. Heparin and protamine dosing

1. Ideal anticoagulation for CPB should minimize activation of the coagulation cascade, be fully reversible, and minimize perioperative bleeding. The most commonly used drug is heparin, which binds to antithrombin to inhibit thrombin and factor Xa. Empiric dosing of heparin (3–4 mg/kg) to achieve an activated clotting time (ACT) >480 seconds has been recommended, although patients with antithrombin deficiency may be heparin-resistant and require FFP or antithrombin (Thrombate) to achieve a satisfactory ACT.[59] Inadequate heparin dosing increases thrombin generation, which in turn activates platelets and can trigger clotting within the CPB circuit. Lower doses of heparin may be used in biocompatible circuits with an acceptable ACT most likely being 400 seconds, although this has not been well defined. A heparin level of 2 units/mL should be achieved.

2. Systems that provide heparin–protamine titration tests to measure circulating heparin concentrations and determine dose-response curves are recommended in order to optimize heparin dosing. Use of these systems may result in more heparin being administered, but usually a lower dose of protamine being necessary to achieve reversal, which is based on heparin levels at the conclusion of CPB. The end result is generally less thrombin and platelet activation, a reduction in fibrinolysis, and a reduction in perioperative bleeding, whether a higher or lower dose of heparin is used than predicted by empiric dosing.[14,60]

3. The major advantage of heparin is that its anticoagulant effect can be reversed with protamine. In contrast, other effective anticoagulants that can be used for CPB, such as bivalirudin in HIT patients, are not reversible.

4. Protamine is usually given in a 1:1 ratio to the dose of heparin. However, using dose-response curves, lower doses of protamine usually suffice to adequately reverse heparin. This may result in less bleeding, because excessive protamine serves as an anticoagulant that directly impairs platelet function and elevates the ACT.[14,60,61]

G. Perfusion considerations to optimize blood conservation include the following (see also Chapter 5):[14,22,62]

1. **Autologous blood withdrawal** before instituting bypass (acute normovolemic hemodilution) protects platelets from the damaging effects of CPB. This blood remains of high quality despite storage during the surgery, preserves red cell mass, and reduces transfusion requirements. However, its efficacy in reducing perioperative bleeding is controversial.[63,64] It can be considered when the calculated on-pump HCT after withdrawal remains satisfactory (>20–22%). This can be calculated using the following equation:

$$\text{amount withdrawn} = \text{EBV} - \frac{0.22(\text{EBV} + \text{PV} + \text{CV})}{\text{HCT}}$$

where:

EBV = estimated blood volume $(70 \times kg)$
PV = priming volume
CV = estimated cardioplegia volume
HCT = prewithdrawal hematocrit

2. **Platelet-rich plasmapheresis** entails the withdrawal of platelet-rich plasma using a plasma separator at the beginning of the operation with its re-administration after protamine infusion. This improves hemostasis and reduces blood loss. Although it might be beneficial in reoperations, it is expensive, time-consuming, and probably of marginal benefit.[65,66]

3. The use of **biocompatible circuits** for CPB (usually heparin-bonded) may reduce activation of platelets and the coagulation cascade with a subsequent reduction in blood loss.[14] These systems usually allow for use of lower doses of heparin to achieve a target ACT of 400 seconds. Despite using lower doses of heparin, which could theoretically increase thrombin generation, there is little evidence that this contributes to a prothrombotic milieu.

4. **Avoidance of cardiotomy suction** may reduce perioperative bleeding. Blood aspirated from the pericardial space has been in contact with tissue factor, contains high levels of factor VIIa, procoagulant particles, fat particles, and activated complement proteins, and exhibits fibrinolytic activity.[22,67] It may be associated with thrombin generation and cause platelet activation resulting in more bleeding. Blood aspirated with cardiotomy suckers drains into a reservoir and mixes directly with the pump blood that is reinfused through the CPB circuit. Most groups use cardiotomy suction routinely and do not find that it has a significant effect on bleeding.

5. **Miniaturized CPB circuits** require low priming volumes (500–800 mL) that limit the degree of hemodilution, thus maintaining a higher HCT on pump. Studies have arguably demonstrated that these systems reduce activation of coagulation and fibrinolysis and minimize blood loss. However, the lack of a cardiotomy reservoir increases the risk of air embolism.[68]

6. **Retrograde autologous priming** of the extracorporeal circuit entails initial withdrawal of crystalloid prime to minimize hemodilution, thus maintaining a higher HCT and colloid oncotic pressure on pump. This also reduces extravascular lung water. In some studies, this has been shown to reduce the rate of transfusion.[69–71]

7. **Intraoperative autotransfusion** of blood that is aspirated from the field into a cell-saving device is recommended as a routine means of salvaging red blood cells whether cardiotomy suction is used or not. It is most helpful in salvaging red cells from dilute fluids (e.g. after cold saline is poured on the heart during cardioplegic arrest). Cell salvage of pump contents at the conclusion of CPB is routinely performed as well. The cells are centrifuged and washed to remove heparin and cytokines and concentrate red cells, but the washing results in loss of coagulation factors and platelets from the blood. Most studies suggest that routine intraoperative cell salvage reduces transfusion requirements, but large reinfusion volumes (>1000 mL) may impair coagulation.[14,72] The routine use of ultrafiltration to remove the pump prime is not recommended, except in patients with large pump primes relative to their blood volume.[22]

H. **Meticulous surgical technique** is the mainstay of hemostasis. Warming the patient to normothermia before terminating bypass improves the function of the coagulation system.

IV. Assessment of Bleeding in the ICU

A. The appropriate assessment of bleeding in the ICU requires the following steps (Table 9.4):[73]

1. Frequent documentation of the amount of blood draining into the collection system and attention to tube patency.

2. Determination of the color (arterial or venous) and pattern of drainage (sudden dump when turned or continuous drainage).

3. Monitoring of hemodynamic parameters with ongoing awareness of the possibility of cardiac tamponade.

4. Identification of potential causative factors by review of coagulation studies.

Table 9.4 • Assessment of Postoperative Mediastinal Bleeding
1. Obtain immediate postoperative chest x-ray as baseline evaluation of the mediastinum and pleural spaces
2. Quantify the degree of bleeding into drainage unit frequently
3. Optimize hemodynamic status while addressing bleeding issues
4. Obtain coagulation studies:
a. PT/INR, PTT, platelet count, fibrinogen level
b. Thromboelastogram, if available
c. Platelet function testing
4. Repeat coagulation studies after blood products are administered if still bleeding
5. Repeat chest x-ray if concerned about tamponade or undrained blood
6. Obtain TEE if concerned about tamponade

5. Suspicion of undrained blood in the mediastinum or pleural spaces by review of a chest x-ray (looking for a widened mediastinum or haziness in the pleural cavity as blood layers posteriorly), auscultating decreased breath sounds on examination, or noting elevation of peak inspiratory pressures on the ventilator.

6. Obtaining an echocardiogram if tamponade is suspected based upon the pattern of bleeding, hemodynamic derangements, or abnormalities on chest x-ray.

B. **Quantitate the amount of chest tube drainage.** Make sure that the chest tubes are patent, because the extent of ongoing hemorrhage may be masked when the tubes have clotted or blood has drained into an open pleural space. **Note:** when patients are turned or moved, they will occasionally drain a significant volume of blood that has been accumulating in the chest for several hours. This may suggest the acute onset of bleeding and the need for surgical exploration. The presence of dark blood and minimal additional drainage are clues that this does not represent active bleeding. Serial chest x-rays may be helpful in identifying residual blood in the pleural space.

1. The amount of bleeding that warrants treatment is somewhat arbitrary. Some have defined "active bleeding" as bleeding occurring at a rate exceeding 1.5 mL/kg/h for six consecutive hours (which would correspond to >100–150 mL/h for the average adult).[74] Other studies suggest that a rate of bleeding exceeding 2 mg/kg/h for three hours (corresponding to >150–200 mL/h for the average adult) is associated with adverse outcomes.[23] Yet another study considered significant bleeding to be a bleeding rate of >3 mL/kg/h (about 250–300 mL/h) for more than two consecutive hours.[75] It may be inferred that persistent bleeding that exceeds 200 mL/h for several hours requires specific treatment. It is worth remembering that there may be more bleeding occurring than is evident from the amount of chest tube drainage.

2. A "universal definition" of perioperative bleeding was proposed in 2014.[76] This defined five classes of bleeding, based on chest tube output, blood and blood component therapy given, the need for delayed sternal closure, and the need for re-exploration. By evaluating the total amount of drainage in 12 hours, moderate bleeding was defined as 801–1000 mL/12h, severe was 1001–2000 mL/12h and massive was >2000 mL/12h. This categorization was retrospective and is not that helpful in making treatment decisions, since it is not predictable whether significant early postoperative bleeding will taper without treatment.

C. Assess hemodynamics with the Swan-Ganz catheter. Maintenance of adequate filling pressures and cardiac output is essential and is generally accomplished using crystalloid or colloid solutions. However, in the bleeding patient, these will produce hemodilution and progressive anemia, and may potentiate a coagulopathy. It should be noted that unstable hemodynamics are frequently seen in the bleeding patient even if filling pressures are maintained.

  1. If filling pressures are decreasing and nonheme fluid is administered, one needs to anticipate a decrease in the HCT from hemodilution, but more so with ongoing bleeding. Five percent albumin will have a dilutional effect on clotting factors and the HCT, but it is the preferred colloid for volume expansion (other than blood or blood component therapy). One should avoid use of any hetastarch (HES) compounds in the bleeding patient. The high-molecular-weight HES-based compounds adversely affect fibrin formation and platelet function (perhaps slightly less with HES in balanced electrolyte solution [Hextend] than HES 6% in saline [Hespan]).[77,78] Although the low-molecular-weight HES compounds, such as pentastarch and tetrastarch, appear to have minimal effect on coagulation, they may still be associated with postoperative bleeding and should probably be avoided.[79]

  2. The administration of volume in the form of clotting factors and platelets promotes hemostasis but must be accompanied by red cell transfusions to maintain a safe HCT. Anemia not only reduces oxygen-carrying capacity of the blood but also reduces blood oncotic pressure and viscosity, which contribute to hypotension.

  3. Evidence of rising filling pressures and decreasing cardiac outputs may suggest the development of cardiac tamponade. Equilibration of intracardiac pressures may be noted with postoperative tamponade, but, more commonly, accumulation of clot adjacent to the right or left atrium or either ventricle will produce variable elevation in intracardiac pressures that may also be consistent with right (RV) or left ventricular (LV) failure, respectively.

  4. If hemodynamic measurements suggest borderline cardiac function and tamponade cannot be ruled out, **transesophageal echocardiography (TEE)** is invaluable in making the correct diagnosis. Tamponade should be suspected when hemodynamic compromise is associated with excessive bleeding, bleeding that has abruptly stopped, or even minimal chest tube drainage caused by clotted tubes or spillage into the pleural space. Although a transthoracic study (TTE) may identify a large effusion, acoustic windows are often not ideal, especially with dressings, ECG leads, chest tubes, and tape on the chest. TEE is more helpful in detecting clot behind the heart and should be considered if the TTE is nondiagnostic.[80]

D. **Coagulation studies** should be obtained after administration of protamine in the OR, and abnormal studies associated with "nonsurgical" coagulopathic bleeding should be promptly treated prior to chest closure. Upon arrival in the ICU, these studies are usually repeated, and serial HCTs should then be obtained if the patient is bleeding. If studies are abnormal, but the patient has an insignificant amount of mediastinal bleeding, use of blood component therapy is **not** indicated.

  1. If hemostasis was difficult to achieve in the OR or hemorrhage persists in the ICU, lab tests may be helpful in assessing whether a coagulopathy is contributing to mediastinal bleeding. Tests for some of the more common nonsurgical causes of bleeding (residual heparin effect, thrombocytopenia, and clotting

factor deficiency [primarily fibrinogen levels]) are readily available, but documentation of platelet dysfunction and fibrinolysis requires additional technology. Although no individual test correlates that well with the amount of bleeding, together they can usually direct interventions in a somewhat scientific manner.

2. No matter what the results of coagulation testing are, clinical judgment remains paramount in trying to ascertain whether the bleeding is more likely to be of a surgical nature (which tends to persist) or due to a coagulopathy (which might improve). If normal coagulation studies are present upon arrival in the ICU, significant bleeding usually requires surgical re-exploration (see pages 446–447). If markedly abnormal coagulation studies are present, yet bleeding persists despite their correction, surgical exploration is also indicated.

3. **Prothrombin time (PT)** measured as the INR assesses the extrinsic coagulation cascade. The INR may be slightly increased after a standard pump run, but clotting factor levels exceeding 30% of normal should allow for satisfactory hemostasis. An abnormal INR is usually corrected with FFP, but administration of PCC may be more effective.[81,82]

4. **Partial thromboplastin time (PTT)** assesses the intrinsic coagulation cascade and can also detect residual or recurrent heparin effect ("heparin rebound"). When an elevated PTT occurs as an isolated abnormality, or with slight elevation of the INR, protamine may be beneficial in correcting the PTT and controlling bleeding. One study found that heparin rebound documented by elevated Xa levels and an abnormal clotting time was present in virtually all patients after surgery and could be abolished by a continuous infusion of 25 mg/h of protamine for six hours.[83] However, another study found little correlation of elevated anti-Xa levels with elevated PTTs, because the latter may be related to clotting factor deficiency or excessive protamine rather than residual heparin.[84] It is sometimes worthwhile obtaining an ACT in the ICU, although it may also be elevated in the absence of residual heparin.

5. **Platelet count.** Although CPB reduces the platelet count by about 30–50% and also produces platelet dysfunction, platelet function is usually adequate to produce hemostasis. Platelet transfusions may be justified in the bleeding patient with thrombocytopenia (generally <100,000/μL) or for suspicion of platelet dysfunction (usually for patients on aspirin or P2Y12 inhibitors) even in the absence of thrombocytopenia.

6. **Fibrinogen** (factor I) levels should be assessed in patients with moderate–severe bleeding. Low levels preoperatively and upon arrival in the ICU are risk factors for bleeding and re-exploration.[29] Fibrinogen is essential for proper platelet function by promoting platelet–platelet interaction leading to platelet aggregation. It is also a cell adhesion molecule that enhances platelet adhesion to endothelial cells. If the patient has significant bleeding and a fibrinogen level <100 mg/dL, transfusion of cryoprecipitate, which is rich in factors I, VIII, and XIII, is helpful. Alternatively, fibrinogen concentrate can be used to increase clot stability, and in combination with platelets, can improve platelet aggregation.[85] One study found that fibrinogen concentrates (about 8 g) were more effective in reducing bleeding than the combination of eight units of FFP and four units of platelets.[86]

7. **Fibrinolysis** is invariably present in all patients having heart surgery, although it may be attenuated by the use of lysine analogues, which exhibit antifibrinolytic properties. Test results consistent with fibrinolysis are non-specific and include elevations in the INR and PTT, decreased levels of factors I and VIII, and elevated fibrin split products (such as D-dimer). The best means of identifying fibrinolysis are thromboelastography (TEG) and a Sonoclot analysis.

8. **Platelet function** can be assessed by a variety of available technologies, including TEG and those that measure whole blood impedance platelet aggregometry.[73,87] Although the correlation of these tests with the occurrence of bleeding is not specific, qualitative platelet abnormalities in the bleeding patient do suggest that platelet transfusions are indicated. One comparative study of TEG and platelet aggregometry found that both were effective in identifying impaired hemostasis, but neither correlated with the amount of blood loss.[87] In most centers, suspicion of platelet dysfunction is based upon preoperative use of antiplatelet agents and prompts platelet transfusions without point-of-care testing.

9. **Thromboelastography (TEG)** and rotational **thromboelastometry (ROTEM)** give a qualitative measurement of clot strength. These tests evaluate the interaction of platelets with the coagulation cascade from the onset of clot formation through clot lysis and have a distinct contour for a variety of coagulation abnormalities, including fibrinolysis (Figure 9.1). Although these tests are very helpful in guiding therapy in patients with coagulopathic bleeding, they do not necessarily identify patients who are going to bleed, and treatment is not indicated for abnormalities noted in the absence of bleeding.[88-91] However, in the bleeding patient, they provide more rapid assessment of hemostatic abnormalities than standard blood coagulation testing, thus allowing for more prompt and effective therapy. Studies have found that use of a TEG-guided protocol reduces blood loss and transfusions.[92] ROTEM has been used to identify platelet dysfunction and also exclude residual heparin as the cause of an elevated ACT.[93]

10. **Sonoclot analysis** (Figure 9.2) is another viscoelastic method of evaluating clot formation and retraction that allows for the assessment of coagulation factors, fibrinogen, and platelet activity. The device measures the changing impedance to movement imposed by the developing clot on a small probe that vibrates at an ultrasonic frequency within a blood sample. Studies have suggested that Sonoclot is more predictive of bleeding than routine coagulation studies.[94] This device has seen limited use but can direct appropriate therapy in patients with persistent bleeding.

E. Repeat a chest x-ray

1. Note the overall width of the mediastinum. A widened mediastinum may suggest undrained clotted blood accumulating within the pericardial cavity that could cause cardiac tamponade. Comparison with preoperative films can be misleading because of differences in technique, but any difference between the immediate postoperative supine film and a repeat film is of concern (Figure 9.3). A widened superior mediastinum is noted when there is significant clot accumulation around the great vessels.

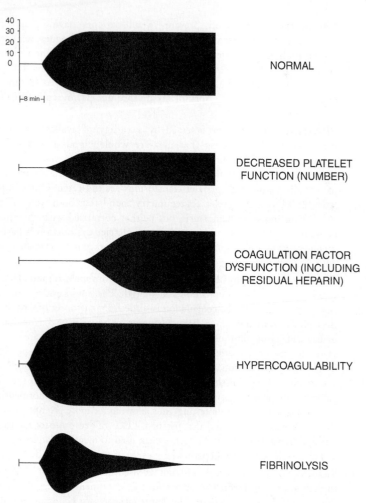

Figure 9.1 • Representative thromboelastogram tracings.

2. Note the distance between the edge of the mediastinal silhouette and the location of the Swan-Ganz catheter in the right atrium or the right atrial pacing wires (if placed on the right atrial free wall). If this distance widens, suspect clot accumulation adjacent to the right atrium.

3. Note any accumulation of blood within the pleural space that has not drained through the pleural chest tubes. This can be difficult to assess since fluid will layer out on a supine film, so a discrepancy in the haziness of the two pleural spaces should be sought.

F. Consider obtaining an **echocardiogram** if any of the above suggests the presence of cardiac tamponade. If the TTE is inconclusive, obtain a transesophageal study.

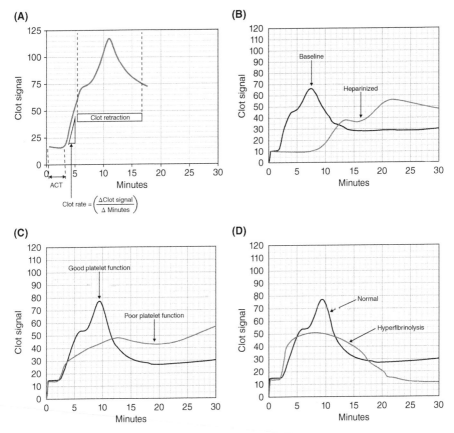

Figure 9.2 • Representative Sonoclot tracings. (A) The Sonoclot signature assesses the liquid phase of initial clot formation, the rate of fibrin and clot formation, further fibrinogenesis and platelet-fibrin interaction, a peak impedance after completion of fibrin formation, and a downward slope as platelets induce contraction of the completed clot. (B) Heparinization. (C) Poor platelet function (slow clot retraction). (D) Hyperfibrinolysis (no tightening associated with clot retraction). (Reproduced with permission from Sienco, Inc.)

V. Management of Mediastinal Bleeding

Although there is no role for prophylactic blood product transfusions in the prevention of bleeding following open-heart surgery, persistent bleeding must be treated immediately and aggressively based on the degree of bleeding and the suspected etiology of hemorrhage (Table 9.5). It is a truism that the longer a patient bleeds, the worse the coagulopathy becomes. In general, the most benign and least invasive treatments should be considered first. If a patient was "dry" at the time of closure and suddenly starts to bleed, the source is usually surgical in nature and requires re-exploration. In contrast, the patient with persistent bleeding may have a surgical or medical cause for the bleeding. When significant mediastinal bleeding persists despite prompt correction of a suspected coagulopathy, earlier re-exploration (within 12 hours)

(A)   **(B)**

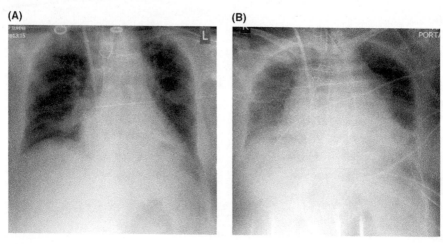

Figure 9.3 • (A) Supine chest x-ray obtained at the conclusion of surgery. (B) Supine chest x-ray obtained six hours later in the same patient with minimal mediastinal bleeding but hemodynamic compromise. Since neither pleural space was entered, blood accumulated primarily around the heart, producing a wide mediastinum consistent with cardiac tamponade.

Table 9.5 • Management of Postoperative Mediastinal Bleeding

1. Explore early for significant ongoing bleeding or tamponade
2. Ensure that chest tubes are patent
3. Warm patient to normothermia
4. Control hypertension, agitation, and shivering
5. Check results of coagulation studies (INR, PTT, platelet count, fibrinogen level, or TEG)
6. Correct ionized calcium to >1.1 mmol/L
7. Protamine 25 mg IV for two doses if elevated PTT or infusion of 25 mg/h × 6 h
8. Consider use of 10 cm PEEP with caution
9. Packed cells if hematocrit <24%
10. Platelets, 1–2 "six packs"
11. Fresh frozen plasma, 2–4 units
12. Cryoprecipitate, 6 units
13. Fibrinogen concentrate 25–75 mg/kg
14. Prothrombin complex concentrate (PCC) 25 units/kg
15. Desmopressin (DDAVP) 0.3 mg/kg IV over 20 minutes (if suspect platelet dysfunction from uremia or aspirin, von Willebrand's factor deficiency)
16. Recombinant factor VIIa 90 mg/kg if severe coagulopathy
17. **Transesophageal echocardiography** if concerned about tamponade
18. **Urgent exploration** for significant ongoing bleeding or tamponade
19. **Emergency exploration** for exsanguinating hemorrhage or near cardiac arrest from tamponade

significantly lowers the mortality rate.[95] Excessive bleeding prompting re-exploration increases the mortality rate two- to fourfold compared with patients with an insignificant amount of bleeding, which reinforces the importance of careful hemostasis at the conclusion of surgery and aggressive management of coagulopathies.[20,21,96,97]

A. Ensure chest tube patency. Ongoing bleeding without drainage leads to cardiac tamponade. Gently milk the tubes to remove clot. Aggressive stripping is not necessary.

B. Warm the patient to 37 °C. Hypothermia produces a generalized suppression of the coagulation mechanism and also impairs platelet function.[98] The use of a heated humidifier in the ventilator circuit and a forced-air warming blanket are beneficial in promoting warming and will reduce the tendency to shiver. All blood products should be delivered through blood-warming devices, if possible.

C. Control hypertension with vasodilators (clevidipine, nitroprusside, nicardipine) or β-blockers (esmolol for the hyperdynamic heart). Higher doses of propofol or morphine can also be used since extubation should not be contemplated in the bleeding patient.

D. Control agitation in the awake patient with short-acting sedatives:

   1. Propofol 25–75 μg/kg/min
   2. Dexmedetomidine 1 mg/kg load over 10 minutes followed by a continuous infusion of 0.2–1.5 μg/kg/h
   3. Midazolam 2.5–5.0 mg IV q1–2h
   4. Morphine 2.5–5 mg IV q1–2h

E. Control shivering with meperidine 25–50 mg IV or dexmedetomidine

F. Use increasing levels of positive end-expiratory pressure (PEEP) to augment mediastinal pressure, which may reduce microvascular bleeding.[22] However, prophylactic PEEP at levels of either 5 or 10 cm H_2O has not been found to be effective in reducing bleeding or transfusion requirements.[99] If it is elected to increase PEEP to control bleeding, careful attention to its effects on hemodynamics is essential.

G. Use blood components to treat early significant bleeding. This should preferably be based on point-of-care testing, but appropriate treatment may initially be based on suspicion of the hemostatic defect. For example, the patient who has received aspirin, a P2Y12 inhibitor, a IIb/IIIa inhibitor, or is uremic is likely to have platelet dysfunction and will benefit primarily from platelet transfusions, even if the platelet count is normal. In some cases, desmopressin may also prove beneficial (see section V.K. on page 439)[100,101] In contrast, the patient who has recently been on warfarin or has hepatic dysfunction is more likely to have clotting factor deficiencies and may benefit more from an initial transfusion of FFP, PCC, cryoprecipitate, or fibrinogen concentrate. Use of multiple products may be necessary in the patient who has had a long duration of CPB (>3 h) or who has received multiple packed red blood cells (PRBCs) during surgery. Aggressive treatment with blood components should be provided promptly for significant bleeding from a suspected coagulopathy, because persistent bleeding causes progressive depletion of clotting factors and platelets ("coagulopathy begets coagulopathy").

H. Once the results of coagulation studies become available, there is more objective information upon which to base therapy. Point-of-care testing in the OR is the most expeditious way of assessing the hemostatic profile (Figure 9.4). Some groups preferentially use the thromboelastogram to identify the exact nature of the hemostatic defect, allowing for more prompt initiation of appropriate therapy. This may result in

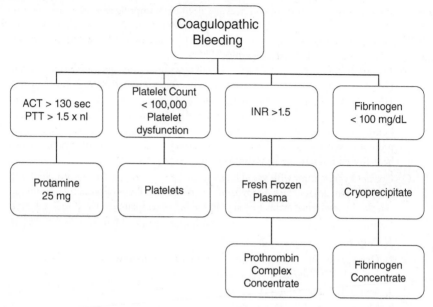

Figure 9.4 • Point-of-care testing of routine coagulation studies to guide treatment of postoperative bleeding.

lower transfusion requirements.[92] The results of routine coagulation studies drawn after CPB is terminated are usually available in the OR or soon after arrival in the ICU. If bleeding persists despite corrective measures, clotting studies can be repeated to reassess the status of the coagulation system.

1. An elevated PT implies the need for clotting factors provided by FFP, PCC, and/ or cryoprecipitate.

2. An elevated PTT or ACT suggests a problem with the intrinsic coagulation cascade or persistent heparin effect. Additional protamine may be given first, with an understanding that an elevated PTT may not be related to heparin, and protamine could exacerbate a coagulopathy. FFP and/or cryoprecipitate may also be indicated.

3. Fibrinogen levels <100 mg/dL warrant administration of cryoprecipitate or fibrinogen concentrate when bleeding is persistent.

4. A platelet count below 100,000/μL suggests the need for platelet transfusions. Because CPB induces platelet dysfunction, suspicion of a qualitative defect in the actively bleeding patient should be treated with platelets even if the platelet count is adequate.

5. **Note:** abnormal results do not need to be treated if the patient has minimal bleeding. Blood samples are frequently drawn from heparinized lines, so they should be repeated if results are markedly abnormal or inconsistent with the amount of bleeding. Platelet transfusions are not indicated in the nonbleeding patient until the platelet count approaches 20,000–30,000/μL, although most patients in the immediate postoperative period will tend to bleed at a platelet count of less than about 60,000/μL.

I. Blood transfusions are often neglected in the bleeding patient when anemia may be progressive and exacerbated by hemodilution from the administration of FFP and platelets. Although a low transfusion trigger (HCT of 21%) might be acceptable in a nonbleeding, stable young patient with no comorbidities, this is **not** safe in the bleeding patient. The patient with ongoing mediastinal bleeding should be transfused to maintain a HCT at a reasonable level (>24%) as a safety margin to maintain satisfactory tissue oxygenation. Furthermore, there are a number of clinical indications for transfusion to a higher HCT, especially those suggestive of an impairment in tissue oxygen supply (see section VI.D on page 441). Notably, platelet function is impaired in the profoundly anemic patient.[102] Red cells increase platelet-to-platelet interaction and facilitate the interaction of platelets with the subendothelium to improve hemostasis. Nonetheless, bleeding does not seem to be exacerbated by HCTs as low as 24% compared with 30%.[103]

J. **Protamine** may be given in a dose of 25–50 mg (5 mg/min) if the PTT is elevated. Generally, the ACT correlates with the PTT but is usually not drawn once the patient leaves the OR. Although the ACT should return to baseline after protamine administration, reinfusion of cell-saver blood may reintroduce a small amount of heparin, and release of heparin from tissue stores can introduce residual unneutralized heparin that contributes to bleeding. This may occur because the half-life of protamine is only about five minutes, with virtual elimination from the bloodstream in about 20–30 minutes.[104] Thus, a continuous infusion of low-dose protamine or a few small additional doses for potential heparin rebound is a feasible approach.[83] However, prolonged ACTs (and inferentially PTTs) may be noted in the absence of circulating heparin, so if additional protamine is given and the PTT remains elevated, unneutralized heparin may not be the problem. In fact, excessive use of protamine will elevate the ACT and cause bleeding. Excess protamine causes platelet dysfunction, enhances fibrinolysis, and decreases clot strength, emphasizing that indiscriminate use of excessive protamine should be avoided.[14,105]

K. **Desmopressin (DDAVP)** has no role in the prophylaxis of postoperative bleeding, but might be considered in patients with documented von Willebrand's disease, aortic stenosis with impaired platelet function associated with acquired von Willebrand's disease, uremia, and possibly drug-induced platelet dysfunction.[100,101]

   1. Bleeding following cardiac surgery is often secondary to an acquired defect in the formation of the platelet plug caused by a deficiency in von Willebrand factor. DDAVP increases the level of factor VIII precursors, von Willebrand factor (by approximately 50%), and tissue-type plasminogen activator by releasing them from vascular endothelium. These factors are responsible for promoting platelet adhesion to the subendothelium.

   2. Patients with aortic stenosis often have acquired type 2A von Willebrand syndrome.[30] This develops due to proteolysis of the largest multimers of von Willebrand factor by shear stress generated on blood as it passes through the stenotic valve. These multimers are important for platelet-mediated hemostasis, so when reduced, they can cause bleeding. Desmopressin given after the induction of anesthesia in patients with abnormal platelet function associated with this syndrome has been shown to significantly reduce perioperative blood loss.[101]

   3. DDAVP is given in a dose of 0.3–0.4 µg/kg IV over 20 minutes. A slow infusion may attenuate the peripheral vasodilation and hypotension that often follows DDAVP infusion. Peak effects are seen in 30–60 minutes.

L. **Calcium chloride 1 g IV** (10 mL of 10% solution) given over 15 minutes may be administered if the patient has received multiple transfusions of CPD preserved blood during a short period of time (e.g. more than 10 units within 1–2 hours). The citrate used as a preservative in CPD blood binds calcium, but hypocalcemia is unusual because of the rapid metabolism of citrate by the liver. However, calcium administration is not necessary when adenine-saline (AS-1) is used as the preservative. If hypocalcemia is present, as it often is following CPB, calcium chloride is preferable to calcium gluconate because it provides three times more ionized calcium.

VI. Blood Transfusions: Red Cells

A. Red cell transfusions are indicated primarily to increase the oxygen-carrying capacity of blood to avoid end-organ ischemia and dysfunction. Tissue oxygen delivery depends on the cardiac output, the hemoglobin level, and the oxygen extraction ratio in tissues. Because the early postoperative period is associated with delayed myocardial metabolic recovery, reduced cardiac output, and significant anemia, oxygen delivery is commonly reduced by at least 25% postoperatively. Tissue oxygenation may be maintained in healthy patients with a hemoglobin as low as 6–7 g/dL (HCT around 18–21%), and the safe lower limit for the HCT in the **stable** postoperative patient is probably around 22%.

B. Nonetheless, the approach to the bleeding patient requires extra vigilance and a margin of safety to ensure adequate tissue oxygenation, minimize myocardial ischemia, and prevent hemodynamic compromise. It is therefore safest to administer blood if the HCT is less than 24% when there is ongoing substantial blood loss with the predictable hemodilution from administration of blood components and platelets. However, there is no indication for transfusing to a HCT greater than 30%.

C. Blood transfusions are not benign, because they are associated with significant postoperative morbidity and compromised short- and long-term survival after open-heart surgery.[9,106] Blood contains cytokines and proinflammatory mediators that are immunomodulatory. Transfusions are associated with numerous potential complications, including, but not limited to:

1. An increased risk of graft occlusion, renal, neurologic, gastrointestinal, and pulmonary morbidity after heart surgery.[8–13,107]

2. Fever associated with hemolytic or nonhemolytic transfusion reactions. The former is caused by circulating antibodies directed against donor leukocytes or HLA antigens. The latter may be related to cytokines in the donor product.

3. Allergic reactions ranging from urticarial to anaphylaxis

4. Viral infections, especially with cytomegalovirus (CMV), which is present in about 50% of donor units. However, HIV, hepatitis B, and hepatitis C are rarely transmitted with effective screening. Bacterial infections are also uncommon, but the risk of pneumonia is increased and may be related to transfusion-related immunomodulation (TRIM). Leukocyte depletion by the blood bank can reduce the risk of infection and may lower mortality rates as well.[14,108]

5. Transfusion-related acute lung injury (TRALI). This may be caused by donor antibody–recipient leukocyte interactions and possibly neutrophil activation by bioactive substances from transfusions, resulting in lung damage and a capillary leak occurring within six hours of a transfusion. Although most patients recover from TRALI in a few days, the associated mortality rate is noted to be 5–15%.[9]

6. Transfusion-related circulatory overload (TACO) is a syndrome of cardiogenic pulmonary edema manifested by hypoxemia, hypertension, and tachycardia occurring within 12 hours of transfusion. This is related to the aggressive administration of too much volume of blood products too rapidly to a patient with preexisting fluid overload from heart failure, LV dysfunction, or chronic kidney

disease.[109] Its occurrence can be avoided by giving a diuretic, such as furosemide, at the same time as a blood transfusion. This is most applicable to the profoundly anemic patient who is somewhat fluid overloaded but not actively bleeding.

D. Transfusion triggers should be determined by clinical criteria, including hemodynamic factors (hypotension, tachycardia, low cardiac output states with low mixed venous oxygen saturation, metabolic acidosis, elevated lactate), or evidence of neurologic impairment, respiratory insufficiency, or renal dysfunction. Despite the fundamental concept that blood will dramatically improve oxygen delivery, it must be recognized that transfusions may provide minimal improvement in oxygen-carrying capacity immediately after transfusion, may reduce microcirculatory flow, and in fact could prove more detrimental than beneficial. This is because the 2,3-diphosphoglycerate (2,3-DPG) level in blood is very low, especially with longer durations of storage, resulting in a leftward shift of the oxyhemoglobin dissociation curve with more avid binding of oxygen to hemoglobin and less release to tissues. Fortunately, 2,3-DPG levels return to 50% of normal within 24 hours after transfusion.

E. Use of blood filters is beneficial in removing microaggregates of blood. Blood filters of at least 170 μm pore size must be used for all blood transfusions. Filters of 20–40 μm pore size are more effective in removing microaggregates of fibrin, platelet debris, and leukocytes that accumulate in stored blood. These filters have been shown to decrease the incidence of nonhemolytic febrile transfusion reactions and may reduce the adverse effects of multiple transfusions on pulmonary function. Blood lines should be primed with isotonic solutions (preferably normal saline), avoiding lactated Ringer's, which contains calcium, and D5W, which is hypotonic and will produce significant red cell hemolysis.

F. **Note:** care should be taken to avoid transfusing cold blood products. Blood warmers should generally be used if the patient receives rapid transfusions. If one unit is to be transfused, it should be allowed to sit at ambient room temperature or under a heating hood for several minutes to warm.

G. **Packed red blood cells (RBCs)** contain approximately 200 mL of red cells and 70 mL of a preservative, most commonly citrate-phosphate-dextrose (CPD) with various additives to extend shelf life. The addition of adenine (CPDA-1) extends shelf life to 35 days, and solutions with more dextrose and adenine and with mannitol (AS-1 [Adsol] and AS-5 [Optisol]) increase shelf life to 42 days. Each unit has an average HCT of 70%, and one unit will raise the HCT of a 70 kg man by 3%. At least 70% of transfused cells survive 24 hours, and these cells have a normal lifespan. Since packed cells contain no clotting factors, administration of FFP should be considered to replace clotting factors if a large number of units (generally more than five) is given over a short period of time.

1. Despite the extended shelf life with improved preservation solutions, significant changes still occur in the red cells with storage. These include increased levels of cytokines, which produce more systemic inflammation, increased lactate with a reduction in pH, loss of deformability, which increases capillary transit time, depletion of 2,3-DPG, which reduces oxygen unloading from hemoglobin, and increased cell lysis leading to hyperkalemia.[110] Although some studies suggest that the risk of infection is greater with prolonged storage, other studies indicate that the storage time of packed RBCs does not affect outcomes.[14,111,112]

2. Leukoreduction of red cells is beneficial in reducing some of the febrile and nonhemolytic transfusion reactions. In some hospitals, this is done routinely.[108]

H. **Fresh whole blood** (less than six hours old) has a HCT of about 35% and contains clotting factors and platelets. One unit has been shown to provide equivalent, if not superior, hemostasis to that of 10 units of platelets.[113] It is probably the best replacement product, but is usually not available since most blood banks fractionate blood into components. Whole blood stored over 24 hours has few viable platelets, but levels of other clotting factors are reasonably well maintained for several days.

I. **Cell-saver blood** (shed and washed in the OR) is rinsed with heparinized saline and is devoid of clotting factors and platelets. A small amount of heparin may be present after centrifugation, but this is not considered clinically significant. The survival, function, and hemolysis of washed red blood cells is equivalent to that of nonprocessed blood.[114]

J. **Hemofiltration blood** is obtained by placing a hemofilter in the extracorporeal circuit. This provides concentrated red cells and also preserves platelets and clotting factors. Studies have shown superior blood salvage and hemostasis with use of a hemofilter than with cell-saving devices, but ultrafiltration of pump blood is generally not recommended.[22]

K. **Autotransfusion** of shed mediastinal blood in the ICU is a controversial means of blood salvage. It has arguably been shown to reduce the need for transfusions, and most systems have been designed for reinfusion through 20–40 μm blood filters without washing. Blood filters do not completely remove lipid particles and blood microaggregates, and the reinfused blood contains low levels of factor I and VIII, a low level of platelets which are dysfunctional, elevated levels of fibrinolytics (fibrin split products), inflammatory cytokines, endotoxin, tissue factor, and free hemoglobin. Washing can remove some of these factors but will also eliminate all clotting factors and platelets. If unwashed blood is returned in moderate amounts (>500 mL), an apparent coagulopathy will be present with an elevation in INR, PTT, and D-dimers, and a reduction in fibrinogen.[115,116] There may also be an increased incidence of wound infections with reinfusion of unwashed shed mediastinal blood.[117] Thus, if autotransfusion is to be used as part of a blood conservation program, blood should be washed in a cell-saving device prior to reinfusion, and the amount of reinfused blood should be limited.[22]

VII. Blood Components, Factor Concentrates, and Colloids

A. **Platelets** should be given to the bleeding patient if the platelet count is less than 100,000/μL. Furthermore, since platelets are dysfunctional in patients receiving antiplatelet medications preoperatively and as a result of CPB, one should not hesitate to administer platelets for ongoing bleeding even if the platelet count exceeds 100,000/μL. Platelets are not indicated in the nonbleeding patient unless the count is perilously low (<20–30,000/μL).

1. Platelets are provided as a pooled preparation from one or several donors, usually as a six-unit bag, which is the usual amount given to an average-sized adult. Each unit contains approximately 8×10^{10} platelets and should increase the platelet count by about 7000–10,000/μL in a 75 kg adult. One unit of platelets contains 70% of the platelets in a unit of fresh blood, but platelets lose some of their functional capacity during storage. Platelets stored at room temperature can be used for up to five days and have a lifespan of eight days. Those stored at 4 °C are useful for only 24 hours (only 50–70% of total platelet activity is present at six hours) and have a lifespan of only 2–3 days.

2. Platelet function is impaired in patients with hypofibrinogenemia and when the HCT is less than 30%. Thus, administration of cryoprecipitate or fibrinogen concentrates along with platelets will improve platelet aggregation and clot stability.[85] Red cell transfusion to raise the HCT to 26% may also improve platelet function.[102]

3. Transfused platelets will be less effective when given within 4–6 hours of a dose of a P2Y12 inhibitor, because the active compound may still be present in the bloodstream.

4. ABO compatibility should be observed for platelets, but it is not essential. For each donor used, there is a similar risk of transmitting hepatitis and HIV as one unit of blood.

5. Platelets should be administered through a 170 μm filter. Several filters are available (such as the Pall LRF 10 filter) that can be used to remove leukocytes from platelet transfusions. Use of these filters may be beneficial in reducing the risk of allergic reactions caused by red and white cells present in platelet packs. Pretreatment with diphenhydramine (50 mg IV), ranitidine (150 mg IV) (H_1 and H_2 blockers), and steroids (hydrocortisone 100 mg IV) might also attenuate these reactions, but is usually not necessary.

6. Despite some claims that platelet transfusions are associated with higher risks of infection, respiratory complications, stroke, and death, it is more likely that the need for platelets is simply a surrogate marker for sicker patients.[118] A study of nearly 33,000 patients from the Cleveland Clinic confirmed increased postoperative morbidity in patients receiving platelets, but after risk adjustment, there was no increase in morbidity or mortality from transfused platelets.[119]

B. **Fresh frozen plasma (FFP)** contains all clotting factors at normal concentrations with a slight reduction in factor V (66% of normal) and factor VIII (41% of normal). It is devoid of red cells, white cells, and platelets. When cryoprecipitate is obtained from the same unit of blood, FFP will contain low levels of factors I, VIII, XIII, von Willebrand factor, and fibronectin. Only 30% of the normal level of most clotting factors is essential to provide hemostasis, and the INR generally has to exceed 1.5 before a clinically significant factor deficiency exists. However, due to the hemodilutional effects of CPB and the progressive loss of clotting factors during ongoing bleeding, one should not hesitate to administer FFP to improve hemostasis in the bleeding patient even if the INR is mildly elevated. Although some degree of coagulopathy with a reduction in clotting factors is present after CPB, there is no documented benefit of prophylactically administering FFP.[120] Because of the importance of factors I and VIII in promoting platelet aggregation and adhesion to the endothelium, the additional transfusion of cryoprecipitate should be considered if fibrinogen levels are low.

1. One unit of FFP contains about 250 mL of volume. The amount given is usually **2–4 units for the average adult**. Four units will increase the level of clotting factors by 10%, which is considered the amount necessary to improve coagulation status.

2. FFP should be ABO compatible and given through a 170 μm filter. FFP is not viral inactivated, and since each unit is derived from one unit of whole blood from one donor, it has a similar risk of transmitting hepatitis or HIV as one unit of blood.

3. FFP may be given to patients with antithrombin (AT) deficiency to achieve adequate anticoagulation for CPB.[59] This may only be recognized when significant heparin resistance is noted in the OR. To minimize the amount of volume infused, a concentrated source of AT is commercially available (Thrombate III).

The amount required is based on an estimate of the level of AT present (see calculation on page 251). Antithrombin is not recommended to reduce bleeding following CPB.

4. **Note:** the administration of FFP and platelets not only provides clotting factors but also raises filling pressures. These blood products will therefore lower the HCT and can precipitate fluid overload. If the HCT is less than 24% or not yet available and the patient is bleeding, anticipate the need for blood if other volume is being administered. Remember that the HCT does not change with acute blood loss until replacement fluids are administered.

C. **Prothrombin complex concentrate (PCC)** contains the vitamin-K-dependent coagulation factors II, IX, and X (three-factor PCC [Profilnine]) and may contain variable amounts of factor VII as well (four-factor PCC [Kcentra]).[121]

1. PCC is able to reduce an elevated INR more rapidly than FFP (usually in less than an hour) and with less volume.[37] It comes in 500- and 1000-unit vials, reflecting units of factor IX. The dosage is calculated based on the patient's weight and INR. It can also be used to offset the anticoagulant effects of the NOACs in the absence of the more expensive antidotes noted on page 426.

2. PCC is very effective in the control of refractory bleeding after cardiac surgery.[122] It is more effective than FFP in reducing blood loss and transfusions when used for postsurgical bleeding, albeit with a slightly increased risk of thromboembolic events and acute kidney injury.[123] Studies comparing three- and four-factor PCC with recombinant factor VII have found them to be equally efficacious in reducing bleeding, but with less renal impairment.[124,125] The preoperative dose used for warfarin reversal is 25 units/kg for an elevated INR <4, 35 units/kg for an INR of 4–6, and 50 units/kg for an INR >6. Postoperatively, the INR is rarely that high, and the dose may be based on thromboelastographic findings. The usual dose is 25–35 units/kg. There is potential benefit in reducing bleeding following surgery in patients taking a NOAC preoperatively.

D. **Cryoprecipitate**

1. Cryoprecipitate represents the cold insoluble portion of plasma that precipitates when FFP is thawed at 1–6 °C. It is then refrozen at 20 °C within one hour. Approximately 15 mL is derived from one unit which is then suspended in 15 mL of plasma and pooled into a concentrate of 5–6 units, containing about 200 mL. Viral inactivation is not performed, so there is a risk of pathogen transmission.[126]

2. Each unit of 10–20 mL provides concentrated levels of factors I, VIII, and XIII. This amounts to about 150–250 mg of fibrinogen, 80–100 units of factor VIII procoagulant activity (VIII:C), 40–50% of the original plasma content of von Willebrand factor, factor XIII (fibrin-stabilizing factor), and fibronectin (a tissue integrin involved in wound healing). Factors I and VIII are essential for proper platelet aggregation and platelet adherence to endothelium.

3. Hypofibrinogenemia can significantly impair hemostasis, and when a patient has significant bleeding and a fibrinogen level <100 mg/dL, cryoprecipitate given with platelets is more effective than FFP in reducing bleeding. Although often utilized empirically for significant bleeding due to slow turnaround times in obtaining fibrinogen levels, TEG may be helpful in determining whether it should be given.

4. The amount given is usually 1 unit/7–10 kg of body weight (e.g. 7 units to a 70 kg patient). One unit will raise the fibrinogen level of a 70 kg man by 7–10 mg/dL. Cryoprecipitate must be thawed before infusion and should be given through a 170 μm filter within 4–6 hours of thawing. ABO compatibility should be observed. One can also calculate the number of units that will be required from the following equations:

$$\text{Blood volume}(\text{BV}) = 70\,\text{mL/kg} \times \text{weight in kg}$$
$$\text{Plasma volume}(\text{PV}) = \text{BV} \times (1 - \text{hematocrit})$$
$$\text{Fibrinogen required}(\text{mg}) = 0.01 \times \text{PV} \times (\text{desired level} - \text{current level})$$
$$\text{Bags of cryo required} = \text{mg fibrinogen required}/250\,\text{mg per bag}$$

For example, to raise the fibrinogen to 200 mg/dL for a 75 kg man with a HCT of 25% and a fibrinogen level of 100 mg/dL, one would give 70 × 75 × (1 - 0.25) × 0.01 × (200 - 100) = about 4000 mg/250 = 15 units.

E. **Fibrinogen concentrate** is derived from pooled human plasma using a cryoprecipitation process. It is viral inactivated and stored as a powder with a standardized amount of fibrinogen for rapid reconstitution. It is commercially available and does not need preparation by the hospital's blood bank. The dose may be based on the current fibrinogen level and usually ranges between 25 and 75 mg/kg. Although it does not contain all of the factors present in cryoprecipitate, it is highly effective in reducing bleeding in patients with low fibrinogen levels, especially when given along with platelets.[85] It is also more effective than the combination of FFP and platelets in reducing postoperative bleeding.[86] The combined use of PCC and fibrinogen concentrates is also more effective than FFP in reducing blood transfusion and thromboembolic events.[127,128] Neither cryoprecipitate nor fibrinogen concentrates appear to increase the risk of thromboembolic events after cardiac surgery.[129]

F. **Recombinant factor VIIa (rFVIIa)** has been used "off-label" quite successfully in arresting bleeding in patients with a severe uncontrollable coagulopathy after various types of open-heart surgery.[75] It combines with tissue factor at the site of vessel injury and to the surface of activated platelets, activating factor X. This results in thrombin generation, platelet activation, and an explosive "thrombin burst" that promotes localized hemostasis at the site of the tissue injury. It produces a prompt improvement in the INR. Because tissue factor and activated platelets are present systemically after CPB, systemic thrombosis may occur, being noted in 5–10% of patients. Thus, rFVIIa is recommended for use only after the full gamut of coagulation factors and platelets has been administered, yet bleeding persists. The recommended "on-label" dose is 90 μg/kg with a second dose given after two hours, if necessary, as the half-life of rFVIIa is 2.9 hours. Whether earlier use of lower doses (<20 μg/kg) given before there is depletion of clotting factors is just as effective in reducing bleeding is speculative, although it may be associated with fewer thrombotic events.[130] Studies have suggested equal efficacy and perhaps fewer thrombotic events with PCC compared with rFVIIa.[124,125]

G. Volume expansion is usually required in the bleeding patient to maintain hemody-namics. Aside from use of blood and blood component therapy, this is best achieved with colloids that are retained within the intravascular space. Five percent **albumin** is the safest solution to use if blood components are not available as it has primarily a dilutional effect on clotting factors. In contrast, the high-molecular-weight HES compounds Hespan and Hextend are best avoided in the bleeding patient because they can produce a coagulopathy by reducing levels of factor VIII, von Willebrand factor and fibrinogen, and impairing fibrin polymerization and clot strength. These issues, as well as reduced availability of the platelet glycoprotein IIb/IIIa receptor, contribute to their antiplatelet effects.[77–79] If the patient is not bleeding, these com-pounds can be safely used by limiting infusion volume to 1500 mL per day (about 20–25 mL/kg).

VIII. Mediastinal Re-exploration for Bleeding or Tamponade

A. The presence of untapering mediastinal bleeding or suspected cardiac tamponade is an indication for urgent mediastinal re-exploration. Emergency re-exploration in the ICU is indicated for exsanguinating hemorrhage or tamponade with incipi-ent cardiac arrest.[131–136] Surgical exploration should be considered when there is the acute onset of rapid bleeding (>300 mL/h) after minimal blood loss, or per-sistent bleeding above arbitrary bleeding threshold levels at various times after surgery. These must take into consideration the extent of coagulopathy that may be in the process of being treated and the hemodynamic effects of ongoing bleed-ing. General guidelines for re-exploration include hourly bleeding rates of:

1. More than 400 mL/h for 1 h (>200 mL/m^2)
2. More than 300 mL/h for 2–3 h (>150 mL/m^2/h × 2–3 h)
3. More than 200 mL/h for 4 h (>100 mL/m^2/h × 4 h)

B. Re-exploration for **bleeding** is associated with increased operative morbidity and a two- to fourfold increase in mortality, primarily because of a delay in returning the patient to the OR, and occasionally because of the necessity for open-chest resuscitation in the ICU.[20,21,95–97] There should be a low threshold for returning a patient to the OR early for bleeding using the guidelines noted above. The bene-fits of doing so greatly outweigh the risks. Surgical bleeding sites are reported to be present in about two-thirds of patients.[19] Early exploration (<12 hours in sev-eral studies) reduces the risk of adverse outcomes because it can mitigate factors that contribute to increased morbidity and mortality. Early exploration can:

1. Minimize the use of multiple transfusions, which are associated with a higher risk of respiratory and renal failure, sepsis, and death.
2. Avert periods of hemodynamic instability and low cardiac output syndrome, which can lead to multisystem organ failure.
3. Reduce the risk of tamponade and cardiac arrest – events that frequently occur in the middle of the night due to reluctance to explore a patient earlier.
4. Lower the risk of wound complications.

C. The diagnosis of **cardiac tamponade** is suggested by hemodynamic compromise with elevated filling pressures, usually in a patient with significant mediastinal bleeding or significant bleeding that has stopped. In the early postoperative period, the following findings alone, but often in combination, should heighten the suspi-cion of cardiac tamponade:

1. Sudden cessation of significant mediastinal bleeding.
2. A persistent low cardiac output state with respiratory variation (either with spontaneous or mechanical ventilation) and narrowing of the pulse pressure noted on the arterial tracing. An increasing requirement for inotropic or vasopressor medications is commonly necessary in response to increasing filling pressures, low blood pressure, and a dwindling cardiac output.
3. Equilibration of intracardiac pressures with RA = PCW = LA pressure resulting from increased intrapericardial pressure. However, it is not unusual for clot to selectively accumulate next to any of the cardiac chambers and cause unequal elevations of right- and left-sided pressures, suggesting that RV or LV failure is the primary problem rather than tamponade.
4. Radiographic findings of an enlarged cardiac silhouette or widened mediastinum compared with an earlier postoperative chest x-ray (Figure 9.3). However, this finding is helpful only if present since it is absent in 80% of patients with tamponade.[137] Displacement of the right heart border from the cardiac silhouette, indicated by an increased distance from the Swan-Ganz catheter or right atrial free wall pacing wires to the edge of the cardiac silhouette, suggests accumulation of clot adjacent to the right atrium. A very large pleural effusion can also cause tamponade.
5. ECG changes, including decreased voltage, a compensatory tachycardia, dysrhythmias, and, terminally, electromechanical dissociation.

D. The diagnosis of tamponade may be obvious on a clinical basis when the typical abnormalities just noted are present. However, occasionally, tamponade may be suspected when in fact ventricular dysfunction is the primary problem. The scenario of hypotension, tachycardia, and elevated filling pressures with moderate mediastinal bleeding is not an uncommon scenario in a patient with marginal myocardial function. If hemodynamics do not improve after volume infusion and inotropic support, tamponade should be suspected and ruled out. If the diagnosis is not clear, and if time allows, an **echocardiogram** should be performed to differentiate ventricular failure from tamponade. Transthoracic echocardiography usually can detect blood compressing the atria and ventricles, but it will fail to provide adequate visualization due to unsatisfactory acoustic windows in up to 60% of patients.[137] Thus, in equivocal situations, a **transesophageal echocardiogram** should be performed to make the proper diagnosis. Even then, an occasional finding is a small, localized effusion producing selective chamber compression without the classic features of tamponade, such as right atrial and RV diastolic collapse. LV diastolic collapse is a reliable sign of tamponade in the postoperative patient.[138]

E. Once tamponade is diagnosed clinically or by echocardiography, or when suspicion remains high despite echocardiographic findings, emergency mediastinal exploration should be performed.[139] CT scanning is also very sensitive in detecting a large hemopericardium, but it cannot provide an assessment of tamponade physiology; furthermore, it requires moving an unstable patient out of the monitoring environment of the ICU.

1. If the patient can be temporarily stabilized, plans should be made for exploration in the OR as soon as possible.
2. If the patient is markedly hypotensive and cardiac arrest is imminent or has occurred, emergency exploration in the ICU is indicated. With appropriate technique, this is associated with low infection rates and excellent survival.

IX. Technique of Emergency Resternotomy

A. Emergency re-exploration is indicated for exsanguinating hemorrhage or tamponade with incipient cardiac arrest. Every member of the house staff must be thoroughly familiar with the location and use of emergency thoracotomy equipment, as they may be the only individual available to perform an emergency sternotomy and save a patient's life. A small subxiphoid incision may initially relieve some of the pressure around the heart in dire circumstances, but it is usually easier to open the entire sternotomy wound.

B. An emergency resternotomy pack must be available and readily accessible in all cardiac surgical ICUs. This must include all the essential equipment to perform the procedure, including gowns, gloves, and masks, antiseptic solutions, and drapes to prep and drape the patient expeditiously, and a preselected assortment of essential instruments. Having a separate small kit with instruments required to open the chest (knife, heavy needle holder and wire cutter, sponges, one-piece retractor) is helpful while the larger pack of instruments is being opened.

C. Technique of emergency resternotomy

1. Remove the dressing over the wound (often not present if wound was sealed with 2-octyl cyanoacrylate tissue adhesive (Dermabond).

2. Pour antiseptic on the skin and then place four towels around the sternotomy incision and other drapes over the rest of the patient. Alternatively, some have recommended use of a one-piece sterile thoracic drape that covers the entire field and may immobilize bacteria.[131] This allows for external compressions to be immediately restarted after the drape is applied. After antiseptic solutions are placed, the wound can be emergently opened, but external compressions have to be applied over a towel since the skin has not dried.

3. Open the wound down to the sternum with a knife. If skin staples are present, make the incision adjacent to the staples. If Dermabond is present, just cut through it.

4. If sternal wires were used, cut with a wire cutter; if a wire cutter is not available, untwist the wires with a heavy needle holder until they fatigue and break. If the sternum was closed with sutures (TiCron or Ethibond), simply cut the sutures with a knife. If other means of sternal reinforcement were used, additional devices should be available at the bedside (e.g. a sterile screwdriver for sternal talons (KLA Martin), or a screwdriver for SternaLock Blu (Zimmer Biomet) plates, which can also be cut with heavy metal cutters across the plate cross-section.

5. Place the sternal retractor to expose the heart (a one-piece retractor is essential).

6. Place a finger over the bleeding site if it can be identified and suction the remainder of the chest to improve exposure.

7. Resuscitate with volume through central or peripheral lines.

8. Initiate internal massage if the chest is opened for cardiac arrest or marginal blood pressure. Commonly, improvement in cardiac activity and blood pressure will be noted upon relief of tamponade (and often from the bolus of epinephrine given as the patient is deteriorating). Performing internal massage mandates attention to the location of bypass grafts, especially the left internal thoracic artery (LITA) graft to the left anterior descending artery (LAD), which can easily be avulsed. An experienced individual can achieve satisfactory

compression using one-hand massage (usually the left hand), placing the fingers behind the heart and compressing the ventricles against the thenar eminence. Use of the right hand may result in perforation of the RV outflow tract and is more difficult to perform. Therefore, it is generally recommended that two hands be used, compressing the heart between the right hand, placed around the LV apex and behind the heart, and the palm and flattened fingers of the left hand anteriorly.

9. Control major and then minor bleeding sites. Manual control of a bleeding site should be obtained while the chest is suctioned and the patient receives volume resuscitation. Only then should specific attention be paid to placing sutures or ties to control bleeding, unless the bleeding site is obvious and easy to control. Manual control can usually minimize bleeding and "buys time" until a more experienced person arrives or the OR can be made available. If the patient remains hemodynamically unstable, it is preferable to resuscitate the patient in the ICU rather than rush the patient to the OR. Invariably the bleeding site can be controlled and the patient stabilized.

10. If the patient has arrested, but tamponade is not present, internal cardiac massage is carried out, an IABP may be placed, and the patient brought back to the OR as soon as possible. Extracorporeal membrane oxygenation can also be considered in dire circumstances once the appropriate equipment and a perfusionist are available.

11. Irrigate the mediastinum extensively with warm saline or antibiotic solution and consider leaving drainage catheters for postoperative antibiotic irrigation.

12. Note that patients who have had cardiac surgery via a right thoracotomy incision or a short left anterior thoracotomy incision cannot be resuscitated with internal massage, although opening of the incision may allow for drainage of tamponade. Either equipment for a full sternotomy must be available in the ICU or the patient will need to be returned to the OR for further resuscitation.

13. Always make sure that someone communicates with the patient's family.

References

1. Despotis GJ, Hogue CW Jr. Pathophysiology, prevention, and treatment of bleeding after cardiac surgery: a primer for cardiologists and an update for the cardiothoracic team. *Am J Cardiol* 1999;83:15B–30B.

2. Khuri SF, Valeri CR, Loscalzo J, et al. Heparin causes platelet dysfunction and induces fibrinolysis before cardiopulmonary bypass. *Ann Thorac Surg* 1995;60:1008–14.

3. Puskas JD, Williams WH, Duke PG, et al. Off-pump coronary artery bypass grafting provides complete revascularization with reduced myocardial injury, transfusion requirements, and length of stay: a prospective randomized comparison of two hundred unselected patients undergoing off-pump versus conventional coronary artery bypass grafting. *J Thorac Cardiovasc Surg* 2003;125:797–808.

4. Murphy GJ, Mango E, Lucchetti V, et al. A randomized trial of tranexamic acid in combination with cell salvage plus a meta-analysis of randomized trials evaluating tranexamic acid in off-pump coronary artery bypass grafting. *J Thorac Cardiovasc Surg* 2006;132:475–80.

5. Bjessmo S, Hylander S, Vedin J, Mohlkert D, Ivert T. Comparison of three different chest drainages after coronary artery bypass surgery: a randomised trial in 150 patients. *Eur J Cardiothorac Surg* 2007;31:372–5.

6. Sakopoulos AG, Hurwitz AS, Suda RW, Goodwin JN. Efficacy of Blake drains for mediastinal and pleural drainage following cardiac operations. *J Card Surg* 2005;20:574–7.

7. Christensen MC, Dziewior F, Kempel A, von Heymann C. Increased chest tube drainage is independently associated with adverse outcome after cardiac surgery. *J Cardiothorac Vasc Anesth* 2012;26:46–51.

8. Vivacqua A, Koch CG, Yousuf AM, et al. Morbidity of bleeding after cardiac surgery: is it blood transfusion, reoperation, or both? *Ann Thorac Surg* 2011;91:1780–90.

9. Kilic A, Whitman GJR. Blood transfusions in cardiac surgery: indications, risks, and conservation strategies. *Ann Thorac Surg* 2014;97:726–34.

10. Engoren M, Schwann TA, Jewell E, et al. Is transfusion associated with graft occlusion after cardiac operations? *Ann Thorac Surg* 2015;99:502–8.

11. Schwann TA, Habib JR, Khalifeh JM, et al. Effects of blood transfusion on cause-specific late mortality after coronary artery bypass grafting: less is more. *Ann Thorac Surg* 2016;102:465–73.

12. Horvath KJ, Acker MA, Chang H, et al. Blood transfusion and infection after cardiac surgery. *Ann Thorac Surg* 2013;95:2194–201.

13. Tantawy J, Li A, Dai F, et al. Association of red cell transfusion and short- and longer-term mortality after coronary artery bypass graft surgery. *J Cardiothorac Vasc Anesth* 2018;32:1225–32.

14. Boer C, Meesters MI, Milojevic M, et al. 2017 EACTS/EACTA guidelines on patient blood management for adult cardiac surgery. *J Cardiothorac Vasc Anesth* 2018;12:88–120.

15. Mazer CD, Whitlock RP, Fergusson DA, et al. Six-month outcomes after restrictive or liberal transfusion for cardiac surgery. *N Engl J Med* 2018;379:1224–33.

16. Chen QH, Wang HL, Liu L, Shao J, Yu J, Zheng RQ. Effects of restrictive red blood cell transfusion on the prognosis of adult patients undergoing cardiac surgery: a meta-analysis of randomized controlled trials. *Crit Care* 2018;22:142.

17. Despotis G, Avidan M, Eby C. Prediction and management of bleeding in cardiac surgery. *J Thromb Haemost* 2009;7(Suppl 1):111–7.

18. Bolliger D, Tanaka KA. Point-of-care coagulation testing in cardiac surgery. *Semin Thromb Hemost* 2017;43:386–96.

19. Biancari F, Kinnunen EM, Kiviniemi T, et al. Meta-analysis of the sources of bleeding after adult cardiac surgery. *J Cardiothorac Vasc Anesth* 2018;32:1618–24.

20. Petrou A, Tzimas P, Siminelakis S. Massive bleeding in cardiac surgery: definitions, predictors, and challenges. *Hippokratia* 2016;20:179–86.

21. Kristensen KL, Rauer LJ, Mortensen PE, Kjeldsen BJ. Reoperation for bleeding in cardiac surgery. *Interact Cardiovasc Thorac Surg* 2012;14:709–13.

22. Society of Thoracic Surgeons Blood Conservation Guideline Task Force, Ferraris VA, Brown JR, Despotis GJ, Hammon JW, Reece TB, Saha SP, Song HK, Clough ER; Society of Cardiovascular Anesthesiologists Special Task Force on Blood Transfusion, Shore-Lesserson LJ, Goodnough LT, Mazer CD, Shander A, Stafford-Smith M, Waters J; International Consortium for Evidence Based Perfusion, Baker RA, Dickinson TA, FitzGerald DJ, Likosky DS, Shann KG. 2011 update to the Society of Thoracic Surgeons and the Society of Cardiovascular Anesthesiologists blood conservation clinical practice guidelines *Ann Thorac Surg* 2011;91:944–82.

23. Vuylsteke A, Pagel C, Gerrard C, et al. The Papworth bleeding risk score: a stratification scheme for identifying cardiac surgery patients at risk of excessive early postoperative bleeding. *Eur J Cardiothorac Surg* 2011;39:924–30.

24. Petricevic M, Kopjar T, Biocina B, et al. The predictive value of platelet function point-of-care tests for postoperative blood loss and transfusion in routine cardiac surgery: a systematic review. *Thorac Cardiovasc Surg* 2015;63:2–20.

25. Ranucci M, Baryshnikova E for the Surgical and Clinical Outcome Research Score Group. The interaction between preoperative platelet count and function and its relationship with postoperative bleeding in cardiac surgery. *Platelets* 2017;28:794–8.

26. Gravlee GP, Hopkins MB, Yetter CR, Buss DH. Heparin content of washed red blood cells from the cardiopulmonary bypass circuit. *J Cardiothorac Vasc Anesth* 1992;6:140–2.

27. Boer C, Meesters MI, Veerhoek D, Vonk ABA. Anticoagulant and side-effects of protamine in cardiac surgery: a narrative review. *Br J Anaesth* 2018;120:914–27.

28. Meesters MI, Verrhoek D, de Lange F, et al. Effect of high or low protamine dosing on postoperative bleeding following heparin anticoagulation in cardiac surgery: a randomized controlled trial. *Thromb Haemost* 2016;116:251–61.

29. Essa Y, Zeynalov N, Sandhaus T, Hofmann M, Lehmann T, Doenst T. Low fibrinogen is associated with increased bleeding-related re-exploration after cardiac surgery. *Thorac Cardiovasc Surg* 2018;66:622–8.

30. Vincentelli A, Susen S, Le Tourneau T, et al. Acquired von Willebrand syndrome in aortic stenosis. *N Engl J Med* 2003;349:343–9.

31. Mahla E, Suarez TA, Bliden KP, et al. Platelet function measurement-based strategy to reduce bleeding and waiting time in clopidogrel-treated patients undergoing coronary artery bypass graft surgery: the timing based on platelet function strategy to reduce clopidogrel-associated bleeding related to CABG (TARGET-CABG) Study. *Circ Cardiovasc Interv* 2012;5:261–9.

32. Williams ML, He X, Rankin JS, Slaughter MS, Gammie JS. Preoperative hematocrit is a powerful predictor of adverse outcomes in coronary artery bypass graft surgery: a report from the Society of Thoracic Surgeons adult cardiac surgery database. *Ann Thorac Surg* 2013;96:1628–34.

33. Karkouti K, Wijeysundera DN, Yau TM, et al. Acute kidney injury after cardiac surgery: focus on modifiable risk factors. *Circulation* 2009;119:495–502.

34. Ghatanatti R, Teli A, Narayan P, et al. Ideal hematocrit to minimize renal injury on cardiopulmonary bypass. *Innovations (Phila)* 2015;10:420–4.

35. Rubin DS, Matsumoto MM, Moss HE, Joslin CE, Tung A, Roth S. Ischemic optic neuropathy in cardiac surgery: incidence and risk factors in the United States from the National Inpatient Sample 1998 to 2013. *Anesthesiology* 2017;126:810–21.

36. Roth S, Moss HE. Update on perioperative ischemic optic neuropathy associated with non-ophthalmic surgery. *Front Neurol* 2018;9:557.

37. Levy JH, Douketis J, Steiner T, Goldstein JN, Milling TJ. Prothrombin complex concentrates for perioperative vitamin K antagonist and non-vitamin K anticoagulant reversal. *Anesthesiology* 2018;129:1171–84.

38. Khorsand N, Kooistra HA, van Hest RM, Veeger NJ, Meijer K. A systematic review of prothrombin complex concentrate dosing strategies to reverse vitamin K antagonist therapy. *Thromb Res* 2015;135:9–19.

39. Htet NN, Barounis D, Knight C, Umunna BP, Hormese M, Lovell E. Protocolized use of Factor Eight Inhibitor Bypassing Activity (FEIBA) for the reversal of warfarin induced coagulopathy. *Am J Emerg Med* 2019;38:539–44.

40. Solo K, Lavi S, Choudhury T, et al. Pre-operative use of aspirin in patients undergoing coronary artery bypass grafting: a systematic review and updated meta-analysis. *J Thorac Dis* 2018;10:3444–59.

41. Hastings S, Myles PA, McIlroy DM. Aspirin and coronary artery surgery: an updated meta-analysis. *Br J Anaesth* 2016;116:716–7.

42. Myles PS, Smith JA, Kasza J, et al. Aspirin in coronary artery surgery: 1-year results of the Aspirin and Tranexamic Acid for Coronary Artery Surgery trial. *J Thorac Cardiovasc Surg* 2019;157:633-40.

43. Gerstein NS, Brierley JK, Windsor J, et al. Antifibrinolytic agents in cardiac and noncardiac surgery: a comprehensive overview and update. *J Cardiothorac Vasc Anesth* 2017;31:2183–2205.

44. McIlroy DR, Myles PS, Phillips LE, Smith JA. Antifibrinolytics in cardiac surgical patients receiving aspirin: a systematic review and meta-analysis. *Br J Anaesth* 2009;102:168–78.

45. Koster A, Faraoni D, Levy JH. Antifibrinolytic therapy for cardiac surgery: an update. *Anesthesiology* 2015;123:214–21.

46. Seese L, Sultan I, Gleason TG, Navid F, Wang Y, Kilic A. The impact of preoperative clopidogrel on outcomes after coronary artery bypass grafting. *Ann Thorac Surg* 2019;108:1114–21.

47. Hansson EC, Jeppson A. Platelet inhibition and bleeding complications in cardiac surgery: a review. *Scand Cardiovasc J* 2016;50:349–54.

48. Rosengart TK, Romeiser JL, White LJ, et al. Platelet activity measured by a rapid turnaround assay identifies coronary artery bypass grafting patients at increased risk for bleeding and transfusion complications after clopidogrel administration. *J Thorac Cardiovasc Surg* 2013;146:1259–66.

49. Kim JY, Kim SH, Myong JP, et al. Outcomes of direct oral anticoagulants in patients with mitral stenosis. *J Am Coll Cardiol* 2019;73:1123–31.

50. Eikelboom JW, Brueckmann M, Van de Werf F. Dabigatran in patients with mechanical heart valves. *N Engl J Med* 2014;370:383–4.

51. Hassan K, Bayer N, Schlingloff F, et al. Bleeding complications after use of novel oral anticoagulants in patients undergoing cardiac surgery. *Ann Thorac Surg* 2018;105:702–8.

52. Chaudhary R, Sharma T, Garg J, et al. Direct oral anticoagulants: a review on the current role and scope of reversal agents. *J Thromb Thrombolysis* 2020;49:271–86.

53. Momin JH, Hughes GJ. Andexanet alfa (Andexxa®) for the reversal of direct oral anticoagulants. *PT* 2019;44:530–2.

54. Bhatt DL, Pollack CV, Weitz JI, et al. Antibody-based ticagrelor reversal agent in healthy volunteers. *N Engl J Med* 2019;380:1825–33.

55. Dager WE, Robert AJ, Nishijima DK. Effect of low and moderate dose FEIBA to reverse bleeding in patients on direct oral anticoagulants. *Thromb Res* 2019;173:71–6.

56. Bizzari F, Scolletta S, Tucci E, et al. Perioperative use of tirofiban hydrochloride (Aggrastat) does not increase surgical bleeding after emergency or urgent coronary artery bypass grafting. *J Thorac Cardiovasc Surg* 2001;122:1181–5.

57. Dyke CM, Smedira NG, Koster A, et al. A comparison of bivalirudin to heparin with protamine reversal in patients undergoing cardiac surgery with cardiopulmonary bypass: the EVOLUTION-ON study. *J Thorac Cardiovasc Surg* 2006;131:533–9.

58. Chaudhary FA, Pervaz Z, Ilyas S, Niaz MN. Topical use of tranexamic acid in open heart surgery. *J Pak Med Assoc* 2018;68:538–42.

59. Beattie GW, Jeffrey RR. Is there evidence that fresh frozen plasma is superior to antithrombin administration to treat heparin resistance in cardiac surgery? *Interact Cardiovasc Thorac Surg* 2014;18:117–20.

60. Runge M, Møller CH, Steinbüchel DA. Increased accuracy in heparin and protamine administration decreases bleeding: a pilot study, *J Extra Corpor Technol* 2009;41:10–4.

61. Shigeta O, Kojima H, Hiramatsu Y, et al. Low-dose protamine based on heparin-protamine titration method reduces platelet dysfunction after cardiopulmonary bypass. *J Thorac Cardiovasc Surg* 1999;118:354–60.

62. Avgerinos DV, DeBois W, Salemi A. Blood conservation strategies in cardiac surgery: more is better. *Eur J Cardiothorac Surg* 2014;46:865–70.

63. Zimmerman E, Zhu R, Ogami T, et al. Intraoperative autologous blood donation leads to fewer transfusions in cardiac surgery. *Ann Thorac Surg* 2019;108:1738–44.

64. Ramnath AN, Naber HR, de Boer A, Leusink JA. No benefit of intraoperative whole blood sequestration and autotransfusion during coronary artery bypass grafting: results of a randomized clinical trial. *J Thorac Cardiovasc Surg* 2003;125:1432–7.

65. Carless PA, Rubens FD, Anthony DM, O'Connell D, Henry DA. Platelet-rich plasmapheresis for minimising peri-operative allogeneic blood transfusion. *Cochrane Database Syst Rev* 2003;2:CD004172. https://doi.org/10.1002/14651858.CD004172.pub2.

66. Rubens FD, Fergusson D, Wells PS, Huang M, McGowan JL, Laupacis A. Platelet-rich plasmapheresis in cardiac surgery: a meta-analysis of the effect on transfusion requirements. *J Thorac Cardiovasc Surg* 1998;116:641–7.

67. Chung JH, Gikakis N, Rao AK, Drake TA, Colman RW, Edmunds LH Jr. Pericardial blood activates the extrinsic coagulation pathway during clinical cardiopulmonary bypass. *Circulation* 1996;93:2014–8.

68. Nollert G, Schwabenland I, Maktav D, et al. Miniaturized cardiopulmonary bypass in coronary artery bypass surgery: marginal impact on inflammation and coagulation but loss of safety margins. *Ann Thorac Surg* 2005;80:2326–32.

69. Trapp C, Schiller W, Mellert F, et al. Retrograde autologous priming as a safe and easy method to reduce hemodilution and transfusion requirements during cardiac surgery. *Thorac Cardiovasc Surg* 2015;63:628–34.

70. Sun P, Ji B, Sun Y, et al. Effects of retrograde autologous priming on blood transfusion and clinical outcomes in adults: a meta-analysis. *Perfusion* 2013;28:238–43.

71. Hofmann B, Kaufmann C, Stiller M, et al. Positive impact of retrograde autologous priming in adult patients undergoing cardiac surgery: a randomized clinical trial. *J Cardiothorac Surg* 2018;13:50.

72. Carless PA, Henry DA, Moxey AJ, O'Connell D, Brown T, Fergusson DA. Cell salvage for minimising perioperative allogeneic blood transfusion. *Cochrane Database Syst Rev* 2010;4:CD001888. https://doi.org/10.1002/14651858.CD001888.pub4.

73. Görlinger K, Shore-Lesserson L, Dirkman D, Hanke AA, Rahe-Meyer N, Tanaka KA. Management of hemorrhage in cardiothoracic surgery. *J Cardiothorac Vasc Anesth* 2013;27(4 suppl):S20–34.

74. Colson PH, Gaudard P, Fellahi JL, et al. Active bleeding after cardiac surgery: a prospective observational multicenter study. *PLoS One* 2016;11:e0162396.

75. Habib AM, Mousa AY, Al-Halees Z. Recombinant factor VII for uncontrolled bleeding postcardiac surgery. *J Saudi Heart Assoc* 2016;28:222–31.

76. Dyke C, Aronson S, Dietrich W, et al. Universal definition of perioperative bleeding in adult cardiac surgery. *J Thorac Cardiovasc Surg* 2014;147:1458–63.

77. Dailey SE, Dysart CB, Langan DR, et al. An *in vitro* study comparing the effects of Hextend, Hespan, normal saline, and lactated Ringer's solution on thromboelastography and the activated partial thromboplastin time. *J Cardiothorac Vasc Anesth* 2005;19:358–61.

78. Moskowitz DM, Shander A, Javidroozi M, et al. Postoperative blood loss and transfusion associated with use of Hextend in cardiac surgery patients at a blood conservation center. *Transfusion* 2008;48:768–75.

79. Haynes GR. Fluid management in cardiac surgery: is one hydroxyethyl starch solution safer than another? *J Cardiothorac Vasc Anesth* 2006;20:916–7.

80. Imren Y, Tasoglu I, Oktar GL, et al. The importance of transesophageal echocardiography in diagnosis of pericardial tamponade after cardiac surgery. *J Card Surg* 2008;23:450–3.

81. Bhatt HV, Subramanian K. PRO: prothrombin complex concentrate should be used in preference to fresh frozen plasma for hemostasis in cardiac surgical patients. *J Cardiothorac Vasc Anesth* 2018;32:1062–7.

82. Roman M, Biancari F, Ahmed AB, et al. Prothrombin complex concentrate in cardiac surgery: a systematic review and meta-analysis. *Ann Thorac Surg* 2019;107:1275–83.

83. Teoh KH, Young E, Blackall MH, Roberts RS, Hirsh J. Can extra protamine eliminate heparin rebound following cardiopulmonary bypass surgery? *J Thorac Cardiovasc Surg* 2004;128:211–9.

84. Taneja R, Marwaha G, Sinha P, et al. Elevated activated partial thromboplastin time does not correlate with heparin rebound following cardiac surgery. *Can J Anaesth* 2009;56:489–96.

85. Shams Hakimi C, Singh S, Hesse C, Jeppsson A. Effects of fibrinogen and platelet transfusion on coagulation and platelet function in bleeding cardiac surgery patients. *Acta Anaesthesiol Scand* 2019;63:475–82.

86. Rahe-Meyer N, Hanke A, Schmidt DS, Hagl C, Pichlmaier M. Fibrinogen concentrate reduces intraoperative bleeding when used as first-line hemostatic therapy during major aortic replacement surgery: results from a randomized, placebo-controlled trial. *J Thorac Cardiovasc Surg* 2013;145(3 Suppl):S178–85.

87. Mengistu AM, Wolf MW, Boldt J, Röhm KD, Lang J, Piper SN. Evaluation of a new platelet function analyzer in cardiac surgery: a comparison of modified thromboelastography and whole-blood aggregometry. *J Cardiothorac Vasc Anesth* 2008;22:40–6.

88. Davidson SJ, McGrowder D, Roughton N, Kelleher AA. Can ROTEM thromboelastometry predict postoperative bleeding after cardiac surgery? *J Cardiothorac Vasc Anesth* 2008;22:655–61.

89. Ghavidel AA, Toutounchi Z, Shahandashti FJ, Mermesdagh Y. Rotational thromboelastometry in prediction of bleeding after cardiac surgery. *Asian Cardiovasc Thorac Ann* 2015;23:525–9.

90. Meesters MI, Burtman D, van de Ven PM, Boer C. Prediction of postoperative blood loss using thromboelastometry in adult cardiac surgery: cohort study and systematic review. *J Cardiothorac Vasc Anesth* 2018;32:141–50.

91. Deppe AC, Weber C, Zimmermann J, et al. Point-of-care thromboelastography/thromboelastometry-based coagulation management in cardiac surgery: a meta-analysis of 8332 patients. *J Surg Res* 2016;203:424–33.

92. Kuiper GJAJM, van Egmond LT, Henskens YMC, et al. Shifts of transfusion demand in cardiac surgery after implementation of rotational thromboelastometry-guided transfusion protocols: analysis of the HEROES-CS (HEmostasis Registry of patiEntS in Cardiac Surgery) observational, prospective open cohort database. *J Cardiothorac Vasc Anesth* 2019;33:307–17.

93. Mittermayr M, Velik-Salchner C, Stalzer B, et al. Detection of protamine and heparin after termination of cardiopulmonary bypass by thrombelastometry (ROTEM): results of a pilot study. *Anesth Analg* 2009;108:743–50.

94. Bischof DB, Ganter MT, Shore-Lesserson L, et al. Viscoelastic blood coagulation management with Sonoclot predicts postoperative bleeding in cardiac surgery after heparin reversal. *J Cardiothorac Vasc Anesth* 2015;29:715–22.

95. Haneya A, Diez C, Kolat P, et al. Re-exploration for bleeding or tamponade after cardiac surgery: impact of timing and indication on outcome. *Thorac Cardiovasc Surg* 2015;63:51–7.

96. Fröjd V, Jeppson A. Reexploration for bleeding and its association with mortality after cardiac surgery. *Ann Thorac Surg* 2016;102:109–17.

97. Biancari F, Mikkola R, Heikkinen J, Lahtinen J, Airaksinen KE, Juvonen T. Estimating the risk of complications related to re-exploration for bleeding after adult cardiac surgery: a systematic review and meta-analysis. *Eur J Cardiothorac Surg* 2012;41:50–5.

98. Valeri CR, Khabbaz K, Khuri SF, et al. Effect of skin temperature on platelet function in patients undergoing extracorporeal bypass. *J Thorac Cardiovasc Surg* 1992;104:108–16.

99. Collier B, Kolff J, Devineni R, Gonzalez LS III. Prophylactic positive end-expiratory pressure and reduction of postoperative blood loss in open-heart surgery. *Ann Thorac Surg* 2002;74:1191–4.

100. Desborough MJ, Oakland KA, Landoni G, et al. Desmopressin for treatment of platelet dysfunction and reversal of antiplatelet agents: a systematic review and meta-analysis of randomized controlled trials. *J Thromb Haemost* 2017;15:263–72.

101. Steinlechner B, Zeidler P, Base E, et al. Patients with severe aortic valve stenosis and impaired platelet function benefit from preoperative desmopressin infusion. *Ann Thorac Surg* 2011;91:1420–6.

102. Fernandez F. Goudable C, Sie P, et al. Low haematocrit and prolonged bleeding time in uremic patients: effect of red cell transfusions. *Br J Haematol* 1985;59:139–48.

103. Laine A, Niemi T, Schramko A. Transfusion threshold of hemoglobin 80 g/L is comparable to 100 g/L in terms of bleeding in cardiac surgery: a prospective randomized study. *J Cardiothorac Vasc Anesth* 2018;32:131–9.

104. Butterworth J, Lin YA, Prielipp RC, Bennett J, Hammon JW, James RL. Rapid disappearance of protamine in adults undergoing cardiac operation with cardiopulmonary bypass. *Ann Thorac Surg* 2002;74:1589–95.

105. Nielsen VG. Protamine enhances fibrinolysis by decreasing clot strength: role of tissue factor-initiated thrombin generation. *Ann Thorac Surg* 2006;81:1720–7.

106. Ganz ML, Wu N, Rawn J, Pashos CL, Strandberg-Larsen M. Clinical and economic outcomes associated with blood transfusions among elderly Americans following coronary artery bypass graft surgery requiring cardiopulmonary bypass. *Blood Transfus* 2014;12(Suppl 1): S90–9.

107. Rawn JD. Blood transfusion in cardiac surgery: a silent epidemic revisited. *Circulation* 2007;116:2523–4.

108. van de Watering LMG, Hermans J, Houbiers JGA, et al. Beneficial effects of leukocyte depletion of transfused blood on postoperative complications in patients undergoing heart surgery: a randomized clinical trial. *Circulation* 1998;97:562–8.

109. Semple JW, Rebetz J, Kapur R. Transfusion-associated circulatory overload and transfusion-related acute lung injury. *Blood* 2019;133:1840–53.

110. Oyet C, Okongo B, Onuthi RA, Muwanguzi E. Biochemical changes in stored donor units: implications on the efficacy of blood transfusion. *J Blood Med* 2018;9:111–5.

111. Koch CG, Li L, Sessler DI, et al. Duration of red cell storage and complications after cardiac surgery. *N Engl J Med* 2008;358:1229–39.

112. Alexander PE, Barty R, Fei Y, et al. Transfusion of fresher vs older red blood cells in hospitalized patients: a systematic review and meta-analysis. *Blood* 2016;127:400–10.

113. Mohr R, Martinowitz U, Lavee J, Amroch D, Ramot B, Goor DA. The hemostatic effects of transfusing fresh whole blood versus platelet concentrates after cardiac operations. *J Thorac Cardiovasc Surg* 1988;96:530–4.

114. Valeri CR, Dennis RC, Ragno G, Pivacek LE, Hechtman HB, Khuri SF. Survival, function, and hemolysis of shed red blood cells processed as nonwashed and washed red blood cells. *Ann Thorac Surg* 2001;72:1598–602.

115. Hartz R, Smith JA, Green D. Autotransfusion after cardiac operation: assessment of hemostatic factors. *J Thorac Cardiovasc Surg* 1988;96:178–82.

116. Griffith LD, Billman GF, Daily PO, Lane TA. Apparent coagulopathy caused by infusion of shed mediastinal blood and its prevention by washing of the infusate. *Ann Thorac Surg* 1989;47:400–6.

117. Body SC, Birmingham J, Parks R, et al. Safety and efficacy of shed mediastinal blood transfusion after cardiac surgery: a multicenter observational study: Multicenter Study of Perioperative Ischemia Research Group. *J Cardiothorac Vasc Anesth* 1999;13:410–6.

118. Spiess BD, Royston D, Levy JH, et al. Platelet transfusions during coronary artery bypass graft surgery are associated with serious adverse outcomes. *Transfusion* 2004;44:1143–8.

119. McGrath T, Koch CG, Xu M, et al. Platelet transfusion in cardiac surgery does not confer increased risk for adverse morbid outcomes. *Ann Thorac Surg* 2008;86:543–53.

120. Desborough M. Sandu R, Brunskill SJ, et al. Fresh frozen plasma for cardiovascular surgery. *Cochrane Database Syst Rev* 2015;7:CD007614. https://doi.org/10.1002/14651858.CD007614.pub2.

121. Tanaka KA, Mazzeffi M, Durila M. Role of prothrombin complex concentrate in perioperative coagulation therapy. *J Intensive Care* 2014;2:60.

122. Hashmi MK, Ghadimi K, Srinivasan AJ, et al. Three-factor prothrombin complex concentrates for refractory bleeding after cardiovascular surgery within an algorithmic approach to haemostasis. *Vox Sang* 2019;114:374–85.

123. Cappabianca G, Mariscalco G, Biancari F, et al. Safety and efficacy of prothrombin complex concentrate as first-line treatment in bleeding after cardiac surgery. *Crit Care* 2016;20:5.

124. Mehringer SL, Klick Z, Bain J, et al. Activated factor 7 versus 4-factor prothrombin complex concentrate for critical bleeding post-cardiac surgery. *Ann Pharmacol* 2018;52:533–7.

125. Harper PC, Smith MM, Brinkman NJ, et al. Outcomes following three-factor inactive prothrombin complex concentrate versus recombinant activated factor VII administration during cardiac surgery. *J Cardiothorac Vasc Anesth* 2018;32:151–7.

126. Nascimento B, Goodnough LT, Levy JH. Cryoprecipitate therapy. *Brit J Anaesth* 2014;113:922–34.

127. Görlinger K, Dirkmann D, Hanke AA, et al. First-line therapy with coagulation factor concentrates combined with point-of-care coagulation testing is associated with decreased allogeneic blood transfusion in cardiovascular surgery: a retrospective, single-center cohort study. *Anesthesiology* 2011;115:1179–91.

128. Smith MM, Ashikhmina E, Brinkman NJ, Barbara DW. Perioperative use of coagulation factor concentrates in patients undergoing cardiac surgery. *J Cardiothorac Vasc Anesth* 2017;31:1810–9.

129. Maeda T, Miyata S, Usui A, et al. Safety of fibrinogen concentrate and cryoprecipitate in cardiovascular surgery: multicenter database study. *J Cardiothorac Vasc Anesth* 2019;33:321–7.

130. Brase J, Finger B, He J, et al. Analysis of outcomes using low-dose and early administration of recombinant activated factor VII in cardiac surgery. *Ann Thorac Surg* 2016;102:35–40.

131. Dunning J, Fabbri A, Kolh PH, et al. Guideline for resuscitation in cardiac arrest after cardiac surgery. *Eur J Cardiothorac Surg* 2009;36:3–28.

132. Ley SJ. Standards for resuscitation after cardiac surgery. *Critical Care Nurse* 2015;35:30–8.

133. The Society of Thoracic Surgeons Task Force on Resuscitation after Cardiac Surgery. The Society of Thoracic Surgeons expert consensus for the resuscitation of patients who arrest after cardiac surgery. *Ann Thorac Surg* 2017;103:1005–20.

134. Ranucci M, Bozzetti G, Ditta A, Cotza M, Carboni G, Ballotta A. Surgical reexploration after cardiac operations: why a worse outcome? *Ann Thorac Surg* 2008;86:1557–62.

135. Karthik S, Grayson AD, McCarron EE, Pullan DM, Desmond MJ. Reexploration for bleeding after coronary artery bypass surgery: risk factors, outcomes, and the effect of time delay. *Ann Thorac Surg* 2004;78:527–34.

136. Choong CK, Gerrard C, Goldsmith KA, Dunningham H, Vuylsteke A. Delayed re-exploration for bleeding after coronary artery bypass surgery results in adverse outcomes. *Eur J Cardiothorac Surg* 2007;31:834–8.

137. Hamid M, Khan MU, Bashour AC. Diagnostic value of chest x-ray and echocardiography for cardiac tamponade in post cardiac surgery patients. *J Pak Med Assoc* 2006;56:104–7.

138. Chuttani K, Pandian NG, Mohanty PK, et al. Left ventricular diastolic collapse: an echocardiographic sign of regional cardiac tamponade. *Circulation* 1991;83:1999–2006.

139. Carmona P, Mateo E, Casanovas I, et al. Management of cardiac tamponade after cardiac surgery. *J Cardiothorac Vasc Anesth* 2012;26:302–11.

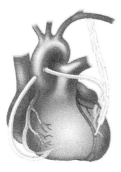

CHAPTER 10

Respiratory Management

♡ **10** Respiratory Management

I. General Comments

A. Virtually all patients undergoing open-heart surgery will have some element of postoperative pulmonary dysfunction.[1] However, in the vast majority of patients, it is well tolerated with minimal impairment in oxygenation and ventilation. Thus, it is possible and desirable in most patients to achieve early endotracheal extubation within the first 4–6 hours after surgery. This reduces pulmonary complications, encourages earlier mobilization, and reduces costs and the hospital length of stay.[2,3] Some centers recommend extubation in the operating room (OR) in lower-risk patients and have documented improved outcomes and lower costs.[4–7]

B. The use of general anesthesia and a median sternotomy incision for most open-heart operations and the use of the internal thoracic artery (ITA) for virtually all coronary bypass operations have significant adverse effects on pulmonary function and chest wall mechanics.[8 10] Although the use of cardiopulmonary bypass (CPB) is associated with a systemic inflammatory response that has been incriminated as the major cause of postoperative pulmonary dysfunction, studies comparing postoperative pulmonary function in patients undergoing on- and off-pump surgery have not demonstrated a significant difference, except perhaps in patients with advanced pulmonary disease.[11–14] Thus, anesthetic management and intensive care unit (ICU) protocols to achieve early extubation should be the goal after both types of operations.

C. Minimally invasive incisions preserve a more stable chest wall and have less impact on chest wall mechanics. Ministernotomies for aortic valve replacement, for example, are associated with less atelectasis than a full sternotomy incision.[15] Both sternotomy and thoracotomy incisions produce moderate pain with splinting, which can be minimized using epidural or intercostal analgesia or a continuous infusion pump (On-Q Avanos Medical Inc).[16–18] Generally, pulmonary function is better preserved with limited incisions. However, the potential adverse influence of CPB on gas exchange will still be noted following minimally invasive valve operations that require CPB.

D. Postoperative respiratory impairment and the likelihood of "delayed extubation" or the need for prolonged ventilatory support can be predicted fairly reliably based on clinical variables.[19–26] Careful preoperative evaluation for obstructive or restrictive pulmonary disease with review of baseline arterial blood gases (ABGs) should identify patients at high risk for pulmonary complications after surgery. However, most patients without severe preoperative respiratory compromise have adequate pulmonary reserve to tolerate the insults imposed by cardiac surgery. Standard protocols for ventilatory management and early extubation can be applied to all but the very highest-risk patients,

Manual of Perioperative Care in Adult Cardiac Surgery, Sixth Edition. Robert M. Bojar.
© 2021 John Wiley & Sons Ltd. Published 2021 by John Wiley & Sons Ltd.

with excellent results. In approximately 5–10% of patients, mechanical ventilatory support beyond 48 hours is necessary because of marked hemodynamic compromise, poor oxygenation, or inadequate ventilation.

E. An understanding of the postoperative changes in pulmonary function, basic concepts in oxygenation and ventilation, routine pulmonary management, and contributing factors to respiratory dysfunction allows for the early identification and treatment of problems to optimize the recovery of pulmonary function.

II. Postoperative Changes in Pulmonary Function

During the early postoperative period, the principal mechanisms underlying poor gas exchange with borderline oxygenation are ventilation/perfusion (V/Q) mismatch and intrapulmonary shunting.[27] Comparison of pre- and postoperative pulmonary function tests has shown a reduction of about 30–50% in many parameters, including the peak expiratory flow rate (PEFR), forced expiratory volume in 1 second (FEV_1), forced vital capacity (FVC), functional residual capacity (FRC), forced expiratory flow at 50% of vital capacity (FEF_{50}), maximum voluntary ventilation, and expiratory reserve volume after surgery.[10] These abnormalities persist in the postoperative period and may only partially recover out to 3.5 months.[8] Contributing factors include the following issues:

A. General anesthetics, neuromuscular relaxants, and narcotics decrease the central respiratory drive and contribute to decreased respiratory muscle function.

B. The median sternotomy incision produces chest wall splinting that reduces alveolar ventilation and most pulmonary function testing variables.

C. The presence of chest tubes for mediastinal or pleural drainage impairs respiratory function, although less so with subxiphoid than intercostal insertion sites for pleural tubes.[28]

D. Harvesting of the ITA is associated with a decrease in chest wall compliance and deterioration of pulmonary function to a greater degree than when no ITA is harvested.[29] Furthermore, pleural entry for ITA harvesting is associated with even more deterioration in pulmonary function in both on- and off-pump surgery,[30–32] and is associated with a higher incidence of bleeding, pleural effusions, and atelectasis.[32] Interestingly, a few studies have shown that the incidence of respiratory complications and the degree of respiratory impairment is no greater if bilateral, rather than just unilateral, ITA harvesting was performed in patients without preexisting lung disease.[33,34]

E. Diaphragmatic dysfunction from phrenic nerve injury may result from direct injury or devascularization during harvesting of the IMA, the latter arguably being more frequent in diabetic patients.[35–38] The use of ice slush without an insulation pad may also contribute to phrenic nerve injury, with an eightfold increase noted in one study.[36]

F. CPB produces numerous problems that can contribute to postoperative respiratory dysfunction.[1,39] It is curious that most studies demonstrate comparable deterioration in pulmonary function after on- and off-pump surgery when all of these factors are taken into consideration.

1. Cardiogenic pulmonary edema may result from hemodilution, fluid overload, and reduction in oncotic pressure. Postcardiotomy left ventricular (LV) dysfunction with elevated pulmonary artery (PA) pressures may contribute to pulmonary edema and lead to impairment of right ventricular (RV) function.

2. Noncardiogenic interstitial pulmonary edema is a manifestation of the "systemic inflammatory response", which produces an increase in endothelial permeability and accumulation of extravascular lung water; this also decreases lung surfactant, contributing to atelectasis. Contributory factors to this syndrome include:

   a. Complement activation

   b. Release of cytokines and other inflammatory mediators

   c. Pulmonary sequestration of neutrophils activated by blood contact with the extracorporeal circuit, resulting in release of proteolytic enzymes, such as neutrophil elastase, that may damage tissue and increase alveolar-endothelial permeability.

3. Hyperoxia may increase oxygen free-radical damage.

4. Pulmonary ischemia-reperfusion injury or failure to ventilate the lungs during CPB may impair pulmonary function.[40] The efficacy of gas exchange post-pump may be improved if the lungs remain inflated with CPAP during CPB.[41]

G. Blood transfusions introduce microemboli and proinflammatory mediators that may elevate pulmonary vascular resistance and PA pressures, increase inspiratory pressures, impair oxygenation, and reduce RV function. Transfusions are associated with an increased risk of pulmonary morbidity that may be also associated with the development of transfusion-related acute lung injury (TRALI), which is considered an immune mediated phenomenon, and transfusion-associated circulatory overload (TACO), caused by rapid transfusion of blood to a patient with preexisting fluid overload (see page 482).[42,43]

H. Preexisting conditions may impair postoperative pulmonary function, such as chronic obstructive pulmonary disease (COPD) with any active bronchitic component, and obesity, which produces V/Q imbalance and impairs oxygenation.[44,45]

III. Routine Ventilator, Sedation, and Analgesia Management

A. For open-heart surgery, patients generally receive a balanced anesthetic regimen consisting of a narcotic (fentanyl, sufentanil, or remifentanil), an inhalational anesthetic, a neuromuscular blocker, and a sedative, such as propofol. Surgical outcomes appear comparable with a balanced technique using "volatile anesthesia" and total intravenous anesthesia.[46] In addition to taking the patient's underlying cardiac disease and comorbidities into consideration, the use and dosing of medications should be modified based upon plans for postoperative extubation. Generally, remifentanil is used only in patients for whom very early extubation is planned because of its rapid offset of action. This allows for very early awakening, and is associated with less respiratory depression and less atelectasis after extubation.

B. If not extubated in the OR, the patient should be placed on a volume-cycled respirator for full ventilator support upon arrival in the ICU, using either the synchronized intermittent mandatory ventilation (SIMV) or assist/control (A/C) mode (Table 10.1). The patient remains anesthetized from the residual effects of narcotics, anxiolytic medications, and muscle relaxants given during surgery. Before the patient can initiate and achieve adequate spontaneous ventilation, controlled ventilation will provide efficient gas exchange and decrease oxygen consumption by reducing the

Table 10.1 • Initial Respiratory Orders

1. Initial ventilator settings
   a. Tidal volume 6–8 mL/kg
   b. Respiratory rate (usually in the IMV mode): 10–12/min
   c. FiO$_2$: 1.0
   d. PEEP: 5 cm H$_2$O
2. Display pulse oximetry on bedside monitor
3. Chest x-ray after arrival in ICU (or in OR)
4. Check ABGs 15–30 minutes after arrival
5. Reduce FiO$_2$ to 0.4 as long as the O$_2$ sat is >95%
6. Adjust ventilator settings to maintain PCO$_2$ >30 torr with pH 7.30–7.50
7. Propofol 25–75 µg/kg/min; gradually decrease dose once standard weaning criteria are present and then initiate weaning when patient is mentally alert with reversal of neuromuscular blockade
8. Utilize dexmedetomidine if propofol weaning is not tolerated

work of breathing. This may be very important during the first few postoperative hours when hypothermia, acid–base and electrolyte disturbances, and hemodynamic instability are most pronounced.

C. Initial ventilator settings are as follows:

- Tidal volume: 6–8 mL/kg
- Intermittent mandatory ventilation (IMV) rate: 10–12 breaths/min
- Fraction of inspired oxygen (FiO$_2$): 1.0
- Positive end-expiratory pressure (PEEP): 5 cm H$_2$O
- Inspiratory : expiratory (I:E) ratio of 1:2–1:3

D. The tidal volume and respiratory rate are selected to achieve a minute ventilation of approximately 100 mL/kg/min. Low tidal volumes may be preferable to higher ones, which have been associated with the development of adult respiratory distress syndrome (ARDS) after surgery.[39] In contrast, patients with COPD often benefit from lower respiratory rates and higher tidal volumes with increased inspiratory flow rates. The latter allows more time for the expiratory phase and can reduce the potential for developing high levels of "auto-PEEP" and air-trapping that may adversely affect hemodynamics. Lower tidal volumes with higher respiratory rates are often beneficial for patients with restrictive lung disease.

E. A low level (5 cm H$_2$O) of PEEP is routinely added to the respiratory circuit to prevent atelectasis. Despite this common practice, studies suggest that this level of PEEP does not reopen atelectatic lung and produces no significant improvement in oxygenation over zero PEEP.[47] A PEEP level of 10 cm H$_2$O or higher is usually necessary to improve lung recruitment, but it must be used judiciously because it may reduce venous return and impair RV and LV function. Caution is required when the patient is hypovolemic from peripheral vasodilation or when RV function is impaired.

F. Continuous pulse oximetry is used during mechanical ventilation with display of the arterial oxygen saturation (SaO$_2$) on the bedside monitor. This can bring attention to abrupt changes in oxygenation and should obviate the need to obtain ABGs on a frequent basis in the stable patient. Concern should be raised when the SaO$_2$ is <95%.

G. Although not commonly used in the ICU, capnography (end-tidal CO_2) can be used to provide a relative assessment of the level of PCO_2, although it is inaccurate when V/Q mismatch is present. For example, the end-tidal CO_2 will be much lower than the PCO_2 when there is an increase in physiologic dead space (increased V/Q). It is also affected by the degree of CO_2 production, the minute ventilation, and the cardiac output. Nonetheless, an abrupt change in the contour of the capnogram signifies an acute problem with the patient's ventilatory status, hemodynamics, or metabolic state.

H. A chest x-ray should be checked after arrival in the ICU. The position of the endotracheal tube, Swan-Ganz catheter or any central line, and intra-aortic balloon pump (IABP) should be identified. The lung fields should be evaluated for lung expansion/atelectasis, pneumothorax, undrained pleural effusion, pulmonary edema, or infiltrates. Attention should be paid to the width of the mediastinum, primarily for later comparison in the event of postoperative hemorrhage.

I. An initial ABG should be checked about 15–20 minutes after arrival in the ICU. The FiO_2 is initially set at 1.0 as a safety margin until the patient's oxygenation is assessed. Then it should be reduced to 0.40 and the tidal volume and respiratory rate adjusted to maintain the ABGs within a normal range. The extent of hypothermia should be taken into consideration when making these adjustments, anticipating that the PCO_2 will rise as the patient warms. The metabolic demand and CO_2 production are decreased 10% for every degree less than 37 °C. Acceptable ABGs include:

- PaO_2 >80 torr (SaO_2 >95%)
- PCO_2 32–48 torr
- pH 7.32–7.48

J. Adequate sedation and analgesia must be provided in the early postoperative period to minimize anxiety, pain, and hemodynamic stress, which may contribute to myocardial ischemia and hypertension. This often seems difficult when the goal is to have a stable and comfortable patient who is awakening from anesthesia with an indwelling endotracheal tube.

1. For patients extubated in the OR, adequate analgesia must be provided while minimizing sedation. Thoracic epidural analgesia, a parasternal injection of bupivacaine (0.5% 2 mg/kg in 50 mL injected prior to sternal closure), or a continuous subcutaneous bupivacaine infusion of 4 mL/h × 48 hours using the On-Q Pain Relief System are beneficial in reducing pain.[16–18,48–51] Patient-controlled IV and thoracic epidural analgesia can also be used with comparable pain relief.[52,53] Nonsteroidal anti-inflammatory drugs or IV acetaminophen are useful nonsedating analgesics that may supplement the use of low-dose narcotics.

2. Most patients will arrive in the ICU sedated from narcotics and short-acting medications, such as propofol (usually at a dose of 25 μg/kg/min), started at the conclusion of surgery. Once standard criteria for weaning are met, the propofol infusion is weaned off over a short period of time. Most patients will awaken within 20 minutes of termination of a propofol infusion, although it may take several more hours before they can be extubated. The offset of propofol is related to its dose, the duration of use, and the patient's body habitus. For example, with light sedation for up to 24 hours, emergence occurs in only 13 minutes, but in heavily sedated patients, it may take up to 25 hours![54]

3. Dexmedetomidine is an α-2 adrenergic agonist that may be used as an alternative to propofol when very early extubation is planned or when weaning of propofol is poorly tolerated. It may be started in the OR or later with a loading dose of 1 μg/kg over 10 minutes followed by a continuous infusion of 0.2–1.5 μg/kg/h. It provides analgesia, anxiolysis, and sympatholysis, but only mild sedation and no amnesia. It allows for use of lower doses of other medications and can be continued after extubation. In comparison with propofol and midazolam, dexmedetomidine is generally associated with earlier extubation, a lower risk of delirium, and also a lower risk of acute kidney injury.[55–61] However, it is associated with more hypotension and bradycardia and more pain. It remains a useful alternative for patients requiring mechanical ventilation for over 24 hours.[62–65]

4. If delayed extubation is anticipated, propofol remains an excellent choice for several days and may be converted to fentanyl for longer-term sedation. Although use of dexmedetomidine has only been recommended for 24 hours, several studies have found it to be comparable to or better than propofol or midazolam for long-term sedation.[62–65]

5. Numerous options can be used to optimize perioperative analgesia.

   a. Most commonly, initial analgesia consists of IV narcotics, which are then transitioned to oral medications. With plans for early extubation, lower doses of narcotics should be selected to minimize respiratory depression. Small doses of IV narcotics or a continuous infusion of narcotics (such as morphine sulfate 0.02 mg/kg/h for patients under age 65 and 0.01 mg/kg/h for patients over age 65) may be given to provide analgesia and blunt the sympathetic response while minimizing respiratory depression associated with the peaks and valleys of bolus doses of narcotics. Use of low-dose narcotics may often be given safely after the patient is extubated, but elderly patients are more prone to persistent respiratory depression and delirium with narcotics.

   b. An alternative approach is to give ketorolac (Toradol) 30 mg IV just before propofol is discontinued to decrease narcotic requirements. Its use should be limited to 72 hours, and it should be avoided in patients with renal dysfunction or concerns about mediastinal bleeding. Other nonsteroidal anti-inflammatory medications, such as indomethacin 50 mg PR or ibuprofen given with a proton-pump inhibitor, may be administered safely as well.[66]

   c. Intravenous acetaminophen may be effective in providing analgesia after cardiac surgery, but a significant benefit of reducing the requirement for opioids for pain control has not been demonstrated.[67] One study did demonstrate that IV acetaminophen given with propofol or dexmedetomidine significantly and equivalently reduced the incidence of delirium.[68]

   d. Epidural narcotics are beneficial in providing analgesia, but there may be reluctance to place these catheters because of concerns about heparinization and the risk of producing an epidural hematoma.

   e. Patient-controlled analgesia (PCA) using narcotics (morphine, fentanyl, or remifentanil) provides adequate analgesia with few side effects in patients with a low pain threshold.[48,69,70]

K. Arterial blood gases should be checked if there is a significant change in the patient's clinical picture or if noninvasive monitoring (pulse oximetry or end-tidal CO_2) suggests a problem. A cautious approach is to check the ABGs after 4–6 hours, before initiating weaning, and just before extubation. Once criteria for weaning have been met, the patient may be given a spontaneous breathing trial (SBT) on continuous positive airway pressure (CPAP) with 5 cm of PEEP. If satisfactory mechanics and ABGs are present, the patient is extubated.

IV. Basic Concepts of Oxygenation

A. The first of the two primary goals of mechanical ventilation is the achievement of satisfactory arterial oxygenation. Although this is usually assessed by the arterial PO_2 (PaO_2), it should be remembered that the PaO_2 is a measurement of the partial pressure of oxygen dissolved in the bloodstream – it indirectly reflects oxygen saturation of hemoglobin (Hb) in the blood and does not measure the oxygen content of the blood.

B. Blood oxygen content is determined primarily by the Hb level and the amount of oxygen bound to Hb (the SaO_2), and to a lesser extent by that dissolved in solution (the PaO_2). Each gram of Hb can transport 1.39 mL of oxygen per 100 mL of blood (vol %), whereas each 100 torr of PaO_2 transports 0.031 vol %. Thus, correction of anemia does significantly more to improve blood oxygen content than does raising the level of dissolved oxygen (PaO_2) by increasing the FiO_2.

1. The oxygen–hemoglobin dissociation curve demonstrates the relationship between PaO_2 and O_2 saturation (Figure 10.1). The amount of oxygen delivered to

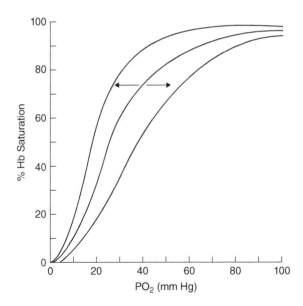

Figure 10.1 • Oxygen–hemoglobin dissociation curve. The sigmoid curve delineates the saturation of hemoglobin at increasing levels of PO_2. Note that a PO_2 of 65 mm Hg (torr) corresponds to a saturation of 90%. Higher levels of O_2 produce only small increments in blood oxygen content, but a PO_2 below this level results in a precipitous fall in O_2 saturation. A shift of the curve to the left, as is noted with alkalosis and hypothermia, increases the affinity of hemoglobin for oxygen and decreases tissue oxygen delivery. A shift to the right occurs with acidosis and improves tissue oxygen delivery.

tissues depends on a number of factors that can affect this relationship. A shift to the left, as noted with hypothermia and alkalosis, indicates more avid binding of oxygen and less release to the tissues, whereas a shift to the right, noted with acidosis, improves tissue oxygen delivery. Blood transfusions have very low levels of 2,3-DPG, which will also result in a leftward shift of the curve, resulting in less tissue oxygen delivery.

2. Note that a PaO_2 of 65 torr corresponds to an O_2 saturation of 90%, but this lies at the shoulder of the sigmoid curve. Below this level, a small decrease in PaO_2 causes a precipitous fall in O_2 saturation. Therefore, although a PaO_2 of 60–70 torr is certainly acceptable, there is little margin of safety in the event of a sudden change in hematocrit (HCT), cardiac output, or ventilator function.

3. The correlation of PaO_2 and oxygen saturation dissociates when methemoglobinemia is present. This occurs when more than 1% of available Hb is in an oxidized form (methemoglobin) and unable to bind oxygen. It has been noted in patients receiving high-dose intravenous nitroglycerin (IV NTG) (over 10 µg/kg/min for several days), especially when hepatic or renal dysfunction is present.[71] When methemoglobinemia is present, the PaO_2 may be high, but the O_2 saturation measured by oximetry is lower than expected because the O_2 saturation of metHb is only 85%. Because some of the hemoglobin is not carrying oxygen, ischemia may be exacerbated by a reduced oxygen-carrying capacity despite the high PaO_2. It should be remembered that the O_2 saturation reported back from the blood gas laboratory is usually calculated from a nomogram based on the PaO_2, pH, and temperature – it is not measured directly.

4. Pulse oximetry is beneficial in measuring O_2 saturations continuously when the PaO_2 is low, but, because it measures several forms of hemoglobin, it will overestimate the oxyhemoglobin content when methemoglobinemia is present.

5. The amount of oxygen available to tissues depends not only on the SaO_2, pH, and the blood Hb content, but also on the cardiac output. An attempt to improve oxygen saturation at the expense of a decrease in cardiac output is counterproductive. This may be noted when increasing levels of PEEP are applied in the hypovolemic patient.

C. The PaO_2 is generally used to assess the adequacy of oxygenation, but its relationship to the FiO_2 should be examined. The PaO_2/FiO_2 ratio is a reliable predictor of pulmonary dysfunction and can also be used to assess whether weaning is feasible. The calculation of the alveolar–arterial oxygen difference $(D(A-a)O_2)$ also takes the FiO_2 into consideration and is a very sensitive index of the efficiency of gas exchange. This is calculated according to the following equation:

$$D(A-a)O_2 = (FiO_2)(713) - PaO_2 - PCO_2/0.8$$

D. In patients with normal pulmonary function, the PaO_2 should usually be greater than 350 torr on 100% oxygen immediately after surgery. The FiO_2 should then be decreased to 0.40 as tolerated to prevent adsorption atelectasis and oxygen toxicity. However, it should not be lowered any further, even if the PaO_2 seems high, in order to maintain a safety margin for oxygenation in the event that hypotension, dysrhythmias, bleeding, or a pneumothorax should suddenly develop.

E. The definitions of ARDS and TRALI include poor oxygenation with a PaO_2/FiO_2 ratio less than 200 and 300, respectively.[39] However, such ratios are not that uncommon following open-heart surgery, especially in patients with significant COPD or in hypertensive smokers with low preoperative PaO_2 levels.[72] Impaired oxygenation may be both cardiogenic and noncardiogenic in etiology, caused by fluid overload and/or a transient capillary leak from CPB. Acute pulmonary dysfunction is of concern when the PaO_2/FiO_2 ratio is <150. This would correspond, for example, to a PaO_2 of 150 torr on an FiO_2 of 1.0 or 75 torr on an FiO_2 of 0.5. This is more likely to occur in patients with advanced age, obesity, pulmonary hypertension, low cardiac output syndromes, surgery requiring very long pump runs, and postoperative renal dysfunction.[72,73]

F. Some patients with chronic pulmonary disease have a relatively "fixed shunt" with a PaO_2 of 60–70 torr despite a high FiO_2 and moderate levels of PEEP. It is best to avoid an FiO_2 greater than 0.5 for more than a few days, if possible, to avoid complications associated with oxygen toxicity. Keep in mind that a PaO_2 of 65 torr corresponds to an O_2 saturation of 90% and is acceptable in these patients.

V. Basic Concepts of Alveolar Ventilation

A. The second goal of mechanical ventilation is that of alveolar ventilation, which regulates the level of PCO_2. This is controlled by setting the tidal volume and the respiratory rate on the ventilator and should provide a minute ventilation of approximately 8 L/min. The level of PCO_2 is determined most reliably from ABGs. Noninvasive monitoring with end-tidal CO_2 gives a reasonably accurate assessment of PCO_2, although the correlation depends on the amount of physiologic dead space.

B. **Hypocarbia**

1. Mild hypocarbia (PCO_2 of 30–35 torr) is quite acceptable in the immediate postoperative period, especially when the patient is hypothermic. It produces a mild respiratory alkalosis that:

   a. Decreases the patient's respiratory drive

   b. Allows for increased CO_2 production to occur from the increased metabolic rate associated with warming and shivering without producing respiratory acidosis. Remember that the metabolic rate is decreased 10% for every degree below 37 °C, and most patients return to the ICU from the OR with a core temperature of around 35–36 °C.

   c. Compensates for the mild metabolic acidosis that frequently develops from hypoperfusion and peripheral vasoconstriction when the patient is still hypothermic.

2. A more profound respiratory alkalosis has potential detrimental effects and must be avoided.

   a. It leads to hypokalemia and may predispose to ventricular arrhythmias.

   b. It shifts the oxygen–hemoglobin dissociation curve to the left, decreasing oxygen release to the tissues.

   c. It induces cerebral vasoconstriction, reducing cerebral blood flow.

   d. **Note:** hypocarbia with a normal or somewhat acidotic pH, sometimes resulting from tachypnea of unclear etiology, may be masking a metabolic acidosis that may need to be evaluated and addressed.

3. **Management** of hypocarbia is best accomplished by lowering the IMV rate. The amount of dead space in the tubing can also be increased. Adding 10% of the tidal volume in mL/kg to the tubing will raise the PCO_2 approximately 5 torr.

    a. Although the addition of PEEP to the ventilator circuit usually prevents alveolar collapse by maintaining volume in the lungs above the critical closing volume, alveolar hypoventilation and atelectasis are best prevented by maintaining an adequate tidal volume, which at the minimum should be 6 mL/kg. The tidal volume should usually not be lowered any further unless the peak inspiratory pressures are excessively high (over 35–40 cm H_2O).

    b. Occasionally, hypocarbia may develop in a patient who is "fighting the ventilator" with repeated triggering. These patients seem to be unable to breathe in synchrony with delivered breaths, such that the phases of respiration vary between the patient and the ventilator. This may be noted in patients with hypoxia, mental confusion, delirium, anxiety, or inadequate sedation. Some patients also become very agitated when spontaneous breaths are initiated against high levels of PEEP. Patient–ventilator dyssynchrony usually occurs in the assist mode when the patient's breath does not trigger the demand valve due to too insensitive a trigger. It may also occur when the tidal volume is set too high with a low inspiratory flow rate, resulting in an increase in the inspiratory time. Thus the patient becomes short of breath and has an increased work of breathing.

       i. It is important to assess the adequacy of ventilation and oxygenation first and ensure that there are no major pleuropulmonary issues (mucus plugs, bronchospasm, tension pneumothorax) or mechanical issues with the ventilator.

       ii. The ventilator settings can be readjusted to increase the inspiratory flow rate or increase the time between the end of inspiration and the beginning of expiration with an end-inspiratory pause.

       iii. If no specific issues can be identified, additional sedation or selection of a different medication (propofol, fentanyl, or dexmedetomidine) and/or paralysis may be necessary to minimize the patient's respiratory drive.

       iv. Full ventilation is then resumed in the controlled mandatory ventilation (CMV) mode. PEEP levels should be decreased to 5 cm H_2O or less if PaO_2 permits.

       v. Pressure support ventilation (PSV) (see page 496) increases the comfort of the spontaneously breathing patient and may reduce the work of breathing.

C. Hypercarbia

1. Hypercarbia indicates that the minute ventilation provided by the ventilator is inadequate to meet ventilatory demands. Adjustment of ventilator settings must accommodate the progressive increase in PCO_2 that occurs during the early postoperative period as the metabolic rate increases from warming and postanesthetic shivering. During the weaning process, a slightly elevated PCO_2 in the range of 48–50 torr is usually acceptable, since the patient is still somewhat sedated. Higher levels of PCO_2 usually mean that the patient is not awake enough to maintain adequate ventilation.

2. A lower tidal volume may be requested by the surgeon to minimize tension on a short ITA pedicle. In these patients, it is preferable to increase the IMV rate rather than the tidal volume to compensate for an elevated PCO_2.

3. During weaning from mechanical ventilation, hypercarbia may represent compensatory hypoventilation in response to a metabolic alkalosis. This frequently results from aggressive diuresis in the early postoperative period. Use of acetazolamide (Diamox) 250–500 mg IV q8–12h in conjunction with other diuretics is beneficial in correcting a primary metabolic alkalosis. However, the metabolic component should only be partially corrected in patients with chronic CO_2 retention.

4. **Manifestations** of significant hypercarbia and respiratory acidosis include tachycardia, increasing PA pressures, hypertension, and arrhythmias.

5. **Treatment**

   a. Moderate hypercarbia in the fully ventilated patient is corrected by increasing either the respiratory rate or the tidal volume, as long as the peak inspiratory pressure is less than 30 cm H_2O.

   b. Significant hypercarbia usually indicates a mechanical problem, such as ventilator malfunction, endotracheal tube malposition, or a pneumothorax. The latter may still be present even when bilateral breath sounds seem to be heard above all the other extraneous noises of the ICU setting. Temporary hand-bag ventilation, adjustment of ventilator settings, repositioning of the endotracheal tube, or insertion of a chest tube will usually resolve the problem.

   c. Sedation can be obtained with short-acting narcotics or other sedatives. These include:

      i. Propofol 25–75 µg/kg/min

      ii. Morphine sulfate 2.5–5 mg IV q1–2 h

      iii. Dexmedetomidine 1 µg/kg over 10 minutes followed by a continuous infusion of 0.2–1.5 µg/kg/h. The loading dose provides sedation within 10–15 minutes after the infusion is started. The mix is 2 mL/50 mL normal saline, which gives a final concentration of 4 µg/mL.

      iv. Fentanyl drip can be used when a more prolonged period of sedation is indicated. The usual dose is a 50–100 µg IV bolus over five minutes with subsequent doses every two hours prn or an infusion of 50–200 µg/h of a 2.5 mg/250 mL mix.

      v. Midazolam 2–4 mg IV q1h or 2–10 mg/h as a continuous infusion is often given along with fentanyl. This can reduce the total narcotic requirement but will delay extubation.

   d. Shivering is best controlled using meperidine 25–50 mg IV or dexmedetomidine.[74] More persistent and refractory shivering that is deleterious to hemodynamics may need to be controlled with pharmacologic paralysis. **It is important never to paralyze an awake patient without also administering sedation.** Paralytic agents, including vecuronium or atracurium, can be used if these medications fail to control shivering (see Appendix 12 for doses).

6. If the patient becomes hypercarbic because of "fighting the ventilator" and is receiving inadequate tidal volumes, the steps noted in section B.3.b (change in ventilator settings, sedation, and conversion to PSV) will allow for improved ventilation.

7. The persistence of hypercarbia during the weaning process requires further investigation. In the absence of preexisting pulmonary dysfunction, concerns such as a neurologic event or phrenic nerve injury should be entertained. Issues related to the management of acute and chronic respiratory insufficiency are presented later in this chapter.

VI. Considerations to Achieve Early Extubation

A. Some centers have standard protocols to extubate patients in the OR and have shown this to be safe with a low incidence of reintubation and a reduction in ICU and postoperative length of stay and costs.[4-7,75,76] Anesthetic protocols often use lower doses of fentanyl or remifentanil combined with propofol and thoracic epidural analgesia for pain control. Identification of favorable factors for early extubation is useful in deciding which patient will benefit from this approach. A predictive risk score was devised which combined factors which independently were found to be associated with successful extubation in the OR. These included younger age, lower BMI, higher albumin, absence of COPD or diabetes, a less invasive approach, isolated CABG (especially OPCAB), elective surgery, and use of lower doses of fentanyl.[6] Predictive factors in other studies included good LV function, shorter pump times, and OPCABs.[76]

B. A more common approach is to transfer the patient to the ICU sedated with propofol or dexmedetomidine with some residual narcotic effect. This provides a brief period for monitoring and observation while the patient warms to normothermia, achieves hemodynamic stability, and has the degree of mediastinal bleeding assessed. Then, either "ultrafast extubation" within 1–3 hours or "early extubation" within 4–6 hours can be achieved. Compared to maintaining a patient on the ventilator for longer periods of time, these approaches decrease pulmonary complications, require less medication, and allow for more rapid mobilization and a faster recovery. Virtually all studies have demonstrated the safety and efficacy of "early extubation" with documentation of decreased length of stay and hospital costs, with probably little difference between the two protocols. Having a multidisciplinary, protocol-driven approach in the ICU is effective in expediting extubation.[2,3]

C. The important concept is that **extubation**, no matter when it is accomplished, **requires that standard criteria be met**. It should never represent "premature" extubation, when discontinuation of mechanical ventilation may prove deleterious to the patient's recovery. Following appropriate protocols, overnight extubation appears to be safe with a very low risk of reintubation.[77,78]

D. The potential disadvantages of very early extubation must always be taken into consideration. These include:

1. Increased sympathetic tone causing tachycardia and hypertension that can adversely affect myocardial recovery and can contribute to myocardial ischemia during the first 4–6 hours in the ICU.

2. Failure to differentiate between comfortable breathing and persistent residual narcotic/sedative effect that may be worsened by additional use of narcotics.

3. Increased risk of bleeding if hypertension develops.

4. More chest pain and splinting if inadequate analgesia is given. This may result in hypoventilation and atelectasis, potentially contributing to oxygen desaturation and the need for reintubation. Ineffective lung expansion is less capable of tamponading chest wall bleeding than positive-pressure ventilation (PPV).

Thus, provision of adequate analgesia without respiratory depression is a critical aspect of an early extubation protocol.

   5. Compromise of ventilatory status if there is significant fluid overload.

E. The selection of patients for early extubation should not be overly restrictive, yet it does depend on an understanding of potential risk factors for pulmonary dysfunction and delayed extubation. Some of these factors can be modified or influenced by therapeutic measures, whereas others cannot. The Society of Thoracic Surgeons (STS) risk model for operative mortality also provides a risk calculator for numerous complications, including prolonged ventilation beyond 48 hours. This can be accessed at the STS website (www.sts.org). One study, in fact, showed that the STS mortality risk had the highest correlation with the need for prolonged ventilation.[23] In addition, several studies have identified risk factors for acute pulmonary dysfunction upon arrival in the ICU and for increased respiratory morbidity and prolonged ventilation (Figure 10.2).[19-26,79-81] All of these factors must be taken into consideration when deciding whether early extubation is feasible or whether more prolonged support will be in the patient's best interest. Generally, about 5–10% of patients require ventilation for over 48 hours.[24,25] Evaluating these risk factors, one can define some exclusion criteria for early extubation (Table 10.2). Factors that delay extubation include:

   1. **Preoperative factors:** older patient age, females, low and high body surface areas, preexisting impairment of cardiac (NYHA class IV/HF, poor LV function, shock),

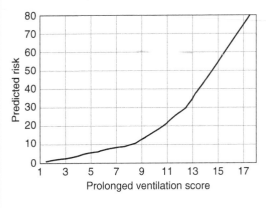

Risk Factor	Score
Age 66–75	2
Age 76–80	5
Age > 80	5.5
$FEV_1 < 70\%$	1.5
Current smoker	1.5
Scr > 125–175 µmol/L (1.4–2 mg/dL)	2
Scr > 175 µmol/L (> 2 mg/dL)	4
PVD	2
EF < 30%	2
MI < 90 days	2
Preop ventilation	4
Reoperation	2.5
Urgent surgery	1.5
Emergent surgery	2
MV surgery	2
Aortic surgery	5.5
CPB	1.5

Figure 10.2 • Logistic model to predict risk of postoperative respiratory failure following cardiac surgery. A score >18 had a greater than 80% risk of requiring prolonged ventilation >48 hours. (Reproduced with permission from Reddy et al. *Ann Thorac Surg* 2007;84:528–36.)[25]

Table 10.2 • Relative Exclusion Criteria for Early Extubation

Preoperative Criteria	Intraoperative Criteria	Postoperative Criteria
Pulmonary edema	Deep hypothermic circulatory arrest	Mediastinal bleeding
Intubated	Coagulopathy	Hemodynamic instability or need for an IABP
Cardiogenic shock	Severe myocardial dysfunction	Respiratory failure or hypoxia
Sepsis	Long pump run >4–6 hours	Stroke

respiratory (smoking, severe COPD, preoperative intubation and ventilation), and renal (elevated creatinine) subsystems, diabetes,[82] urgent or emergent surgery with hemodynamic instability, and active endocarditis.

2. **Intraoperative factors:** reoperations, long duration of CPB (often for combined valve-CABGs or double valve operations), requirement for multiple blood products, significant fluid administration, elevated blood glucose on CPB, poor hemodynamic performance requiring inotropes or IABP support, and perioperative MI.

3. **Postoperative factors:** hypothermia upon arrival in the ICU,[83] excessive mediastinal bleeding, re-exploration for bleeding or use of multiple blood products, low cardiac output syndromes, sepsis, pneumonia, renal dysfunction, stroke, or depressed level of consciousness, and GI bleeding.

F. The pharmacologic protocol for postoperative sedation should be similar for most patients, since propofol or dexmedetomidine can be used for several days if prolonged support is necessary. However, use of a longer-acting medication (such as fentanyl) can be considered. Lorazepam has been used successfully as well, but it is associated with a higher incidence of delirium and is not recommended.[84] Use of standard protocols and criteria for weaning should allow for extubation when clinically indicated, even if it takes a little longer than desired. The duration of intubation should not be based on risk factors alone or dictated by a rigid time schedule. Of interest, although smoking is a significant risk factor for postoperative morbidity, one study showed that it is advantageous to extubate smokers earlier rather than later to reduce the risk of respiratory complications.[85]

VII. Therapeutic Interventions to Optimize Postoperative Respiratory Performance and Early Extubation

A. Recognition of risk factors for pulmonary dysfunction can direct attention to potential therapeutic steps that can be taken to optimize postoperative respiratory performance. The treatment of modifiable factors, performance of a proficient operation, and aggressive postoperative management of all subsystems are essential to achieve early extubation and minimize the risk of postoperative respiratory failure.

B. Preoperative considerations

1. Pulmonary function testing (PFTs) with room air ABGs should be considered in patients with respiratory symptoms that cannot be attributed to their cardiac disease. Although the patient's clinical limitations (climbing stairs, walking short distances) often supersede abnormal PFTs in determining operability, markedly abnormal PFTs can provide an indication of the patient's risk for pulmonary complications and mortality. Patients with a PO_2 <60 torr or PCO_2 >50 torr on room air, and those who are oxygen-dependent or on chronic steroids for advanced lung disease, should be considered at very high risk for respiratory complications. Alternative procedures, such as coronary stenting or transcatheter approaches for valve pathology, should be considered.

2. Attempt to convince the patient to stop cigarette smoking at least one month prior to surgery. Recommend use of nicotine patches or start the patient on varenicline (Chantix) or bupropion HCL (Wellbutrin, Zyban).

3. Treat all active cardiopulmonary disease processes, such as pneumonia, bronchospasm, or CHF, to optimize oxygenation and ventilatory status.

4. Consider intensive inspiratory muscle training in patients at high risk for pulmonary complications.[86]

5. Transfuse profoundly anemic patients to a HCT of at least 28% prior to surgery to minimize the degree of hemodilution during surgery and the requirement for blood and blood components.

6. Optimize hemodynamic performance and renal function as best as possible prior to surgery.

C. Intraoperative considerations

1. Modify the CPB circuit to minimize the inflammatory response, hemodilution, and bleeding: use membrane oxygenators, centrifugal pumps, biocompatible circuits, or miniaturized circuits, if available; avoid cardiotomy suction; consider retrograde autologous priming and perhaps use of leukocyte-depleting filters. Use of steroids to potentially minimize the inflammatory response has not been shown to improve outcomes and cannot be recommended.[39,87,88]

2. Process shed mediastinal blood at the conclusion of CPB through a cell saving device to eliminate fat, particulate matter, and vasoactive mediators. This has been shown to improve cardiopulmonary hemodynamics and may reduce ventilatory requirements after surgery.[89]

3. Minimize fluid administration during CPB or off-pump surgery.

4. Perform an expeditious, technically proficient operation with excellent myocardial protection to achieve complete revascularization or satisfactory valve function.

5. Use inotropic and/or vasopressor support or an IABP as necessary to achieve satisfactory hemodynamic performance (cardiac index >2 L/min/m²) and avoid excessively high filling pressures. Avoidance of hypotension and low cardiac output syndromes may also reduce the risk of acute kidney injury, allowing for more effective diuresis after surgery. Pharmacologic intervention shown to reduce this risk is limited, with only fenoldopam showing some promise.[90]

6. Use antifibrinolytic therapy to minimize perioperative bleeding.

7. Pay fastidious attention to hemostasis.

8. Minimize use of blood and blood components.[91]

9. Maintain blood glucose <180 mg/dL on CPB with IV insulin.

10. Consider ventilating the lungs during bypass (shown to improve post-pump oxygenation).[40]

11. Consider hemofiltration to remove fluid in patients with preoperative CHF or renal dysfunction and to remove inflammatory mediators[92]

12. Use short-acting narcotics, inhalational anesthetics, and propofol or dexmedetomidine for sedation to allow for early extubation.

D. **Postoperative considerations**

1. Select medications to provide short-acting anxiolysis and sedation that either allow the patient to awaken and be extubated within hours of its discontinuation (propofol) or while still being given (dexmedetomidine).

2. Provide adequate analgesia without producing respiratory depression (continuous low-dose IV morphine, ketorolac, IV acetaminophen, epidural analgesia, ON-Q bupivacaine).

3. Use antihypertensive medications (clevidipine, nitroprusside), rather than sedatives, to control hypertension.

4. Administer volume judiciously to optimize hemodynamics, and then use diuresis once hemodynamics have stabilized to eliminate extravascular lung water.

5. Have a restrictive threshold for blood transfusions (HCT in the low 20s) except for patients with hemodynamic compromise (hypotension, tachycardia), oxygenation issues, or end-organ dysfunction (usually renal) in whom a higher HCT may be beneficial. Although it may seem logical to transfuse profoundly anemic patients in these situations, blood transfusions are initially not that effective in improving oxygen-carrying capacity and carry multiple potential risks which can worsen pulmonary function.[91]

6. Initiate aggressive management of postoperative bleeding, yet have a low threshold for re-exploration to minimize use of blood products, which can increase pulmonary morbidity, including the risk of TRALI.[42,43,93,94] Avoid transfusing blood products to correct abnormal coagulation parameters when bleeding is insignificant.

VIII. Ventilatory Weaning and Extubation in the Immediate Postoperative Period

A. **Criteria for weaning.** Weaning a patient from the ventilator depends on the ability and desire of the nursing and medical staffs to identify when the patient is ready to be weaned, and their willingness to initiate weaning when indicated, no matter what time of the day or night, not when it is convenient to do so. The criteria for weaning are noted in Table 10.3.

B. **Method of weaning after short-term ventilation**

1. Minimize sedation or use dexmedetomidine.

2. Maintain the FiO_2 at 0.5 or below with PEEP of no more than 5–7.5 cm H_2O. If the patient still requires a higher level of PEEP, weaning is usually not indicated. If oxygenation is satisfactory, lower the PEEP in 2.5–5 cm H_2O increments to 5 cm H_2O and initiate weaning.

3. If the patient is alert with good respiratory efforts and meets the criteria listed in Table 10.3, they may be immediately placed on CPAP of 5 cm H_2O for a SBT.

Table 10.3 • Weaning Criteria from Mechanical Ventilation

Initial Postoperative Period
1. Awake with stimulation
2. Adequate reversal of neuromuscular blockade
3. Chest tube drainage <50 mL/h
4. Core temperature >35.5 °C
5. Hemodynamic stability
   a. Cardiac index >2.2 L/min/m²
   b. BP stable at 100–140 systolic on/off meds
   c. Heart rate <120 bpm
   d. No arrhythmias
6. Satisfactory ABGs on full ventilation
   a. PaO_2/FiO_2 >150 (PO_2 >75 torr on FiO_2 of 0.5)
   b. PCO_2 <50 torr
   c. pH 7.30–7.50

Prolonged Ventilation
1. Underlying disease process has resolved
2. Awake, oriented with adequate mental alertness to initiate an inspiratory effort and maintain an airway
3. Hemodynamic stability on no vasoactive drugs
4. Hemoglobin and metabolic status are optimized
5. Satisfactory ABGs as above (many studies recommend PaO_2/FiO_2 >200) with respiratory rate <35/min
6. Rapid shallow breathing index (respiratory rate/tidal volume in liters) <100

Table 10.4 • Failure Criteria During Weaning from the Ventilator

1. Somnolence, agitation, or diaphoresis
2. Systolic BP increases by more than 20 mm Hg or to over 160 mm Hg
3. Heart rate changes by more than 20% in either direction or to over 120 bpm
4. Acute need for vasoactive medication
5. Arrhythmias develop or become more frequent
6. Respiratory rate increases more than 10 breaths/min or to over 35/min for five minutes
7. PaO_2 falls to less than 60 torr on FiO_2 of 0.5 or SaO_2 falls to less than 90%
8. PCO_2 rises above 50 torr with respiratory acidosis (pH <7.30)

Gradual reduction in the IMV rate to "wean" the patient off the ventilator is usually not necessary in the early postoperative period. If the ABGs are acceptable after a 30–60 minute SBT on either T-piece or CPAP of 5 cm H_2O (see extubation criteria below), the endotracheal tube is removed. Obtaining respiratory mechanics may be helpful, but usually is not necessary in the "routine" patient.

4. Weaning should be stopped and ventilation resumed at a higher rate when there are clinical signs that it is not being tolerated. These signs are noted in Table 10.4.

5. **Note:** a rise in PA pressures is often the first hemodynamic abnormality noted in the patient who is not tolerating weaning very well. Tachypnea is the first clinical sign of ineffective weaning.

Table 10.5 • Extubation Criteria

Initial Postoperative Period
1. Awake without stimulation
2. Acceptable respiratory mechanics
   a. Negative inspiratory force >25 cm H_2O
   b. Tidal volume >5 mL/kg
   c. Vital capacity >10–15 mL/kg
   d. Spontaneous respiratory rate <24/min
3. Acceptable ABGs on 5 cm or less of CPAP or PSV
   a. PaO_2 >70 torr on FiO_2 of 0.5 or less
   b. PCO_2 <48 torr
   c. pH 7.32–7.45

Prolonged Ventilation
1. Comfortable breathing pattern without diaphoresis, agitation, or anxiety; respiratory rate <35/min
2. Adequate mental status to protect the airway, initiate a cough, and raise secretions
3. Hemodynamic tolerance of the weaning process as delineated in Table 10.3
4. Respiratory mechanics and ABGs as above
5. A cuff leak >110 mL with the cuff deflated

C. Extubation criteria include the weaning criteria listed in Table 10.3 as well as the additional considerations noted in Table 10.5.

D. Extubation may be accomplished from CPAP or T-piece. Although oxygenation may be slightly better during a CPAP than a T-piece trial, postextubation oxygenation is frequently better in patients weaned with T-piece, because the PaO_2 declines less than in patients who were extubated from CPAP.[95]

E. Additional considerations

   1. Some patients get very agitated when sedatives are weaned. Even though adequate ABGs may be maintained, agitated patients are frequently given more sedation throughout the night with another attempt at weaning in the morning. Steps noted on page 468 may be taken if the patient is breathing dyssynchronously with the ventilator. Gradual weaning of sedation, substituting dexmedetomidine for propofol, assurance from the nurses that "you're doing well", and then a very rapid wean to CPAP and extubation is often the best course for these patients.

   2. If the patient was very difficult to intubate in the OR, it is essential to ensure that the ABGs and respiratory mechanics are satisfactory before extubation. Extubation in the middle of the night should be performed cautiously in these patients. An individual experienced in difficult intubations should be present. A flexible laryngoscope, video laryngoscope (GlideScope [Verathon]), or bronchoscope should also be available.

   3. Elderly patients and those with more advanced cardiac disease or hepatic dysfunction often take longer to awaken from anesthesia, even if sedatives are not administered. This may reflect slow metabolism of medications administered intraoperatively or may occasionally represent transient obtundation from borderline cerebral hypoperfusion during surgery or other causes. It is important to

resist the temptation to reverse narcotic effect with naloxone. This medication can precipitate severe pain, anxiety, hypertension, dysrhythmias, and bleeding, and may result in recurrent respiratory depression when its effects have worn off. Similarly, flumazenil to reverse benzodiazepines should be avoided early in the postoperative period. Keep in mind that the offset of propofol is significantly greater when doses producing deep sedation are used.[54]

4. However, if a patient fails to awaken after 24–36 hours and the question arises as to whether this represents a stroke, encephalopathy, or simply residual sedation, one might consider the cautious use of a reversal agent to sort out the nature of the problem. Naloxone (Narcan) may be given by administering 1–2 mL/min of a mix of a 1 mL vial containing 0.4 mg/mL in 9 mL of NS (0.04–0.08 mg/min) to a total dose of 0.4 mg. Flumazenil is given in a dose of 0.2 mg IV over 30 seconds, followed by additional doses of 0.2 mg to a maximum of 1 mg. To address resedation, additional doses may be given up to a maximum of 3 mg in one hour.

5. Many patients, especially those who have received supplemental narcotics, will demonstrate excellent respiratory mechanics when stimulated, but then drift off to sleep and become apneic. Constricted pupils may be noted in patients with persistent narcotic effect. These patients are not yet ready for weaning and extubation. Do not confuse comfortable breathing with a persistent narcotic or sedative effect. These tend to be the patients who require reintubation.

IX. Postextubation Respiratory Care (Table 10.6)

A. After extubation, the patient's breathing pattern, SaO_2, and hemodynamics must be observed carefully. Occasionally, especially in the patient who was difficult to intubate, laryngeal stridor may be prominent and may require use of racemic epinephrine, steroids, or even reintubation. Failure to demonstrate a "cuff leak" during PPV when the cuff is deflated usually indicates laryngotracheal edema, which may cause upper airway obstruction after extubation. This phenomenon is uncommon after short-term intubation, but it may be noted after several days of mechanical ventilation, especially if the patient is fluid overloaded (see page 498).

Table 10.6 • Postextubation Respiratory Care

1. Monitor pulse oximetry
2. Place on facemask or nasal cannula to achieve SaO_2 >90%
3. Consider high-flow nasal cannula (Oxymizer®) or a BPAP mask for patients with borderline hypoxemia or hypercarbia
4. Administer adequate analgesia while minimizing sedation (ketorolac, low-dose narcotics, IV acetaminophen)
5. Chest x-ray after pleural tubes are removed
6. Incentive spirometer/deep breaths q1–2h; use cough pillow
7. Mobilize as soon as possible; frequent repositioning in bed
8. Compression stockings (T.E.D.) for VTE prophylaxis; consider Venodyne boots or SC heparin if high-risk
9. Aggressive diuresis once hemodynamically stable
10. Bronchodilators for bronchospasm (consider steroids if severe COPD)
11. Antibiotics for a positive sputum culture

B. Because the median sternotomy incision is associated with moderate discomfort and decreased chest wall compliance, patients tend to splint, take shallow breaths, and cough poorly. Oxygenation may be compromised by fluid overload and atelectasis from poor inspiratory effort. It is advisable to supply 40–70% humidified oxygen by facemask for a few days.

C. If the patient has borderline oxygenation, higher levels of oxygen or some form of noninvasive ventilation (NIV) may be utilized to improve oxygenation and avoid reintubation.[96,97]

1. Use of a high-flow oxygen system is preferable in the patient with moderate hypoxemia or hypercarbia.[98,99] It produces more comfortable breathing, reduces the respiratory rate, and improves gas exchange. The oxygen is heated and humidified and supplied at up to 60 L/min and the FiO_2 is kept at a constant level. The system decreases anatomic dead space, improves alveolar ventilation, decreases the work of breathing, minimizes atelectasis, improves mucociliary clearance, and reduces airway resistance. Because there is some resistance to expiratory flow, there is an increase in airway pressure, producing some degree of PEEP with an increase in end-expiratory lung volume.

2. A nonrebreather mask covers the patient's nose and mouth and is attached to a reservoir bag, which is continuously filled with oxygen at a rate of 8–15 L/min. The patient inhales oxygen from the reservoir bag and then exhales through a one-way valve to the atmosphere, thus ensuring that little exhaled gas or room air is inspired during the next breath. Partial rebreather masks lack the one-way valve, but ensure a higher FiO_2 than a simple facemask because of a tighter fit and the oxygen reservoir bag.

3. Bilevel positive airway pressure (BPAP) is a form of NIV during which the patient breathes spontaneously and each breath is supported by positive pressure. BPAP provides preset inspiratory and expiratory positive airway pressure at two different levels, with the inspiratory pressure usually set at 8–12 cm H_2O and expiratory pressure set at 3–5 cm H_2O. The pressure difference determines the tidal volume delivered. It is superior to incentive spirometry in improving oxygenation in the first few postoperative days.[100] It has also been shown to prevent the increase in extravascular lung water associated with the weaning process that is noted in patients placed on nasal cannula after extubation.[101] Although often abbreviated as BiPAP, that is actually the name of a ventilator manufactured by Respironics. Inc.

4. Continuous positive airway pressure (CPAP) provides a continuous level of positive airway pressure without any ventilatory support. Nasal CPAP masks are helpful in patients with cardiogenic pulmonary edema by preventing alveolar collapse, redistributing intra-alveolar fluid, improving pulmonary compliance, and reducing the pressure of breathing.[102] A study of prophylactic nasal CPAP of 10 cm H_2O for at least six hours showed that it improved oxygenation better than CPAP for 10 minutes every four hours, with a lower incidence of pneumonia and reintubation.[103] However, another study found noninvasive pressure support ventilation (NIPSV) superior to CPAP in preventing atelectasis after surgery.[104]

5. Another useful mode of NIV is airway pressure release ventilation, which cycles between high and low CPAPs. This may decrease peak airway pressures, improve alveolar recruitment and oxygenation, and increase the ventilation of dependent lung zones. Demonstration of the clinical benefits of this modality are not uniform.[105]

D. Upon transfer to the floor, most patients benefit from the use of supplemental oxygen via nasal cannula for a few days. Monitoring of SaO_2 by pulse oximetry is helpful in patients with borderline oxygenation, especially during ambulation. The patient should be mobilized and encouraged to cough and take deep breaths. A cooperative patient who can actively participate in these maneuvers can generally prevent atelectasis and pulmonary complications, but additional support is commonly necessary in elderly patients and those with significant chest wall discomfort. A "cough pillow" should be used to brace the chest during deep breathing and coughing to minimize discomfort and splinting.

1. An incentive spirometer is very beneficial in maintaining the FRC and preventing atelectasis, although its effectiveness in preventing postoperative pulmonary complications is unclear.[106] A literature review showed that CPAP, BPAP, or intermittent positive-pressure breathing (IPPB) produced better pulmonary function and oxygenation than incentive spirometry, although the incidence of complications was comparable. However, none of these was more effective than preoperative patient education.[107] One study showed that the same benefit could be derived from taking 30 deep breaths without mechanical assistance as from use of a blow bottle device or inspiratory resistance positive expiratory pressure mask.[108]

2. Chest physical therapy may be helpful in patients with significant underlying lung disease, borderline pulmonary function, or copious secretions, but otherwise is of little additional benefit.[109] Albuterol administered via nebulizer is frequently beneficial in patients with bronchospasm.

E. Although dysphagia with difficulty swallowing foods is unusual in patients intubated for less than 24 hours, it is not uncommon following a longer duration of intubation. Careful attention must be paid to the patient's initial oral intake to observe for potential aspiration. Patients who require longer periods of intubation usually require a full swallowing evaluation before initiating oral intake (see pages 804–805). The risk of dysphagia is greater in patients intubated >24 hours, with a twofold increase for every 12 hours of intubation, and it is also related to the duration of sedative use, prolonged nasogastric tube drainage, use of TEE during surgery, and a history of a remote stroke or perioperative stroke.[110,111]

F. Once the patient is hemodynamically stable and no longer requires volume administration to maintain intravascular volume, aggressive diuresis with IV furosemide, either with intermittent bolus doses or a continuous infusion, should be initiated to eliminate excess extravascular lung water. Diuretics are continued until the patient has approached their preoperative weight and can be weaned from nasal cannula with an acceptable SaO_2 (>90% on room air).

G. Satisfactory analgesia is very helpful in improving the patient's respiratory effort. A few doses of ketorolac are given initially after extubation, and most patients are then given oral narcotics such as oxycodone or hydrocodone with acetaminophen. Patients with significant pain issues may benefit from PCA pumps that provide morphine, fentanyl, or remifentanil.[69,70] Alternatively, a fentanyl patch (Duragesic) can be used in patients with persistent pain despite opioid use. A common dose is 25 µg/h, which is the dose delivered by a 10 cm^2 patch. Note that the fentanyl plasma concentration is increased by amiodarone. There is a delicate balance between achieving adequate analgesia and minimizing opiate use.

H. Venous thromboembolism (VTE) is rarely detected, but not that uncommon, following cardiac surgery. A literature review found the incidence of symptomatic deep venous thrombosis (DVT), pulmonary embolism (PE), and fatal PE to be 3.2, 0.6, and 0.3%, respectively.[112] In the early postoperative period, patients may be prothrombotic, with contributory factors including elevated fibrinogen levels, thrombin generation, tissue factor activation, reduced fibrinolysis, return of normal platelet aggregation, and aspirin resistance.[113,114] Thus, it is recommended that elastic graduated compression (anti-embolism) stockings (GCS) should be used routinely for patients after surgery to reduce the risk of VTE. Mobilization is probably more important in reducing this risk, so once the patient is stable, getting them out of bed and ambulating is very important. For patients remaining in the ICU who may be sedated on mechanical ventilation and poorly mobilized, sequential or intermittent pneumatic compression (IPC) devices, such as the Venodyne system, should be used. Most patients are started on aspirin 81 mg daily after surgery, although higher doses might be necessary to reduce the risk of VTE because of early aspirin resistance. However, the ICU patient may also benefit from pharmacologic prophylaxis (see also pages 750–752).[112]

1. The literature remains contentious on whether early initiation of pharmacologic prophylaxis with either SQ heparin (5000 units SC q12h) or low-molecular-weight heparin (40 mg SC daily) should be considered in selected patients and when it should be started. If so chosen, it may be considered once mediastinal bleeding has tapered off, but the risk of developing a hemopericardium and delayed tamponade must always be taken into consideration.

2. A systematic literature review published in 2015 noted an increased risk for VTE associated with older age, obesity, heart failure, a history of VTE, prolonged bed rest, and mechanical ventilation.[112] The 2018 European guidelines also identified age >70, transfusion of more than four units of RBC concentrate/fresh frozen plasma/cryoprecipitate/fibrinogen concentrate, mechanical ventilation >24 hours, or a postoperative complication (e.g. acute kidney injury, infection/sepsis, neurological complication), as placing a patient at higher risk for VTE.[115] For these patients, early initiation of pharmacologic prophylaxis was "highly" recommended, even as soon as the first postoperative day, once bleeding becomes insignificant. However, the earlier 2012 American College of Chest Physicians guidelines concluded that the risk of bleeding exceeded that of VTE in cardiac surgery patients and therefore only recommended pharmacologic therapy for patients with prolonged hospitalization postsurgery.[116]

X. Acute Respiratory Insufficiency/Short-term Ventilatory Support

A. Prolonged mechanical ventilation beyond 48 hours is necessary in about 5–10% of patients undergoing open-heart surgery on CPB.[24,25,73] The STS database defines "prolonged ventilation" as the requirement for ventilation for over 24 hours from the time of exit from the OR. This usually results from a significant perioperative cardiopulmonary insult (such as a long duration of CPB or postcardiotomy low cardiac output syndrome) that is superimposed on preexisting lung disease. Mechanical ventilation may be required until hemodynamic issues, significant mediastinal bleeding, or transient pleuropulmonary insults, such as pulmonary edema, have resolved. It may also be indicated for patients without intrinsic pulmonary problems who are sedated, obtunded, or sustain neurologic insults. These patients may have adequate gas exchange but need an endotracheal tube for airway protection.

B. Acute respiratory insufficiency is usually characterized by inadequate oxygenation (PaO_2 <60 torr with an FiO_2 of 0.5 or PaO_2/FiO_2 ≤120) or ventilation (PCO_2 >50 torr). Predisposing factors to acute pulmonary dysfunction are fairly comparable to those that are predictive of the need for prolonged ventilatory support (see pages 471–472). One study found that the STS mortality risk score was the best predictor of the need for prolonged ventilation.[23]

1. Preoperative risk factors include a critical preoperative state (HF), advanced age, significant COPD or renal dysfunction, endocarditis, active smoking history, reoperative surgery, obesity (BMI >30 kg/m²), diabetes, a mean PA pressure ≥20 mm Hg, depressed LV function (stroke volume index ≤30 mL/m²), low serum albumin, and a history of cerebrovascular disease.[19–26,79–81,117]

2. Intraoperative factors include emergency surgery and CPB time ≥140 minutes. The latter is often associated with a significant inflammatory response, with patients usually receiving a significant amount of volume during and after surgery.

3. The development of acute respiratory insufficiency is associated with more renal dysfunction, gastrointestinal and neurologic complications, and an increased risk of nosocomial infections. The development of multisystem organ problems explains the high mortality rate of postoperative respiratory failure, which averages 20–25%.

4. Several logistic models have been created which are predictive of prolonged ventilatory failure (>72 hours).[24–26] A sophisticated bedside model is noted in Figure 10.2.[25]

C. "Acute lung injury" defined by poor oxygenation is a clinical spectrum that ranges from a transient phenomenon with low risk to that of ARDS, which carries a very high mortality rate. In most patients with a PaO_2/FiO_2 ratio <200–300 immediately after surgery, a short period of ventilatory support while the patient is stabilized hemodynamically and diuresed usually results in improvement in oxygenation and the need for very short-term ventilation. However, acute lung injury may progress to a chronic phase of ventilatory dependence in about 5% of patients. This is more likely to occur in older patients with preexisting pulmonary, cardiac, or renal problems that compromise postoperative recovery or when postoperative care is complicated by stroke, bleeding, and multiple blood transfusions.[24,25] Chronic respiratory insufficiency/ventilator dependence is discussed in section XI (pages 488–494).

D. **Etiology.** During the first 48 hours, oxygenation problems predominate and can produce tissue hypoxia. Inadequate ventilation (hypercapnia) at this time is usually the result of a mechanical problem.

1. Inadequate O_2 delivery and ventilation (mechanical problems)
   a. Ventilator malfunction
   b. Improper ventilator settings: low FiO_2, inspiratory flow rate, tidal volume, or respiratory rate
   c. Endotracheal tube problems: cuff leak, incorrect endotracheal tube placement (larynx, mainstem bronchus, esophagus), kinking or occlusion of the tube

2. Low cardiac output states leading to mixed venous desaturation, venous admixture, and hypoxemia

3. Pulmonary problems
   a. Atelectasis or lobar collapse, possibly associated with diaphragmatic paralysis from phrenic nerve injury
   b. Pulmonary edema
      i. Cardiogenic from fluid overload and/or LV dysfunction, hemodilution on pump with reduced colloid oncotic pressure
      ii. Noncardiogenic from pulmonary endothelial injury with increased microvascular permeability. This may be related to activation of complement, neutrophils, and macrophages with release of inflammatory mediators associated with extracorporeal circulation. This problem is more prominent as the duration of CPB lengthens and is more common in patients receiving multiple blood transfusions.
   c. Pneumonia
   d. Intrinsic pulmonary disease (COPD), bronchospasm, or air trapping
   e. Blood transfusions: microembolization, transfusion of proinflammatory mediators, TRALI, TACO
4. Intrapleural problems
   a. Pneumothorax
   b. Hemothorax or pleural effusion
5. Metabolic problems: shivering leading to increased peripheral oxygen extraction
6. Pharmacologic causes: drugs that inhibit hypoxic pulmonary vasoconstriction (nitroglycerin, nitroprusside, calcium channel blockers, ACE inhibitors)[118]

E. **Transfusion-related acute lung injury (TRALI)** is a problem of acute respiratory distress with hypoxemia ($PaO_2/FiO_2 <300$) and pulmonary infiltrates on chest x-ray that occurs within six hours of a blood or blood product transfusion when other risk factors for acute lung injury, such as sepsis or aspiration, are not present. It is most likely an immune-mediated phenomenon with interaction between donor plasma antibodies and recipient leukocyte antigens that causes release of cytotoxic substances that damage lung tissue and causes noncardiogenic pulmonary edema from increased microvascular permeability. It is more common in older patients and those with longer durations of CPB. This is an acute phenomenon that rarely progresses to an ARDS picture and has a more favorable prognosis, although the mortality rate is still quite high at around 15–30%. Although transfusions per se are associated with increased pulmonary morbidity and increased mortality, TRALI appears to be a distinct entity.[42,43,94,119,120]

F. TRALI is to be differentiated from **TACO (transfusion-associated circulatory overload)**, which is another cause of acute respiratory distress that occurs within 12 hours of a blood transfusion. This is not immune-mediated, but rather a phenomenon that occurs when a patient with preexisting fluid overload, often with LV dysfunction, HF, or chronic kidney disease, receives too large a volume of blood products or is transfused too rapidly. The patient may become hypertensive, tachycardic, and hypoxemic when the circulatory system is "overwhelmed" by the transfusion volume. It therefore represents a picture of cardiogenic pulmonary edema that should be preventable by administering diuretics at the time of blood transfusion or treatable with short-term ventilatory support and diuresis.[120]

G. The acute development of shortness of breath after extubation or an abrupt change in ABGs during or after extubation should raise suspicion of the following problems:
   1. Pneumothorax, possibly tension
   2. Atelectasis or lobar collapse from poor inspiratory effort or mucus plugging

3. Aspiration pneumonia
4. Acute pulmonary edema (from myocardial ischemia, LV dysfunction, new ventricular septal defect, worsening mitral regurgitation, or undetected renal insufficiency)
5. Delayed tamponade causing a low cardiac output syndrome
6. Compensation for an evolving metabolic acidosis
7. Pulmonary embolism

H. **Manifestations**

1. Tachypnea (rate >30 breaths/min) with shallow breaths
2. Paradoxical inward movement of the abdomen during inspiration ("abdominal paradox")
3. Agitation, diaphoresis, obtundation, or mental status changes
4. Tachycardia or bradycardia
5. Arrhythmias
6. Hypertension or hypotension

I. **Assessment and management** of acute respiratory insufficiency during mechanical ventilation (Table 10.7)

1. **Examine the patient:** auscultate for bilateral breath sounds and listen over the stomach to make sure the tube has not slipped into the larynx or been placed in the esophagus.

Table 10.7 • Management of Acute Ventilatory Insufficiency

1. Examine patient, ventilator settings and function, ABGs, and chest x-ray
2. Hand ventilate with 100% oxygen; increase FiO_2 on ventilator until problem is sorted out
3. Ensure alveolar ventilation by correcting mechanical problems (adjust ventilator, reposition endotracheal tube, insert chest tube)
4. Assess and optimize hemodynamics
5. Add PEEP in 2.5–5 cm H_2O increments while decreasing FiO_2 to 0.5 or less; serially evaluate cardiac outputs at higher levels of PEEP to ensure optimal systemic oxygen delivery
6. Consider sedation or paralysis if patient–ventilator dyssynchrony is not improved by a change in ventilator settings
7. Treat identifiable problems:
   a. Diuretics for pulmonary edema
   b. Antibiotics for pneumonia
   c. Bronchodilators for bronchospasm
   d. Transfusion for low HCT (<24%)
   e. Stop amiodarone which might contribute to a hypersensitivity ARDS picture
8. Chest physiotherapy
9. Begin nutritional supplementation
10. For severe hypoxemia:
    a. Use low tidal volume ventilation
    b. Tolerate SaO_2 of 88–92% with moderate hypercapnia
    c. Neuromuscular blockade
    d. Prone positioning
    e. Inhaled nitric oxide or epoprostenol (Flolan) 10–40 ng/kg via ventilator
    f. Extracorporeal membrane oxygenation (ECMO)

2. **Increase the FiO$_2$ to 1.0** until the causative factors have been identified. **Manually ventilate** with a resuscitation bag (Ambu) if ventilator malfunction is suspected. This not only provides ventilation but also permits an assessment of pulmonary compliance. **Note:** make sure the gas line on the bag is attached to the oxygen (green) and not the room air (yellow) connector and the gas has been turned on.

3. **Ensure adequate alveolar ventilation**

   a. **Check ventilator function** and settings and optimize the following:

      i. Tidal volume

      ii. Ventilator trigger sensitivity

      iii. Inspiratory flow rate. Patients with COPD may have significant air trapping which produces an auto-PEEP effect. This is noted when inspiration commences before expiratory airflow is completed, resulting in positive airway pressure at the end of expiration. It can exacerbate the adverse hemodynamic effects of PPV, cause barotrauma, and impair patient triggering of assisted ventilation. Steps that can be taken to eliminate this problem are discussed on page 497.

      iv. Consider using PSV to minimize the risk of high airways pressures.

   b. **Obtain a chest x-ray** to look for any of the potential etiologic factors listed above; specifically note any mechanical problems that can be corrected by simple repositioning of the endotracheal tube or chest tube insertion.

   c. **Repeat the ABGs**

   d. **Note:** an acute increase in peak inspiratory pressure may signify the development of a pneumothorax, although it can also result from severe bronchospasm, flash pulmonary edema, mainstem intubation, or an obstructed airway (copious secretions, the patient biting the endotracheal tube).

4. **Assess and optimize hemodynamic status.** A Swan-Ganz PA catheter is useful in assessing the patient's fluid status and cardiac output. The latter can also be assessed less invasively using other noninvasive monitoring systems, including the FloTrac device, which uses pulse wave analysis from the arterial line to calculate continuous cardiac outputs, although it is not helpful when the patient is in atrial fibrillation. A low cardiac output reduces oxygen delivery, lowers the mixed venous oxygen saturation, and increases venous admixture, further decreasing the PaO$_2$. Inotropic support or diuresis may be indicated to improve oxygenation. An echocardiogram may be helpful in identifying a contributory problem, such as significant LV or RV dysfunction, cardiac tamponade, mitral regurgitation, or a new or recurrent ventricular septal defect.

5. **Alveolar recruitment** maneuvers that increase the mean airway pressure can open previously closed alveoli to increase the surface area for oxygen exchange and prevent early airway closure. This will decrease intrapulmonary shunting by improving ventilation to perfused areas. It will also redistribute lung water from the alveoli to the perivascular interstitial space, although it does not decrease extravascular lung water content.

   a. A baseline level of 5 cm H$_2$O of **PEEP** is usually added to the circuit for all patients admitted to the ICU. This substitutes for the loss of the "physiologic PEEP" of normal breathing caused by the endotracheal tube. This level of PEEP is well tolerated by the heart, but probably does little to improve oxygenation.

b. PEEP is added in increments of 2.5–5 cm H_2O up to 10 cm H_2O or greater to improve oxygenation and allow for weaning of the FiO_2 to less than 0.5. With low mean airway pressures, intrapulmonary shunting may result from inadequate ventilation of perfused alveoli, and increasing the FiO_2 alone will often be ineffective in improving oxygenation if the shunt exceeds 20%. This problem can be overcome by increasing the tidal volume and the level of PEEP. Furthermore, using an FiO_2 >0.5 for several days can produce alveolar-capillary damage, alveolar collapse, and stiff, noncompliant lungs (so-called oxygen toxicity).

c. Caution must be exercised when using high levels of PEEP because it will accentuate the adverse effects of PPV on hemodynamics by creating high positive airway and intrathoracic pressures. Increasing levels of PEEP reduce venous return, increase pulmonary vascular resistance which can depress RV performance, and will lead to decreased LV filling and a reduced cardiac output in the hypovolemic patient. Thus, adding PEEP could be counterproductive because it may actually reduce oxygen transport and tissue oxygenation, lower the mixed venous oxygen saturation, and increase admixture, further decreasing the PaO_2. Volume infusion is necessary to counteract these effects before increasing the level of PEEP. The optimal level of PEEP can be determined by observation of the arterial waveform and serial assessments of cardiac function while adjustments are being made.

d. Adding high levels of PEEP to patients with severe COPD results in increased transmission of airway pressure to the lungs, resulting in overdistention of alveoli that are highly compliant and poorly perfused. This may result in increased V/Q shunting, possibly producing endothelial damage, and progressive hypoxia.

e. In patients with intrinsic pulmonary disease, and especially ARDS, the pulmonary vascular resistance may be elevated and the lungs less compliant. Increasing levels of PEEP may produce RV failure and dilatation, shifting the interventricular septum and compromising filling and compliance of the LV. In these patients, volume infusion must be given cautiously.

f. High levels of PEEP can result in "barotrauma" (pneumothorax, subcutaneous emphysema, or pneumomediastinum), which can compromise ventilation and produce acute hemodynamic embarrassment. Barotrauma is caused by alveolar overdistention, and is attributable more directly to the severity of the underlying lung disease than to the peak airway pressure. Nonetheless, modes of ventilation that provide lower tidal volumes have been used in patients with ARDS to improve oxygenation and are now recommended routinely during early ventilatory support.[39,121]

g. Note: care must be exercised when suctioning a patient on high levels of PEEP. Oxygenation can become very marginal when PEEP has been temporarily discontinued. A PEEP valve should be used during manual ventilation if the patient's oxygenation is dependent on PEEP.

h. The interpretation of pressure tracings from a Swan-Ganz PA catheter is influenced by PEEP. The measured CVP, PA, and left atrial pressures are elevated, but transmural filling pressures, which determine the gradient for venous return, are decreased, because pressure is transmitted through the lungs to the pleural space. A general rule is that the true pulmonary capillary wedge pressure (PCWP) is equal to the measured pressure minus one-half of the PEEP level at end-expiration (minus one-quarter if lung compliance is decreased). Another way of assessing the PCWP is the "index of transmission":

$$\text{Index of transmission} = (\text{end-inspiratory PCWP} - \text{end-expiratory PCWP})/$$
$$(\text{plateau airway pressure} - \text{total PEEP})$$
$$\text{Transmural PCWP} = \text{end-expiratory PCWP}$$
$$- (\text{index of transmission} \times \text{total PEEP})$$

   i. In situations in which the alveolar pressure exceeds that in the pulmonary vessels (e.g. during hypovolemia), the PCWP will reflect the intra-alveolar pressure and not the left atrial pressure.

6. **Sedation** with/without paralysis often improves gas exchange by improving the efficiency of ventilation.[122] It can relax the diaphragm and chest wall and reduce the energy expenditure or "oxygen cost" of breathing. It is generally preferable to use propofol or dexmedetomidine if it is anticipated that a short additional period of ventilatory support is required. Otherwise, fentanyl may be used to reduce pain and anxiety. Very few patients require additional neuromuscular blockade, usually only if they cannot be satisfactorily oxygenated or ventilated. Commonly used drugs include vecuronium (Norcuron) given in a dose of 0.1 mg/kg followed by an infusion of 1 µg/kg/min, or cisatracurium (Nimbex) given in a dose of 0.15 mg/kg IV followed by an infusion of 3 µg/kg/min. A sedation protocol (Figure 10.3) with titration of drug effect using a sedation scale, such as the Ramsay scale or

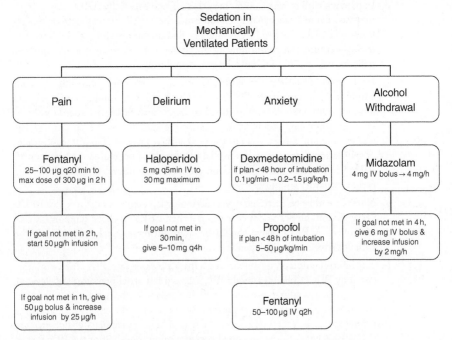

Figure 10.3 • Algorithm for sedation in the ICU.

Sedation Level	Description
Table 10.8 • Ramsay Scale	
1	Anxious and agitated
2	Cooperative, tranquil, oriented
3	Responds only to verbal commands
4	Asleep with brisk response to light stimulation
5	Asleep without response to light stimulation
6	Nonresponsive

the Richmond Agitation Sedation Scale (RASS) (Tables 10.8 and 10.9), should be utilized to optimize patient comfort.

7. Additional supportive measures include the following:

   a. **Diuresis** (usually with IV furosemide) usually improves oxygenation in the early postoperative period when pulmonary interstitial edema may impair gas exchange. Depending on the patient's hemodynamic stability and renal function, a continuous infusion of IV furosemide (10–20 mg/h) can be used to promote a steady diuresis.

   b. The patient's chest x-ray should be reviewed and cultures obtained of pulmonary secretions. Indiscriminate use of antibiotics should be discouraged, but broad-spectrum antibiotics can be initiated if there is suspicion of an infectious component to the patient's borderline pulmonary function. The antibiotics should then be modified depending on culture sensitivities.

   c. **Bronchodilators,** such as albuterol, are useful for patients with increased airway resistance that may be compromising their ventilatory or hemodynamic status. Steroids may be useful for the patient with severe COPD (see page 504).

   d. **Blood transfusions** can be given to treat anemia if the HCT is less than 24%. Despite the intuitive logic that blood transfusions should improve blood oxygen content and tissue oxygen delivery and should potentially reduce the duration of mechanical ventilation, transfused red cells have a low level of 2,3-DPG and initially have poor oxygen-carrying capacity, transmit proinflammatory mediators that can worse pulmonary function, and are immunosuppressive, increasing the risk of nosocomial infection.[91,123] There is little evidence that a liberal transfusion policy (transfusing for a Hb <9.5 g/dL) rather than a restrictive one (transfusion for a Hb <7.5 g/dL) decreases the duration of mechanical ventilation. However, most studies show noninferiority of a restrictive policy in regards to the incidence of renal failure, stroke, MI, or death, but they often fail to specifically address pulmonary issues.[124,125]

Table 10.9 • Richmond Agitation Sedation Scale (RASS)	
Target RASS	**RASS Description**
+4	Combative, violent, danger to staff
+3	Pulls or removes tubes or catheters; aggressive
+2	Frequent nonpurposeful movement, fights ventilator
+1	Anxious, apprehensive, but not aggressive
0	Alert and calm
−1	Awakens to voice (eye opening/contact) >10 sec
−2	Light sedation, briefly awakens to voice (eye opening/ contact) <10 sec
−3	Moderate sedation, movement, or eye opening; no eye contact
−4	Deep sedation, no response to voice, but movement or eye opening to physical stimulation
−5	Unarousable, no response to voice or physical stimulation

    e. **Bronchoscopy** may be beneficial when postural drainage and suctioning are unable to resolve atelectasis because of the presence of tenacious secretions.

    f. If the patient has refractory hypoxemia, use of low tidal volume ventilation, as recommended in the management of ARDS, should be utilized. Prone position, neuromuscular blockade, tolerating an SaO_2 of 88–92%, and use of either inhaled nitric oxide or epoprostenol may improve oxygenation.[126–129]

    g. Patients with COPD or postoperative respiratory failure are more predisposed to the development of atrial fibrillation, which can compromise hemodynamic performance and the ability to wean from the ventilator.[130–132] Cardioselective ß-blockers can be used safely even in patients with bronchospasm. Short-term use of amiodarone is rarely associated with idiosyncratic acute respiratory failure and should not deter its use in patients with COPD.[133]

  8. Methods of mechanical ventilation for patients requiring prolonged ventilatory support are discussed in section XII (pages 494–497).

XI. Chronic Respiratory Failure/Ventilator Dependence

    A. **Etiology.** The inability to wean the patient from the ventilator within a few days after surgery may be caused by problems that impair oxygenation ("hypoxemic respiratory failure)" and/or produce primary ventilatory insufficiency ("hypercapneic respiratory failure"). Although many patients can be weaned after a few days of additional ventilatory support once contributing factors have been treated, a few will progress to a phase of ventilator dependence. Nonetheless, any patient who cannot be weaned within a few days of surgery should be managed so as to achieve extubation as soon as is feasible. The mortality rate associated with the need for prolonged ventilation for just five days after cardiac surgery is approximately 20–25%, with death commonly resulting from multisystem organ failure.

1. **Hypoxia.** The persistence of oxygenation problems beyond 48 hours usually indicates severe hemodynamic compromise or an acute parenchymal lung problem. These are frequently superimposed on preexisting problems, such as preoperative acute pulmonary edema, pulmonary hypertension, or COPD, often in a deconditioned patient with frailty. The primary causes of hypoxemia are:

   a. Hemodynamic instability, especially a low cardiac output state that requires multiple pressors. This increases the oxygen cost of breathing and can produce both hypoxemia and hypercarbia.

   b. Pulmonary issues

      i. Interstitial pulmonary edema, either noncardiogenic (capillary leak or sepsis) or cardiogenic (HF)

      ii. Pneumonia

      iii. Lower airway obstruction (bronchitis, secretions, bronchospasm) often associated with COPD

      iv. Pulmonary embolism, occasionally precipitated by deep venous thrombosis from heparin-induced thrombocytopenia

2. **Hypercarbia.** Primary ventilatory failure is caused by an imbalance between ventilatory capacity and demand and is the most common reason for failure to wean from the ventilator.[134] The patient is incapable of generating the respiratory effort necessary to sustain the "work of breathing", a term that refers to the work necessary to overcome the impedance to ventilation produced by the disease process and the resistance of the ventilator circuitry. Contributory factors include:

   a. Increased ventilatory demand with increased CO_2 production and O_2 demand

      i. Sepsis (which also impairs oxygen uptake), fever, chills

      ii. Pain, anxiety

      iii. Catabolic states

      iv. Carbohydrate overfeeding

      v. Increased dead space (COPD)

      vi. Reduced lung compliance – pneumonia, pulmonary edema

      vii. Increased resistance – bronchospasm, airway inflammation

   b. Decreased respiratory drive

      i. Altered mental status from medications, stroke, delirium, or encephalopathy

      ii. Sleep deprivation

   c. Decreased respiratory muscle function

      i. Significant obesity

      ii. Ventilatory muscle weakness from protein malnutrition, medications (neuromuscular blockers, aminoglycosides, steroid myopathy), dynamic hyperinflation, disuse myopathy, or critical illness polyneuropathy

      iii. Metabolic abnormalities (hypophosphatemia, hyper- or hypomagnesemia, hypokalemia, hypocalcemia, hypothyroidism)

      iv. Diaphragmatic paralysis from phrenic nerve injury. This may be caused by the use of iced slush within the pericardial well during cardioplegic arrest.

Unilateral paralysis usually does not cause ventilatory insufficiency unless there is severe underlying lung disease. Bilateral paralysis may require prolonged ventilatory support, although recovery can usually be anticipated within a year.[135] Diaphragmatic plication can improve pulmonary function when the patient is severely compromised by this problem.[136]

d. The transition from mechanical to spontaneous ventilation with conversion from positive to negative intrapleural pressure increases LV afterload. This increases metabolic and cardiac demands and may not be tolerated by patients with limited cardiac reserve.

3. **Adult respiratory distress syndrome (ARDS)** represents a nonspecific diffuse acute lung injury with inflammation of the lung parenchyma. It is associated with noncardiogenic pulmonary edema from increased microvascular permeability. The lungs become stiff and noncompliant with severe impairment to gas exchange from alveolar-capillary damage, interstitial edema, and atelectasis. ARDS can produce both oxygenation and ventilatory failure. The mortality rate for ARDS after cardiac surgery is substantial, ranging between 18% in some studies[137] to as high as 80%.[138]

a. CPB has been implicated as a causative factor of ARDS because it produces a systemic inflammatory response with increased pulmonary vascular permeability. Neutrophil-initiated pulmonary dysfunction from pulmonary ischemic-reperfusion injury with oxygen free-radical generation is suspected to be the mechanism of this injury.

b. Although the pathophysiology of ARDS appears to be noncardiogenic in nature, most patients developing the syndrome have compromised cardiac function. The major risk factors for the development of postoperative ARDS are reoperative or emergency surgery, longer bypass times, aortic surgery, use of deep hypothermic circulatory arrest, increasing number of blood transfusions, poor LV function, advanced NYHA class, and perioperative shock.[39,137,138] It might be inferred that the capillary leak associated with CPB may be worse in patients in poor clinical condition, especially if there is perioperative hemodynamic compromise, and these patients are more prone to develop this highly lethal syndrome. Subsequently, any additional insult, such as pneumonia, sepsis, cardiogenic pulmonary edema from LV dysfunction or renal failure, or multiple transfusions, will lead to progressive respiratory deterioration, multisystem organ failure, and death.

c. ARDS is usually managed by low tidal volume ventilation and may benefit from inhaled nitric oxide or inhaled epoprostenol.[126–129] In extreme cases, ECMO may be considered.

B. **Clinical manifestations** of ventilator dependence that often indicate inability to wean include:

1. Tachypnea (rate >30 breaths/min) with shallow breaths

2. Paradoxical inward movement of the abdomen during inspiration ("abdominal paradox")

C. **Management** involves selecting an appropriate means of ventilation (see section XII, pages 494–497) while identifying the factors that may be contributing to ventilator dependence. Measures should be taken to optimize cardiac performance, improve

---

Table 10.10 • Supportive Measures in Patients with Chronic Ventilatory Failure

1. Select appropriate mode of ventilatory support – use low tidal volume ventilation (tidal volume of 6 mL/kg with plateau pressures <30 cm H_2O)
2. Suction prn and prevent aspiration
3. Optimize hemodynamic status
4. Avoid excessive fluid management and diurese as tolerated
5. Avoid unnecessary transfusions
6. Remove invasive catheters as soon as possible to prevent ICU-acquired infections
7. Have protocol to reduce risk of ventilator-associated pneumonia
8. Provide adequate analgesia but avoid oversedation and neuromuscular blockers; use intermittent interruption of sedatives rather than a continuous infusion
9. Provide adequate nutrition, preferably with low carbohydrate enteral feedings
10. Optimize metabolic and electrolyte status (thyroid, HCT, glucose, magnesium, phosphate)
11. Specific considerations:
    a. Bronchodilators/steroids for bronchospasm
    b. Antibiotics for infections/antipyretics for fever
    c. Diuresis for fluid overload
    d. Drain any pleural effusions
    e. Specific measures to prevent ventilator-associated pneumonia
    f. VTE prophylaxis
12. Physical therapy and repositioning to prevent decubitus ulcers
13. Stress ulcer prophylaxis with sucralfate or a proton-pump inhibitor
14. Consider tracheostomy if anticipate prolonged ventilatory support >2 weeks

---

the respiratory drive and neuromuscular competence, and reduce the respiratory load by improving intrinsic pulmonary function and reducing the minute ventilation requirement (Table 10.10). Efforts must be made to reduce the risk of ICU-acquired infections and pneumonia. As these issues are being addressed, it is important to identify when a patient is ready for weaning or discontinuation of ventilatory support. One study suggested that there was a trigger point of recovery usually related to an improvement in respiratory mechanics that indicates when fairly rapid weaning is feasible in patients with chronic respiratory failure.[139]

1. **Improve hemodynamic status** with inotropic support while avoiding fluid overload. Pulmonary vasodilators, such as nitroprusside and nitroglycerin, should generally be avoided because they can increase intrapulmonary shunting by preventing hypoxic vasoconstriction. Milrinone is beneficial by providing inotropic, lusitropic (relaxant), and vasodilator effects that can improve RV and LV function. Selective inhaled pulmonary vasodilators, such as nitric oxide or epoprostenol (Flolan), may be helpful in patients with RV dysfunction.

2. **Improve respiratory drive and neuromuscular competence**
    a. Avoid oversedation and neuromuscular blockers. Daily interruption of sedation is associated with more rapid weaning from ventilatory support than a continuous sedative infusion.[140–142]

b. Provide adequate nutrition to achieve positive nitrogen balance and improve respiratory muscle strength and immune competence. Most patients fare well with standard tube feedings, but in patients with significant hypercarbia, low-carbohydrate tube feedings (Pulmocare, Abbott Nutrition) should be considered. Overfeeding with carbohydrates or fats can increase CO_2 production and the respiratory quotient (RQ), which will add to the ventilatory burden. The RQ represents the CO_2 output/O_2 uptake and is normally 0.8.

c. Select the appropriate mode of ventilatory support to reduce the work of breathing and train the respiratory muscles to support spontaneous ventilation. Use of low tidal volume ventilation provides the best lung-protective ventilation in patients at risk for or with ARDS.[39,121] Avoid prolonged periods of spontaneous ventilation until the patient appears ready for a weaning trial. In patients with severe oxygen desaturation, prone positioning may improve oxygenation and allow for earlier weaning.[143]

d. Optimize acid–base, electrolyte, and endocrine (thyroid) status. Metabolic alkalosis and hypothyroidism inhibit the central respiratory drive. Correct potassium, magnesium, and phosphate levels. Correct profound anemia.

e. Initiate physical therapy.

f. Evaluate diaphragmatic motion during fluoroscopy ("sniff test"). Diaphragmatic plication may improve respiratory function in patients with ventilator dependence caused by unilateral diaphragmatic dysfunction.[136]

3. **Reduce the respiratory load**

a. Reduce impedance to ventilation

i. Give bronchodilators or steroids for bronchospasm (see pages 503–504)

ii. Employ chest physical therapy, frequent repositioning, and suctioning to mobilize and aspirate secretions and prevent atelectasis

iii. Consider tracheostomy (see pages 493–494)

b. Improve lung compliance

i. Antibiotics for pneumonia

ii. Diuretics for fluid overload and pulmonary edema

iii. Thoracentesis or tube thoracostomy for pleural effusions

iv. Prevent abdominal distention with nasogastric suction or metoclopramide.

c. Reduce the minute ventilation requirement

i. Provide adequate analgesia for pain and use sedatives for anxiety. Excessive sedation must be avoided, because it inhibits the central respiratory drive.

ii. Administer antipyretics for fever to reduce metabolic demand.

iii. Treat infections (sepsis, pneumonia) with appropriate antibiotics to minimize antibiotic resistance.

iv. Avoid overfeeding to lower CO_2 production.

4. Take steps to prevent line sepsis and **ventilator-associated pneumonia (VAP)** or initiate appropriate treatment once they develop.[144–147]

a. VAP is more common in patients who are older, and those who are undergoing reoperative, emergency, or aortic surgery, receive more blood transfusions, require re-exploration, are taking steroids, require inotropic support, or have a prolonged duration of ventilation.

b. Invasive catheters, including central lines and arterial lines, should be removed when no longer necessary.

c. Basic strategies involve oral intubation and using appropriate sedation and weaning protocols to achieve extubation as soon as feasible, adequate hand washing by the healthcare team, keeping the patient semi-recumbent with the head of the bed elevated 30 degrees, draining condensates from the ventilator circuit, maintaining adequate cuff pressure to prevent aspiration, avoiding gastric overdistention, using oro- rather than nasogastric tubes, initiating enteral feedings when feasible to provide adequate nutritional support, using frequent subglottic secretion aspiration, and optimizing oropharyngeal hygiene with 0.12–2% chlorhexidine rinses.

d. The benefit of stress ulcer prophylaxis in critically ill ventilated patients is controversial.[148] Sucralfate is more effective in reducing the risk of VAP than H_2 antagonists, which raise gastric pH, but shows little effect on the incidence of bleeding or mortality.[149] Although proton-pump inhibitors (PPIs) may reduce the risk of bleeding, they do increase the risk of pneumonia, more so than with the use of H_2 blockers.[150] The SUP-ICU study found that use of pantoprazole actually increased mortality compared with placebo.[151,152]

e. The use of selective digestive decontamination to reduce the incidence of lower respiratory tract infection is controversial and not routinely recommended. There is evidence that the combination of topical oropharyngeal agents, drugs given down the nasogastric tube (tobramycin, polymyxin, amphotericin), and IV antibiotics (broad-spectrum cephalosporins) can reduce the incidence of VAP in surgical patients, but this strategy may lead to the emergence of antibiotic-resistant strains.[153]

f. Organisms causing early- and late-onset VAP are usually different. Early-onset VAP often responds to empiric monotherapy (such as ceftriaxone) until specific culture results are available. Late-onset VAP is commonly caused by *Enterobacter*, *Pseudomonas*, or MRSA, and usually requires an initial combination of ceftazidime, ciprofloxacin, and vancomycin (see empiric recommendations in the 2016 guidelines).[147]

5. **Tracheostomy** should be performed to reduce the risk of laryngeal damage and swallowing dysfunction if it is anticipated that the patient will require mechanical ventilatory support for more than two weeks. A tracheostomy reduces airway resistance and glottic trauma, improves the ability to suction the lower airways, lowers the risk of sinusitis (although it probably does not reduce the risk of VAP), improves patient comfort and mobility, often allows the patient to eat, and generally makes the patient look and feel better. It commonly leads to earlier decannulation than standard endotracheal intubation. Mortality rates in patients requiring a tracheostomy are quite high (40–50%), usually indicative of more advanced cardiac and respiratory disease, and often related to neurologic dysfunction.[154] If it is anticipated that the patient will require prolonged ventilatory support, early tracheostomy (within 10 days vs. after 14 days) has been shown to decrease hospital mortality.[155]

a. Avoidance of tracheostomy is reasonable when it is anticipated that extubation will be accomplished within 7–10 days. One study of patients on ventilatory support for three days found that the absence of major organ system problems was predictive of successful weaning by the 10th postoperative day.

Favorable criteria included a Glasgow coma score of 15, urine output >500 mL/24 h, absence of acidosis (bicarbonate ≥20 mmol/L), no requirement for epinephrine or norepinephrine, and absence of lung injury.[156]

b. The traditional concept has been that tracheostomy should be delayed for at least 2 weeks after a median sternotomy to decrease the risk of deep sternal wound infection (DSWI). However, some studies suggest that performing a tracheostomy within 10 days of surgery is associated with better outcomes without an increased risk of mediastinitis.[155] Other studies have shown that although the risk of mediastinitis may be increased in patients having a tracheostomy, it is not related to when the tracheostomy is performed.[157,158] Most likely, it is related to the severity of illness producing respiratory failure and other associated complications rather than the tracheostomy itself.

c. A percutaneous dilatational tracheostomy performed at the bedside has a low complication rate that may include bleeding, posterior tracheal laceration, tube obstruction from hematoma or tracheal edema of the posterior wall, and stomal infection. The incidence of late tracheal stenosis is lower than that of a surgical tracheostomy.

XII. Methods of Ventilatory Support

A. Full ventilatory support is required when the patient remains anesthetized and sedated after surgery. It is also required for the patient with acute or chronic respiratory failure while underlying disease processes are treated and nutrition is optimized. Ventilatory support is initially provided using volume- or pressure-controlled ventilation.[105] Inadequate support may lead to ventilatory muscle fatigue, whereas excessive support may lead to muscle atrophy, so settings for each patient must be individualized.

B. Positive-pressure ventilation (PPV) improves V/Q matching to increase the efficiency of gas exchange. It also reduces the work of breathing in the sedated and/or paralyzed patient. Weaning from ventilatory support should be initiated as soon as feasible to minimize the potential complications of prolonged ventilatory support that contribute to its high mortality. These include:

1. Pulmonary effects (barotrauma, acute lung injury, ventilator-associated pneumonia), diaphragmatic atrophy, respiratory muscle weakness (polyneuropathy), and diminished mucociliary clearance

2. Hemodynamic compromise

3. Gastrointestinal issues: stress ulceration, hypomotility and intolerance of tube feedings, splanchnic hypoperfusion, swallowing difficulties after extubation

4. Renal dysfunction and fluid retention

5. Increased intracranial pressure (from reduced cerebral venous flow)

6. Disordered sleep and delirium

7. Development of heparin-induced thrombocytopenia from use of heparin for VTE prophylaxis

C. **Volume-limited modes.** Most patients are initially placed on volume ventilators that deliver a preset tidal volume. A limit is set on the peak pressure to avoid barotrauma. Patients with noncompliant stiff lungs or bronchospastic airways can be difficult to ventilate in this mode because some of the preset tidal volume may not be delivered once the peak pressure limit is reached. This system is best for patients with normal or increased compliance (emphysema).

1. Ventilator settings should be selected to provide a minute ventilation of about 8 L/min. These include a respiratory rate of 10–12/min and a tidal volume of 6–8 mL/kg. This tidal volume is preferred as a means of minimizing the risk of developing ARDS after surgery.[39] PEEP of 5 cm H_2O is routinely added. Adjustments may be made based upon ABGs, but the plateau airway pressure should ideally be maintained at <30 cm H_2O.

2. **Assist/control (A/C) ventilation** delivers a preset tidal volume when triggered by the patient's inspiratory effort (a demand valve senses a negative airway deflection) or at preset intervals if no breath is taken. The rate should generally be set about four breaths below the patient's spontaneous rate or at 10–12 breaths/min before the patient begins spontaneous breathing. If the patient is out of synchrony with the ventilator or hyperventilates, a significant respiratory alkalosis or acidosis may occur. This mode of ventilation is best used only when the patient requires significant ventilator support and should not be used for weaning. In fact, the patient's efforts may persist despite the machine's superimposed breath, leading to increased respiratory muscle fatigue.

3. **Controlled mandatory ventilation (CMV)** will provide a positive-pressure breath to the patient at a preset tidal volume and rate. This should also be used only during the temporary period of full ventilator support, because it will lead to respiratory muscle deconditioning.

4. **Intermittent mandatory ventilation (IMV).** In the IMV mode, the patient's spontaneous inspiration will generate a tidal volume consistent with their effort and the machine will deliver a full tidal volume at a designated rate.

5. **Synchronized intermittent mandatory ventilation (SIMV).** In the SIMV mode, the patient breathes spontaneously and, at preset intervals, the next spontaneous breath is augmented by a full tidal volume from the ventilator. Since the ventilator's breath is synchronized to the patient's efforts, high peak pressures are avoided and breathing is more comfortable. Flow-by triggering is used such that the ventilator provides a breath when the return flow is less than the delivered flow. This results in decreased work of breathing. Because many of the patient's efforts are not augmented, SIMV should not be used during the early phase of chronic ventilatory support, because it increases the work of breathing more than A/C ventilation. However, it is an excellent mode for ventilatory weaning in that it produces good patient–ventilator synchrony, preserves respiratory muscle function, and produces a low airway pressure. A low level of pressure support can be added to decrease the work of spontaneous breathing.

D. **Pressure-limited (cycled) ventilation.** Pressure ventilators deliver gas flow up to a set peak airway pressure limit at a preset respiratory rate. The amount of gas flow delivered (the tidal volume) depends upon the compliance of the lungs, airway resistance, and tubing resistance. This ensures delivery of a more consistent tidal volume to patients with increased airway resistance (bronchospasm, restrictive lung disease). It is best avoided in patients with emphysema, in whom overinflation of the lungs can occur at low pressures. The peak airway pressure is constant but generally lower than with volume-limited ventilation. It may produce more homogeneous gas distribution, improved gas exchange, better patient–ventilator synchrony, and perhaps earlier weaning from mechanical ventilation than volume-limited ventilation. However, there is little evidence that it improves oxygenation or the work of breathing. Pressure-limited ventilation can be delivered in A/C, CMV, or IMV (SIMV) mode.

1. **Pressure-limited A/C** allows the patient's inspiratory effort to trigger pressure-limited breaths in addition to those delivered at the set respiratory rate and pressure.

2. **Pressure-limited CMV** (pressure-controlled ventilation or PCV) is a time-cycled mode of ventilation that provides no additional ventilation above that delivered by the preset peak airway pressure and respiratory rate. PCV at a level of 20 cm H_2O provides full ventilatory support with a tidal volume of about 8–10 mL/kg. This is used in a similar manner to volume-controlled CMV in the patient who is not initiating any spontaneous breaths.

3. **Pressure-limited IMV** allows the patient to take spontaneous unassisted breaths in addition to ventilation provided at the set rate and pressure limit.

E. **Pressure support ventilation (PSV)** is a patient-triggered, pressure-limited system that will deliver ventilation only as triggered by the patient's inspiratory efforts. The system will then deliver inspiratory pressure and gas flow to the circuit until the inspiratory flow falls below about 25% of its peak value, and exhalation will then occur passively. The patient's effort determines the respiratory rate, inspiratory time and flow rate (tidal volume/inspiratory time), and the expiratory time. The tidal volume delivered depends on the patient's inspiratory effort, the selected level of pressure support and resistance in the patient's lungs (compliance and airway resistance), and circuitry.

1. With PSV, airway pressure remains constant by automatic adjustment of the flow rate as long as the patient maintains an inspiratory effort. There is no gas flow provided if the patient does not breathe spontaneously. Modifications of this system include "volume support", with which the PSV level is automatically adjusted to provide a preset tidal volume, and "volume-assured pressure support", with which additional volume is given to provide a preset tidal volume, even if the pressure rises.

2. PSV results in lower peak airway pressures, slower respiratory rates, and higher tidal volumes than other modes of ventilation. Thus, it is beneficial for the patient who is out of synchrony with the ventilator ("fighting the ventilator"). However, if the patient has COPD, the inspiratory phase may be prolonged and the patient may try to expire during late inspiration from the ventilator. This may induce patient discomfort but can be counteracted by reducing the level of pressure support or converting to pressure control to provide a shorter inspiratory phase.

F. No matter which mode of ventilation is selected, attention must be paid to avoiding high peak inspiratory pressures, which will produce barotrauma as well as hemodynamic compromise by impeding venous return and impairing ventricular function. The inspiratory plateau pressure (IPP), which is the peak pressure at the end of inspiration, should be maintained at less than 35 cm H_2O. Means of lowering the IPP include lowering of the level of PEEP, lowering the tidal volume, or decreasing the inspiratory flow rate to increase the I:E ratio.

1. Low tidal volume ventilation has been used in patients with ARDS. It is believed that alveolar overdistention can produce changes in endothelial cell permeability

and produce barotrauma and noncardiogenic pulmonary edema. Low tidal volume ventilation (5–6 mL/kg) may improve oxygenation with permissive hypercapnia, and has been associated with reduced mortality in patients with ARDS.[121]

2. Decreasing the inspiratory flow rate increases the inspiratory flow time and may decrease peak pressures. However, if the expiratory time is too short to allow for full exhalation, as may occur in patients with bronchospastic airways, the next breath may be "stacked" on top of the previous one, producing lung hyperinflation and the auto-PEEP effect. Inspiration will commence before expiratory airflow is completed, resulting in positive airway pressure at the end of expiration. This may impair patient triggering of assisted ventilation. This problem can be overcome by taking steps to improve the expiratory phase of ventilation:

   a. Increasing the inspiratory flow rate (tidal volume/inspiratory flow time)

   b. Decreasing the I:E ratio

   c. Treating conditions that increase expiratory flow resistance, such as bronchospasm

   d. Decreasing the respiratory rate or tidal volume

   e. Adding PEEP to the ventilator settings

3. Patient–ventilator dyssynchrony occurs when the phase of respiration differs between the patient and the ventilator. The patient appears to be fighting the ventilator, becomes short of breath, and tires out from the increased work of breathing. Although patient-related factors, such as delirium, may be contributory, ventilator adjustments can usually overcome the problem. For example, ineffective triggering or too long an inspiratory time (i.e. the tidal volume is too high for the inspiratory flow rate) may cause dyssynchrony.

G. **Noninvasive ventilation (NIV)** can be used as a means of avoiding intubation in patients with acute respiratory decompensation (see section IX.C on page 478).[96,97,159] It can also support earlier extubation in patients in whom standard criteria are not quite met. The primary advantage is the avoidance of some of the risks of intubation, including laryngotracheal trauma, sinusitis, and respiratory tract infections.

   1. Generally, an oronasal mask with a soft silicone seal is used to improve patient comfort, although it can make the patient feel claustrophobic. Standard ICU or portable ventilators are connected to the mask with tubing that provides positive pressure with heated, humidified oxygen. Bilevel NIV (BPAP) and CPAP are the modes most commonly utilized. The former is preferable, as it is leak-tolerant, allows for rebreathing, and is more effective in treating hypercarbia than CPAP, which does not increase alveolar ventilation. The oxygen flow rate is adjusted to achieve an SaO_2 >90%. Generally, it is not possible to exceed an FiO_2 of 0.5, so if the patient is severely hypoxic, intubation will usually be necessary.

   2. If the patient cannot tolerate either BPAP or CPAP, the A/C and PSV modes can also be delivered noninvasively. For the PSV mode, the ventilator is set in a pressure-limited mode with an initial pressure of 8–10 cm H_2O that is gradually increased to a maximum of 20 cm H_2O. This limits the maximal inspiratory time and improves patient–ventilator synchrony. The expiratory pressure is set at 5 cm H_2O.

   3. Use of dexmedetomidine is very helpful in reducing patient agitation during NIV for hypoxia, because it does not produce respiratory depression.[160]

XIII. Weaning from the Ventilator

A. Once it is decided that a patient has improved sufficiently to no longer require full ventilatory support, a means of weaning the patient from the ventilator should be selected.[161–165] For patients requiring short-term ventilation, SBTs using CPAP or low-level pressure support are the most expeditious means of weaning. For patients requiring more prolonged durations of mechanical support, PSV weaning appears to be best.

B. **Practical aspects of weaning and extubation**

1. It is essential to address and treat all the potentially correctable causes of respiratory failure. Once this has been accomplished, weaning can be initiated if the criteria noted in Table 10.3 are met. Generally, weaning should not be considered if the patient has insufficient oxygenation (PaO_2 <55 torr).

2. The use of sedatives during mechanical ventilation is usually necessary to reduce the patient's anxiety and minute ventilation requirements. However, continuous IV sedation depresses the patient's sensorium and respiratory drive and can delay the weaning process. Thus, a sedation protocol with daily awakening and administering sedatives only as necessary should expedite the weaning process.[140–142] Sedatives should be withheld prior to initiating a SBT.

3. No matter which technique is used for weaning (T-piece, SIMV, or PSV), a SBT should be attempted using a T-piece or a low level of CPAP or PSV for 30 minutes and no more than two hours. All of these techniques are associated with fairly comparable extubation outcomes.[166]

   a. If the patient appears to be weaning satisfactorily with a comfortable breathing pattern and mental status, adequate hemodynamics and ABGs (Tables 10.3 and 10.5), extubation can be accomplished. Additional concerns include the ability to protect the airway, initiate a cough, and raise secretions. The necessity to suction more than every two hours for excessive secretions may preclude extubation.

   b. One of the criteria often used to predict the possibility of postextubation stridor and the need for reintubation is the "cuff leak" test. This is most applicable to patients who have been intubated for a long period of time. A crude way of doing this is to deflate the endotracheal tube cuff and feel how much of the delivered breath exits around the tube. One objective method involves recording the difference between the inspiratory tidal volume and the average of six expiratory tidal volumes with the cuff deflated. A cuff leak <110 mL may be predictive of postextubation stridor, although some studies have not found this assessment a very sensitive and accurate predictor of stridor.[167,168] One of the problems with this method is that some of the inspiratory volume may also leak with the cuff down, so the cuff leak volume may be spuriously high since it may measure both inspiratory and expiratory leaks.[169] A third method is the "percent cuff leak", which measures the difference between the exhaled tidal volume with the cuff up and down, divided by the exhaled volume with the cuff up. Values of less than 10% are predictive of stridor and the need for reintubation.[170]

   c. If there are concerns about postextubation stridor, especially in patients intubated >6 days, steroids may be of benefit in reducing laryngeal edema. Most studies suggest that this should be started at least four hours and preferably 12–24 hours prior to planned extubation. Regimens include methylprednisolone 20–40 mg IV q4–6h or dexamethasone 5 mg IV q6h.[171-173]

d. If the patient does not satisfy extubation criteria after a SBT, 24 hours of full ventilation is recommended before another attempt at weaning. If the next attempt is unsuccessful, pressure-support weaning is probably better than T-piece or SIMV weaning. It is estimated that about 10% of patients will still require reintubation even if they meet extubation criteria.

4. Noninvasive PPV using BPAP can improve oxygenation in many patients after extubation. It may be used to provide ventilatory support if the patient is extubated even though standard criteria are not met. If the patient has evidence of pulmonary edema, mask CPAP usually suffices.[159] High-flow oxygen systems are useful when hypoxia is the primary problem after extubation.

C. Predictors of weaning success

1. Several predictors of weaning success have been evaluated, but the easiest and arguably most sensitive predictor of a successful ventilatory wean is a "rapid shallow breathing index" (RSBI) of less than 100 breaths/min.[174] The RSBI is the ratio of the respiratory rate/tidal volume in liters during spontaneous ventilation for one minute. If the RSBI is <100, a weaning trial should be attempted because the estimated rate of successful weaning is greater than 80%. A RSBI >100 does not preclude weaning, since about 50% of such patients can be weaned and extubated. Generally, however, if the RSBI exceeds 100 and the patient's respiratory rate is greater than 38 during a brief SBT, the likelihood of a successful wean is quite low. One study found that extubation failure was most likely when the RSBI was >57, the patient was in positive fluid balance within the 24 hours before extubation, or pneumonia was present at the time of extubation.[175]

2. Nonetheless, the best method to determine whether extubation can be accomplished successfully is to perform a SBT once readiness criteria are met. Maintenance of satisfactory oxygenation with comfortable breathing usually predicts successful extubation. These include markers such as a PaO_2 >60 torr on an FiO_2 <0.35, a PaO_2/FiO_2 ratio >200, or A-a gradient <350 torr on 100% oxygen.

3. Careful observation of the patient's breathing pattern is very important in assessing weaning success. Evidence of tachypnea, increased respiratory effort, or change in hemodynamics (especially an increase in PA pressure if a Swan-Ganz catheter is in place) often suggest that the patient is not tolerating the weaning process (Table 10.4).

D. T-piece or CPAP weaning

1. T-piece or CPAP weaning is usually used to achieve early extubation. Once standard criteria are met, especially adequate mental status, the patient is placed on a T-piece or CPAP of 5 cm H_2O and then extubated if the SBT is well tolerated. Use of a low level of pressure support during a SBT is most beneficial in patients with small high-resistance endotracheal tubes. For patients receiving more prolonged ventilatory support, alternating periods of full support (rest) with increasing periods of independent spontaneous ventilation (stress) can theoretically increase the strength and endurance of the respiratory muscles. However, the sudden transition to a complete workload may not be well tolerated in the early phase of recovery from severe ventilatory failure and may result in profound respiratory muscle fatigue.

2. However, once contributing factors to a patient's ventilatory dependence have been addressed and it is decided that an attempt at weaning should be made, an SBT of 30 minutes can be used to see if the patient satisfies the criteria for extubation. If the patient fails a 30 minute trial, they should be returned to full ventilatory support for 24 hours and a 2 hour SBT should be attempted the following day.

E. **Synchronized intermittent mandatory ventilation (SIMV) weaning**

1. With SIMV, the mandatory breaths are patient-triggered, thus avoiding over-inflation and improving the patient's comfort. During the weaning process, the IMV rate is gradually decreased and the patient assumes a greater proportion of the minute ventilation. Since the energy expenditure of the respiratory muscles increases as the IMV rate is lowered, lowering of the IMV rate during the day can be coupled with complete rest at night to avoid muscle fatigue.

2. Patient effort increases in proportion to both the ventilator-assisted breaths and spontaneous breaths. Respiratory muscle rest does not occur during the mandatory breath, and this may induce respiratory muscle fatigue. Although SIMV uses a demand trigger valve, use of a flow-by system provides adequate gas flow to minimize the work of breathing. When the patient can maintain spontaneous ventilation for a prolonged period of time and satisfies standard criteria, extubation can be accomplished.

3. The use of pressure support concomitantly with IMV can also reduce the work of breathing during the patient's spontaneous respirations. Weaning can be accomplished by initially reducing the IMV rate and subsequently reducing the level of pressure support. The duration of spontaneous ventilation on progressively lower levels of pressure support or CPAP is then extended and the patient is extubated.

4. Rapid SIMV weaning can be used immediately after surgery to achieve early extubation, although most patients do well with a SBT with T-piece or CPAP directly from full ventilation once standard weaning criteria are met. For the chronically ventilated patient, most studies suggest that SIMV weaning is the least effective means of weaning.[161–165,176]

F. **Pressure support ventilation (PSV) weaning**

1. PSV is best used to provide partial support as the patient is weaned from the ventilator, since it cannot provide any support unless the patient triggers a breath. As long as the inspiratory flow is adequate (i.e. the patient makes adequate inspiratory efforts), a higher level of support will reduce the work of breathing, especially since it can overcome any impedance in the system (small endotracheal tube, bronchospasm, secretions) to initiate ventilation. Thus, PSV generally results in more comfortable breathing for the patient. By reconditioning the respiratory muscles to assume more spontaneous ventilation without producing excessive energy expenditure, PSV may expedite the weaning process. Weaning is accomplished by progressively lowering the levels of PSV and observing the patient for fatigue and other parameters indicative of intolerance of the weaning process (Table 10.4). Weaning options include:

   a. Increasing the duration of spontaneous ventilation with lower levels of PSV during the daytime ("sprinting") with full support of higher levels of PSV at night. If the patient tolerates PSV for 12 hours, the level of PSV is gradually reduced by 2 cm H_2O intervals daily or every other day, and the tidal volume and respiratory rate are assessed. Extubation is accomplished when the patient is able to breathe comfortably for two hours at low levels of PSV (around 6–8 cm H_2O support).

b. PSV with IMV. A level of partial PSV support is selected and the IMV rate is gradually decreased. When the IMV rate has been reduced to fewer than four breaths/min, the PSV level is decreased as noted.

c. If the failure criteria noted in Table 10.4 are noted, PSV should be titrated to achieve a respiratory rate <25/min, and an additional period of support should be provided before another attempt at weaning.

2. Potential disadvantages of PSV

a. PSV requires an intact respiratory drive to trigger the ventilator. Inadequate ventilation will result if the patient is apneic or has an unstable neurologic status, respiratory drive, or mechanics.

b. Cardiac output may be compromised because airway pressure is always positive. With IMV weaning, there is a phase of negative intrathoracic pressure that can augment venous return.

c. Shallow tidal volumes from poor inspiratory effort may lead to atelectasis.

d. A gas leak in the system may prevent PSV from being terminated, producing persistently high airway pressures and hemodynamic compromise.

e. In-line nebulizers (for bronchodilators) are in the inspiratory limb and may make it difficult for the patient to initiate a breath to trigger PSV.

XIV. Other Respiratory Complications

A. Respiratory complications can occur during the period of mechanical ventilation, soon after extubation, or later during convalescence on the postoperative floor. The management of these complications must be individualized, taking the patient's overall medical condition, the extent and nature of the surgical procedure, the precipitating factors, and the phase of recovery into consideration. The management of pneumothorax, pleural effusions, chylothorax, and bronchospasm are discussed here. Pulmonary embolism, diaphragmatic dysfunction, and pneumonia are discussed in Chapter 13.

B. **Pneumothorax.** If the pleural space is entered at the time of surgery, a chest tube should be placed for evacuation of air and fluid. Occasionally, a small pneumothorax will be noted on an early postoperative chest x-ray, often related to passage of a sternal wire through the pleura. If small, this may be managed conservatively, but it may potentially enlarge with the use of PPV and therefore must be carefully reassessed. A chest tube should be placed for a larger pneumothorax. Less commonly, a pneumothorax will be absent on the initial x-ray but will be evident on subsequent films. A small pneumothorax noted after extubation or after chest tube removal can generally be observed and monitored by serial x-rays if the patient is asymptomatic.

1. Always consider the possibility of a pneumothorax (possibly tension) when ABGs deteriorate or hemodynamic instability develops for no obvious reason after several hours of stability. The first sign is often a sudden increase in the peak inspiratory pressure, indicated by repeated alarming of the ventilator.

2. Evidence of an air leak in the chest drainage system may indicate loose connections, rather than a leak from the lung. However, chest tubes should never be

removed until it is confirmed that an air leak is not the result of an intrapleural or parenchymal problem. Air leaks gradually resolve in the vast majority of patients within a few days. If not, placement of a new pleural tube should be considered. A small 8 Fr chest tube (a "dart") is usually effective when appropriately placed and is less traumatic to the patient. Often a persistent air leak on suction will abate on water seal, allowing for the removal of the tube without the development of a recurrent pneumothorax. Clamping the tube to prevent air escape and repeating a chest x-ray with the tube clamped is more assuring that there is no ongoing leak if a pneumothorax is not present on a subsequent chest x-ray. Use of a Heimlich valve may allow the patient to be discharged with an active air leak.

3. Progressive subcutaneous emphysema may develop if air exits under positive pressure where the pleura has been violated. In patients with severe emphysema or bronchospastic airways, it may result from alveolar rupture. However, it may result from visceral pleural injury at the time of surgery, no matter how small. Subcutaneous emphysema may occur when the chest tubes are still in place (usually when they are kinked), but it more commonly occurs after they have been removed. A pneumothorax may or may not be present. Management usually requires placement of unilateral or bilateral chest tubes, and, if the emphysema is severe, performing decompressing skin incisions in the upper chest or neck.

4. Proper positioning of any chest tube is critical. Often the skin site will appear to be fairly high but is actually close to the diaphragm. There are a number of potentially serious complications associated with tube thoracotomy placement that need to be kept in mind, especially damage to intra-abdominal structures and the lung itself.[177]

5. A chest x-ray should always be performed after the removal of pleural chest tubes. A small pneumothorax (<20%) can be observed with serial films. However, aspiration of the pleural space or placement of a new chest tube is indicated for a larger pneumothorax or if the patient is symptomatic.

C. **Pleural effusions** are noted postoperatively in approximately 60% of patients undergoing cardiac surgery and are more common when the pleural cavity has been entered for ITA takedown.[178] This usually results from oozing of blood and serous fluid from the chest wall. However, a hemothorax may also develop if blood spills over from the pericardial space. An effusion developing on the right side is more commonly serous in nature from fluid overload.

1. **Prevention.** Adequate drainage of opened pleural cavities at the time of surgery should reduce the incidence of bloody effusions, but optimal positioning of chest tubes in the most dependent portion of the pleural space is often not accomplished. This is especially true after minimally invasive procedures. Leaving a silicone Blake drain (or probably any type of tube) in the pleural cavity for several days after surgery has been shown to lower the incidence of late pleural effusions.[179]

2. A hemothorax may develop if significant mediastinal bleeding drains into an opened pleural cavity. This may prove beneficial in avoiding cardiac tamponade, but should be suspected in the patient with hemodynamic instability, a falling HCT, cardiac filling pressures that fail to rise with volume (although they may rise if tamponade is also developing), and increasing peak inspiratory pressures on the ventilator. A portable chest x-ray may demonstrate more opacification on one side than the other, but the degree of hemothorax may be difficult to determine with

the patient lying supine. CT scans are more sensitive in detecting pleural effusions, but they tend to overestimate the size of an effusion that may be clinically insignificant. Echocardiography can also identify a large left pleural effusion.

3. A large pleural effusion can produce atrial or ventricular diastolic collapse and cardiac tamponade even in the absence of a pericardial effusion.[180,181] These findings can be confirmed by echocardiography.

4. Most patients with pleural effusions are asymptomatic, and in the vast majority of cases, small effusions resolve within a few months, either with use of diuretics (especially right-sided effusions) or spontaneously. However, patients with underlying lung disease or moderate effusions may develop dyspnea. In these situations, a thoracentesis is indicated either in the hospital or during a follow-up visit. This can usually be performed safely based upon evaluation of a chest x-ray, but CT or ultrasound-guided thoracentesis may be helpful in improving localization for needle placement.[182] Chest tube placement is preferable for large effusions in the early postoperative period, when blood is more likely to have accumulated.

5. Postpericardiotomy syndrome may contribute to the development of recurrent serous or serosanguineous pleural and pericardial effusions. This should be managed initially by use of NSAIDs, colchicine, or steroids, but may require a thoracentesis (and pericardiocentesis) for symptom relief.

D. **Chylothorax** is a rare complication of surgery caused by interruption of lymphatic tributaries of the thoracic duct in the left upper mediastinum. It is most likely to occur during proximal mobilization of the left ITA near the subclavian vessels or during aortic arch surgery.

1. **Manifestations.** If early drainage is significant, turbulent milky fluid may be noted in the chest tubes that is exacerbated by dietary fat. More commonly, an enlarging left pleural effusion will be noted after the chest tubes have been removed.

2. **Diagnosis.** Examination of the pleural fluid will reveal chyle, which is sterile, with large quantities of lymphocytes and a high level of triglycerides (>110 mg/dL). Staining with Sudan III can distinguish chyle from purulent fluid.

3. **Treatment.** Conservative treatment with chest tube drainage, elimination of fat from the diet, and use of medium-chain triglycerides (which comes as an oral oil to be mixed with fruit juices) is recommended initially. If drainage persists for more than a few days, use of octreotide (Sandostatin) 100 µg SC q8h is usually successful in terminating the leak.[183,184] If this fails, thoracoscopic clipping, coagulation, or ligation of the thoracic duct can be performed.

E. **Bronchospasm** can occur at the termination of surgery and can produce difficulty with sternal closure. Severe bronchospasm and air trapping developing in the ICU can produce difficulties with mechanical ventilation as well as hemodynamic problems that can mimic cardiac tamponade. Modification of the ventilator circuit to increase the inspiratory flow rate will decrease the inspiration : expiration (I:E) ratio, allowing more time for exhalation, and should decrease the auto-PEEP effect. Bronchospasm can be precipitated by fluid overload, drug reactions, blood product transfusions, or the use of β-blockers, and it can occur in patients with or without known COPD or bronchospastic airways. Treatment involves the following:

1. Inhalational bronchodilators delivered by metered-dose inhaler (MDI) or nebulizer are helpful during mechanical ventilation as well as after extubation. They can reduce bronchospasm and reduce dynamic hyperinflation of the

lung, the latter perhaps contributing more to symptomatic improvement. Short-acting β_2-agonists combined with anticholinergic (muscarinic) medications (such as ipratroprium) provide superior benefit to individual medications alone.[185]

2. Commonly used fast-acting bronchodilators:[186]

   a. Short-acting β_2-agonists (SABAs)

      i. Albuterol (Ventolin, Proventil) 0.5 mL of 0.5% solution (2.5 mg) in 3 mL normal saline q6h or two puffs q6h

      ii. Levalbuterol (Xopenex) 0.63 mg in 3 mL normal saline q8h (three times a day); it can also be given as two inhalations q4–6h through a pressured MDI

   b. Anticholinergics: ipratroprium (Atrovent) 2.5 mL of 0.02% (0.5mg) in 2.5 mL normal saline q6–8h or two puffs q4–6h

   c. Combination preparations of albuterol and ipratroprium provide the best bronchodilation.[185] DuoNeb contains albuterol 3 mg/ipratropium bromide 0.5 mg given in 3 mL normal saline up to four times a day. The Combivent MDI provides 100 mg of albuterol and about 20 µg of ipratroprium with two inhalations given four times a day.

3. Other bronchodilators

   a. Racemic epinephrine can be used in patients with laryngospasm around the time of endotracheal extubation. It is usually given as 0.5 mL of a 0.25% solution in 3.5 mL normal saline and can be given every four hours.

   b. An IV infusion of low-dose epinephrine is an excellent choice for inotropic support for low cardiac output syndrome because it provides bronchodilatory effects. Since it is also a strong positive chronotrope, it must be used cautiously when sinus tachycardia is present.

   c. Phosphodiesterase inhibitors (aminophylline preparations) have potential cardiac toxicity at higher doses (arrhythmias, tachycardia) and are therefore best avoided, unless the patient has refractory bronchospasm.

4. Inhaled corticosteroids: budesonide-formoterol (Symbicort) may be given along with short-acting SABAs to prevent exacerbations of bronchospasm.

5. Systemic corticosteroids are frequently beneficial when bronchospasm is refractory to the above measures. They may increase airway responsiveness to other β_2-agonists. Dosing regimens involve no more than two weeks of treatment. Two of these protocols are the following:

   a. Methylprednisolone (Solu-Medrol) 0.5 mg/kg IV q6h × 3 days, then prednisone 0.5 mg/kg q12h × 3 d, then 0.5 mg/kg qd × 4 days (10-day total course)

   b. Methylprednisolone 125 mg IV q6h × 3 d, then prednisone 60 mg qd × 4 d, then 40 mg qd × 4 d, then 20 mg qd × 3 days (14-day total course)

6. Note: β-blockers are generally contraindicated during episodes of bronchospasm. However, patients with a history of bronchospastic airways can frequently tolerate the selective β-blockers, such as esmolol, metoprolol, and atenolol. Furthermore, use of β-blockers appears to improve survival in patients with COPD undergoing CABG, with comparable rates of COPD exacerbation as patients not taking β-blockers.[187]

References

1. Apostolakis E, Filos KS, Koletsis E, Dougenis D. Lung dysfunction following cardiopulmonary bypass. *J Card Surg* 2010;25:47–55.

2. Cove ME, Ying C, Taculod JM, et al. Multidisciplinary extubation protocol in cardiac surgical patients reduces ventilation time and length of stay in the intensive care unit. *Ann Thorac Surg* 2016;102:28–34.

3. Chan JL, Miller JG, Murphy M, Greenberg A, Iraola M, Horvath KA. A multidisciplinary protocol-driven approach to improve extubation times after cardiac surgery. *Ann Thorac Surg* 2018;105:1684–90.

4. Nagre AS, Jambures NP. Comparison of immediate extubation versus ultrafast tracking strategy in the management of off-pump coronary artery bypass surgery. *Ann Card Anaesth* 2018;21:129–33.

5. Totonchi Z, Azarfarin R, Jafari L, et al. Feasibility of on-table extubation after cardiac surgery with cardiopulmonary bypass: a randomized clinical trial. *Anesth Pain Med* 2018;24:e80158.

6. Subramaniam K, DeAndrade D, Mendell DR, et al. Predictors of operating room extubation in adult cardiac surgery. *J Thorac Cardiovasc Surg* 2017;154:1656–65.

7. Badhwar V, Esper S, Brooks M, et al. Extubating in the operating room after adult cardiac surgery safely improves outcomes and lowers costs. *J Thorac Cardiovasc Surg* 2014;148:3101–9.

8. Shenkman Z, Shir Y, Weiss YG, Bleiberg B, Gross D. The effects of cardiac surgery on early and late pulmonary functions. *Acta Anaesth Scand* 1997;41:1193–9.

9. Weissman C. Pulmonary function after cardiac and thoracic surgery. *Curr Opin Anaesthesiol* 2000;13:47–51.

10. Urell C, Westerdahl E, Hedenström H, Janson C, Emtner M. Lung function before and two days after open-heart surgery. *Crit Care Research and Practice* 2012;article ID 291628.

11. Çetin E, Altinay L. Effects of cardiopulmonary bypass on pulmonary function in COPD patients undergoing beating heart coronary artery bypass surgery. *Cardiovasc J Afr* 2019;30:1–5.

12. Chiarenza F, Tsoutsouras T, Cassisi C, et al. The effects of on-pump and off-pump coronary artery bypass surgery on respiratory function in the early postoperative period. *J Intensive Care Med* 2019;34:126–32.

13. Izzat MB, Almohammad F, Raslan AF. Off-pump grafting does not reduce postoperative pulmonary dysfunction. *Asian Cardiovasc Thorac Ann* 2017;25:113–7.

14. Reddy SL, Grayson AD, Oo AY, Pullan MD, Poonacha T, Fabri BM. Does off-pump surgery offer benefit in high respiratory risk patients? A respiratory risk stratified analysis in a propensity-matched cohort. *Eur J Cardiothorac Surg* 2006;30:126–31.

15. Foghsgaard S, Gazi D, Bach K, Hansen H, Schmidt TA, Kjaergard HK. Minimally invasive aortic valve replacement reduces atelectasis in cardiac intensive care. *Acute Card Care* 2009;11:169–72.

16. Wheatley GH 3rd, Rosenbaum DH, Paul MC, et al. Improved pain management outcomes with continuous infusion of a local anesthetic after thoracotomy. *J Thorac Cardiovasc Surg* 2005;130:464–8.

17. Ogus H, Selimoglu O, Basaran M, et al. Effect of intrapleural analgesia on pulmonary function and postoperative pain in patients with chronic obstructive pulmonary disease undergoing coronary artery bypass graft surgery. *J Cardiothorac Vasc Anesth* 2007;21:816–9.

18. Toutonchi Z, Ghavidel AA. Continuous local infusion of bupivacaine with ON-Q pump system for pain management after median sternotomy. *Multidiscip Cardio Annal* 2009;2:e8722.

19. Rajakaruna C, Rogers CA, Angelini GD, Ascione R. Risk factors for and economic implications of prolonged ventilation after cardiac surgery. *J Thorac Cardiovasc Surg* 2005;130:1270–7.

20. Cislaghi F, Condemi AM, Corona A. Predictors of prolonged mechanical ventilation in a cohort of 5123 cardiac surgical patients. *Eur J Anaesthesiol* 2009;26:396–403.

21. Legare JF, Hirsch GM, Buth KJ, MacDougall C, Sullivan JA. Preoperative prediction of prolonged mechanical ventilation following coronary artery bypass grafting. *Eur J Cardiothorac Surg* 2001; 20:930–6.

22. Suematsu Y, Sato H, Ohtsuka T, Kotsuka Y, Araki S, Takamoto S. Predictive risk factors for delayed extubation in patients undergoing coronary artery bypass grafting. *Heart Vessels* 2000;15:214–20.

23. Branca P, McGaw P, Light R. Factors associated with prolonged mechanical ventilation following coronary artery bypass surgery. *Chest* 2001;119:537–46.

24. Filsoufi F, Rahmanian PB, Castillo JG, Chikwe J, Adams DH. Logistic risk model predicting postoperative respiratory failure in patients undergoing valve surgery. *Eur J Cardiothorac Surg* 2008;34:953–9.

25. Reddy SLC, Grayson AD, Griffiths EM, Pullan DM, Rashid A. Logistic risk model for prolonged ventilation after adult cardiac surgery. *Ann Thorac Surg* 2007;84:528–36.

26. Dunning J, Au J, Kalkat M, Levine A. A validated rule for predicting patients who require prolonged ventilation post cardiac surgery. *Eur J Cardiothorac Surg* 2003;24:270–6.

27. Hachenberg T, Tenling A, Nyström SO, Tyden H, Hedenstierna G. Ventilation-perfusion inequality in patients undergoing cardiac surgery. *Anesthesiology* 1994;80:509–19.

28. Hagl C, Harringer W, Gohrbandt B, Haverich A. Site of pleural drain insertion and early postoperative pulmonary function following coronary artery bypass grafting with internal mammary artery. *Chest* 1999;115:757–61.

29. Hurlbut D, Myers ML, Lefcoe M, Goldbach M. Pleuropulmonary morbidity: internal thoracic artery versus saphenous vein graft. *Ann Thorac Surg* 1990;50:959–64.

30. Guizilini S, Gomes WJ, Faresin SM, et al. Influence of pleurotomy on pulmonary function after off-pump coronary artery bypass grafting. *Ann Thorac Surg* 2007;84:817–22.

31. Iyem H, Islamoglu F, Yagdi T, et al. Effects of pleurotomy on respiratory sequelae after internal mammary artery harvesting. *Tex Heart Inst J* 2006;33:116–21.

32. Uzun A, Yener AU, Kocabeyoglu S, et al. Effects of pleural opening on respiratory function tests in cardiac surgery: a prospective study. *Eur Rev Med Pharmacol Sci* 2013;17:2310–7.

33. Taggart DP. Respiratory dysfunction after cardiac surgery: effects of avoiding cardiopulmonary bypass and the use of bilateral internal mammary arteries. *Eur J Cardiothorac Surg* 2000;18:31–7.

34. Daganou M, Dimopoulou I, Michalopoulos N, et al. Respiratory complications after coronary artery bypass surgery with unilateral or bilateral internal mammary artery grafting. *Chest* 1998;113:1285–9.

35. O'Brien JW, Johnson SH, VanSteyn SJ, et al. Effects of internal mammary artery dissection on phrenic nerve perfusion and function. *Ann Thorac Surg* 1991;52:182–8.

36. Dimopoulou I, Daganou M, Dafni U, et al. Phrenic nerve dysfunction after cardiac operations: electrophysiologic evaluation of risk factors. *Chest* 1998;113:8–14.

37. Yamazaki K, Kato H, Tsujimoto S, Kitamura R. Diabetes mellitus, internal thoracic artery grafting, and the risk of an elevated hemidiaphragm after coronary artery bypass surgery. *J Cardiothorac Vasc Anesth* 1994;8:437–40.

38. Tripp HF, Bolton JW. Phrenic nerve injury following cardiac surgery: a review. *J Card Surg* 1998;13:218–23.

39. Stephens RS, Shah AS, Whitman GJR. Lung injury and acute respiratory distress syndrome after cardiac surgery. *Ann Thorac Surg* 2013;95:1122–9.

40. Ng CS, Arifi AA, Wan S, et al. Ventilation during cardiopulmonary bypass: impact on cytokine response and cardiopulmonary function. *Ann Thorac Surg* 2008;85:154–62.

41. Wang YC, Huang CH, Tu YK. Effects of positive airway pressure and mechanical ventilation of the lungs during cardiopulmonary bypass on pulmonary adverse events after cardiac surgery: a systematic review and meta-analysis. *J Cardiothorac Vasc Anesth* 2018;32:748–59.

42. Voelker MT, Spieth P. Blood transfusion associated lung injury. *J Thorac Dis* 2019;11:3609–15.

43. Vlaar AP, Hofstra JJ, Determann RM, et al. The incidence, risk factors, and outcome of transfusion-related acute lung injury in a cohort of cardiac surgery patients: a prospective nested case-control study. *Blood* 2011;117:4218–25.

44. Yamagishi T, Ishikawa S, Ohtaki A, Takahashi T, Ohki S, Morishita Y. Obesity and postoperative oxygenation after coronary artery bypass grafting. *Jpn J Thorac Cardiovasc Surg* 2000;48:632–6.

45. Akdur H, Yigit Z, Sözen AB, Cagatay T, Güven O. Comparison of pre- and postoperative pulmonary function in obese and non-obese female patients undergoing coronary artery bypass graft surgery. *Respirology* 2006;11:761–6.

46. Landoni G, Lomivorotov VV, Neto CN, et al. Volatile anesthetics versus total intravenous anesthesia for cardiac surgery. *N Engl J Med* 2019;380:1214–25.

47. Michalopoulos A, Anthi A, Rellos K, Geroulanos S. Effects of positive end-expiratory pressure (PEEP) in cardiac surgery patients. *Respir Med* 1998;92:858–62.

48. Hansdottir V, Philip J, Olsen MF, Eduard C, Houltz E, Ricksten SE. Thoracic epidural versus intravenous patient-controlled analgesia after cardiac surgery: a randomized controlled trial of length of hospital stay and patient-perceived quality of recovery. *Anesthesiology* 2006;104:142–51.

49. Rahman SU, Siddiqi TA, Husain A, et al. Efficacy of parasternal injection of bupivacaine on postoperative pain for early extubation in patients undergoing coronary artery bypass surgery. *J Cardiol Curr Res* 2016;6:00210.

50. White PF, Rawal S, Latham P, et al. Use of a continuous local anesthetic infusion for pain management after median sternotomy. *Anesthesiology* 2003;99:918–23.

51. Koukis I, Argiriou M, Dimakopoulou A, Panagiotakopoulos V, Theakos N, Charitos C. Use of continuous subcutaneous anesthetic infusion in cardiac surgical patients after median sternotomy. *J Cardiothorac Surg* 2008;3:2.

52. Turker G, Goren S, Sahin S, Korfali G, Sayan E. Combination of intrathecal morphine and remifentanil infusion for fast-track anesthesia in off-pump coronary artery bypass surgery. *J Cardiothorac Vasc Anesth* 2005;19:708–13.

53. Lena P, Balarac N, Lena D, et al. Fast-track anesthesia with remifentanil and spinal analgesia for cardiac surgery: the effect on pain control and quality of recovery. *J Cardiothorac Vasc Anesth* 2008;22:536–42.

54. Barr J, Egan TD, Sandoval NF, et al. Propofol dosing regimens for ICU sedation based upon an integrated pharmacokinetic-pharmacodynamic model. *Anesthesiology* 2001;95:324–33.

55. Cheng H, Li Z, Young N, et al. The effect of dexmedetomidine on outcomes of cardiac surgery in elderly patients. *J Cardiothorac Vasc Anesth* 2016;30:1502–8.

56. Wu M, Liang Y, Dai Z, Wang S. Perioperative dexmedetomidine reduces delirium after cardiac surgery: a meta-analysis of randomized controlled trials. *J Clin Anesth* 2018;50:33–42.

57. Ji F, Li Z, Nguyen H, et al. Perioperative dexmedetomidine improves outcomes of cardiac surgery. *Circulation* 2013;127:1576–84.

58. Wanat M, Fitousis K, Boston F, Masud F. Comparison of dexmedetomidine versus propofol for sedation in mechanically ventilated patients after cardiovascular surgery. *Methodist Debakey Cardiovasc J* 2014;10:111–7.

59. Riker RR, Shehabi Y, Bokesch PM, et al. Dexmedetomidine vs midazolam for sedation of critically ill patients: a randomized trial. *JAMA* 2009;301:489–99.

60. Liu Y, Sheng B, Wang S, Lu F, Zhen J, Chen W. Dexmedetomidine prevents acute kidney injury after adult cardiac surgery: a meta-analysis of randomized controlled trials. *BMC Anesthesiol* 2018;18:7.

61. Nguyen J, Nacpil N. Effectiveness of dexmedetomidine versus propofol on extubation times, length of stay, and mortality rates in adult cardiac surgery patients: a systematic review and meta-analysis. *JBI Database System Rev Implement Rep* 2018;16:1220–39.

62. Ruokonen E, Parviainen I, Jakob SM, et al. Dexmedetomidine versus propofol/midazolam for long-term sedation during mechanical ventilation. *Intensive Care Med* 2009;35:282–90.

63. Abuhasna S, Al Jundi A, Abdelatty W, Urrahman M. Evaluation of long-term infusion of dexmedetomidine in critically ill patients: a retrospective analysis. *Int J Crit Illn Inj Sci* 2012;2:70–4.

64. Jakob SM, Ruokonen E, Grounds RM, et al. Dexmedetomidine vs midazolam or propofol for sedation during prolonged mechanical ventilation: two randomized controlled trials. *JAMA* 2012;307:1151–60.

65. Jakob SM, Ruokonen E, Takata J. Efficacy of dexmedetomidine compared with midazolam for sedation in adult intensive care patients. *Br J Anaesth* 2014;112:581–2.

66. Qazi SM, Sindby EJ, Nørgaard MA. Ibuprofen: a safe analgesic during recovery? A randomized controlled trial. *J Cardiovasc Thor Res* 2015;7:141–8.

67. Mamoun MF, Lin P, Zimmerman NM, et al. Intravenous acetaminophen analgesia after cardiac surgery: a randomized, blinded controlled superiority trial. *J Thorac Cardiovasc Surg* 2016;152:881–9.

68. Subramaniam B, Shankar P, Shaefi S, et al. Effect of intravenous acetaminophen vs placebo combined with propofol or dexmedetomidine on postoperative delirium among older patients following cardiac surgery: the DEXACET randomized clinical trial. *JAMA* 2019;321:686–96.

69. Gurbet A, Goren S, Sahin S, Uchunkaya N, Korfali G. Comparison of analgesic effects of morphine, fentanyl, and remifentanil with intravenous patient-controlled analgesia after cardiac surgery. *J Cardiothorac Vasc Anesth* 2004;18:755–8.

70. Baltali S, Turkoz A, Bozdogan N, et al. The efficacy of intravenous patient-controlled remifentanil versus morphine anesthesia after coronary artery surgery. *J Cardiothorac Vasc Anesth* 2009;23:170–4.

71. Bojar RM, Rastegar H, Payne DD, et al. Methemoglobinemia from intravenous nitroglycerin: a word of caution. *Ann Thorac Surg* 1987;43:332–4.

72. Suematsu Y, Sato H, Ohtsuka T, Kotsuka Y, Araki S, Takamoto S. Predictive risk factors for pulmonary oxygen transfer in patients undergoing coronary artery bypass grafting. *Jpn Heart J* 2001;42:143–53.

73. Rady MY, Ryan T, Starr NJ. Early onset of acute pulmonary dysfunction after cardiovascular surgery: risk factors and clinical outcome. *Crit Care Med* 1997;25:1831–9.

74. Liu ZX, Xu FY, Liang X, et al. Efficacy of dexmedetomidine on postoperative shivering: a meta-analysis of clinical trials. *Can J Anaesth* 2015;62:816–29.

75. Dajani GN, Ali M, Heinrich L, et al. Ultra-fast-track anesthetic technique facilitates operating room extubation in patients undergoing off-pump coronary revascularization surgery. *J Cardiothorac Vasc Anesth* 2001;15:152–7.

76. Rodriguez Bianco YF, Candiotti K, Gologorsky A, et al. Factors which predicts safe extubation in the operating room following cardiac surgery. *J Card Surg* 2012;27:275–80.

77. Gershengorn HB, Wunsch H, Hua M, Bavaria JE, Gutsche J. Association of overnight extubation with outcomes after cardiac surgery in the intensive care unit. *Ann Thorac Surg* 2019;108:432–42.

78. Krebs EG, Hawkins RB, Mehaffey JH, et al. Is routine extubation overnight safe in cardiac surgery patients? *J Thorac Cardiovasc Surg* 2019;157:1533–42.

79. Canver CC, Chanda J. Intraoperative and postoperative risk factors for respiratory failure after coronary bypass. *Ann Thorac Surg* 2003;75:853–8.

80. Yende S, Wunderink R. Causes of prolonged mechanical ventilation after coronary artery bypass surgery. *Chest* 2002;122:245–52.

81. Murthy SC, Arroliga AC, Walts PA, et al. Ventilatory dependency after cardiovascular surgery. *J Thorac Cardiovasc Surg* 2007;134:484–90.

82. Lauruschkat AH, Arnrich B, Albert AA, et al. Diabetes mellitus as a risk factor for pulmonary complications after coronary bypass surgery. *J Thorac Cardiovasc Surg* 2008;135:1047–53.

83. Insler SR, O'Connor MS, Leventhal MJ, Nelson DR, Starr NJ. Association between postoperative hypothermia and adverse outcome after coronary artery bypass surgery. *Ann Thorac Surg* 2000;70:175–81.

84. Pandharipande PP, Pun BT, Herr DL, et al. Effect of sedation with dexmedetomidine vs lorazepam on acute brain dysfunction in mechanically ventilated patients: the MENDS randomized controlled trial. *JAMA* 2007;298:2644–53.

85. Ngaage DL, Martins E, Orkell E, et al. The impact of the duration of mechanical ventilation on the respiratory outcome in smokers undergoing cardiac surgery. *Cardiovasc Surg* 2002;10:345–50.

86. Hulzebos EHJ, Helders PJM, Favié NJ, De Bie RA, de la Riviere AB, Van Meeteren NLU. Preoperative intensive inspiratory muscle training to prevent postoperative pulmonary complications in high-risk patients undergoing CABG surgery: a randomized clinical trial. *JAMA* 2006;296:1851–7.

87. Apostolakis EE, Koletsis EN, Baikoussis NG, Siminelakis SN, Papadopoulos GS. Strategies to prevent intraoperative lung injury during cardiopulmonary bypass. *J Cardiothorac Surg* 2010;5:1.

88. Karaiskos TE, Palatianos GM, Triantafillou CD, et al. Clinical effectiveness of leukocyte filtration during cardiopulmonary bypass in patients with chronic obstructive pulmonary disease. *Ann Thorac Surg* 2004;78:1339–44.

89. Boodhwani M, Nathan HJ, Mesana TG, Rubens FD, on behalf of the Cardiotomy Investigators. Effects of shed mediastinal blood on cardiovascular and pulmonary function: a randomized, double-blind study. *Ann Thorac Surg* 2008;86:1167–74.

90. Landoni G, Biondi-Zaccai GG, Marino G, et al. Fenoldopam reduces the need for renal replacement therapy and in-hospital death in cardiovascular surgery: a meta-analysis. *J Cardiothorac Vasc Anesth* 2008;22:27–33.

91. Koch C, Li L, Figueroa P, Mihaljevic T, Svensson L, Blackstone EH. Transfusion and pulmonary morbidity after cardiac surgery. *Ann Thorac Surg* 2009;88:1410–8.

92. Huang H, Yao T, Wang W, et al. Continuous ultrafiltration attenuates the pulmonary injury that follows open heart surgery with cardiopulmonary bypass. *Ann Thorac Surg* 2003;76:136–40.
93. Marik PE, Corwin HL. Acute lung injury following blood transfusion: expanding the definition. *Crit Care Med* 2008;36:3080–4.
94. Toy P, Popovsky MA, Abraham E, et al. Transfusion-related acute lung injury: definition and review. *Crit Care Med* 2005;33:721–6.
95. Jones DP, Byrne P, Morgan C, Fraser I, Hyland R. Positive end-expiratory pressure vs T-piece: extubation after mechanical ventilation. *Chest* 1991;100:1655–9.
96. De Santo LS, Bancone C, Santarpino G, et al. Noninvasive positive-pressure ventilation for extubation failure after cardiac surgery: pilot safety evaluation. *J Thorac Cardiovasc Surg* 2009;137:342–6.
97. Hyzy RC, McSparron JI. Noninvasive ventilation adults with acute respiratory failure: practical aspects of initiation. 2020 www.uptodate.com.
98. Nishimura M. High-flow nasal cannula oxygen therapy in adults: physiological benefits, indication, clinical benefits, and adverse effects. *Respiratory Care* 2016;61:529–41.
99. Frat JP, Coudroy R, Marjanovic N, Thille AW. High-flow nasal oxygen therapy and noninvasive ventilation in the management of acute hypoxemic respiratory failure. *Ann Transl Med* 2017;5:297.
100. Matte P, Jacquet L, Van Dyck M, Goenen M. Effects of conventional physiotherapy, continuous positive airway pressure and non-invasive ventilatory support with bilevel positive airway pressure after coronary artery bypass grafting. *Acta Anaesthesiol Scand* 2000;44:75–81.
101. Gust R, Gottschalk A, Schmidt H, Bottiger BW, Bohrer H, Martin E. Effects of continuous (CPAP) and bi-level positive airway pressure (BiPAP) on extravascular lung water after extubation of the trachea in patients following coronary artery bypass grafting. *Intensive Care Med* 1996;22:1345–50.
102. Vital FM, Saconato H, Ladeira MT, et al. Non-invasive positive pressure ventilation (CPAP or bilevel NPPV) for cardiogenic pulmonary edema. *Cochrane Database Syst Rev* 2008;3.CD005351. https://doi.org/10.1002/14651858.CD005351.pub2.
103. Zarbock A, Mueller E, Netzer S, Gabriel A, Feindt P, Kindgen-Milles D. Prophylactic nasal continuous positive airway pressure following cardiac surgery protects from postoperative pulmonary complications: a prospective, randomized, controlled trial in 500 patients. *Chest* 2009;135:1252–9.
104. Pasquina P, Merlani P, Granier JM, Ricou B. Continuous positive airway pressure versus noninvasive pressure support ventilation to treat atelectasis after cardiac surgery. *Anesth Analg* 2004;99:1001–8.
105. Hyzy RC. Modes of mechanical ventilation. 2019 www.uptodate.com.
106. Overend TJ, Anderson CM, Lucy SD, Bhatia C, Jonsson BI, Timmermans C. The effect of incentive spirometry on postoperative pulmonary complications: a systematic review. *Chest* 2001;120:971–8.
107. Freitas ER, Soares BG, Cardoso JR, Atallah AN. Incentive spirometry for preventing pulmonary complications after coronary artery bypass graft. *Cochrane Database Syst Rev* 2012 Sep 12 (9):CD004466. https://doi.org/10.1002/14651858.CD004466.pub3.
108. Westerdahl E, Lindmark B, Eriksson T, Hedenstierna G, Tenling A. The immediate effects of deep breathing exercises on atelectasis and oxygenation after cardiac surgery. *Scand Cardiovasc J* 2003;37:363–7.
109. Pasquina P, Tramèr MR, Walder B. Prophylactic respiratory physiotherapy after cardiac surgery: systematic review. *BMJ* 2003;327:1379–81.
110. Barker J, Martino R, Reichardt B, Hickey EJ, Ralph-Edwards A. Incidence and impact of dysphagia in patients receiving prolonged endotracheal intubation after cardiac surgery. *Can J Surg* 2009;52:119–24.
111. Zhou XD, Dong WH, Zhao CH, et al. Risk scores for predicting dysphagia in critically ill patients after cardiac surgery. *BMC Anesthesiol* 2019;19:7.
112. Ho KM, Bham E, Pavey W. Incidence of venous thromboembolism and benefits and risks of thromboprophylaxis after cardiac surgery: a systematic review and meta-analysis. *J Am Heart Assoc* 2015;4:e002652.
113. Van Poucke S, Stevens K, Wetzels R, et al. Early platelet recovery following cardiac surgery with cardiopulmonary bypass. *Platelets* 2016;27:751–7.
114. Bednar F, Osmancik P, Hlavicka J, Jedlickova V, Paluch Z, Vanek T. Aspirin is insufficient in inhibition of platelet aggregation and thromboxane formation early after coronary artery bypass surgery. *J Thromb Thrombolysis* 2009;27:394–9.

115. Ahmed AB, Koster A, Lance M, et al. European guidelines on perioperative venous thromboembolism prophylaxis: cardiovascular and thoracic surgery. *Eur J Anaesthesiology* 2018;3:84–9.

116. Gould MK, Garcia DA, Wren SM, et al. Prevention of VTE in nonorthopedic surgical patients: antithrombotic therapy and prevention of thrombosis, 9th ed: American College of Chest Physicians evidence-based clinical practice guidelines. *Chest* 2012;141(2 Suppl):e227S–77S.

117. Bailey ML, Richter SM, Mullany DV, Tesar PJ, Fraser JF. Risk factors and survival in patients with respiratory failure after cardiac operations. *Ann Thorac Surg* 2011;92:1573–9.

118. Tsai BM, Wang M, Turrentine MW, Mahomed Y, Brown JW, Meldrum DR. Hypoxic pulmonary vasoconstriction in cardiothoracic surgery: basic mechanisms to potential therapies. *Ann Thorac Surg* 2004;78:360–8.

119. Cho MS, Sharma S. Transfusion-related acute lung injury (TRALI) [Updated 2019 Jun 4]. In: StatPearls [Internet]. Treasure Island (FL): StatPearls Publishing; 2020 Jan. https://www.ncbi.nlm.nih.gov/books/NBK507846.

120. Semple JW, Rebetz J, Kapur R. Transfusion-associated circulatory overload and transfusion-related acute lung injury. *Blood* 2019;133:1840–53.

121. Malhotra A. Low-tidal-volume ventilation in the acute respiratory distress syndrome. *N Engl J Med* 2007;357:1113–20.

122. Hariharan U, Garg R. Sedation and analgesia in critical care. *J Anesth Crit Care Open Access* 2017;7:00262. doi: 10.15406/jaccoa.2017.07.00262.

123. Hébert PC, Blajchman MA, Cook DJ, et al. Do blood transfusions improve outcomes related to mechanical ventilation? *Chest* 2001;119:1850–7.

124. Kheiri B, Abdalla A, Osman M, et al. Restrictive versus liberal red blood cell transfusions for cardiac surgery: a systematic review and meta-analysis of randomized controlled trials. *J Thromb Thrombolysis* 2019;47:179–85.

125. Estcourt LJL, Roberts DJ. Six-month outcomes after restrictive or liberal transfusion for cardiac surgery (TRICS III trial). *Transfus Med* 2019;29:77–9.

126. Chiumello D, Brioni M. Severe hypoxemia: which strategy to choose. *Crit Care* 2016;20:132.

127. Tabrizi MB, Schinco MA, Tepas JJ 3rd, Hwang J, Spiwak E, Kerwin AJ. Inhaled epoprostenol improves oxygenation in severe hypoxemia. *J Trauma Acute Care Surg* 2012;73:503–6.

128. Torbic H, Szumita PM, Anger KE, Nuccio P, LaGamvina S, Weinhouse G. Inhaled epoprostenol vs inhaled nitric oxide for refractory hypoxemia in critically ill patient. *J Crit Care* 2013;28:844–8.

129. Ammar MA, Bauer SR, Bass SN, Sasidhar M, Mullin R, Lam SW. Noninferiority of inhaled epoprostenol to inhaled nitric oxide for the treatment of ARDS. *Ann Pharmacother* 2015;49:1105–12.

130. Mariscalco G, Biancari F, Zanobini M, et al. Bedside tool for predicting the risk of postoperative atrial fibrillation after cardiac surgery: the POAF score. *J Am Heart Assoc* 2014;3:e000752. doi: 10.1161/JAHA.113.000752.

131. Aydogdu M, Hanazay C, Aldag Y, Bahs A, Bilgin S, Gürsel G. Atrial fibrillation in critical care patients with respiratory failure: incidence and clinical effects. *Eur Resp J* 2012;40:P2014.

132. Tseng YH, Ko HK, Tseng YC, Lin YH, Kou YR. Atrial fibrillation on intensive care unit admission independently increases the risk of weaning failure in nonheart failure mechanically ventilated patients in a medical intensive care unit: a retrospective case-control study. *Medicine (Baltimore)* 2016;95:e3744.

133. Kaushik S, Hussain A, Clarke P, Lazar HL. Acute pulmonary toxicity after low-dose amiodarone therapy. *Ann Thorac Surg* 2001;72:1760–1.

134. MacIntyre NR, Epstein SK, Carson S, Scheinhorn D, Christopher K, Muldoon S. Management of patients requiring prolonged mechanical ventilation: report of a NAMDRC Consensus Conference. *Chest* 2005;128:3937–54.

135. Elefteriades J, Singh M, Tang P, et al. Unilateral diaphragm paralysis: etiology, impact, and natural history. *J Cardiovasc Surg (Torino)* 2008;49:289–95.

136. Versteegh MI, Braun J, Voigt PG, et al. Diaphragm plication in adult patients with diaphragm paralysis leads to long-term improvement of pulmonary function and level of dyspnea. *Eur J Cardiothorac Surg* 2007;32:449–56.

137. Milot J, Perron J, Lacasse Y, Létourneau L, Cartier PC, Maltais F. Incidence and predictors of ARDS after cardiac surgery. *Chest* 2001;119:884–8.

138. Asimakoipoulos G, Taylor KM, Smith PL, Ratnatunga CP. Prevalence of acute respiratory distress syndrome after cardiac surgery. *J Thorac Cardiovasc Surg* 1999;117:620–1.

139. Herlihy JP, Koch SM, Jackson R, Nora H. Course of weaning from prolonged mechanical ventilation after cardiac surgery. *Tex Heart Inst J* 2006;33:122–9.

140. Kollef MH, Levy NT, Ahrens TS, Schaiff R, Prentice D, Sherman G. The use of continuous IV sedation is associated with prolongation of mechanical ventilation. *Chest* 1998;114:541–8.

141. Schweickert WD, Gehlbach BK, Pohlman AS, Hall JB, Kress JP. Daily interruption of sedative medications and complications of critical illness in mechanically ventilated patients. *Crit Care Med* 2004;32:1272–6.

142. Mehta S, Burry L, Martinez-Motta JC, et al. A randomized trial of daily awakening in critically ill patients managed with a sedation protocol: a pilot trial. *Crit Care Med* 2008;36:2092–9.

143. Maillet JM, Thierry S, Brodaty D. Prone positioning and acute respiratory distress syndrome after cardiac surgery: a feasibility study. *J Cardiothorac Vasc Anesth* 2008;22:414–7.

144. Spalding MC, Cripps MW, Minshall CT. Ventilator-associated pneumonia: new definitions. *Crit Care Clin* 2017;33:277–92.

145. Keyt H, Faverio P, Restrepo MI. Prevention of ventilator-associated pneumonia in the intensive care unit: a review of the clinically relevant recent advancements. *Ind J Med Res* 2014;139:814–21.

146. Li Bassi G, Senussi T, Aguilera Xiol E. Prevention of ventilator-associated pneumonia. *Curr Opin Infect Dis* 2017;30:214–20.

147. Kalil AC, Metersky ML, Klompas M, et al. Management of adults with hospital-acquired and ventilator-associated pneumonia: 2016 Clinical Practice Guidelines by the Infectious Diseases Society of America and the American Thoracic Society. *Clin Infect Dis* 2016;63:e61–111.

148. Alhazzani W, Alshamsi F, Belley-Cote E, et al. Efficacy and safety of stress ulcer prophylaxis in critically ill patients: a network meta-analysis of randomized trials. *Intensive Care Med* 2018;44:1–11.

149. Alquraini M, Alshamsi F, Møller MH, et al. Sucralfate versus histamine 2 receptor antagonists for stress ulcer prophylaxis in adult critically ill patients: a meta-analysis and trial sequential analysis of randomized trials. *J Crit Care* 2017;40:21–30.

150. Miano TA, Reichert MG, Houle TT, MacGregor DA, Kincaid EH, Bowton DL. Nosocomial pneumonia risk and stress ulcer prophylaxis: a comparison of pantoprazole vs ranitidine in cardiothoracic surgery patients. *Chest* 2009;136:440–7.

151. Krag M, Marker S, Perner A, et al. Pantoprazole in patients at risk for gastrointestinal bleeding in the ICU. *N Engl J Med* 2018;379:2199–208.

152. Marker S, Perner A, Wetterslev J, et al. Pantoprazole prophylaxis in ICU patients with high severity of disease: a post hoc analysis of the placebo-controlled SUP-ICU trial. *Intensive Care Med* 2019;45:609–18.

153. Kollef MH. Selective digestive decontamination should not be routinely employed. *Chest* 2003; 123:464S–8S.

154. Ballotta A, Kandil H, Generali T, et al. Tracheostomy after cardiac operations: in-hospital and long-term survival. *Ann Thorac Surg* 2011;92:528–34.

155. Devarajan J, Vydyanathan A, Xu M, et al. Early tracheostomy is associated with improved outcomes in patients who require prolonged ventilation after cardiac surgery. *J Am Coll Surg* 2012;214:1008–16.

156. Trouillet JL, Combes A, Vaissier E, et al. Prolonged mechanical ventilation after cardiac surgery: outcome and predictors. *J Thorac Cardiovasc Surg* 2009;138:948–53.

157. Curtis JJ, Clark NC, McKenney CA, et al. Tracheostomy: a risk factor for mediastinitis after cardiac operation. *Ann Thorac Surg* 2001;72:731–4.

158. Rahmanian PB, Adams DH, Castillo JG, Chikwe J, Filsoufi F. Tracheostomy is not a risk factor for deep sternal wound infection after cardiac surgery. *Ann Thorac Surg* 2007;84:1984–92.

159. Zhu G, Huang Y, Wei D, Shi Y. Efficacy and safety of noninvasive ventilation in patients after cardiothoracic surgery: a PRISMA-compliant systematic review and meta-analysis. *Medicine (Baltimore)* 2016;95:e4734.

160. Takasaki Y, Kido T, Semba K. Dexmedetomidine facilitates induction of noninvasive positive pressure ventilation for acute respiratory failure in patients with severe asthma. *J Anesth* 2009;23:147–50.

161. Epstein SK, Walkey A. Methods of weaning from mechanical ventilation. www.uptodate.com 2019.

162. McConville JF, Kress JP. Weaning patients from the ventilator. *N Engl J Med* 2012;367:2233–9.

163. Schmidt GA, Girard TD, Kress JP, et al. Official Executive Summary of an American Thoracic Society/American College of Chest Physicians Clinical Practice Guideline: liberation from mechanical ventilation in critically ill adults. *Am J Respir Crit Care Med* 2017;195:115–9.

164. MacIntyre N. Discontinuing mechanical ventilatory support. *Chest* 2007;132:1049–56.

165. MacIntyre NR. The ventilator discontinuation process: an expanding evidence base. *Respir Care* 2013;58:1074–82.

166. Esteban E, Alía I, Tobin MJ, et al. Effect of spontaneous breathing trial duration on outcome of attempts to discontinue mechanical ventilation: Spanish Lung Failure Cooperative Group. *Am J Respir Crit Care Med* 1999;159:512–8.

167. Engoren M. Evaluation of the cuff-leak test in a cardiac surgery population. *Chest* 1999;116:1029–31.

168. Kriner EJ, Shafazand S, Colice GL. The endotracheal tube cuff-leak test as a predictor for postextubation stridor. *Respir Care* 2005;50:1632–8.

169. Prinianakis G, Alexopoulou C, Mamidakis E, Kondili E, Georgopoulos D. Determinants of the cuff-leak test: a physiological study. *Crit Care* 2005;9:R24–31.

170. Sandhu RS, Pasquale MD, Miller K, Wasser TE. Measurement of endotracheal tube cuff leak to predict postextubation stridor and need for reintubation. *J Am Coll Surg* 2000;190:682–7.

171. Jaber S, Jung B, Chanques G, Bonnet F, Marret E. Effects of steroids on reintubation and postextubation stridor in adults: meta-analysis of randomized controlled trials. *Crit Care* 2009;13:R49.

172. Roberts RJ, Welch SM, Devlin JW. Corticosteroids for prevention of postextubation laryngeal edema in adults. *Ann Pharmacother* 2008;42:686–91.

173. Lee CH, Peng MJ, Wu CL. Dexamethasone to prevent postextubation airway obstruction in adults: a prospective, randomized, double-blind, placebo-controlled trial. *Crit Care* 2007;11:R72.

174. Yang KL, Tobin MJ. A prospective study of indexes predicting the outcome of trials of weaning from mechanical ventilation. *N Engl J Med* 1991;324:1445–50.

175. Frutos-Vivar F, Ferguson ND, Esteban A, et al. Risk factors for extubation failure in patients following a spontaneous breathing trial. *Chest* 2006;130:1664–71.

176. Meade M, Guyatt G, Sinuff T, et al. Trials comparing alternative weaning modes and discontinuation assessments. *Chest* 2001;120:425S–37S.

177. Kwiatt M, Tarbox A, Seamon MJ, et al. Thoracostomy tubes: A comprehensive review of complications and related topics. *Int J Crit Illn Inj Sci* 2014;4:43–55.

178. Light RW, Rogers JT, Moyers JP, et al. Prevalence and clinical course of pleural effusions at 30 days after coronary artery and cardiac surgery. *Am J Respir Crit Care Med* 2002;166:1567–71.

179. Payne M, Magovern GJ Jr, Benckart DH, et al. Left pleural effusion after coronary artery bypass decreases with a supplemental pleural drain. *Ann Thorac Surg* 2002;73:149–52.

180. Kopterides P, Lignos M, Papanikolaou S, et al. Pleural effusion causing cardiac tamponade: report of two cases and review of the literature. *Heart Lung* 2006;35:66–7.

181. Bilku RS, Bilku DK, Rosin MD, Been M. Left ventricular diastolic collapse and late regional cardiac tamponade postcardiac surgery caused by large left pleural effusion. *J Am Soc Echocardiogr* 2008;21:978.

182. Cao W, Wang Y, Zhou N, Xu B. Efficacy of ultrasound-guided thoracentesis catheter drainage for pleural effusion. *Onco Lett* 2016;12:4445–8.

183. Aljazairi AS, Bhuiyan TA, Alwadai AH, Almehizia RA. Octreotide use in post-cardiac surgery chylothorax: a 12-year perspective. *Asian Cardiovasc Thorac Ann* 2017;25:6–12.

184. Kilic D, Sahin E, Gulcan O, Bolat B, Turkoz R, Hatipoglu A. Octreotide for treating chylothorax after cardiac surgery. *Tex Heart Inst J* 2005;32:437–9.

185. The COMBIVENT Inhalation Solution Study Group. Routine nebulized ipratropium and albuterol together are better than either alone in COPD. *Chest* 1997;112:1514–21.

186. Global Initiative for Asthma. Pocket guide for asthma management and prevention. 2019 Ginasthma. org/pocket-guide.

187. Angeloni E, Melina G, Roscitano A, et al. ß-blockers improve survival of patients with chronic obstructive pulmonary disease after coronary artery bypass grafting. *Ann Thorac Surg* 2013;95:525–32.

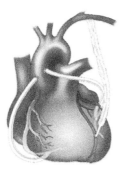

CHAPTER 11

Cardiovascular Management

♡ 11 Cardiovascular Management

The achievement of satisfactory hemodynamic performance is the primary objective of postoperative cardiac surgical management. Optimal cardiac function ensures adequate perfusion and oxygenation of other organ systems and improves the chances for an uneventful recovery from surgery. Even brief periods of cardiac dysfunction can lead to impairment of organ system function, leading to potentially life-threatening complications. This chapter presents the basic concepts in cardiovascular management and then reviews the evaluation and management of low cardiac output syndrome, hypertension, perioperative myocardial infarction, coronary spasm, cardiac arrest, and rhythm disturbances that can contribute to compromised cardiovascular function.

I. Basic Principles

The important concepts of postoperative cardiac care are those of cardiac output, tissue oxygenation, and the ratio of myocardial oxygen supply and demand. Ideally, one should strive to obtain a cardiac index greater than 2.2 L/min/m² with a normal mixed venous oxygen saturation, reflecting adequate oxygen delivery to meet metabolic needs, while optimizing the myocardial oxygen supply:demand ratio.[1–4]

A. **Cardiac output** is determined by the stroke volume and heart rate (CO = SV × HR). The stroke volume is equal to the left ventricular end-diastolic volume (LVEDV) minus the left ventricular end-systolic volume (LVESV) and is calculated by dividing the cardiac output by the heart rate. The three major determinants of stroke volume are preload, afterload, and contractility.

　　1. **Preload** refers to the LV end-diastolic fiber length and is generally considered to reflect the LVEDV. Although this can be estimated best by echocardiography, preload in the postoperative patient is more commonly assessed by a measurement of left-sided filling pressures using a Swan-Ganz pulmonary artery catheter. These include the pulmonary artery diastolic (PAD) pressure and pulmonary capillary wedge pressure (PCWP). Thus, these pressure measurements acts as surrogates for the assessment of preload. The left atrial pressure (LAP) provides a more precise approximation of the left ventricular end-diastolic pressure (LVEDP), but requires placement of a catheter directly into the left atrium at the time of surgery. The relationship between filling pressures and volumes is determined by ventricular compliance.

　　　　a. The PAD and PCW pressures generally correlate with each other, and in most patients "wedging" of the catheter is unnecessary. However, the PAD may be

Manual of Perioperative Care in Adult Cardiac Surgery, Sixth Edition. Robert M. Bojar.
© 2021 John Wiley & Sons Ltd. Published 2021 by John Wiley & Sons Ltd.

higher than the PCW pressure in patients with preexisting precapillary pulmonary hypertension (PH) or intrinsic pulmonary disease, in whom there is an increased transpulmonary gradient (equal to the PA mean pressure minus the PCW pressure). In these patients, the PAD pressure will underestimate the LV volume status, yet wedging of the catheter is not recommended because of an increased risk of PA rupture.

   i. Filling pressures must be interpreted cautiously in the early postoperative period.[5-7] The PAD and PCW pressures often correlate poorly with the LVEDV early after surgery and tend to be elevated relative to the intracardiac volume status due to altered ventricular compliance from myocardial edema resulting from cardiopulmonary bypass (CPB) and the use of cardioplegia solutions. Furthermore, the release of various inflammatory substances during bypass and the administration of blood products may increase the pulmonary vascular resistance (PVR), increasing the PAD out of proportion to actual left-sided filling. A stiff, hypertrophied left ventricle noted in patients with hypertension or aortic stenosis has reduced ventricular compliance and frequently manifests diastolic dysfunction coming off bypass. These patients usually require high filling pressures to achieve adequate ventricular filling. In contrast, the dilated, volume-overloaded heart may be highly compliant, with an elevated LVEDV at lower pressures.

   ii. Elevated filling pressures measured by a Swan-Ganz catheter are somewhat insensitive to the status of intracardiac volume and in predicting fluid responsiveness.[7-9] Numerous studies have shown that goal-directed therapy (GDT) using alternative monitoring techniques, such as pulse pressure and stroke volume variation, is more accurate in predicting fluid responsiveness. GDT is designed to optimize fluid administration with subsequent use of inotropic medications to improve the cardiac output. GDT may increase volume administration, but it reduces vasopressor use, the duration of ventilation, and complications, producing a shorter hospital length of stay, but with no impact on mortality.[4,10-14]

  b. For patients with relatively normal ventricular function, many centers do not use Swan-Ganz catheters, and they rely upon central venous pressure (CVP) measurements to assess preload. Although this is a less accurate means of assessing preload in the diseased heart, it gives a fairly good approximation of left-heart filling in the normal heart.[15,16] One study showed that use of a Swan-Ganz catheter provided no mortality benefit in low-risk patients and, in fact, increased mortality in high-risk patients, although patient selection for use of the catheter had to be taken into consideration.[17] Generally, if the CVP exceeds 15–18 mm Hg, inotropic support is indicated. If the patient has other signs of low cardiac output (poor oxygenation, tapering urine output, acidosis), additional monitoring, whether it be by transpulmonary thermodilution (PiCCO, Pulsion Medical Systems), pulse contour analysis (FloTrac/Vigileo, Edwards Lifesciences),[18] or insertion of a Swan-Ganz catheter, will allow for a more objective evaluation of the problem.

  c. Despite the invasiveness of the Swan-Ganz catheter and concerns about its precise value in most patients, most anesthesiologists and cardiac surgeons still use it for perioperative management, since it is a less-expensive, time-proven means of providing scientific information about trends in hemodynamic management to those managing the patient in the critical early postoperative period.[19] Its use actually supports the theory that GDT is beneficial, especially for the patient with tenuous hemodynamics after surgery.

2. **Afterload** refers to the left ventricular systolic wall tension, which is related to the intraventricular systolic pressure and wall thickness. It is determined by both the preload (Laplace's law relating radius to wall tension) and the systemic vascular resistance (SVR) against which the heart must eject after the period of isovolumic contraction. The SVR can be calculated from measurements obtained from the Swan-Ganz catheter (Table 11.1) and should be indexed to the patient's size. The use of vasodilators to lower the SVR may improve the stroke volume, often in combination with volume infusions and inotropic agents.

Table 11.1 • Hemodynamic Formulas

Formula	Normal values
Cardiac output (CO) and Index (CI) $CO = SV \times HR$ $CI = CO/BSA$	4–8 L/min 2.2–4.0 L/min/m²
Stroke volume (SV) $SV = CO(L/min) \times \dfrac{1000(mL/L)}{HR}$	60–100 mL/beat (1 mL/kg/beat)
Stroke volume index (SVI) $SVI = SV/BSA$	33–47 mL/beat/m²
Mean arterial pressure (MAP) $MAP = DP + \dfrac{(SP - DP)}{3}$	70–100 mm Hg
Systemic vascular resistance (SVR) $SVR = \dfrac{MAP - CVP}{CO} \times 80$	800–1200 dyn-s/cm⁵
Pulmonary vascular resistance (PVR) $PVR = \dfrac{PAP - PCWP}{CO} \times 80$	50–250 dyn-s/cm⁵
Left ventricular stroke work index (LVSWI) $LVSWI = SVI \times (MAP - PCWP) \times 0.0136$	45–75 g/M/m²/beat

BSA, body surface area; HR, heart rate; DP, diastolic pressure; SP, systolic pressure; CVP, central venous pressure; PAP, mean pulmonary artery pressure; PCWP, pulmonary capillary wedge pressure

3. **Contractility** is the intrinsic strength of myocardial contraction at constant preload and afterload. However, it can be improved by increasing preload or heart rate, decreasing the afterload, or using inotropic medications.

   a. Contractility generally reflects systolic function as assessed by the ejection fraction (EF), but it is only indirectly related to the cardiac output. For example, the cardiac output generated by a dysfunctional dilated ventricle with a poor EF may be comparable to or greater than that generated by a normal sized heart with a normal EF, especially if a significant tachycardia is present. Furthermore, a low cardiac output does not necessarily imply that ventricular function is impaired. It may be noted with slow heart rates, hypovolemia, and with a small, hypertrophied ventricle.

   b. Nonetheless, the state of contractility is usually inferred from an analysis of the cardiac output and filling pressures, based upon which steps can be taken to optimize hemodynamic performance. In cardiac surgery patients, the cardiac output is usually obtained by thermodilution technology using a Swan-Ganz catheter and bedside computer. A measured aliquot of volume is infused into the CVP port of the catheter and the thermistor near the tip measures the pattern of temperature change from which the computer calculates the cardiac output. A continuous cardiac output catheter is frequently used during off-pump surgery and can provide frequent in-line assessments of the cardiac output. The FloTrac device calculates the cardiac output from the energy of the arterial pressure waveform and is helpful when thermodilution assessment appears inaccurate or the Swan-Ganz PA catheter has been removed.[18] There are numerous other less-invasive hemodynamic monitoring system available, many of which have been used in the GDT studies.

B. **Tissue oxygenation**

1. Oxygen delivery to tissues is the basic principle upon which hemodynamic support should be based. It is determined by the cardiac output (CO), the hemoglobin (Hb) level, and the arterial oxygen saturation (SaO_2). This is represented by the equation:

$$O_2 \text{ delivery} = CO\,(Hb \times \%\ \text{sat}\,)(1.39) + (PaO_2)(0.0031)$$

   where 1.39 is the mL of oxygen transported per gram of Hb and 0.0031 is the solubility coefficient of oxygen dissolved in solution (mL/torr of PaO_2).

2. It should be noted in this equation that the majority of oxygen transported to the tissues is in the form of oxygen bound to Hb, not that dissolved in solution. Thus, one of the major factors lowering O_2 delivery in the postoperative period is a low hemoglobin (Hb) or hematocrit (HCT). Increasing the Hb level by 1 g/dL can increase blood oxygen content by 1.39 vol%, whereas an increase in PaO_2 of 100 torr will only transport an additional 0.3 vol% of oxygen. However, in the profoundly anemic patient, dissolved oxygen represents a greater proportion of the oxygen delivered to tissues. Therefore, it is important to maintain the arterial oxygen

saturation as close to 100% and to normalize the cardiac output to achieve adequate O_2 delivery. However, trying to achieve supranormal cardiac outputs with excessive volume infusions and inotropes is probably more harmful than beneficial to myocardial metabolism.

3. Due to concerns that blood transfusions are not benign, numerous studies have attempted to identify the safe lower limit for hematocrit to establish an appropriate transfusion trigger. Transfused blood contains proinflammatory cytokines and low levels of 2,3-DPG with increased Hb affinity for oxygen, which reduces tissue oxygen delivery. Transfusions are associated with an increased risk of myocardial infarction (MI), respiratory complications, stroke, renal failure, infections, and mortality.[20-22] Thus, the transfusion trigger should be based on evidence of impaired oxygen delivery to tissues or hemodynamic issues. Numerous studies have demonstrated comparable outcomes using either a restrictive (transfuse if Hb <7–7.5 g/dL) and liberal (transfuse if Hb <9 g/dL) strategy.[23,24] Thus, it is reasonable to accept a hematocrit of 21% in the stable postoperative patient and to prescribe iron supplements or, on occasion, even erythropoietin. However, it is also reasonable to transfuse patients to a hematocrit over 25% when they are elderly, frail and deconditioned, have poor ventricular function, borderline respiratory function, hypotension, tachycardia, ischemic ECG changes, oliguria, or a metabolic acidosis.

4. **Mixed venous oxygen saturation (SvO_2)** can be used to assess the adequacy of tissue perfusion and oxygenation, aiming for an SvO_2 >60%. Swan-Ganz PA catheters using reflective fiberoptic oximetry are available to monitor the SvO_2 in the pulmonary artery on a continuous basis. Intermittent SvO_2 measurements can be obtained from blood samples from the distal PA port of the Swan-Ganz catheter. A change of 10% in the SvO_2 can occur before any change is noted in hemodynamic parameters. Despite its theoretical benefit, several studies have suggested that the SvO_2 is an unreliable and insensitive predictor of the cardiac output since it is really measuring the balance between oxygen delivery and consumption.[25,26] However, since it does reflect the adequacy of tissue oxygenation, it should indicate whether the cardiac output is sufficient to meet tissue needs. When analyzed in conjunction with other hemodynamic parameters, trends in the SvO_2 offer insight into both cardiac performance and tissue oxygen delivery.

   a. In the postoperative cardiac surgical patient, a fall in SvO_2 generally reflects decreased oxygen delivery or increased oxygen extraction by tissues and is suggestive of a reduction in cardiac output. However, other constantly changing factors that affect oxygen supply and demand may also influence SvO_2 and must be taken into consideration. These include shivering, pain, agitation, temperature, anemia, alteration in FiO_2, and the efficiency of alveolar gas exchange. The Fick equation, which uses the arteriovenous oxygen content difference to determine cardiac output, can be rearranged as follows:

$$SvO_2 = SaO_2 - \frac{VO_2}{Hb \times 1.39 \times CO} \times 10$$

where:

SvO_2 = mixed venous oxygen saturation

SaO_2 = arterial oxygen saturation

VO_2 = oxygen consumption

normal PvO_2 = 40 torr and SvO_2 = 75%

normal PaO_2 = 100 torr and SaO_2 = 99%

b. This equation indicates that a decrease in SvO_2 may result from a decrease in SaO_2, cardiac output, or hemoglobin level, or an increase in oxygen consumption.

c. When the arterial O_2 saturation is normal (SaO_2 >95%), an SvO_2 <60% suggests the presence of a decreased cardiac output and the need for further assessment and therapeutic intervention. Conversely, a high SvO_2 may reflect less oxygen extraction, as seen with hypothermia, sepsis, or intracardiac or significant peripheral arteriovenous shunting. When this is noted, oxygen delivery or utilization may be impaired and an otherwise "normal" cardiac output may be insufficient to provide adequate tissue oxygenation.

d. Studies have also analyzed whether the central venous oxygen saturation ($ScvO_2$) has value in perioperative management. Many GDT protocols do utilize this parameter and have found that its use improved outcomes. Although a very low $ScvO_2$ is most likely associated with a low cardiac output, the $ScvO_2$ is not as accurate as the SvO_2 in assessing either tissue oxygenation or cardiac output.[26,27]

5. When the cardiac index exceeds 2.2 L/min/m² and the arterial oxygen saturation is adequate (>95%), it may be inferred that oxygen delivery to the tissues is satisfactory. Thus, SvO_2 measurements to assess oxygen delivery are not necessary. However, there are a few situations in which calculation of tissue oxygenation may be valuable in assessing cardiac function:

a. When the thermodilution cardiac output is unreliable (tricuspid regurgitation, improperly positioned Swan-Ganz catheter) or cannot be obtained (Swan-Ganz catheter has not been placed or cannot be placed, such as in the patient with a mechanical tricuspid valve or central venous thrombosis, or has been removed).[28]

b. When the thermodilution cardiac output may seem spuriously low and inconsistent with the clinical scenario (malfunctioning Swan-Ganz catheter or incorrect calibration of computer). A normal SvO_2 indicates that the cardiac output is sufficient to meet tissue metabolic demands.

c. When the cardiac output is marginal, in-line assessment of trends in the mixed venous oxygen saturation can provide up-to-date information on the relative status of cardiac function.

C. **Myocardial oxygen supply and demand**

1. **Myocardial O_2 demand (mvO_2)** is influenced by factors similar to those that determine the cardiac output (afterload, preload, heart rate, contractility). Reducing afterload will generally improve cardiac output with a decrease in mvO_2, whereas an increase in any of the other three factors will improve cardiac output at the expense of an increase in mvO_2. Preoperative management of the patient with ischemic heart disease is primarily directed towards minimizing O_2 demand.[29]

2. **Myocardial O$_2$ supply** is determined by coronary blood flow, the duration of diastole, coronary perfusion pressure, the Hb level, and the arterial oxygen saturation When complete revascularization has been achieved, postoperative management is directed towards optimizing factors that improve O$_2$ supply and, to a lesser degree, minimize an increase in O$_2$ demand.

   a. A heart rate of 80–90 bpm should be achieved and excessive tachycardia and arrhythmias must be avoided.

   b. An adequate perfusion pressure (mean arterial pressure [MAP] >70 mm Hg) should be maintained, taking care to avoid both hypotension and hypertension.

   c. Ventricular distention and wall stress (i.e. afterload) should be minimized by avoiding excessive preload, reducing the SVR, and using inotropic medications to improve contractility.

   d. The hematocrit should be maintained at a safe level. Although an increased level of Hb should improve oxygen delivery, transfusions carry inherent risks. In general, myocardial ischemia should not occur in the well-protected, revascularized heart unless the hematocrit drops into the low 20s.

   e. Ischemic ECG changes suggest that coronary blood flow may not be adequate. This may result from stenosis, thrombus, or spasm in a native vessel, anastomotic stenosis, kinking, thrombus or spasm in a bypass graft, or incomplete revascularization. If ECG changes are noted, immediate attention and possible reevaluation by catheterization are indicated.

II. Low Cardiac Output Syndrome

A. The achievement of a satisfactory cardiac output to achieve adequate tissue oxygenation is the primary objective of postoperative cardiovascular management. Hemodynamic norms for the patient recovering uneventfully from cardiac surgery are a cardiac index (CI) greater than 2.0 L/min/m^2, a PAD or PCW pressure below 20 mm Hg, and a heart rate below 100 bpm with an SvO$_2$ >65%. The patient should have warm, well-perfused extremities with an excellent urine output.

B. **Risk factors** for low cardiac output states include:[4,16,30,31]

   1. Preoperative clinical factors: advanced age, malnutrition, diabetes with chronic kidney disease, LV systolic dysfunction, (e.g. low EF or cardiac output), and diastolic dysfunction (e.g. low cardiac output often with a hyperdynamic ventricle and an LVEDP >20 mm Hg).

   2. Preoperative abnormal lab values including anemia and elevated BNP levels

   3. Operative factors: longer durations of aortic cross-clamping or CPB, emergency surgery and reoperations, CABG with incomplete revascularization, concomitant CABG-valve operations, mitral valve surgery.

   4. Diastolic dysfunction. After weaning from CPB, this is a particularly difficult problem to treat and usually requires pharmacologic support for a low output state despite normal systolic function.[32]

   5. Increased lactate release after five minutes of reperfusion is an independent predictor of a low cardiac output. It suggests that there is delayed recovery of aerobic metabolism, perhaps as a result of inadequate myocardial protection.[33]

C. **Pathophysiology.** A basic principle of cardiac surgery is to prevent myocardial damage while a corrective procedure is being performed. Although this has led to the concept of off-pump bypass surgery or even beating heart surgery, the vast majority of open-heart operations involve use of CPB with cardioplegic arrest. Despite adherence to basic principles and with improvements in cardioplegic solutions, including the more recent adoption of del Nido cardioplegia, myocardial protection is never perfect, and more myocardial injury tends to occur with longer cross-clamp times. In general, myocardial function declines for about 6–8 hours following surgery, presumably from ischemia/reperfusion injury with use of cardioplegic arrest, and from the systemic inflammatory response. It then usually returns to baseline within 24 hours in the absence of significant myocardial injury (see section VIII, pages 586–589, on perioperative myocardial infarction).[34]

1. Temporary inotropic support is often required during this period to optimize hemodynamic performance. Drugs used at the conclusion of CPB should generally be continued for this brief period of time and can be weaned once the cardiac output is satisfactory. Although use of low-dose inotropes for several hours is fairly common in most practices, even independent of LV function, studies do suggest that patients who receive inotropes after surgery have a higher mortality rate.[35]

2. When marginal ventricular function is present in the anesthetized or sedated patient, the compensatory mechanisms that can augment cardiac output in the awake patient are blunted. These include sympathetic autonomic stimulation and endogenous catecholamine production that can increase heart rate, contractility, and arterial and venous tone, elevating both preload and afterload. All of these factors may improve cardiac output or systemic blood pressure, but they may also increase myocardial oxygen demand at a time when asymptomatic ischemia may be present.

3. When these compensatory mechanisms are not present in the sedated patient, therapeutic intervention is necessary to improve the cardiac output. It is imperative to intervene before or at the first sign of clinical manifestations of a low cardiac output syndrome. These include:

   a. Poor peripheral perfusion with pale, cool extremities, and diaphoresis

   b. Pulmonary congestion and poor oxygenation

   c. Impaired renal perfusion and oliguria

   d. Metabolic acidosis

4. The use of invasive monitoring to continuously evaluate a patient's hemodynamic status allows for appropriate therapeutic interventions to be undertaken before these clinical signs become apparent. Nonetheless, subtle findings, such as a progressive tachycardia or cool extremities, should alert the astute clinician to the fact that the patient needs more intensive management. Intervention is indicated for a low cardiac output state, defined as a cardiac index below 2.0 L/min/m², usually associated with left-sided filling pressures exceeding 20 mm Hg and an SVR exceeding 1500 dyn-s/cm⁵. It cannot be overemphasized that observing trends in hemodynamic parameters, rather than absolute numbers, is important when evaluating a patient's progress or deterioration.

5. A general scheme for the management of postoperative hemodynamic problems is presented in Table 11.2.

Table 11.2 • Management of Hemodynamic Problems

BP	PCW	CO	SVR	Plan
↓	↓	↓	↓	Volume
N	↑	N	↑	Venodilator or diuretic
↓	↑	↓	↑	Inotrope
↑	↑	↓	↑	Vasodilator
↑↓	↑	↓	↑	Inotrope/vasodilator/IABP
↓	N	N ↑	↓	α-agent

↑ increased; ↓ decreased; N normal; ↑↓ variable

D. **Etiology.** A low cardiac output state is usually associated with impaired left or right systolic function and may result from abnormal preload, contractility, heart rate, or afterload. However, a variety of other factors may be contributory. It may also be noted in patients with satisfactory systolic function but marked left ventricular hypertrophy (LVH) and diastolic dysfunction.[1-4,16,36]

1. Decreased left ventricular preload
   a. Hypovolemia (bleeding, vasodilation from warming, narcotics, or sedatives)
   b. Cardiac tamponade
   c. Positive-pressure ventilation and PEEP
   d. Right ventricular dysfunction (RV infarction, PH)
   e. Tension pneumothorax
2. Decreased contractility
   a. Low ejection fraction
   b. Myocardial "stunning" from transient ischemia/reperfusion injury or myocardial ischemia; perioperative infarction
      i. Poor intraoperative myocardial protection
      ii. Incomplete myocardial revascularization
      iii. Anastomotic complications/graft thrombosis
      iv. Native coronary artery or graft spasm
      v. Evolving infarction at time of surgery
   c. Hypoxia, hypercarbia, acidosis
3. Tachy- and bradyarrhythmias
   a. Tachycardia with reduced cardiac filling time
   b. Bradycardia
   c. Atrial arrhythmias with loss of atrial contraction

   d. Ventricular arrhythmias

   e. Second- or third-degree heart block

4. Increased afterload

   a. Vasoconstriction

   b. Fluid overload and ventricular distention

   c. Left ventricular outflow tract obstruction following mitral valve repair or replacement (from struts or retained leaflet tissue or uncorrected hypertrophic obstructive cardiomyopathy)

5. Diastolic dysfunction with impaired relaxation and high filling pressures[37]

6. Syndromes associated with cardiovascular instability and hypotension

   a. Sepsis (hypotension from a reduction in SVR; hyperdynamic with a high cardiac output early and myocardial depression at a later stage)

   b. Anaphylactic reactions (blood products, drugs)

   c. Adrenal insufficiency (primary or in the patient on preoperative steroids)

   d. Protamine reactions

E. **Assessment** (abnormalities of concern noted in parentheses)

1. Bedside physical examination: breath sounds, jugular venous distention, murmurs, warmth of extremities, and peripheral pulses (cool extremities, weak pulses, distended neck veins)

2. Hemodynamic measurements: assess filling pressures and determine the cardiac output with a Swan-Ganz catheter; calculate SVR; measure SvO_2 (low cardiac output, high filling pressures, high SVR, low SvO_2)

3. Arterial blood gases (hypoxia, hypercarbia, acidosis/alkalosis) hematocrit (anemia), and serum potassium (hypo- or hyperkalemia)

4. ECG (ischemia, arrhythmias, conduction abnormalities)

5. Chest x-ray (pneumothorax, hemothorax, position of the endotracheal tube or intra-aortic balloon)

6. Urinary output (oliguria)

7. Chest tube drainage (mediastinal bleeding)

8. Two-dimensional echocardiography is very helpful when the cause of a low cardiac output syndrome is unclear. Along with hemodynamic measurements, it can help identify whether it is related to LV systolic or diastolic dysfunction, RV systolic dysfunction, or cardiac tamponade.

9. **Transesophageal echocardiography (TEE)** provides better and more complete information than a transthoracic study and can be readily performed in the intubated patient. It should always be considered when the clinical picture is consistent with tamponade but a transthoracic study is inconclusive.[38]

F. **Treatment** (Table 11.3)

1. Ensure satisfactory **oxygenation** and **ventilation** (see Chapter 10).

2. Treat **ischemia** or **coronary spasm** if suspected to be present due to ECG changes. Myocardial ischemia often responds to intravenous nitroglycerin (IV NTG) but may require further investigation if it persists. Coronary spasm (see section IX, pages 589–591) can be difficult to diagnose but usually responds to IV NTG and/or a calcium channel blocker (CCB), such as sublingual nifedipine or IV diltiazem.

Table 11.3 • Management of Low Cardiac Output Syndrome
1. Look for noncardiac correctable causes (respiratory, acid–base, electrolytes)
2. Treat ischemia or coronary spasm
3. Optimize preload (PAD/PCW or LA pressure of 18–20 mm Hg)
4. Optimize heart rate at 90 bpm with pacing
5. Control arrhythmias
6. Assess cardiac output and start an inotrope if cardiac index is less than 2.0 L/min/m²
• Epinephrine unless arrhythmias or tachycardia
• Dobutamine (if high SVR)
• Milrinone along with a catecholamine
7. Calculate SVR and start a vasodilator if SVR over 1500
• Clevidipine or nitroprusside if moderate–high filling pressures, SVR, and BP
• IV NTG if high filling pressures or evidence of coronary ischemia or spasm
8. If SVR is low
• Norepinephrine if marginal cardiac output
• Phenylephrine if satisfactory cardiac output
• Vasopressin 0.01–0.1 units/min if satisfactory cardiac output
9. Blood transfusion if hematocrit less than 22%
10. IABP if refractory to pharmacologic intervention
11. Ventricular assist device if no response to the above

3. Optimize **preload** by raising filling pressures with volume infusion to a PAD or PCW pressure of about 18–20 mm Hg. Despite concerns that these pressures are insensitive measures of preload, their trends generally indicate when additional measures may be required to optimize cardiac output. Most times, a volume infusion that raises the PAD is all that is necessary to achieve a satisfactory cardiac output. This can initially be achieved using crystalloid or colloid solutions (see Chapter 12, page 678). Volume infusion is preferable to atrial pacing for improving cardiac output because it produces less metabolic demand on the recovering myocardium.[39]

a. Again, because left-sided filling pressures are only surrogates for ventricular volume, the correlation between the two is best assessed from a review of pre- and intra-operative hemodynamic data and an understanding of the patient's cardiac pathophysiology. Filling pressures will differ once the patient is anesthetized due to alterations in loading conditions and autonomic tone. They will subsequently be affected by reduced ventricular compliance at the termination of CPB. Direct visual inspection of the heart, evaluation of TEE images to correlate ventricular end-diastolic dimensions with filling pressures, and measurement of cardiac outputs at the same time will usually indicate the appropriate filling pressures for optimal ventricular filling and cardiac performance in the early postoperative period.

b. For example, a PAD or PCW pressure around 15–18 mm Hg is usually best for patients with preserved LV function. In contrast, a pressure in the low 20s may be necessary to achieve adequate preload in the patient with poor LV function, a stiff hypertrophied ventricle with diastolic dysfunction, a small LV chamber (mitral or aortic stenosis or after resection of a left ventricular aneurysm), or preexisting PH from mitral valve disease. Ventricular size and compliance should be kept in mind when deciding whether additional volume is the next appropriate step in the patient with marginal cardiac function.

c. The response to volume infusion may be variable (see the postoperative scenario described on pages 377–380). Failure of filling pressures to rise with volume may result from the capillary leak that is present during the early postoperative period. It may also result from vasodilation associated with rewarming or the use of medications with vasodilator properties, such as propofol or narcotics. It is more common in the volume-overloaded compliant ventricle. However, it may also reflect the beneficial attenuation of peripheral vasoconstriction that is attributable to an improvement in cardiac output caused by the volume infusion. As the SVR and afterload gradually decrease, the cardiac output may improve further without an increase in preload.

d. A rise in filling pressures without improvement in cardiac output may adversely affect myocardial performance as well as the function of other organ systems. At this point, inotropic support is usually necessary. Thus, careful observation of the response to volume infusion is imperative.

   i. Excessive preload increases left ventricular wall tension and may exacerbate ischemia by increasing myocardial oxygen demand and decreasing the transmyocardial gradient (aortic diastolic minus LV diastolic pressure) for coronary blood flow. It may also impair myocardial contractility.

   ii. Excessive preload may lead to interstitial edema of the lungs, resulting in increased extravascular lung water, ventilation/perfusion (V/Q) abnormalities, and hypoxemia.

   iii. Excessive preload in the patient with right ventricular dysfunction may impair myocardial blood flow to the RV, resulting in progressive ischemia. A distended RV may contribute to left ventricular dysfunction because of overdistention and septal shift that impairs LV distensibility and filling.

   iv. The presence of RV or biventricular dysfunction may also cause systemic venous hypertension which may reduce perfusion pressure to other organ systems. This may affect the kidneys (causing oliguria), the gastrointestinal (GI) tract (causing splanchnic congestion, jaundice, or ileus), or the brain (contributing to altered mental status).

   v. Thus, the temptation must be resisted to administer additional volume to the failing heart with high filling pressures. Excessive preload **must** be avoided because it may lead to deterioration, rather than improvement, in hemodynamic performance. Once a satisfactory cardiac output has been achieved, volume infusions can be minimized.

4. Stabilize the **heart rate and rhythm**. All attempts should be made to achieve atrioventricular (AV) synchrony with a heart rate around 90 bpm. This may require atrial (AOO or AAI) or AV (DDD or DVI) pacing. These modalities take advantage of the 20–30% improvement in cardiac output provided by atrial contraction that will not be achieved with ventricular pacing alone. This is especially important in the hypertrophied ventricle. Temporary biventricular pacing may be beneficial in improving hemodynamics (both systolic and diastolic function) in patients with impaired ventricular function, especially with prolonged AV conduction (wide QRS complex).[40–43] Antiarrhythmic drugs should be used as necessary to control ventricular ectopy or slow the response to atrial fibrillation (AF).

5. **Improve contractility** with inotropic agents.[1-4,16,44] This should be based on an understanding of the α, β, or nonadrenergic hemodynamic effects of vasoactive medications and their anticipated effects on preload, afterload, heart rate, and contractility. These medications and a strategy for their selection are noted in section III, starting on page 535.

   a. The use of inotropic agents in the early postoperative period may seem paradoxical in that augmented cardiac output is being achieved at the expense of an increase in oxygen demand (e.g. increased heart rate and contractility). However, the major determinant of oxygen demand is the pressure work that the left ventricle must perform. This is reflected by the afterload, which is determined by preload and SVR. Inotropic drugs that increase contractility do not necessarily increase oxygen demand in the failing heart, because they may reduce preload, afterload, and frequently the heart rate as a result of improved cardiac function.

   b. If the cardiac output remains low despite pharmacologic support, physiologic support with an **intra-aortic balloon pump (IABP)** should be strongly considered. If the patient cannot be weaned from bypass or has hemodynamic evidence of severe ventricular dysfunction despite maximal medical therapy and the IABP, use of a **circulatory assist device** should be considered.

6. **Reduce afterload** with vasodilators if the cardiac output is marginal while carefully monitoring systemic blood pressure to avoid hypotension. Vasodilators must be used cautiously when the cardiac index is very poor, because an elevated SVR from intense vasoconstriction is often a compensatory mechanism in low cardiac output states to maintain central perfusion. If the calculated SVR exceeds 1500 dyn-s/cm^5, vasodilators may be indicated either alone or in combination with inotropic medications.

7. It is essential to integrate all hemodynamic parameters when determining whether a patient is or is not doing well. For example, the blood pressure may be high when the heart is not performing well, the cardiac output may be acceptable when the heart is struggling, and the cardiac output can be low even when ventricular function is normal.

   a. The presence of a satisfactory or elevated blood pressure is not necessarily a sign of good cardiac performance. Blood pressure is related directly to both the cardiac output and the systemic vascular resistance (BP = CO × SVR). In the early postoperative period, myocardial function may be marginal despite normal or elevated blood pressures because of an elevated SVR resulting from augmented sympathetic tone and peripheral vasoconstriction. Vasodilators can be used to reduce afterload in the presence of elevated filling pressures, thus reducing myocardial ischemia and improving myocardial function. However, **withdrawal of inotropic support in the hypertensive patient should be considered only after a satisfactory cardiac output has been documented.** Otherwise, acute deterioration may ensue.

   b. One should not be deceived into concluding that myocardial function is satisfactory when the cardiac output is "adequate" but is being maintained by fast heart rates at low stroke volumes.

      i. Although sinus tachycardia is often related to the use of catecholamines or even milrinone, it is often an ominous sign of acute myocardial ischemia or infarction, and it may render the borderline heart ischemic. The stroke volume index (SVI) is an excellent method of assessing myocardial function, because it assesses how much blood the heart is pumping each beat, indexed for the patient's size. Once hypovolemia has been corrected, a low SVI (less than 30 mL/beat/m²) indicates poor myocardial function for which inotropic support is usually indicated. Although β-blockers would theoretically be beneficial to control tachycardia in the injured or ischemic heart, they are poorly tolerated in the presence of LV or RV dysfunction and should be use cautiously, if at all. A potential role for ivabradine in this situation to lower the heart rate without affecting the inotropic effects of catecholamines is not clear.[45]

ii. Sinus tachycardia may represent a beneficial compensatory mechanism for a small stroke volume in a patient with a small left ventricular chamber (following LV aneurysm resection or mitral valve replacement for mitral stenosis). In these situations, an attempt to slow the heart rate pharmacologically may compromise the cardiac output significantly. Not infrequently, sinus tachycardia is a means of compensating for hypovolemia and quickly resolves after fluid administration. It may also be present in the profoundly anemic patient.

iii. Tachycardia may also be present in patients with marked LVH and diastolic dysfunction, especially after aortic valve replacement (AVR) for aortic stenosis. In these situations, the cardiac output may be low despite preserved ventricular function because of a small noncompliant LV chamber. β-blockers or CCBs can be used to slow the heart rate after adequate volume replacement has been achieved, but they must be used with extreme caution. Use of a medication with lusitropic (relaxant) properties, such as milrinone, may be helpful.

iv. Tachycardia accompanying a large stroke volume is often seen in young patients with preserved ventricular function. It can be treated safely with a β-blocker, such as esmolol or IV metoprolol.

c. The cardiac output may be marginal despite normal LV systolic and diastolic function when the patient is hypovolemic but does not develop a compensatory tachycardia. This is noted in patients who were well β-blocked prior to surgery, require pacing at the conclusion of the operation, or are receiving other medications that slow the heart rate, such as dexmedetomidine. Pacing up to a rate of 90 bpm and moderate volume infusion are invariably successful in improving the cardiac output in these situations. If the cardiac output is not acceptable once the filling pressures are satisfactory, an inotrope should be added. The common temptation to continue to administer fluid once the filling pressures are elevated may do more harm than good to the struggling heart.

8. **Maintain blood pressure**

a. Tissue perfusion may be impaired when the systemic pressure is low despite a satisfactory cardiac output. The mean arterial pressure is the average pressure during each cardiac cycle, and generally represents the perfusion pressure to organ systems. In addition to optimizing cardiac output and oxygenation, the mean arterial pressure should be maintained at a level exceeding at least 70 mm Hg to ensure adequate tissue perfusion.

b. If the patient has **a satisfactory cardiac output but a low systemic resistance and low blood pressure**, the filling pressures are often low, and a moderate volume infusion should improve the blood pressure. This scenario is common in sedated patients receiving medications that have potent vasodilator properties. It is also common in patients who had been taking certain medications up to the time of surgery, including ACE inhibitors, angiotensin receptor blockers (ARBs), CCBs, and amiodarone (which blocks sympathetic stimulation by α and β blockade).

   i. If hypotension persists after volume infusion, an α-agent should be used to increase the SVR. Norepinephrine is the preferred drug when the cardiac output is marginal because it has β-agonist properties, whereas phenylephrine is a pure α-agonist and should be used only if the cardiac output is satisfactory. Some patients respond better to norepinephrine than phenylephrine, and others just the reverse.

   ii. Although norepinephrine does induce renal vasoconstriction, it generally has little adverse effect on renal function.[46] Furthermore, unless used in high doses, norepinephrine is effective in raising the systemic pressure without adversely affecting intestinal mucosal perfusion or the splanchnic oxygen supply:demand ratio.[47] Thus, unless the patient remains hypotensive in a low cardiac output state, concerns about impaired regional perfusion are mitigated.

   iii. When catecholamine-resistant hypotension persists despite a satisfactory cardiac output, it may represent a condition of autonomic failure termed "vasoplegia". This may be a consequence of the systemic inflammatory response (although it has been noted after off-pump surgery as well) and may be related to vasodilation induced by nitric oxide. Levels of vasopressin are low in most normotensive patients after bypass but are inappropriately low in patients with "vasodilatory shock". **Arginine vasopressin** acts on vasomotor V_1 and renal V_2 receptors and, given in a dose of 0.01–0.1 units/min, can restore blood pressure in these patients and may be preferable to use of norepinephrine.[48,49] Such low doses may suffice because patients with vasodilatory shock tend to be hypersensitive to its effects. It induces intestinal and gastric mucosal vasoconstriction and also reduces renal blood flow while increasing renal oxygen consumption. Thus, if the cardiac output remains marginal, mesenteric and renal ischemia are more likely to occur.[50,51]

   iv. When there is a poor response to vasopressin, **methylene blue** 1.5 mg/kg should be considered. It inhibits guanylate cyclase activation by nitric oxide and has been reported to reduce morbidity and mortality in patients with postbypass vasoplegia, especially when given early.[52] Another alternative is **hydroxocobalamin** (5 g IV), which can be used in patients taking serotonergic antidepressants (citalopram, sertraline, fluoxetine), in whom methylene blue is contraindicated.[53]

c. **If the patient has a persistently low blood pressure and cardiac output** despite volume infusions and adequate filling pressures, inotropic support should be initiated or increased, anticipating a rise in systemic blood pressure. If this does not occur, an IABP may be required to improve the cardiac output. Frequently, an α-agent must also be added simultaneously to augment the blood pressure, and norepinephrine is preferable because it provides some β effects. Sometimes, use of an α-agent to improve coronary perfusion pressure leads to an improvement in cardiac output. Vasopressin and phenylephrine are best avoided when the cardiac output is marginal because they are pure vasoconstrictors with no inotropic properties and may compromise renal and splanchnic blood flow.

d. Correct **anemia** with blood transfusions. The hematocrit is usually maintained above 21% in the postoperative period, but transfusions should be considered for persistent hypotension, ongoing bleeding, hemodynamic instability, metabolic acidosis, or evidence of myocardial ischemia.

G. **Right ventricular failure and pulmonary hypertension (PH)** (also see pages 382 and 396–397)[14,16,54,55]

1. **Mechanisms.** Right ventricular dysfunction results from decreased RV contractility and may be exacerbated by excessive RV preload, elevated RV afterload (PH), or right coronary ischemia or infarction.

a. Volume overload (elevated preload) may occur with tricuspid regurgitation or excessive fluid administration.

b. Pressure overload (elevated afterload) may result from any condition causing PH, whether pulmonary (ARDS, positive pressure ventilation, pulmonary embolism) or left-sided cardiac disease (LV dysfunction, left-sided valve disease).

c. The right ventricle functions in a low-pressure circuit, so when any of the above factors is present, the RV will dilate, causing an increase in RV end-diastolic pressure, which will reduce right coronary perfusion pressure. RV dilatation will also shift the interventricular septum leftward, impairing LV distensibility and filling, which will reduce the cardiac output. Progressive LV dysfunction will then create a vicious cycle by reducing systemic perfusion pressure, causing RV ischemia, and raising PA pressures and RV afterload, which will worsen RV function.

2. **Risk factors**

a. Preoperative risk factors

i. Proximal RCA occlusion with possible RV infarction

ii. PH of any cause: most commonly, this is "postcapillary" and associated with mitral/aortic disease or severe LV dysfunction, but it may result from severe lung disease (cor pulmonale) or primary PH ("precapillary").

b. Intraoperative and postoperative contributing factors:

i. Poor myocardial protection, usually due to poor collateral circulation with an occluded RCA or due to exclusive use of retrograde cardioplegia, which provides suboptimal RV protection

ii. Prolonged ischemic times/myocardial stunning

iii. Inadvertent RCA distribution ischemia (obstruction of a coronary ostium during AVR, kinking of the RCA ostial button in aortic root replacements)

iv. Coronary embolism from air (usually in valve operations), thrombi, or particulate matter (in reoperative CABG or valve operations)

v. Systemic hypotension causing RV hypoperfusion

vi. Acute PH (increased PVR and RV afterload) from:
- Vasoactive substances associated with blood product transfusions and CPB
- Severe LV dysfunction
- Protamine reaction ("catastrophic pulmonary vasoconstriction")
- Hypoxemia and acidosis
- Tension pneumothorax

vii. RV pressure overload from intrinsic pulmonary disease, ARDS, pulmonary embolism

3. **Assessment**

a. Echocardiography is the best way to identify RV dysfunction, which is usually associated with RV dilatation. Markers of RV dysfunction include an RV fractional area change <35% or a tricuspid annular plane systolic excursion (TAPSE – the distance traveled between end-diastole and end-systole at the lateral corner of the tricuspid annulus) <16 mm.[56] These findings may be identified by TEE during surgery, but are uncommonly assessed in the ICU.

b. Specially designed Swan-Ganz catheters can measure RVEF and RVEDV, but the correlation with contractility is not that precise. The EF may increase with increased preload or decreased afterload without any change in contractility since, by definition, the EF only reflects contractility at constant preload and afterload. The presence of significant tricuspid regurgitation will render thermodilution cardiac outputs unreliable. Alternative means of assessing the cardiac output, directly by using the FloTrac system or indirectly by measuring the SvO_2, may be helpful, although the former cannot be relied upon if atrial fibrillation is present.

c. CVP measurements alone often do not accurately reflect the RVEDV, but trends in the CVP with volume challenges along with cardiac output measurements are valuable in dictating the best course of action. If the CVP rises above 15–18 mm Hg without an improvement in cardiac output, further volume infusions should not be given, and steps to reduce RV afterload and increase contractility are indicated. Although isolated RV dysfunction is best characterized by a high RA/PCW pressure ratio, this is unreliable when LV dysfunction is also present.

d. RV afterload is generally assessed by the mean PA pressure and less commonly by the PVR, since the latter is not influenced by RV dilatation and will be higher when the cardiac output is lower (mean PA = PVR × CO). However, sometimes a low PA pressure is encountered when the RV is failing, because the RV is simply incapable of generating an adequate PA pressure, yet the PVR will remain unchanged.

4. **Treatment.** The goals of treatment are to optimize RV preload, ensure AV conduction, maintain systemic and coronary perfusion pressures, improve RV contractility, reduce RV afterload by reducing PVR, and optimize LV function (Table 11.4).

a. **RV preload** must be raised cautiously to avoid the adverse effects of RV dilatation on RV myocardial blood flow and LV function. It is generally taught that cardiac output can be improved by volume infusions in patients sustaining an RV infarction with compromised RV function. However, the CVP (RA

Table 11.4 • Management of Right Ventricular Failure

1. Optimize preload with CVP of 18–20 mm Hg
2. Ensure AV conduction
3. Maintain adequate systemic perfusion pressure with vasoactive medications or an IABP
4. Reduce RV afterload (PVR) and improve RV contractility
   a. Correct hypothermia, hypoxemia, hypercarbia, acidosis
   b. Select inotropes with vasodilator properties (milrinone, low-dose epinephrine, dobutamine, isoproterenol)
   c. Use a pulmonary vasodilator
      • Inhaled nitric oxide (iNO)
      • Inhaled epoprostenol
      • Inhaled iloprost
5. Optimize LV function
6. Mechanical circulatory assist (RVAD or ECMO) if no response to the above

pressure) should not be increased to more than 18–20 mm Hg, which indirectly indicates RV volume overload. If no improvement in cardiac output ensues when volume is given to reach this level, additional volume infusions should be avoided. Volume overload of the right ventricle contributes to progressive deterioration of RV function, impairment of LV filling, and systemic venous hypertension.

b. **AV conduction** is essential if it can be achieved.

c. Systemic perfusion pressure must be maintained while trying to avoid medications that can also increase PVR. Maintaining adequate perfusion of the RV might benefit from IABP support.

d. Correction of hypothermia, hypoxemia, and respiratory acidosis by hyperventilation will decrease the PVR (acidosis rather than hypercarbia is most deleterious).

e. **Inotropic medications** that can support RV and LV function and also reduce the pulmonary artery pressure should be selected, and they may be combined with a pulmonary vasodilator.

   i. Milrinone is a phosphodiesterase (PDE) inhibitor that is very beneficial in improving RV contractility and reducing PA pressures, although it usually causes systemic hypotension that requires an α-agent to support the SVR. Unfortunately, the use of α-agents may also increase the PVR. The combination of IV milrinone with oral sildenafil produces a synergistic reduction in PVR.[55]

   ii. Isoproterenol may be the most effective drug to improve RV contractility. Its use must be tempered by the possibility of inducing a significant tachycardia.

   iii. Dobutamine is an effective inotrope that improves RV contractility in patients with RV failure, although it has little effect on pulmonary hemodynamics. It has fairly similar effects to milrinone and acts synergistically with it, but it does cause more tachycardia.

iv. If RV function remains depressed, addition of epinephrine may be considered. Norepinephrine may be necessary to maintain SVR in the hypotensive patient, although it will also increase PVR.

v. Levosimendan (see section III.L.2, pages 544–545) exhibits similar inotropic effects to dobutamine but is more effective in reducing RV afterload.[57]

f. **Pulmonary vasodilators** should also be considered to reduce RV afterload.[58]

  i. **Intravenous nitroso dilators**, including NTG and nitroprusside, may be effective in reducing PA pressures, but NTG is usually associated with a reduction in cardiac output, and nitroprusside primarily reduces the SVR. Thus, they may be beneficial in patients with moderate PH and RV dysfunction, but they have relatively limited application in patients with severe RV dysfunction. They have been supplanted by other more potent and selective pulmonary vasodilators.

  ii. **Inhaled nitric oxide (iNO)** is a selective pulmonary vasodilator that can decrease RV afterload and augment RV performance with minimal effect on SVR, thus maintaining systemic perfusion pressure. Despite these benefits, a meta-analysis reported that iNO did not reduce the duration of mechanical ventilation or mortality when used for postoperative RV dysfunction.[59]

- It does not increase intrapulmonary shunting and may reverse the hypoxic vasoconstriction that is frequently noted with other pulmonary vasodilators (such as nitroprusside) and may improve the PaO_2/FiO_2 ratio.[60]

- The usual dose is 10–40 ppm administered via the ventilatory circuit. The circuit must be designed to optimally mix O_2 and NO to generate a low level of NO_2, which is toxic to lung tissue. Measurements of the concentration of iNO in the inhalation limb and NO_2 in the exhalation limb of the ventilatory circuit by chemiluminescence are essential during delivery. Ideally, a scavenger system should be attached to the exhaust port of the ventilator. Once in the bloodstream, iNO is rapidly metabolized to methemoglobin, which rarely causes methemoglobinemia in adults but can be a significant problem in young children.

- iNO should be weaned slowly to prevent a rebound increase in PVR. A general guideline is to decrease the dose no more than 20% every 30 minutes. Inhalation can be stopped once 6 ppm is reached.

- Comparative studies in patients with postoperative PH have shown that iNO is comparable to inhaled epoprostenol, but not quite as effective as iloprost, in lowering PA pressures and improving RV function.[61,62] In comparison with IV milrinone, iNO is associated with lower heart rates, better RVEF, and less requirement for vasopressor support.[63]

  iii. **Prostaglandin and prostacyclin analogues** are potent pulmonary vasodilators that have been used primarily to assess vascular reactivity in patients awaiting heart transplantation. However, they are also beneficial in reducing PA pressure and improving RV function in patients with severe PH during and after various types of cardiac surgery, including mitral valve surgery and heart transplantation. These medications can optimize the PVR/SVR ratio and maintain RV contractility without affecting systemic perfusion pressure.

- **Epoprostenol** (prostacyclin, PGI_2 [Flolan]) is both a pulmonary and very strong systemic vasodilator when administered intravenously because it is not inactivated by the lungs. However, inhaled PGI_2 is a very effective short-acting selective pulmonary vasodilator that can improve RV performance without affecting SVR. It may also improve oxygenation by decreasing V/Q mismatch. A single 60 μg inhalation in the operating room may initially be used, but a continuous inhalation setup in the ICU, using either a weight-based protocol (up to 50 ng/kg/min, at which dose some systemic vasodilation may occur) or a concentration-based protocol, giving 8 mL/h of a 20 μg/mL solution, can be recommended. There is complete reversal of effect about 25 minutes after inhaled PGI_2 is stopped. It is as effective as iNO while being less expensive and less cumbersome to administer.[61]

- **Iloprost** (Ventavis) is a synthetic prostacyclin analogue that also reduces PVR and increases cardiac output with little effect on blood pressure or SVR. It can be given in an aerosolized dose of 25–50 μg during and after surgery. Its hemodynamic effect lasts 1–2 hours after a single administration. Comparative studies have shown it to be more effective than iNO in reducing PVR,[62,63] with the combination of iNO and iloprost having additive effects on the pulmonary vasculature.[64]

iv. **Inhaled milrinone** has shown comparable effects to IV milrinone in reducing PA pressures while demonstrating more pulmonary selectivity by not influencing the SVR and mean arterial pressure.[65] It also improves oxygenation by reducing intrapulmonary shunting and V/Q mismatch.[66] Studies have found it to be less effective than iNO or inhaled iloprost,[66,67] but to have an additive effect in reducing PA pressures and the requirement for vasoactive support when used with inhaled prostacyclin.[68] The dose is 50 μg/kg when given as an inhalation, but a 5 mg bolus into the endotracheal tube might be just as effective in reducing PA pressures and improving RV function.[69] Studies of preemptive pre-CPB inhaled milrinone have shown some pulmonary vasodilatory effect without any effect on clinical outcome.[70] Despite individual reports of efficacy, a meta-analysis failed to show clinical benefits of inhaled milrinone.[71]

v. **Sildenafil** is a PDE type V inhibitor that prevents the degradation of cGMP and reduces pulmonary vascular tone without any effect on the systemic vasculature. Studies have shown a significant pulmonary vasodilatory effect postoperatively when given for 24 hours before surgery (25 mg q8h),[72] 10 minutes before induction (50 mg),[73] and when given in the ICU through an NG tube (20 mg every eight hours in one study[74] and 0.5 mg/kg in another).[75] It is also beneficial when given along with iNO.[76] It may be helpful in weaning patients off intravenous or inhaled pulmonary vasodilator support.

g. If RV dysfunction persists despite use of inotropic support, pulmonary vasodilators, and an IABP, implementation of mechanical assistance with a right ventricular assist device may be necessary. Commonly used systems are the Impella RP, the CentriMag device, TandemHeart RVAD, Protek Duo, or veno-arterial ECMO (see pages 559–560).

H. **Diastolic dysfunction** is a common cause of congestive heart failure (HF) in hypertensive patients, and can pose hemodynamic problems after surgery when ventricular compliance is affected by the use of CPB and cardioplegia. It is most prominent after a prolonged period of cardioplegic arrest, especially with small hypertrophied hearts.

1. Diastolic dysfunction is caused by decreased diastolic compliance, often with an inappropriate tachycardia.[77] The end result is a low cardiac output syndrome with low end-diastolic volumes yet high left-sided filling pressures. The stiffness of the heart is usually evident on echocardiogram, which may confirm normal systolic function even though the patient is in a low output state.

2. This problem can be difficult to manage and often results in end-organ dysfunction, such as renal failure, that progresses until the diastolic dysfunction improves (see pages 381–382). Although inotropic drugs are frequently given, they are of little benefit. In contrast, ACE inhibitors may improve diastolic compliance; lusitropic drugs, such as the CCBs, magnesium, and milrinone, may improve ventricular relaxation; and bradycardic drugs, such as β-blockers or CCBs, can be used for an inappropriate tachycardia. Aggressive diuresis may also be beneficial in reducing myocardial edema that might contribute to reduced compliance.

III. Inotropic and Vasoactive Drugs

A. General comments

1. A variety of vasoactive medications are available to provide hemodynamic support for the patient with marginal myocardial function.[1–4,16,44] They should be chosen carefully to achieve a satisfactory cardiac index (>2.2 L/min/m^2) and blood pressure (MAP >70 mm Hg) once adequate filling pressures have been achieved. The selection of a particular drug depends on an understanding of its mechanism of action and limitations to its use (see section M, page 545 for recommendations on drug selection). The catecholamines exert their effects on α- and β-adrenergic receptors. They elevate levels of intracellular cyclic AMP (cAMP) by β-adrenergic stimulation of adenylate cyclase. In contrast, the PDE inhibitors (milrinone) elevate cAMP levels by inhibiting cAMP hydrolysis. Elevation of cAMP augments calcium influx into myocardial cells and increases contractility.

   a. α_1 and α_2 stimulation result in increased systemic and pulmonary vascular resistance. Cardiac α_1-receptors increase contractility and decrease the heart rate.

   b. β_1 stimulation results in increased contractility (inotropy), heart rate (chronotropy), and conduction (dromotropy).

   c. β_2 stimulation results in peripheral vasodilation and bronchodilation.

2. The net effects of medications that share α and β properties usually depend on the dosage level and are summarized in Table 11.5.

3. The concomitant use of several medications with selective effects may minimize the side effects of higher doses of individual medications. For example:

   a. Inotropes with vasoconstrictive (α) properties can be combined with vasodilators to improve contractility while avoiding an increase in SVR (e.g. norepinephrine with clevidipine, propofol, or nitroprusside).

   b. Inotropes with vasodilator properties can be combined with α-agonists or other vasoconstrictors to maintain SVR (e.g. milrinone with phenylephrine, norepinephrine, or vasopressin).

Table 11.5 • Hemodynamic Effects of Vasoactive Medications

Medication	SVR	HR	PCW	CI	MAP	MvO$_2$
Epinephrine	↓↑	↑↑	↓↑	↑	↑	↑
Dobutamine	↓	↑↑↑	↓	↑	↓↔↑	↑↔
Milrinone	↓↓	↑	↓	↑	↓	↓↑
Dopamine	↓↑	↑↑↑	↓↑	↑	↓↑	↑
Isoproterenol	↓↓	↑↑↑↑	↓	↑	↓↑	↑↑
Norepinephrine	↑↑	↑↑	↑↑	↑	↑↑↑	↑
Phenylephrine	↑↑	↔	↑	↔	↑↑↑	↔↑
Vasopressin	↑↑	↔	↑	↔	↑↑↑	↔↑
Calcium chloride	↑	↔	↑	↑	↑↑	↑

↑ increased; ↓ decreased; ↔ no change; ↓↑ variable effect. The relative effect is indicated by the number of arrows.

Note: the effect may vary with dosage level (particularly dopamine and epinephrine, in which case the effect seen at low dose is indicated by the first arrow). For some medications, an improvement in MAP may occur from the positive inotropic effect despite a reduction in SVR. The effects of milrinone and calcium are not mediated by α and β receptors.

    c. Catecholamines can be combined with a PDE inhibitor to provide synergistic inotropic effects while achieving pulmonary and systemic vasodilation (e.g. epinephrine or dobutamine with milrinone).

    d. α-agents can be infused directly into the left atrium to maintain SVR while a pulmonary vasodilator is infused into the right heart.

  4. The benefits of most vasoactive medications are noted when adequate blood levels are achieved in the systemic circulation. Thus, these medications should be given into the central circulation via controlled infusion pumps rather than peripherally. Although higher levels can be reached by drug infusion into the left atrium to avoid pulmonary vascular effects and reduce drug inactivation by the lungs, this is an uncommon practice.

  5. The standard mixes and dosage ranges are listed in Table 11.6.

  6. Inotropic drugs should be used to normalize the cardiac output after steps have been taken to improve preload, afterload, and rhythm issues. Although numerous studies have suggested that the use of inotropes is associated with increased morbidity and mortality after cardiac surgery, it is difficult to conclude that the patients who needed such support would have done better without hemodynamic support.[78–80]

B. Epinephrine

  1. Hemodynamic effects

    a. Epinephrine is a potent β$_1$-inotropic agent that increases cardiac output by an increase in heart rate and contractility, generally increasing myocardial oxygen

Table 11.6 • Mixes and Dosage Ranges for Vasoactive Medications

Medication	Mix	Dosage Range
Epinephrine	1 mg/250 mL	1–4 µg/min (0.01–0.05 µg/kg/min)
Dobutamine	500 mg/250 mL	5–20 µg/kg/min
Milrinone	20 mg/200 mL	50 µg/kg bolus, then 0.25–0.75 µg/kg/min
Dopamine	400 mg/250 mL	2–20 µg/kg/min
Isoproterenol	1 mg/250 mL	0.5–10 µg/min (0.0075–0.1 µg/kg/min)
Norepinephrine	4 mg/250 mL	1–30 µg/min (0.01–0.3 µg/kg/min)
Phenylephrine	40 mg/250 mL	5–150 µg/min (0.05–1.5 µg/kg/min)
Vasopressin	40 units/80 mL	0.01–0.1 units/min

Note: × milligrams placed in 250 mL gives an infusion rate of × micrograms (mg divided by 100) in 15 drops of solution. For example, a 200 mg/250 mL mix gives a drip of 200 µg in 15 drops. 60 microdrops = 1 mL. 15 drops/min = 15 mL/h.

demand. At doses of less than 2 µg/min (<0.02–0.03 µg/kg/min), it has a β_2 effect that produces mild peripheral vasodilation, but the blood pressure is usually maintained or elevated by the increase in cardiac output. At doses greater than 2 µg/min (>0.03 µg/kg/min), α effects will increase the SVR and raise the blood pressure. Metabolic acidosis may also be noted at low doses of epinephrine when α effects are not evident, but this is not related to reduced tissue perfusion.[81]

b. Epinephrine has strong β_2 properties that produce bronchodilation.

c. Although epinephrine may contribute to arrhythmias or tachycardia, studies have shown that epinephrine given at a dose of 2 µg/min causes less tachycardia than dobutamine given at a dose of 5 µg/kg/min.[82]

2. **Indications**

a. Epinephrine may be considered a first-line drug for a **borderline cardiac output** in the absence of tachycardia or ventricular ectopy. Some authors state that it should be considered a second-line inotrope because of the risk of tachycardia and arrhythmias, an increase in myocardial oxygen consumption, a decrease in splanchnic blood flow, and the risk of lactic acidosis.[16] It is very helpful in the hypertrophied heart that often takes a while to recover adequate systolic function after cardioplegic arrest. Epinephrine is extremely effective and has very low cost.

b. It is especially helpful in **stimulating the sinus node** mechanism when the intrinsic heart rate is slow. It is frequently beneficial in improving the atrium's responsiveness to pacing at the conclusion of bypass.

c. **Bronchospasm** may respond well to epinephrine, especially when an inotrope is also required.

    d. Anaphylaxis (protamine reaction)

    e. Resuscitation from cardiac arrest

  3. **Starting dose** is 1 µg/min (about 0.01 µg/kg/min) with a mix of 1 mg/250 mL. Dosage can be increased to 4 µg/min (about 0.05 µg/kg/min). Higher doses are rarely indicated in patients following cardiac surgery.

C. Dobutamine

  1. **Hemodynamic effects**

    a. Dobutamine is a positive inotropic agent with a strong β_1 effect that increases heart rate in a dose-dependent manner and also increases contractility. Although it has a mild vasoconstrictive α_1 effect, this is offset by its mild vasodilatory β_2 effect, resulting in reduced filling pressures, a reduction in SVR, but maintenance of blood pressure due to improved cardiac performance. Although the increased heart rate may increase myocardial oxygen demand, this is mostly offset by augmented myocardial blood flow and a reduction in preload and afterload, reducing LV wall stress.[83] This is particularly evident in volume-overloaded hearts (valve replacement for mitral or aortic regurgitation).[84]

    b. Dobutamine may cause more tachycardia than low-dose epinephrine, so switching from one inotrope to another may be considered to minimize any increase in oxygen demand that could trigger ischemia.[82]

    c. Dobutamine and the PDE inhibitors (milrinone) provide comparable hemodynamic support, although dobutamine is associated with more hypertension, tachycardia, and a greater chance of triggering atrial fibrillation.[85]

  2. **Indications**

    a. Dobutamine is most useful when the **cardiac output is marginal and there is a mild elevation in SVR.** Its use is usually restricted by development of a tachycardia. Some groups consider this the best first-line drug for inotropic support.

    b. It is a moderate **pulmonary vasodilator** and may be helpful in improving RV function and lowering RV afterload.

    c. It has a synergistic effect in improving cardiac output when used with a PDE inhibitor (milrinone). This combination is commonly used in patients awaiting cardiac transplantation.

  3. **Starting dose** is 5 µg/kg/min using a mix of 500 mg/250 mL. Dosage can be increased to 20 µg/kg/min.

D. Milrinone (Primacor)

  1. **Hemodynamic effects**

    a. Milrinone is a phosphodiesterase (PDE) III inhibitor best described as an "inodilator".[86] It improves cardiac output by reducing systemic and pulmonary vascular resistance, lowers coronary vascular resistance,[87] and exerts a moderate positive inotropic effect. There is usually a modest increase in heart rate, a lowering of filling pressures, and a moderate reduction in systemic blood pressure despite the improvement in myocardial contractility. This is generally associated with a reduction in myocardial oxygen demand. Although the unloading effect produced by the decrease in SVR may contribute a great deal to its efficacy, an α-agent (phenylephrine or norepinephrine) is frequently required to maintain systemic blood pressure.

b. Milrinone increases cyclic AMP levels, which causes relaxation of myofilaments. Although this lusitropic effect improves ventricular compliance after bypass, some studies suggest that milrinone has no effect on diastolic function and does not have lusitropic properties.[88-92]

c. Additive effects on ventricular performance are noted when milrinone is combined with one of the catecholamines, such as epinephrine or dobutamine, due to differing mechanisms of action.

d. Milrinone may produce a tachycardia, especially in the hypovolemic patient. However, in comparison with dobutamine, it generally produces a comparable increase in cardiac output with less increase in heart rate, suggesting strong inotropic properties, and is associated with a lower incidence of arrhythmias, although one study found that milrinone was an independent risk factor for atrial fibrillation.[93] Since it is generally used in addition to a catecholamine in patients with poor RV or LV dysfunction, it is not clear if the risk of AF might still have been high without its use.

e. Although it would seem counterintuitive to use a β-blocker (with its negative inotropic properties) with a PDE inhibitor, one study did show that β-blockers could offset the tachycardia produced by a PDE inhibitor without compromising the beneficial inotropic effects.[94]

f. Prior to the availability of milrinone, inamrinone (known at the time as amrinone or Inocor) was the preferred PDE inhibitor. Both drugs had comparable effects, but inamrinone was associated with thrombocytopenia, so its use has declined.[95]

g. Several meta-analyses have found that milrinone use in cardiac surgery is associated with similar or higher mortality rates than use of other or no inotropes at all.[96,97] However, it is difficult to justify using no inotropic support in a low cardiac output state. Thus, when milrinone is added due to inadequate response to a catecholamine, it is most likely beneficial in reducing the need for an IABP, optimizing organ system function, and improving outcomes in the early postoperative period.

h. Inhaled milrinone has selective pulmonary vasodilator effects that can reduce PA pressures and improve RV function without any systemic effects. The literature provides conflicting evidence of its efficacy and benefits.[66-71]

2. **Indications**

a. Milrinone is generally the second medication selected for a **persistent low cardiac output state** despite use of one of the catecholamines or when their use is limited by tachycardia. However, a preemptive bolus of milrinone given on pump significantly reduces the need for any catecholamine in the immediate perioperative period.[98]

b. It is particularly valuable in patients with **right ventricular dysfunction** associated with an elevation in PVR, such as patients with PH from mitral valve disease or those awaiting and following cardiac transplantation. Use of inhaled or intratracheal milrinone shows selective pulmonary vasodilatory effects without influencing systemic hemodynamics, but is of unclear benefit.

c. The lusitropic (relaxant) property may be of value in patients with significant **diastolic dysfunction** that may contribute to a low output state, even with preserved systolic function.

    d. Milrinone is effective in dilating arterial conduits and may be beneficial when there is suspected coronary or graft spasm and the need for inotropic support.[87]

  3. Advantages and disadvantages

    a. Milrinone has a long elimination half-life of 1.5–2 hours that increases to 2.3 hours in patients with low cardiac output states or HF. Thus, an intraoperative bolus can be used to terminate bypass and provide a few hours of additional inotropic support without the need for a continuous infusion.

    b. Because the hemodynamic effects persist for several hours after the drug infusion is discontinued (in contrast to the short duration of action of the catecholamines), the patient must be observed carefully for deteriorating myocardial function for several hours as the hemodynamic effects wear off. The dose is generally sequentially halved, and if hemodynamic performance remains adequate, it is then stopped.

  4. Starting dose is a 50 µg/kg IV bolus over 10 minutes, followed by a continuous infusion of 0.25–0.75 µg/kg/min of a 20 mg/200 mL solution. Note that, because of its long half-life, it takes up to six hours to reach a steady-state level if not given with a loading dose. The inhalational dose is comparable to the IV bolus dose.

E. Dopamine

  1. The hemodynamic effects of dopamine vary with increasing doses, but reports of adverse effects have significantly reduced its usage. It tends to cause a tachycardia and arrhythmias, accelerates AV conduction in atrial fibrillation,[99] will depress ventilation due to inhibition of peripheral chemoreceptors causing V/Q mismatch, and may worsen renal function despite producing an improvement in urine output.[16,100]

    a. Renal dose dopamine (2–3 µg/kg/min) is effective in improving urine output, but it has adverse effects on renal function if used during surgery and does not alter the natural history of acute kidney injury if it develops.[101,102]

    b. At moderate doses of 3–8 µg/kg/min, dopamine exhibits a β_1 inotropic effect that improves contractility, and, to a variable degree, a chronotropic effect that increases heart rate and the potential for arrhythmogenesis.

    c. At doses greater than 8 µg/kg/min, there are increasing inotropic effects, but also a predominant α effect that occurs directly and by endogenous release of norepinephrine. This raises the SVR, systemic blood pressure, and filling pressures, and may adversely affect myocardial oxygen consumption and ventricular function. Concomitant use of a vasodilator, such as nitroprusside, to counteract these α effects allows for the best augmentation of cardiac output.

  2. Indications

    a. Dopamine may be considered for a **low cardiac output state**, especially when the SVR is low and the blood pressure is marginal, but its use is usually limited by the development of a profound tachycardia and other potential adverse effects, so the other inotropes listed above are preferable.

    b. It does **improve urine output** in patients with or without preexisting renal dysfunction, but has no demonstrable benefit in preserving renal function, and may in fact worsen renal function if used intraoperatively.[101]

F. Isoproterenol

1. Hemodynamic effects

    a. Isoproterenol has a strong β_1 effect that increases cardiac output by a moderate increase in contractility and a marked increase in heart rate with a slight β_2 effect that lowers SVR. The increased myocardial O_2 demand caused by the tachycardia limits its usefulness in coronary bypass patients. Isoproterenol may produce ischemia out of proportion to its chronotropic effects, and it also predisposes to ventricular arrhythmias.

    b. Isoproterenol's β_2 effect lowers PVR and reduces RV afterload.

    c. There is a strong β_2 bronchodilator effect.

2. Indications

    a. **Right ventricular dysfunction** associated with an elevation in PVR. Isoproterenol is both an inotrope and a pulmonary vasodilator and thus is helpful in supporting RV function following mitral valve surgery in patients with PH. Because it causes a profound tachycardia, it has generally been replaced by the PDE inhibitors and dobutamine. However, it is still used following heart transplantation to reduce PVR, improve RV function, and produce ventricular relaxation.

    b. **Bronchospasm** when an inotrope is required.

    c. **Bradycardia** in the absence of functioning pacemaker wires. It may be used after heart transplantation to maintain a heart rate around 100 bpm.

3. Starting dose is 0.5 µg/min with a mix of 1 mg/250 mL. It can be increased to about 10 µg/min (usual dosage range is 0.0075–0.1 mg/kg/min).

G. Norepinephrine (Levophed)

1. Hemodynamic effects

    a. Norepinephrine is a powerful catecholamine with both α- and β-adrenergic properties. Its predominant α effect raises SVR and blood pressure, while the β_1 effect increases both contractility and heart rate.

    b. By increasing afterload and contractility, norepinephrine increases myocardial oxygen demand and may prove detrimental to the ischemic or marginal myocardium. Although it may also cause regional redistribution of blood flow, studies suggest that renal and intestinal perfusion are maintained if the systemic blood pressure improves. Furthermore, the addition of dobutamine has been shown to improve gastric mucosal perfusion in patients receiving norepinephrine.[103]

    c. **Note:** there is a tendency to think that norepinephrine is providing only an α effect, but it does possess strong β properties. Thus, it should be anticipated that both the stroke volume and heart rate will fall when the drug is weaned.

2. Indications

    a. Norepinephrine is primarily indicated when the patient has a marginally **low cardiac output with a low blood pressure caused by a low SVR**. This is often noted when the patient warms and vasodilates. Use of a pure α-agent is feasible if the cardiac index exceeds 2.5 $L/min/m^2$, but norepinephrine can provide some inotropic support if the cardiac index is borderline. If the cardiac index is below 2.0 $L/min/m^2$, another inotrope should probably be used in addition to norepinephrine.

b. It is frequently effective in raising the blood pressure when little effect has been obtained from phenylephrine (and vice versa).

c. It has been used as an inotrope to improve cardiac output in conjunction with a vasodilator to counteract its α effects.

3. **Starting dose** is 1 μg/min (about 0.01 μg/kg/min) with a mix of 4 mg/250 mL. The dose may be increased as necessary to achieve a satisfactory blood pressure. Higher doses (probably >20 μg/min or >0.2 μg/kg/min) most likely will reduce visceral and peripheral blood flow and may produce a metabolic acidosis.

H. **Phenylephrine** (Neo-Synephrine)

1. **Hemodynamic effects**

a. Phenylephrine is a pure α-agent that increases SVR and may cause a reflex decrease in heart rate. Myocardial function may be compromised if an excessive increase in afterload results. However, it is frequently improved by an elevation in coronary perfusion pressure that resolves myocardial ischemia.

b. Phenylephrine has no direct cardiac effects.

2. **Indications**

a. Phenylephrine is indicated only to **increase the SVR when hypotension coexists with a satisfactory cardiac output.** This is commonly noted at the termination of bypass or in the ICU when the patient warms and vasodilates. If the blood pressure remains low after volume infusions yet the cardiac output is satisfactory, phenylephrine can be used to maintain a systolic blood pressure around 100–110 mm Hg. Significantly higher pressures should be avoided to minimize the adverse effects of an elevated SVR on myocardial function.

b. Phenylephrine can be used **preoperatively to treat ischemia** by maintaining perfusion pressure, while IV NTG is used to reduce preload. It is beneficial in maintaining the blood pressure in patients with hypertrophic obstructive cardiomyopathy in whom inotropes will accentuate the outflow tract gradient and is useful in patients who exhibit systolic anterior motion (SAM) after mitral valve repair.

3. **Advantages and disadvantages**

a. Patients often become refractory to the effects of phenylephrine after several hours, necessitating a change to norepinephrine. Conversely, some patients respond very poorly to norepinephrine and have an immediate blood pressure response to low-dose phenylephrine.

b. By providing no cardiac support other than an increase in central perfusion pressures, phenylephrine has limited indications.

c. **Note:** be very careful when administering an α-agent to the patient whose entire revascularization procedure is based on arterial grafts, as it may provoke spasm and causes profound ischemia, which can be fatal.

4. Starting dose is 5 μg/min with a mix of 40 mg/250 mL. The dosage can be increased as necessary to maintain a satisfactory blood pressure. The usual dosage range is 0.05–1.5 μg/kg/min.

I. **Vasopressin**

1. **Hemodynamic effects**

a. Vasopressin acts on vasomotor V_1 and renal V_2 receptors to increase SVR. It has no direct cardiac effects, so any improvement in cardiac function is related to an improvement in perfusion pressure.

   b. It may improve renal perfusion in that it constricts the efferent rather than the afferent arterioles, in contradistinction to the effects of α-agents on renal perfusion. However, one study suggested that it reduced renal blood flow, increased renal oxygen extraction, and impaired renal oxygenation.[50]

   c. It induces intestinal and gastric mucosal vasoconstriction; thus if the cardiac output remains marginal, mesenteric ischemia is more likely to occur.[51]

   d. It is beneficial in patients with a low SVR and PH as it does not produce a significant alteration in PA pressures.

   e. It may induce vasospasm in internal thoracic artery (ITA) and radial artery grafts.

2. Indications

   a. Low blood pressure that is poorly responsive to phenylephrine or norepinephrine.

   b. Vasodilatory shock ("vasoplegia") after CPB associated with a satisfactory cardiac output that is not responsive to norepinephrine or phenylephrine. Norepinephrine is preferable in patients with a compromised cardiac output.

3. Dosage is an infusion of 0.01–0.1 units/min.

J. Calcium chloride

1. Hemodynamic effects

   a. The primary effect of calcium chloride ($CaCl_2$) is an increase in SVR that improves the mean arterial pressure.[104] It has little effect on the heart rate. It produces a transient improvement in systolic function at the termination of CPB, although it may increase ventricular stiffness, suggesting it produces transient diastolic dysfunction.[105]

   b. One study showed that $CaCl_2$ produces a transient inotropic effect if hypocalcemia is present and a more sustained increase in SVR, independent of the calcium level.[106]

   c. A study that compared epinephrine and calcium chloride upon emergence from CPB showed that both increased the mean arterial pressure, but only epinephrine increased the cardiac output, suggesting that calcium did not provide any inotropic support.[107] Although this study did not find any beneficial or negative effects of combining these two medications, another one did suggest that calcium salts may attenuate the cardiotonic effects of catecholamines, such as dobutamine or epinephrine, but have little effect on the efficacy of inamrinone (and presumably milrinone).[108]

2. Indications

   a. Frequently used **at the termination of CPB to augment systemic blood pressure** by either a vasoconstrictive or positive inotropic effect. This is a common practice despite concerns that calcium influx during reperfusion may contribute to myocardial dysfunction.[109,110]

   b. **To support myocardial function or blood pressure on an emergency basis** until further assessment and intervention can be undertaken. **Note:** calcium is not recommended for routine use during a cardiac arrest.

   c. **Hyperkalemia** ($K^+ > 6.0$ mEq/L).

3. Usual dose is 0.5–1 g slow IV bolus.

K. Triiodothyronine (T_3)

1. Hemodynamic effects

a. Thyroid hormone (triiodothyronine or T_3) exerts a positive inotropic effect by increasing aerobic metabolism and synthesis of high-energy phosphates. It causes a dose-dependent increase in myocyte contractile performance that is independent of and additive to β-adrenergic stimulation.[111]

b. A low T_3 level preoperatively is associated with low cardiac output syndrome and increased mortality after CABG.[112] Most patients have reduced levels of free T_3 for up to three days following operations on CPB.[113,114] Routine administration of T_3 to maintain normal levels produces a transient improvement in cardiac output, lowers troponin release, reduces SVR, and may reduce the need for inotropes, but it does not appear to influence outcomes.[115–117] However, a significant improvement in hemodynamics has been noted in patients with impaired ventricular function, many of whom could not be weaned from bypass on multiple inotropes until T_3 was administered.[118]

c. **Note:** CCBs have been shown to interfere with the action of T_3.

d. There is some evidence that postoperative atrial fibrillation is more common in patients with subclinical hypothyroidism and low T_3 levels, and administration of T_3 may reduce the incidence of postoperative AF.[119,120]

2. Indications

a. T_3 may be indicated to provide inotropic support as a salvage step when CPB cannot be terminated with maximal inotropic support and an IABP.

b. T_3 is helpful in improving donor heart function in brain-dead patients when ventricular function is depressed.

3. Usual dose is 10–20 µg, although some studies have used a bolus of 0.8 µg/kg followed by an infusion of 0.12 µg/kg/h for six hours.[116]

L. Other modalities to treat low cardiac output

1. Glucose–insulin–potassium (GIK) has been demonstrated to have an inotropic effect on the failing myocardium after cardioplegic arrest. It provides metabolic support to the myocardium by increasing anaerobic glycolysis, lowering free fatty acid levels, preserving intracellular glycogen stores, and stabilizing membrane function. It has been shown to reduce myocardial injury and improve hemodynamic performance.[121] The mixture contains 50% glucose, 80 units/L of regular insulin, and 100 mEq/L of potassium infused at a rate of 1 mL/kg/h.

2. Levosimendan is a calcium-sensitizing "inodilator" that has been used for patients with decompensated HF and has been further evaluated in the management of cardiac surgical patients. There is vast literature suggesting that its administration before initiating CPB may improve myocardial function after revascularization, with a reduced requirement for additional inotropes, less IABP usage, and a reduction in mortality.[122–124] However, several additional studies have not shown any survival benefit independent of the extent of LV dysfunction.[125–129]

a. **Mechanisms and effects.** Levosimendan improves cardiac function by both inotropic and vasodilatory effects. The positive inotropic effect results from sensitizing myofilaments to calcium without increasing intracellular calcium levels. It also has coronary, pulmonary, and systemic vasodilator effects by opening

ATP-dependent potassium channels in vascular smooth muscle. Thus, it improves cardiac output by increasing stroke volume with little increase in heart rate, by reducing afterload from its vasodilating effects, and to a slight degree by lusitropic effects. Given at high doses, it may require use of an α-agent to counteract systemic vasodilation. The one major difference between levosimendan and other inotropes is the enhancement of contractility without an increase in myocardial oxygen demand. At low doses, it is not arrhythmogenic. The half-life is 70–80 hours, so it has a long-lasting effect after administration.

b. **Indications.** Levosimendan is useful in improving hemodynamics in patients with anticipated postcardiotomy RV and LV dysfunction and in facilitating weaning from bypass. In patients with RV dysfunction, it decreases PVR and improves RV contractility (better than dobutamine in one study).[57] An infusion started prior to bypass (with or without a loading dose of 24 μg/kg) is very effective in reducing troponin leakage, suggesting a cardioprotective effect, and in maintaining an improved cardiac output without the need for additional inotropic support. In view of numerous studies suggesting no significant impact on outcomes, the role for levosimendan in cardiac surgical patients remains undefined.

c. **Starting dose.** It is given as a 12–24 μg/kg loading dose over 10 minutes, followed by a continuous infusion of 0.1 μg/kg/min.

M. **Recommended strategy for selection of vasoactive medications**

1. The selection of a vasoactive medication should be based on several factors:

    a. An adequate understanding of the underlying cardiac pathophysiology derived from hemodynamic measurements and echocardiography.

    b. Knowledge of the α, β, or nonadrenergic hemodynamic effects of the medications and their anticipated influence on preload, afterload, heart rate, and contractility.

    c. Assessment of intravascular volume, since preload should be optimized before inotropic drugs are initiated. However, it is common practice to initiate low-dose inotropic support at the termination of CPB, which may or may not need to be continued depending on volume status and cardiac performance.

2. Vasoactive medications are usually started in the operating room and maintained for about 6–12 hours while the heart recovers from the period of ischemia/reperfusion. The doses are adjusted as the patient's hemodynamic parameters improve. Occasionally, when the heart demonstrates persistent "stunning" or has sustained a perioperative infarction, pharmacologic support and/or an IABP may be necessary for several days.

3. When the cardiac index is satisfactory (>2.2 L/min/m²) but the blood pressure is low, an α-agent should be selected. Phenylephrine is commonly used in the operating room, but norepinephrine is probably a better drug to use in that it provides some β effects that are beneficial during the early phase of myocardial recovery. Systolic blood pressure need only be maintained around 100 mm Hg (mean pressure >70 mm Hg) to minimize the increase in afterload. If neither of these medications suffices, vasopressin should be utilized. Occasionally, a simple bolus of 1–2 units of vasopressin overcomes the initial vasoplegic state after pump and minimizes the subsequent need for an α-agent.

4. When the cardiac index remains marginal (<2.0 L/min/m^2) after optimizing volume status, heart rate, and rhythm, an inotropic agent should be selected. The first-line drugs are usually epinephrine or dobutamine. The major limitation to their use is the development of tachycardia, which tends to be less prominent with low-dose epinephrine. At inotropic levels, epinephrine tends to raise SVR, whereas dobutamine's effect on SVR is variable but usually not significant. If a satisfactory cardiac output has been achieved and the blood pressure is elevated, addition of a vasodilator is beneficial. If the blood pressure is low, an α-agent can be added.

5. If the cardiac output still remains suboptimal despite moderate doses of drugs (epinephrine 2–3 µg/min [0.03–0.04 µg/kg/min] or dobutamine 10 µg/kg/min), a second drug should be added. The PDE inhibitor milrinone exhibits additive effects to those of the catecholamines and should be selected. This will lower the SVR and may cause a modest tachycardia. It commonly requires the use of norepinephrine to maintain SVR, although blood pressure may be maintained by the improvement in cardiac function. If norepinephrine is used, its β effect may further improve contractility, but it can also increase the heart rate. Its α effect usually has minimal effect on organ system perfusion if a satisfactory cardiac output can be achieved, but it can compromise flow in arterial conduits (such as the ITA or radial artery). If the cardiac index remains marginal despite the use of two medications, an IABP should be inserted.

6. If the patient cannot be weaned from bypass and has hemodynamic evidence of persistent cardiogenic shock (CI <1.8 L/min/m^2, PCWP >20 mm Hg) despite medications and the IABP, a circulatory assist device should be considered.

7. **Note:** it is not uncommon for the cardiac output to fall to below 1.8–2.0 L/min/m^2 during the first 4–6 hours after surgery, which represents the time of maximal myocardial depression. After optimizing fluid status, the dose of an inotrope may need to be increased transiently or, less frequently, another one added if the cardiac output does not improve. Such goal-directed hemodynamic management usually improves outcomes. However, it is the **persistence of a low output state** beyond this time that raises concerns, especially if there is any evidence of myocardial ischemia on ECG, a low SvO$_2$, rising filling pressures out of proportion to fluid administration, oliguria, or a progressive metabolic acidosis. An IABP may need to be inserted in the ICU if these problems are present. However, in the absence of any specific identifiable problem, most patients will gradually improve, and one should not be overly alarmed by transient drops in cardiac output and respond too aggressively. If there is any concern, echocardiography is helpful in assessing whether ventricular dysfunction or cardiac tamponade is causing the low output state, and can direct management appropriately.

8. **Note:** use of α-agents can be dangerous in patients receiving radial artery grafts or when multiple grafts are based on ITA inflow. It is preferable to reduce the dose of the vasodilating drug (diltiazem or IV NTG used to prevent spasm), rather than increase the dose of a vasoconstricting medication if hypotension is noted.

N. Vasoactive medications provide specific hemodynamic benefits, but their use may be limited by the development of adverse effects. Nearly all of the catecholamines will increase myocardial oxygen demand by increasing heart rate and contractility. Other side effects that may necessitate changing to or addition of another medication include:

1. Arrhythmogenesis and tachycardia (epinephrine, dobutamine, isoproterenol)
2. Vasoconstriction and poor renal, splanchnic, and peripheral perfusion (norepinephrine, phenylephrine, vasopressin)
3. Vasodilation requiring α-agents to support systemic blood pressure (milrinone)
4. Excessive urine output (dopamine)
5. Thrombocytopenia (inamrinone)
6. Cyanide and thiocyanate toxicity (nitroprusside)
7. Methemoglobinemia (IV NTG)

O. **Weaning of vasoactive medications**

1. Once the cardiac output and blood pressure have stabilized for a few hours, vasoactive medications should be weaned. α-agents should generally be weaned first. Their use should ideally be restricted to increasing the SVR to support blood pressure when the cardiac output is satisfactory. However, there are circumstances when α-agents are required to maintain cerebral and coronary perfusion in the face of a poor cardiac output. In these desperate life-saving situations, the resultant intense peripheral vasoconstriction can compromise organ system and peripheral perfusion, causing renal, mesenteric, and peripheral ischemia, acidosis, and frequently death.

   a. In the routine patient, SVR and blood pressure increase when myocardial function improves, narcotic effects abate, and sedatives, such as propofol or dexmedetomidine, have been discontinued. As the patient awakens and develops increased intrinsic sympathetic tone, α-agents can be stopped.

   b. When milrinone or an IABP is used to support myocardial function, an α-agent is frequently required to counteract the unloading effect and decreased SVR that is achieved. It may not be possible to wean the α-agent before the patient has been weaned from milrinone or the IABP, because the patient may become hypotensive despite an excellent cardiac output. It is usually necessary to wean the α-agent in conjunction with the weaning of the other modalities.

   c. An occasional patient who has sustained a small perioperative infarction will have an excellent cardiac output but a low SVR. This requires temporary vasoconstrictor support until the blood pressure improves spontaneously. Such support may be required for several days.

2. The stronger positive inotropes with the most potential detrimental effects on myocardial metabolism should be weaned next. Those that possess α properties should be decreased to doses at which these effects do not occur. If an IABP is present, it should not be removed until the patient is on a low dose of only one inotrope, unless complications of the IABP develop. Otherwise, weaning of the IABP should usually be deferred.

   a. The catecholamines should be weaned first to low doses. If the patient is on multiple drugs, epinephrine should be weaned to a low dose (2 μg/min or less) to avoid any α effects. Dobutamine (which lacks a significant α effect) should be weaned to doses of less than 10 μg/kg/min.

   b. Milrinone is usually weaned off with the patient still supported by low doses of catecholamines. However, since it has few deleterious effects on myocardial function, and catecholamines may cause a tachycardia, it is not unreasonable to continue the milrinone while the catecholamine is weaned off. Because of its long half-life, it should be withdrawn slowly, usually halving the dose and then discontinuing it if the patient remains hemodynamically stable. Occasionally, deterioration in myocardial function may occur several hours later and require the reinstitution of inotropic support.

   c. IABP removal may be performed once the patient is on low doses of inotropic support, such as epinephrine at 1 µg/min, dobutamine <10 µg/kg/min, or milrinone at ≤0.5 µg/kg/min.

   d. The requirement for vasoactive medications in patients on circulatory assist devices depends on the extent of support provided and the function of the unsupported ventricle. In patients receiving univentricular support, inotropic medications may be necessary to improve the function of the unassisted ventricle. Patients with biventricular support are usually given only α-agents or vasopressin to support systemic resistance. If the device is being used for temporary support, rather than as a bridge to transplantation, inotropes may be given to assess cardiac reserve when flows are transiently reduced. If ventricular function is recovering, an inotrope, such as milrinone, can be given to provide support after removal of the device, if necessary. With the use of ECMO, it is beneficial to support some LV contraction to minimize the risk of LV thrombus formation.

3. Vasodilators are commonly used during the early phase of postoperative recovery to reduce blood pressure when the patient is hypothermic, vasoconstricted, and hypertensive. They are weaned when the patient vasodilates to maintain a systolic blood pressure of 100–120 mm Hg.

   a. Vasodilators may also be used alone or in conjunction with inotropic medications to improve myocardial function by lowering the SVR. In this situation, they are weaned concomitantly with the inotropes, depending on the cardiac output and the blood pressure. Sodium nitroprusside and clevidipine have half-lives of only two and one minute, respectively, but nicardipine has a duration of action of 4–6 hours.

   b. In patients with preexisting hypertension, conversion from intravenous antihypertensives to oral agents can be tricky. Some patients require significant doses of multiple drugs to control their blood pressure, only to become hypotensive when the drugs take effect and sympathetic stimulation and the hormonal response to surgery abate. The initial drug is usually a β-blocker (unless the patient is bradycardic), which is routinely used for prophylaxis of atrial fibrillation. An ACE inhibitor or ARB is then added, starting at a low dose if not used before or at a lower dose than used preoperatively. Amlodipine is another option, especially if the patient is bradycardic. Intravenous hydralazine can be used on a prn basis until higher doses of medications take effect.

IV. Intra-aortic Balloon Counterpulsation

Intra-aortic balloon counterpulsation provides hemodynamic support and/or control of ischemia both before and after surgery.[130-132] In contrast to the inotropic drugs, the IABP provides physiologic assistance to the failing heart by decreasing myocardial oxygen demand and improving coronary perfusion. Although it is an invasive device with several potential complications, it has proven invaluable in improving the results of surgery in high-risk patients and allowing for the survival of many patients with postcardiotomy ventricular dysfunction.

A. Indications

1. Ongoing ischemia refractory to medical therapy or hemodynamic compromise prior to urgent or emergent surgery.

2. Prophylactic placement prior to surgery for high-risk patients with critical coronary disease (usually left main disease) or severe LV dysfunction – usually following cardiac catheterization, but occasionally at the beginning of surgery.[133–136]

3. Unloading for mechanical complications of myocardial infarction (acute mitral regurgitation, ventricular septal rupture) prior to emergent surgery.

4. High-risk patients undergoing off-pump surgery to maintain hemodynamic stability during lateral wall or posterior wall grafting.[137]

5. Acute myocardial infarction primarily with, but occasionally without, cardiogenic shock. This remains a common indication for use of an IABP, yet most studies have not demonstrated any mortality benefit even when percutaneous coronary intervention (PCI) is performed.[138–143] In this situation, use of a mechanical circulatory assist device may be preferable.[144]

6. Prophylactic use during high-risk PCI[145]

7. Postcardiotomy low cardiac output syndrome unresponsive to moderate doses of multiple inotropic agents. One study devised a clinical risk score to predict the need for an IABP after CABG. These factors included older age, poor LV function, redo and emergency procedures, left main disease, recent MI, and class 3–4 symptoms.[146] Although this study reported a 19% mortality rate in this situation, others have reported mortality rates of 30–50%.[147,148]

8. Postoperative myocardial ischemia

9. Acute deterioration of myocardial function (refractory heart failure) to provide temporary support or serve as a bridge to transplantation.

B. Contraindications

1. Aortic regurgitation (unless mild)

2. Aortic dissection/extensive aneurysmal disease

3. Severe aortic and peripheral vascular atherosclerosis (balloon can be inserted via the ascending aorta during surgery)

4. Sepsis

C. Principles

1. The IABP reduces the impedance to LV ejection ("unloads the heart") by rapid deflation just before ventricular systole.

2. It increases diastolic coronary perfusion pressure by rapid inflation just after aortic valve closure with improvement in native coronary, ITA, and graft diastolic flow.

3. This sequence reduces the time–tension index (systolic wall tension) and increases the diastolic pressure–time index, favorably altering the myocardial oxygen supply:demand ratio.

4. The IABP may also improve left ventricular diastolic function after surgery.[149]

5. In patients with RV failure, the IABP may improve RV function by improving right coronary perfusion pressure and reducing RV afterload by decreasing LV filling pressures. However, the benefit of an IABP for severe RV failure is limited and further mechanical circulatory assist may be necessary.[54,150–153]

D. Insertion techniques

1. The IABP is placed through the femoral artery with the balloon situated just distal to the left subclavian artery so as not to impair flow into the left internal thoracic artery (LITA) (Figure 11.1). Generally, a 50 mL balloon is selected for patients >162 cm (5'4") tall, using smaller balloons with shorter lengths (the Datascope 25 mL or 34 mL or Arrow 40 mL balloons) for smaller patients.

2. Percutaneous insertion is performed by the Seldinger technique, placing the balloon over a guide wire and either through a sheath or without a sheath ("sheathless"). The catheter is usually 7.5 Fr in diameter. The sheath can be left in place or removed from the artery, especially if the femoral artery is small. Smaller-caliber systems can minimize the reduction in flow that could cause distal ischemia, and are preferable in patients with peripheral vascular disease and diabetes. Sheathless insertion may cause shearing of the balloon during placement if significant iliofemoral disease is present. Although insertion of the IABP can be performed blindly in the OR or at the bedside, preoperative placement is usually performed in the cardiac cath lab using fluoroscopy to visualize the wire and the eventual location of the balloon. This may allow for placement through a tortuous iliofemoral system, which otherwise might be fraught with danger. During surgery, the position of the balloon catheter can be identified by TEE.

3. Surgical insertion can be accomplished by exposing the femoral artery and placing the balloon through a sidearm graft or directly into the vessel through a purse-string suture. This is rarely required with current systems.

4. Alternative cannulation sites in patients with severe aortoiliac disease include the ascending aorta during surgery and the subclavian or brachial artery.[154,155] For

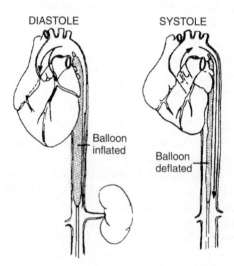

DIASTOLE   SYSTOLE

Balloon inflated

Balloon deflated

Figure 11.1 • The intra-aortic balloon (IABP) is positioned just distal to the left subclavian artery. Balloon inflation occurs in early diastole and improves coronary perfusion pressure. Deflation occurs just before systole to reduce the impedance to left ventricular ejection. (Reproduced with permission from Maccioli et al., *J Cardiothorac Anesth* 1988;2:365–73.)

patients in whom long-term IABP support is considered prior to transplantation, percutaneous insertion into the left axillary/subclavian artery can be used.[156]

E. **IABP timing** is performed from the ECG or the arterial waveform.

1. ECG: input to the balloon console is provided from skin leads or the bedside monitor. Inflation is set for the peak of the T wave at the end of systole with deflation set just before or on the R wave. The use of bipolar pacing eliminates the interpretation of pacing spikes as QRS complexes by the console.

2. Arterial waveform: inflation should occur at the dicrotic notch with deflation just before the onset of the aortic upstroke. This method is especially useful in the operating room, where electrocautery may interfere with the ECG signal.

3. A typical arterial waveform during a 1:2 ratio of IABP inflation is demonstrated in Figures 11.2 and 11.3. This shows the systolic unloading (decrease in the balloon-assisted systolic pressure and end-diastolic pressure) and the diastolic augmentation (increase in the balloon-assisted diastolic pressure) that are achieved with the IABP.

4. Appropriate timing of inflation and deflation is essential. Proper timing should improve stroke volume and reduce LVESV and pressure. Early inflation may decrease stroke volume due to the abrupt increase in LV afterload during late systolic ejection. Late deflation will increase afterload during early ejection and decrease afterload during late ejection. This may increase stroke volume but also increase stroke work.

5. During a cardiac arrest, ballooning may be synchronized to cardiac contractions using the pressure trigger mode. Without cardiac massage, an internal trigger at 100 inflations/minute should be used.

F. **IABP problems and complications**

1. **Inability to balloon.** Once the balloon is situated properly and has unwrapped, satisfactory ballooning should be achieved by proper timing of inflation and deflation. However, unsatisfactory ballooning can occur in the following situations.

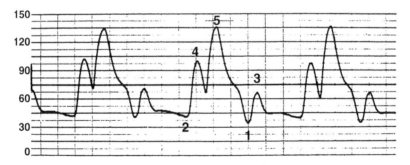

Figure 11.2 • IABP tracing at 1:2 inflation ratio. Note that the balloon aortic end-diastolic pressure (1) is lower than the patient's aortic end-diastolic pressure (2), and that the balloon-assisted peak systolic pressure (3) is lower than the systolic pressure that is generated without a preceding assisted beat (4). These changes reflect a decreased impedance to ejection during systole. Coronary perfusion pressure is increased by diastolic augmentation achieved by balloon inflation (5).

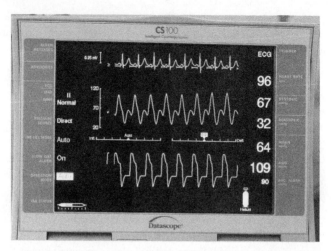

Figure 11.3 • IABP monitor showing the ECG, arterial pressure tracing with balloon augmentation, and balloon inflation/deflation pattern.

a. Unipolar atrial pacing. This produces a large atrial pacing spike that can be interpreted by the console as a QRS complex leading to inappropriate inflation. Use of bipolar pacing eliminates this problem. Most monitoring equipment suppresses pacing signals.

b. Rapid rates. Some balloon consoles are unable to inflate and deflate fast enough to accommodate heart rates over 150 (usually when there is a rapid ventricular response to atrial fibrillation). Augmentation can be performed with a 1:2 ratio.

c. Arrhythmias. Atrial and ventricular ectopy can disrupt normal inflation and deflation patterns and must be treated.

d. Volume loss from the balloon detected by the console monitor alarms. This indicates a leak in the system, either at the connectors or from the balloon itself. Volume loss may also indicate that the balloon has not unwrapped properly, preventing proper inflation.

e. Balloon rupture. When blood appears in the balloon tubing, the balloon has perforated. Escape of gas (usually helium) from the balloon into the bloodstream can occur. **The balloon must be removed immediately.** Difficulty with removal (balloon entrapment) may be encountered if thrombus has formed within the balloon, and this tends to occur extremely quickly. Most consoles have alarms that will call attention to this problem and prevent the device from inflating.

2. **Vascular complications**

a. Catastrophic complications, such as aortic dissection, usually from inadvertent advancement of the guide wire into the vessel wall creating a false lumen, or rupture of the iliac artery or aorta, are very uncommon. Paraplegia can result from development of a periadventitial aortic hematoma or embolization of atherosclerotic debris.[157] Bleeding around the balloon cable may occur if placed into a diseased vessel and can be problematic upon percutaneous removal.

b. Embolization to visceral vessels, especially the mesenteric and renal arteries, can occur in the presence of significant aortic atherosclerosis, although balloon placement usually does not affect mesenteric flow.[158] Cerebral embolization can occur if there are mobile atheromas in the proximal descending thoracic aorta.[159] Renal ischemia may occur if the balloon is situated too low and inflates below the level of the diaphragm.[160]

c. Distal ischemia is the most common complication of indwelling balloons, occurring in 8–18% of patients.[161–163] It is more likely to occur with use of larger catheter sizes, so sheathless techniques are preferable. Ischemia is more likely when the IABP remains in place longer, and when the patient has impaired ventricular function, often requiring inotropic or vasopressor support.[164] Additional risk factors include female gender (small femoral arteries), comorbidities (including diabetes, hypertension, obesity, and smoking), and peripheral vascular disease, especially involving the iliofemoral system. Thrombosis near the insertion site or distal thromboembolism can also occur and is related more to the duration of IABP usage. Use of intravenous heparin (maintaining a PTT of 1.5–2 times control) is advisable to minimize ischemic and thromboembolic problems if the balloon remains in place for more than a few days after surgery. Otherwise, patients have a low-grade coagulopathy in the early postoperative period and anticoagulation is not necessary.

d. The presence of distal pulses or Doppler signals **must be assessed frequently** in all patients with an IABP. This should be compared with a preoperative peripheral pulse examination. Not infrequently, cool extremities with weak signals are noted in the early postoperative period from peripheral vasoconstriction that may be associated with a low cardiac output state, hypothermia, or use of vasopressors. This should resolve when the patient warms and myocardial function improves. However, persistent ischemia jeopardizes the viability of the distal leg and could also lead to a compartment syndrome. Options at this time include:

  i. Removing the sheath from the femoral artery if the balloon has been placed percutaneously.

  ii. Removing the balloon if the patient appears to be hemodynamically stable. If adequate distal perfusion cannot be obtained, femoral exploration is indicated.

  iii. Removing the balloon and placing it in the contralateral femoral artery (if that leg has adequate perfusion) if the patient is IABP-dependent. Using as small a caliber balloon as possible with sheath removal is essential.

  iv. Considering placement of the balloon through another site, such as the axillary/subclavian artery.[156]

3. **Thrombocytopenia.** Persistent inflation and deflation of the IABP will destroy circulating platelets, with thrombocytopenia being noted in about 50% of patients. It is not always clear whether progressive thrombocytopenia is caused by the IABP or by medications that the patient may be receiving, such as heparin. Platelet counts must be checked on a daily basis.

4. **Sepsis** may occur with longer duration of IABP usage.

G. Weaning of the IABP

1. IABP support can be withdrawn when the cardiac output is satisfactory on minimal inotropic support (usually 1 μg/min of epinephrine, 5 μg/kg/min of dobutamine, or ≤0.5 μg/kg/min of milrinone). However, earlier removal may be indicated if complications develop, such as leg ischemia, balloon malfunction, thrombocytopenia, or infection.

2. Weaning is initiated by decreasing the inflation ratio from 1:1 to 1:2 for about 2–4 hours, and then to 1:3 or 1:4 (depending on which console device is used) for 1–2 more hours. If the patient is not heparinized, the duration at a low inflation ratio should be minimized. Once it is determined that the patient can tolerate a low inflation ratio with stable hemodynamics, the IABP should be removed. Recovery of LV function is usually suggested when the arterial tracing suggests a good stroke volume with a systolic pressure that approaches or exceeds the diastolic augmentation pressure on the monitor. Remember that the IABP produces efficient unloading, and the blood pressure noted on the monitor is lower during balloon assistance than with an unassisted beat (actually the diastolic pressure is higher, but the true systolic pressure is lower). Thus, visual improvement in blood pressure with weaning of the IABP is not, by itself, a sensitive measure of the patient's progress. If there is an anticipated delay in removal of more than a few hours for manpower reasons or because of the need to correct a coagulopathy, the ratio should be maintained at 1:1 or 1:2 to prevent thrombus formation on the balloon.

H. IABP removal techniques

1. Balloons inserted by the percutaneous technique can usually be removed percutaneously. This is performed by compressing the groin distal to the insertion site as the balloon is removed, allowing blood to flush out the skin wound for 1–2 heart beats, and then compressing just proximal to the skin hole where the arterial puncture site is located (Figure 11.4). Pressure must be maintained for at least 45 minutes to ensure satisfactory sealing at the puncture site. This may on occasion cause thrombosis of the vessel, so a distal pulse examination during and after compression is essential. **Note:** it is important to resist the temptation to remove manual pressure

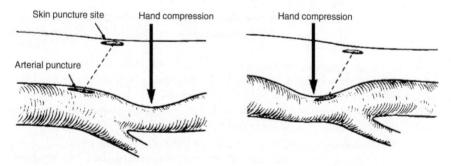

Figure 11.4 • Technique of percutaneous balloon removal. Initial compression is held below the level of the arterial puncture site to allow for flushing of blood. However, subsequent pressure should be maintained over the arterial puncture site to prevent bleeding. Note that the hole in the artery lies more cephalad than the hole in the skin. (Modified from Rodigas and Finnegan, *Ann Thorac Surg* 1985;40:80–1.)

and peek to see if hemostasis is achieved. This can be counterproductive and flush away immature clot that is sealing the vessel. Improved hemostasis may be obtained using the D-STAT Dry (Teleflex) or QuikClot (Z-Medica) hemostatic pads.

2. **Note:** coagulation parameters must be checked and corrected before percutaneous removal or the patient may require groin exploration for persistent hemorrhage or a false aneurysm.

3. Surgical removal should be considered in patients with small or diseased vessels and in those with very weak pulses or Doppler signals with the balloon in place. The need for a thrombectomy and embolectomy may be anticipated in these patients. If the IABP has been in place for more than five days, percutaneous removal can be performed, but there is a greater chance that surgical repair of the femoral artery may be required.

I. **Results of IABP usage**

1. The indications for placement of an IABP are virtually all high-risk situations with high mortality rates despite some benefits of the IABP. Preoperative placement for cardiogenic shock or active ischemia is associated with high operative mortality. Results are the best when an IABP is placed prophylactically in the cath lab or prior to surgery in "high risk" patients, specifically those with threatening anatomy and/or poor LV function who are hemodynamically stable. In these situations, use of an IABP has been shown to lower the likelihood of postoperative low cardiac output syndrome and operative mortality.[133–136] Patients receiving an IABP for postcardiotomy support have already demonstrated failure of pharmacologic management to achieve satisfactory hemodynamics, and most studies have shown a 30–50% mortality in such patients, which is greatest if the IABP is placed postoperatively.[146–148]

2. One study showed that the most significant correlate of operative mortality in patients requiring an IABP was a serum lactate level >10 mmol/L during the first eight hours of support (100% mortality). Additional poor prognostic signs were a metabolic acidosis (base deficit >10 mmol/L), mean arterial pressure <60 mm Hg, urine output <30 mL/h for two hours, and the requirement for high doses of epinephrine or norepinephrine (>10 µg/min) during the early postoperative period.[165]

V. Mechanical Circulatory Support

A. If a patient cannot be weaned from CPB despite maximal pharmacologic support and use of an IABP, consideration should be given to use of extracorporeal membrane oxygenation (ECMO) or placement of a circulatory assist device for mechanical circulatory support (MCS). These devices provide flow to support the systemic and/or pulmonary circulation while resting the heart, allowing it to undergo metabolic and functional recovery. In some cases, weaning and removal of the device may be possible after several days of recovery. In others, weaning is not possible, and conversion to a long-term device as a bridge to transplantation or for destination therapy must be considered.

B. **Clinical conditions** that may benefit from MCS include:

1. Postcardiotomy ventricular dysfunction refractory to maximal medical therapy and an IABP. Although left ventricular and right ventricular assist devices (LVADs and RVADs) may be used, biventricular failure is not uncommon and is often

associated with hypoxemic respiratory failure from a long pump run. Therefore, short-term ECMO is often the easiest way to provide initial support.[166,167]

2. Acute myocardial infarction with cardiogenic shock. Percutaneous LVADs can provide superior hemodynamic support to that which can be achieved with an IABP, but only the use of MCS prior to PCI improves results.[142,168–171]

3. Supporting high-risk interventions in the cath lab. Studies comparing Impella- and IABP-supported procedures showed improved event-free survival with use of an Impella, but not with IABPs.[172–174]

4. Resuscitation from cardiac arrest[175]

5. Patients with class IV heart failure and deteriorating clinical status in INTERMACS classes 1–5. Bridging to transplantation or destination therapy with long-term devices may be indicated for patients with HF from advanced cardiomyopathies, but temporary support may also be useful in patients with myocarditis, which may have a self-limited course.

C. **Basic principles of VADs**

1. VADs are preload-dependent, so their output is reduced with low filling pressures either from hypovolemia or cardiac tamponade, which restricts atrial filling and decreases cardiac output. The centrifugal and axial pumps are also afterload-sensitive, such that an increase in blood pressure will decrease pump flow/output.

2. VADs decompress an overdistended ventricle to allow it to recover some function, although unloading of the left ventricle with an LVAD can precipitate RV failure. Unloading is comparable with nonpulsatile continuous flow devices and earlier pulsatile devices.[176,177] ECMO does not unload the left ventricle or reduce oxygen demand as well as VADs and can exacerbate myocardial ischemia or precipitate pulmonary edema, but additional support with an IABP or LVAD can address that concern.[178]

3. VADs provide pulmonary (RVAD) or systemic (LVAD) flow, in contrast to the IABP, which supports ventricular function only by systolic unloading. The improvement in systolic flow, independent of pulsatility, usually allows organ system function to improve.[179]

4. VADs function independently of the ECG and can keep a patient alive during ventricular fibrillation (VF).

5. They require an energy source.

6. They require anticoagulation despite attempts at biocompatibility.

7. They are associated with multiple major complications, including infection, bleeding, stroke, and device malfunction.

D. **Left ventricular assist devices (LVADs)**

1. **Technique and hemodynamics.** Drainage of oxygenated blood from the left atrium or ventricle passes through the pump and is returned to the ascending aorta. This will provide systemic perfusion while decompressing the left ventricle. LV wall stress is reduced by about 80% with a 40% decrease in myocardial oxygen demand. LVAD flow is dependent on adequate intravascular volume and right ventricular function. Although volume unloading might be superior with the early generation pulsatile pumps, left ventricular pressure unloading is generally considered comparable with nonpulsatile (centrifugal or axial flow) pumps.[176,177]

Table 11.7 • Indications for Mechanical Circulatory Support

1. Complete and adequate cardiac surgical procedure
2. Correction of all metabolic problems (ABGs, acid–base, electrolytes)
3. Inability to wean from bypass despite maximal pharmacologic therapy and use of an IABP
4. Cardiac index <1.8 L/min/m²

LVAD	RVAD	BiVAD
Systolic BP <90 mm Hg	Mean RAP >20 mm Hg	LAP >20 mm Hg
LAP >20 mm Hg	LAP <15 mm Hg	RAP >20–25 mm Hg
SVR >2100 dyn-s/cm⁵	No tricuspid regurgitation	No tricuspid regurgitation
Urine output <20 mL/h		Inability to maintain LVAD flow >2.0 L/min/m² with RAP >20 mm Hg

LVAD, left ventricular assist device; RVAD, right ventricular assist device; BiVAD, biventricular assist device; RAP, right atrial pressure; LAP, left atrial pressure

2. **Indications** (Table 11.7). The general indications for LVAD insertion are the presence of a cardiac index <1.8 L/min/m² with a systolic blood pressure <90 mm Hg and a PCW pressure or LAP >20 mm Hg on maximal medical support and an IABP. In the postcardiotomy patient, an extensive delay in initiating VAD support increases the risk of multisystem organ failure and death.[180] Any of the clinical situations listed in section V.B with primarily LV failure may benefit from LVAD insertion.

3. **Contraindications** to the use of an LVAD vary depending on the access and drainage sites of the particular device.

    a. General contraindications include aortic regurgitation, a mechanical aortic valve, aortic aneurysm/dissection, left heart thrombus (atrial or ventricular), iliofemoral disease for percutaneous systems, and sepsis.

    b. When the indications for LVAD placement are present, critical elements of decision-making include whether there is a reasonable chance of recovery, whether the patient is a candidate for transplantation or destination therapy if there is little chance for recovery, whether RVAD placement is also indicated, and whether placement is contraindicated based upon noncardiac comorbidities. Generally, one must consider the patient's age and general medical condition, the status of RV function, noncardiac organ system function (neurologic, pulmonary, renal, hepatic), and other medical issues (infectious, vascular disease, diabetes), in making this critical decision, whether for postcardiotomy support or for heart failure patients. Risk models to assess survivability after LVAD implantation in heart failure patients are helpful in reaching the appropriate decision.[181]

4. **Devices to provide LVAD support** (see sections H and I, pages 565–571)

   a. Postcardiotomy support is most readily achieved using systems that use central cannulation sites that are exposed during open-heart surgery via a sternotomy. The CentriMag system (Abbott) can be used for LVAD support using left atrial (LA) or left ventricular (LV) and aortic cannulation, for RVAD support using right atrial and pulmonary artery cannulation, and for ECMO using right atrial and aortic cannulation with an oxygenator added to the circuit.[182–184] An alternative is the Impella LD (Abiomed), which is inserted directly through the ascending aorta into the left ventricle.[185]

   b. Percutaneous devices are used for procedures performed in the cath lab or hybrid operating room, and can be placed in a postcardiotomy patient. These include the Impella series and the TandemHeart (TandemLife, LivaNova).[186] The Impella can also be inserted through the subclavian/axillary artery, either via a cutdown or percutaneously.

   c. Long-term devices for bridging and destination therapy include the second-generation HeartMate II (HM II) and HeartWare, and the third-generation HeartMate 3 (HM 3) (Abbott).

5. **Management** during LVAD support

   a. LVAD flow is initiated to achieve a systemic flow of 2.2 L/min/m² with an LA pressure of 10–15 mm Hg. The flow rate of centrifugal or axial flow devices can be preset on a console, with limitations to flow being hypovolemia, improper position of the drainage catheter, or RV failure. Adequacy of tissue perfusion can be assessed by mixed venous oxygen saturations.

   b. To decrease myocardial oxygen demand and allow for ventricular recovery, vasoactive medications should be used only as necessary to support RV function or increase systemic resistance to maintain a MAP >75 mm Hg. α-agents or vasopressin may be necessary because LVAD patients commonly manifest "vasodilatory shock".[187]

   c. Heparinization is recommended to achieve a PTT of 2–2.5 times normal or an ACT of 185–200 seconds for most short-term assist devices once perioperative bleeding has ceased. An infusion of 500 units/h of heparin usually suffices, although most patients become heparin-resistant. For pump flows <3 L/min or during weaning attempts, the PTT and ACT should be increased to 2.5–3 times normal and 250–300 seconds, respectively. Anticoagulation is also required in patients with bioprosthetic or mechanical valves.

   d. When used for temporary postcardiotomy support, LV function is assessed by TEE after at least 48 hours of support. However, weaning is rarely possible before five days of support. Flow is reduced in 0.5 L/min intervals every five minutes to 2 L/min with careful observation of regional and global wall motion, filling pressures, and systemic pressure. Low-dose inotropic support can be initiated during the weaning process. If adequate recovery has occurred, the device may be explanted.

   e. Note that external compressions during VF are feasible with percutaneous and continuous flow devices, but generally are not recommended, because they can cause displacement of the devices.[188]

6. **Overall results.** The mortality rate associated with VAD usage for postcardiotomy support depends on how aggressively one manages a low output syndrome. Because

of the high incidence of bleeding and other organ system problems associated with VADs, there is often a reluctance to insert the device "prematurely", because in many cases, the heart will gradually improve with time on pharmacologic and IABP support without organ system sequelae. Although there are concerns that complications associated with premature VAD insertion could compromise outcomes, an early, aggressive approach to VAD insertion may lower mortality rates, not just because the patient might have survived without it, but because it might avoid the adverse sequelae of a prolonged low cardiac output syndrome in some patients.

a. In general, it has been estimated that about 50% of patients receiving LVADs for postcardiotomy support are discharged from the hospital.[189] The RECOVER I study noted a 93% hospital survival with use of the Impella 5.0/LD for postcardiotomy circulatory support.[185] Improved survival may be noted in patients with preserved RV function, no evidence of a perioperative MI, and recovery of LV function within 48–72 hours.

b. If ventricular function does not recover after a week of support with a short-term device, a longer-term device should be considered for destination therapy or as a bridge to transplantation. Survival following transplantation is similar to that of patients not requiring bridging with mechanical circulatory support.[190]

E. **Right ventricular assist devices (RVADs)**[142,191–197]

1. **Technique and hemodynamics.** Deoxygenated blood is drained from the right atrium and returned to the pulmonary artery, thus providing pulmonary blood flow while decompressing the right ventricle. Achieving satisfactory systemic flow rates depends on having adequate intravascular volume and satisfactory LV function. Although isolated RV failure may occur, it is more commonly associated with LV failure and often with oxygenation issues in the postcardiotomy period that might benefit preferentially from ECMO.

2. **Indications** (Table 11.7). RVAD insertion is indicated when there is evidence of severe RV dysfunction with a high CVP (usually >20mmHg) and inability to maintain a satisfactory cardiac output despite maximal pharmacologic therapy (usually epinephrine/milrinone and an IABP). RV failure may result from an RV infarction, worsening of preexisting RV dysfunction caused by PH or correction of severe tricuspid regurgitation, or poor intraoperative protection. RV dysfunction is exacerbated by an elevation in PVR, which can often be attributed to proinflammatory cytokines due to CPB, noncardiogenic or cardiogenic pulmonary edema, and microembolization from multiple blood product transfusions. Evidence of severe RV dysfunction with vasopressor-refractory low cardiac output syndrome, hypotension, oliguria, and lactic acidosis is highly predictive of mortality; therefore, early RVAD placement should be considered in such a patient. LVAD placement may also lead to RV failure, for which RVAD support may also be required.

3. **Available systems for RV assist**

a. Postcardiotomy support is best provided by the CentriMag system using cannulas placed directly into the right atrium and pulmonary artery. The percutaneously placed systems can be used, but they require a hybrid OR with appropriate radiographic imaging for placement.

b. The **Impella RP** is an 11 Fr catheter with a 22 Fr pump motor (Figure 11.5) that is placed via the femoral vein and propels blood from the right atrium

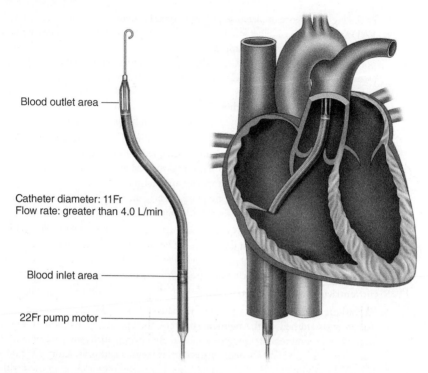

Blood outlet area

Catheter diameter: 11 Fr
Flow rate: greater than 4.0 L/min

Blood inlet area

22Fr pump motor

Figure 11.5 • (A, B) The Impella RP device is advanced from the femoral vein into the right atrium, across the tricuspid valve into the pulmonary artery. The inlet area lies in the inferior vena cava near the IVC–right atrial junction and the outlet lies in the pulmonary artery.

directly into the PA at a rate of up to 4 L/min, resulting in a reduction in RA pressure and an increase in mean PA pressure. The device will increase LV preload, so it can only be used when there is satisfactory LV function; otherwise, increased LV preload and afterload may result in pulmonary edema.[191–195]

c. The TandemHeart RVAD has been used to provide RV support by placing one 62 cm cannula into the RA through the femoral vein to drain blood into the pump, with blood return via a 72 cm cannula placed through the contralateral femoral vein and positioned in the PA. This produces similar hemodynamic benefits as the Impella RP, but it leaves the patient bedbound with femoral cannulas and has been replaced by the Tandem Protek Duo system.

d. The TandemLife Protek Duo system uses a dual lumen catheter placed via the right internal jugular vein that drains blood from the right atrium, passes it through the TandemHeart pump, and returns it to the pulmonary artery at a rate of up to 4.5 L/min (Figure 11.6). An oxygenator can also be placed in the circuit to improve systemic oxygenation.[196,197]

e. RV and LV support can also be achieved using a veno-arterial ECMO circuit.

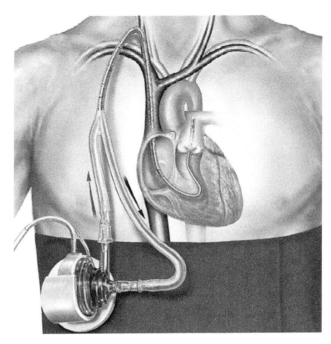

Figure 11.6 • The Tandem Heart Protek Duo system to provide RV support uses a dual lumen catheter that drains blood from the right atrium and returns it to the pulmonary artery. This can be combined with an oxygenator to provide ECMO support as well.

4. **Management** during RVAD support

a. RVAD flow is initiated to achieve a flow rate of 2.2 L/min/m², increasing the LA pressure to 15 mm Hg while maintaining an RA pressure of 5–10 mm Hg. The flow rate of centrifugal or axial flow devices can be preset on a console. Inability to achieve satisfactory flow rates may indicate hypovolemia, improper position of the drainage catheter, or cardiac tamponade that compresses the right atrium. If intravascular volume is adequate and tamponade is not present, systemic hypotension may result from systemic vasodilation that requires use of an α-agent or vasopressin. If impaired LV function is present, additional inotropic, IABP, LVAD, or ECMO support may be necessary. TEE is helpful in evaluating the status of LV function in patients on RVAD support.

b. Pulmonary vasodilators, including IV milrinone, inhaled NO, epoprostenol, iloprost, or milrinone, or oral sildenafil, may be beneficial in reducing pulmonary artery pressures and RV afterload, allowing for recovery of RV function.

c. The requirement for heparinization is similar to that for LVADs.

d. Assessment of myocardial recovery by TEE and weaning of the device are similar to LVADs.

5. **Overall results.** Patients receiving isolated RVADs for acute RV failure have about a 70% one-month survival.[191–193] However, patients requiring RVAD support for postcardiotomy support fair much worse, with limited data suggesting survival rates of only 25%.[194]

F. **Biventricular assist devices (BiVADs)**

1. **Technique and hemodynamics.** BiVADs incorporate the drainage sites of both RVAD and LVAD systems. They provide support of both the pulmonary and systemic circulations but do not provide oxygenation, and can function during periods of VF. In the postcardiotomy patient, ECMO is more readily accomplished using the cannulas already in place for CPB and is used for short-term support.

   a. In patients receiving continuous flow LVADs, RV failure is noted in about 15–20% of patients and can often be managed with pulmonary vasodilators and inotropic support. However, RVAD support will be necessary in about 4–5% of these patients. This is less than previously noted with pulsatile devices as complete LV unloading can be avoided, resulting in less septal shift with better preservation of RV mechanics.[198] Generally, an acute increase in LV unloading with an increase in RV preload may distort RV geometry and unmask RV dysfunction.[199]

   b. Numerous studies have evaluated predictors for RV failure and the necessity for additional RVAD assist in patients receiving LVADs.[200–204] These predictors include:

      i. A higher severity of global illness: patients in INTERMACS I-II, preop ECMO or renal replacement therapy, severe tricuspid regurgitation, reoperative surgery, and concomitant procedures other than TV repair at the time of LVAD implantation.

      ii. Hemodynamic instability: high RA pressures (specifically an RA/PCW ratio >0.63), reduced pulmonary artery pulse pressure, stroke volume, stroke work index, and cardiac output, and the requirement for multiple vasoactive drugs to maintain flow.

      iii. End-organ dysfunction: preoperative ventilatory support, hepatic or renal dysfunction.

      iv. One study proposed an echo score which was predictive of RV failure to identify patients who might benefit from RVAD support. These included a higher RA pressure, lower RV fractional area change, and lower LA volume.[203] Another study designed an RV failure risk score based on vasopressor requirement, abnormal LFTs, and abnormal renal function.[204]

2. **Available devices**

   a. Postcardiotomy BiVAD support can be achieved using two CentriMag devices using RA/PA and LA/aortic cannulation through a median sternotomy. Percutaneous systems combining an Impella RP or Protek Duo with a left-sided Impella device can also be used.[205,206]

   b. If the patient requires longer-term BiVAD support, the HM II, HM 3, or the HeartWare system (Medtronic) is implanted and is combined with either an Impella RP inserted via the axillary artery or the TandemHeart Protek Duo inserted via the internal jugular vein.

3. **Management** during BiVAD support

   a. Sequential manipulations of RVAD and LVAD flow are used to achieve a systemic flow rate of 2.2 L/min/m². The RVAD flow is increased to raise the LA pressure to 15–20 mm Hg, and then the LVAD flow is increased to reduce the LA pressure to 5–10 mm Hg. Inability to achieve satisfactory flow rates usually indicates hypovolemia, tamponade, or catheter malposition on either side. Left- and right-sided flow rates may differ because of varying contributions of the native ventricles to pulmonary or systemic flow.

   b. Heparin requirements are similar to those noted above for LVADs.

   c. Assessment of recovery and weaning are similar to the methods described for RVAD and LVAD devices.

4. **Overall results.** The requirement for biventricular support has an adverse effect on survival. However, one report on BiVAD support for postcardiotomy low cardiac output syndrome with the CentriMag system showed a 56% 30-day survival.[182]

G. **Extracorporeal membrane oxygenation (ECMO)**[207,208]

   1. ECMO is a form of extracorporeal life support (ECLS) that serves as an alternative to ventricular assist devices. The system employs a membrane oxygenator, centrifugal pump, heat exchanger, oxygen blender, and a heparin-coated circuit. The latter provides a more biocompatible surface that minimizes platelet activation and the systemic inflammatory response, and reduces the heparin requirement. This allows the ECMO circuit to be used for several days.

   2. **Indications.** ECMO is indicated for the short-term treatment of severe postcardiotomy ventricular dysfunction with or without hypoxemia. Criteria for use are similar to those for left ventricular or biventricular assist. In many patients requiring VAD support, the duration of CPB is quite long due to the delay in deciding to proceed with VAD support, often resulting in both cardiogenic and noncardiogenic pulmonary edema that impairs oxygenation. ECMO can also be used emergently in patients sustaining a cardiac arrest and in patients with severe hypoxemic ARDS, while the lung recovers from the inciting pathologic insult. Veno-venous ECMO is used for pulmonary support alone (see Figure 5.12, page 314).

   3. **Technique.** At the conclusion of surgery, the same cannulation setup used for CPB is maintained (right atrium and aorta). If ECMO is considered subsequently, it may be established with venous drainage from the internal jugular vein or femoral vein with return of blood to the femoral, axillary, or carotid artery (Figure 11.7). Steps should be taken to ensure distal perfusion with the use of femoral arterial cannulation (see page 312). Because ECMO does not produce LV unloading, it may cause ventricular distention with rising filling pressures and will worsen myocardial oxygen demand. Therefore, either an IABP or preferably an Impella should be considered to unload the LV.[178] Percutaneous femorofemoral bypass may be used to resuscitate a patient from cardiac arrest.

   4. **Management.** Maximal medical support is essential to optimize the results of ECMO. Some of the essential elements are:

   a. Optimizing preload to provide pulmonary perfusion.

   b. Supporting SVR with α-agents or vasopressin; however, elevated SVR and bronchial venous return to the left ventricle can elevate LV pressures and cause

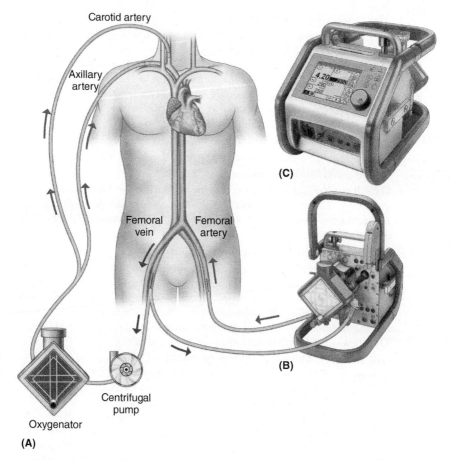

Figure 11.7 • Cannulation sites for veno-arterial ECMO. (A) Venous return from the femoral vein is pumped via a centrifugal pump through an oxygenator and returned to the femoral artery, axillary/subclavian artery, or the carotid artery. (B) The Cardiohelp system is a portable unit for ECMO that includes a centrifugal pump and oxygenator which allows for easy transport. At the conclusion of surgery, right atrial and aortic cannulation sites may be used instead of peripheral cannulation. (C) Close-up of the front of the Cardiohelp console.

LV thrombus formation or pulmonary edema. Since the LV is not unloaded, additional support (IABP or Impella) may be indicated to prevent pulmonary edema and worsening of LV function.

c. Use of femoral artery–femoral vein ECMO may cause coronary or cerebral ischemia if there is any cardiac ejection.[142]

d. Aggressive use of pulmonary vasodilators for PH.

e. Early and aggressive use of renal replacement therapy.

f. Use of low tidal volume ventilation.

g. Minimizing bleeding by initiating anticoagulation after mediastinal bleeding is at a minimum and use of low ACTs in the heparin-coated circuit.

5. If the patient has suffered a severe neurologic insult or is not considered a candidate for transplantation, ECMO is usually terminated after 48 hours. If the heart does not recover after up to one week of ECMO support, a clinical decision must be made about conversion to long-term support. Detailed assessment of neurologic, pulmonary, hepatic, and renal status is essential. It is sometimes difficult to ascertain whether the patient has survivable or nonsurvivable organ system dysfunction that might contraindicate LVAD implantation.

6. **Results.** The results of ECMO depend on the indication for its use and the degree of organ system failure at the time it is initiated.

   a. About one-third of patients receiving ECMO for postcardiotomy support will survive for 30 days, but most would have died without support.[166,167,209–212] A study of ECMO vs. VAD support for postcardiotomy cardiogenic shock found better survival in patients receiving VADs, and in that study only 16% of patients on ECMO support survived the hospital stay.[213]

   b. A large multicenter study provided a postcardiotomy ECMO score to quantify the mortality risk. This included female gender (1 point), advanced age (60–69, 2 points, >70, 4 points), prior cardiac surgery (1 point), lactate >6 mmol/L prior to ECMO (2 points), aortic arch surgery (2 points), and preoperative stroke/coma (5 points). Mortality rate was 45–57% for 1–3 points, but increased to 70% or greater for ≥4 points.[210] Another study confirmed that older age, an elevated lactate level (>4 mmol/L after 48 hours), and hepatic and renal failure were associated with higher mortality.[211]

   c. One study reported a 31% survival in patients undergoing emergent ECMO for prolonged cardiac arrest.[214]

   d. Complications are not insignificant with ECMO. A meta-analysis reported a 17% need for dialysis, 43% reoperations for bleeding, 15% mediastinal wound infections, 11% neurologic events, and an 11% incidence of lower limb ischemia.[212]

H. **Short-term devices to provide ventricular assist**

   1. **Short-term support for high-risk PCI or cardiogenic shock** is best provided with percutaneous systems that require fluoroscopic imaging for their insertion. This is usually performed in the cath lab or hybrid operating room.

      a. The **Impella** series includes LVAD devices, such as the Impella 2.5, CP, and 5.0 devices, which provide increasing amounts of systemic flow, and the Impella RP, which provides RV support.

         i. The Impella 5.0 is a 9 Fr catheter with a 21 F pump motor that is inserted through the femoral artery and positioned across the aortic valve into the left ventricle (Figure 11.8). This axial-flow device withdraws blood from the distal end of the catheter in the LV and pumps it into the ascending aorta. The Impella CP is a 9 Fr catheter with a 14 Fr pump motor that can provide 4L/min flow and is preferred during high-risk PCI.

         ii. The Impella RP is designed for RVAD support.

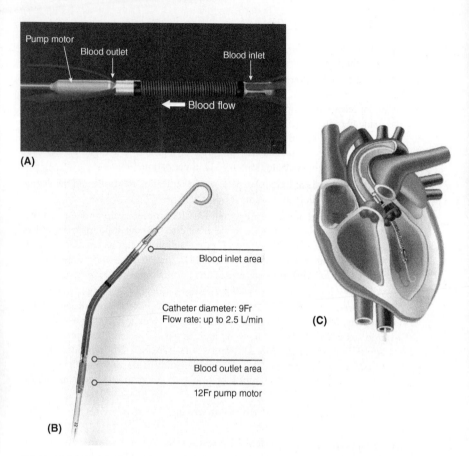

Figure 11.8 • The Impella devices. (A) The basic design of the catheter with an inlet that lies within the left ventricle and an outlet within the ascending aorta, next to which is located the rotary pump. (B, C) The Impella 2.5 device (12 Fr pump motor diameter), Impella CP (14 Fr diameter), and Impella 5 (21 Fr pump motor diameter) devices have similar designs and are placed percutaneously to lie across the aortic valve.

b. The **TandemHeart (PTVA)** system (LivaNova) is a continuous-flow centrifugal pump that can provide up to 5 L/min flow (Figure 11.9). It consists of a 21 Fr transseptal cannula placed percutaneously through the femoral vein and positioned across the atrial septum into the left atrium. Blood drains into a dual-chamber pump which uses a magnetically driven impeller to pump the blood back to the patient through 15 or 17 Fr cannulas placed into one or both femoral arteries. Anticoagulation with heparin to achieve a PTT of 2.5–3 times normal (65–80 seconds) or an ACT >200 seconds is recommended. This device can also be used for postcardiotomy LVAD support with direct LA or LV and aortic cannulation, or as an RVAD for postcardiotomy support or cardiogenic

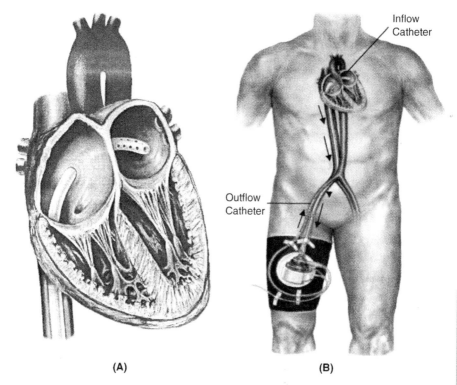

(A) **(B)**

Figure 11.9 • The Tandem Heart percutaneous ventricular assist (PTVA) system. A cannula is introduced into the femoral vein and passed transseptally into the left atrium. The arterial return cannula is placed in the femoral artery.

shock from an RV infarct with percutaneous or direct placement of cannulas into the RA and PA. Use of the TandemLife Protek Duo allows for RV support through a cannula placed through the right internal jugular vein.[196,197]

2. **Short-term postcardiotomy support** can be achieved using continuous-flow (centrifugal, axial) devices that can implanted during surgery. These are the most readily available, easy-to-use systems for uni- or biventricular short-term support. Their use is usually limited to several weeks, at which time conversion to long-term devices may be necessary if recovery does not occur.

a. The **CentriMag** is a centrifugal pump that uses standard cannulation techniques and can provide RVAD, LVAD, or ECMO support by placing a membrane oxygenator in the circuit. This pump uses a magnetically levitated rotor to propel blood forward at a rate of up to 10L/min (Figure 11.10). This avoids friction to minimize blood trauma and hemolysis and can be used for several months of support, although the pump head and external circuit may need to be changed after six weeks. Heparinization to achieve a PTT of 60–100 seconds is recommended.

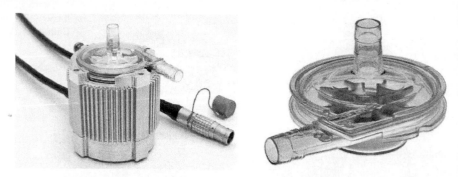

Figure 11.10 • The CentriMag centrifugal motor and pump and a larger image of the pump head.

b. In the absence of an approved device, the **Bio-Medicus** (Medtronic) centrifugal pump that is routinely used for CPB can be used successfully to provide a brief period of uni- or biventricular support until other devices can be implanted. These systems can also be used in ECMO circuits.

c. The Impella LD device is inserted directly through a graft in the ascending aorta.

d. The Impella 5.0 device can be inserted through an axillary/subclavian approach usually via a cutdown.[215]

e. ECMO can be established using the right atrial and aortic cannulas from CPB. Several systems, including the CentriMag device with a oxygenator spliced into the system (Quadrox, MAQUET), and the Cardiohelp system (Getinge), which uses the MAQUET Rotaflow magnetically levitated centrifugal pump that produces minimal hemolysis, can be used to provide ECMO support (Figure 11.7). The latter is a fairly compact system that allows for transport to tertiary care hospitals.[216,217]

3. If myocardial recovery does not occur, a clinical decision must be made as to whether a device capable of longer-term support should be implanted either as a bridge to transplantation or destination therapy, based primarily upon the patient's neurologic function and organ system recovery. Thus, these devices are implanted as a "bridge to decision".[218]

I. **Long-term devices** have evolved from bulky, paracorporeal, and intracorporeal pulsatile systems to smaller, intracorporeal, nonpulsatile, continuous flow devices that are more biocompatible and have improved durability with newer designs. These systems are valve-less and designed with a permanent magnetic field that rapidly spins a simple impeller supported by mechanical bearings. They are preload- and afterload-sensitive and can provide unloading comparable to that of pulsatile devices. However, the degree of unloading can be prescribed, such that excessive LV unloading that can lead to RV failure can be minimized. These devices are effective in maintaining organ system perfusion and can be used as long-term bridges to transplantation or for destination therapy

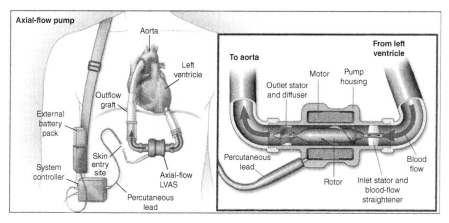

Figure 11.11 • The HeartMate II device is a continuous-flow pump interposed between a cannula placed into the left ventricular apex and a graft sewn to the ascending aorta. (Reproduced with permission of Slaughter et al., *N Engl J Med* 2009;361:2241–51. © 2009 Massachusetts Medical Society.)[219]

in patients who are not considered transplant candidates. Technologic advances in newer generation systems have resulted in smaller devices with improved biocompatibility, more durability, and fewer complications, including device thrombosis.

1. The **Impella 5.0** can be used for long-term support as a bridge to transplantation. It can flow up to 5 L/min. It is inserted through the axillary artery, thus enabling the patient to ambulate.[215]

2. The **HeartMate II** (HM II) is a continuous axial flow device with a rotary pump that can provide up to 10 L/min flow.[219] The inflow cannula is placed through the LV apex, and the outflow cannula is sewn to the ascending aorta (Figure 11.11). The pump is inserted in a preperitoneal pocket with a drive line exiting the right upper quadrant. Early anticoagulation with heparin has been used, but it can contribute to bleeding and is probably not essential. The patient is then maintained on warfarin with a target INR of around 2.0. This device is an excellent bridge to transplantation and has also been used for destination therapy.

3. The **HeartWare** device (HVAD) (Medtronic) is a very small 160 g device implanted through the left ventricular apex which consists of a small centrifugal pump that relies on magnetic and hydrodynamic rotor levitation to generate up to 10 L/min of flow that is returned to the aorta through a 10 mm graft (Figure 11.12).[220] It has one moving part and no mechanical bearings. It can be used as a bridge or for destination therapy.

4. The **HeartMate 3** (HM 3) is a continuous flow centrifugal pump that is partially inserted into the left ventricular apex with return of up to 10 L/min of flow through a graft sewn to the ascending aorta (Figure 11.13). The technological advance is the use of "Full MagLev™" (magnetically levitated) technology that allows the device's

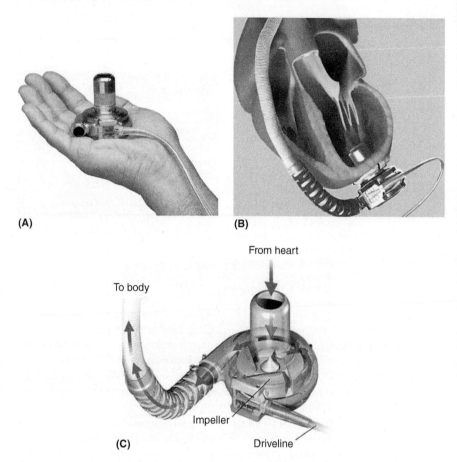

(A)

(B)

From heart

To body

Impeller

Driveline

(C)

Figure 11.12 • (A, B) The HeartWare device is a 160 g device inserted into the LV apex. (C) The blood enters the device and is propelled by a magnetic hydrodynamically levitated propeller back to the aorta. (Image courtesy of Medtronic, Inc. (A), Rogers JG, et al., *N Engl J Med* 2017;376:451–60. Copyright © 2017 Massachusetts Medical Society. All rights reserved.[220] (B), HeartWare® Ventricular Assist System, link for reference: https://www.heartware.com/sites/default/files/uploads/docs/ifu00184_rev08_patientmanual_uspma.pdf © 2020 HeartWare (C).)

rotor to be suspended by magnetic forces. Since the parts "float", there is no friction and therefore less wear and tear on the rotor. This contact-free environment is designed to optimize hemocompatibility and reduce blood trauma through gentle blood handling. There is also "artificial pulse technology" designed to promote washing of the pump to prevent the formation of zones of recirculation and stasis.[221] It can be used as a bridge to transplantation or for destination therapy.

5. Other axial/rotary flow pumps that have been used successfully as bridges to transplantation and for destination therapy include the **Jarvik 2000** (Jarvik Heart) and **Heart Assist 5** (Reliant Heart) devices.[222,223]

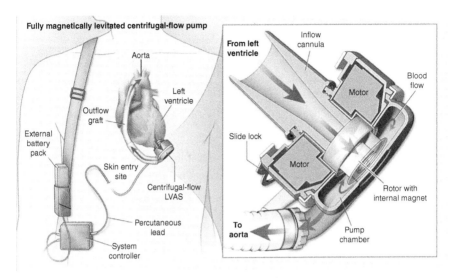

Figure 11.13 • The Heartmate 3 device is a magnetically levitated centrifugal pump implanted through the LV apex with return of blood to the ascending aorta. (Reproduced with permission of Mehra MR, et al., *N Engl J Med* 2017;376(5):440–50. © 2017 Massachusetts Medical Society.)

6. The **HeartWare miniaturized VAD** (MVAD) uses hydrodynamic levitation with a layer of blood to lift the rotor. Blood flow follows the axis of rotation of the impeller, but exits perpendicular to inflow. This lowers shear stress on the impeller and optimizes blood flow paths, which is expected to improve hemodynamic performance. The system also incorporates a pulsatility algorithm called the qPulse™ Cycle individualized for each patient to enhance aortic valve function and reduce chronic bleeding. This device was not approved as of mid-2020.[224]

7. Total artificial hearts (TAHs) potentially hold promise for destination therapy, but are only approved as bridges to transplantation. The most commonly implanted TAH is the **SynCardia** system, which is an offshoot of the Jarvik 7 heart, first implanted in 1988 (Figure 11.14). It consists of two artificial ventricles with mechanical valves, and a pneumatic drive line that compresses a polyurethane diaphragm and can generate up to 9 L/min of flow.[225–227]

8. A number of other devices have been developed and evaluated for long-term ventricular assist with the objective of minimizing complications and improving durability. Advances include technology to provide pulsatility, enable physiologic feedback to control flow, and reduce shear stress to improve biocompatibility, which should reduce platelet activation, hemolysis, and von Willebrand factor degradation, which contributes to bleeding. Some of these advances are present in the HM 3 and HeartWare MVAD devices. Improved transcutaneous energy transmission systems should reduce the risk of infection.

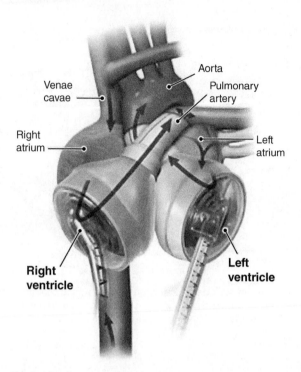

Figure 11.14 • The SynCardia total artificial heart.

J. **Complications.**[188,199] The evolution from early-generation pulsatile pumps (Novacor, Thoratec, Abiomed BV, HeartMate XVE) to axial and continuous flow pumps has reduced but not eliminated the many complications associated with the use of MCS. The most common morbidities with use of short-term assist devices are bleeding, stroke, and organ system failure, the latter usually due to hypoperfusion or hypotension before circulatory assist is initiated. Other complications associated with these devices include the following:

1. **Bleeding.** Despite reversal of anticoagulation, a substantial percentage of patients (up to 60%) require re-exploration for evacuation of mediastinal clot that can cause tamponade (manifested by inadequate drainage into the device). Contributing factors include coagulopathies related to a long duration of CPB in postcardiotomy patients, the large amount of dead space around the catheters in the mediastinum, often an open chest, and the use of early postoperative anticoagulation to minimize thrombus formation within the devices. Although early anticoagulation is desirable, it must be withheld until bleeding is at minimum.

    a. Gastrointestinal bleeding is noted in 15–30% of patients due to the use of anticoagulation, low pulsatility, development of AV malformations, and acquired von Willebrand factor (vWF) deficiency. The latter is caused by the high sheer stress that causes degradation of vWF high-molecular-weight multimers and may be less common with the HM 3 system because of lower sheer stress.[228]

b. Hemolysis, fibrinolysis, and platelet dysfunction are common with LVADs.[229]

c. Heparin-induced thrombocytopenia (HIT) was noted in 26% of patients in one report.[230] Use of warfarin for device thromboprophylaxis and an alternative anticoagulant at the time of transplantation may be necessary unless the time from the diagnosis of HIT to transplantation exceeds three months.

2. **Mediastinitis and sepsis.** With the use of implantable devices, infection is usually related to the drive lines for energy transmission, which exit through the skin. About 20% of patients will develop drive line infections and 15–20% will develop mediastinitis or sepsis.[231,232] Because long-term antibiotic usage is commonplace, resistant organisms are often identified. In addition, many patients are debilitated and malnourished and have numerous intravascular and other invasive catheters that can become colonized. The most common organisms are *Staphylococcus aureus* and coagulase-negative staph, *Candida*, and *Pseudomonas aeruginosa*. Infection is associated with a significantly increased mortality, especially so in the case of fungal endocarditis, which occurs in about 20% of patients. If this develops, antifungal therapy along with either device removal and replacement or urgent transplantation may lead to a successful result. Generally, however, infections are controllable and do not influence the results of transplantation.

3. **Neurologic complications** are noted in 10–20% of patients and are more commonly ischemic than hemorrhagic in nature, although the latter is associated with higher mortality.[233] Ischemic strokes are related to device/graft thrombosis, whereas hemorrhagic strokes are related to anticoagulation, acquired von Willebrand syndrome, endocarditis, hypertension, and hemorrhagic conversion of ischemic cerebral infarcts. The ENDURANCE trial found that the stroke rate was 2.5 times higher with the HeartWare device compared with the HM II (30% vs. 12%),[220] but was comparable with both devices at around 12–15% at two years with good blood pressure control.[234] The MOMENTUM trial showed a 50% reduction in stroke with the HM 3 compared with the HM II devices (19% vs 10%).[221] Patients with mechanical aortic valves should have them covered with tissue or sewn shut to prevent thromboembolism.

4. **Malignant ventricular arrhythmias** may develop as a result of myocardial ischemia, infarction, or the use of catecholamines.[235] BiVADs function during VF, as can LVADs as long as the PVR is not high. If LVAD flow cannot be maintained, the patient may require placement of an RVAD. VF may foster thrombus formation in the ventricles and should be treated aggressively. Early cardioversion should also be considered to prevent RV injury from prolonged VF. Chest compressions can be used for percutaneous and continuous flow devices, but are usually not necessary nor recommended.[188]

5. **Renal failure** is usually caused by prolonged episodes of hypotension or low cardiac output prior to insertion of a VAD. Serum creatinine generally returns to the patient's baseline after VAD implantation, except when there is evidence of other organ system failure (especially hepatic) or infection. Early aggressive treatment with renal replacement therapy (usually continuous veno-venous hemofiltration)

should be considered. The mortality rate for patients with persistent renal failure on VAD support is very high.

6. **Respiratory failure** is usually attributable to a prolonged duration of CPB, sepsis, and use of multiple blood products.

7. **Vasodilatory shock** due to inappropriately low levels of vasopressin is not uncommon in patients requiring placement of VADs. In fact, vasopressin hypersensitivity may be noted. Use of arginine vasopressin in doses up to 0.1 units/min is effective in increasing the mean arterial pressure in these patients.[187]

8. **Worsening heart failure** may result from:

   a. **De novo aortic regurgitation**, which has been noted in 30% of patients with HM II devices after two years. This may be the result of excessive unloading and lack of valve opening, which may lead to cusp remodeling and commissural fusion. Maintaining some degree of pulsatility may minimize this problem.[236]

   b. The development of **RV failure**, which occurs in 15–25% of patients early after LVAD implantation and may require an RVAD in 4%.[194,201] This is usually caused by excessive LV unloading which increases RV preload and unmasks preexisting RV dysfunction. Signs of RV dysfunction by catheterization (high PVR, high PCW/CVP) or echocardiography, ventilator dependence, and renal dysfunction are predictors of the need for RVAD support (as noted in section F.1.b, page 562). The risk of right heart failure was greater with the HeartWare than the HM II device in the ENDURANCE trial.[220]

   c. **Pump thrombosis** related to turbulent flow, device geometry, or underanticoagulation. This has become less common with newer device designs, with only a 1% incidence in the HM 3 studies.[221]

9. Patients receiving LVADs become immunologically sensitized and have a reduced rate of transplantation due to crossmatch issues. Furthermore, they have a higher risk of rejection. However, after transplantation, survival appears to be similar to that of nonbridged recipients who are not sensitized. Immunomodulatory treatment with intravenous immunoglobulins and cyclophosphamide may be beneficial in offsetting the problems associated with sensitization.[237]

VI. Systemic Hypertension

A. General comments

1. Systemic hypertension is fairly common after open-heart surgery, even in patients with no prior history of hypertension. In the immediate postoperative period, it usually results from vasoconstriction due to systemic hypothermia, enhanced sympathetic tone, and altered baroreceptor sensitivity. Postoperative hypertension is more common in patients with chronic hypertension, diabetes, vascular disease, and chronic kidney disease.

2. Hypertension more commonly results from elevated SVR than from hyperdynamic myocardial performance. Therefore, it is imperative that cardiac hemodynamics be assessed before therapeutic interventions are initiated. **One should never assume that hypertension is the result of hyperdynamic cardiac performance.** Withdrawal of inotropic support when hypertension is caused by intense

vasoconstriction may precipitate rapid hemodynamic deterioration if the cardiac output is marginal.

3. Treatment is indicated to maintain the systolic blood pressure <130 mm Hg or the MAP <90 mm Hg. Aggressive treatment is warranted to minimize the potential adverse effects of hypertension. These include an increase in afterload, which increases systolic wall stress and can precipitate myocardial ischemia and impair ventricular function, and the potential for mediastinal bleeding, suture-line disruption, aortic dissection, and stroke.

B. **Etiology**

1. The hormonal milieu of CPB which raises levels of norepinephrine and vasopressin and alters the renin-angiotensin system, increasing autonomic tone and inducing a hyperadrenergic state

2. Vasoconstriction from hypothermia, vasopressors, or a low cardiac output state

3. Fever, anxiety, pain, agitation, and awakening when sedatives wear off

4. Abnormal ABGs (hypoxia, hypercarbia, acidosis)

5. Pharyngeal manipulation (readjusting an endotracheal tube, placing a nasogastric tube or echo probe)

6. A hyperdynamic LV, especially in patients with LVH

7. Altered baroreceptor function following combined CABG carotid endarterectomy

8. Severe acute hypoglycemia

C. **Assessment**

1. Careful patient examination, especially for breath sounds and peripheral perfusion

2. Assessment of cardiac hemodynamics

3. Measurement of ABGs, serum potassium, HCT

4. Review of a chest x-ray and 12-lead ECG

5. Note: don't forget to check the chest drainage unit for the amount of mediastinal bleeding!

D. **Treatment.** Systolic pressure should be maintained between 100 and 130 mm Hg (MAP around 80 mm Hg). The objective is to reduce the SVR sufficiently enough to lower myocardial oxygen demand without compromising coronary perfusion pressure. A secondary benefit is frequently an improvement in myocardial function. Ideally, an antihypertensive agent should prevent myocardial ischemia without adversely affecting heart rate, AV conduction, or myocardial contractility. When used in the early postoperative period, it should have rapid onset and offset of action in the event of changes in hemodynamics.

1. Ensure satisfactory oxygenation and ventilation.

2. Use vasodilator medications if the cardiac output is satisfactory (see section VII, starting on page 576).

3. Provide inotropic support along with vasodilators if the cardiac output is marginal (CI <2.0 L/min/m^2).

4. Sedate with propofol 25–75 μg/kg/min, dexmedetomidine 0.5–1.5 μg/kg/h, midazolam 2.5–5.0 mg IV, or morphine 2.5–5.0 mg IV. Sedation is usually an

appropriate first step in the fully ventilated patient when extubation is not imminently planned. However, antihypertensive drugs rather than sedatives are preferable to allow for early extubation.

5. Control shivering with meperidine 25–50 mg IV, dexmedetomidine 0.75–1.0 µg/kg/h, or pharmacologic paralysis (always with sedation).[238]

VII. Vasodilators and Antihypertensive Medications in the ICU

A. General comments

1. A variety of medications can be used to control systemic hypertension (Table 11.8). Their hemodynamic effects depend on the patient's intravascular volume and myocardial function and the site at which they exert their antihypertensive action. Vasodilators may reduce blood pressure by increasing venous capacitance (which reduces preload) or decreasing arterial resistance (which reduces afterload and usually preload as well). Other antihypertensive medications reduce blood pressure by inhibiting central adrenergic discharge or exerting a

Table 11.8 • Mixes and Dosage Ranges for Common Intravenous Antihypertensive Medications

Medication	Mix	Dosage range
Nitroprusside	50 mg/250 mL	0.1–8 µg/kg/min
Nitroglycerin	50 mg/250 mL	0.1–5 µg/kg/min
Calcium channel blockers		
Clevidipine	50 mg/100 mL	1–21 mg/h
Nicardipine	50 mg/250 mL	5–15 mg/h
Diltiazem	100 mg/100 mL D5W	0.25 mg/kg over 2 min, then 0.35 mg/kg over 2 min, then 5–15 mg/h
Verapamil	120 mg/250 mL	0.1 mg/kg bolus over 2 min, then 2–5 µg/kg/min
Beta-blockers		
Esmolol	2.5 g/250 mL	0.25–0.5 mg/kg/min bolus then 50–200 µg/kg/min
Labetalol	200 mg/200 mL	1–4 mg/min
Hydralazine		10–20 mg IV q6h
Fenoldopam	10 mg/250 mL	0.05–0.1 µg/kg/min initial infusion, up to 0.8 µg/kg/min

negative inotropic effect, a property also shared by several of the vasodilators. Thus, a careful cardiac assessment is required to ensure that the appropriate medication is selected.

2. Antihypertensive medications are most commonly used during the early phase of postoperative recovery when the patient is hypothermic, vasoconstricted, and hypertensive. They are weaned off as the patient vasodilates in order to maintain a systolic blood pressure in the 100 to 130 mm Hg range. Vasodilators may also be used alone or in conjunction with inotropic medications to improve myocardial function by lowering SVR.

3. The most commonly used intravenous antihypertensives in the ICU are sodium nitroprusside and clevidipine, which are both short-acting medications. Other IV medications, such as NTG, CCBs (nicardipine), β-blockers (intermittent IV boluses of metoprolol or continuous infusions of esmolol or labetalol), hydralazine, or fenoldopam can also be considered in selected situations.

4. Most patients without chronic hypertension will exhibit only transient hypertension after surgery and usually do not require antihypertensive therapy after 24 hours. For those with a history of hypertension, oral medications must be initiated before transfer from the ICU. The appropriate choice depends on the patient's hemodynamic status and renal function (see pages 585–586).

B. **Sodium nitroprusside (SNP)**

1. **Hemodynamic effects**

   a. SNP primarily relaxes arterial smooth muscle and reduces SVR and PVR. It has a lesser effect on venous capacitance that will also reduce preload. The overall effect is a reduction in systemic blood pressure and filling pressures, often resulting in an improvement in LV function. Maintenance or improvement in cardiac output usually requires a modest volume infusion to restore filling pressures to an optimal level. The approach is: "optimize preload → reduce afterload → restore preload". The development of a reflex tachycardia during SNP infusion usually reflects hypovolemia.

   b. SNP is a very dangerous drug which always requires close monitoring with an indwelling arterial cannula. It has a very rapid onset of action (within seconds) and can lower the blood pressure precipitously. Fortunately, its effects dissipate within 1–2 minutes.

2. **Indications**

   a. **To control systemic hypertension** caused by an increase in SVR. SNP is an excellent drug to use if cardiac function is marginal, filling pressures are elevated, and SVR is high.

   b. **To improve myocardial function** when the SVR is elevated, usually when systemic hypertension is present. The best results are often obtained with concomitant inotropic support.

3. The usual **starting dose** is 0.1 µg/kg/min with a mix of 50 mg/250 mL. The bottle must be wrapped in aluminum foil to prevent metabolic breakdown from light. The dose is gradually increased to a maximum of 8 µg/kg/min.

4. Adverse effects

a. Potentiation of myocardial ischemia by:

   i. A reduction in diastolic perfusion pressure. If filling pressures do not decrease when systemic perfusion pressure falls, the diastolic transmyocardial gradient for coronary blood flow will be reduced, potentially producing myocardial ischemia.

   ii. Producing a coronary steal syndrome by dilating resistance vessels in the coronary circulation and shunting of blood away from ischemic zones.

   iii. Causing a reflex tachycardia.

b. Reflex increase in contractility and dp/dt. In the patient with an aortic dissection, SNP should generally not be given prior to administering a β-blocker unless the patient is bradycardic.

c. Inhibition of hypoxic vasoconstriction, which produces V/Q mismatch and hypoxia.

d. Tachyphylaxis to its vasodilating effects

e. **Cyanide toxicity.** Nitroprusside is metabolized to cyanide, which is then converted to thiocyanate in the liver. Cyanide toxicity, manifested by metabolic acidosis and an elevated mixed venous PO_2, may occur when large doses (>8 μg/kg/min) are given for several days (cumulative dose >1 mg/kg over 12–24 hours) or if hepatic dysfunction is present. Hemolysis and free Hb release during CPB may accelerate the release of free cyanide from SNP.[239] Moderate cyanide toxicity is treated by converting the cyanide to thiocyanate for its excretion by the kidneys:

   i. Sodium bicarbonate for metabolic acidosis in doses of 1 mEq/kg

   ii. Sodium thiosulfate 150 mg/kg IV (approximately 12.5 g in a 50 mL D5W solution given over 10 minutes)

f. **Thiocyanate toxicity** (level >5 mg/dL) may develop from chronic use of SNP especially when there is impaired renal excretion of this metabolite. It is manifested by dyspnea, vomiting, and mental status changes with dizziness, headache, and loss of consciousness. **Treatment** of both severe cyanide and thiocyanate toxicity involves use of nitrite preparations to induce methemoglobin formation. The methemoglobin combines with cyanide to form cyanmethemoglobin, which is nontoxic.

   i. Amyl nitrite inhalation of 1 ampule over 15 seconds

   ii. Sodium nitrite 5 mg/kg IV slow push. This is usually given at a rate of 2.5 mL/min of a 3% solution to a total of 10–15 mL. One-half of this dose can be used subsequently if toxicity recurs.

   iii. Sodium thiosulfate in the dose noted just above can then be administered to convert the cyanide, which is gradually dissociated from cyanmethemoglobin, into thiocyanate for excretion.

C. Nitroglycerin (NTG)

1. Hemodynamic effects

a. NTG is primarily a venodilator that lowers blood pressure by reducing preload, filling pressures, stroke volume, and cardiac output. If filling pressures are satisfactory, NTG will maintain aortic diastolic perfusion pressure, although at high doses some arterial vasodilation does occur. In the presence of hypovolemia or a marginal cardiac output, NTG should be avoided, because it will lower cardiac output further and produce a reflex tachycardia.

 b. NTG dilates coronary conductance vessels and improves blood flow to ischemic zones.[240]

 c. IV NTG is rapid-acting with an onset of action of 2–5 minutes and a duration of action of 10–20 minutes.

2. Indications

 a. **Hypertension** in association with myocardial ischemia or high filling pressures

 b. ECG changes of **myocardial ischemia**. NTG is useful prior to surgery in conjunction with phenylephrine which is used to maintain coronary perfusion pressures.

 c. **Coronary spasm**

 d. **Pulmonary hypertension**, to reduce RV afterload and improve RV function

3. Starting dose is 0.1 µg/kg/min with a mix of 50 mg/250 mL. The dose can be titrated up to 5 µg/kg/min. The dose used prophylactically to prevent radial artery spasm is only 5–10 µg/min. NTG must be administered through non-polyvinyl chloride tubing, which absorbs up to 80% of the NTG.

4. Adverse effects. NTG is metabolized by the liver to nitrites, which oxidize Hb to methemoglobin. Methemoglobinemia and impaired oxygen transport can occur if the patient receives extremely high doses of IV NTG (over 10 µg/kg/min) for several days or has renal or hepatic dysfunction. The diagnosis is suggested by the presence of chocolate-brown blood and a lower oxygen saturation measured by oximetry than one would expect from the PaO_2. It can be confirmed by an elevated methemoglobin level (>1% of total Hb). Symptoms (cyanosis, progressive weakness, and acidosis) are usually not noted until the methemoglobin level exceeds 15–20%. The treatment is IV methylene blue 1 mg/kg of a 1% solution.[241]

D. Calcium channel blockers (CCBs)

1. Hemodynamic and electrophysiologic effects

 a. CCBs control hypertension by relaxing vascular smooth muscle and producing peripheral vasodilation. The various CCBs have differing effects on cardiovascular hemodynamics and electrophysiology (Table 11.9). Use of these medications during the perioperative period has been shown to reduce the incidence of MI, ischemia, and supraventricular arrhythmias, and may also improve survival.[242]

 b. Other effects may include coronary vasodilation, negative inotropy, a reduction in sinoatrial (SA) nodal automaticity (slowing the sinus mechanism), and slowing of AV nodal conduction (decreasing the ventricular rate response to atrial tachyarrhythmias).

2. Indications

 a. Use as a first-line drug for control of **postoperative hypertension**. IV clevidipine and nicardipine lack a negative inotropic effect and can be used

Table 11.9 • Effects of Calcium Channel Blockers

	Clevidipine	Nicardipine	Diltiazem	Verapamil	Nifedipine	Amlodipine
Inotropy	0	0	↓	↓↓	0↑	0
Heart rate	0	0↑	↓↓	↓↓	↑	0
AV conduction	0	0	↓↓	↓↓	0	0
Systemic resistance	↓↓↓	↓↓↓	↓↓	↓↓	↓↓	↓↓
Coronary vascular resistance	↓↓	↓↓↓	↓↓	↓↓	↓↓	↓↓

0, no effect; ↑ increased; ↓ decreased. The relative effect is indicated by the number of arrows.

independent of the cardiac output; in contrast, other CCBs, which might be used for other indications (vasospasm or rate control in AF), have negative inotropic properties.

    b. Treatment of **coronary vasospasm**

    c. Prevention of **radial artery spasm**

    d. **Slowing the ventricular response** to AF/flutter (diltiazem)

3. **Clevidipine** is a very short-acting CCB that relaxes arterial vascular smooth muscle without producing myocardial depression. It does not reduce preload but may improve LV function by reducing afterload. It reduces the blood pressure within 2–4 minutes and has a half-life of one minute with a duration of action of 5–15 minutes. It is metabolized by blood and tissue esterases and therefore is safe to use in patients with renal or hepatic dysfunction.[243,244]

    a. **Indications.** An excellent first-line drug for control of early postoperative hypertension because it has a rapid onset of action with achievement of a target blood pressure usually within six minutes. It minimizes blood pressure fluctuations and has rapid offset of action in the event of hemodynamic problems. It is commonly used during TAVR procedures due to the rapid changes in hemodynamics that occur around the time of valve deployment. It is an excellent drug to supplement use of β-blockers in the initial medical management of aortic dissections.[245,246]

    b. **Dosage.** It is given in an initial dose of 1–2 mg/h; if the blood pressure remains elevated, the dose can be doubled every 90 seconds; as the blood pressure approaches the target range, the dose should be adjusted in smaller increments every 5–10 minutes. The usual maintenance dose is 4–6 mg/h, but doses up to 21 mg/h can be given. It comes premixed with a concentration of 0.5 mg/mL in 50 mL or 100 mL bottles.

    c. Advantages. The ECLIPSE trial showed that clevidipine was more effective than SNP or NTG in maintaining the blood pressure within a target range, and when the blood pressure range was narrowed, it was also more effective than nicardipine in minimizing blood pressure excursions.[247]

4. **Nicardipine** selectively relaxes arterial smooth muscle, reducing the SVR. It lacks a negative inotropic effect, produces a minimal increase in heart rate, and has no effect on AV conduction. It has a rapid onset of action, but a half-life of about 45 minutes and a duration of action of 4–6 hours.

   a. **Indications**

      i. An excellent first-line drug for control of hypertension in the hemodynamically stable patient because of a rapid onset of action, selective arterial vasodilation, and minimal cardiac effects. The only concern is its long duration of action in the event of hemodynamic changes.

      ii. Radial artery spasm prophylaxis in a dose of 0.25 µg/kg/min.[248] Prophylaxis may be optimized by combining nicardipine with IV NTG.[249] However, one study of preexisting vasospasm in coronary artery conduits found that nicardipine added to NTG caused no more vasodilation than NTG alone.[250]

   b. **Dosage.** It is given with an initial dose of 5 mg/h using a mix of 50 mg/250 mL; the rate is then increased by 2.5 mg/h every 5–15 minutes to a maximum dose of 15 mg/h.

   c. Advantages over SNP include more stable blood pressure control and avoidance of a reduction in preload, a reflex tachycardia, and coronary steal. It is a potent coronary vasodilator that can improve distribution of blood to ischemic zones. It has been shown to decrease the extent and duration of postoperative ischemia more than NTG.[251]

   d. Disadvantages include having a long offset of action that can be problematic in a hemodynamically unstable patient, and an increase in V/Q mismatch that can produce hypoxemia.

5. **Diltiazem** reduces systemic blood pressure by lowering the SVR, but it has significant cardiac effects that limit its use as an antihypertensive agent. It depresses systolic function by a negative inotropic effect, slows the heart rate, and suppresses AV conduction. A reduction in blood pressure is a benefit when used for other indications, but it can be deleterious when the blood pressure is not elevated in those situations.

   a. **Indications**

      i. **Slowing the ventricular response** to AF. Diltiazem slows AV conduction and can produce heart block; therefore, pacemaker backup should be available when it is administered intravenously. **Note:** the patient's blood pressure and cardiac output are often marginal when AF develops and there is often some reluctance to use diltiazem for rate control. However, a reduction in ventricular response will usually improve stroke volume and blood pressure. If the blood pressure is marginal, a pure α-agent may be given along with diltiazem. If the blood pressure is unacceptably low, then cardioversion should be performed.

      ii. Prevention of **radial artery spasm**

      iii. Treatment of **coronary artery spasm** (diltiazem is a potent coronary vasodilator)

        iv. **Systemic hypertension** when there is another indication for its use (such as radial artery prophylaxis or slowing the ventricular response to AF).

    b. **Dosage.** An IV bolus of 0.25 mg/kg IV is given over two minutes, which may be followed by a repeat bolus of 0.35 mg/kg 15 minutes later. A continuous infusion is then started at a rate of 5–15 mg/h with a 100 mg/100 mL mix.

  6. **Verapamil** reduces systemic blood pressure by lowering the SVR, but it also has significant cardiac effects that depress contractility, slow the heart rate, and depress AV conduction. In the early postoperative period, indications for its use are similar to those for diltiazem, which is preferentially used. The IV dosage is a 0.1 mg/kg IV bolus followed by a 2–5 μg/kg/min continuous infusion of a 120 mg/250 mL mix.

  7. **Nifedipine** is a potent arterial vasodilator that lowers blood pressure by reducing SVR, and may also increase cardiac output because of a baroreceptor-mediated reflex tachycardia and a slight reflex increase in cardiac inotropy and AV conduction. It is also a potent coronary vasodilator and is beneficial in treating coronary spasm. Although it has been shown to be an effective antihypertensive drug, it has a long duration of action (6–8 hours) and is rarely used in the ICU.

  8. **Amlodipine** is an oral CCB that reduces SVR and blood pressure and may improve cardiac output due to a decrease in afterload. It has no negative inotropic effects and no effect on the SA node or AV nodal conduction. It produces a gradual decrease in blood pressure that persists for 24 hours after an oral dose. Thus, it is indicated for the long-term control of blood pressure. Because it is an effective antispasmodic agent, it is frequently used for the prevention of radial artery spasm in a 5 mg daily dose. It is useful in controlling hypertenson when given in addition to a β-blocker or when a β-blocker is contraindicated due to bradycardia.

E. **β-blockers**

  1. **Hemodynamic effects**

    a. In contrast to the vasodilating drugs, β-blockers reduce blood pressure primarily by their negative inotropic and chronotropic effects. They reduce contractility, lowering the stroke volume and cardiac output, and also slow the heart rate by depressing the SA node. Their antihypertensive activity may also be attributable to a decrease in central sympathetic outflow and suppression of renin activity.

    b. β-blockers slow AV conduction and can precipitate heart block. Pacemaker backup should be available when IV β-blockers are given. This electrophysiologic effect is beneficial in reducing the ventricular rate response to atrial tachyarrhythmias.

  2. **Indications**

    a. β-blockers can be used to control postoperative systolic hypertension associated with a satisfactory cardiac output. They are especially beneficial in the hyperdynamic, tachycardic heart that is often noted in patients with normal LV function and/or LVH. **Note:** intravenous β-blockers should be avoided in hypertensive patients with compromised cardiac output.

b. They are routinely used for prophylaxis (usually oral metoprolol or carvedilol) or treatment (usually IV metoprolol) of AF and will provide the additional benefit (or disadvantage) of reducing blood pressure.

c. They are the treatment of choice for both hypertension and heart rate control during the initial evaluation and treatment of patients with suspected acute aortic dissection.

3. **Esmolol** is a cardioselective, ultrafast, short-acting β-blocker with an onset of action of two minutes, reaching a steady-state level in five minutes, with reversal of effect in 10–20 minutes. Because of its very short duration of action, esmolol is the β-blocker of choice in the ICU for transient **hypertension control** in high cardiac output states, and is also beneficial in the initial management of **acute aortic dissection**.

a. Esmolol is contraindicated in the hypertensive patient with a low cardiac output. Frequently, blood pressure and cardiac output are maintained by fast heart rates at low stroke volumes. Use of esmolol in this circumstance will often reduce blood pressure and cardiac output by a negative inotropic effect with little reduction in heart rate. Even in patients with an excellent cardiac output, the reduction in blood pressure is generally more pronounced than the decrease in heart rate.

b. Esmolol can be used safely in the patient with a history of bronchospasm because of its cardioselectivity.

c. **Dosage.** Because patients tend to be very sensitive to esmolol in the immediate postoperative period, an initial dose of 0.25 mg/kg or less can be given to determine its effect on heart rate and blood pressure. If an adequate antihypertensive effect is not achieved, a repeat bolus dose of up to 0.5 mg/kg can be given and a maintenance infusion of 50–100 µg/kg/min started. Additional bolus doses can be given with an increase in the infusion rate by 50 µg/kg/min to a maximum infusion rate of 200 µg/kg/min of a 2.5 g/250 mL mix.

4. **Labetalol** has both α- and β-blocking properties as well as a direct vasodilatory effect. The ratio of β:α effects is 3:1 for the oral form and 7:1 for the intravenous form. In the postoperative cardiac surgical patient, IV labetalol reduces blood pressure primarily by its negative inotropic and chronotropic effects. The α-blocking effect prevents reflex vasoconstriction.[252]

a. The onset of action for IV labetalol is rapid with a maximum blood pressure response in five minutes for a bolus injection and in 10–15 minutes for a continuous infusion. Since the approximate duration of action is six hours, labetalol is useful when a **longer-acting antihypertensive drug** is desired. It is a very useful medication for the patient with an **aortic dissection**, both pre- and postoperatively.

b. **Dosage.** Labetalol is given as a 0.25 mg/kg bolus over two minutes with subsequent doses of 0.5 mg/kg every 15 minutes until effect is achieved (to a total dose of 300 mg). Alternatively, a continuous IV infusion can be given at a rate of 1–4 mg/min, mixing 40 mL of the 5 mg/mL solution in 160 mL (200 mg/200 mL).

5. **Metoprolol** is a cardioselective β-blocker that is given routinely in oral form for AF prophylaxis (starting at 12.5–25 mg bid). It can be supplemented by 2.5–5 mg doses IV every five minutes for three doses for a rapid ventricular response to AF. With IV usage, the onset of action is 2–3 minutes with a peak effect in 20 minutes and a duration of action of up to five hours. Although effective in reducing the blood pressure, which is often not desirable when being given for rapid AF, IV metoprolol is usually not selected for hypertension management in the ICU unless the patient is tachycardic. However, it is quite beneficial in reducing systolic hypertension postoperatively in increasing oral doses, as long as the heart rate remains above 60 bpm and the patient has adequate cardiac function.

F. **Hydralazine**

1. Hydralazine is a direct arteriolar vasodilator that decreases SVR and systemic blood pressure. The reduction in afterload may improve myocardial function, but it is usually accompanied by a compensatory tachycardia.

2. **Indication.** Hydralazine is most commonly used as a prn drug when adequate blood pressure control has not been achieved as the patient is being converted from IV to oral antihypertensive medications. Often patients are started back on lower doses of their preoperative medications yet still have persistent hypertension for a few days that subsequently abates. Use of prn hydralazine allows the clinician to avoid being too aggressive with the reinstitution of higher-dose or multiple medications that might otherwise precipitate hypotension when the transient hyperadrenergic state improves.

3. **Dosage.** The usual dose is 10 mg IV q15 min until effect and them q6h prn. Less commonly it is given in a dose of 20–40 mg IM. The onset of action after IV injection is about 5–10 minutes with a peak effect at 20 minutes and a duration of action of 3–4 hours.

G. **Fenoldopam mesylate**

1. Fenoldopam is a dopamine (DA_1) receptor agonist that is a rapid-acting peripheral and renal vasodilator with an onset of action of five minutes and a duration of action of less than 30 minutes. Its antihypertensive effect is accompanied by a reflex tachycardia and an increase in stroke volume, which both increase the cardiac output.[253] It also lowers PVR, with potential benefits in patients with preexisting RV dysfunction. A beneficial effect on renal function is related to dilatation of renal afferent arterioles, resulting in an increase in renal blood flow. It also produces hypokalemia, either through a direct drug effect or enhanced $K^+–Na^+$ exchange.

2. **Indication.** This drug is rarely used for postoperative hypertension, but, if used for renoprotection during surgery, the dose could be increased to control severe hypertension when rapid onset of effect is necessary.

3. **Dosage.** A continuous infusion is given starting at 0.05–0.1 μg/kg/min using a 10 mg/250 mL mix. The dose may be increased in 0.05–0.1 μg/kg/min increments every 15 minutes until effect is achieved to a maximum rate of 0.8 μg/kg/min. The dose used to provide a renoprotective effect (0.1 μg/kg/min) generally does not produce systemic hypotension.

H. **Selection of the appropriate antihypertensive medication in the postoperative cardiac surgical patient**

1. When filling pressures are normal or slightly elevated and the cardiac output is adequate or marginal, a selective arterial vasodilator with minimal cardiac effects is the best selection.

   a. **Clevidipine** is a very short-acting arterial vasodilator that is able to achieve a target blood pressure fairly rapidly and has a rapid offset of action in the event of hemodynamic compromise. It is preferentially used during and following TAVR procedures and may be added to propofol at the conclusion of cardiac surgery procedures if the patient remains hypertensive.

   b. **Nitroprusside** is both an arterial and a venous dilator, so it will reduce elevated filling pressures and improve cardiac output while lowering the blood pressure. In patients with low filling pressures, volume infusion may be necessary to prevent a precipitous drop in blood pressure. Because SNP is so powerful, caution is necessary in initiating the infusion to avoid excessive blood pressure reduction, and thus it tends to take longer than clevidipine to achieve the target blood pressure. Extreme care with its administration is necessary during patient transfer to the ICU.

   c. It is best to avoid longer-acting drugs, such as nicardipine, immediately after surgery because hypertension is often transient and hypotension might ensue before its effects dissipate.

   d. With any of these medications, use of additional inotropic support must be considered if the cardiac output is marginal or low and does not improve with optimization of preload and a reduction in afterload.

2. When filling pressures are high and the cardiac output is satisfactory, a venodilator, such as **IV nitroglycerin**, may be beneficial. This will reduce venous return, filling pressures, stroke volume, cardiac output, and blood pressure. It may be beneficial if there is evidence of myocardial ischemia. However, IV NTG is best avoided when hypovolemia or a marginal cardiac output is present.

3. When the heart is hyperdynamic with adequate filling pressures, a high cardiac output, and frequently a tachycardia, a β-blocker with negative inotropic and chronotropic properties, such as **esmolol**, should be selected. Any of the CCBs, including those with negative chronotropic properties, such as **diltiazem**, can also be selected in that they may improve myocardial oxygen metabolism, especially when there is evidence of ischemia. Tachycardia at the conclusion of surgery is often worrisome: it may be related to catecholamine infusions or hypovolemia, and thus easily remedied; however, it may be a sign of myocardial injury or ischemia, and the cause should be identified and corrected if possible. β-blockers must be avoided in the tachycardic patient with compromised RV or LV function.

4. Once the patient is able to tolerate oral medications, the IV medications should be weaned while monitoring the blood pressure response to oral medications. It is appropriate to restart the medications the patient was taking before surgery, but other medications should be considered under certain circumstances.

   a. β-blockers (**metoprolol** 12.5–75 mg PO bid) are initiated in virtually all patients to reduce the incidence of AF, are effective in treating a sinus tachycardia, and may also control the blood pressure. They can be used effectively if the patient is not bradycardic. In patients with impaired LV function, but in the absence of a low cardiac output syndrome or pressor dependence, **carvedilol**, which is an α- and β-blocker, can be started at a dose of 3.125 mg twice daily and increased up to 25 mg twice daily as tolerated.

b. The next choice is usually an **ACE inhibitor**, such as lisinopril 5–10 mg PO qd. This should be considered for all patients with poor ventricular function (EF <40%) and is not contraindicated in the presence of chronic kidney disease.[254] However, in the early postoperative period, it must be used cautiously in patients with acute kidney injury in whom a higher blood pressure may improve renal perfusion. As an alternative, or if the patient cannot tolerate an ACE inhibitor (usually because of a cough), an **ARB** can be chosen, such as losartan 25–50 mg daily or valsartan 80 mg daily.

c. The third choice is usually a **calcium channel blocker (CCB)**, such as amlodipine (Norvasc), which has no effects on cardiac inotropy or heart rate. Diltiazem may be useful when primarily used for heart rate control in AF or for spasm prophylaxis in patients receiving radial artery grafts.

d. Long-acting **nitrates** are alternative coronary vasodilators that can be used in patients receiving radial artery grafts and may also provide an antihypertensive benefit.

VIII. Perioperative Myocardial Infarction

Despite advances in myocardial protection, use of off-pump procedures, and refinements in surgical technique, a small percentage of patients will sustain a perioperative myocardial infarction (PMI). Virtually all patients undergoing on-pump surgery with cardioplegic arrest will have an elevation in cardiac biomarkers consistent with periprocedural myocardial injury, so the threshold for defining a PMI is somewhat arbitrary. The relevance lies in whether the degree of myocardial necrosis compromises the patient's outcome. In the short-term, a PMI may lead to a low cardiac output state, HF, or malignant arrhythmias; in the long-term, it may compromise the patient's survival.[255,256]

A. **Predisposing factors**

1. Left main or diffuse three-vessel disease
2. Preoperative ischemia or infarction. This includes ST-elevation infarctions (STEMIs), other acute coronary syndromes, or evidence of ongoing ischemia, often following a failed PCI.
3. Poor LV systolic and diastolic function (low EF, HF, LVEDP >15 mm Hg, LVH)
4. Reoperations, which predispose to atheroembolism of debris or to graft thrombosis
5. Poor surgical targets; requirement for a coronary endarterectomy
6. Uncontrolled diabetes

B. **Mechanisms**

1. Prolonged ischemia during anesthetic induction or before the establishment of coronary reperfusion. This is usually caused by tachycardia, hypertension,

hypotension, or ventricular distention, but may occasionally result from damage to grafts during reoperation or embolization down a stenotic vein graft.

2. Prolonged aortic cross-clamp time/CPB time

3. Inadequate myocardial protection or ischemia/reperfusion injury following cardioplegic arrest

4. Incomplete revascularization

5. Acute graft flow problems from anastomotic stenosis, graft spasm, or thrombosis; poor graft quality, small ITA

6. Native coronary vasospasm, plaque rupture, thrombosis

7. Coronary air or particulate embolization (usually from patent but atherosclerotic vein grafts during reoperations)

8. Other problems causing impaired hemodynamics or oxygenation: tachyarrhythmias, shock, respiratory failure, severe anemia

C. **Diagnosis.** A PMI can be difficult to diagnose since many groups do not routinely assess cardiac biomarkers after surgery because they are nearly always elevated. Management is dictated by hemodynamic performance, not biomarker elevation. Nonetheless, there is a spectrum of perioperative myocardial damage, and the definition of a **significant** PMI is based on the premise that enzyme levels beyond a certain threshold level are associated with more myocardial necrosis and adverse outcomes.

1. The Fourth Universal Definition of Myocardial Infarction from 2018 considers a CABG-related MI to be a type 5 MI.[257] This is defined as:

   a. cTn (troponin) >10 × the 99th percentile URL (the upper reference limit) within 48 hours of surgery with normal baseline values. If the preoperative cTn is elevated, the post-procedure cTn must rise by >20% and must also be >10 times the 99th percentile URL. In addition, one of the following elements is required:

      i. Development of new pathological Q waves

      ii. Angiographic documentation of new graft occlusion or new native coronary artery occlusion

      iii. Imaging evidence of loss of viable myocardium that is presumed to be new and in a pattern consistent with an ischemic etiology

   b. In some cases, marked isolated elevation of cTn values may be noted within the initial 48 h postoperative period in the absence of ECG/angiographic or other imaging evidence of an MI. Levels of cTnT >7 × URL or cTnI >20 × URL are considered consistent with a prognostically significant cardiac procedural myocardial injury, especially when there was difficulty coming off pump, technical concerns during surgery, low cardiac output states, ECG changes, or recurrent ventricular arrhythmias. Such levels should prompt further evaluation to see whether a graft-related failure is present and whether further revascularization, preferably by PCI, would be indicated.

2. Although low cardiac output states and regional wall motion abnormalities on echocardiogram may be consistent with a PMI, in many cases they represent a

period of reversible myocardial depression ("stunning") that can recover after several days of pharmacologic or mechanical support. However, the persistence of new regional wall motion abnormalities on serial evaluations is more consistent with the occurrence of a PMI.

3. Significant ST elevation on a postoperative ECG suggests a problem with graft flow and an evolving infarction. Differentiation from acute pericarditis on ECG can be difficult, the latter being suggested not just by the ECG abnormalities but by the absence of hemodynamic or echocardiographic abnormalities (see Figures 8.2 and 8.3, pages 384 and 385). New Q waves on the ECG are noted in about 5% of patients after surgery, but in many cases they are not associated with significant enzyme elevation and therefore may be of little consequence. These "false positive" Q waves may be associated with areas of altered depolarization or unmasking of old infarcts.[258] The persistence of ST segment depression, deep T wave inversions, ventricular tachyarrhythmias, or a new bundle branch block for over 48 hours suggests some degree of myocardial injury, especially if associated with new regional wall motion abnormalities. T wave inversions are commonly noted days to weeks after surgery when there has been no other evidence of a PMI.

D. **Presentations and treatment**

1. **Intraoperative ischemia.** Identification of new regional wall motion abnormalities by TEE is a sensitive means of assessing intraoperative myocardial ischemia. These changes precede evidence of ischemia noted with Swan-Ganz monitoring (elevation of PA pressures) or the ECG (ST segment elevation). Aggressive treatment to reduce myocardial oxygen demand and maintain perfusion pressure is essential to lower the risk of PMI. Placement of an IABP prior to going on bypass can often reduce the risk of PMI in patients with ongoing ischemia or poor LV function.[259] In patients undergoing reoperative surgery, avoiding manipulation of patent but diseased grafts is essential to prevent atheroembolism.

2. **Postcardiotomy low cardiac output syndrome with/without ECG evidence of ischemia.** Although enzyme elevation is more common with a longer duration of aortic clamping, fastidious attention to myocardial protection should offset the adverse effects of prolonged cross-clamping. The occurrence of severe postcardiotomy ventricular dysfunction, whether caused by ischemia, "stunning", or an infarction, requires careful evaluation and treatment.

   a. If myocardial dysfunction or ischemia is noted in the operating room at the conclusion of CPB, the adequacy of the operative procedure should be assessed. Supplemental grafts or graft revision may be necessary during bypass surgery, and other potential etiologies may have to be considered and addressed following valve surgery. An IABP or MCS may be indicated in addition to pharmacologic support.

   b. If ECG changes are detected upon arrival in the ICU (especially ST elevations), IV NTG or CCBs (if spasm is suspected) should be given. Emergency coronary angiography with possible PCI or surgical graft revision should be strongly considered.[260,261] An IABP is helpful in temporarily improving coronary perfusion and reducing the workload of the heart.

c. Management of a hemodynamically significant MI involves supportive care until arrhythmias and hemodynamic instability resolve. Cardiac output should be optimized in standard fashion, but care must be taken to avoid excessive volume infusions and tachycardia that may increase myocardial oxygen demand and worsen the ischemic insult. Use of milrinone or placement of an IABP will minimize oxygen consumption. It is difficult to treat the sinus tachycardia that frequently accompanies a low cardiac output state because it usually represents a compensatory mechanism to maintain cardiac output. Sinus tachycardia is frequently a sign of an "injured heart" and can perpetuate myocardial ischemia and damage. It can only be treated once the cardiac output improves.

3. **Good cardiac output but low SVR.** The patient sustaining a small PMI may have a normal cardiac output accompanied by systemic hypotension. This syndrome usually requires use of an α-agent for several days to maintain an adequate systemic blood pressure until the SVR returns to normal.

4. **Persistent ventricular ectopy** may reflect ischemia, infarction, or reperfusion of previously ischemic muscle. It may be treated short-term with lidocaine or amiodarone. β-blockers are generally used for their antiarrhythmic effect and are beneficial regardless of LV function, but they are contraindicated in low output states or with profound bradycardia. Nonsustained or sustained ventricular tachycardia occurring in patients with impaired ventricular function often requires electrophysiologic testing, use of amiodarone, and/or use of a LifeVest (ZOLL Medical Corporation) or placement of an ICD.

5. Some patients will have an infarction diagnosed by electrocardiographic, enzymatic, or functional criteria but will have no clinical or hemodynamic sequelae. These patients do not require any special treatment, but should be maintained on β-blockers.

E. **Prognosis**

1. An uncomplicated PMI generally does not influence operative mortality or long-term survival. Despite a return of ventricular function to baseline, the heart may fail to demonstrate functional improvement during exercise.

2. However, significant enzyme elevation as well as the occurrence of a hemodynamically significant MI (i.e. one presenting as a low cardiac output syndrome or malignant arrhythmias) do increase operative mortality and decrease long-term survival.[262–265]

3. The prognosis following a perioperative infarction is determined primarily by the adequacy of revascularization and the residual EF. One study reported that the prognosis for patients sustaining an MI with an EF >40% and with complete revascularization was comparable to patients not developing a perioperative infarction.[266]

IX. Coronary Vasospasm

A. Vasospasm has become increasingly recognized as a cause of postoperative morbidity and mortality following CABG. It can affect normal coronary arteries, bypassed vessels, saphenous vein grafts, or arterial grafts (ITA, radial, gastroepiploic artery).[249,250,267,268]

B. **Etiology** may be related to mechanical or endothelial vein damage during harvesting, enhanced α-adrenergic tone, use of α-agents such as phenylephrine to support blood pressure, endothelial dysfunction from reduced nitric oxide production, hypothermia, hypomagnesemia, or CCB withdrawal.[269,270] It has also been associated with the administration of 5-HT$_3$ antagonists, such as ondansetron (Zofran), which is commonly prescribed for postoperative nausea.[271]

C. **Diagnosis** of vasospasm can be extremely difficult to confirm and requires further evaluation to differentiate it from other more common clinical conditions with similar manifestations. The usual presentation is ST elevation consistent with ischemia, often with a low cardiac output state, hypotension, ventricular arrhythmias, or heart block.

D. **Evaluation**

1. An ECG will usually show localized, and occasionally diffuse, ST elevations, although these findings are more commonly associated with an anatomic compromise in graft flow, usually at an anastomosis. As noted, spasm may occur in native coronary arteries (unbypassed or beyond an anastomosis) as well as in arterial and rarely venous conduits. Spasm is most common in radial artery grafts, but is usually mitigated by the prophylactic use of perioperative vasodilators.

2. Echocardiography will usually demonstrate an area of hypokinesis which corresponds to the ECG changes, but it is not diagnostic of spasm.

3. Coronary angiography may be necessary to make the appropriate diagnosis if there is no response to IV therapy with coronary vasodilators. It will usually demonstrate sluggish flow through grafts, diffuse spasm, and poor flow into distal native vessels. Resolution of spasm with intracoronary NTG or a CCB (verapamil) confirms the diagnosis. Differentiation from technical problems at the anastomosis can be difficult to make due to poor flow. If there is little response to pharmacologic intervention, re-exploration may be indicated.

E. **Treatment** involves hemodynamic support and initiation of medications that can reverse the vasospasm. Improvement in ECG changes is consistent with spasm, but it does not eliminate the possibility of some compromise of graft flow from surgical issues.

1. Optimize oxygenation and correct acidosis.

2. Optimize hemodynamic parameters. If an inotrope is indicated, a PDE inhibitor (milrinone) is the best choice because it is a potent vasodilator of the ITA and perhaps of native vessels as well.

3. Correct hypomagnesemia (IV **magnesium sulfate** 1–2 g in 10 mL of D5W).

4. Although several vasodilators are effective in preventing or treating native coronary, arterial and vein graft spasm, the most effective approach may be the combination of IV nitroglycerin with a CCB.[268]

   a. Start IV **nitroglycerin** at 0.5 μg/kg/min and raise as tolerated.

   b. **Diltiazem** drip: 0.25 mg/kg IV bolus over two minutes, followed by a repeat bolus of 0.35 mg/kg 15 minutes later. A continuous infusion is then given at a rate of 5–15 mg/h using a 100 mg/100 mL mix.

   c. IV nicardipine 5 mg/h with a mix of 50 mg/250 mL; the dose can be increased by 2.5 mg/h every 5–15 minutes to a maximum dose of 15 mg/h, if tolerated.

d. IV verapamil drip: 0.1 mg/kg bolus, followed by a 2–5 µg/kg/min infusion of a 120 mg/250 mL mix (most likely to cause hypotension).

5. If the patient does not improve and/or ECG changes persist, emergency cardiac catheterization is indicated to identify and possibly correct the problem. During catheterization, intracoronary NTG and verapamil are usually successful in reversing spasm.

6. Once the patient has stabilized, an oral coronary vasodilator is recommended. These include isosorbide mononitrate sustained release (Imdur) 20 mg qd, nifedipine 30 mg q6h, diltiazem CD 180 mg qd, or amlodipine 5 mg qd.

7. Statins may prove of benefit in reducing spasm.[272]

8. Emergency ECMO has been utilized in patients with cardiogenic shock from diffuse spasm.[273]

X. Cardiac Arrest

A. Cardiac arrest is a serious and dreaded complication of any cardiac operation that can occur unexpectedly at the conclusion of surgery, during transport from the operating room, in the ICU, or later during convalescence on the floor. The three leading causes of a postoperative cardiac arrest are ventricular fibrillation, cardiac tamponade, and mediastinal bleeding, with survival being least likely with VF since it is often caused by an MI or pump failure. The mortality rate for patients sustaining a cardiac arrest after cardiac surgery averages about 50%.[274,275]

1. For patients suffering a cardiac arrest in the ICU, protocols adapted for cardiac surgical patients, presented by the European Association for Cardio-Thoracic Surgery in 2009, the European Resuscitation Council in 2015, and the Society of Thoracic Surgeons in 2017, should be followed.[275–277] The two basic principles which differ from standard ACLS teachings are a one-minute delay in initiating external compressions to establish pacing or perform defibrillation, and performance of a redo sternotomy within five minutes if the resuscitation is unsuccessful (Figure 11.15). A resternotomy addresses most contributory causes (especially bleeding or tamponade) and allows for the performance of internal cardiac massage, which is nearly twice as effective as external compressions in increasing the cardiac output and coronary perfusion pressure.[278]

2. In patients arresting outside of an ICU setting, basic and ACLS recommendations should be followed, with plans for an early resternotomy if resuscitation is unsuccessful and the patient is within 10 days of surgery. If the arrest is witnessed, the one-minute rule of an initial defibrillation should be considered.

B. Resuscitation from cardiac arrest is a team approach with seven key roles: airway and breathing, external cardiac massage, defibrillation/pacing, drug administration, a team leader to coordinate management, an ICU coordinator to coordinate peripheral activities, and individuals to perform an open sternotomy. In brief, the basic ABCD steps are the follows:

1. **AIRWAY & BREATHING:** manually ventilate the patient at 8–10/min

2. **CIRCULATION:** initiate external chest compressions (100–120/min) **only after** three serial attempts at defibrillation for ventricular tachycardia (VT) or ventricular fibrillation (VF) or attempted pacing for asystole in ICU patients within the first minute after arrest.

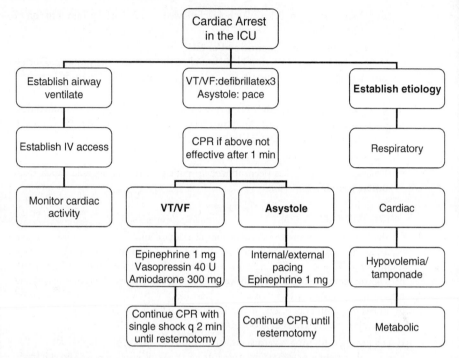

Figure 11.15 • A simplified algorithm for the management of a cardiac arrest in the ICU. Note that up to three defibrillations for VF or pacing for asystole should be attempted within the first minute prior to initiating external compressions in a patient with a witnessed arrest in the ICU.

3. **DEFIBRILLATE** for pulseless VT/VF or **PACE** for asystole or bradycardia

4. **DRUGS** (see Table 11.10)

C. **Etiology/assessment/management.** While resuscitation is under way, an evaluation should be undertaken to determine the possible cause of the cardiac arrest (Table 11.11). The most common causes of non-VF arrests in cardiac surgical patients are cardiac tamponade, marked hypovolemia from bleeding, asystole from pacing failure, and tension pneumothorax. All of these can be addressed with reopening of the sternotomy incision once adequate ventilation has been achieved.

1. Listen to the chest, check the ventilator function, ABGs, and recent acid–base and electrolyte status. If the patient is not intubated, secure an airway first, administer oxygen, and then intubate. Do **not** try to intubate before delivering oxygen by face mask because this may prolong the period of hypoxemia. This assessment may indicate whether the patient has:

   a. Severe ventilatory or oxygenation disturbance (hypoxia, hypercarbia from pneumothorax, endotracheal tube displacement, acute pulmonary embolism)

   b. Severe acid–base and electrolyte disturbances (acidosis, hypo- or hyperkalemia)

Table 11.10 • Drug Doses Used During Cardiac Arrest

Vasopressin	40 units IV push × 1 dose
Epinephrine (1:1000)	1 mg IV push, repeat doses q3–5 min
Amiodarone	300 mg IV push; can give 150 mg q5 min to total 2.2 g/24h
Lidocaine	1–1.5 mg/kg bolus, followed by 0.5–0.75 mg/kg boluses every 5–10 min to total dose of 3 mg/kg
Magnesium sulfate	1–2 g in 10 mL D5W
Atropine	1 mg IV push with repeat doses of 1 mg q3–5 min to total dose of 0.04 mg/kg

Table 11.11 • Most Common Causes of Postoperative Cardiac Arrest

Cause	Treatment
Hypovolemia	Volume infusions
Hypoxia	Hand ventilation with 100% O_2
Hydrogen ion acidosis	Sodium bicarbonate
Hyperkalemia	Calcium chloride, glucose/insulin/bicarbonate drip
Hypokalemia	KCl infusion
Hypothermia	Warming blankets
Tamponade	Pericardiocentesis, subxiphoid exploration, or emergency sternotomy
Tension pneumothorax	Needle decompression, chest tube
Thrombosis (myocardial infarction)	IABP, emergency cardiac catheterization
Thrombosis (pulmonary embolism)	Anticoagulation, embolectomy, IVC umbrella

Tablets
  Drug overdose
  Digoxin toxicity
  β-blockers, calcium channel blockers
	Gastric lavage, activated charcoal
	Digibind
	Inotropic support, pacing

2. Examine the cardiac monitor and ECG. These may reveal:
   a. Third-degree heart block (may occur spontaneously or if AV pacing fails in a patient with complete heart block)
   b. Acute ischemia (graft thrombosis, coronary spasm)
   c. Ventricular tachyarrhythmias (VT or VF)
3. Check the chest tube drainage and review the chest x-ray. These may indicate whether there is:
   a. Acute impairment of venous return (tension pneumothorax, cardiac tamponade, occasionally with sudden cessation of massive bleeding)
   b. Acute hypovolemia (massive mediastinal bleeding)
4. Assess whether inotropes, vasopressors, or vasodilators are being administered at the correct rate. Because there may have been inadvertent cessation of inotropic support or profound vasodilation from bolusing of a vasodilator, it is recommended that **all medication infusions should be stopped** to clarify matters until the patient is resuscitated.

D. **Treatment.** Cardiac surgery patients are usually extensively monitored in the ICU, and ventilation can be provided immediately by Ambu bags present at the bedside. Many patients are still intubated and most arrests are "witnessed". Thus, immediate resuscitation using an ICU protocol should be used. On the floor, most patients are only monitored by telemetry and many arrests are not "witnessed". Immediate resuscitation using standard ACLS protocols should be used for those patients.

1. Disconnect the patient from the ventilator and **hand ventilate** with an Ambu bag with 100% oxygen at a rate of 8–10/min and listen for bilateral breath sounds. If not already intubated, intubate after establishing an adequate airway after a brief period of satisfactory manual ventilation. Perform endotracheal suctioning for a potential tube or airway obstruction. If the latter is present, it is best to remove the tube, hand ventilate, and have an experienced individual reintubate the patient. If breath sounds are not heard on one side and a tension pneumothorax is suspected, a large-bore needle can be placed in the second intercostal space for immediate decompression and a chest tube may subsequently be placed. When the patient is reconnected to the ventilator, do not use PEEP.

2. In any patient sustaining a cardiac arrest after cardiac surgery, emergency **resternotomy for open-chest resuscitation** should always be considered from the outset and performed within five minutes of the arrest if the resuscitation is unsuccessful (see below).

3. **Ventricular tachycardia or fibrillation** can be identified on a monitor and confirmed by lack of a pulse.
   a. **ICU patients. Three attempts at defibrillation** with 200 joules (biphasic) or 360 joules (monophasic) should be performed, all **within one minute of arrest**. If the patient remains in VT/VF or has severe hypotension after one minute, **then external chest compressions** at a rate of 100–120/min should be commenced. Preparations should be made for an emergency resternotomy, which should then be performed within five minutes of the onset of the arrest. The rationale for delaying external massage is that it can cause disruption of the sternal closure, injury to bypass grafts, or damage to the ventricular myocardium from prosthetic valves. This potential damage can be minimized if

compressions are **delayed for a very short period of time (one minute)** to prepare and use the defibrillator for VT/VF or attach the pacing wires to a pacemaker (or turn the pacemaker on if already attached) for asystole or bradycardia. After subsequent defibrillations, it is advisable to continue CPR briefly since the initial rhythm may be slow and may not generate an adequate perfusion pressure.

b. **Floor patients or unwitnessed arrests. External compressions** should be started **immediately** because the onset of the arrest may not be known and it is less likely that defibrillation can be performed within one minute of the onset of arrest. External compressions are started and **defibrillation** should be done as soon as possible and then repeated every two minutes, if necessary. It is recommended that CPR be resumed immediately after each defibrillation, with assessment of the rhythm on the monitor and palpation for a pulse during CPR and for no more than 10 seconds with CPR stopped. If the patient is not monitored, CPR should be continued for two minutes before checking for a pulse. After two minutes of CPR, defibrillation should be attempted again. A postoperative cardiac floor should always be equipped with a "crash cart" and preparations started immediately for opening the sternotomy incision after five minutes.

c. Initial medications are given after three unsuccessful shocks within the first minute in ICU patients or after two attempts for floor patients (Table 11.10). All drug infusions the patient was receiving prior to the arrest should be stopped. It is recommended in both the European and STS guidelines that neither vasopressin nor epinephrine should be given routinely except by those experienced with cardiac surgical management, because they may cause severe hypertension once cardiac activity resumes.

- **Vasopressin** 40 units IV as a single dose provides comparable or superior efficacy to epinephrine in promoting return of spontaneous circulation.[279]

- **Epinephrine** 1 mg IV push (10 mL of 1:10,000 solution) should be given if VT/VF persists or recurs after defibrillation. It may be repeated every 3–5 minutes. In a patient with a pending arrest, smaller doses are usually recommended (50–300 µg).

- If the cardiac arrest occurs outside of the ICU setting and intravenous access is not immediately available, epinephrine, vasopressin, and lidocaine are effective when given down an endotracheal tube at 2–2.5 times the usual IV dose diluted in 10 mL of normal saline. Note that ACLS protocols recommend the intraosseous route as second choice, but this requires a special rigid needle from an access kit.

d. Antiarrhythmic drugs may improve the success of defibrillation and should be used for persistent/recurrent VT/VF despite three shocks. Defibrillation should be repeated after each dose of medication.

- **Amiodarone** should be given first in a bolus dose of 300 mg; a dose of 150 mg may be repeated every 3–5 minutes. It is then given as an infusion of 1 mg/min for six hours, then 0.5 mg/min for 18 hours with conversion to oral dosing if necessary. The maximum dose is 2.2 g IV/24 h.

- **Lidocaine** may be given for refractory VT/VF as a 1–1.5 mg/kg bolus followed by 0.5–0.75 mg/kg boluses twice every 5–10 minutes to a total dose of 3 mg/kg.

- **Magnesium sulfate** 1–2 g in 10 mL of D5W IV may be helpful for torsades de pointes, especially if hypomagnesemia is suspected.

4. **Asystole or pulseless electrical activity (PEA)** (pacing spikes or QRS complex with no detectable pulse)

   a. **Note that a patient being "paced" who develops suspected PEA may actually have underlying VF, which is not easily recognizable on a monitor.** The pacer may need to be turned off to identify this rhythm.

   b. Initiate immediate epicardial pacing by connecting the patient's ventricular pacing wires to a pacing box, which should be available at the bedside or nearby. The default emergency setting of VOO can be used initially at a rate of 80–100/min. However, most patients in the ICU have both atrial and ventricular pacing wires connected to the box, and DDD pacing should be initiated, which will also function if there is an adequate sinus mechanism and no atrial wires.

   c. With a witnessed arrest, CPR may be delayed for one minute while the pacing wires are connected. If successful **pacing with a documented pulse** cannot be achieved **within one minute** of a witnessed arrest, **external compressions must be started.** Compressions should be started immediately in patients with an unwitnessed arrest, since it takes some effort to set this up.

   d. **Epinephrine** bolus 1 mg IV (10 mL of a 1:10,000 solution) every 3–5 minutes; an infusion of 2–10 μg/min can be used for bradycardia.

   e. **Vasopressin** one dose of 40 units IV can be given instead of epinephrine.

   f. **Atropine** is not recommended for asystole or extreme bradycardia per the STS guidelines. In ACLS protocols, the recommended dose is 1 mg IV with repeat doses of 1 mg every 3–5 minutes to a total dose of 0.04 mg/kg.

5. **Bradycardia** that is unresponsive to epicardial pacing

   a. Attempt **transcutaneous** pacing

   b. **Epinephrine** 2–10 mg/min (1 mg/250 mL mix)

6. **Tachycardia with pulses** may be well tolerated at a rate of less than 150 bpm, but at higher rates the patient may develop chest pain, altered mental status, or hypotension.

   a. If unstable, perform synchronized cardioversion with 200–360 joules.

   b. **Stable with narrow QRS** usually represents a supraventricular mechanism.

      - **Regular rhythm:** give adenosine 6 mg IV push with two repeat doses of 12 mg IV; if conversion occurs, this probably represents a reentry supraventricular tachycardia (SVT); if the rhythm does not convert, it may represent atrial flutter, ectopic atrial tachycardia, or junctional tachycardia that should be managed with diltiazem and/or β-blockers.

      - **Irregular rhythm** may be AF/flutter or multifocal atrial tachycardia that should be managed with IV diltiazem and/or β-blockers.

   c. **Stable with wide complex QRS** is usually VT or AF with aberrancy.

      - **Regular rhythm** is most likely VT and should be treated by amiodarone 150 mg IV over 10 minutes and then a synchronized cardioversion if persistent; if it represents SVT with aberrancy, it should be treated with adenosine.

- **Irregular rhythm** is most commonly AF with aberrancy, to be treated with diltiazem and/or β-blockers; less common are AF with Wolff-Parkinson-White (WPW) syndrome (use amiodarone), polymorphic VT, or torsades de pointes (give magnesium).

7. **Emergency sternotomy**

   a. The potential need for an open sternotomy should be considered immediately when a cardiac arrest occurs and should be performed within five minutes if resuscitation is unsuccessful. It usually takes at least that long to get everybody and everything organized to accomplish an open sternotomy. The team leader who is coordinating the resuscitation is most likely the best individual to keep track of time. During the stress of a cardiac arrest, sometimes one minute seems like five minutes, or vice versa. If defibrillation for VT/VF or pacing for asystole is unsuccessful in restoring a rhythm, uninterrupted chest compressions are essential to optimize perfusion and should be performed as long as necessary or until the chest can be opened. If one cannot achieve a systolic pressure >60 mm Hg with compressions, it is likely that tamponade or severe hypovolemia is present, and emergency resternotomy should be performed.

   b. Emergency resternotomy is a life-saving procedure in patients with bleeding or tamponade as it will allow for evacuation of blood and control of bleeding. If the cardiac surgeon is not available to open the chest, manual control of the bleeding site by a less experienced person can often be achieved, allowing the surgeon to subsequently precisely control the bleeding site. Invariably, immediate hemodynamic improvement will be noted if the patient has been fluid resuscitated. In patients with other causes of cardiac arrest, such as myocardial ischemia from graft occlusion or primary arrhythmic events, internal massage is much more effective than external compressions.

   c. Emergency resternotomy is still feasible up to 10 days after surgery and may be considered later based on an experienced surgeon's judgment.

   d. Emergency re-exploration for cardiac arrest can be problematic in patients whose surgery was performed through an approach other than a full sternotomy. A full sternotomy is usually required to perform effective internal cardiac massage, and it has been recommended that a sternal saw be available in the ICU for use by an experienced surgeon in these situations. Equipment to remove rigid fixation devices (sternal talons, plates) should be available at the bedside for patients whose sternums were reapproximated with these systems after a full sternotomy.

   e. Internal cardiac massage for most "first responders" requires two-handed massage, with the right hand placed behind the heart after identifying the grafts (primarily the LITA graft) and the left hand placed anteriorly with the fingers flat to minimize cardiac damage. Massage should occur at 100–120/min. With experience, excellent internal massage can be carried out with the left hand alone.

   f. If the patient cannot be resuscitated successfully, placement of a transfemoral IABP may improve myocardial perfusion in cases of a primary cardiac event. A more supportive measure is the establishment of CPB through the open sternotomy incision to rest the heart. Peripheral ECMO can also be considered and may be beneficial for nonbleeding/tamponade arrests in patients without a full sternotomy incision or for those who require prolonged support.

8. **Persistent hypotension.** Reestablishment of satisfactory myocardial blood flow is the most important element in a successful resuscitation. Because coronary perfusion occurs during compression "diastole" (i.e. when the aortic pressure exceeds the right atrial pressure), elevation of SVR and coronary perfusion pressure is critical. This is best achieved with medications that have predominantly α effects (epinephrine in high doses) or strong vasoconstrictor properties (vasopressin). Patients with a cardiac etiology to their arrest will often benefit from placement of an IABP.

9. **Other situations**

   a. **Intra-aortic balloon counterpulsation**

      i. The IABP will respond to a pacing spike, so in the presence of asystole or PEA, the monitor tracing may identify the spike and give the false impression of cardiac activity. Lack of pulsatility in other waveforms and no cardiac component to the IABP tracing are clues to the presence of asystole or very weak cardiac contractions.

      ii. The IABP should be set in the pressure trigger mode that will respond to external cardiac massage. If there is a prolonged period of no massage, the internal trigger at 100/min should be used.

   b. **Minimally invasive incisions.** As noted, a full sternotomy would need to be made to initiate internal massage if the patient had a hemisternotomy or limited thoracotomy incision for the original surgery.

   c. **Cardiac assist devices:** external compressions can be performed in patients with implantable centrifugal or axial flow pumps, but generally are not recommended, as they can displace the devices.

10. **Controversial medications**

    a. **Epinephrine and vasopressin** are the two recommended drugs in ACLS protocols for intractable VF as well as asystole. When given as a bolus dose, they may cause a hypertensive crisis after cardiac recovery, and therefore routine use has been discouraged in cardiac surgical patients.

    b. **Sodium bicarbonate** should not be given routinely for the attended arrest during which excellent ventilation and cardiac compressions are achieved. Administration of $NaHCO_3$ reduces SVR and compromises cerebral perfusion, creates extracellular alkalosis that shifts the oxygen–hemoglobin dissociation curve to the left, inhibiting oxygen release to tissues, exacerbates central venous acidosis, inactivates catecholamines administered during an arrest, and can produce hypernatremia and hyperosmolarity. Its use should be guided by the results of ABGs drawn every 10 minutes during the arrest. If not drawn and there are questions about the timing of the arrest and the initiation of CPR or its adequacy, it is not unreasonable to presume that the patient is acidotic and give $NaHCO_3$ in doses of 1 mEq/kg, with half that dose re-administered 10 minutes later.

    c. **Calcium chloride** is not routinely recommended during a cardiac arrest as it may contribute to intracellular damage. Doses of 5–10 mL of a 10% solution can be given for hyperkalemia, hypocalcemia, or CCB toxicity.

d. **Atropine** is not recommended for bradycardia or asystole in the STS guidelines, as it has not been shown to improve outcomes.[275] Pacing should be utilized instead, using the epicardial wires or transcutaneous pacing.

11. **Post-arrest care.** Virtually all patients following an arrest should be monitored and assessed in the ICU. Most will stabilize if an immediately treatable cause has been identified. If the chest has been opened, it may be closed in the ICU if provisions are available. Otherwise, it is beneficial to return the patient to the operating room for further evaluation and chest closure. The risk of wound infection is quite low despite opening the chest in the ICU under emergency circumstances.[280]

   a. Most patients will require mechanical ventilatory support, and use of sedatives can confound a neurologic evaluation. Although there may be some benefit to a hypothermia protocol, early weaning of sedation is feasible once the patient's hemodynamics, ABGs, acid-base balance, electrolyte and and glucose status have improved.

   b. Myocardial "stunning" is common, and an immediate post-arrest assessment of myocardial function by echocardiography may be misleading as to whether the arrest was caused by a primary cardiac event. Similarly, cardiac biomarkers may be elevated from ischemia and defibrillation and may not necessarily reflect myocardial damage preceding the arrest. However, placement of an IABP is very beneficial when a myocardial insult is suspected, and cardiac catheterization should be considered if there are any associated ECG changes prior to or following the arrest. Patients suffering VF/VT arrests with known impairment of LV function should be further evaluated by an electrophysiologist, and implantation of an ICD should be considered.

   c. The long-term outcome of a patient sustaining a postoperative arrest is suboptimal. One study found that at a mean follow-up of 7.5 years, the mortality rate was twice as high in those who arrested and survived the hospital stay compared with those who did not sustain an arrest.[274]

XI. Pacing Wires and Pacemakers

A. General comments[281,282]

1. The use of cold cardioplegic arrest is commonly associated with temporary sinus node or AV node dysfunction. Placement of two temporary right atrial and two right ventricular epicardial pacing wire electrodes is beneficial in these situations to optimize hemodynamics at the conclusion of bypass and for several hours in the ICU (Figure 11.16). Pacing wires are also useful in the event that medications used to control atrial fibrillation precipitate advanced AV block. They can also be used for overdrive pacing and have diagnostic utility in delineating unusual rhythm problems.

2. Reluctance to routinely place epicardial wires during surgery is based on concerns that bleeding and tamponade may complicate their removal. This is nearly always associated with the removal of ventricular wires and, although very uncommon, can be life-threatening. Nonetheless, although most surgeons will place ventricular wires, many tend to avoid placement of atrial pacing wires. Bleeding is rare with their removal unless they are directly sewn to the right atrium. Placing the wires into a plastic button sewn low on the right atrial free wall will virtually never result

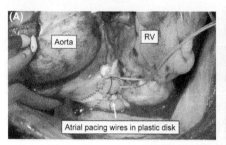

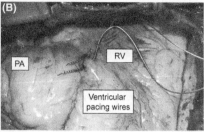

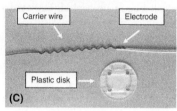

Figure 11.16 • (A) Atrial pacing wires (Medtronic 6500) are placed into a plastic disk that is sewn low on the right atrial free wall, permitting contact of the electrodes with the atrial wall. (B) The two ventricular wires are sewn superficially over the right ventricular free wall or inferiorly in the muscle. (C) Close up of the pacing wire demonstrating the plastic carrier wire adjacent to the electrode and the plastic disk into which the atrial wires are placed. PA, pulmonary artery; RV, right ventricle.

in bleeding with wire removal (Medtronic model 6500 wires). The benefits of atrial pacing in bradycardic patients with LVH or LV dysfunction can be significant.

3. To assess whether pacing wire placement should be performed routinely, one study found that 15% of patients needed pacing to terminate bypass, but less than 10% of patients required temporary pacing postoperatively.[283] However, it is not always predictable which patients may require subsequent pacing, and it is recommended that at least one ventricular pacing wire (with a skin ground) should be placed; the risk:benefit ratio of atrial pacing wires suggests that they should be placed routinely as well.

B. **Diagnostic uses.** When the exact nature of an arrhythmia cannot be ascertained from a 12-lead ECG, atrial electrograms (AEGs) are helpful in making the appropriate diagnosis. Atrial pacing wires can be used to record atrial activity in both unipolar and bipolar modes. With suitably equipped monitors, these recordings can be obtained simultaneously with standard limb leads to distinguish among atrial and junctional arrhythmias and differentiate them from more life-threatening ventricular arrhythmias. Simultaneous ECG and AEG tracings for each of the most commonly encountered postoperative arrhythmias are provided in section XII, starting on page 611. The technique for obtaining atrial wire tracings is either of the following:

1. A multichannel recorder can be used to print simultaneous monitor ECGs and AEGs. Most monitoring systems have cartridges with three leads for recording the AEG: two of them represent the arm leads and are connected with alligator clips to the atrial pacing wires; the third represents a left leg lead and is attached to an electrode pad over the patient's flank. When the monitor channel for the

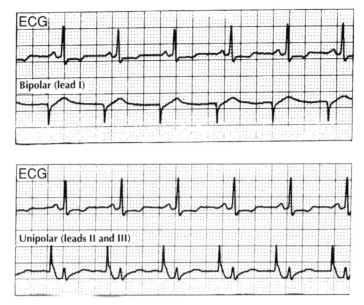

Figure 11.17 • Sinus rhythm in simultaneous monitor leads and AEGs. In the upper tracing, note that the bipolar AEG (lead I) produces predominantly an atrial complex with essentially no visible ventricular complex. In contrast, the unipolar tracing (leads II and III) at the bottom shows both a large atrial wave and a smaller ventricular complex.

AEG is set on lead I, a bipolar AEG is obtained (Figure 11.17). This shows a large atrial complex and a very small or undetectable ventricular complex. When the AEG monitor channel is set on leads II or III, a unipolar AEG is obtained. This demonstrates a large atrial and slightly smaller ventricular complex.

2. When a standard ECG machine is used, the two arm leads are connected to the atrial wires with alligator clips, and the leg leads are attached to the right and left legs. A bipolar AEG will be recorded in lead I and a unipolar AEG in leads II or III. Alternatively, the atrial wires can be connected to the V leads. Bipolar AEGs give a better assessment of atrial activity than unipolar AEGs and can distinguish between sinus tachycardia and atrial arrhythmias. However, because the AEG and standard ECG tracings are not obtained simultaneously, a unipolar tracing is required to differentiate sinus from junctional tachycardia because it can demonstrate the relationship between the larger atrial and smaller ventricular complexes.

C. **Therapeutic uses**

1. Optimal hemodynamics are achieved at a heart rate of around 90 bpm in the immediate postoperative period. Use of temporary pacing wires attached to an external pulse generator (Figure 11.18) to increase the heart rate is preferable to the use of positive chronotropic agents that have other effects on myocardial function. Atrial pacing with normal conduction will nearly always demonstrate superior hemodynamics to AV pacing, which in turn is superior to ventricular pacing. Since AV delay is often prolonged after bypass, shortening it artificially using AV

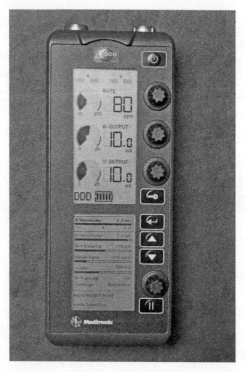

Figure 11.18 • The Medtronic model 5392 external pacemaker. This device can be used to provide pacing in a variety of modes, including AAI, DVI, DDD, and VVI pacing. It also has rapid atrial pacing capabilities.

pacing can improve hemodynamics, especially in patients with impaired ventricular function.[284]

2. Some, but not all, studies have showed that biventricular pacing with leads placed during surgery will improve LV systolic and diastolic function compared with RA or RA–RV pacing in patients with AV block who have LV dysfunction. Benefit is greatest in patients who also have a wide QRS complex.[40–43]

3. Reentrant rhythms can be terminated by rapid pacing. Rapid atrial pacing can terminate type I atrial flutter (flutter rate of less than 350/min) and other paroxysmal supraventricular tachycardias. Rapid ventricular pacing can terminate VT.

D. Pacing nomenclature

1. The sophistication and reprogrammability of permanent pacemaker systems led to the establishment of a joint nomenclature by the North American Society of Pacing and Electrophysiology (NASPE) and the British Pacing and Electrophysiology Group (BPEG). This nomenclature classifies pacemakers by their exact mode of function (Table 11.12).

2. Use of the first three letters is helpful in understanding the temporary pacemaker systems that are used after cardiac surgical procedures (Table 11.13). The most

Table 11.12 • Pacemaker Identification Codes

			Code Positions	
I	**II**	**III**	**IV**	**V**
Chamber paced	Chamber sensed	Response to sensing	Programmability/rate response	Antitachyarrhythmia functions
O – none	O – none	O – none	O – none	O – none
A – atrium	A – atrium	T – triggers pacing	R – rate-responsive	P – antitachycardia pacing
V – ventricle	V – ventricle	I – inhibits pacing	P – simple programmable	S – shock
D – dual	D – dual	D – triggers and inhibits pacing	M – multiprogrammable	D – dual (pace and shock)
S – single chamber	S – single chamber		C – communicating	

Table 11.13 • Temporary Pacing Modes Used After Heart Surgery

Code positions			Description
I	II	III	
A	O	O	Asynchronous atrial pacing
A	A	I	Atrial demand pacing
V	V	I	Ventricular demand pacing
D	V	I	AV sequential pacing (ventricular demand)
D	D	D	AV sequential pacing (both chambers sensed)
A, atrium; V, ventricle; D, both chambers; I, inhibits; O, does not apply			

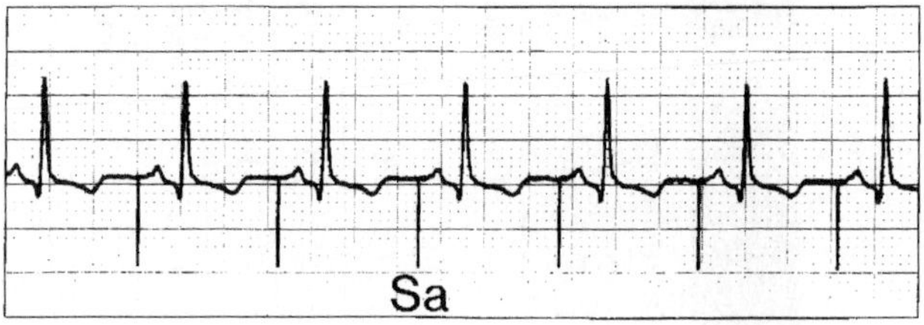

Figure 11.19 • Atrial pacing at a rate of 95 bpm. The atrial pacing stimulus artifact (Sa) is well seen in this tracing but is frequently difficult to identify on the monitor. The height of the atrial pacing spike may be increased on the monitor for better visualization, or it may be decreased to prevent problems with ECG interpretation or IABP tracking.

common modes are AOO (asynchronous atrial pacing), VVI (ventricular demand pacing), DVI (AV sequential pacing), and DDD (AV sequential demand pacing).

E. **Atrial pacing**

1. Atrial bipolar pacing is achieved by connecting both atrial electrodes to the pacemaker. This produces a smaller pacing stimulus artifact on a monitor than unipolar pacing and can often be difficult to detect even in multiple leads (Figure 11.19). It does, however, prevent IABP consoles from misinterpreting large pacing spikes as QRS complexes.

2. Atrial pacing can also be achieved using transesophageal electrodes or a pacing catheter placed through Swan-Ganz Paceport catheters. These are particularly beneficial during minimally invasive surgery.[285]

3. Pacing is usually accomplished in the AOO or AAI mode. The usual settings include a pulse amplitude of 10–20 mA in the asynchronous mode (insensitive to the ECG signal), set at a rate faster than the intrinsic heart rate. With the Medtronic 5392 External Dual-Chamber Pacemaker, AAI demand pacing may be accomplished if atrial sensing is satisfactory.

4. **Indications.** Atrial pacing requires the ability to capture the atrium as well as normal conduction through the AV node. It is ineffective during atrial fibrillation/flutter (AF/flutter).

    a. Sinus bradycardia or desire to increase the sinus rate to a higher level

    b. Suppression of premature ventricular complexes (PVCs): set at a rate slightly faster than the sinus mechanism

    c. Suppression of premature atrial complexes or prevention of AF (with dual-site atrial pacing)

    d. Slow junctional rhythm

    e. Overdriving supraventricular tachycardias (atrial flutter, paroxysmal atrial or AV junctional reentrant tachycardia). Rapid atrial pacing can interrupt a reentrant circuit and convert it to sinus rhythm or a nonsustained rhythm, such as AF, which may allow for better rate control and which may terminate spontaneously.

5. Technique of overdrive pacing

    a. Overdrive pacing is accomplished using pacemakers that can produce rates as high as 800/min. When attaching pacemaker wires to the generator, **be absolutely certain** that the atrial wires, not the ventricular wires, are being attached. Pacing initially 10–15 beats/min above the ventricular rate will allow one to determine whether the ventricle is inadvertently being paced, which can occur when atrial pacing wires are placed close to the ventricle.

    b. The patient must be attached to an ECG monitor during rapid atrial pacing. Bipolar pacing should be used to minimize distortion of the atrial complex. Pacing spikes are often best identified by evaluation of lead II.

    c. Turn the pacer to full current (20 mA) and to a rate about 10 beats faster than the tachycardia or flutter rate. When the atrium has been captured, increase the rate slowly until the morphology of the flutter waves changes (atrial complexes become positive). This is usually about 20–30% above the atrial flutter rate. Pacing for up to one minute may be required.

    d. The pacer should be turned off abruptly. Sinus rhythm, a pause followed by sinus rhythm, atrial fibrillation, or recurrent flutter may be noted (Figure 11.20). If severe bradycardia develops, the pacemaker may be turned on at a rate around 60 until the sinus mechanism recovers.

F. **Atrioventricular (AV) pacing**

1. AV pacing is achieved by connecting both atrial wires to the atrial inlets and both ventricular wires to the ventricular inlets of a dual-chamber pacer (Figure 11.21). If two ventricular wires are not available or not functioning, a skin lead can be used as a ground (the positive electrode) for ventricular pacing. The atrial and ventricular outputs are both set at 10–20 mA with a PR interval of 150 ms. Cardiac output can often be improved by increasing or decreasing the PR interval to alter ventricular filling time.[284] The ECG will demonstrate both pacing spikes, although the atrial spike is often difficult to detect.

2. Current external pacemakers, such as the Medtronic 5392 model, can pace in a variety of modes. The DDD mode senses atrial activity, following which the ventricle contracts at a preset time interval after the atrial contraction. This mode reduces the risk of triggering atrial, junctional, and pacemaker-induced

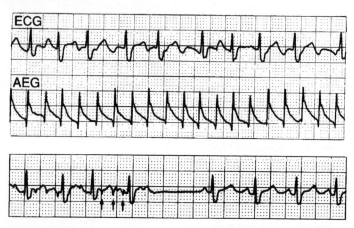

Figure 11.20 • Rapid atrial bipolar pacing of atrial flutter in sequential ECG tracings. The upper tracings confirm the rhythm as type I atrial flutter (rate 300/min) with variable AV block. In the lower tracing, rapid atrial pacing at a slightly faster rate entrains the atrium; the pacer is turned off and sinus rhythm resumes after a brief pause. The arrows indicate the atrial pacing stimulus artifact.

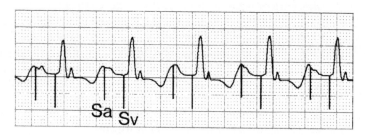

Figure 11.21 • Atrioventricular (AV) pacing at a rate of 75 bpm with a PR interval of about 220 ms. The P wave is often very poorly seen between the pacing stimulus artifacts (Sa, atrial; Sv, ventricular).

arrhythmias. Careful monitoring is necessary in the event that the pacemaker tracks the atrial signal in atrial fibrillation/flutter, resulting in a very fast ventricular response. However, setting an appropriate upper rate limit on these pacemakers usually prevents this complication. Occasionally, a pacemaker-mediated tachycardia can develop from repetitive retrograde conduction from premature ventricular complexes, producing atrial deflections that are sensed and tracked.

3. If atrial activity is absent, either the DDD or DVI mode can be used. The DVI mode senses only the ventricle, so if a ventricular beat does not occur, both chambers are paced. This may lead to competitive atrial activity if the atrium is beating at a faster rate.

4. **Indications**

   a. Complete heart block

   b. Second-degree heart block to achieve 1:1 conduction

    c. First-degree heart block if 1:1 conduction cannot be achieved at a faster rate because of a long PR interval

5. Additional comments

    a. Sequential AV pacing is ineffective during AF/flutter.

    b. AV pacing is always preferable to ventricular pacing because of the atrial contribution to ventricular filling. This is especially important in noncompliant ventricles, for which atrial contraction contributes up to 20–30% of the cardiac output. Atrial pacing alone in patients with normal conduction is superior to AV pacing by ensuring virtually simultaneous biventricular activation. Biventricular pacing usually provides superior hemodynamics to RA–RV pacing in patients with impaired LV function, especially with a prolonged QRS interval.[40–43]

    c. If sudden hemodynamic deterioration occurs during AV pacing, consider the possibility that atrial fibrillation has occurred with loss of atrial contraction. If AV conduction is slow, the ECG will demonstrate two pacing spikes with a QRS complex suggesting AV sequential pacing, although only ventricular pacing is occurring. This may be noted in the DDD mode with undersensing of AF or in the DVI mode in which the atrium is not sensed. If the patient has no detectable blood pressure despite pacing spikes on the monitor, VF may be present.

G. Ventricular pacing

1. Ventricular pacing is achieved by connecting the two ventricular wires to the pulse generator for bipolar pacing or connecting one ventricular wire to the negative pole and an indifferent electrode (skin wire or an atrial wire) to the positive pole for unipolar pacing.

2. The pacemaker is used in the VVI mode. The ventricular output is set at 10–20 mA in the synchronous (demand) mode. The rate selected depends on whether the pacemaker is being used for bradycardia backup, pacing at a therapeutic rate, or for overdrive pacing (Figure 11.22). Ventricular pacing in the VOO mode or in the VVI mode with undersensing of native R waves may result in the delivery of an inappropriate spike on the T wave at a time when the ventricle is vulnerable, inducing ventricular tachyarrhythmias.

3. **Indications**

    a. A slow ventricular response to AF/flutter

    b. Failure of atrial pacing to maintain heart rate

    c. Ventricular tachycardia (overdrive pacing)

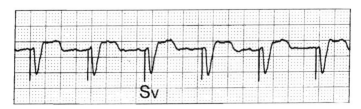

Figure 11.22 • Ventricular pacing at a rate of 80 bpm, demonstrating the wide ventricular complex. Since the patient's own ventricular rate is slower, the pacemaker produces all of the ventricular complexes. Sv, ventricular pacing stimulus artifact.

4. If a patient is dependent on AV or ventricular pacing, the pacing threshold must be tested. Gradually lower the mA until there is no capture. If the current necessary to generate electrical activity is rising or exceeds 10 mA, consideration should be given to placement of a transvenous pacing system (temporary or permanent).

5. If the pacemaker is in the demand mode, the sensing threshold should be checked. This represents the least sensitive mV at which the pacemaker can detect an ECG signal. Since demand pacing relies on the native rhythm to determine when to pace, undersensing will result in inappropriate pacing, while oversensing will inhibit pacing. To determine the sensing threshold, set the pacemaker to the VVI or DDD mode and turn the outputs to a very low level. Decrease the sensitivity (which increases the mV) until the sense indicator stops flashing and the pace indicator starts flashing. Then increase the sensitivity (which decreases the mV) until the sense indicator flashes again. This represents the sensing threshold. **Ventricular tachycardia can be triggered by inappropriately sensing ventricular pacing wires.**

H. Potential problems with epicardial pacing wire electrodes

1. **Failure to function** may result from:
   a. Faulty connections of the connecting cord to the pacing wires or to the pulse generator
   b. A defective pacing cord
   c. Faulty pulse generator function (low battery)
   d. Electrodes located in areas of poor electrical contact and high threshold
   e. Undetected detachment of the wire electrode from the atrial or ventricular epicardium
   f. Undetected development of AF/flutter causing failure of atrial capture

2. Options to restore pacemaker function and/or reestablish a rhythm include:
   a. Checking all connections; changing the connecting cord
   b. Increasing the output of the pulse generator to maximal current (20 mA)
   c. Using a different wire electrode as the negative (conducting) electrode (reversing polarity)
   d. Unipolarizing the pacemaker by attaching the positive lead to a surface ECG electrode or skin pacing wire
   e. Converting to ventricular pacing if the atrial stimulus fails to produce capture
   f. Using a chronotrope (any of the catecholamines) to increase the intrinsic rate or possibly increase atrial sensitivity to the pacing stimulus
   g. Placing a transvenous pacing wire if the patient has heart block or severe bradycardia and is pacer-dependent
   h. Attaching transcutaneous pacing pads

3. **Change in threshold.** The pacing threshold rises from the time of implantation because of edema, inflammation, thrombus, or the formation of scar tissue near the electrodes. If an advanced degree of heart block persists for more than a few days, consideration should be given to the placement of a permanent transvenous pacemaker system.

4. **Oversensing problems.** If the atrial activity of AF/flutter is sensed during DDD pacing, a very fast ventricular response will be noted. The upper rate limit should

be programmed (i.e. lowered) to prevent this. If this is not possible, the pacemaker should be converted to the VVI mode. Oversensing of T waves may lead to inhibition of VVI pacing.

5. **Competition with the patient's own rhythm.** When atrial or ventricular ectopy occurs during asynchronous pacing, suspect that the pacemaker is set at a rate similar to the patient's intrinsic mechanism. Turning off the pacemaker will eliminate the problem.

6. **Inadvertent triggering of VT or VF.** Use of ventricular pacing in the asynchronous mode can potentially trigger ventricular ectopy by competing with the patient's own mechanism. Appropriate sensing should always be confirmed if the pacemaker generator is left attached to the patient and is turned on. Ventricular pacing must always be accomplished in a demand mode (DVI, VVI, DDD). Pacing wires that are not being used should be electrically isolated to prevent stray AC or DC current near the wires from triggering VF. Wires should be placed in needle caps and left in accessible locations.

7. **Mediastinal bleeding** can occur if a pacing wire or the plastic carrier wire beyond the electrode (on Medtronic 6500 pacing wires) is placed close to bypass grafts, shearing them by intermittent contact during ventricular contractions. During epicardial wire removal, bleeding from vessels in the RV epicardial fat, muscle, the RV chamber, or even an adjacent graft can occur, especially if the wire was secured with sutures. This may occur despite easy removal or when excessive traction is applied. Bleeding is unlikely to occur when the atrial wires are placed in a plastic sleeve producing superficial contact with the atrial wall.

   a. Pacing wires should be removed with the patient off heparin, before a therapeutic INR has been achieved in patients receiving warfarin, and off of a NOAC for about 12 hours. The patient should remain at bedrest and be observed carefully for signs of tamponade with frequent vital signs for several hours after removal of epicardial wires.

   b. Some surgeons prefer that pacing wires be removed fairly early when chest tubes are still present, so any bleeding will be quickly detected. When wires are removed with chest tubes no longer present, progressive hemodynamic instability may warrant an echocardiogram to assess for a developing pericardial effusion. However, significant bleeding causing **cardiac tamponade can also occur within minutes** of pacing wire removal, for which arrangements for emergency sternotomy, commonly at the bedside, may be necessary.

8. **Inability to remove the wire electrodes from the heart.** The wire can be caught beneath a tight suture on the heart or, more likely, between the sternal halves or within a subcutaneous suture. Constant gentle traction, allowing the heart to "beat the wire loose", should be applied. A lateral chest x-ray may reveal where the wires are entrapped. If the wires cannot be removed, they should be pulled out as far as possible, cut off at the skin level, and allowed to retract. Infection can occur in pacing wire tracts, but it is unusual.

I. Other temporary pacing modalities

   1. Current monitor/defibrillators can provide transcutaneous pacing through gel pads attached to the patient's chest and back. This is most useful in emergency situations when epicardial pacing wires fail to function. This should not be relied

upon for more than a few hours, because ventricular capture frequently deteriorates over time. This type of pacing is also very uncomfortable for the patient.

2. Placement of a 5 Fr temporary transvenous ventricular pacing wire is indicated if
the patient is pacemaker-dependent and the threshold of the epicardial wires is
high or the wires fail to function. These wires are usually placed through an introducer in the internal jugular or subclavian vein, but can also be placed through the
femoral vein. The latter is routinely performed during TAVR procedures and may
be left in place for advanced heart block or significant bradycardia. These wires
have balloon tips that assist in floating the pacing wire into the apex of the right
ventricle, although fluoroscopy may occasionally be required.

3. Some Swan-Ganz catheters have extra channels that open into the right atrium
and ventricle (Paceport catheters) through which pacing catheters can be placed.
This is convenient during and following minimally invasive cardiac operations. It
is also helpful in emergency situations since central venous access has already been
achieved. These pacing leads should not be relied upon for chronic pacing in the
pacemaker-dependent patient.

4. Transesophageal atrial pacing is valuable during minimally invasive procedures
and can be used in the intensive care unit on a temporary basis if AV conduction
is preserved.[285]

J. **Indications for permanent pacemakers**

1. Although the temporary use of epicardial pacing is not uncommon after surgery,
most patients with preoperative sinus rhythm will achieve a satisfactory sinus rate
within a few days and can receive β-blockers for AF prophylaxis. Conduction
abnormalities such as first-degree block and bundle branch blocks are the most
common abnormalities noted after CABG, but they have not been shown to
affect long-term outcome.[286]

2. About 1–2% of patients require placement of a PPM after cardiac surgery. This is
more likely in older patients, those with pulmonary hypertension or a preexisting
left bundle branch block (LBBB), surgery that involves valve replacements (tricuspid > aortic > mitral), complex operations requiring a long cross-clamp time,
and reoperations.[287–289]

a. Tricuspid valve replacement involves suturing in close proximity to the AV
node, and evidence of complete heart block should prompt placement of permanent epicardial pacing leads.

b. Mitral valve procedures performed through the superior transseptal approach
are twice as likely to require a PPM, primarily for sinus node dysfunction.[290]
PPM placement is also more common following mitral annular reconstructive
surgery and Maze procedures.[287]

c. AVR has about a 5% risk of requiring a PPM, more commonly when surgery
is performed for endocarditis, aortic regurgitation, and with extensive calcification. The need for a PPM compromises the prognosis after a surgical AVR.[291,292]

3. The risk of requiring a PPM after TAVR is greater with self-expanding valves
than balloon-expandable valves, but newer designs and higher positioning have
reduced the risk to less than 5%. Baseline conduction disturbances, especially a
right bundle branch block (RBBB) with first-degree block, increase the risk of
complete heart block and the need for a PPM.[293] In fact, a baseline RBBB also

increases the risk of high-grade AV block and sudden cardiac death after hospital discharge.[294] A new LBBB leads to deterioration in LV function, increases the risk of requiring a PPM, and, in most studies, compromises intermediate-term survival.[295–298]

4. If a PPM is being considered in the postoperative patient, oral anticoagulation with warfarin should be withheld or given in low doses, with use of IV heparin for AF or valve thromboprophylaxis, when indicated. If the patient's INR is already in therapeutic range, the dose should be reduced to achieve an INR at the low therapeutic range if the patient is at high thromboembolic risk, at which point PPM implantation can be safely performed. It is preferable to avoid a heparin bridge, which is associated with more periprocedural bleeding.[299]

5. PPM placement is indicated postoperatively for the following conditions:
   a. Complete heart block
   b. Symptomatic or significant sinus node dysfunction
   c. Slow ventricular response to AF (usually at rates of less than 50 bpm) that persists despite cessation of potentially contributory medications, including β-blockers, sotalol, amiodarone, CCBs, and digoxin.
   d. Tachycardia-bradycardia syndrome: when medications used to control a fast response to AF produce a very slow sinus mechanism upon conversion
   e. Advanced second-degree heart block with a slow ventricular response

6. The optimal timing for placement of a PPM has not been determined. In some patients, the indication may be a transient phenomenon, and waiting a few extra days may obviate its need. However, it often seems more cost-effective to implant a pacemaker after 3–4 days to expedite the patient's discharge from the hospital. A study from the Mayo Clinic showed that 40% of patients were not pacer-dependent at follow-up, although about 85% of patients who required implantation for complete heart block had become pacer-dependent.[300] A follow-up study of patients receiving PPMs after TAVR found that only 40% of patients receiving a PPM within 10 days were pacer-dependent at one year.[301]

XII. Cardiac Arrhythmias

The development of cardiac arrhythmias following open-heart surgery is fairly common. Supraventricular arrhythmias, especially atrial fibrillation, are noted in about 25% of patients. Ventricular arrhythmias are less common and usually reflect some degree of myocardial injury. Whereas AF is usually benign, ventricular arrhythmias may warrant further evaluation and treatment because of their potentially life-threatening nature. The mechanisms underlying the development of most arrhythmias are those of altered automaticity (impulse formation) and conductivity (impulse conduction). An understanding of these mechanisms and the electrophysiologic effects of the antiarrhythmic drugs has provided a rational basis for their use. The treatment of arrhythmias commonly noted after open-heart surgery is summarized in Table 11.14.

A. **Etiology.** Although the factors that contribute to the development of various cardiac arrhythmias may differ, there are several common causes that should be considered.
   1. Cardiac problems
      a. Underlying heart disease
      b. Preexisting arrhythmias

Table 11.14 • Treatment of Common Arrhythmias

Arrhythmia	Treatment
1. Sinus bradycardia	Pacing: atrial or AV > ventricular Catecholamine infusion
2. Third-degree heart block	Pacing: AV > ventricular Catecholamine infusion
3. Sinus tachycardia	Address cause β-blocker
4. Premature atrial complexes	No treatment Atrial pacing (preferably dual-site) Magnesium sulfate β-blocker Amiodarone Calcium channel blockers
5. Atrial fibrillation	Cardioversion if hemodynamically compromised Rate control: 　ß-blocker 　Diltiazem 　Amiodarone Convert: 　Amiodarone 　Propafenone/ibutilide 　Electrical cardioversion V-pace if slow response
6. Atrial flutter	Cardioversion if compromised Rapid atrial pacing See treatment for atrial fibrillation
7. Paroxysmal supraventricular tachycardia (PAT or AVNRT)	Atrial overdrive pacing Cardioversion Adenosine Verapamil/diltiazem β-blocker Digoxin
8. Slow junctional rhythm	Pacing: atrial > AV > ventricular Chronotropic medication
9. Nonparoxysmal AV junctional tachycardia	Not on digoxin: beta-blocker 　CCB (diltiazem, verapamil) 　propafenone or flecainide if no structural heart disease On digoxin: stop digoxin 　Potassium 　Phenytoin
10. Premature ventricular complexes	Treat hypokalemia Atrial overdrive pacing Lidocaine Amiodarone
11. Ventricular tachycardia/fibrillation	Defibrillation Amiodarone Lidocaine

    c. Myocardial ischemia or infarction

    d. Poor intraoperative myocardial protection

    e. Pericardial inflammation

2. Respiratory problems

    a. Endotracheal tube irritation or misplacement

    b. Hypoxia, hypercarbia, acidosis

    c. Pneumothorax

3. Electrolyte imbalance (hypo- or hyperkalemia, hypomagnesemia)

4. Intracardiac monitoring lines (Swan-Ganz PA catheter)

5. Surgical trauma (atriotomy or ventriculotomy incisions), dissection near the conduction system (aortic valves) or suture placement near the AV node (tricuspid valve surgery)

6. Drugs (vasoactive drugs, proarrhythmic effects of antiarrhythmic medications)

7. Hypothermia

8. Fever, anxiety, pain

9. Gastric dilatation

B. Assessment

1. Check the ABGs, ventilator function, position of the endotracheal tube, and chest x-ray for mechanical problems.

2. Check serum electrolytes (especially potassium).

3. Review a 12-lead ECG for ischemia and a more detailed examination of the arrhythmia. If the diagnosis is not clear-cut, obtain an AEG. This is frequently beneficial in differentiating among some of the more common arrhythmias by providing an amplified tracing of atrial activity.

C. Sinus bradycardia

1. Sinus bradycardia is present when the sinus rate is less than 60 bpm. It is frequently caused by persistent β-blockade, dexmedetomidine, and the use of narcotics, and may result in atrial, junctional, or ventricular escape rhythms.

2. Because sinus bradycardia reduces cardiac output, the heart rate should be maintained around 90 bpm following the termination of CPB to optimize hemodynamics. An increase in heart rate can improve myocardial contractility and cardiac output.

3. **Diagnosis.** See Figure 11.23.

4. **Treatment**

    a. Atrial pacing should be used to take advantage of the 20–30% increase in stroke volume that results from the contribution of atrial filling. This is particularly helpful in the early postoperative period when reperfusion and myocardial edema impair ventricular compliance and cause diastolic dysfunction. Atrial contraction is especially important in patients with LVH, such as those with aortic valve disease or systemic hypertension, in whom loss of atrial "kick" reduces stroke volume by 25–30%.

    b. AV pacing should be used if abnormal AV conduction is present with a slow ventricular rate (second- or third-degree AV block).

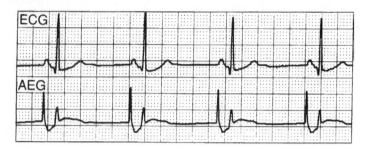

Figure 11.23 • Sinus bradycardia at a rate of 54 bpm recorded simultaneously in lead I and a unipolar AEG. The AEG demonstrates the larger atrial complex, a PR interval of 0.18 seconds, and the smaller ventricular complex.

    c. If atrial pacing wires were not placed at the conclusion of surgery or if they fail to function, one of the catecholamines can be used to stimulate the sinus mechanism. Epinephrine 1–2 µg/min, dobutamine 5–10 µg/kg/min, or isoproterenol 1–2 µg/min may be useful. However, these medications not only increase the heart rate but have other hemodynamic effects as well. Atropine 0.01 mg/kg IV (usually 0.5–1 mg IV) can be used for severe symptomatic bradycardia on an emergency basis.

    d. Ventricular pacing can be used if the atrium fails to capture or there is little response to pharmacologic management. It will nearly always produce less effective hemodynamics than a supraventricular mechanism. If the ventricular pacing wires fail to function, the other pacing modes listed on pages 609–610 can be considered.

    e. If sinus bradycardia is induced by medications used to either prevent or treat atrial fibrillation, lower doses or cessation of those medications should be considered if the heart rate remains <60 bpm. Patients with known sick sinus or tachycardia-bradycardia syndrome often have problems with slow heart rates postoperatively when medications are used to slow the response to AF, and they may require placement of a PPM.

D. Conduction abnormalities and heart block

    1. Transient disturbances of conduction at the AV node are noted in about 25–45% of patients following coronary bypass surgery. They are more frequent when cold cardioplegic arrest is used for myocardial protection.

        a. Conduction abnormalities are more common in patients with compromised LV function, hypertension, severe coronary disease (especially involving the right coronary artery in a right-dominant system), long aortic cross-clamp times, and extremely low myocardial temperatures. These findings suggest that ischemic or cold injury to the conduction system may be responsible for these problems. Although most will resolve within 24–48 hours, the persistence of a new LBBB suggests the possible occurrence of a perioperative infarction. The presence of a new LBBB after CABG does not appear to influence the long-term prognosis.[286]

b. Conduction abnormalities occurring after an AVR may be caused by hemorrhage, edema, suturing, or debridement near the AV node and bundle of His. A new LBBB, as well as the need for a PPM, is an ominous prognostic sign after both surgical and transcatheter AVRs, and has been found to compromise long-term survival.[291,295-298,302]

c. Algorithms for the management of conduction abnormalities following TAVRs were provided by a JACC scientific expert panel in 2019.[303] Telemetry overnight was recommended for all patients following TAVR. PPM implantation was recommended for those who developed high-grade AV block or complete heart block (CHB). If there was a new LBBB or persistent increase of >20 ms in the PR or QRS duration with a preexisting conduction disturbance (RBBB, LBBB, intraventricular conduction delay [IVCD] with QRS >120 ms, or first degree AV block), it was recommended that the pacemaker wire be left in overnight. If these changes persisted or the PR interval was >240 ms or the QRS duration was >150 ms with or without a LBBB, the patient was at higher risk of developing high-grade AV block or CHB and may require monitoring for an additional 24 hours. In these patients, the options were implanting a PPM, continuous ECG monitoring after discharge, or invasive electrophysiologic evaluation to guide the decision about a PPM, with the presence of an infra-Hisian block during atrial pacing or spontaneous HV interval >100 ms prompting consideration of a PPM.

d. Exposure of the mitral valve by the biatrial transseptal approach involves division of the sinus node artery and anterior internodal pathways. Although some studies have not documented a higher incidence of postoperative rhythm disturbances, others have shown a high incidence of sinus node dysfunction with ectopic atrial rhythms, junctional rhythms, and varying degrees of heart block. About 10% of patients may require a PPM for bradycardia or complete heart block when this approach is used.[290]

2. **Diagnosis.** See Figures 11.24–11.28.

3. **Treatment**

a. Conduction abnormities are best treated using both atrial and ventricular pacing wires placed at the conclusion of surgery.

b. **First-degree AV block** is characterized by prolongation of the PR interval to greater than 200 ms and usually does not require treatment. If the PR interval is markedly prolonged, attempts to achieve faster atrial pacing will not achieve 1:1 conduction because the AV node will remain refractory when the next impulse arrives. This will produce functional second-degree heart block. AV pacing in the DDD or DVI mode can be used in this situation. Shortening a prolonged AV interval can significantly improve hemodynamics, especially in patients with impaired LV function.[284]

c. **Second-degree AV** block is caused by intermittent failure of AV conduction.

i. Mobitz type I (Wenckebach) is characterized by progressive PR interval prolongation culminating in a nonconducted P wave with no QRS complex (Figure 11.25). This usually does not require treatment unless the ventricular rate is slow. In this situation, it can be treated by AV pacing

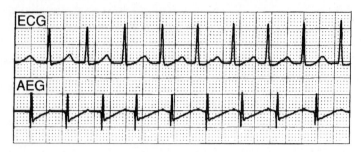

Figure 11.24 • First-degree AV block recorded simultaneously in lead II and a bipolar AEG. The PR interval is approximately 0.26 seconds (260 ms).

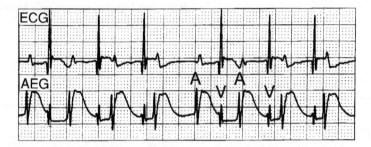

Figure 11.25 • Mobitz type I (Wenckebach) second-degree block. The unipolar AEG demonstrates a constant atrial rate of 120 bpm with progressive lengthening of the A–V (PR) intervals until the ventricular complex is dropped. In the AEG, the atrial activity is represented by the larger of the two complexes (A, atrial complex; V, ventricular complex).

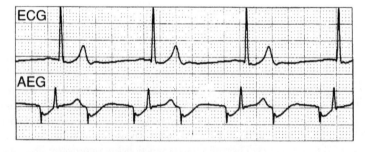

Figure 11.26 • Second-degree block. Atrial activity is present at a rate of 100/min with 2:1 block, producing a ventricular rate of 50/min.

(DVI) at a slightly faster rate. If the atrial rate is too fast to overdrive, it can be treated by DDD pacing.

    ii. Mobitz type II is characterized by constant PR intervals and intermittent dropped QRS complexes. The P–P and R–R intervals remain unchanged. This reflects block in the His-Purkinje system and therefore is associated with a wide QRS complex. If the ventricular rate is too slow,

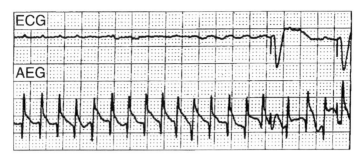

Figure 11.27 • Complete AV block. The AEG demonstrates type I atrial flutter, but the monitor ECG shows no ventricular complex until ventricular pacing is initiated.

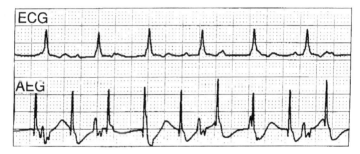

Figure 11.28 • Complete AV block with AV dissociation. The unipolar AEG demonstrates an atrial rate of 140/min (large spikes) with no clear-cut relationship to the QRS complex, which represents a junctional mechanism at a rate of 100/min.

AV pacing in the DVI or DDD mode should be used. If this rhythm persists, a PPM should usually be implanted because it is likely to progress to complete heart block.

    iii. 2:1 AV block entails a constant PR interval with a dropped QRS complex every other beat (Figure 11.26). It is treated in a similar fashion to Mobitz type II block with AV pacing.

    iv. High-grade second-degree heart block is evident when there is a constant PR interval but two or more consecutive atrial impulses do not conduct to the ventricle. It is treated by AV pacing and may require a PPM if persistent.

  d. Third-degree (complete) heart block is characterized by failure of AV conduction of any atrial activity. Thus, there will usually be variable rates for the P waves and QRS complexes, which may be absent or represent escape rhythms at various rates (Figures 11.27 and 11.28). This usually requires AV pacing in either the DDD or DVI mode. If the atrial rate is acceptable, the DDD mode should be used to track the atrial rate and then provide a sequential ventricular contraction. If there is atrial inactivity or a slow atrial rate, either DDD or

DVI pacing can be used. Ventricular pacing should be used if AF/flutter is present. Pacing is usually not necessary when there is an adequate junctional or idioventricular rate. However, AV pacing can be accomplished in the DVI mode or the DDD mode if the atrial rate is not too fast to take advantage of the atrial contribution to filling.

   e. If the patient is dependent on AV or ventricular pacing, the pacing threshold must be tested. Gradually lower the mA until there is no capture. If the current necessary to generate electrical activity is rising or exceeds 10 mA, consideration should be given to placement of a transvenous pacing system (temporary or permanent).

   f. If advanced degrees of heart block persist, the patient's medications should be reviewed. Those that might accentuate AV block (β-blockers, amiodarone, CCBs, or digoxin) should be withheld to assess the patient's intrinsic rate and conduction. If complete heart block persists for more than a few days with the patient off these medications, a PPM should be placed. The most significant predictor of pacemaker dependency is its insertion for complete heart block.

E. Sinus tachycardia

1. Sinus tachycardia is present when the sinus rate exceeds 100 bpm. It generally occurs at rates of less than 130. A faster and regular ventricular rate suggests atrial flutter with 2:1 block or paroxysmal supraventricular (atrial or junctional) tachycardia.

2. Fast heart rates are detrimental to myocardial metabolism. They can exacerbate myocardial ischemia by increasing oxygen demand and decreasing the time for diastolic coronary perfusion. They also reduce the time for ventricular filling and can reduce stroke volume, especially in patients with LVH and diastolic dysfunction.

3. **Etiology**

   a. Benign hyperdynamic reflex response related to sympathetic overactivity:
      • Pain, anxiety, fever
      • Adrenergic rebound (patient on β-blockers preoperatively)
      • Drugs (catecholamines)
      • Gastric dilatation
      • Anemia
      • Hypermetabolic states (sepsis)

   b. Compensatory response to myocardial injury or impaired cardiorespiratory status:
      • Hypoxia, hypercarbia, acidosis
      • Hypovolemia or low stroke volumes noted with small, stiff left ventricles with LVH and diastolic dysfunction
      • Myocardial ischemia or infarction
      • Cardiac tamponade

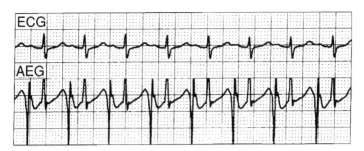

Figure 11.29 • Sinus tachycardia at a rate of 130 bpm on simultaneous recordings of monitor lead II and a unipolar AEG. Note the larger atrial and smaller ventricular complex in the unipolar AEG tracing, which demonstrates the 1:1 AV conduction.

- Tension pneumothorax
- Pulmonary embolism

c. Once a patient is transferred from the ICU and is clinically stable, sinus tachycardia is usually caused by pain, anemia, hypovolemia, or respiratory issues. However, the possibility of delayed tamponade should always be kept in mind. Some patients have higher sympathetic activity and a higher baseline heart rate with no other identifiable cause.

4. **Diagnosis.** See Figure 11.29.

5. **Treatment**

   a. Correction of the underlying cause

   b. Sedation and analgesia in the ICU setting; adequate analgesia subsequently on the postoperative floor

   c. β-blockers can be used if the heart is hyperdynamic with an excellent cardiac output. They must be used cautiously, however, when cardiac function is marginal. Tachycardia is a compensatory mechanism to maintain cardiac output when the stroke volume is low, and attempts to slow the heart rate may prove detrimental. Even when the cardiac output is satisfactory, β-blockers often lower the blood pressure significantly more than they reduce the heart rate.

      i. Esmolol 0.25–0.5 mg/kg IV over one minute followed by a continuous infusion of 50–200 μg/kg/min. A trial bolus of 0.125 mg/kg is recommended to determine whether the patient can tolerate esmolol.

      ii. Metoprolol 2.5–5 mg IV increments every five minutes for three doses

      iii. Increasing doses of oral metoprolol (25–100 mg bid) are usually used to control a postoperative sinus tachycardia on the floor. Some patients are refractory to its effects and respond better to atenolol (25–100 mg qd).

   d. CCBs have mild negative chronotropic effects on the SA node, but they do not play a major role in the treatment of sinus tachycardia.

   e. **Note:** both IV β-blockers and CCBs are safe to administer, but their simultaneous use must be done cautiously if functional pacing wires are not present.

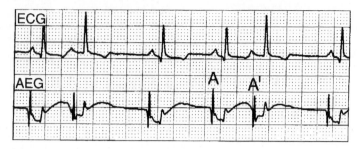

Figure 11.30 • Premature atrial complexes (PACs) in monitor lead II and a unipolar AEG. Note the slightly different morphology of the normal (A) and premature (A′) atrial complexes and the slightly different PR interval following the PACs that indicates a focus different from the sinus node. The PR interval exceeds 120 ms, thus differentiating these beats from premature junctional complexes.

F. **Premature atrial complexes (PACs)**

1. PACs are premature beats arising in the atrium that generally have a different configuration than the normal P wave and produce a PR interval that exceeds 120 ms. Although benign, they often herald the development of AF or flutter, and this occurrence can be very difficult to prevent.

2. Magnesium sulfate may be beneficial in reducing the incidence of PACs in the immediate postoperative period. The dose is 2 g in a 100 mL solution.

3. **Diagnosis.** See Figure 11.30.

4. **Treatment**

   a. PACs generally do not need to be treated, but because they frequently precede the development of AF, medications that can alter atrial automaticity and conduction or slow the ventricular response to AF can be considered. These include β-blockers, CCBs, and amiodarone.

   b. Digoxin is useful in decreasing the frequency of PACs and slows conduction through the AV node if AF does develop. However, by increasing conduction velocity in the atrium, digoxin can theoretically increase the risk of developing AF if PACs are present. It is rarely used in cardiac surgery patients anymore.

   c. Temporary right atrial pacing at a faster rate ("overdrive pacing") may suppress PACs, but it may also trigger atrial arrhythmias and induce AF. This may occur even in the AAI mode when there is difficulty sensing atrial activity leading to inappropriate pacing. This problem generally does not occur with permanent dual-chamber pacemakers. If PACs occur during atrial pacing, one should suspect competition with the patient's own rhythm. Dual-site atrial pacing may suppress PACs and also prevent AF.

G. **Atrial fibrillation or flutter**

1. Atrial fibrillation (AF) (atrial rate >380) and atrial flutter (atrial rate generally <380) are the most common arrhythmias noted after open-heart surgery. Despite various prophylactic measures to decrease their incidence, they still occur in about

25–30% of patients. There is probably a reversible trigger that causes AF in postoperative patients in whom there is an underlying substrate for its development, such as increased dispersion of atrial refractoriness with nonuniform atrial conduction.

2. Numerous **risk factors** for the development of AF have been identified, and their presence may indicate the aggressiveness with which prophylactic antiarrhythmic therapy should be used. Several models have been used to predict the risk of postoperative AF, although with limited success.

   a. Risk models include the following:[304–308]

      i. CHA$_2$DS$_2$-VASc score: HF, hypertension, older age, diabetes, stroke/TIA, PVD, female gender

      ii. POAF score: age >60 in increments, COPD, dialysis, emergency surgery, preoperative IABP, EF <30%

      iii. AF risk index: older age, COPD, concurrent valve surgery, prior history of AF, withdrawal of β-blockers and ACE inhibitors

      iv. HATCH score: HF, stroke/TIA, age >75, COPD

      v. CHARGE-AF score: age, race, height/weight, blood pressure, and use of antihypertensive medications, smoking, diabetes, history of MI or HF

   b. The most consistent risk factors in these models are those of older age, heart failure (systolic or diastolic), poor LV function, COPD, and withdrawal of β-blockers. Other studies have shown an increased risk in patients undergoing mitral valve surgery, especially those with an enlarged left atrium, and with LVH, a baseline heart rate >100 bpm, or increased P-wave duration.[309–312]

   c. Comparative studies of risk models suggest that some may be better than others in predicting the risk of AF. One analysis showed that the CHA$_2$DS$_2$-VASc score, which was devised to predict the risk of stroke in nonanticoagulated patients with AF, may be more discriminative than the POAF and HATCH scoring systems in predicting the risk of postoperative AF.[305] Another study found that, other than the CHARGE-AF score, which is a predictor of AF in the general population, the best predictor of postoperative AF was the patient's age.[308]

3. AF can compromise cardiac hemodynamics and also increases the risk of systemic thromboembolism and stroke from LA thrombus by two- to threefold.[313] AF prolongs the hospital length of stay and increases hospital costs. Although it has not been shown consistently to influence operative mortality, its occurrence has been shown to increase the risk of early AF recurrence (28% within one month in one study),[314] increase the risk of later AF eightfold, and reduce long-term survival by twofold after coronary and valve surgery.[315–320] The longer the duration of postoperative AF, the greater the impact on late survival.[321]

4. AF occurs most commonly on the second and third postoperative day. By that time, myocardial function has recovered to baseline and few adverse hemodynamic effects are noted. However, when atrial tachyarrhythmias occur during the first 24 hours, especially when the patient is hemodynamically unstable, or in patients with noncompliant hypertrophied ventricles, a rapid ventricular response can

precipitate ischemia and lower the cardiac output by eliminating the atrial contribution to ventricular filling, leading to hypotension. Although slowing the ventricular response rate may improve the blood pressure, it may remain low because most drugs used to slow the rate tend to reduce the blood pressure as well (ß-blockers and CCBs).

5. After the initial 24 hours, AF is frequently an incidental finding on the ECG monitor, and many patients do not even notice that it is present. Symptoms such as palpitations, nausea, fatigue, or lightheadedness may occur, especially in patients with LVH or poor ventricular function.

6. **Etiology**

   a. Enhanced sympathetic activity following surgery (intrinsic or with use of catecholamines) or adrenergic rebound in patients taking β-blockers preoperatively, but not started postoperatively.[322] However, it still occurs in those in whom β-blockers are started the morning after surgery.

   b. Atrial ischemia from poor myocardial preservation during aortic crossclamping. Since AF is associated with more complex procedures (redos, valve-CABGs) during which there is a longer cross-clamp time, inadequate protection of the atria and systemic hypothermia are likely to be contributory. Nonetheless, a reduced incidence of AF following off-pump surgery has not been documented in most studies.[323,324]

   c. Acute atrial distention from fluid shifts and chronic atrial dilatation from preexisting structural heart disease, including hypertension, ischemic or valvular heart disease. These create the substrate that leads to the occurrence and persistence of postoperative AF.

   d. Surgical trauma, inflammation (pericarditis), or oxidative stress

   e. Metabolic derangements (hypoxia, hypokalemia, hypomagnesemia)

7. **Diagnosis.** See Figures 11.31 and 11.32.

8. **Prevention.** Prophylactic therapy can reduce the risk of AF by approximately 50% with a trend towards a reduction in stroke.[309–312,325–328]

   a. The only class I pharmacologic recommendation is the initiation of a lowdose ß-blocker, which has shown to reduce the incidence of AF by up to 65%. It should be given to all patients after surgery whether taken prior to

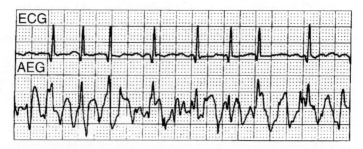

Figure 11.31 • Atrial fibrillation (AF) with a ventricular response of 130 bpm. The AEG demonstrates the chaotic atrial activity that is characteristic of AF.

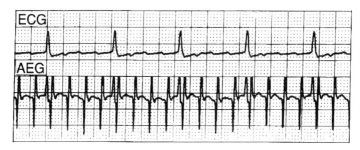

Figure 11.32 • Atrial flutter with 4:1 AV block. The unipolar AEG demonstrates an atrial rate of about 300 bpm with a ventricular response of about 75 bpm.

surgery or not, unless contraindicated by bradycardia, hypotension, pressor dependence, or a low cardiac output state. Metoprolol 12.5–50 mg bid and atenolol 25 mg qd are most commonly used. Numerous studies have reported that carvedilol, an α- and β-blocker with oxidative-stress reducing properties, commonly used in patients with depressed LV function, is superior to metoprolol in reducing the incidence of AF.[329–331]

b. **Amiodarone** (class IIa indication) is a class III antiarrhythmic with some class I, II, and IV properties that is effective in reducing the incidence of AF by 50%, either when given alone or in conjunction with β-blockers.[309,327,328,332–337]

   i. The timing (pre-, intra-, or postoperative), route (IV vs. PO), and dosage of amiodarone which provides the best prophylaxis has not been clarified, because different protocols have been used in virtually every study. Optimal benefit requires adequate dosing to achieve electrophysiologic effects at the time of highest risk for AF. Thus, regimens of preoperative oral loading must be long enough or use high enough doses to be effective since it takes several days to achieve effect.

   ii. The vast majority of studies have shown that amiodarone reduces the incidence of postoperative AF. Whether amiodarone should be used for all patients or only in those at higher risk has yet to be determined. It has been recommended for patients with the commonly identified risk factors noted in section 2.a, but most specifically for older patients, whether >age 60 or 70. Amiodarone may be particularly beneficial in patients with COPD, in whom the incidence and morbidity of AF are greater.[338] However, the potential for acute amiodarone toxicity that can produce hypoxemia must be kept in mind.[339]

   iii. In general, for patients at higher risk of AF, it is recommended that oral loading be started prior to surgery. In the classic PAPABEAR trial, a 50% reduction in postoperative AF was noted using a six-day preoperative load of 10 mg/kg daily and a 13-day total course.[335] This benefit was independent of age, but was greater in patients >age 65. Other recommended regimens for patients undergoing elective surgery include:[312]

      • 200 mg tid × 5 days prior to surgery, then 400 mg bid × 4–6 days postoperatively

- 400 mg qid × 1 day prior to surgery, then 600 mg bid on day of surgery, then 400 mg bid × 4–6 days after surgery (if surgery scheduled within 1–5 days)

iv. Logistic considerations in patients requiring more urgent surgery suggest that an alternative approach must be used. Protocols have included:

- 150 mg IV load over 15 minutes given at the end of CPB, followed by a 1 mg/min infusion × 6 hours, then 0.5 mg/min × 18 hours (which would correspond to 1,050 mg over 24 hours) with conversion to oral dosing starting at 400 mg bid × 4 days and reduced to 200 mg daily for a few weeks.
- 300 mg IV over 20 minutes on POD #1, then 600 mg bid × 5 days[336]
- 0.73 mg/min starting on call to the operating room and continuing for 48 hours with conversion to 400 mg q12h for three days[337]

v. The benefits of continuing amiodarone after hospital discharge are uncertain. Amiodarone can probably be stopped at the time of discharge if effective for prophylaxis since it will have persistent electrophysiologic effects for weeks. If the patient does develop intermittent AF and converts, it is usually continued for about one month, with the dosage being weaned down to 200 mg qd. Some have argued that one week of therapy is adequate if the patient is discharged home in sinus rhythm.[340]

c. **Ranolazine** is used primarily for patients with refractory angina, but it is a very effective antiarrhythmic medication with properties similar to amiodarone. It is effective in reducing the incidence and recurrence of postoperative AF by about 60%.[341–343] Concomitant use of IV amiodarone enhances efficacy and shortens the time to AF conversion, and this combination may be more effective in patients with a reduced EF.[344] One study found that ranolazine produced more than a fourfold reduction in postoperative AF compared with use of a β-blocker.[345] One recommended dosing regimen is 1 g PO preoperatively, then 1 g PO bid × 7 days.

d. **Sotalol** is a β-blocker with class III antiarrhythmic properties that is equally if not more effective than standard β-blockers and as effective as amiodarone in preventing supraventricular tachyarrhythmias when used at a dose of 80 mg bid.[327,328,346] However, it is a negative inotrope and is not tolerated in about 20% of patients, in whom hypotension, bradycardia, or AV block may develop. Sotalol may also cause QT prolongation and polymorphic ventricular arrhythmias, including torsades de pointes. It is excreted by the kidneys and should be avoided in patients with renal dysfunction. It is available in IV form (75 mg IV = 80 mg oral) if the patient cannot take the oral dose.

e. **Magnesium sulfate** (2 g in 100 mL) is often effective in decreasing the occurrence and number of episodes of postoperative AF, although a meta-analysis could not demonstrate much benefit.[347] It appears to be most effective when given with sotalol and when the serum magnesium level is low.[348,349] Since it is benign and of potential benefit, it is worthwhile administering to all patients during surgery and on the first postoperative day in addition to β-blockers.

f. Although standard right-atrial pacing may increase atrial ectopy and does not reduce the incidence of AF, **dual-site atrial pacing** has been shown in numerous studies to reduce the incidence of AF, especially when given with a β-blocker.[350,351] It is theorized that intra-atrial conduction delays may contribute to AF. Dual-site pacing alters the atrial activation sequence and may achieve more uniform electrical activation of the atria. It may also overdrive/suppress PACs, eliminate compensatory pauses after PACs, and reduce the dispersion of refractoriness that may contribute to AF.

g. A number of other medications and substances have been evaluated for their effectiveness in reducing the incidence of postoperative AF. Those that have few side effects might be considered routinely, but medications with potential morbidity are not commonly utilized with the more routine use of β-blockers and amiodarone.

   i. **Dofetilide** is effective in reducing the incidence of AF (by 50% in one study), but other medications are preferable due to its cost and risk of causing QT prolongation.[352]

   ii. **Propafenone** 300 mg PO bid is also effective and was found comparable to atenolol in one study.[353]

   iii. **Colchicine** (class IIb indication) has an anti-inflammatory effect and is useful in reducing the incidence of post-pericardiotomy syndrome. A meta-analysis found that it reduced the incidence of AF by 30%.[354]

   iv. **Steroids** (class IIb indication) may reduce inflammation and possibly the risk of AF, but commonly cause hyperglycemia and may increase the risk of infection.[355] Study protocols include use of hydrocortisone 100 mg prior to surgery followed by 100 mg q8h × 3 days[356] or methylprednisolone 1 g before surgery followed by dexamethasone 4 mg q6h x 4 doses after surgery.[357]

   v. **Statins** given in high doses (atorvastatin 40–80 mg) in statin-naive patients have been found in some studies to reduce AF by 50%, but meta-analyses have not demonstrated any benefit.[358–362] Nonetheless, virtually all patients undergoing cardiac surgery receive statins for other reasons, so a reduction in AF would be an incidental benefit.

   vi. **Ascorbic acid** (vitamin C) 2 g before surgery and 1 g daily for five days has been shown to enhance the benefits of β-blockers in reducing AF.[363] One meta-analysis showed a 60% reduction in AF with use of vitamin C,[364] but some trials have not found any benefit.[365,366]

   vii. **N-3 fatty acids** (fish oils) 2 g/day started preoperatively have been shown to reduce AF in CABG patients, but only when the EPA/DHA ratio was <1.[367] However, the OPERA study published in 2012 failed to show this benefit.[368]

   viii. A combination of multiple antioxidants, including vitamin C, vitamin E, and polyunsaturated fatty acids produced a 22% absolute reduction (nearly threefold) in AF.[369]

   ix. **N-acetylcysteine** is an antioxidant medication has been shown in several studies to reduce the incidence of AF by about 30%.[364,370] The protocol is 50 mg/kg after the induction of anesthesia with additional doses on the first and second postoperative days.

   x. CCBs, including diltiazem and verapamil, as well as digoxin, have not been uniformly efficacious in preventing AF.

xi. The presence of pericardial blood is considered to create a pro-inflammatory and pro-oxidant milieu in the pericardial space that may contribute to AF. Placement of a posterior mediastinal pericardial tube may improve drainage, and performing a posterior pericardiotomy to allow blood to drain into the pleural space has been shown to reduce the incidence of AF.[371,372]

9. **Management** of the unstable patient developing AF initially involves cardioversion, whereas the strategy for the stable patient involves rate control, anticoagulation if AF persists, and attempts to achieve conversion to sinus rhythm (Table 11.15 and Figure 11.33). Although conversion to sinus rhythm will occur in 50–80% of patients before hospital discharge with use of ß-blockers,[373] additional pharmacologic intervention is usually recommended to promote conversion and avoid the requirement for anticoagulation. Although it has been presumed that most patients will subsequently remain in sinus rhythm, follow-up studies have shown a recurrence rate of up to 30%, which may be one factor that increases long-term mortality in patients who develop postoperative AF.[314] This approach is in contradistinction to medical patients in whom a rate-controlled strategy is considered acceptable due to comparable survival, potentially fewer adverse effects from medications, yet worse functional outcome.[374]

a. Electric **cardioversion** with 50–100 joules can be used in a variety of circumstances.

   i. Cardioversion should always be considered first if there is evidence of significant hemodynamic compromise. This is more common in the early postoperative period, when a very rapid ventricular response may be present and myocardial function is moderately depressed from surgery. AF is also more likely to have adverse effects in patients with significant LVH.

   ii. If a patient fails to convert to normal sinus rhythm with medications within 48 hours, one strategy is to perform cardioversion to avoid the necessity for anticoagulation. The administration of amiodarone may increase the likelihood of successful cardioversion.[375] If the patient is recurrently going in and out of AF, it will most likely occur again, so cardioversion is probably not worthwhile. If AF has been present or recurrent for more than 48 hours and the patient has not been anticoagulated, a preliminary TEE must be performed to rule out LA thrombus before performing cardioversion.[376,377] The decision to prescribe anticoagulation for one month after delayed cardioversion may be considered, because de novo thrombus may form due to mechanical atrial inactivity after electrical cardioversion.[378]

   iii. If the patient cannot be converted pharmacologically or electrically, anticoagulation should be given for three weeks and then elective cardioversion attempted. If successful, anticoagulation is continued for an additional four weeks.

b. **Rapid atrial overdrive pacing** should be attempted to convert atrial flutter (see Figure 11.20 and page 605 for technique of rapid atrial pacing). It is usually successful in converting only type I flutter (atrial rate of less than 350/min). Several medications, such as propafenone and ibutilide, increase the efficacy of rapid atrial pacing by prolonging the atrial flutter cycle length.[379,380]

Table 11.15 • Management Protocols for Atrial Fibrillation/Flutter

1. Prophylaxis
   a. Magnesium sulfate 2 g IV after CPB and on first postoperative morning
   b. β-blocker
      - Metoprolol 12.5–50 mg PO (per NG tube) bid starting eight hours after surgery
      - Carvedilol 3.125–12.5 mg PO bid
   c. Alternatives
      - Amiodarone started either PO preoperatively or IV the day of surgery
      - Ranolazine 1 g preoperatively followed by 1 g bid × 7 days
      - Sotalol 80 mg PO bid
      - Dual-site atrial pacing
2. Treatment
   a. Cardioversion with 50–100 joules if unstable
   b. Rapid atrial pace if atrial flutter
   c. Increase prophylactic oral β-blocker dose if hemodynamically stable (heart rate <100)
   d. Rate control if heart rate >100
      - IV **metoprolol** 5 mg IV q5 min × 3 doses
      - IV **amiodarone**: give initial bolus or rebolus if received prior dosing; 150 mg over 30 min, followed by an infusion of 1 mg/min × 6 h, then 0.5 mg/min × 18 h, then 400 mg orally bid
      - IV **diltiazem** 0.25 mg/kg IV over two minutes, followed 15 minutes later by 0.35 mg/kg over two minutes, followed by a continuous infusion of 10–15 mg/h, if necessary
   e. Conversion to sinus rhythm and anticoagulation
      - Magnesium sulfate 2 g IV
      - Option #1: Amiodarone in the dose noted above
         → If successful, continue amiodarone for 1–4 weeks
         → If unsuccessful, consider cardioversion at 36–48 hours without heparin or subsequently on heparin; consider TEE to rule out LA thrombus
         → If unsuccessful, continue anticoagulation and β-blockers, but stop amiodarone
      - Option #2: heparin/warfarin or NOAC after 48 hours; await spontaneous conversion on β-blockers and discharge home in either SR or AF
      - Option #3: consider alternative pharmacologic management if cardioversion is not attempted or is unsuccessful; anticoagulation after 48 hours
         ○ **Sotalol** 80 mg q4h × 4 doses, then 80 mg bid and stop other β-blockers
         ○ **Propafenone** 1 mg/kg IV over two minutes, followed 10 minutes later by another 1 mg/kg dose; if IV not available, give one oral dose of 600 mg
         ○ **Ibutilide** 1 mg infusion over 10 minutes (0.01 mg/kg if <60 kg) with a second infusion 10 minutes later
         ○ **Dofetilide** 500 μg PO bid

c. **Rate control** can be achieved most readily with one of the rapid-acting IV medications. Once the rate has been controlled, the IV medications can be converted to oral ones. One study showed that 80% of patients who received only "rate control" drugs, such as β-blockers and CCBs, converted to sinus rhythm within 24 hours, suggesting either some conversion efficacy or possibly spontaneous conversion.[373] It is not uncommon to require use of multiple medications to achieve rate control and pharmacologic conversion.

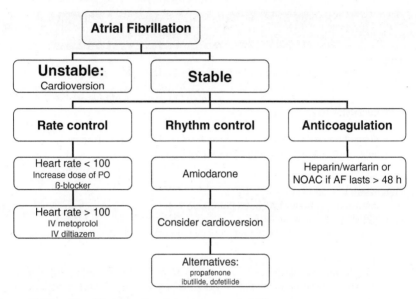

Figure 11.33 • Simplified algorithm for management of AF.

i. **ß-blockers** are very effective in achieving rate control and have the advantage of converting about 50% of patients to sinus rhythm (whether considered spontaneous or not). If an oral β-blocker has already been given, it can be supplemented by an IV dose if the ventricular response is rapid. If the patient has a relatively slow heart rate (whether already receiving a β-blocker or not) and then develops AF, amiodarone or diltiazem is a better selection to avoid the bradycardia that may occur after conversion.

- **Metoprolol** is the preferred β-blocker in that it can be given in the ICU or on the postoperative floor. It is a negative inotrope, so it must be used cautiously in patients with significantly compromised LV function or hypotension. For fairly rapid rates (>100 bpm), it is given in 2.5–5 mg IV increments q5 min up to a total dose of 15 mg. The onset of action is 2–3 minutes with a peak effect noted at 20 minutes. The duration of action is approximately five hours. Slower rates (<100 bpm) can be managed with increasing doses of oral metoprolol.

- **Esmolol** can be used in the operating room or ICU setting with arterial line monitoring, but it is a very dangerous drug due to its tendency to produce hypotension. It has a rapid onset of action of two minutes with rapid reversal of effect in 10–20 minutes. Thus, it may be safer to use than longer-acting drugs in the immediate perioperative period in case adverse effects develop, such as bronchospasm, conduction disturbances, excessive bradycardia, or LV dysfunction. The dose is 0.125–0.5 mg/kg IV over one minute, followed by an infusion of 50–200 μg/kg/min.[381]

ii. **Amiodarone** is effective in reducing the ventricular response to AF due to its multiple mechanisms of action (β-blockade, class III effects), but the rapidity and degree of slowing is less than with the β-blockers and CCBs. It is especially useful in the patient with borderline hemodynamics and more compromised LV function because it lacks negative inotropic effects. Thus, it can be recommended as a first-line therapy if the ventricular response is not excessively rapid or β-blockers and CCBs are contraindicated; otherwise, it should be added after rate control has been achieved, primarily in an attempt to achieve conversion to sinus rhythm.

iii. **Diltiazem** is an excellent alternative for patients with rapid AF and mildly to moderately compromised LV function in that it is a fairly weak negative inotrope. It must be used cautiously in hypotensive patients because of its vasodilatory effects, but blood pressure commonly improves with rate control. Concomitant use of an α-agent may be helpful if the blood pressure remains marginal. Diltiazem is also preferable to ß-blockers to control very rapid ventricular rates if the antecedent sinus mechanism was slow. It is less effective in slowing the ventricular response to atrial flutter and it is also less effective than β-blockers and amiodarone in converting AF back to sinus rhythm.

- **Dosage.** It is given in a dose of 0.25 mg/kg IV over two minutes, followed 15 minutes later by 0.35 mg/kg over two minutes, followed by a continuous infusion of 10–15 mg/h, if necessary. Heart rate response is noted in about three minutes with a peak effect within seven minutes. The reduction in heart rate lasts 1–3 hours after a bolus dose. The median duration of action is seven hours after a 24-hour continuous infusion.

- **Note:** caution must be used when administering any IV CCB concomitantly with an IV β-blocker because of the risk of inducing complete AV block. Availability of functional pacing wires is essential.

d. **Anticoagulation.** Heparinization should be considered for patients with recurrent or persistent AF to minimize the risk of stroke from embolization of LA thrombus. The risk : benefit ratio of initiating anticoagulation has to be individualized for every patient, balancing the risk of stroke with the risk of mediastinal bleeding. Understandably, guidelines have provided inconsistent information as to when anticoagulation should be started and how aggressive to be in achieving a therapeutic level of anticoagulation (such as starting warfarin without concomitant heparin).[382,383] One report suggested that transient self-limited postoperative AF is not a high-risk situation, and aggressive anticoagulation was not warranted.[384] However, another study found that AF preceded the occurrence of stroke in 36% of patients at a mean time of only 21.3 hours.[385] Furthermore, an echo study found that 14% of patients developed thrombus and 39% had spontaneous echo contrast in the left atrium within three days of the development of AF.[386]

i. It is generally recommended that anticoagulation should be initiated after 48 hours of persistent or intermittent AF.[313] If AF develops within the first few days of surgery, the risk of bleeding may supersede concerns about the risk of stroke. Use of the CHA$_2$DS$_2$-VASc score to assess the risk of stroke and the HAS-BLED score (see Appendices 10A and 10B) to predict the risk of bleeding might be of some value in deciding when to initiate anticoagulation and whether to continue it, but neither one has been evaluated in postoperative cardiac surgical patients.[387] If the patient is to receive warfarin (patients with mechanical valves), heparinization should be initiated. Otherwise, it is not unreasonable to select a NOAC, which can provide adequate thromboprophylaxis from the outset and may be continued after discharge. A strategy of early cardioversion may avert the need for anticoagulation. However, anticoagulation is essential before later cardioversion to reduce the risk of thromboembolism. Alternatively, a TEE can be performed to rule out LA appendage thrombus prior to attempting cardioversion.

ii. If the patient remains in AF and is to be discharged on warfarin rather than a NOAC, bridging with low-molecular-weight heparin should be considered in patients at high risk (older patients, low EF, valve surgery).

iii. Whether continuation of anticoagulation is warranted for the patient who converts back to sinus rhythm after several days is controversial. One rationale would be that it provides protection against stroke if the patient develops recurrent AF after discharge, which in one study was noted in nearly 30% of patients.[314] It is not unreasonable to utilize the CHA_2DS_2-VASc score in making that determination, although this has not been validated for such patients.

e. **Conversion to sinus rhythm.** Conversion to sinus rhythm is fairly common with the use of β-blockers or amiodarone and, as noted, nearly 80% of patients receiving either β-blockers or CCBs, but not given type I or III anti-arrhythmics, will convert back to sinus rhythm without additional medications.[373] Nonetheless, numerous medications can be used to achieve pharmacologic conversion. However, if a patient cannot be converted pharmacologically, a strategy of anticoagulation, rate control, and subsequent cardioversion is a viable and cost-effective alternative strategy.

i. **Magnesium sulfate** 2 g IV over 15 minutes is a benign and relatively effective means of converting patients back to sinus rhythm, with a conversion rate of 60% within four hours in one study.[388]

ii. **β-blockers** are effective for both rate control and conversion, more so than diltiazem.[381] The dosage of the prophylactic dose can be increased if the patient's blood pressure and heart rate are acceptable. Substitution of sotalol (80 mg bid) for the selective β-blockers may be considered, because it is slightly more successful in producing conversion. However, many patients cannot tolerate sotalol because of bradycardia or hypotension.

iii. **Amiodarone** is probably the most effective drug for conversion of AF and produces adequate rate control, although not as promptly or as effectively as β-blockers. Because it lacks other significant cardiac effects, it has an excellent safety profile. Hypotension is usually seen only with rapid IV infusion, and QTc prolongation, although common, is usually not accompanied by a proarrhythmic effect. Note that the QT interval adjusted for heart rate (QTc) is normally <450–470 ms. For rapid effect, amiodarone is given with the standard IV load (150 mg IV over 15–30 minutes, followed by a 60 mg/h infusion × 6 hours, then 30 mg/h × 18 hours), followed by an oral taper (400 mg bid for 1 week, 400 mg qd × 1 week,

200 mg qd × 2 weeks). If AF develops despite the use of prophylactic amiodarone, an additional 150 mg bolus can be given over 30 minutes. Alternatively, an oral load of 400 mg tid × 1 week may be given and then reduced to 200 mg/day.

iv. The type IC and other type III antiarrhythmics have been successful in converting 50–70% of patients with recent-onset AF back to sinus rhythm. They generally cause less hypotension than amiodarone and produce more rapid conversion.

- **Propafenone** (class IC) is effective in slowing the ventricular response and in rapidly converting patients to sinus rhythm within a few hours. Because it is a negative inotrope, it is contraindicated in the presence of LV dysfunction. Comparative studies reported equivalent efficacy to amiodarone in converting patients back to SR, but with more rapid conversion.[389–391] Similar conversion rates have been noted with IV and oral dosing, although conversion takes longer with oral dosing.[392] The IV dose is 1–2 mg/kg IV over 15 minutes, followed 10 minutes later by another 1 mg/kg dose. The oral dose is 600 mg given once. IV propafenone is not available in the USA.

- **Ibutilide** (class III) is an effective medication for conversion of AF and especially atrial flutter.[393] It is given as a 1 mg infusion over 10 minutes (0.01 mg/kg if <60 kg) with a second infusion 10 minutes later, if necessary. Most patients will convert within one hour. Because of the proarrhythmic risk (VT and torsades), careful monitoring is required, and the infusion should be stopped as soon as the arrhythmia has terminated, VT occurs, or there is marked prolongation of the QT interval. Although safe in patients with moderately impaired LV function, it is best avoided in patients with very low EFs. In comparative studies, ibutilide was found to be just as effective as amiodarone in converting AF/flutter to sinus rhythm.[394]

- **Dofetilide** (class III) has no negative inotropic effects and is beneficial when there are contraindications to class I drugs (i.e. LV dysfunction) or β-blockers (i.e. bradycardia and COPD). It is usually given in a dose of 500 μg PO bid. One study using IV dofetilide (up to 8 μg/kg over 15 minutes) found that it was more successful in converting atrial flutter (70%) than fibrillation (30%) within one hour.[395] It also causes QT prolongation and is proarrhythmic. The dosage must be adjusted by creatinine clearance and the baseline QTc. One study showed that the addition of magnesium did not affect dofetilide conversion of AF, but did double the efficacy of electrical cardioversion.[396] IV dofetilide is not approved for use in the USA.

- **Flecainide** (class IC) is effective in converting AF to sinus rhythm, and in one study was found to be more effective than IV propafenone or amiodarone.[391] Although it is contraindicated in patients with structural heart disease, it is not unreasonable to consider in patients who are completely revascularized if other drugs are ineffective.

v. **Vernakalant** (class III) is an atrial-selective potassium- and sodium-channel blocking agent which has been shown to convert about 50% of patients with new-onset postoperative AF to sinus rhythm at a median time of just over 10 minutes. The dosage is 3 mg/kg infused over 10 minutes with a subsequent 2 mg/kg infusion over 10 minutes if AF is still present after 15 minutes. The drug received approval by the European Union in September 2010, but was not approved for use in the USA as of mid-2020.[397–400]

vi. **Low-energy internal cardioversion** using epicardial defibrillation wires sewn to the left and right atria at the time of surgery is 90% successful in restoring sinus rhythm.[401]

H. Other supraventricular tachycardias (SVTs)

1. This designation refers to a tachycardia of sudden onset that arises either in the atrium (paroxysmal atrial tachycardia, PAT) or in the AV nodal region (atrioventricular nodal reentrant tachycardia, AVNRT), or uses the AV node as an integral part of the reentrant circuit (atrioventricular reentrant tachycardia, AVRT). These rhythms usually occur at a rate of 150–250/min and are uncommon after cardiac surgery. PAT with AV block may be associated with ischemic heart disease and commonly results from digoxin toxicity. As with any arrhythmia causing a rapid ventricular response, immediate treatment is indicated because of potential adverse effects on myocardial metabolism and function.

2. **Diagnosis.** Differentiation among sinus tachycardia, PAT, AVNRT, AVRT, and atrial flutter with 2:1 block may require examination of an AEG (Figure 11.34). Carotid sinus massage is often recommended as a diagnostic modality to differentiate among various arrhythmias by slowing the ventricular response to atrial tachyarrhythmias. However, it must be used cautiously in patients with coronary artery disease, not only because it may precipitate asystole, but because it may produce an embolic stroke in patients with coexistent carotid artery disease.

3. **Treatment**[402]

   a. Rapid atrial overdrive pacing may capture the atrium and cause reversion to sinus rhythm.

   b. Cardioversion should be considered if there is evidence of hemodynamic compromise.

   c. Vagal stimulation will often break a reentrant rhythm involving the AV node. Carotid sinus massage must be used cautiously as noted above.

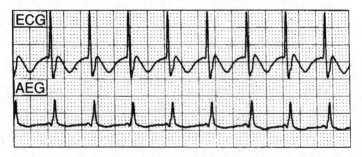

Figure 11.34 • AV junctional tachycardia at a rate of about 140 bpm recorded in simultaneous monitor and bipolar AEGs. Note the nearly simultaneous occurrence of retrograde atrial activation in the AEG and the antegrade ventricular activation in the monitor lead.

d. Adenosine produces transient high-grade AV block and is successful in terminating SVT caused by AVNRT.[403] It is given as a 6 mg rapid IV injection via a central line followed by a saline flush. A repeat dose of 12 mg may be given two minutes later. The half-life of adenosine is only 10 seconds. Adenosine can help distinguish AVRT and AVNRT, in which it terminates the circuit, from atrial flutter or fibrillation, in which it transiently slows AV conduction and the ventricular rate.

e. Medications used for AVNRT that slow SA node and AV conduction include:

- Verapamil 5–10 mg (0.075–0.15 mg/kg) IV push over two minutes, followed 30 minutes later by an additional 10 mg (0.15 mg/kg), then start an infusion of 5 μg/kg/min.

- Diltiazem given in standard doses (0.25 mg/kg IV over two minutes, followed 15 minutes later by 0.35 mg/kg, then an infusion of 10–15 mg/min if necessary) is effective in converting AVNRT to sinus rhythm in about 90% of patients.[404] The dose usually given is 20 mg IV, followed by a 10 mg/min infusion.

- Metoprolol 5 mg q5 min to a total dose of 15–25 mg

f. PAT with block is usually associated with digoxin toxicity and treatment should be provided accordingly:

- Digoxin should be withheld and a digoxin level obtained

- Administration of potassium chloride (KCl)

- Digibind (digoxin immune Fab [ovine]) starting at a dose of 400 mg (10 vials) over 30 minutes if severe digoxin toxicity

- Phenytoin (Dilantin) 250 mg IV over five minutes

I. **AV junctional rhythm and nonparoxysmal AV junctional tachycardia**[402]

1. An AV junctional rhythm occurs when junctional tissue has a faster intrinsic rate than the sinus node. This generally occurs at a rate of less than 60 bpm and is termed a junctional escape rhythm.

2. Nonparoxysmal AV junctional tachycardia occurs at a rate of 70–130/min and usually results from enhanced automaticity in the bundle of His or from triggered activity. In the postoperative patient, this rhythm may reflect digitalis toxicity, pericarditis, or an inferior infarction. Its presence may be suggested by a regularized ventricular rate in a patient with underlying AF and can be confirmed with an AEG.

3. As with any nonatrial rhythm, cardiac output is diminished by lack of synchronous atrial and ventricular contractions.

4. **Diagnosis.** See Figures 11.34 and 11.35. The focus may be localized by the relationship of the P wave to the QRS on a surface ECG (short PR interval if high-nodal, invisible P wave if mid-nodal, and P wave following the QRS if low-nodal). The P–QRS relationship is more evident on an AEG.

5. **Treatment**

a. Slow junctional rhythm (junctional escape rhythm)

i. Atrial pacing if AV conduction is normal.

ii. AV pacing if AV conduction is depressed.

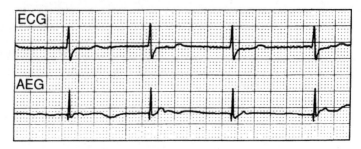

Figure 11.35 • Slow junctional rhythm at a rate of 54 bpm. Note the simultaneous occurrence of atrial and ventricular activation.

      iii. Use of a vasoactive drug with chronotropic β_1 action to stimulate the sinus mechanism; any drug the patient is receiving that might slow the sinus mechanism should be stopped.

   b. Nonparoxysmal junctional tachycardia[402]

      i. Overdrive pacing at a faster rate may establish AV synchrony.

      ii. If the patient is receiving digoxin, it should be stopped. Severe digoxin toxicity may be treated with digoxin immune fab (ovine) (Digibind). Use of potassium, lidocaine, phenytoin, or a β-blocker may be helpful.

      iii. If the patient is not on digoxin, a β-blocker or CCB (diltiazem or verapamil) can be considered to slow the junctional focus (class IIa indication), with use of atrial or AV pacing to establish AV synchrony. Flecainide or propafenone are helpful as well (class IIb indication), but both are rarely used after surgery since they are negative inotropes and contraindicated in patients with LV dysfunction.

J. Premature ventricular complexes (PVCs)

   1. Despite complete revascularization with good myocardial protection, the occurrence of PVCs after surgery is quite common. One study, in fact, identified PVCs and couplets in 100 and 82% of postoperative patients, respectively, but they were of relative insignificance as they rarely led to sustained ventricular tachyarrhythmias.[405]

   2. PVCs commonly reflect transient perioperative phenomena, such as augmented adrenergic tone or increased levels of catecholamines (endogenous or exogenous), inflammation and oxidative stress, myocardial stretch (as they are more common in patients with any degree of mitral regurgitation), irritation from a Swan-Ganz catheter or endotracheal tube, abnormal acid–base status, or hypoxemia. Thus, most PVCs are self-limited, benign, and not predictive of more serious or life-threatening arrhythmias. Ventricular ectopy is also fairly common preoperatively in the postinfarction patient and may persist after surgery, although ischemia-induced ectopy may be improved.

   3. Nonetheless, PVCs developing de novo may also reflect poor intraoperative myocardial protection or myocardial ischemia or infarction, and may herald

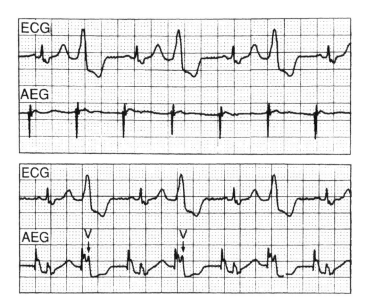

Figure 11.36 • Premature ventricular complexes (ventricular bigeminy) recorded simultaneously from monitor lead II and bipolar (upper) and unipolar (lower) AEGs. Note the wide QRS complex of unifocal morphology representing the PVC on the ECG. The bipolar AEG shows that the interval between atrial complexes is maintained despite the PVCs. The unipolar tracing shows that the PVC directly follows the sinus beat but leaves the ventricle refractory to the following beat, producing a full compensatory pause. V, premature ventricular complex.

malignant ventricular arrhythmias. Therefore, some surgical groups believe that even occasional PVCs should never be ignored in the early postoperative period. During the first 24 hours after surgery, when a multitude of cardiac and noncardiac precipitating factors may be present, it is of potential benefit and little risk to treat any ventricular ectopy.

4. **Diagnosis.** See Figure 11.36.

5. **Treatment**

   a. Correct the serum potassium with an intravenous KCl infusion at a rate up to 10–20 mEq/h through a central line. Some patients require potassium levels between 4.5 and 5.0 mEq/L to eliminate ventricular ectopy.

   b. Atrial pace at a rate exceeding the current sinus rate (overdrive pacing) unless tachycardia is present.

   c. Magnesium sulfate (2 g in 100 mL IV) administered at the termination of CPB has been shown to reduce the incidence of ventricular ectopy.[406]

   d. In patients with impaired LV function, recent infarction, or ongoing ischemia, PVCs are more likely to lead to VT or VF, although both are still uncommon. Nonetheless, in these and potentially all patients, it is not unreasonable to pharmacologically suppress ventricular ectopy. Commonly used drugs include:

    i. Lidocaine 1 mg/kg with 1–2 repeat doses of 0.5 mg/kg 10 minutes apart. A continuous infusion of 1–2 mg/min of a 1 g/250 mL mix should be started and continued for 12–24 hours. Do not exceed 4 mg/min to avoid seizure activity. Consider the patient's weight, hepatic function, and any underlying congestive heart failure when calculating a maximum dose. Several studies have shown about a 50% reduction in PVCs with less VT/VF with a strategy of prophylactic lidocaine, albeit with little evidence that this influences outcomes.[407,408] Another study showed that lidocaine may reduce myocardial injury in patients undergoing OPCAB.[409] Note that lidocaine is the major component of del Nido cardioplegia, which does provide excellent myocardial protection during surgery.

    ii. Amiodarone 150 mg IV load over 15 minutes, followed by a 60 mg/h infusion × 6 hours, then 30 mg/h × 18 hours. Control of ventricular ectopy is an added benefit when amiodarone is used prophylactically to prevent AF.

K. Ventricular tachycardia (VT) and ventricular fibrillation (VF)

  1. Etiology

    a. VT/VF occur postoperatively in about 1–3% of patients undergoing open-heart surgery and carry a mortality rate of about 20–30%.[410–412] Risk factors include prior infarction, an EF <40%, NYHA class III–IV, unstable angina, pulmonary and systemic hypertension, long pump times, low cardiac output syndromes, use of an IABP, and when bypass grafts are placed to infarct zones or noncollateralized occluded vessels, especially the left anterior descending artery. One study of patients undergoing CABG with an EF <50% (20% of whom had concomitant procedures) reported a much higher incidence of VT/VF of 15%, but a lower mortality rate of 7.6%. In addition to LV dilatation and remodeling following an infarction, this study reported that chronic kidney disease, an EF <30% and not being on a preoperative β-blocker increased the risk of VT/VF.[413]

    b. Ventricular tachyarrhythmias result from disorders of impulse formation or propagation. When they are present preoperatively on the basis of ischemia, resolution may be anticipated with revascularization of the ischemic zones. However, reperfusion of zones of ischemia or infarction can trigger de novo malignant ventricular arrhythmias. Potential triggers include residual ischemia or development of a PMI secondary to incomplete revascularization, anastomotic problems, or acute graft closure. Elevated levels of catecholamines and autonomic imbalance early in the postoperative periods may be contributory.

      i. Nonsustained ventricular tachycardia (NSVT) (VT lasting less than 30 seconds) may be encountered for reasons similar to those of PVCs and may occur in patients with normal or abnormal ventricular function.

      ii. Sustained monomorphic VT (VT lasting over 30 seconds) is usually noted in patients with a previous MI and depressed LV function, often with formation of a left ventricular aneurysm. The border zone between scar and viable tissue provides the electrophysiologic substrate for a reentry mechanism that passes through myocyte bands surviving within the infarct.[414–416]

iii. Sustained polymorphic VT with a normal QT interval is usually caused by increased dispersion of repolarization in areas of reperfused ischemia or infarction. Triggered activity in the form of delayed afterdepolarizations and occasionally enhanced automaticity are the mechanisms involved. Polymorphic VT may be facilitated by perioperative phenomena such as ischemia, hemodynamic instability, use of catecholamines or intrinsic sympathetic activity, withdrawal of β-blockers, and other metabolic problems. VF may be triggered by an acute ischemic insult.

iv. Polymorphic VT with QT prolongation is called **torsades de pointes**. The mechanism involves early afterdepolarizations, which is a form of triggered activity. It may complicate the use of type IA and III antiarrhythmic agents, especially if hypokalemia is present. Other medications that can contribute to torsades are metoclopramide, droperidol (for nausea), and high-dose haloperidol (>35 mg/day) used for agitation in the ICU.[417]

c. If the patient has a VVI or DDD pacemaker, the use of electrocautery during surgery can inactivate the sensing circuit, converting it to the VOO mode. This may result in bizarre-appearing arrhythmias and may trigger VF. These pacemakers must be evaluated upon arrival in the ICU and reprogrammed if necessary.[418]

2. **Diagnosis.** See Figures 11.37–11.40. An arrhythmia commonly confused with VT is AF with a rate-dependent conduction block (aberrancy) that produces a wide QRS complex. This should be distinguished by its irregularity, although it may be difficult to detect at fast heart rates.

3. **Evaluation and treatment** depend on the status of LV function, the nature of the arrhythmia (nonsustained vs. sustained, monomorphic vs. polymorphic VT), and whether the VT is inducible.[419]

a. Any potential triggering factors should be identified and managed. These include acid–base and electrolyte abnormalities, intracardiac catheters, myocardial ischemia or infarction, HF, and potentially proarrhythmic medications.

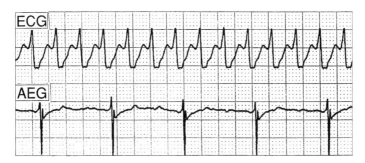

Figure 11.37 • Ventricular tachycardia recorded simultaneously in lead II and a bipolar AEG. There is dissociation between the sinus tachycardia at a rate of 72 bpm noted in the AEG and the wide complex ventricular tachycardia occurring at a rate of 210 bpm noted in the monitor lead.

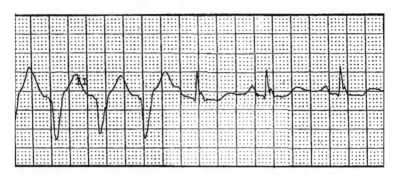

Figure 11.38 • Nonsustained ventricular tachycardia at a rate exceeding 130 bpm that spontaneously reverted to a sinus mechanism at a rate of 75 bpm.

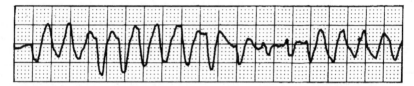

Figure 11.39 • Ventricular fibrillation on monitor lead.

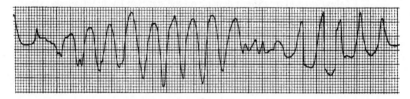

Figure 11.40 • Torsades de pointes on monitor lead. Note how the QRS complex appears to twist around the isoelectric baseline. Torsades usually has a pause-dependent onset initiated by a premature ventricular complex discharging at the end of a T wave, usually associated with a long QT interval.

    b. NSVT with preserved LV function has a favorable prognosis. Although lidocaine or amiodarone may be considered when this rhythm develops, β-blockers alone should suffice if evaluation reveals an EF >35%.[420]

    c. NSVT in patients with depressed LV function may be associated with a poor prognosis without treatment. Extrapolating from the MADIT and MUSTT trials, an electrophysiology study and ICD placement should be considered if NSVT develops after surgery in these patients.

    d. Sustained VT occurring without hemodynamic compromise can be managed by:

    i. Ventricular overdrive pacing to terminate the reentry circuit

    ii. Cardioversion if VT persists or hemodynamic compromise develops

    iii. Amiodarone 150 mg over 15 minutes, then 1 mg/min (60 mg/h) × 6 hours, then 0.5 mg/min (30 mg/h) × 18 hours

e. Any patient developing **VF or sustained VT that is pulseless or associated with hemodynamic instability** requires immediate defibrillation per ACLS protocol (see pages 591–595). If unsuccessful, emergency resternotomy and open-chest massage are indicated.

f. Electrophysiologic evaluation is essential for patients with sustained VT and impaired ventricular function to improve the long-term prognosis. In general, ICD placement can be justified in any patient with an EF <35%, using a LifeVest device upon hospital discharge if one wants to await the 90-day moratorium after revascularization recommended in the ICD trials.[419]

    i. **Monomorphic VT** is inducible in 80% of patients with spontaneous VT and is usually associated with a remote infarct and an arrhythmogenic substrate causing a reentry mechanism. This usually requires antiarrhythmic therapy (usually amiodarone) as well as the placement of an ICD.

    ii. **Polymorphic VT** is usually associated with an MI, ischemia, or reperfusion, and should prompt further evaluation for ongoing ischemia. This may involve coronary arteriography to identify potential graft occlusion or an anastomotic stenosis, which may be a correctable problem. It is often transient and therapy must be individualized.

g. **Torsades de pointes**[421]

    i. Cardiovert immediately for hemodynamic compromise or prolonged episodes (usually because VF is suspected to be present).

    ii. Administer potassium chloride, unless hyperkalemia is present, to shorten the QT interval.

    iii. Ventricular pace at 90–100 beats/min or start an isoproterenol infusion at 1–4 µg/min.[422] This will shorten the action potential to prevent early afterdepolarizations and triggered activity.

    iv. Magnesium 1–2 g and β-blockers may eliminate triggered activity to prevent recurrence, but do not shorten the QT interval.

XIII. Antiarrhythmic Medications

A variety of medications are available for the control of supraventricular and ventricular arrhythmias. A basic understanding of their mechanism of action is critical to the appropriate selection of these drugs for the treatment of various arrhythmias, as noted in the preceding sections. In this section, drugs that may be used in patients undergoing cardiac surgery are presented. The reader is referred to any of the major cardiology textbooks or websites for more detailed information.

A. The Vaughan-Williams classification of antiarrhythmic medications has been updated and modified with further understanding of their mechanisms of action and the development of newer medications (Table 11.16).[423,424]

Table 11.16 • Modernized Classification of Antiarrhythmic Drugs

Class 0	**HCN channel blocker**	Ivabradine
Class I	**Na+ channel blockers**	
	Class IA	Procainamide Disopyramide
	Class IB	Lidocaine Mexiletine
	Class IC	Propafenone Flecainide
	Class ID	Ranolazine
Class II	**Autonomic inhibitors and activators**	
	Class IIA: Autonomic inhibitors (β-adrenergic blockers)	Metoprolol Atenolol Carvedilol
	Class IIB: β-adrenergic activators	Isoproterenol
	Class IIC: Muscarinic M2 receptor inhibitors	Atropine
	Class IID: Muscarinic M2 receptor activators	Digoxin
	Class IIE: Adenosine A1 receptor activators	Adenosine
Class III	**K+ channel blockers and openers**	
	Class IIIA: voltage dependent K+ channel blockers	
	Nonselective K+ channel blockers	Amiodarone Dronedarone
	Kv11.1 (HERG) channel-mediated rapid K+ current (I_{Kr}) blockers	Dofetilide Ibutilide Sotalol
	Kv1.5 channel-mediated, ultrarapid K+ current (I_{Kur}) blockers	Vernakalant
Class IV	**Calcium handling modulators**	
	Class IVA: surface membrane CCBs $Ca_v1.2$ and $Ca_v1.3$ channel-mediated L-type Ca^{2+} current (ICaL) blockers	Diltiazem Verapamil
	Class IVB: intracellular CCBs SR RyR2-Ca^{2+} channel blockers	Flecainide Propafenone

Reproduced with permission of Lei et al., *Circulation* 2018;138:1879–96.[424]

Table 11.17 • Electrophysiologic Properties of Commonly Used Antiarrhythmic Drugs

Property		Class 0	Class IA	Class IB	Class IC	Class II	Class III	Class IV
Automaticity								
SA node		↓	—	—	—	↓	↓	↓
Vent ectopic foci (Purkinje)		↓	↓	↓	↓	↓	—	—
Delayed Afterdepolarizations		—	—	↓	↓	↓	—	↓
Conduction								
Atria	CV	—	↓	—	↓	—	↓	—
	ERP	—	↑	—	↑	—	↑	—
AV node	CV	—	↓	—	↓	↓	↓	↓
	ERP	—	—	—	↑	↑	↑	↑
His-Purkinje	CV	—	↓	↓	↓	—	—	—
	ERP	—	↓	↑	↑	↑	—	—
Ventricle	CV	—	↓	↓	↓	—	—	—
	ERP	—	↑	↓	↑	—	↑	—

CV = conduction velocity; ERP = effective refractory period
Many antiarrhythmic medications have properties of several classes of drugs

B. Table 11.17 shows the effects of the various classes of antiarrhythmic drugs on automaticity, conduction velocity (CV), and the effective refractory period (ERP). Some medications have multiple properties (such as amiodarone and sotalol), so they may have additional electrophysiologic effects. The appropriate classes of antiarrhythmic drug that can be selected for the management of the common arrhythmias are as follows:

1. Alterations in automaticity
   a. Sinus tachycardia (sinus node): class 0, II, IV
   b. Ventricular ectopy (Purkinje and ventricular fibers): class IA, IB, IC, II, III
   c. Digoxin-toxic ectopy (delayed afterdepolarizations: class IB (phenytoin)
2. Alterations in conduction velocity and ERP
   a. Conversion of AF (atrium): class IA, IC, II, III. IV
   b. To slow the response to AF (AV node): class II, III, IV, digoxin
   c. Conversion of AVNRT or AVRT: class II, IV, digoxin
   d. Ventricular tachycardia (interrupt reentrant circuits in His-Purkinje fibers or ventricle): class IA, IB, III

C. **Note:** the clinical indications listed below for each of the antiarrhythmic medications are those for which there is documented efficacy. US Food and Drug Administration (FDA) approval has not necessarily been provided for each of these indications.

D. Drugs that may be used in cardiac surgery patients are listed below in order from class 0 to class IV drugs.

E. **Ivabradine:** class 0

1. Clinical indications: inappropriate sinus tachycardia; to slow the heart rate in ischemic heart disease if contraindications to ß-blockers

2. Dose: 2.5–5 mg PO bid

3. Metabolism: >50% hepatic (CYP3A4); contraindicated with use of a CYP3A4 inhibitor (diltiazem, verapamil)

4. Therapeutic level: unknown

5. Hemodynamic effects: none, unless related to a slower heart rate

6. Electrophysiologic effects and contraindications

   a. Direct inhibitory effect on the Na+–K+ inward pacemaker currents that slows the sinus node mechanism without any effect on contractility

   b. May increase risk of AF

   c. Contraindicated in acute decompensated heart failure, hypotension, sick sinus syndrome, SA block, complete heart block, significant bradycardia

7. Noncardiac side effects: sensation of bright lights, headache, dizziness

F. **Procainamide:** class IA

1. Clinical indications (used infrequently due to the superiority of amiodarone)

   a. Prevention/conversion of AF

   b. Suppression of premature atrial and ventricular complexes and sustained ventricular tachyarrhythmias

   c. WPW syndrome (slows conduction over accessory pathways)

2. Doses

   a. IV: 100 mg q5 min up to 1000 mg (never more than 50 mg/min), then a 2–4 mg/min drip (1 g/250 mL mix)

   b. PO procainamide is no longer available

3. Metabolism: hepatic to active metabolite N-acetylprocainamide (NAPA) and then excreted by the kidneys

4. Therapeutic level: 4–10 µg/mL of procainamide and 2–8 µg/mL of NAPA

5. Hemodynamic effects: decreases SVR, negative inotrope in high doses

6. Electrophysiologic effects

   a. Slows conduction and decreases automaticity and excitability of the atrium and ventricle

   b. Slows the atrial rate in atrial flutter, but vagolytic effects on AV conduction may increase the ventricular response to AF/flutter. Medications that prevent accelerated AV conduction must be given first.

      c. Evidence of toxicity

         i. QT prolongation and polymorphic VT

         ii. Myocardial depression

         iii. NAPA may accumulate in patients with heart and renal failure. It has a longer half-life than procainamide (7 h vs. 4 h) and can lead to cardiac toxicity, including early afterdepolarizations, triggered activity, and ventricular arrhythmias, including torsades de pointes.

         iv. Amiodarone increases procainamide levels, so doses have to be reduced by 20–33%, but preferentially, procainamide should not be used.

    7. Noncardiac side effects: GI (nausea, anorexia), CNS (insomnia, hallucinations, psychosis, depression), rash, drug fever, agranulocytosis, lupus-like syndrome with long-term use

G. Disopyramide: class IA

    1. Clinical indications

      a. Suppression of ventricular and supraventricular arrhythmias

      b. Termination and prevention of recurrence of AVNRT

      c. Prevention/conversion of AF

      d. WPW syndrome (slows conduction over accessory pathways)

    2. Dose: 100–200 mg PO q6h

    3. Metabolism: 65% renal, 35% hepatic

    4. Therapeutic level: 2–5 μg/mL

    5. Hemodynamic effects: strong negative inotrope (thus useful in patients with hypertrophic obstructive cardiomyopathy)

    6. Electrophysiologic effects

      a. Reduces ventricular automaticity, slows conduction in the AV node, and prolongs the action potential

      b. May cause torsades de pointes or other ventricular tachyarrhythmias associated with QT prolongation

    7. Noncardiac side effects: anticholinergic (urinary retention, constipation, blurred vision), nausea, dizziness, insomnia

H. Lidocaine: class IB

    1. Clinical indications: premature ventricular complexes and ventricular tachyarrhythmias

    2. Doses

      a. 1 mg/kg IV followed by a continuous infusion of 2–4 mg/min (1 g/250 mL mix); a dose of 0.5 mg/kg may be given 15 minutes later to achieve a stable plasma concentration.

      b. A rebolus of 0.5 mg/kg should be given to increase plasma levels if the infusion rate is increased.

    3. Metabolism: hepatic; half-life is 15 minutes after one dose and two hours with constant infusion (often longer with hepatic impairment)

4. Therapeutic level: 1–5 µg/mL

5. Hemodynamic effects: none in the absence of severe LV dysfunction

6. Electrophysiologic effects: benefits are derived from suppression of abnormal automaticity in ventricular fibers

7. Noncardiac side effects: CNS (dizziness, delirium, tremors, seizures), GI (nausea)

I. **Propafenone:** class IC

1. Clinical indication: conversion of AF

2. Doses

   a. PO: 600 mg load, then 150–300 mg q8h (intermediate release) or 225–425 mg bid (extended-release)

   b. IV: 1 mg/kg IV over two minutes, followed 10 minutes later by another 1 mg/kg dose (used for conversion of AF) (not approved for use in the USA in 2020)

3. Metabolism: hepatic

4. Therapeutic level: 0.2–3.0 µg/mL

5. Hemodynamic effects: negative inotrope and generally contraindicated in patients with structural heart disease and LV dysfunction

6. Electrophysiologic effects

   a. Slows conduction in the atria (prolongs PR interval), AV node (can produce AV block), His-Purkinje system, and ventricle (widens the QRS), and prolongs atrial refractoriness

   b. Has some β-blocker activity and can produce AV block and sinus node depression

   c. Proarrhythmic effects are noted in 5% of patients

   d. Doubles the digoxin level; warfarin dose should be decreased

7. Noncardiac side effects are noted in 15% of patients: CNS (dizziness, diplopia), unusual taste, asthma, GI upset

J. **Flecainide:** class IC

1. Clinical indications: prevention/treatment of AF; maintenance of sinus rhythm

2. Doses:

   a. Loading dose: 200–300 mg PO

   b. Maintenance dose: 50–150 mg PO bid

3. Metabolism: primarily renal (reduce dose by 50% if GFR <50 mL/min) with some hepatic elimination; elimination half-life 20 hours

4. Therapeutic level: 0.2–1.0 µg/mL

5. Hemodynamic effects: negative inotrope that can exacerbate and increase mortality in HF; generally contraindicated with structural heart disease, although could be used after revascularization with normal LV function

6. Electrophysiologic effects

  a. Prolongs PR and QRS intervals; QT prolongation; prolongs AV conduction; can slow the atrial flutter rate but cause 1:1 AV conduction, necessitating use of an AV nodal blocking drug (ß-blocker, digoxin)

  b. Blocks inward sodium and potassium channels

  c. Proarrhythmic even without QT prolongation

  d. Although generally not recommended to use a β-blocker with flecainide to avoid bradycardia, its use with metoprolol in selected patients has been shown to reduce AF recurrence.[425]

7. Noncardiac side effects: dizziness, tremors, blurred vision, headache, shortness of breath, fatigue, nausea

K. **Ranolazine:** class ID

  1. Clinical indications: prevention/treatment of AF; primarily used in ischemic heart disease

  2. Dose: 500–1000 mg PO preoperatively, then 1 g PO bid × 7 days

  3. Metabolism: hepatic by the CYP3A enzyme; dosage should be reduced when drugs that inhibit CYP3A are used (diltiazem, verapamil)

  4. Therapeutic level: unknown

  5. Hemodynamic effects: reduces intracellular calcium levels and myocardial wall tension, reducing myocardial oxygen demand and reducing ischemia

  6. Electrophysiologic effects

    a. Blocks the inward sodium and potassium currents; this prevents calcium overload, which stabilizes membranes and reduces excitability; it also increases the atrial effective refractory period and atrial conduction velocity.[426]

    b. Slows the SA node, prolongs action potential duration, and prolongs the QT interval

  7. Noncardiac side effects: dizziness, constipation, nausea, headache; contraindicated with liver disease

L. **β-adrenergic blockers:** class IIA

  1. Clinical indications

    a. Prevention/treatment of postoperative of AF/flutter

    b. Sinus tachycardia

    c. Ventricular arrhythmias associated with digoxin toxicity, myocardial ischemia, or QT prolongation

    d. AVNRT and reciprocating tachycardias in WPW syndrome

  2. Doses

    a. Metoprolol (relative potency is 2.5:1 for IV:PO)

      i. IV: 5 mg q5 min for three doses

      ii. PO: 25–100 mg q12h

    b. Atenolol: 25–100 mg PO qd

    c. Esmolol: IV: 500 µg/kg load, then 50–200 µg/kg/min drip

3. Metabolism: hepatic (metoprolol), renal (atenolol), blood (esmolol)

4. Hemodynamic effects: negative inotropes (worsening of HF), hypotension

5. Electrophysiologic effects

   a. Reduces automaticity at all levels, slowing the heart rate

   b. Decreases AV conduction (increases AV node refractoriness) and can cause heart block

6. Noncardiac side effects: bronchospasm (less with the cardioselective β-blockers atenolol and metoprolol), fatigue, diarrhea, impotence, depression, claudication

M. **Adenosine:** class IIE

   1. Clinical indication: paroxysmal supraventricular tachycardias with AV nodal reentry (AVNRT or AVRT)

   2. Dose: 6 mg rapid IV injection through a peripheral line followed by a saline flush; a second dose of 12 mg may be given two minutes later if necessary.

   3. Metabolism: rapidly degrades in blood, with a half-life of less than 10 seconds

   4. Electrophysiologic effects: negative effects on SA and AV nodes; can produce asystole and transient high-grade AV block; the latter effect can unmask atrial activity to differentiate the causes of narrow and wide complex tachycardias.

   5. Side effects: flushing, dyspnea, or chest pressure of very brief duration

N. **Amiodarone:** class III

   1. Clinical indications

      a. Prevention/conversion of postoperative AF

      b. Pulseless VT/VF (first choice to facilitate defibrillation success)

      c. Sustained ventricular tachyarrhythmias

   2. Doses

      a. PO: 400 mg tid, weaned down to 200 mg qd over several weeks (onset of action takes several days); 10 g should be given before reducing to the lower dose.

      b. IV: 150 mg over 15–30 min (300 mg during cardiac arrest), then 1 mg/min × 6 h, 0.5 mg/min × 18 h, then 1 g/day. Onset of action occurs within several hours, but serum levels fall within 30 minutes after infusion is stopped. Repeat bolus doses of 150 mg can be given over 30 min for recurrent AF.

   3. Metabolism: hepatic (half-life of 58 days) and clinical effect dissipates after three months.

   4. Therapeutic level: 1.0–2.5 µg/mL

   5. Hemodynamic effects: β-blocker (class II); coronary and peripheral vasodilator

   6. Electrophysiologic effects

      a. Has class I, II, and IV properties as well

      b. Initial effects of IV infusion are prolongation of AV conduction and refractoriness, to some degree related to class II (β-blocking) and class IV (calcium channel blocking) effects. This accounts for its early benefit in slowing the ventricular response to AF. With the initial infusion, there is less effective prolongation of repolarization in the atria and ventricles. It also slows the sinus rate, so it may produce bradycardia and heart block.

   c. Prolongs the QT interval but rarely causes ventricular arrhythmias; lengthens the PR interval, and may increase the QRS duration

7. Reduces clearance (and therefore increases serum levels) of drugs metabolized by the liver. These include **digoxin, procainamide, and warfarin.** Doses of these medications should be reduced by about one-half. Due to the increased risk of rhabdomyolysis, no more than 20 mg of **simvastatin** should be given to patients on amiodarone.

8. Noncardiac side effects are noted in more than 50% of patients, especially during chronic therapy. Minor problems include corneal microdeposits, elevated liver function tests (LFTs), photosensitivity, and alteration in thyroid function.[427]

9. Baseline and follow-up LFTs and thyroid function tests should be performed. Peripheral neuropathy and myopathy may produce an unstable gait. The most serious complication is pulmonary toxicity, which is more common in patients on high-dose chronic amiodarone therapy, especially with abnormal chest x-rays or pulmonary function tests prior to surgery. Acute pulmonary toxicity, which probably represents a hypersensitivity reaction, can also occur but is rare.[339] Baseline PFTs are also recommended for any patient in whom amiodarone will be used for more than one month.

O. **Dofetilide:** class III

1. Clinical indications: conversion of AF/flutter

2. Dose: 125–500 µg PO bid (based on renal function and QT prolongation): first five doses must be given in hospital with an ECG obtained 2–3 hours after each dose to monitor for QT prolongation. An IV preparation has been used in numerous studies, but is not available in the USA.

3. Metabolism: 50% renal, 50% hepatic

4. Therapeutic level: unknown

5. Hemodynamic effects: no negative inotropic effects, so can be used with structural heart disease

6. Electrophysiologic effects

   a. Slightly decreases the sinus rate, but no effect on AV conduction

   b. Proarrhythmic effect from QT prolongation, so contraindicated if QT interval >440 ms (or if creatinine clearance <20 mL/min); torsades occurs in 4%

   c. Has drug interaction with verapamil, which contraindicates its use

   d. All class I or III antiarrhythmic medications should be stopped for three half-lives before it is given.

   e. Amiodarone must be stopped for three months (or a level <0.3 mg/L) before it is given.

P. **Sotalol:** class III

1. Clinical indications

   a. Prevention/treatment of postoperative AF

   b. Suppression of ventricular tachyarrhythmias

2. Doses
   a. 80–160 mg PO bid
   b. 75–150 mg IV bid (administered over five hours)
3. Metabolism: excreted unchanged in the urine (so give once daily if GFR <60 mL/min and contraindicated if GFR <40 mL/min)
4. Hemodynamic effects: causes bradycardia; negative inotropic effect can cause hypotension, fatigue, and HF.
5. Electrophysiologic effects
   a. Prolongs atrial and ventricular action potential and refractory periods (slows SA node, increases AV node refractoriness); QT prolongation
   b. Exhibits class II (β-blocking) and class III effects
   c. Produces torsades de pointes or proarrhythmic effects in about 4% of patients. Torsades de pointes is dose-related and predictable from the QT interval (avoid if QT >500 ms).
6. Noncardiac side effects: fatigue, dyspnea, dizziness, heart failure exacerbation, nausea, and vomiting

Q. **Ibutilide:** class III
1. Clinical indication: conversion of recent-onset AF/flutter
2. Dose: 1 mg IV over 10 minutes (0.01 mg/kg if <60 kg) with a second dose if no response
3. Metabolism: hepatic
4. Therapeutic level: unknown
5. Hemodynamic effects: no significant hemodynamic effects, but not recommended if severely depressed LV function
6. Electrophysiologic effects
   a. Increases refractoriness of atrium, AV node, and ventricle
   b. Dose-related prolongation of the QT interval (avoid if the QT interval exceeds 440 ms). QT prolongation may contribute to torsades de pointes, but sustained polymorphic VT may occur even in the absence of a prolonged QT interval.
   c. Monomorphic or polymorphic VT (sustained or nonsustained) is noted in about 10% of patients; careful monitoring in the ICU is essential for four hours after an administered dose (half-life is six hours) or until the QT interval has returned to baseline.
7. Noncardiac side effects: headache, nausea

R. **Vernakalant:** class III
1. Clinical indications: conversion of AF
2. Doses: 3 mg/kg infused over 10 minutes with a subsequent 2 mg/kg infusion over 10 minutes if AF is still present after 15 minutes. Not approved for use in the USA as of mid-2020.
3. Metabolism: hepatic > renal; half-life of 3–4 hours
4. Therapeutic level: unknown
5. Hemodynamic effects: none

6. Electrophysiologic effects

a. Blocks atrial sodium channels and the cardiac transient outward potassium current influencing atrial repolarization, such that it is beneficial at very fast heart rates.

b. May cause bradycardia, hypotension, torsades de pointes and other ventricular arrhythmias.

7. Noncardiac side effects: altered taste, sneezing, paresthesia, nausea and pruritus

S. **Calcium channel blockers** (verapamil and diltiazem): class IV

1. Clinical indications

a. Control rapid ventricular response to AF/flutter

b. Treat supraventricular tachycardias including AVNRT, reciprocating tachycardias of WPW syndrome (AVRT), and multifocal atrial tachycardia; contraindicated for AF in WPW syndrome

c. Ischemic ventricular ectopy

2. Doses

a. Diltiazem

i. IV: 0.25 mg/kg IV bolus over two minutes, with a repeat bolus of 0.35 mg/kg 15 minutes later; then a continuous infusion of 10–15 mg/h (100 mg/100 mL mix)

ii. PO: 30–90 mg q8h (or 180–360 mg qd of long-acting preparation)

iii. Conversion from IV to PO: (rate [mg/h] x 3 + 3) x 10 = PO dose in mg/day

b. Verapamil

i. 5–10 mg (0.075–0.15 mg/kg) IV push over two minutes, followed 30 minutes later by an additional 10 mg (0.15 mg/kg), then start an infusion of 2–5 µg/kg/min (120 mg/250 mL mix)

ii. PO: 80–160 mg q8h

3. Metabolism: hepatic

4. Therapeutic level: 0.1–0.15 µg/mL (verapamil)

5. Hemodynamic effects: negative inotropes and vasodilators (verapamil more than diltiazem); cause hypotension and can worsen HF

6. Electrophysiologic effects

a. Slows sinus rate, prolongs PR interval, slows AV conduction; can precipitate bradycardia, asystole, or heart block when used concomitantly with IV β-blockers.

b. Verapamil reduces clearance of digoxin and increases the digoxin level by about 35%.

7. Noncardiac side effects: GI (constipation, nausea), headache, dizziness, elevation in LFTs

T. **Digoxin**

1. Clinical indications

a. Slowing ventricular response to AF/flutter. Since it is much less effective than CCBs or β-blockers and has been shown to increase mortality, it no longer has much of a role in the postoperative cardiac surgical patient.[428]

b. Prevention of AVNRT

2. Doses
   a. IV: 0.5 mg, then 0.25 mg q4–6h to total dose of 1.0–1.25 mg, then 0.125 mg qd
   b. PO: 0.5 mg, then 0.25 mg q4–6h to total dose of 1.25 mg, then 0.25 mg qd (dosing without a load will take 7–10 days to reach a steady-state level).
      i. Maintenance dose depends on serum level and therapeutic effect.
      ii. Dose is 0.125 mg qd for patients in renal failure.
      iii. IV dose is two-thirds of the PO dose.
3. Metabolism: hepatic (but renal failure prolongs its half-life and decreases its distribution)
4. Therapeutic level: 1–2 ng/mL (drawn not less than six hours after an oral dose or four hours after an IV dose)
   a. Serum levels are increased by medications that reduce its clearance or volume of distribution; thus digoxin dosing should be reduced accordingly.
   b. **Levels are increased by amiodarone** (by 70–100%) and verapamil (by 35%)
5. Hemodynamic effects: slight inotropic effect, peripheral vasodilation
6. Electrophysiologic effects: enhances vagolytic activity which reduces sinus node automaticity (slows the heart rate) and prolongs AV conduction and refractoriness (controls ventricular response to AF)
7. Noncardiac side effects: GI (anorexia, nausea, vomiting), CNS (headache, fatigue, confusion, seizures), visual symptoms

U. **Comments on digoxin toxicity**[429]
   1. Digoxin is used primarily to slow the ventricular response to AF/flutter by virtue of its vagotonic effect (at low dose) and a direct effect (high dose) on the AV node. It is less effective than other medications in slowing the ventricular response to AF in the early postoperative period when a high adrenergic state is present. Thus, it is not the drug of choice for acute rate control. However, it can provide additional rate control, especially when AF is persistent.
   2. Aggressive digitalization for rapid AF is usually not successful in achieving rate control and can lead to digoxin toxicity for a number of reasons in the early postoperative period.
      a. There is increased sensitivity to digoxin related to augmented sympathetic tone, myocardial ischemia, electrolyte imbalance (hyper- or hypokalemia, hypercalcemia, hypomagnesemia), acid–base imbalance, or use of vasoactive or antiarrhythmic drugs (verapamil).
      b. Large doses need to be given to achieve effect because digoxin's vagotonic effects are offset by increased sympathetic tone. IV doses are usually given to provide 1.25 mg within the first 24 hours, but subsequent IV doses should be two-thirds of the oral doses to avoid toxicity.
      c. The volume of distribution is less in many elderly patients with decreased lean body mass.
      d. Hypokalemia from postoperative diuresis and hypomagnesemia predispose to digoxin toxicity.

e. Renal excretion may be impaired in patients with chronic kidney disease. Elderly patients have reduced GFRs and excrete digoxin less efficiently.

3. Digoxin toxicity should be considered in any patient receiving digoxin who develops a change in rhythm. These include, in decreasing order of frequency:

   a. Premature ventricular complexes (multiform and bigeminy)

   b. Nonparoxysmal AV junctional tachycardia

   c. AV block: first-degree or Wenckebach second-degree block

   d. Paroxysmal atrial tachycardia with 2:1 block

   e. Ventricular tachycardia (especially bidirectional VT at a rate of 140–180 bpm)

   f. Sinus bradycardia or SA block

4. Digoxin toxicity in a patient with AF is usually manifested by:

   a. Slow ventricular response (<50 bpm)

   b. AV dissociation with AV junctional escape or accelerated junctional rhythm. Regularization of the ventricular rate in the presence of AF should always raise concern about the development of complete heart block with a junctional escape rhythm.

5. **Treatment**

   a. Bradyarrhythmias are treated by atrial, AV, or ventricular pacing, depending on the underlying atrial rhythm and the status of AV conduction. Atropine can be used, but isoproterenol should be avoided because it may induce malignant ventricular arrhythmias.

   b. Tachyarrhythmias

      i. Potassium chloride, except in the presence of high-grade AV block, because hyperkalemia can potentiate the depressant effect of digoxin on AV conduction.

      ii. Lidocaine in usual doses

      iii. Phenytoin (Dilantin), 100 mg IV every five minutes to a maximum of 1 g, then 100–200 mg PO q8h

   c. Digibind (digoxin immune Fab [Ovine]) 400 mg (10 vials) IV, which may be repeated after several hours, can be used for life-threatening digoxin toxicity.

6. Special concerns

   a. Digoxin toxicity decreases the threshold for postcardioversion malignant arrhythmias. This may be exacerbated when hypokalemia or hypercalcemia is present. Use of lidocaine, phenytoin, or lower energy levels should be considered.

   b. Dialysis is ineffective in removing digoxin. Its half-life is 36–48 hours.

References

1. Griffin MJ, Hines RL. Management of perioperative ventricular dysfunction. *J Cardiothorac Vasc Anesth* 2001;15:90–106.

2. Mebazaa A, Pitsis A, Ridiger A, et al. Clinical review: practical recommendations on the management of perioperative heart failure in cardiac surgery. *Crit Care* 2010;14:201.

3. Stephens RS, Whitman GJR. Postoperative critical care of the adult cardiac surgical patient: part I: routine postoperative care. *Crit Care Med* 2015;49:1477–97.

4. Carl M, Alms A, Braun J, et al. S3 guidelines for intensive care in cardiac surgery patients: hemodynamic monitoring and cardiocirculatory system. *Ger Med Sci* 2010;8:Doc12.

5. Hansen RM, Viquerat CE, Matthay MA, et al. Poor correlation between pulmonary arterial wedge pressure and left ventricular end-diastolic volume after coronary artery bypass surgery. *Anesthesiology* 1986;64:764–70.

6. St. André AC, Del Rossi A. Hemodynamic management of patients in the first 24 hours after cardiac surgery. *Crit Care Med* 2005;33:2082–93.

7. Buhre W, Weyland A, Schorn B, et al. Changes in central venous pressure and pulmonary capillary wedge pressure do not indicate changes in right and left heart volume in patients undergoing coronary artery bypass surgery. *Eur J Anaesthesiol* 1999;16:11–17.

8. Hoeft A, Schorn B, Weyland A, et al. Bedside assessment of intravascular volume status in patients undergoing coronary bypass surgery. *Anesthesiology* 1994;81:76–86.

9. Kramer A, Zygun D, Hawes H, Easton P, Ferland A. Pulse pressure variation predicts fluid responsiveness following coronary artery bypass surgery. *Chest* 2004;126:1563–8.

10. Li P, Qu LP, Qi D, et al. Significance of perioperative goal-directed hemodynamic approach in preventing postoperative complications in patients after cardiac surgery: a meta-analysis and systematic review. *Ann Med* 2017;49:343–51.

11. Kapoor PM, Kakani M, Chowdhury U, Choudhury M, Lakshmy R, Kiran U. Early goal-directed therapy in moderate to high risk cardiac surgery patients. *Ann Card Anaesth* 2008;11:27–34.

12. Goepfert MS, Reuter DA, Akyol D, Lamm P, Kilger E, Goetz AE. Goal-directed fluid management reduces vasopressor and catecholamine use in cardiac surgery patients. *Intensive Care Med* 2007; 33:96–103.

13. Giglio M, Dalfino L, Puntillo F, Rubino FG, Manucci M, Brienza N. Haemodynamic goal-directed therapy in cardiac and vascular surgery: a systematic review and meta-analysis. *Interact Cardiovasc Thorac Surg* 2012;15:878–87.

14. Osawa EA, Rhodes A, Landoni G, et al. Effect of perioperative goal-directed hemodynamic resuscitation therapy on outcomes following cardiac surgery: a randomized clinical trial and systematic review. *Crit Care Med* 2016;44:724–33.

15. Schwann TA, Zacharias A, Riordan CJ, Durham SJ, Engoren M, Habib RH. Safe, highly selective use of pulmonary artery catheters in coronary artery bypass grafting: an objective patient selection method. *Ann Thorac Surg* 2002;73:1394–401.

16. Lomivorotov VV, Efremov SM, Kirov MY, Fominskiy EV, Karaskov AM. Low-cardiac-output after cardiac surgery. *J Cardiothorac Vasc Anesth* 2017;31:291–308.

17. Chiang Y, Hosseinian L, Rhee A, Itagaki S, Cavallaro P, Chikwe J. Questionable benefit of the pulmonary artery catheter after cardiac surgery in high risk patients. *J Cardiothorac Vasc Anesth* 2015;29:76–81.

18. Zimmermann A, Kufner C, Hofbauer S, et al. The accuracy of the Vigileo/FloTrac continuous cardiac output monitor. *J Cardiothorac Vasc Anesth* 2008;22:388–93.

19. Judge O, Ji F, Fleming N, Liu H. Current use of the pulmonary artery catheter in cardiac surgery: a survey study. *J Cardiothorac Vasc Anesth* 2015;29:69–75.

20. Rawn J. The silent risks of blood transfusion. *Curr Opin Anaesthesiol* 2008;21:664–8.

21. Society of Thoracic Surgeons Blood Conservation Guideline Task Force, Ferraris VA, Brown JR, Despotis GH, et al. 2011 update to the Society of Thoracic Surgeons and the Society of Cardiovascular Anesthesiologists blood conservation clinical practice guidelines. *Ann Thorac Surg* 2011;91:944–82.

22. Scott BH, Seifert FC, Grimson R. Blood transfusion is associated with increased resource utilisation, morbidity and mortality in cardiac surgery. *Ann Card Anaesth* 2008;11:15–9.

23. Murphy GJ, Pike K, Rogers CA, Wordsworth S. Liberal or restrictive transfusion after cardiac surgery. *N Engl J Med* 2015;372:997–1008.

24. Mazer CD, Whitlock RP, Fergusson DA, et al. Six-month outcomes after restrictive or liberal transfusion for cardiac surgery. *N Engl J Med* 2018;379:1224–33.

25. Sommers MS, Stevenson JS, Hamlin RL, Ivey TD, Russell AC. Mixed venous oxygen saturation and oxygen partial pressure as predictors of cardiac index after coronary artery bypass grafting. *Heart Lung* 1993;22:112–20.
26. Shepherd SJ, Pearse RM. Role of central and mixed venous oxygen saturation measurement in perioperative care. *Anesthesiology* 2009;111:649–56.
27. Walley KR. Use of central venous oxygen saturation to guide therapy. *Am J Resp Crit Care Med* 2011;184:514–20.
28. Balik M, Pachl J, Hendl J, Martin B, Jan P, Jan H. Effect of the degree of tricuspid regurgitation on cardiac output measurements by thermodilution. *Intensive Care Med* 2002;28:1117–21.
29. Ardehali A, Ports TA. Myocardial oxygen supply and demand. *Chest* 1990;98:699–705.
30. Maganti MD, Rao V, Borger MA, Ivanov J, David TE. Predictors of low cardiac output syndrome after isolated aortic valve surgery. *Circulation* 2005;112(9 Suppl):I–448–52.
31. Rao V, Ivanov J, Weisel RD, Ikonimidis JS, Christakis GT, David TE. Predictors of low cardiac output syndrome after coronary artery bypass. *J Thorac Cardiovasc Surg* 1996;112:38–51.
32. Bernard F, Denault A, Babin D, et al. Diastolic dysfunction is predictive of difficult weaning from cardiopulmonary bypass. *Anesth Analg* 2001;92:291–8.
33. Rao V, Ivanov J, Weisel RD, Cohen G, Borger MA, Mickle DA. Lactate release during reperfusion predicts low cardiac output syndrome after coronary bypass surgery. *Ann Thorac Surg* 2001;71:1925–30.
34. Breisblatt WM, Stein KL, Wolfe CJ, et al. Acute myocardial dysfunction and recovery: a common occurrence after coronary bypass surgery. *J Am Coll Cardiol* 1990;15:1261–9.
35. Shahin J, DeVarennes B, Tse CW, Amarica DA, Dial S. The relationship between inotrope exposure, six-hour postoperative physiological variables, hospital mortality, and renal dysfunction in patients undergoing cardiac surgery. *Crit Care* 2011;15:R162.
36. Geisen M, Spray D, Fletcher SN. Echocardiography-based hemodynamic management in the cardiac surgical intensive care unit. *J Cardiothorac Vasc Anesth* 2014;28:733–44.
37. Casthely PA, Shah C, Mekhjian H, et al. Left ventricular diastolic function after coronary artery bypass grafting: a correlative study with three different myocardial protection techniques. *J Thorac Cardiovasc Sug* 1997;114:254–60.
38. Imren Y, Tasoglu I, Oktar GL, et al. The importance of transesophageal echocardiography in diagnosis of pericardial tamponade after cardiac surgery. *J Card Surg* 2008;23:450–3.
39. Weisel RD, Burns RJ, Baird RJ, et al. A comparison of volume loading and atrial pacing following aortocoronary bypass. *Ann Thorac Surg* 1983;36:332–44.
40. Muehlschlegel JD, Peng YG, Lobato EB, Hess PJ Jr, Martin TD, Klodell DT Jr. Temporary biventricular pacing postcardiopulmonary bypass in patients with reduced ejection fraction. *J Card Surg* 2008;23:324–30.
41. Eberhardt F, Heringlake M, Massalme MS, et al. The effect of biventricular pacing after coronary artery bypass grafting; a prospective randomized trial of different pacing modes in patients with reduced left ventricular function. *J Thorac Cardiovasc Surg* 2009;137:1461–7.
42. Wang DY, Richmond ME, Quinn A, et al. Optimized temporary biventricular pacing acutely improves intraoperative cardiac output after weaning from cardiopulmonary bypass: a substudy of a randomized clinical trial. *J Thorac Cardiovasc Surg* 2011;141:1002–8.
43. Gielgens RCW, Herold IHF, van Straten AHM, et al. The hemodynamic effects of different pacing modalities after cardiopulmonary bypass in patients with reduced left ventricular function. *J Cardiothorac Vasc Anesth* 2018;32:259–66.
44. Francis GS, Bartos JA, Adatya S. Inotropes. *J Am Coll Cardiol* 2014;63:2069–78.
45. Cavusoglu Y, Mert U, Nadir A, Mutlu F, Morrad B, Ulus T. Ivabradine treatment prevents dobutamine-induced increase in heart rate with acute decompensated heart failure. *J Cardiovasc Med (Hagerstown)* 2015;16:603–9.
46. Morimatsu H, Uchino S, Chung J, Bellomo R, Raman J, Buxton B. Norepinephrine for hypotensive vasodilatation after cardiac surgery: impact on renal function. *Intensive Care Med* 2003;29:1106–12.
47. Nygren A, Thorén A, Ricksten SE. Norepinephrine and intestinal mucosal perfusion in vasodilatory shock after cardiac surgery. *Shock* 2007;28:536–43.

48. Hajjar LA, Vincent JL, Barbosa Gomes Galas FR, et al. Vasopressin versus norepinephrine in patients with vasoplegic shock after cardiac surgery: the VANCS randomized controlled trial. *Anesthesiology* 2017;126:85–93.

49. Busse LW, Barker N, Petersen C. Vasoplegic syndrome following cardiothoracic surgery – review of pathophysiology and update of treatment options. *Crit Care* 2020;24:36.

50. Bragadottir G, Redfors B, Nygren A, Sellgren J, Ricksten SE. Low-dose vasopressin increases glomerular filtration rate, but impairs renal oxygenation in post-cardiac surgery patients. *Acta Anaesthesiol Scand* 2009;53:1052–9.

51. Nygren A, Thorén A, Ricksten SE. Vasopressin decreases intestinal mucosal perfusion: a clinical study on cardiac surgery patients in vasodilatory shock. *Acta Anaesthesiol Scand* 2009;53:581–8.

52. Mehaffey JH, Johnston LE, Hawkins RB, et al. Methylene blue for vasoplegic syndrome after cardiac operation: early administration improves survival. *Ann Thorac Surg* 2017;104:36–41.

53. Roderique JD, VanDyck K, Holman B, Tang D, Chui B, Speiss BD. The use of high-dose hydroxocobalamin for vasoplegic syndrome. *Ann Thorac Surg* 2014;97:1785–6.

54. Lahm T, McCaslin CA, Wozniak TC, et al. Medical and surgical treatment of right ventricular failure. *J Am Coll Cardiol* 2010;56:1435–46.

55. Forrest P. Anaesthesia and right ventricular failure. *Anaesth Intensive Care* 2009;37:370–85.

56. Wu VCC, Takeuchi M. Echocardiographic assessment of right ventricular systolic function. *Cardiovasc Diag Ther* 2018;8:70–9.

57. Kerbaul F, Rondelet B, Demester JP, et al. Effects of levosimendan versus dobutamine on pressure load-induced right ventricular failure. *Crit Care Med* 2006;34:2814–9.

58. Elmi-Sarabi M, Deschamps A, Delisle S, et al. Aerosolized vasodilators for the treatment of pulmonary hypertension in cardiac surgical patients: a systematic review and meta-analysis. *Anesth Analg* 2017;125:393–402.

59. Sardo S, Osawa EA, Finco G, et al. Nitric oxide in cardiac surgery: a meta-analysis of randomized controlled trials. *J Cardiothorac Vasc Anesth* 2018;32:2512–9.

60. Frostell CG, Blomqvist H, Hedenstierna G, Lundberg J, Zapol WM. Inhaled nitric oxide selectively reverses human hypoxic pulmonary vasoconstriction without causing systemic vasodilation. *Anesthesiology* 1995;78:427–35.

61. McGinn K, Reichert M. A comparison of inhaled nitric oxide versus inhaled epoprostenol for acute pulmonary hypertension following cardiac surgery. *Ann Pharmacother* 2016;50:22–6.

62. Winterhalter M, Simon A, Fischer S, et al. Comparison of inhaled iloprost and nitric oxide in patients with pulmonary hypertension during weaning from cardiopulmonary bypass in cardiac surgery: a prospective randomized trial. *J Cardiothorac Vasc Anesth* 2008;22:406–13.

63. Yin N, Kaestel S, Yin J, et al. Inhaled nitric oxide versus aerosolized iloprost for the treatment of pulmonary hypertension with left heart disease. *Crit Care Med* 2009;37:980–6.

64. Antoniou T, Koletsis EN, Prokakis C, et al. Hemodynamic effects of combination therapy with inhaled nitric oxide and iloprost in patients with pulmonary hypertension and right ventricular dysfunction after high-risk cardiac surgery. *J Cardiothorac Vasc Anesth* 2013;27:459–66.

65. Wang H, Gong M, Zhou B, Dai A. Comparison of inhaled and intravenous milrinone in patients with pulmonary hypertension undergoing mitral valve surgery. *Adv Ther* 2009;26:462–8.

66. Solina A, Papp D, Ginsberg S, et al. A comparison of inhaled nitric oxide and milrinone for the treatment of pulmonary hypertension in adult cardiac surgery patients. *J Cardiothorac Vasc Anesth* 2000;14:12–7.

67. Theodoraki K, Thanopoulos A, Rellia P, et al. A retrospective comparison of inhaled milrinone and iloprost in post-bypass pulmonary hypertension. *Heart Vessels* 2017;32:1488–97.

68. Laflamme M, Perrault LP, Carrier M, Elmi-Sarabi M, Fortier A, Denault AY. Preliminary experience with combined inhaled milrinone and prostacyclin in cardiac surgical patients with pulmonary hypertension. *J Cardiothorac Vasc Anesth* 2015;29:38–45.

69. Denault AY, Bussières JS, Arellano R, et al. A multicentre randomized-controlled trial of inhaled milrinone in high-risk cardiac surgical patients. *Can J Anaesth* 2016;63:1140–53.

70. Gebhard CE, Desjardins G, Gebhard C, Gavra P, Denault AY. Intratracheal milrinone bolus administration during acute right ventricular dysfunction after cardiopulmonary bypass. *J Cardiothorac Vasc Anesth* 2017;31:489–96.

71. Rong LQ, Rahouma M, Abouarab A, et al. Intravenous and inhaled milrinone in adult cardiac surgery patients: a pairwise and network meta-analysis. *J Cardiothorac Vasc Anesth* 2019;33:663–73.

72. Shim JK, Choi YS, Oh YJ, Kim DH, Hong YW, Kwak YL. Effect of oral sildenafil citrate on intraoperative hemodynamics in patients with pulmonary hypertension undergoing valvular heart surgery. *J Thorac Cardiovasc Surg* 2006;132:1420–5.

73. Ram E, Sternik L, Klempfner R, et al. Sildenafil for pulmonary hypertension in the early postoperative period after mitral valve surgery. *J Cardiothorac Vasc Anesth* 2019;33:1648–56.

74. Gandhi H, Shah B, Patel R, et al. Effect of preoperative oral sildenafil on severe pulmonary artery hypertension in patients undergoing mitral valve replacement. *Indian J Pharmacol* 2014;46:281–5.

75. Jiang G, Li B, Zhang G, Xu E, Liu Y, Xu Z. Effects of sildenafil on prognosis in patients with pulmonary hypertension after left-sided valvular surgery. *Heart Lung Circ* 2014;2:680–5.

76. Matamis D, Pampori S, Papathanasiou A, et al. Inhaled NO and sildenafil combination in cardiac surgery patients with out-of-proportion pulmonary hypertension: acute effects on postoperative gas exchange and hemodynamics. *Circ Heart Fail* 2012;5:47–53.

77. Brutsaert DL, Sys SU, Gillebert TC. Diastolic dysfunction in post-cardiac surgical management. *J Cardiothorac Vasc Anesth* 1993;7(Suppl 1):18–20.

78. Fellahi JL, Parienti JJ, Hanouz JJ, Plaud B, Biou B, Ouattara A. Perioperative use of dobutamine in cardiac surgery and adverse cardiac outcome: propensity adjusted analyses. *Anesthesiology* 2008;108:979–87.

79. Schumann J, Henrich EC, Strobl H, et al. Inotropic agents and vasodilator strategies for the treatment of cardiogenic shock or low cardiac output syndromes. *Cochrane Database Syst Rev* 2018;1:CD009669. https://doi.org/10.1002/14651858.CD009669.pub3.

80. Belletti A, Castrol ML, Silvetti S, et al. The effect of inotropes and vasopressors on mortality: a meta-analysis of randomized clinical trials. *Br J Anaesth* 2015;115:656–75.

81. Totaro RJ, Raper RF. Epinephrine-induced lactic acidosis following cardiopulmonary bypass. *Crit Care Med* 1997;25:1693–9.

82. Butterworth JF IV, Prielipp RC, Royster RL, et al. Dobutamine increases heart rate more than epinephrine in patients recovering from aortocoronary bypass surgery. *J Cardiothorac Vasc Anesth* 1992;6:535–41.

83. Fowler MB, Alderman EL, Oesterle SN, et al. Dobutamine and dopamine after cardiac surgery: greater augmentation of myocardial blood flow with dobutamine. *Circulation* 1984;70(suppl I): I–103–11.

84. DiSesa VJ, Brown E, Mudge GH Jr, Collins JJ Jr, Cohn LH. Hemodynamic comparison of dopamine and dobutamine in the postoperative volume-loaded, pressure-loaded, and normal ventricle. *J Thorac Cardiovasc Surg* 1982;83:256–63.

85. Feneck RO, Sherry KM, Withington PS, Oduro-Dominah A, and the European Milrinone Multicenter Trial Group. Comparison of the hemodynamic effects of milrinone with dobutamine in patients after cardiac surgery. *J Cardiothorac Vasc Anesth* 2001;15:306–15.

86. Levy JH, Bailey JM, Deeb GM. Intravenous milrinone in cardiac surgery. *Ann Thorac Surg* 2002;73:325–30.

87. Liu JJ, Doolan LA, Xie B, Chen JR, Buxton BF. Direct vasodilator effect of milrinone, an inotropic drug, on arterial coronary bypass grafts. *J Thorac Cardiovasc Surg* 1997;113:108–13.

88. Yano M, Kohno M, Ohkusa T, et al. Effect of milrinone on left ventricular relaxation and Ca(2+) uptake function of cardiac sarcoplasmic reticulum. *Am J Physiol Heart Circ Physiol* 2000;279: H1898–905.

89. Tanigawa T, Yano M, Kohno M, et al. Mechanism of preserved positive lusitropy by cAMP-dependent drugs in heart failure. *Am J Physiol Heart Circ Physiol* 2000;278:H313–20.

90. Lobato EB, Gravenstein N, Martin TD. Milrinone, not epinephrine, improves left ventricular compliance after cardiopulmonary bypass. *J Cardiothorac Vasc Anesth* 2000;14:374–7.

91. Lobato EB, Willert JL, Looke TD, Thomas J, Urdaneta F. Effects of milrinone versus epinephrine on left ventricular relaxation after cardiopulmonary bypass following myocardial revascularization: assessment by color M-mode and tissue Doppler. *J Cardiothorac Vasc Anesth* 2005;19:334–9.

92. Couture P, Denault AY, Pellerin M, Tardif JC. Milrinone enhances systolic, but not diastolic function during coronary artery bypass grafting surgery. *Can J Anaesth* 2007;54:509–22.

93. Fleming GA, Murray KT, Yu C, et al. Milrinone use is associated with postoperative atrial fibrillation after cardiac surgery. *Circulation* 2008;118:1619–25.

94. Alhashemi JA, Hooper J. Treatment of milrinone-associated tachycardia with beta-blockers. *Can J Anaesth* 1998;45:67–70.

95. Rathmell JP, Prielipp RC, Butterworth JF, et al. A multicenter, randomized blind comparison of amrinone with milrinone after elective cardiac surgery. *Anesth Analg* 1998;86:683–90.

96. Zangrillo A, Biondi-Zoccai G, Ponschab M, et al. Milrinone and mortality in adult cardiac surgery: a meta-analysis. *J Cardiothorac Vasc Anesth* 2012;26:70–7.

97. Majure DT, Greco T, Greco M, et al. Meta-analysis of randomized trials of effect of milrinone on mortality in cardiac surgery: a meta-analysis. *J Cardiothorac Vasc Anesth* 2013;27:220–9.

98. Kikura M, Sato S. The efficacy of preemptive milrinone or amrinone therapy in patients undergoing coronary artery bypass grafting. *Anesth Analg* 2002;94:22–30.

99. Gelfman DM, Ornato JP, Gonzalez ER. Dopamine-induced increase in atrioventricular conduction in atrial fibrillation-flutter. *Clin Cardiol* 1987;10:671–3.

100. Hiemstra B, Koster G, Wettersley J, et al. Dopamine in critically ill patients with cardiac dysfunction: a systematic review with meta-analysis and trial sequential analysis. *Acta Anaesthesiol Scand* 2019;63:424–37.

101. Lassnigg A, Donner E, Grubhofer G, Presterl E, Druml W, Hiesmayr M. Lack of renoprotective effects of dopamine and furosemide during cardiac surgery. *J Am Soc Nephrol* 2000;11:97–104.

102. Savluk OF, Guzelmeric F, Yavuz Y, et al. N-acetylcysteine versus dopamine to prevent acute injury after cardiac surgery in patients with preexisting moderate renal insufficiency. *Braz J Cardiovasc Surg* 2017;32:8–14.

103. Duranteau J, Sitbon P, Teboul JL, et al. Effects of epinephrine, norepinephrine, or the combination of norepinephrine and dobutamine on gastric mucosa in septic shock. *Crit Care Med* 1999;27: 893–900.

104. Shapira N, Schaff HV, White RD, Pluth JR. Hemodynamic effects of calcium chloride injection following cardiopulmonary bypass: response to bolus injection and continuous infusion. *Ann Thorac Surg* 1984;37:133–40.

105. Dehert SG, Ten Broecke PW, De Mulder PA, et al. The effects of calcium on left ventricular function early after cardiopulmonary bypass. *J Cardiothorac Vasc Anesth* 1997;11:864–9.

106. Drop LJ, Scheidegger D. Plasma ionized concentration: important determinant of the hemodynamic response to calcium infusion. *J Thorac Cardiovasc Surg* 1980;79:425–31.

107. Royster RL, Butterworth JF 4th, Prielipp RC, et al. A randomized, blinded, placebo-controlled evaluation of calcium chloride and epinephrine for inotropic support after emergence from cardiopulmonary bypass. *Anesth Analg* 1992;74:3–13.

108. Butterworth JF 4th, Zaloga GP, Prielipp RC, Tucker WY Jr, Royster RL. Calcium inhibits the cardiac stimulating properties of dobutamine but not of amrinone. *Chest* 1992;101:174–80.

109. DiNardo JA. Pro: calcium is routinely indicated during separation from cardiopulmonary bypass. *J Cardiothorac Vasc Anesth* 1997;11:906–7.

110. Prielipp R, Butterworth J. Con: calcium is not routinely indicated during separation from cardiopulmonary bypass. *J Cardiothorac Vasc Anesth* 1997;11:908–12.

111. Walker JD, Crawford FA Jr, Mukherjee R, Spinale FG. The direct effects of 3,5,3'-triiodo-L-thyronine (T3) on myocyte contractile processes: insights into mechanisms of action. *J Thorac Cardiovasc Surg* 1995;110:1369–80.

112. Cerillo AG, Storti S, Kallushi E, et al. The low triiodothyronine syndrome; a strong predictor of low cardiac output and death in patients undergoing coronary artery bypass grafting. *Ann Thorac Surg* 2014;97:2089–95.

113. Batra YK, Singh B, Chavan S, Chari P, Dhaliwal RS, Ramprabu K. Effects of cardiopulmonary bypass on thyroid function. *Ann Card Anaesth* 2000;3:3–6.

114. Reinhardt W, Mocker V, Jockenhovel F, et al. Influence of coronary artery bypass surgery on thyroid hormone parameters. *Horm Res* 1997;47:1–8.

115. Ranasinghe AM, Quinn DW, Pagano D, et al. Glucose-insulin-potassium and tri-iodothyronine individually improve hemodynamic performance and are associated with reduce troponin I release after on-pump coronary artery bypass grafting. *Circulation* 2006;114(1 Suppl):I–245–50.

116. Bennett-Guerrero E, Jimenez JL, White WD, D'Amico EB, Baldwin BI, Schwinn DA. Cardiovascular effects of intravenous triiodothyronine in patients undergoing coronary artery bypass graft surgery. A randomized, double-blind, placebo-controlled trial: Duke T3 Study Group. *JAMA* 1996;275:687–92.

117. Vohra HA, Bapu D, Bahrami T, Gaer JA, Satur CM. Does perioperative administration of thyroid hormone improve outcome following coronary artery bypass grafting? *J Card Surg* 2008;23:92–6.

118. Mullis-Jansson S, Argenziano M, Corwin S, et al. A randomized double-blind study of the effect of triiodothyronine on cardiac function and morbidity after coronary bypass surgery. *J Thorac Cardiovasc Surg* 1999;117:1128–35.

119. Park YJ, Yoon JW, Kim KI, et al. Subclinical hypothyroidism might increase the risk of transient atrial fibrillation after coronary artery bypass grafting. *Ann Thorac Surg* 2009;87:1846–52.

120. Klemperer JD, Klein IL, Ojamaa K, et al. Triiodothyronine therapy lowers the incidence of atrial fibrillation after cardiac operations. *Ann Thorac Surg* 1996;61:1323–9.

121. Fan Y, Zhang AM, Xiao YB, Weng YG, Hetzer R. Glucose-insulin-potassium therapy in adult patients undergoing cardiac surgery: a meta-analysis. *Eur J Cardiothorac Surg* 2011;40:192–9.

122. Harrison RW, Hasselblad V, Mehta RH, Levin R, Harrington RA, Alexander JH. Effect of levosimendan on survival and adverse events after cardiac surgery: a meta-analysis. *J Cardiothorac Vasc Anesth* 2013;27:1224–32.

123. Erickson HI, Jalonen JR, Heikkinen LO, et al. Levosimendan facilitates weaning from cardiopulmonary bypass in patients undergoing coronary artery bypass grafting with impaired left ventricular function. *Ann Thorac Surg* 2009;87:448–54.

124. Wang B, He B, Gong Y, et al. Levosimendan in patients with left ventricular dysfunction undergoing cardiac surgery: an update meta-analysis and trial sequential analysis. *Biomed Res Int* 2018:7563083. doi: 10.1155/2018/7563083.

125. Guarracino F, Heringlake M, Cholley B. Use of levosimendan in cardiac surgery: an update after the LEVO-CTS, CHEETAH, and LICORN trials in the light of clinical practice. *J Cardiovasc Pharmacol* 2018;71:1–9.

126. Landoni G, Lomivorotov VV, Alvaro G, et al. Levosimendan for hemodynamic support after cardiac surgery. *N Engl J Med* 2017;376:2021–31.

127. Elbadawi A, Elgendy IY, Saad M, et al. Meta-analysis of trials on prophylactic use of levosimendan in patients undergoing cardiac surgery. *Ann Thorac Surg* 2018;105:1403–10.

128. Mehta RH, Leimberger JD, van Diepen S, et al. Levosimendan in patients with left ventricular dysfunction undergoing cardiac surgery. *N Engl J Med* 2017;376:2032–42.

129. Toller W, Heringlake M, Guarracino F, et al. Preoperative and perioperative use of levosimendan in cardiac surgery: European expert opinion. *Int J Cardiol* 2015;184:323–36.

130. Jannati M, Attar A. Intra-aortic balloon pump postcardiac surgery: a literature review. *J Res Med Sci* 2019;24:6.

131. Papaioannou TG, Stefanadis C. Basic principles of the intraaortic balloon pump and mechanisms affecting its performance. *ASAIO J* 2005;51:296–300.

132. Santa-Cruz RA, Cohen MG, Ohman EM. Aortic counterpulsation: a review of the hemodynamic effects and indications for use. *Catheter Cardiovasc Interv* 2006;67:68–77.

133. Hou D, Yang F, Hou X. Clinical application of intra-aortic balloon counterpulsation in high-risk patients undergoing cardiac surgery. *Perfusion* 2018;33:178–84.

134. Pilarcyzk K, Boening A, Jakob H, et al. Preoperative intra-aortic counterpulsation in high-risk patients undergoing cardiac surgery: a meta-analysis of randomized controlled trials. *Eur J Cardiothorac Surg* 2017;49:5–17.

135. Ferreira GSR, de Almeida JP, Landoni G, et al. Effect of a perioperative intra-aortic balloon pump in high-risk cardiac surgery patients: a randomized clinical trial. *Crit Care Med* 2018;46:e742–50.

136. Miceli A, Fiorani B, Danesi TH, Melina G, Sinatra R. Prophylactic intra-aortic balloon pump in high-risk patients undergoing coronary artery bypass grafting: a propensity score analysis. *Interact Cardiovac Thorac Surg* 2009;9:291–4.

137. Etienne PY, Papadatos S, Glineur D, et al. Reduced mortality in high-risk coronary patients operated off pump with preoperative intraaortic balloon counterpulsation. *Ann Thorac Surg* 2007;84:498–502.

138. Gao ZW, Huang YZ, Zhao HM, et al. Impact of intra-aortic balloon counterpulsation on prognosis of patients with acute myocardial infarction: a meta-analysis. *Acta Cardiol Sin* 2017;33:567–77.

139. Su D, Yan B, Guo L, et al. Intra-aortic balloon pump may grant no benefit to improve the mortality of patients with acute myocardial infarction in short and long term: an updated meta-analysis. *Medicine (Baltimore)* 2015;94:e876.

140. Unverzagt S, Machemer MT, Solms A, et al. Intra-aortic balloon pump counterpulsation (IABP) for myocardial infarction complicated by cardiogenic shock. *Cochrane Database Syst Rev* 2015;3:CD007398. https://doi.org/10.1002/14651858.CD007398.pub3.

141. Zhou M, Yu K, Wang XH, et al. Analysis of application timing of IABP in emergency PCI treatment of patients with combined acute myocardial infarction and cardiac shock. *Cur Rev Med Pharmacol Sci* 2017;21:2934–9.

142. Mandawat A, Rao SV. Percutaneous mechanical circulatory support in cardiogenic shock. *Circ Cardiovasc Interv* 2017;10:e004337.

143. Ahmad Y, Sen S, Shun-Shin MJ, et al. Intra-aortic balloon pump therapy for acute myocardial infarction a meta-analysis. *JAMA Intern Med* 2015;175:931–9.

144. Seyfarth M, Sibbing D, Bauer I, et al. A randomized clinical trial to evaluate the safety and efficacy of a percutaneous left ventricular assist device versus intra-aortic balloon pumping for the treatment of cardiogenic shock caused by myocardial infarction. *J Am Coll Cardiol* 2008;52:1584–8.

145. Perera D, Sables R, Thomas M, et al. Elective intra-aortic balloon counterpulsation during high-risk percutaneous coronary intervention: a randomized controlled trial. *JAMA* 2010;304:867–74.

146. Miceli A, Duggan SMJ, Capoun R, Romeo F, Caputo M, Angelini GD. A clinical score to predict the need for intraaortic balloon pump in patients undergoing coronary artery bypass grafting. *Ann Thorac Surg* 2010;90:522–7.

147. Pivatto Júnior R, Tagliari AP, Luvizetto AB, et al. Use of intra-aortic balloon pump in cardiac surgery: analysis of 80 consecutive cases. *Rev Bras Cir Cardiovasc* 2012;27:251–9.

148. Parissis H, Leotsinidis M, Akbar MT, Apostolakis E, Dougenis D. The need for intra aortic balloon pump support following open heart surgery: risk analysis and outcome. *J Cardiothorac Surg* 2010;5:20.

149. Khir AW, Price S, Henein MY, Parker KH, Pepper JR. Intra-aortic balloon pumping: effects on left ventricular diastolic function. *Eur J Cardiothorac Surg* 2003;24:277–82.

150. Vanden Eynden F, Mets G, De Somer F, Bouchez S, Bove T. Is there a place for intra-aortic balloon counterpulsation support in acute right ventricular failure by pressure-overload? *Int J Cardiol* 2015;197:227–34.

151. Boeken U, Feindt P, Litmathe J, Kurt M, Gams E. Intraaortic balloon pumping in patients with right ventricular insufficiency after cardiac surgery: parameters to predict failure of IABP support. *Thorac Cardiovasc Surg* 2009;57:324–8.

152. Kapur NK, Esposito ML, Bader Y, et al. Mechanical circulatory support devices for acute right ventricular failure. *Circulation* 2017;136:314–26.

153. Krishnamoorthy A, De Vore AD, Sun JL, et al. The impact of a failing right heart in patients supported by intra-aortic balloon counterpulsation. *Eur Heart J Acute Cardiovasc Care* 2017;6:709–18.

154. Onorati F, Impiombato B, Ferraro A, et al. Transbrachial intraaortic balloon pumping in severe peripheral atherosclerosis. *Ann Thorac Surg* 2007;84:264–6.

155. Marcu CB, Donohue TJ, Ferneini A, Ghantous AE. Intraaortic balloon pump insertion through the subclavian artery: subclavian artery insertion of IABP. *Heart Lung Circ* 2006;15:148–50.

156. Estep JD, Cordero-Reyes AM, Bhimaraj A, et al. Percutaneous placement of an intra-aortic balloon pump in the left axillary/subclavian position provides safe, ambulatory long-term support as bridge to heart transplantation. *JACC Heart Fail* 2013;1:382–8.

157. Hurlé A, Llamas P, Meseguer J, Casillas JA. Paraplegia complicating intraaortic balloon pumping. *Ann Thorac Surg* 1997;63:1217–8.

158. Shimamoto H, Kawazoe K, Kito H, Fujita T, Shimamoto Y. Does juxtamesenteric placement of intra-aortic balloon interrupt superior mesenteric flow? *Clin Cardiol* 1992;15:285–90.

159. Ho AC, Hong CL, Yang MW, Lu PP, Lin PJ. Stroke after intraaortic balloon counterpulsation associated with mobile atheroma in thoracic aorta diagnosed using transesophageal echocardiography. *Chang Gung Med J* 2002;25:612–6.

160. Swartz MT, Sakamoto T, Arai H, et al. Effects of intraaortic balloon position on renal artery blood flow. *Ann Thorac Surg* 1992;53:604–10.

161. Arafa OE, Pedersen TH, Svennevig JL, Fosse E, Geiran OR. Vascular complications of the intraaortic balloon pump in patients undergoing open heart operations: a 15-year experience. *Ann Thorac Surg* 1999;67:645–51.

162. Meharwal ZS, Trehan N. Vascular complications of intra-aortic balloon insertion in patients undergoing coronary revascularization: analysis of 911 cases. *Eur J Cardiothorac Surg* 2002;21:741–7.

163. Parissis H, Soo A, Al-Alao B. Intra aortic balloon pump: literature review of risk factors related to complications of the intraaortic balloon pump. *J Cardiothorac Surg* 2011;6:147.

164. Christenson JT, Sierra J, Romand JA, Licker M, Kalangos A. Long intraaortic balloon treatment time leads to more vascular complications. *Asian Cardiovasc Thorac Ann* 2007;15:408–12.

165. Davies AR, Bellomo R, Raman JS, Gutteridge GA, Buxton BF. High lactate predicts the failure of intraaortic balloon pumping after cardiac surgery. *Ann Thorac Surg* 2001;71:1415–20.

166. Khorsandi M, Dougherty S, Sinclair A, et al. A 20-year multicentre outcome analysis of salvage mechanical circulatory support for refractory cardiogenic shock after cardiac surgery. *J Cardiothorac Surg* 2018;11:151.

167. Khorsandi M, Dougherty S, Bouamra O, et al. Extra-corporeal membrane oxygenation for refractory cardiogenic shock after adult cardiac surgery: a systematic review and meta-analysis. *J Cardiothorac Surg* 2017;12:55.

168. O'Neill WW, Grines C, Schreiber T, et al. Analysis of outcomes for 15,259 US patients with acute myocardial infarction cardiogenic shock (AMICS) supported with the Impella device. *Am Heart J* 2018;202:33–8.

169. Schurtz G, Laine M, Delmas C, et al. Mechanical support in cardiogenic shock complicating acute coronary syndrome: ready for prime time? *Curr Vasc Pharmacol* 2018;16:418–26.

170. Loehn T, O'Neill WW, Lange B, et al. Long term survival after early unloading with Impella CP® in acute myocardial infarction complicated by cardiogenic shock. *Eur Heart J Acute Cardiovasc Care* 2020;9:149–57.

171. Shishenbor MH, Moazami N, Tongt MZY, Unai S, Tang WHW, Soltesz EG. Cardiogenic shock: from ECMO to Impella and beyond. *Cleveland Clin J Med* 2017;84:287–95.

172. O'Neill WW, Kleiman NS, Moses J, et al. A prospective, randomized clinical trial of hemodynamic support with Impella 2.5 versus intra-aortic balloon pump in patients undergoing high-risk percutaneous coronary interventions: the PROTECT II study. *Circulation* 2012;126:1717–27.

173. Dangas GD, Kini AS, Sharma SK, et al. Impact of hemodynamic support with Impella 2.5 versus intra-aortic balloon pump on prognostically important clinical outcomes in patients undergoing high-risk percutaneous coronary intervention (from the PROTECT II randomized trial). *Am J Cardiol* 2014;113:222–8.

174. Alli OO, Singh IM, Holmes DR Jr, Pulido JN, Park SJ, Rihal CS. Percutaneous left ventricular assist device with TandemHeart for high-risk percutaneous coronary intervention: the Mayo Clinic experience. *Catheter Cardiovasc Interv* 2012;80:728–34.

175. Vase H, Christensen S, Christiansen A, et al. The Impella CP device for acute mechanical circulatory support in refractory cardiac arrest. *Resuscitation* 2017;112:70–4.

176. Garcia S, Kandar R, Boyle A, et al. Effects of pulsatile- and continuous flow left ventricular assist devices on left ventricular unloading. *J Heart Lung Transplant* 2008;27:271–7.

177. Klotz S, Deng MC, Stypmann J, et al. Left ventricular pressure and volume unloading during pulsatile versus nonpulsatile left ventricular assist device support. *Ann Thorac Surg* 2004;77:143–50.

178. Russo JJ, Aleksova N, Pitcher I, et al. Left ventricular unloading during extracorporeal membrane oxygenation in patients with cardiogenic shock. *J Am Coll Cardiol* 2019;73:654–62.

179. Kamdar F, Boyle A, Liao K, Colvin-Adams M, Joyce L, John R. Effects of centrifugal, axial, and pulsatile left ventricular assist device support on end-organ function in heart failure patients. *J Heart Lung Transplant* 2009;28:352–9.

180. Samuels LE, Kaufman MS, Thomas MP, Holmes EC, Brockman SK, Wechsler AS. Pharmacological criteria for ventricular assist device insertion following cardiogenic shock: experience with the Abiomed BVS system. *J Card Surg* 1999;14:288–93.

181. Rao V, Oz M, Flannery MA, Catanese KA, Argenziano M, Naka Y. Revised screening scale to predict survival after insertion of a left ventricular assist device. *J Thorac Cardiovasc Surg* 2003;125:855–62.

182. Borisenko O, Wylie G, Payne J, et al. Thoratec CentriMag for temporary treatment of refractory cardiogenic shock or severe cardiopulmonary insufficiency: a systematic literature review and meta-analysis of observational studies. *ASAIO J* 2014;60:487–97.

183. Mikus E, Tripodi A, Calvi S, Giglio MD, Cavallucci A, Lamarra M. CentriMag venoarterial extracorporeal membrane oxygenation support as treatment for patients with refractory postcardiotomy cardiogenic shock. *ASAIO J* 2013;59:18–23.

184. Mohamedali B, Bhat G, Yost G, Tatooles A. Survival on biventricular mechanical support with the CentriMag® as a bridge to decision: a single-center risk stratification. *Perfusion* 2015;30:201–8.

185. Griffith BP, Anderson MB, Samuels LE, Pae WE Jr, Naka Y, Frazier OH. The RECOVER I: a multicenter prospective study of Impella 5.0/LD for postcardiotomy circulatory support. *J Thorac Cardiovasc Surg* 2013;145:548–54.

186. Kar B, Adkins LE, Civitello AB, et al. Clinical experience with the TandemHeart percutaneous ventricular assist device. *Texas Heart Inst J* 2006;33:111–5.

187. Morales DL, Gregg D, Helman DN, et al. Arginine vasopressin in the treatment of 50 patients with postcardiotomy vasodilatory shock. *Ann Thorac Surg* 2002;69:102–6.

188. Sen A, Larson JS, Kashani KB, et al. Mechanical circulatory assist devices: a primer for critical care and emergency physicians. *Critical Care* 2016;20:153.

189. Potopov EV, Loforte A, Weng Y, et al. Experience with over 1000 implanted ventricular assist devices. *J Cardiac Surg* 2008;23:185–94.

190. Suarez-Pierre A, Zhou X, Fraser CD 3rd, et al. Survival and functional status after bridge-to-transplant with a left ventricular assist device. *ASAIO J* 2019;65:661–7.

191. Anderson MB, Goldstein J, Milano C, et al. Benefits of a novel percutaneous ventricular assist device for right heart failure: the prospective RECOVER RIGHT study of the Impella RP device. *J Heart Lung Transplant* 2015;34:1549–60.

192. Anderson MB, Morris DL, Tang D, et al. Outcomes of patients with right ventricular failure requiring short-term hemodynamic support with the Impella RP device. *J Heart Lung Transplant* 2018;37:1448–58.

193. Cheung AW, White CW, Davis MK, Freed DH. Short-term mechanical circulatory support for recovery from acute right ventricular failure: clinical outcomes. *J Heart Lung Transplant* 2014;33:794–9.

194. Kapur NK, Paruchuri V, Jagannathan A, et al. Mechanical circulatory support for right ventricular failure. *JACC Heart Fail* 2013;1:127–34.

195. Pieri M, Pappalardo F. Impella RP in the treatment of right ventricular failure: what we know and where to go. *J Cardiothorac Vasc Anesth* 2018;32:2339–43.

196. Ravichandran AK, Baran DA, Stelling K, Cowger JA, Salerno CT. Outcomes with the Tandem Protek Duo dual-lumen percutaneous right ventricular assist device. *ASAIO J* 2018;64:570–2.

197. Kazui T, Tran PL, Echeverria A, et al. Minimally invasive approach for percutaneous CentriMag right ventricular assist device support using a single PROTEKDuo cannula. *J Cardiothorac Surg* 2016;11:123.

198. Patel ND, Weiss ES, Schaffer J, et al. Right heart dysfunction after left ventricular assist device implantation: a comparison of the pulsatile HeartMate I and axial-flow HeartMate II devices. *Ann Thorac Surg* 2008;86:832–40.

199. Han JJ, Acker MA, Atluri P, et al. Left ventricular assist devices: synergistic model between technology and medicine. *Circulation* 2018;138:2841–51.

200. Fitzpatrick JR 3rd, Frederick JR, Hsu WM, et al. Risk score derived from pre-operative data analysis predicts the need for biventricular mechanical circulatory support. *J Heart Lung Transplant* 2008;27:1286–92.

201. Kormos RL, Teuteberg JJ, Pagani FD, et al. Right ventricular failure in patients with the HeartMate II continuous-flow left ventricular assist device: incidence, risk factors, and effect on outcomes. *J Thorac Cardiovasc Surg* 2010;139:1316–24.

202. Kiernan MS, Grandin EW, Brinkley M Jr, et al. Early right ventricular assist device utilization in patients undergoing continuous-flow left ventricular assist device implantation: incidence and risk factors from INTERMAC. *Circ Heart Fail* 2017;10:e003863.

203. Raina A, Rammohan HRS, Gertz ZM, Rame JE, Woo YJ, Kirkpatrick JN. Postoperative right ventricular failure after left ventricular assist device placement is predicted by preoperative echocardiographic structural, hemodynamic, and functional parameters. *J Card Fail* 2013;19:16–24.

204. Matthews JC, Koelling TM, Pagani FD, Aaronson KD. The right ventricular failure risk score: a pre-operative tool for assessing the risk of right ventricular failure in left ventricular assist device candidates. *J Am Coll Cardiol* 2008;51:2163–72.

205. Patel NJ, Verma DR, Gopalan R, Heuser RR, Pershad A. Percutaneous biventricular mechanical circulatory support with Impella CP and Protek Duo Plus TandemHeart. *J Invasive Cardiol* 2019;31:E46.

206. Khorsandi M, Schroder J, Daneshmand M, et al. Outcomes after extracorporeal right ventricular assist device combined with durable left ventricular assist device support. *Ann Thorac Surg* 2019;107:1768–74.

207. Keebler ME, Haddad EV, Choi CW, et al. Venoarterial extracorporeal membrane oxygenation in cardiogenic shock. *JACC Heart Fail* 2018;6:503–16.

208. Guglin M, Zucker MJ, Bazan VM, et al. Venoarterial ECMO for adults: JACC Scientific Expert Panel. *J Am Coll Cardiol* 2019;73:698–716.

209. Rastan AJ, Dege A, Mohr M, et al. Early and late outcomes of 517 consecutive adult patients treated with extracorporeal membrane oxygenation for refractory postcardiotomy cardiogenic shock. *J Thorac Cardiovasc Surg* 2010;139:302–11.

210. Biancari F, Dalén M, Fiore A, et al. Multicenter study on postcardiotomy venoarterial extracorporeal membrane oxygenation. *J Thorac Cardiovasc Surg* 2020;159:1844–54.

211. Rubino A, Costanzo D, Stanzus D, et al. Central veno-arterial extracorporeal membrane oxygenation (C-VA-ECMO) after cardiothoracic surgery: a single-center experience. *J Cardiothorac Vasc Anesth* 2018;32:1169–74.

212. Biancari F, Perrotti A, Dalén M, et al. Meta-analysis of the outcome after postcardiotomy venoarterial extracorporeal membrane oxygenation in adult patients. *J Cardiothorac Vasc Anesth* 2018;32:1178–82.

213. Mohite PN, Sabashnikov A, Koch A, et al. Comparison of temporary ventricular assist devices and extracorporeal life support in post-cardiotomy cardiogenic shock. *Interact Cardiovasc Thorac Surg* 2018;27:863–9.

214. Chen YS, Chao A, Yu HY, et al. Analysis and results of prolonged resuscitation in cardiac arrest patients rescued by extracorporeal membrane oxygenation. *J Am Coll Cardiol* 2003;41:197–203.

215. Schibilsky D, Lausberg H, Haller C, et al. Impella 5.0 support in INTERMACS II cardiogenic shock using right and left axillary artery access. *Artif Organs* 2015;39:660–3.

216. Mahboub-Ahari A, Heidari F, Sadeghi-Ghyassi F, Asadi M. A systematic review of effectiveness and economic evaluation of Cardiohelp and portable devices for extracorporeal membrane oxygenation (ECMO). *J Artif Organs* 2019;22:6–13.

217. Alwardt CM, Wilson DS, Alore ML, Lanza LA, Devaleria PA, Pajaro OE. Performance and safety of an integrated portable extracorporeal life support system for adults. *J Extra Corpor Technol* 2015;47:38–43.

218. John R, Liao K, Lietz K, et al. Experience with the Levitronix CentriMag circulatory support system as a bridge to decision in patients with refractory acute cardiogenic shock and multisystem organ failure. *J Thorac Cardiovasc Surg* 2007;134:351–8.

219. Slaughter MS, Rogers JG, Milano CA, et al. Advanced heart failure treated with continuous-flow left ventricular assist device. *N Engl J Med* 2009;361:2241–51.

220. Rogers JG, Pagani FD, Tatooles AJ, et al. Intrapericardial left ventricular assist device for advanced heart failure. *N Engl J Med* 2017;376:451–60.

221. Mehra MR, Naka Y, Uriel N, et al. A fully magnetically levitated circulatory pump for advanced heart failure. *N Engl J Med* 2017;376:440–50.

222. Selzman CH, Koliopoulou A, Glotzbach JP, McKellar SH. Evolutionary improvement in the Jarvik 2000 left ventricular device. *ASAIO J* 2018;64:827–30.

223. Kohno H, Matsumiya G, Sawa Y, et al. The Jarvik 2000 left ventricular assist device as a bridge to transplantation: Japanese Registry for Mechanically Assisted Circulatory Support. *J Heart Lung Transplant* 2018;37:71–8.

224. Cheung A, Chorpenning K, Tamez D, et al. Design concepts and preclinical results of a miniaturized HeartWare platform. *Innovations (Phila)* 2015;10:151–6.

225. Cook JA, Shah KB, Quader MA, et al. The total artificial heart. *J Thorac Dis* 2015;7:2172–80.

226. Arabia A. SynCardia total artificial heart opportunities and challenges moving forward. *Artif Organs* 2019;43:1051–2.

227. Goodwin ML, Mokadam NA. Total artificial heart implantation: how I teach it. *Ann Thorac Surg* 2019;108:1271–6.

228. Netuka I, Kvasnička T, Kvasnička J, et al. Willebrand's factor with a fully magnetically levitated centrifugal continuous-flow left ventricular assist device in advanced heart failure. *J Heart Lung Transplant* 2016;35:860–7.

229. Steinlechner B, Dworschak M, Birkenberg B, et al. Platelet dysfunction in outpatients with left ventricular assist devices. *Ann Thorac Surg* 2009;87:131–8.

230. Shroder JN, Daneshmand MA, Villamizar NR, et al. Heparin-induced thrombocytopenia in left ventricular assist device bridge-to-transplant patients. *Ann Thorac Surg* 2007;84:841–6.

231. Morgan JA, Park Y, Oz MC, Naka Y. Device related infections while on left ventricular assist device support do not adversely impact bridging to transplant or posttransplant survival. *ASAIO J* 2003;49:748–50.

232. Zierer A, Melby SJ, Voeller RK, et al. Late-onset driveline infections: the Achilles' heel of prolonged left ventricular assist device support. *Ann Thorac Surg* 2007;84:515–21.

233. Willey JZ, Gavalas MV, Trinh PN, et al. Outcomes after stroke complicating left ventricular assist device. *J Heart Lung Transplant* 2016;35:1003–9.

234. Milano CA, Rogers JG, Tatooles AJ, et al. HVAD: the ENDURANCE supplemental trial. *JACC Heart Fail* 2018;6:792–802.

235. Oz MC, Rose EA, Slater J, Kuiper JJ, Catanese KA, Levin HR. Malignant ventricular arrhythmias are well tolerated in patients receiving long-term left ventricular assist devices. *J Am Coll Cardiol* 1994;24:1688–91.

236. Jorde UP, Uriel N, Nahumi N, et al. Prevalence, significance, and management of aortic insufficiency in continuous flow left ventricular assist device recipients. *Circ Heat Fail* 2014;7:310–9.

237. John R, Lietz K, Schuster M, et al. Immunologic sensitization in recipients of left ventricular assist devices. *J Thorac Cardiovasc Surg* 2003;125:578–91.

238. Kim YS, Kim YI, Seo KH, Kang HR. Optimal dose of prophylactic dexmedetomidine for preventing postoperative shivering. *Int J Med Sci* 2013;10:1327–32.

239. Cheung AT, Cruz-Shiavone GE, Meng QC, et al. Cardiopulmonary bypass, hemolysis, and nitroprusside-induced cyanide production. *Anesth Analg* 2007;105:29–33.

240. Fremes SE, Weisel RD, Mickle DAG, et al. A comparison of nitroglycerin and nitroprusside: I: treatment of postoperative hypertension. *Ann Thorac Surg* 1985;39:53–60.

241. Bojar RM, Rastegar H, Payne DD, et al. Methemoglobinemia from intravenous nitroglycerin: a word of caution. *Ann Thorac Surg* 1987;43:332–4.

242. Wijeysundera DN, Beattie WS, Rao V, Karski J. Calcium antagonists reduce cardiovascular complications after cardiac surgery: a meta-analysis. *J Am Coll Cardiol* 2003;41:1496–505.

243. Espinosa A, Ripollés-Melchor J, Casans-Francés R, et al. Perioperative use of clevidipine: a systematic review and meta-analysis. *PLoS One* 2016;11:e0150625.

244. Aronson S. Clevidipine in the treatment of perioperative hypertension: assessing safety events in the ECLIPSE trials. *Expert Rev Cardiovasc Ther* 2009;7:465–72.

245. Ulici A, Jancik J, Lam TS, Reidt S, Calcaterra D, Cole JB. Clevidipine versus sodium nitroprusside in acute aortic dissection: a retrospective chart review. *Am J Emerg Med* 2017;35:1514–8.

246. Alviar CL, Gutierrez A, Cho L, et al. Clevidipine as a therapeutic and cost-effective alternative to sodium nitroprusside in patients with acute aortic syndromes. *Eur Heart J Acute Cardiovasc Care* 2018;Jun 1:2048872618777919.

247. Aronson S, Dyke CM, Stierer KA, et al. The ECLIPSE trials: comparative studies of clevidipine to nitroglycerin, sodium nitroprusside, and nicardipine for acute hypertension treatment in cardiac surgery patients. *Anesth Analg* 2008;107:1110–21.

248. Grigore AM, Castro JL, Swistel D, Thys DM. Nicardipine infusion for the prevention of radial artery spasm during myocardial revascularization. *J Cardiothorac Vasc Anesth* 1998;12:556–7.

249. Chanda J, Brichkov I, Canver CC. Prevention of radial artery graft vasospasm after coronary bypass. *Ann Thorac Surg* 2000;70:2070–4.

250. Chanda J, Canver CC. Reversal of preexisting vasospasm in coronary artery conduits. *Ann Thorac Surg* 2001;72:476–80.

251. Apostolidou IA, Despotis GJ, Hogue CW Jr. Antiischemic effects of nicardipine and nitroglycerin after coronary artery bypass grafting. *Ann Thorac Surg* 1999;67:417–22.

252. Sladen RN, Klamerus KJ, Swafford MW, et al. Labetalol for the control of elevated blood pressure following coronary artery bypass grafting. *J Cardiothorac Anesth* 1990;4:210–21.

253. Gombotz H, Plaza J, Mahla E, Berger J, Metzler H. DA1-receptor stimulation by fenoldopam in the treatment of postcardiac surgical hypertension. *Acta Anaesthesiol Scand* 1998;42:834–40.

254. Kulik A, Ruel M, Jneid J, et al. Secondary prevention after coronary artery bypass graft surgery: a scientific statement from the American Heart Association. *Circulation* 2015;131:927–64.

255. Jain U. Myocardial infarction during coronary artery bypass surgery. *J Cardiothorac Vasc Anesth* 1992;6:612–23.

256. Thielmann M, Sharma V, Al-Attar N, et al. ESC Joint Working Groups on cardiovascular surgery and the cellular biology of the heart position paper: peri-operative myocardial injury and infarction in patients undergoing coronary artery bypass graft surgery. *European Heart Journal* 2017;38:2392–411.

257. Thygesen K, Alpert JS, Jaffe AS, et al. Fourth universal definition of myocardial infarction (2018). *J Am Coll Cardiol* 2018;72:2231–64.

258. Svedjeholm R, Dahlin LG, Lundberg G, et al. Are electrocardiographic Q-wave criteria reliable for diagnosis of perioperative myocardial infarction after coronary surgery? *Eur J Cardiothorac Surg* 1998;13:655–61.

259. Zangrillo A, Pappalardo F, Dossi R, et al. Preoperative intra-aortic balloon pump to reduce mortality in coronary artery bypass graft: a meta-analysis of randomized controlled trials. *Crit Care* 2015;19:10.

260. Gaudino M, Nesta M, Burzotta F, et al. Results of emergency postoperative re-angiography after cardiac surgery procedures. *Ann Thorac Surg* 2015;99:1576–82.

261. Alqahtani F, Ziada KM, Badhwar V, Sandhu G, Rihal CS, Alkhouli M. Incidence, predictors, and outcomes of in-hospital percutaneous coronary intervention following coronary artery bypass grafting. *J Am Coll Cardiol* 2010;73:415–23.

262. Croal BL, Hillis GS, Gibson PH, et al. Relationship between postoperative cardiac troponin I levels and outcome of cardiac surgery. *Circulation* 2006;114:1468–75.

263. Steuer J, Horte LG, Lindahl B, Stahle E. Impact of perioperative myocardial injury on early and long-term outcome after coronary artery bypass grafting. *Eur Heart J* 2002;23:1219–27.

264. Riedel BJ, Grattan A, Martin CB, Gal J, Shaw AD, Royston D. Long-term outcome of patients with perioperative myocardial infarction as diagnosed by troponin I after routine surgical coronary artery revascularization. *J Cardiothorac Vasc Anesth* 2006;20:781–7.

265. Petäjä L, Salmenperä M, Pulkki K, Pettilä V. Biochemical injury markers and mortality after coronary artery bypass grafting: a systematic review. *Ann Thorac Surg* 2009;87:1981–92.

266. Force T, Hibberd P, Weeks G, et al. Perioperative myocardial infarction after coronary artery bypass surgery: clinical significance and approach to risk stratification. *Circulation* 1990;82:903–12.

267. He GW, Taggart DP. Spasm in arterial grafts in coronary artery bypass grafting surgery. *Ann Thorac Surg* 2016;101:1222–9.

268. He FW, Taggart DP. Antispastic management in arterial grafts. *Ann Thorac Surg* 2016;102:659–68.

269. Gaudino M, Benedetto U, Fremes SE, et al. Effect of calcium-channel blocker therapy on radial artery grafts after coronary bypass surgery. *J Am Coll Cardiol* 2019;73:2299–306.

270. Minato NM, Katayama Y, Sakaguchi M, Itoh M. Perioperative coronary artery spasm in off-pump coronary artery bypass grafting and its possible relationship with perioperative hypomagnesemia. *Ann Thorac Cardiovasc Surg* 2006;12:32–6.

271. Havrilla PL, Kane-Gill SL, Verrico MM, Seybert AL, Reis SE. Coronary vasospasm and atrial fibrillation associated with ondansetron therapy. *Ann Pharmacother* 2009;43:532–6.

272. Piao ZH, Jeong MH, Li Y, Jin L, Kim HK. Benefit of statin therapy in patients with coronary spasm-induced acute myocardial infarction. *Cardiol* 2016;68:7–12.

273. Lorusso R, Crudeli E, Lucà F, et al. Refractory spasm of coronary arteries and grafted conduits after isolated coronary artery bypass surgery. *Ann Thorac Surg* 2012;93:545–51.

274. Vakil K, Kealhofer JV, Alraies MC, et al. Long-term outcomes of patients who had cardiac arrest after cardiac operations. *Ann Thorac Surg* 2016;102:512–7.

275. The Society of Thoracic Surgeons Task Force on Resuscitation After Cardiac Surgery. The Society of Thoracic Surgeons Expert Consensus for the resuscitation of patients who arrest after cardiac surgery. *Ann Thorac Surg* 2017;103:1005–20.

276. Dunning J, Fabbri A, Kolh PH, et al. Guideline for resuscitation in cardiac arrest after cardiac surgery. *Eur J Cardiothorac Surg* 2009;36:3–28.

277. Truhlář A, Deakin CD, Soar J, et al. European Resuscitation Council guidelines for resuscitation 2015: section 4: cardiac arrest in special circumstances. *Resuscitation* 2015;95:148–201.

278. Twomey D, Das M, Subramanian H, Dunning J. Is internal massage superior to external massage for patients suffering a cardiac arrest after cardiac surgery? *Interact Cardiovasc Thorac Surg* 2008;7:151–6.

279. Aung K, Htay T. Vasopressin for cardiac arrest: a systematic review and meta-analysis. *Arch Intern Med* 2005;165:17–24.

280. Reser D, Biefer HRC, Plass A, et al. Incidence of sternal wound infection after reexploration in the intensive care unit and the use of local gentamycin. *Ann Thorac Surg* 2012;94:2033–7.

281. Reade MC. Temporary epicardial pacing after cardiac surgery: a practical review: part 1: general considerations in the management of epicardial pacing. *Anaesthesia* 2007;62:264–71.

282. Reade MC. Temporary epicardial pacing after cardiac surgery: a practical review: part 2: selection of epicardial pacing modes and troubleshooting. *Anaesthesia* 2007;62:364–73.

283. Bethea BT, Salazar JD, Grega MA, et al. Determining the utility of temporary pacing wires after coronary artery bypass surgery. *Ann Thorac Surg* 2005;79:104–7.

284. Broka SM, Ducart AR, Collard EL, et al. Hemodynamic benefit of optimizing atrioventricular delay after cardiopulmonary bypass. *J Cardiothorac Vasc Anesth* 1997;11:723–8.

285. Atlee JL III, Pattison CZ, Mathews EL, Hedman AG. Transesophageal atrial pacing for intraoperative sinus bradycardia or AV junctional rhythm: feasibility as prophylaxis in 200 anesthetized adults and hemodynamic effects of treatment. *J Cardiothorac Vasc Anesth* 1993;7:436–41.

286. Kumbhani DJ, Sharma GV, Khuri SF, Kirdar JA. Fascicular conduction disturbances after coronary artery bypass surgery: a review with a meta-analysis of their long-term significance. *J Card Surg* 2006;21:428–34.

287. Gordon RS, Ivanov J, Cohen G, Ralph-Edwards AL. Permanent cardiac pacing after a cardiac operation: predicting the use of permanent pacemakers. *Ann Thorac Surg* 1998;66:1698–704.

288. Al-Ghamdi B, Mallawi Y, Shafquat A, et al. Predictors of permanent pacemaker implantation after coronary artery bypass grafting and valve surgery in adult patients in current surgical era. *Cardiol Res* 2016;7:123–9.

289. Meri O, Ilan M, Oren A, et al. Permanent pacemaker implantation following cardiac surgery: indications and long-term follow-up. *Pacing Clin Electrophysiol* 2009;32:7–12.

290. Lukac P, Hjortdal VE, Pedersen AK, Mortensen PT, Jensen HK, Hansen PS. Superior transseptal approach to mitral valve is associated with a higher need for pacemaker implantation than the left atrial approach. *Ann Thorac Surg* 2007;83:77–82.

291. Mahaffey JH, Haywood NS, Hawkins RB, et al. Need for permanent pacemaker after surgical aortic valve replacement reduces long-term survival. *Ann Thorac Surg* 2018;106:460–5.

292. Dawkins S, Hobson AR, Kalra PR, Tang ATM, Monro JL, Dawkins KD. Permanent pacemaker implantation after isolated aortic valve replacement: incidence, indications, and predictors. *Ann Thorac Surg* 2008;85:108–12.

293. Siontis GC, Juni P, Pilgrim T, et al. Predictors of permanent pacemaker implantation in patients with severe aortic stenosis undergoing TAVR: a meta-analysis. *J Am Coll Cardiol* 2014;64:129–40.

294. Auffret V, Webb JG, Eltchaninoff H, et al. Clinical impact of baseline right bundle branch block in patients undergoing transcatheter aortic valve replacement. *JACC Cardiovasc Interv* 2017;10:1564–74.

295. Urena M, Webb JG, Tamburino C, et al. Permanent pacemaker implantation after transcatheter aortic valve implantation: impact on late clinical outcomes and left ventricular function. *Circulation* 2014;129:1233–43.

296. Regueiro A, Abdul-Jawad Altisent O, Del Trigo M, et al. Impact of new-onset left bundle branch block and periprocedural permanent pacemaker implantation on clinical outcomes in patients undergoing transcatheter aortic valve replacement: a systematic review and meta-analysis. *Circ Cardiovasc Interv* 2016;9:e003635.

297. Chamandi C, Barbanti M, Munoz-Garcia A, et al. Long-term outcomes in patients with new-onset persistent left bundle branch block following TAVR. *JACC Cardiovasc Interv* 2019;12:1175–84.

298. Nazif TM, Chen S, George I, et al. New-onset left bundle branch block after transcatheter aortic valve replacement is associated with adverse long-term clinical outcomes in intermediate-risk patients: an analysis from the Partner II trial. *Eur Heart J* 2019;40:2218–27.

299. Birnie DH, Healey JS, Essebag V. Management of anticoagulation around pacemaker and defibrillator surgery. *Circulation* 2014;129:2062–5.

300. Glikson M, Dearani JA, Hyberger LK, Schaff HV, Hammill SC, Hayes DL. Indications, effectiveness, and long-term dependency in permanent pacing after cardiac surgery. *Am J Cardiol* 1997;80:1309–13.

301. Kaplan RM, Yadlapati A, Cantey EP, et al. Conduction recovery following pacemaker implantation after transcatheter aortic valve replacement. *Pacing Clin Electrophysiol* 2019;42:146–52.

302. Thomas JL, Dickstein RA, Parker FB Jr, et al. Prognostic significance of the development of left bundle conduction defects following aortic valve replacement. *J Thorac Cardiovasc Surg* 1982;84:382–6.

303. Rodés-Abau J, Ellenbogen KA, Krahn AD, et al. Management of conduction disturbances associated with transcatheter aortic valve replacement: JACC Scientific Expert Panel. *J Am Coll Cardiol* 2019;74:1086–106.

304. Cameron MJ, Tran DTT, Abboud J, Newton EK, Rashidian H, Dupuis JY. Prospective external validation of three preoperative risk scores for prediction of new onset atrial fibrillation after cardiac surgery. *Anesth Analg* 2018;126:33–8.

305. Burgos LM, Seoane L, Parodi JB, et al. Postoperative atrial fibrillation is associated with higher scores on predictive indices. *J Thorac Cardiovasc Surg* 2019;157:2279–86.

306. Mariscalco G, Biancari F, Zanobini M, et al. Bedside tool for predicting the risk of postoperative atrial fibrillation after cardiac surgery: the POAF score. *J Am Heart Assoc* 2014;3:e000752.

307. Mathew JP, Fontes ML, Tudor IC, et al. A multicenter risk index for atrial fibrillation after cardiac surgery. *JAMA* 2004;291:1720–9.

308. Pollock BD, Filardo G, da Graca B, et al. Predicting new-onset post-coronary artery bypass graft atrial fibrillation with existing risk scores. *Ann Thorac Surg* 2018;105:115–21.

309. Burrage PS, Low YH, Campbell NG, O'Brien B. New-onset atrial fibrillation in adult patients after cardiac surgery. *Current Anesth Reports* 2019;9:174–93.

310. Lomivorotov VV, Efremov SM, Pokushalov EA, Karaskov AM. New-onset atrial fibrillation after cardiac surgery: pathophysiology, prophylaxis, and treatment. *J Cardiothorac Vasc Anesth* 2016;30:200–16.

311. Muehlschlegel JD, Burrage PS, Ngai JY, et al. Society of Cardiovascular Anesthesiologists/European Association of Cardiothoracic Anaesthetists practice advisory for the management of perioperative atrial fibrillation in patients undergoing cardiac surgery. *Anesth Analg* 2019;128:33–42.

312. DiDomenico RJ, Massad MG. Pharmacologic strategies for prevention of atrial fibrillation after open heart surgery. *Ann Thorac Surg* 2005;79:728–40.

313. Anderson E, Dyke C, Levy JH. Anticoagulation strategies for the management of postoperative atrial fibrillation. *Clin Lab Med* 2014;34:537–61.

314. Lowres N, Mulcahy G, Jin K, Gallagher R, Neubeck L, Freedman B. Incidence of postoperative atrial fibrillation recurrence in patients discharged in sinus rhythm after cardiac surgery: a systematic review and meta-analysis. *Interact Cardiovasc Thorac Surg* 2018;26:504–11.

315. Lee SH, Kang DR, Uhm JS, et al. New-onset atrial fibrillation predicts long-term newly developed atrial fibrillation after coronary artery bypass graft. *Am Heart J* 2014;167:593–600.

316. Park YM, Cha MS, Park CH, et al. Newly developed post-operative atrial fibrillation is associated with an increased risk of late recurrence of atrial fibrillation in patients who underwent open heart surgery: long-term follow up. *Cardiol J* 2017;24:633–41.

317. Phan K, Ha HS, Phan S, Medi C, Thomas SP, Yan TD. New-onset atrial fibrillation following coronary bypass surgery predicts long-term mortality: a systematic review and meta-analysis. *Eur J Cardiothorac Surg* 2015;48:817–24.

318. Kaw R, Hernandez AV, Masood I, Gillinov AM, Saliba W, Blackstone EH. Short- and long-term mortality associated with new-onset atrial fibrillation after coronary artery bypass grafting: a systematic review and meta-analysis. *J Thorac Cardiovasc Surg* 2011;141:1305–12.

319. Lin MH, Kamel HM, Singer DE, Wu YL, Lee M, Ovbiagele B. Perioperative/postoperative atrial fibrillation and risk of subsequent stroke and/or mortality. *Stroke* 2019;50:1364–71.

320. Filardo G, Hamilton C, Hamman B, Hebeler RF Jr, Adams J, Grayburn P. New-onset postoperative atrial fibrillation and long-term survival after aortic valve replacement surgery. *Ann Thorac Surg* 2010;90:474–80.

321. Sigursson MI, Longford NT, Heydarpour M, et al. Duration of postoperative atrial fibrillation after cardiac surgery is associated with worsened long-term survival. *Ann Thorac Surg* 2016;10:2018–26.

322. Yadava M, Hughey AB, Crawford TC. Postoperative atrial fibrillation: incidence, mechanisms, and clinical correlates. *Heart Fail Clin* 2016;12:299–306.

323. Bohatch Júnior MS, Matkovski PD, et al. Incidence of postoperative atrial fibrillation in patients undergoing on-pump and off-pump coronary artery bypass grafting. *Rev Bras Cir Cardiovasc* 2015;30:316–24.

324. Lewicki L, Siebert J, Rogowski J. Atrial fibrillation following off-pump versus on-pump coronary artery bypass grafting: incidence and risk factors. *Cardiol J* 2016;223:518–23.

325. January CT, Wann LS, Calkins H, et al. 2019 AHA/ACC/HRS focus update on the 2014 AHA/ACC/HRS guideline for the management of patients with atrial fibrillation. *J Am Coll Cardiol* 2019;74:104–32.

326. Kirchof P, Benussi S, Kotecha D, et al. 2016 ESC guidelines for the management of atrial fibrillation developed in collaboration with EACST. *Eur Heart J* 2016;37:2893–2962.

327. Arsenault KA, Yusuf AM, Crystal E, et al. Interventions for preventing post-operative atrial fibrillation in patients undergoing heart surgery. *Cochrane Database Syst Rev* 2013;31:CD003611. https://doi.org/10.1002/14651858.CD003611.pub3.

328. Burgess DC, Kilborn MJ, Keech AC. Interventions for prevention of post-operative atrial fibrillation and its complications after cardiac surgery: a meta-analysis. *Eur Heart J* 2006;27:2846–57.

329. DiNicolantonio JJ, Beavers CJ, Menezes AR, et al. Meta-analysis comparing carvedilol versus metoprolol for the prevention of postoperative atrial fibrillation following coronary artery bypass grafting. *Am J Cardiol* 2014;113:565–9.

330. Wang JS, Wang ZW, Yin ZT. Carvedilol for prevention of atrial fibrillation after cardiac surgery: a meta-analysis. *PLoS One* 2014;9:e954005.

331. Acikel S, Bozbas J, Gultekin B, et al. Comparison of the efficacy of metoprolol and carvedilol for preventing atrial fibrillation after coronary bypass surgery. *Int J Cardiol* 2008;126:108–13.

332. Solomon AJ, Greenberg MD, Kilborn MJ, Katz NM. Amiodarone versus a beta-blocker to prevent atrial fibrillation after cardiovascular surgery. *Am Heart J* 2001;142:811–5.

333. Bagshaw SM, Galbraith PD, Mitchell LB, Sauve R, Exner DV, Ghali WA. Prophylactic amiodarone for prevention of atrial fibrillation after cardiac surgery: a meta-analysis. *Ann Thorac Surg* 2006;82:1927–37.

334. Beaulieu Y, Denault AY, Couture P, et al. Perioperative intravenous amiodarone does not reduce the burden of atrial fibrillation in patients undergoing cardiac valvular surgery. *Anesthesiology* 2010;112:128–37.

335. Mitchell LB, Exner DV, Wyse G, et al. Prophylactic oral amiodarone for the prevention of arrhythmias that begin early after revascularization, valve replacement, or repair: PAPABEAR: a randomized controlled trial. *JAMA* 2005;294:3093–100.

336. Zebis LR, Christensen TD, Thomsen HF, et al. Practical regimen for amiodarone use in preventing postoperative atrial fibrillation. *Ann Thorac Surg* 2007;83:1326–31.

337. Kerstein J, Soodan A, Qamar M, et al. Giving IV and oral amiodarone perioperatively for the prevention of postoperative atrial fibrillation in patients undergoing coronary artery bypass surgery: the GAP study. *Chest* 2004;126:716–24.

338. Kuralay E, Cingöz F, Kiliç S, et al. Supraventricular tachyarrhythmia prophylaxis after coronary artery surgery in chronic obstructive pulmonary disease patients (early amiodarone prophylaxis trial). *Eur J Cardiothorac Surg* 2004;25:224–30.

339. Teerakanok J, Tantrachoti P, Chariyawong P, Nugent K. Acute amiodarone pulmonary toxicity after surgical procedures. *Am J Med Sci* 2016;352:646–51.

340. Izhar U, Ad N, Rudis E, et al. When should we discontinue antiarrhythmic therapy for atrial fibrillation after coronary artery bypass grafting? A prospective randomized study. *J Thorac Cardiovasc Surg* 2005;129:401–6.

341. Trivedi C, Upadhyay A, Solanki K. Efficacy of ranolazine in preventing atrial fibrillation following cardiac surgery: results from a meta-analysis. *J Arrhythm* 2017;33:161–6.

342. Patel N, Kluger J. Ranolazine for prevention of atrial fibrillation after cardiac surgery: a systematic review. *Cureus* 2018;10:e2584.

343. De Vecchis R, Ariano C, Giasi A, Cioppa C. Antiarrhythmic effects of ranolazine used both alone for prevention of atrial fibrillation and as an add-on to intravenous amiodarone for its pharmacological cardioversion: a meta-analysis. *Minerva Cardangiol* 2018;66:349–59,

344. Sımopoulos V, Hevas A, Hatziefthimiou A, et al. Amiodarone plus ranolazine for conversion of post-cardiac surgery atrial fibrillation: enhanced effectiveness in reduced versus preserved ejection fraction patients. *Cardiovasc Drugs Ther* 2018;32:559–65.

345. Tagarakis CI, Aidonidis I, Daskalopoulou SS, et al. Effect of ranolazine in preventing postoperative atrial fibrillation in patients undergoing coronary revascularization surgery. *Curr Vasc Pharmacol* 2013;11:988–91.

346. Wurdeman RL, Mooss AN, Mohiuddin SM, Lenz TL. Amiodarone vs. sotalol as prophylaxis against atrial fibrillation/flutter after heart surgery: a meta-analysis. *Chest* 2002;121:1203–10.

347. Cook RC, Yamashita MH, Kearns M, Ramanathan K, Gin K, Humphries KH. Prophylactic magnesium does not prevent atrial fibrillation after cardiac surgery: a meta-analysis. *Ann Thorac Surg* 2013;95:533–41.

348. Forlani S, De Paulis R, de Notaris S, et al. Combination of sotalol and magnesium prevents atrial fibrillation after coronary artery bypass grafting. *Ann Thorac Surg* 2002;74:720–6.

349. Shepherd J, Jones J, Frampton GK, Tanajewski L, Turner D, Price A. Intravenous magnesium sulphate and sotalol for prevention of atrial fibrillation after coronary artery bypass surgery: a systematic review and economic evaluation. *Health Technol Assess* 2008;12:iii–iv, ix–95.

350. Archbold RA, Schilling RJ. Atrial pacing for the prevention of atrial fibrillation after coronary artery bypass graft surgery: a review of the literature. *Heart* 2004;90:129–33.

351. Debrunner M, Naegeli B, Genoni M, Turina M, Bertel O. Prevention of atrial fibrillation after cardiac valvular surgery by epicardial, biatrial synchronous pacing. *Eur J Cardiothorac Surg* 2004;25:16–20.

352. Seraminovski N, Burke P, Khawaja O, Sekulic M, Machado C. Usefulness of dofetilide for the prevention of atrial tachyarrhythmias (atrial fibrillation or flutter) after coronary artery bypass grafting. *Am J Cardiol* 2008;101:1574–9.

353. Merrick AF, Odom NJ, Keenan DJ, Grotte GJ. Comparison of propafenone to atenolol for the prophylaxis of postcardiotomy supraventricular tachyarrhythmias: a prospective trial. *Eur J Cardiothorac Surg* 1995;9:146–9.

354. Lennerz C, Barman M, Tantaway M, Sopher M, Whittaker P. Colchicine for primary prevention of atrial fibrillation after open-heart surgery: systematic review and meta-analysis. *Int J Cardiol* 2017;249:127–37.

355. Dvirnik N, Belley-Cote EP, Hanif H, et al. Steroids in cardiac surgery: a systematic review and meta-analysis. *Br J Anaesth* 2018;120:657–67.

356. Halonen J, Halonen P, Järvinen O, et al. Corticosteroids for the prevention of atrial fibrillation after cardiac surgery: a randomized controlled trial. *JAMA* 2007;297:1562–7.

357. Prasongsukarn K, Abel JG, Jamieson WRE, et al. The effects of steroids on the occurrence of postoperative atrial fibrillation after coronary artery bypass grafting surgery: a prospective randomized trial. *J Thorac Cardiovasc Surg* 2005;130:93–8.

358. Kouliouros A, Valencia O, Hosseini MT, et al. Preoperative high-dose atorvastatin for prevention of atrial fibrillation after cardiac surgery: a randomized controlled trial. *J Thorac Cardiovasc Surg* 2011;141:244–8.

359. Rezaei Y, Gholami-Fesharaki M, Dehghani MR, Arya A, Haghjoo M, Arjmand N. Statin antiarrhythmic effect on atrial fibrillation in statin-naive patients undergoing cardiac surgery: a meta-analysis of randomized controlled trials. *J Cardiovasc Pharmacol Ther* 2016;21:167–76.

360. Karimi A, Biheni LM, Rezvanfard M, et al. The effect of high dose of atorvastatin on the occurrence of atrial fibrillation after coronary artery bypass grafting. *Ann Thorac Surg* 2012;94:8–14.

361. Kuhn EW, Liakopoulos OJ, Stange S, et al. Preoperative statin therapy in cardiac surgery: a meta-analysis of 90,000 patients. *Eur J Cardiothorac Surg* 2014;45:17–26.

362. Putzu A, Capelli B, Belletti A, et al. Perioperative statin therapy in cardiac surgery: a meta-analysis of randomized controlled trials. *Crit Care* 2016;20:395.

363. Eslami M, Badkoubeh RS, Mousavi M, et al. Oral ascorbic acid in combination with beta-blockers is more effective than beta-blockers alone in the prevention of atrial fibrillation after coronary artery bypass grafting. *Tex Heart Inst J* 2007;34:268–74.

364. Ali-Hasan-Al-Saegh S, Mirhosseini SJ, Tahernejad M, et al. Impact of antioxidant supplementations on cardio-renal protection in cardiac surgery: an updated and comprehensive meta-analysis and systematic review. *Cardiovasc Ther* 2016;34:360–70.

365. Antonic M, Lipovec R, Gregorcic F, Juric P, Kosir G. Perioperative ascorbic acid supplementation does not improve the incidence of postoperative atrial fibrillation in on-pump coronary artery bypass graft patients. *J Cardiol* 2017;69:98–102.

366. Mirmohammadsadeghi M, Mirmohammadsadeghi A, Mahmouian M. Preventive use of ascorbic acid for atrial fibrillation after coronary artery bypass graft surgery. *Heart Surg Forum* 2018;21: E415–7.

367. Wang H, Chen J, Zhao L. N-3 polyunsaturated fatty acids for prevention of postoperative atrial fibrillation: an updated meta-analysis and systematic review. *J Interv Card Electrophysiol* 2018;51:105–15.

368. Mozaffarian D, Marchioli R, Macchia A, et al. Fish oil and postoperative atrial fibrillation: the Omega-3 fatty acids for prevention of post-operative atrial fibrillation (OPERA) randomized trial. *JAMA* 2012;308:2001–11.

369. Rodrigo R, Korantzopoulos P, Cereceda M, et al. A randomized controlled trial to prevent postoperative atrial fibrillation by antioxidant reinforcement. *J Am Coll Cardiol* 2013;62:1457–65.

370. Soleimani A, Habibi MR, Kiabi FH, et al. The effect of intravenous N-acetylcysteine on the prevention of atrial fibrillation after coronary artery bypass graft surgery: a double-blind, randomised, placebo-controlled trial. *Kardiol Pol* 2018;76:99–106.

371. St. Onge S, Perrault LP, Demers P, et al. Pericardial blood as a trigger for postoperative atrial fibrillation after cardiac surgery. *Ann Thorac Surg* 2018;105:321–8.

372. Biancari F, Mahar MAA. Meta-analysis of randomized trials on the efficacy of posterior pericariotomy in preventing atrial fibrillation after coronary artery bypass surgery. *J Thorac Cardiovasc Surg* 2010;139:1158–61.

373. Soucier RJ, Mirza S, Abordo MG, et al. Predictors of conversion of atrial fibrillation after cardiac operations in the absence of class I or III antiarrhythmic medications. *Ann Thorac Surg* 2001;72:694–8.

374. Chung MK, Shemanski L, Sherman DG, et al. Functional status in rate- versus rhythm-control strategies for atrial fibrillation: results of the Atrial Fibrillation Follow-up Investigation of Rhythm Management (AFFIRM) functional status substudy. *J Am Coll Cardiol* 2005;46:1891–9.

375. Samuels LE, Holmes EC, Samuels FL. Selective use of amiodarone and early cardioversion for postoperative atrial fibrillation. *Ann Thorac Surg* 2005;79:113–6.

376. Klein AL, Grimm RA, Murray RD, et al. Use of transesophageal echocardiography to guide cardioversion in patients with atrial fibrillation. *N Engl J Med* 2001;344:1411–20.

377. Black IW, Fatkin D, Sagar KB, et al. Exclusion of atrial thrombus by transesophageal echocardiography does not preclude embolism after cardioversion of atrial fibrillation: a multicenter study. *Circulation* 1994;89:2509–13.

378. Harjai KJ, Mobarek SK, Cheirif J, Boulos LM, Murgo JP, Abi-Samra F. Clinical variables affecting recovery of left atrial mechanical function after cardioversion from atrial fibrillation. *J Am Coll Cardiol* 1997;30:481–6.

379. Stambler BS, Wood MA, Ellenbogen KA. Comparative efficacy of intravenous ibutilide versus procainamide for enhancing termination of atrial flutter by atrial overdrive pacing. *Am J Cardiol* 1996;77:960–6.

380. D'Este D, Bertaglia E, Mantovan R, Zanocco Z, Franceschi M, Pascotto P. Efficacy of intravenous propafenone in termination of atrial flutter by overdrive transesophageal pacing previously ineffective. *Am J Cardiol* 1997;79:500–2.

381. Hilleman DE, Reyes AP, Mooss AN, Packard KA. Esmolol versus diltiazem in atrial fibrillation following coronary artery bypass graft surgery. *Curr Med Res Opin* 2003;19:376–82.

382. Eagle KA, Guyton RA, Davidoff R, et al. ACC/AHA 2004 guideline update for coronary artery bypass graft surgery (summary article: a report of the American College of Cardiology/American Heart Association Task Force on Practice Guidelines [Committee to Update the 1999 Guidelines for coronary artery bypass graft surgery]). *J Am Coll Cardiol* 2004;44:1146–54.

383. Epstein AE, Alexander JC, Gutterman DD, Maisel W, Wharton JM. Anticoagulation: American College of Chest Physicians guidelines for the prevention and management of atrial fibrillation after cardiac surgery. *Chest* 2005;128(2 Suppl):24S–7S.

384. Kollar A, Lick SD, Vasquez KN, Conti VR. Relationship of atrial fibrillation and stroke after coronary artery bypass graft surgery: when is anticoagulation indicated? *Ann Thorac Surg* 2006;82:515–23.

385. Lahtinen J, Biancari F, Salmela E, et al. Postoperative atrial fibrillation is a major cause of stroke after on-pump coronary artery bypass surgery. *Ann Thorac Surg* 2004;77:1241–4.

386. Stoddard MF, Dawkins PR, Prince CR, Ammash NM. Left atrial appendage thrombus is not uncommon in patients with acute atrial fibrillation and a recent embolic event: a transesophageal echocardiographic study. *J Am Coll Cardiol* 1995;25:452–9.

387. Zhu W, He W, Guo L, Wang X, Hong K. The HAS-BLED score for predicting major bleeding risk in anticoagulated patients with atrial fibrillation: a systematic review and meta-analysis. *Clin Cardiol* 2015;38:555–61.

388. Gullestad L, Birkeland K, Molstad P, Hoyer MM, Vanberg P, Kjekshus J. The effect of magnesium versus verapamil on supraventricular arrhythmias. *Clin Cardiol* 1993;16:429–34.

389. Kochiadakis GE, Igoumenidis NE, Simantirakis EN, et al. Intravenous propafenone versus intravenous amiodarone in the management of atrial fibrillation of recent onset: a placebo-controlled study. *Pacing Clin Electrophysiol* 1998;21:2475–9.

390. Nemati MH, Astenah B. Amiodarone versus propafenone to treat atrial fibrillation after coronary artery bypass grafting: a randomized double blind controlled trial. *Korean J Thorac Cardiovasc Surg* 2016;49:177–84.

391. Martinez-Marcos FJ, Garcia-Garmendia JL, Ortega-Carpio A, Fernández-Gómez JM, Santos JM, Camacho C. Comparison of intravenous flecainide, propafenone, and amiodarone for conversion of acute atrial fibrillation to sinus rhythm. *Am J Cardiol* 2000;86:950–3.

392. Boriani G, Capucci A, Lenzi T, Sanguinetti M, Magnani B. Propafenone for conversion of recent-onset atrial fibrillation: a controlled comparison between oral loading dose and intravenous administration. *Chest* 1995;108:355–8.

393. VanderLugt KT, Mattioni T, Denker S, et al. Efficacy and safety of ibutilide fumarate for the conversion of atrial arrhythmias after cardiac surgery. *Circulation* 1999;100:369–75.

394. Bernard EO, Schmid ER, Schmidlin D, Scharf C, Candinas R, Germann R. Ibutilide versus amiodarone in atrial fibrillation: a double-blinded, randomized study. *Crit Care Med* 2003;31:1031–4.

395. Lindeboom JE, Kingma JH, Crijns HJGM, Dunselman PHJM. Efficacy and safety of intravenous dofetilide for rapid termination of atrial fibrillation and flutter. *Am J Cardiol* 2000;85:1031–3.

396. Coleman CI, Sood N, Chawla D, et al. Intravenous magnesium sulfate enhances the ability of dofetilide to successfully cardiovert atrial fibrillation or flutter: results of the Dofetilide and Intravenous Magnesium Evaluation. *Europace* 2009;11:892–5.

397. Camm AJ, Capucci A, Honloser SH, et al. A randomized active-controlled study comparing the efficacy and safety of vernakalant to amiodarone in recent-onset atrial fibrillation. *J Am Coll Cardiol* 2011;57:313–21.

398. Kowey PR, Dorian P, Mitchell LB, et al. Vernakalant hydrochloride for the rapid conversion of atrial fibrillation after cardiac surgery: a randomized, double-blind placebo-controlled trial. *Circ Arrhythm Electrophysiol* 2009;2:652–9.

399. Savelieva I, Grayn R, Camm AJ. Pharmacological cardioversion of atrial fibrillation with vernakalant: evidence in support of the ESC guidelines. *Europace* 2014;16:162–73.

400. Dalyanogu H, Mehdiani A, Minol JP, et al. Conversion of atrial fibrillation after cardiosurgical procedures by vernakalant as an atrial repolarization delaying agent (ARDA). *Heart Surg Forum* 2018;21:E201–8.

401. Patel AN, Hamman BL, Patel AN, et al. Epicardial atrial defibrillation: successful treatment of postoperative atrial fibrillation. *Ann Thorac Surg* 2004;77:831–5.

402. Page RL, Joglar JA, Caldwell MA, et al. 2015 ACC/AHA/HRS guideline for the management of adult patients with supraventricular tachycardia: a Report of the American College of Cardiology/ American Heart Association Task Force on Clinical Practice Guidelines and the Heart Rhythm Society. *Circulation* 2016;133:e506–74.

403. Wilbur SL, Marchlinski FE. Adenosine as an antiarrhythmic agent. *Am J Cardiol* 1997;79:30–7.

404. Dougherty AH, Jackman WM, Naccarelli GV, Friday KJ, Dias VC, for the IV Diltiazem Study group. Acute conversion of paroxysmal supraventricular tachycardia with intravenous diltiazem. *Am J Cardiol* 1992;70:587–92.

405. Mouws EMJP, Yaksh A, Knops P, et al. Early ventricular tachyarrhythmias after coronary artery bypass grafting surgery: is it a real burden? *Jpn J Cardiol* 2017;70:263–70.

406. England MR, Gordon G, Salem M, Chernow B. Magnesium administration and dysrhythmias after cardiac surgery: a placebo-controlled, double-blind, randomized trial. *JAMA* 1992;268:2395–402.

407. Johnson RG, Goldberger AL, Thurer RL, Schwartz M, Sirois C, Weintraub RM. Lidocaine prophylaxis in coronary revascularization patients: a randomized, prospective trial. *Ann Thorac Surg* 1993;55:1180–4.

408. King FG, Addetia AM, Peters SD, Peachey GO. Prophylactic lidocaine for postoperative coronary artery bypass patients, a double-blind, randomized trial. *Can J Anaesth* 1990;37:363–8.

409. Lee EH, Lee HM, Chung CH, et al. Impact of intravenous lidocaine on myocardial injury after off-pump coronary artery surgery. *Brit J Anesth* 2011;106:487–93.

410. Steinberg JS, Gaur A, Sciacca R, Tan E. New-onset sustained ventricular tachycardia after cardiac surgery. *Circulation* 1999;99:903–8.

411. Ascione R, Reeves BC, Santo K, Khan N, Angelini GD. Predictors of new malignant ventricular arrhythmias after coronary surgery: a case-control study. *J Am Coll Cardiol* 2004;43:1630–8.

412. Yeung-Lai-Wah JA, Qi A, McNeill E, et al. New-onset sustained ventricular tachycardia and fibrillation early after cardiac operations. *Ann Thorac Surg* 2004;77:2083–8.

413. Cheng N, Gao C, Wang R, Yang M, Zhang L. New-onset ventricular arrhythmias in patients with left ventricular dysfunction after coronary surgery: incidence, risk factors, and prognosis. *Heart Surg Forum* 2018;21:E117–23.

414. Azar RR, Berns E, Seecharran B, Veronneau J, Lippman N, Kluger J. De novo monomorphic and polymorphic ventricular tachycardia following coronary artery bypass grafting. *Am J Cardiol* 1997;80:76–8.

415. Saxon LA, Wiener I, Natterson PD, Laks H, Drinkwater D, Stevenson WG. Monomorphic versus polymorphic ventricular tachycardia after coronary artery bypass grafting. *Am J Cardiol* 1995;75:403–5.

416. Stevenson WG, Tedrow UB, Koplan BA. Management of ventricular tachycardia complicating cardiac surgery. *Heart Rhythm* 2009;6:S66–9.

417. Sharma ND, Rosman HS, Padhi ID, Tisdale JE. Torsades de pointes associated with intravenous haloperidol in critically ill patients. *Am J Cardiol* 1998;81:238–40.

418. Lamas GA, Antman EM, Gold JP, Braunwald NS, Collins JJ. Pacemaker backup-mode reversion and injury during cardiac surgery. *Ann Thorac Surg* 1986;41:155–7.

419. Al-Khatib SM, Stevenson WG, Ackerman MJ, et al. 2017 AHA/ACC/HRS guideline for management of patients with ventricular arrhythmias and the prevention of sudden cardiac death: a report of the American College of Cardiology/American Heart Association Task Force on Clinical Practice Guidelines and the Heart Rhythm Society. *Circulation* 2018;138:e272–391.

420. Pinto RP, Romerill DB, Nasser WK, Schier JJ, Surawicz B. Prognosis of patients with frequent premature ventricular complexes and nonsustained ventricular tachycardia after coronary artery bypass surgery. *Clin Cardiol* 1996;19:321–4.

421. Roden DM. A practical approach to torsade de pointes. *Clin Cardiol* 1997;20:285–90.

422. Laub GW, Muralidharan S, Janeira L, et al. Refractory postoperative torsades de pointes syndrome successfully treated with isoproterenol. *J Cardiothorac Vasc Anesth* 1993;7:210–2.

423. Kowey PR, Marinchak RA, Rials SJ, Bharucha DB. Classification and pharmacology of antiarrhythmic drugs. *Am Heart J* 2000;140:12–20.

424. Lei M, Wu L, Terrar DA, Huang CL. Modernized classification of cardiac antiarrhythmic drugs. *Circulation* 2018;138:1879–96.

425. Capucci A, Piangerelli L, Bicciotti J, Gabrielli D, Guerra G. Flecainide-metoprolol combination reduces atrial fibrillation clinical recurrences and improves tolerability at 1-year follow-up for persistent symptomatic atrial fibrillation: randomized controlled trial. *Europace* 2016;18:1698–704.

426. Verrier RL, Kumar K, Nieminen T, Belardinelli L. Mechanisms of ranolazine's dual protection against atrial and ventricular fibrillation. *Europace* 2013;15:317–24.

427. Piga M, Serra A, Boi F, Tanda ML, Martino E, Mariotti S. Amiodarone-induced thyrotoxicosis: a review. *Minerva Endocrinol* 2008;33:213–28.

428. Lopez RD, Rordorf R, De Ferrari GM, et al. Digoxin and mortality in patients with atrial fibrillation. *J Am Coll Cardiol* 2018;71:1063–74.

429. Bhatia SJS, Smith TW. Digitalis toxicity: mechanisms, diagnosis, and management. *J Card Surg* 1987;2:453–65.

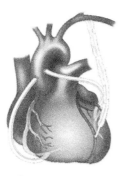

CHAPTER 12

Fluid Management, Renal, Metabolic, and Endocrine Problems

12 Fluid Management, Renal, Metabolic, and Endocrine Problems

Perioperative renal dysfunction is a major determinant of both operative and long-term mortality following cardiac surgery.[1-3] Even patients with mild renal dysfunction prior to surgery are more likely to experience acute kidney injury (AKI) afterwards, with compromised short- and long-term outcomes.[4,5] Therefore, it is essential to identify patients at high risk for developing postoperative AKI who may benefit from specific interventions aimed at optimizing renal function. Although many risk factors for AKI cannot be modified, measures can be taken preoperatively, during cardiac catheterization procedures, during surgery, and in the postoperative period to minimize the risk of developing AKI.[6] If it does develop, careful medical management and, if necessary, early aggressive use of renal replacement therapy may reduce the high mortality associated with postoperative AKI.

I. Body Water Distribution

An understanding of body water distribution is important when administering fluids to patients after open-heart surgery. Approximately 60% of the body's weight (50% in women) is water, with two-thirds of this residing in the intracellular space and one-third in the extracellular space. In the latter, two-thirds is in the interstitial space (the so-called third space), and one-third constitutes the intravascular volume.

A. Water moves freely among all three compartments and shifts so as to normalize serum osmolality (which generally reflects the serum sodium concentration).

B. Sodium moves freely between the intravascular and interstitial spaces but does not move passively into cells. Therefore, if a patient receives a hypotonic sodium load (e.g. 0.45% saline) which would lower the serum osmolality and sodium concentration, water will move from the extracellular space into the intracellular space to normalize these values. The presence of **a low serum sodium concentration in the postoperative patient usually indicates total body water overload.**

C. Starling's law governs the influence of hydrostatic and oncotic pressures on fluid shifts. The primary determinant of oncotic pressure is serum protein, which remains within the intravascular space. Elevated hydrostatic pressure (e.g. increased pulmonary capillary wedge pressure, PCWP) or lower intravascular colloid oncotic pressure (e.g. very low serum albumin, usually <2 g/dL) will shift fluid from the intravascular space into the interstitial space, contributing to lung and tissue edema. Conversely, raising the intravascular oncotic pressure with colloid (e.g. 25% albumin) in patients with hypoalbuminemia will tend to draw fluid from the lung interstitium back into the intravascular space.

Manual of Perioperative Care in Adult Cardiac Surgery, Sixth Edition. Robert M. Bojar.
© 2021 John Wiley & Sons Ltd. Published 2021 by John Wiley & Sons Ltd.

D. It should be kept in mind that Starling's law describes fluid shifts in the absence of abnormalities in membrane integrity. However, extracorporeal circulation is associated with a systemic inflammatory response, characterized by increased membrane permeability and a transient capillary leak. When this leak is present, administered fluid will shift more readily into the interstitial space. Clinically, one may note impaired oxygenation and decreased pulmonary compliance (higher peak pressures on the ventilator) associated with increased extravascular lung water. This can produce the picture of noncardiogenic pulmonary edema. Expansion of the interstitial space may also contribute to cerebral edema (mental obtundation), hepatic congestion (jaundice), and splanchnic congestion (ileus).

E. Because of the capillary leak associated with cardiopulmonary bypass (CPB), patients will be total body fluid overloaded, but can have low filling pressures with compromised cardiac output. Thus, until the capillary leak ceases, which is generally within 12 hours of surgery, fluid administration, whether colloid or crystalloid, will be required to optimize preload to maintain the cardiac output.

II. Effects of CPB and Off-Pump Surgery on Renal Function

A. The influence of CPB on renal function is multifactorial.[7–11] It involves nonpulsatile perfusion with hemodilution and variable degrees of hypothermia. A number of factors can adversely affect renal vasomotor tone, triggering a reduction in renal blood flow (RBF). The longer the duration of CPB, the more protracted the exposure to these adverse elements, increasing the risk of AKI.

1. CPB increases levels of hormones (endogenous catecholamines, vasopressin) and induces the renin–angiotensin–aldosterone cascade, altering vascular tone, RBF, glomerular filtration rate (GFR), filtration fraction, and electrolyte balance.

2. Hemodilution reduces the hematocrit (HCT) and oxygen-carrying capacity of blood.[12–15]

3. Vasodilation may also lower blood pressure during CPB, increasing fluid requirements and the need for vasopressor support to maintain an adequate mean arterial pressure. ACE inhibitors and ARBs may attenuate the effects of vasoconstrictors such as norepinephrine, so stopping them just prior to surgery may reduce the risk of hypotension during bypass and arguably will lower the risk of AKI.[16–21] Judicious use of other vasodilators during surgery (propofol, narcotics, inhalational anesthetics, nitroglycerin) may minimize hypotension during surgery as well.

4. Extracorporeal circulation evokes an inflammatory response with activation of complement and neutrophils, release of cytokines, and production of oxygen free radicals ("oxidative stress").

5. Aortic cannulation and clamping can generate atheroembolism.

6. Low-grade hemolysis from CPB may cause release of iron leading to oxidation from reactive oxygen species.[22]

B. CPB is associated with an increase in virtually all kidney-specific proteins that are markers for tubular damage.[23] Some of these, such as neutrophil gelatinase-associated lipocalin (NGAL), cystatin C, Kidney Injury Molecule-1 (KIM-1), and interleukin-18 (IL-18), have been shown to be early biomarkers of AKI that correlate with the severity and duration of AKI.[24–26] However, very few centers routinely evaluate renal function other than by serum creatinine (SCr) levels, and in the vast majority of cases, there is little significance to subtle changes in tubular function as long as the kidneys produce a satisfactory urine output with or without diuretics with minimal change in the SCr.

C. The potential benefit of avoiding CPB by performing off-pump coronary artery surgery (OPCAB) to reduce the risk of postoperative AKI is controversial.

1. Some studies have reported a reduction in AKI with OPCAB, but with no clear impact on the requirement for renal replacement therapy.[27–31] Others suggest that OPCAB reduces the incidence of postoperative AKI only in patients with normal renal function, but not those with preexisting chronic kidney disease (CKD).[32,33]

2. In theory, avoidance of CPB might preserve RBF and glomerular function better by maintaining a higher systemic pressure. Tubular epithelial function may be better preserved because of decreased complement activation and a lessened inflammatory response.[34] However, off-pump surgery is associated with significant fluid administration, use of comparable anesthetic and vasoactive medications, cytokine release that can damage proximal tubules, and alterations in perfusion pressure (lower systemic pressures with elevated venous pressures during exposure of the posterior heart and lower systemic pressures during construction of proximal anastomoses), all of which can adversely affect renal function.

3. Because postoperative renal dysfunction is related more to preexisting renal disease or significant hemodynamic alterations than to the inflammatory response, particular attention to fluid and hemodynamic management remains paramount no matter whether CPB is used or not.

III. Routine Fluid Management in the Early Postoperative Period

A. Hemodilution on CPB produces a state of total body sodium and water overload, expanding the body weight by about 5% (estimated at 800 mL/m^2/h, but quite variable in amount). Cardiac filling pressures usually do not reflect this state of fluid overload because of a capillary leak from the systemic inflammatory response, decreased plasma colloid osmotic pressure, impaired myocardial relaxation (diastolic dysfunction) from ischemia/reperfusion after cardioplegic arrest, and vasodilation.

1. Low filling pressures are consistent with hypovolemia despite the presence of body water overload, and additional fluid administration may be necessary to maintain satisfactory hemodynamics.

2. High filling pressures may suggest hypervolemia or ventricular dysfunction, but they may also be noted in the presence of hypovolemia, especially in patients with diastolic dysfunction or marked vasoconstriction, and additional fluid administration may be indicated in that situation. Use of Swan-Ganz monitoring (and its correlation with echocardiographic findings) is helpful in providing a scientific basis for fluid management after surgery, especially in patients with significant right or left ventricular dysfunction or after very complex operations with long durations of CPB, although it may not be necessary in low-risk patients.

B. Giving fluids to optimize preload and cardiac output in the early postoperative period may be required whether urine output is adequate or marginal (<1 mL/kg/h). During the first 4–6 hours after surgery, cardiac output is often depressed, and the achievement of satisfactory hemodynamics to optimize renal perfusion is dependent on both preload and inotropic support. Thus, fluid must invariably be administered to maintain intravascular volume and cardiac hemodynamics at the expense of expansion of the interstitial space. It should be noted that early extubation is helpful in reducing fluid requirements because it eliminates the adverse effects of positive-pressure ventilation on venous return and ventricular function.

C. It can be difficult to decide which fluid to administer to maintain filling pressures. Clearly, any fluid infused during a period of altered capillary membrane integrity will expand the interstitial space, but those that can more effectively expand the intravascular space while minimizing expansion of the interstitial space are preferable. Nonetheless, clinical outcomes are fairly comparable with colloid or crystalloid administration in critically ill patients, and this most likely holds true in most cardiac surgery patients who exhibit a systemic inflammatory response.[35,36] Most patients have enough pulmonary reserve to tolerate the volume overload until it can be diuresed, but those developing AKI with oliguria will have a more tenuous course.

1. Blood and colloids are superior to hypotonic or even isotonic crystalloid solutions in expanding the intravascular volume.[37,38] Although a rapid infusion of crystalloid is effective in increasing intravascular volume acutely, this benefit is transient.[39] For example, in the absence of a capillary leak, after a five-minute infusion of one liter of lactated Ringer's, the intravascular volume expands approximately 630 mL. Yet, due to rapid redistribution into the interstitial space, barely 20% of this volume is retained within the intravascular compartment after an hour. Similarly, only 25% (250 mL) of one liter of infused normal saline (NS) is retained in the intravascular compartment after one hour. In contrast, after a five-minute infusion of one liter of 6% hetastarch, the intravascular volume expands by 1123 mL with more long-lasting effects. Five percent albumin can expand the plasma volume five times more than a comparable volume of normal saline.[40]

2. In general, it is reasonable to initially administer a moderate amount of inexpensive crystalloid (up to a liter) if the patient is oxygenating well. Infusing greater amounts may contribute to tissue edema, commonly impairing oxygenation. Colloids should be selected if additional volume is required, although at some centers, they are given first. The selection of colloid should be based on the patient's pulmonary and renal function and the extent of mediastinal bleeding.

a. **Albumin (5%)** provides excellent volume expansion (approximately 400 mL retained per 500 mL bottle administered), has a half-life of 16 hours, and leaves the bloodstream at a rate of about 5–8 g/h. It has primarily dilutional effects on clotting parameters and preserves coagulation better than the hydroxyethyl starches.[41] It has oxygen free-radical scavenging and anti-inflammatory properties, which may exert protective effects on the kidney. However, it will leak into the interstitial space due to the capillary leak and may cause movement of fluid out of the intracellular space. Furthermore, 5% albumin is a saline-based colloid with a high chloride load, and studies suggest that use of albumin increases the risk of AKI in a dose-dependent manner after cardiac surgery.[42] Therefore, although some groups use 5% albumin as the preferential fluid after surgery, it can be inferred that large volumes of 5% albumin must be used with caution.

b. **Hydroxyethyl starch (HES)** preparations are nonprotein colloid volume expanders that provide excellent volume expansion in excess of the volume infused.

    i. The high-molecular-weight solutions, Hespan (6% hetastarch in saline) and Hextend (6% hetastarch in balanced electrolyte solution), maintain volume expansion for about 24 hours, but may cause renal dysfunction and produce a coagulopathy by binding to the von Willebrand/factor VIII complex, causing platelet dysfunction, and also by causing fibrinolysis.[43] This risk may be slightly less with Hextend.[44–46] Thus, despite a recommended maximum infusion of 20 mL/kg, their use has been discouraged in the early postoperative period and should absolutely be avoided in the bleeding patient.[37,38,43]

    ii. The low-molecular-weight solutions include pentastarch (Pentaspan [DuPont Pharma]), tetrastarch in 0.9% saline (Volvuven), and tetrastarch in a balanced electrolyte solution (Volulyte [Fresenius Kabi, Canada]). These also produce excellent volume expansion, but for shorter periods of time (18–24 hours for pentastarch, six hours for tetrastarch). The risks of renal dysfunction and coagulopathy may be slightly less than with the high-molecular-weight solutions, but they are still present.[47] Therefore, these products are also not recommended in the bleeding patient. Otherwise, infusion volumes should be limited to 28 mL/kg (2 L/day maximum) for pentastarch and 50 mL/kg for tetrastarch (3.5 L/day maximum).

  c. **Note:** there is concern that saline-based solutions (0.9% saline, 5% albumin, Hespan, Pentaspan and tetrastarch in saline) provide a high chloride load that, given in high doses, can produce progressive renal vasoconstriction, a decrease in GFR, and a hyperchloremic metabolic acidosis. Studies show that use of chloride-restricted solutions, such as lactated Ringer's, tetrastarch in balanced electrolyte solution, and Plasma-Lyte, is associated with a lower risk of AKI.[48–51] The development of a metabolic acidosis related to the use of high chloride solutions might raise the specter of poor tissue perfusion, prompting unnecessary interventions.

  d. Hypertonic solutions are effective in augmenting intravascular volume by extracting fluid from the interstitial and intracellular spaces. They may reduce the amount of fluid required to maintain intravascular volume when there is total body fluid overload. **Twenty-five percent albumin** can increase the intravascular volume by 450 mL for every 100 mL administered. Other solutions are available that may increase intravascular volume without providing excessive free water, but they are usually used only in the setting of hyponatremia. **Hypertonic saline** (3%) can produce neurologic problems if it causes acute hypernatremia. Studies from Europe have shown that hypertonic saline (7.5%) can produce renal vasodilation, increase GFR, and produce a diuresis.[52] It should be noted that use of these hypertonic colloids can produce hyperoncotic renal failure in dehydrated patients because the glomerular filtration of hyperoncotic colloid molecules may cause hyperviscosity and stasis of tubular flow, resulting in tubular obstruction. This effect may also be one of the mechanisms of high-molecular-weight HES-induced renal dysfunction.

D. An ideal solution for volume expansion would be a commercially available hemoglobin (Hb) based oxygen carrier. Thromboelastographic studies of Oxyvita, a polymerized bovine-Hb-based oxygen carrier, have shown similar effects on the coagulation profile as Hespan at doses up to 23 mL/kg, but with minimal coagulopathic effects at the recommended dose of 2–3 mL/kg.[53] These products enhance fibrinolysis and must be avoided in the bleeding patient.[54]

E. It cannot be overemphasized that the objective of postoperative fluid management is to maintain **adequate** intravascular volume to ensure **satisfactory** cardiac output and tissue perfusion. Administration of excessive volume to maintain high filling pressures and the highest possible cardiac output will increase extravascular water, which will be primarily manifested by pulmonary edema that will delay extubation. The amount of fluid to administer can be confusing in patients with diastolic dysfunction who already have high filling pressures, but often a marginal cardiac output. In addition, the hemodilution caused by intravascular volume expansion may decrease the hematocrit and also reduce the level of clotting factors, possibly precipitating bleeding and necessitating homologous blood or blood product transfusions.

F. When cardiac function is satisfactory, but there is an ongoing volume requirement to maintain filling pressures or blood pressure, often from a combination of the capillary leak, vasodilation, and an excellent urine output, "flooding" the patient with volume should be resisted. After 1.5–2 L of fluid is given, norepinephrine or vasopressin should be used to maintain filling pressures and improve the systemic blood pressure. Norepinephrine may provide some cardiac support, will improve RBF, and may lower renal vascular resistance by lowering renal sympathetic tone.[55,56] Vasopressin (0.01–0.1 units/min) is very effective in restoring the blood pressure to within the renal autoregulatory range (generally a mean pressure >80 mmHg) in the vasodilated "vasoplegic" patient with a good cardiac output.[57,58] In conditions of low cardiac output, however, it may cause splanchnic vasoconstriction, inducing bowel ischemia. Phenylephrine should be utilized only when the cardiac output is satisfactory, because it provides a pure α effect on systemic vascular tone, causing renal arteriolar vasoconstriction.

G. If both cardiac output and urine output remain marginal after adequate filling pressures have been achieved, inotropic support must be considered first, with use of vasoconstrictor drugs only if systemic resistance remains low. Use of α-agents at substantial doses is always of concern with a marginal cardiac output because they may produce renal vasoconstriction and compromise renal function.

H. Generally, diuretics are best avoided in the first six hours after surgery unless pulmonary edema with borderline oxygenation is present. They may be beneficial if the pulmonary edema is cardiogenic in origin, but noncardiogenic pulmonary edema may be present even if the patient is hypovolemic. When the patient has achieved a stable core temperature and the capillary leak has ceased, usually after the first 6–12 hours, filling pressures will stabilize or rise with little fluid administration. By this time, myocardial function has usually recovered, inotropic support can be gradually withdrawn, and the patient can be extubated. Diuresis may then be initiated to excrete the excess salt and water administered during CPB and the early postoperative period. Patients who have undergone operations that require long periods of CPB (usually >3 hours) or who have persistent low output syndromes may experience a longer period of "capillary leak" that requires further fluid administration to maintain filling pressures. In either circumstance, if the patient has low filling pressures despite fluid overload, initiation of diuretics should probably be delayed.

I. **Diuresis** can be augmented most efficiently by the use of loop diuretics.[59,60]

1. Loop diuretics inhibit sodium reabsorption in the ascending limb of the loop of Henle and increase solute (sodium) presentation to the distal tubules. By inhibiting tubular sodium and chloride reabsorption, they increase natriuresis and diuresis. To a lesser extent, they may also act as renal vasodilators, increasing RBF and GFR, and they may improve medullary oxygenation.

2. Most patients with preserved renal function respond to furosemide (Lasix) 10–20 mg IV. In the absence of renal insufficiency, furosemide has a half-life of 1.5–2 hours, and thus it can be repeated every four hours, if necessary. Not infrequently, the diuresis persists after one dose. Some patients with advanced CKD appear to respond better to bumetanide 1–2 mg IV and then may be given torsemide 10–20 mg orally (10–20 mg can be given IV, but this preparation is not available in the USA).

3. A gentle continuous diuresis may be obtained in patients with significant fluid overload and hemodynamic instability using a 40–60 mg IV bolus dose of furosemide followed by a continuous infusion of 0.1–0.5 mg/kg/h (usually 10–20 mg/h).[61] This may decrease the total dosage requirements and usually improves the diuretic response, especially in patients who are diuretic "tolerant". This benefit is also seen in patients with CKD. The addition of a thiazide (chlorothiazide 500 mg IV) is beneficial in overcoming this problem of tolerance, which may be caused by compensatory hypertrophy of the distal nephron segments in response to increased exposure to solute from chronic use of loop diuretics.

4. Diuretics are continued in IV or oral form until the patient has achieved their preoperative weight. This is a common practice, although most patients with normal renal function will auto-diuresis several days after surgery in the absence of diuretics. One study did in fact show no clinical benefit to initiating early diuresis in low-risk patients with normal renal function.[62] Another study suggested that not only intraoperative furosemide but also use of any diuretic postoperatively increased the risk of AKI.[63]

J. "Renal-dose" dopamine (2–3 μg/kg/min) increases RBF and GFR in patients with normal renal function, resulting in effective diuresis and natriuresis and possibly reducing the need for diuretics. However, dopamine initiated during surgery and continuing afterwards for 24 hours is not renoprotective and, in fact, may cause a deterioration in renal function. This has led to the recommendation that dopamine should not be used in postoperative cardiac surgical patients.[64–67]

K. Guidelines for the hemodynamic and fluid management of typical postoperative scenarios are presented in Chapter 8.

IV. Identifying Risk for Acute Kidney Injury

A. The risk of developing postoperative AKI is very low when a patient with normal renal function undergoes an uneventful operation and maintains satisfactory postoperative hemodynamics. In contrast, the presence of any degree of preoperative renal dysfunction increases the risk of postoperative AKI and mortality.[1–5] Therefore, it is important to identify patients with preoperative renal dysfunction and those with other risk factors for developing postoperative AKI.

B. **Definition of preoperative renal dysfunction.** The staging of CKD should be based on GFR, rather than SCr, as GFR provides a better estimate of renal reserve and the ability of the kidneys to tolerate surgical stress. It also correlates with both in-hospital mortality and the long-term prognosis.[68,69] SCr may be in the normal range even when there is a greater than 50% reduction in GFR, which reflects the number of functional neurons. The stages of CKD are defined as follows (in mL/min/1.73 m²)

Stage I	>90
Stage 2	60–89
Stage 3A	45–59
Stage 3B	30–44
Stage 4	15–29
Stage 5	<15 or on dialysis

1. A GFR <60 mL/min/1.73 m² (CKD stages 3–5) represents evidence of significant CKD and is the level below which there is an increased risk of postoperative AKI and increased mortality.[1] However, a higher risk of adverse outcomes, including the need for renal replacement therapy and mortality has even been confirmed in patients with "occult" kidney disease (i.e. a low GFR but normal SCr), who account for about 13% of patients with a normal SCr.[4,5] In fact, one study showed that patients with a normal GFR but impaired renal functional reserve demonstrated after a high oral protein load are also at risk for postoperative AKI.[70]

2. A 24-hour urine collection to precisely measure the creatinine clearance is considered to be no more reliable than an estimate based on formulas using the SCr.

   a. Using the Cockcroft-Gault equation, the GFR can easily be calculated at the bedside and is indexed to the patient's age and weight. This may be the best GFR equation to predict in-hospital mortality.[68]

$$C_{Cr} = \frac{(140 - age) \times wt\ (kg) \times (0.85\ if\ female)}{72 \times Scr\ (mg\,/\,dL)}$$

   b. Other formulas include the Modification of Diet in Renal Disease (MDRD) formula and the 2009 Chronic Kidney Disease Epidemiology Collaboration (CKD-EPI) equation which may be more accurate in calculating GFR, especially at higher levels of GFR.[71,72] Hospital laboratories utilize one of these equations to provide GFR results routinely.

C. **Risk factors for postoperative AKI and predictive models (Table 12.1)**[3,8–11,73–77]

1. The basic pathophysiology of postoperative AKI involves renal ischemia and other phenomena related to CPB, including inflammation, reperfusion injury, oxidative stress, and hemoglobinuria. Hemodynamic compromise in the pre-, intra-, or postoperative period will also heighten the risk of AKI and potentially affect its duration. Thus, more complex procedures requiring longer durations of CPB and the use of vasoactive drugs to support a low cardiac output are the major perioperative factors predisposing to AKI.

2. AKI is usually categorized as prerenal (reduced renal perfusion), renal (intrinsic renal insults), or postrenal (obstructive uropathy). Mechanisms contributing to the first two categories in the perioperative period are noted in Table 12.1. When the

Table 12.1 • Factors Contributing to Pre- and Postoperative Acute Kidney Injury	
Preoperative factors	Demographics: advanced age, female gender Comorbidities: CKD stage 3+, diabetes, vascular disease, hypertension, hyperlipidemia Low cardiac output states/hypotension (cardiogenic shock from acute MI, mechanical complications of MI) Medications that interfere with renal autoregulation (ACE inhibitors, NSAIDs) Nephrotoxins (contrast-induced nephropathy, especially in diabetics), medications (aminoglycosides) Diuretics Anemia Renal atheroembolism (catheterization, IABP) Interstitial nephritis (antibiotics, NSAIDs, furosemide) Glomerulonephritis (endocarditis)
Intraoperative factors	Cardiopulmonary bypass (nonpulsatile, low flow, low pressure perfusion with reduced renal perfusion, systemic hypotension, impairment of autoregulation) Low cardiac output syndrome/hypotension after CPB Blood transfusions Profound anemia (hematocrit <21%) Hemolysis and hemoglobinuria from prolonged duration of CPB
Postoperative factors	Low cardiac output states (decreased contractility, hypovolemia, absent AV synchrony in hypertrophied hearts) Hypotension Blood transfusions Intense vasoconstriction (low flow states, α-agents) Atheroembolism (IABP) Sepsis Medications (cephalosporins, aminoglycosides, ACE inhibitors)

kidneys have sustained an acute preoperative insult, either from a cardiac catheterization or more ominously from decompensated heart failure (HF) or cardiogenic shock from an acute ischemic event, they seem to be particularly sensitive to the abnormal physiology of CPB and to tenuous postcardiotomy hemodynamics. This is especially true in patients with "acute on chronic" renal dysfunction. The BUN and SCr should therefore be allowed to return towards baseline, if possible, before proceeding with surgery.

3. Most predictive models for AKI include similar risk factors, although several additional risk factors, such as a long duration of CPB and recent use of contrast, have been identified in other studies but are not included in many of the risk models.[3,75–78] Common risk factors include:

   a. Older age (2.5-fold increase in risk for each 10-year increment in one study)[79]

   b. Pre-existing comorbidities (CKD, diabetes, hypertension, vascular disease)

   c. Use of preoperative diuretics, nephrotoxic drugs, or medications that interfere with renal vasomotor tone

    d. More tenuous hemodynamic status (shock, recent myocardial infarction, preoperative IABP, low EF), reoperations, and urgent or emergent surgery

4. One simple risk model found that four factors were able to predict AKI with great accuracy (age >65, GFR <80 mL/min/m2, cross-clamp time >50 minutes, and more complex surgery).[80]

5. In virtually all of the risk models predicting AKI and the need for dialysis, the most significant risk factor is that of preexisting renal dysfunction, and most models use SCr rather than GFR as the marker of CKD.[73] Risk models are useful to individualize the risks of AKI and RRT based upon an assessment of multiple contributing risk factors.

    a. Figure 12.1 provides an estimate of the risk of developing severe AKI in patients with occult CKD.[81]

    b. Figure 12.2 provides a model to predict AKI (defined as SCr >2.0 mg/dL and a 50% increase in SCr) based upon pre-, intra-, and postoperative parameters.[82]

    c. Figures 12.3 and 12.4 provide the Cleveland Clinic and STS risk models for the prediction of RRT after cardiac surgery.[83,84]

6. These models do not predict operative mortality, which may be related to other contributing factors. For example, patients undergoing urgent or emergent operations of high complexity will have a higher predicted mortality at any level of SCr. It is best to use the STS short-term risk calculator available online at www.sts.org to incorporate other parameters to determine the risk of AKI and mortality. Generally, mortality risk is greater with increasing SCr levels, correlates with the degree and duration of oliguria,[85] and averages about 10% for patients with non-dialysis-dependent CKD.[1]

7. The development of postoperative AKI is associated with about a fourfold increase in operative mortality.[73,86] Although patients already on dialysis have an operative

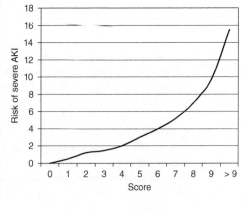

Risk Factor	Score
Age 70–74	1.5
Age 75–79	2.0
Age ≥ 80	2.5
Female	1.5
Diabetes	1.5
WBC > 12,000	1.5
Prior CABG	2.0
CHF	2.5
PVD	1.5
Hypertension	1.5
Preop IABP	3.0

Figure 12.1 • Multivariate risk predictor for severe postoperative renal insufficiency in patients with normal or near normal preoperative renal function (GFR >60 mL/min/1.73 m²). (Data from Brown et al. *Circulation* 2007;116(11 Suppl):I-139–43.)[81]

Risk factor	Points
Preop factors	
NYHA class III-IV	3.2
Scr > 1.2 mg/dL	3.1
Age > 65	2.3
Preop BS > 140 mg/dL	1.7
Intra- and postop factors	
Combined surgery	3.7
CPB time > 120 min	1.8
Low cardiac output	2.5
CVP > 14 cm H$_2$O	1.7

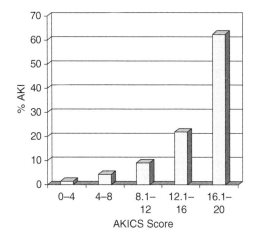

Figure 12.2 • Predictive model of acute kidney injury after cardiac surgery (AKICS) score. Risk of developing postoperative AKI is defined as a serum creatinine (SCr) >2.0 mg/dL and a 50% increase in SCr. (Reproduced with permission from Palomba et al., *Kidney Int* 2007;72:624–31.)[82]

Risk Factor	Points
Female	1
CHF	1
EF < 35%	1
Preop IABP	2
COPD	1
Insulin-DM	1
Reoperation	1
Emergency surgery	2
Isolated valve surgery	1
CABG + Valve	2
Other non-CABG cardiac surgery	2
Preop Scr 1.2–2.0 mg/dL	2
Preop Scr > 2.0 mg/dL	5

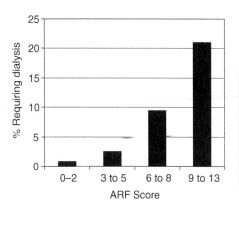

Figure 12.3 • Cleveland Clinic model to predict the risk of acute renal failure requiring dialysis. The risk is divided into four quartiles depending on the risk score. (Reproduced with permission from Thakar et al., *Am J Soc Nephrol* 2005;16:162–8.)[83]

mortality of about 10–15% in most series,[87–89] but as high as 37% in others,[90] the operative mortality for patients who develop AKI that requires de novo dialysis is quite high, ranging from 25–58% in a few series.[91,92] One study even estimated that the risk of dialysis exceeded 30% if the preoperative SCr exceeded 2.5 mg/dL.[89]

Risk Factor	Points
Creatinine (mg/dL) x 10	5–40
Age: 1 point for each 5 yrs > 55	Up to 10
AVR	2
AVR-CABG	5
MV Surgery	4
MV-CABG	7
Diabetes – oral meds	2
Diabetes – insulin	5
MI < 3 weeks	3
Non-white race	2
COPD	3
Reoperation	3
NYHA class IV	3
Cardiogenic shock	7

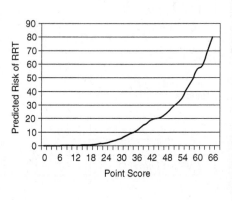

Figure 12.4 ● Bedside model for predicting the risk of dialysis (STS model). (Data from Mehta et al., *Circulation* 2006;114:2208–16.)[84]

8. These alarming statistics emphasize the crucial importance of taking any steps possible to minimize renal insults and preserve renal function in the perioperative period, especially in patients at increased risk. The presence of any degree of preoperative renal insufficiency should therefore lead to a search for potentially treatable causes that might lower the risk of AKI postoperatively. Identifying and correcting these contributing factors before surgery and using measures during and after surgery to optimize renal perfusion and tubular function to try to prevent AKI may ameliorate the complications associated with the development of oliguric renal failure. These may include electrolyte abnormalities, pulmonary and cardiac dysfunction, bleeding, delayed return of gastrointestinal (GI) function affecting nutrition, and infection from immune dysfunction, not to mention the possibility of requiring dialysis and its attendant complications.

V. Prevention of Acute Kidney Injury

A. Preoperative measures

1. Prior to and during cardiac catheterization, consider the following interventions (Table 12.2):

   a. Avoid medications the day of the catheterization that may have adverse effects on renal function, including diuretics.

   b. Adequately hydrate with normal saline before, during, and after catheterization. Leaving a patient NPO all day and performing a catheterization late in the day without hydration is a set-up for contrast-induced nephropathy. When this occurs, studies have shown a fourfold increase in operative mortality.[93] Fluid administration may be based on the patient's estimated left ventricular end-diastolic pressure (LVEDP).

Table 12.2 • Preoperative and Intraoperative Measures to Reduce the Risk of Acute Kidney Injury

A. Preoperative measures
1. Hydrate before, during, and after cardiac catheterization
2. Use low-volume, low-osmolar contrast
3. Avoid preoperative use of diuretics unless clinically indicated
4. Repeat SCr if preoperative CKD, especially in diabetics, and defer surgery, if possible, until it has returned to baseline
5. Delay surgery if feasible at least 24 hours after catheterization
6. Withhold use of ACE inhibitors and ARBs the day of surgery; stop NSAIDs several days in advance
7. Optimize hemodynamic status
8. Treat profound anemia: erythropoietin plus iron for elective cases and preoperative transfusions for more urgent cases
9. Perform emergency surgery, if feasible, for cardiogenic shock to reverse organ system dysfunction or consider mechanical circulatory support in very high-risk patients
10. Correct all acid–base and metabolic problems
11. Perform hemodialysis the day prior to surgery in dialysis-dependent patients and consider preoperative dialysis in patients with stage 4–5 CKD

B. Intraoperative measures
1. Perform off-pump surgery if possible
2. Optimize hemodynamics prebypass
3. Use antifibrinolytics (ε-aminocaproic [Amicar] or tranexamic acid) to minimize bleeding
4. Pharmacologic renoprotection: possible use of fenoldopam or diltiazem
5. Considerations during CPB
   a. Use heparin-coated circuits, miniaturized if possible
   b. Prime pump with non-potassium-containing crystalloid (NS rather than lactated Ringer's, Normosol or Plasma-Lyte)
   c. Consider use of a leukocyte-reducing filter
   d. Maintain a high perfusion pressure (75–80 mm Hg) on bypass
   e. Minimize extent of hypothermia and do not overwarm
   f. Keep the pump run as short as possible
   g. Maintain a hematocrit at least >20%
   h. Be conservative with high-potassium cardioplegia; consider using del Nido cardioplegia
   i. Control hyperglycemia
   j. Use hemofiltration to remove excess fluid

C. Postbypass measures
1. Optimize postbypass hemodynamics (drugs, IABP)
2. Use dexmedetomidine for sedation
3. Treat bleeding with factor concentrates, desmopressin (if suspect uremic platelet dysfunction) to minimize volume
4. Consider placement of a dialysis catheter for patients at high risk for requiring dialysis

c. A common protocol is to give:

Preprocedure:		3 mL/kg × 1 h
During procedure:	LVEDP <13 mm Hg	5 mL/kg/h
	LVEDP 13–18 mm Hg	3 mL/kg/h
	LVEDP >18 mm Hg	1.5 mL/kg/h
Postprocedure:		1.5 mL/kg/h × 4 h or 1 mg/kg × 6 h

d. Although some studies have shown benefits of sodium bicarbonate or n-acetylcysteine alone or together in minimizing the risk of contrast-induced nephropathy, most groups have found hydration protocols to be the most beneficial.[94–96]

e. Use low volumes of iso- or low-osmolar nonionic contrast

2. Repeat the SCr after contrast studies and defer surgery, if possible, until it has returned to baseline. Unfortunately, it can take up to 24–36 hours for the SCr to rise, so even delaying on-pump (but probably not off-pump) surgery for 24 hours after catheterization may not be sufficient to reduce the risk of postoperative AKI in patients with preexisting CKD.[78,97–99] Some studies suggest that surgery should be delayed for five days after coronary angiography, especially when high-contrast doses (>1.4 mL/kg) are used.[100–102] However, surgery should not be delayed in critically ill patients with hemodynamic compromise and worsening renal function, since delay will often lead to less-reversible renal failure and multisystem organ failure.

3. Stop any medication with potential nephrotoxic effects, such as the NSAIDs, which impair autoregulation of RBF. Whether ACE inhibitors and ARBs should be withheld the morning of surgery remains controversial. They may cause refractory hypotension on CPB, which could contribute to kidney injury. However, studies have shown differing effects on the incidence of AKI, with evidence of both higher and lower risks of AKI in patients taking ACE inhibitors prior to surgery.[16–21]

4. Fluid overload should be avoided as it is associated with a higher risk of AKI and worse surgical outcomes, most likely because of its association with decompensated HF and hemodynamic instability.[103] In these patients, diuretics may need to be given to improve the clinical picture. Generally, in stable patients, diuretics should be withheld and consideration given to some preoperative hydration in patients with CKD.[104]

5. Statins are routinely given to patients undergoing coronary bypass surgery, and often to those undergoing valvular surgery as well. There is some evidence that they lower levels of kidney biomarkers after surgery, suggesting that they might provide some degree of renoprotection.[105] Although some individual studies show this benefit,[106] a meta-analysis and subsequent studies of high-dose atorvastatin failed to do so.[107,108] A study of rosuvastatin actually showed it increased the risk of AKI.[109] Another meta-analysis suggested that statin use did not influence the risk of AKI but did reduce the need for RRT.[110] One review suggested continuation of statins might be beneficial for renoprotection, but starting them in statin-naive patients may not.[111]

6. Optimize hemodynamic status. Patients with poor cardiac function, fluid overload, and decompensated HF will often achieve substantial improvement in renal

function with appropriate medical care which should lower the risk of surgery. Patients in cardiogenic shock have a high mortality rate, which might be lessened by emergency surgical intervention. Consideration may be given to mechanical circulatory support if multisystem organ failure has developed, and this may allow for improvement in renal function. If surgery is performed in these high-risk cases, postoperative AKI is inevitable but hopefully transient and reversible.

7. Preoperative anemia is associated with an increased risk of AKI as is the use of multiple transfusions.[6,112-114] Erythropoietin plus iron can be recommended to improve the hematocrit in patients undergoing elective surgery.[115] In other patients in whom the calculated on-pump hematocrit will be less than 21% based on the patient's size and blood volume, it is not unreasonable to transfuse patients preoperatively. It has been suggested that this strategy may be associated with a lower risk of AKI.[116]

8. Correct acid–base and metabolic abnormalities that are often seen in patients with CKD. These patients are more susceptible to fluid overload, metabolic abnormalities (hyponatremia, hyperkalemia, hypomagnesemia, and hyperphosphatemia), and metabolic acidosis or alkalosis (from diuretics) in the perioperative period.

9. Patients on chronic dialysis should be dialyzed within the 24 hours before and after surgery. The overall mortality rate for patients on chronic dialysis undergoing open-heart surgery is approximately 10–15%, but even higher in those with advanced NYHA class and those undergoing urgent or emergent surgery and requiring complex surgery.

10. Preoperative dialysis should also be considered in non-dialysis-dependent renal failure (stages 4–5). This approach to patients with a preoperative SCr ≥2.5 mg/dL has been shown to reduce the need for postoperative dialysis, with less morbidity and significantly less mortality.[117-119]

B. **Intraoperative measures** should be taken to try to augment renal reserve by improving RBF, enhancing the GFR, and preventing tubular damage in patients with known renal dysfunction or risk factors for its development (Table 12.2).

1. Consider performing off-pump coronary surgery, especially in diabetic patients with preoperative renal dysfunction. Whether this reduces the risk of AKI is controversial.[27-33]

2. Maintain optimal hemodynamic performance before CPB. This may require fluid administration, treatment of ischemia, or use of vasoactive drugs to support myocardial function or systemic resistance.

3. Use dexmedetomidine for sedation during surgery and afterwards. This may produce more hemodynamic stability and has been shown to reduce the incidence of AKI.[67,120,121]

4. Use antifibrinolytic drugs to minimize the bleeding diathesis that commonly accompanies renal dysfunction (uremic platelet dysfunction). ε-aminocaproic acid (Amicar) is commonly used and is generally safe, although it is associated with some degree of renal tubular dysfunction without a significant change in creatinine clearance.[122] Tranexamic acid is a good alternative.

5. Pharmacologic means to optimize renal perfusion have been studied with variable results.[121,123]

a. **Fenoldopam** (0.03–0.1 μg/kg/min) may reduce the risk of AKI without any reduction in the need for renal replacement therapy or mortality, but this has not been uniformly demonstrated.[123,124]

b. **Diltiazem** (0.1 mg/kg bolus followed by an infusion of 2 μg/kg/min) reduces renal vascular resistance by dilating afferent arterioles, resulting in an increase in RBF and GFR. It may limit calcium influx into renal tubular cells, preserving their integrity. It has been shown to increase sodium excretion and improve SCr and free water clearance by a direct effect on tubular reabsorption. However, the vasodilatory effect of diltiazem may adversely affect renal function during CPB, and in some studies has increased the risk of AKI.[79] Studies do suggest that diltiazem is more likely to improve rather than reduce glomerular function in patients with mild–moderate renal dysfunction.[125] One study showed that not using a calcium-channel blocker perioperatively increased the risk of AKI.[126] Another showed that the combination of dopamine and diltiazem started 24 hours before surgery and continued for 72 hours afterwards improved SCr and free water clearance compared with use of either drug alone.[127]

c. Regimens using sodium bicarbonate, N-acetylcysteine, and statins have shown mixed results and none can be recommended.[10,121,123,128,129] Specifically, renal-dose dopamine (3 μg/kg/min) may increase urine output during CPB, but is not renoprotective.[65,66] Spironolactone, a mineralocorticoid receptor blocker, may reduce ischemia-reperfusion injury, but has also not been shown to reduce the risk of AKI.[130]

d. **Mannitol** is commonly added to the pump to increase tubular flow and produce a diuresis. It increases oncotic pressure, reduces tissue edema, and may reduce cell swelling after cardioplegic arrest. Usually 25–50 g is added to the pump prime. However, mannitol has not been demonstrated to provide any benefit in preserving renal function in patients with both normal and abnormal preoperative renal function.[131,132]

e. **Furosemide** is often given during surgery to augment urine output and is beneficial in treating patients with significant volume overload, severe oliguria, or hyperkalemia. However, although it may increase urine output, most studies have not demonstrated a renoprotective effect.[66,133-135] There is one study that showed some benefit in patients with more than mild CKD.[136] Although a lower urine output during CPB may be associated with an increased risk of AKI, this does not necessarily imply that pharmacologically increasing the urine output will reduce that risk.[137]

6. **Considerations during CPB**

a. Use heparin-coated and/or miniaturized circuits, and leukodepletion during the pump run, which may lower the incidence of postoperative AKI by reducing the systemic inflammatory response.[138-140]

b. Use a non-potassium-containing crystalloid prime to reduce the risk of hyperkalemia induced by use of cardioplegia.

c. Maintain a higher mean perfusion pressure on bypass (around 80 mm Hg) by increasing the systemic flow rate. If this does not raise the blood pressure to adequate levels, a vasopressor (phenylephrine, norepinephrine, or vasopressin) can be added. Autoregulation of RBF occurs down to a pressure of about 80 mm Hg, but below that, flow is pressure-dependent.[141] Nonetheless, one study did indicate that the incidence of postoperative AKI was no different whether mean pressures <60, 60–69, or >70 mm Hg were used during CPB, although urine output was less at lower pressures.[77]

d. Avoid more than mild hypothermia for routine cases and do not overwarm the patient prior to terminating CPB. Mild–moderate hypothermia probably has little impact on renal function, but rewarming to 37 °C may be deleterious.[142,143] Therefore, it is generally recommended that patients only be warmed to 36.5 °C since the duration of a rewarming temperature above 37 °C contributes to AKI.[144] This may occur because the kidneys may rewarm more rapidly than other organs, including the brain, resulting in hyperthermia-related exacerbation of renal injury. For procedures involving deep hypothermic circulatory arrest, the incidence of AKI correlates with the duration of DHCA.[145]

e. Keep the "pump run" as short as possible. Do what needs to be done and do it expeditiously. Generally, the longer the duration of CPB, the greater the incidence of AKI.[75–77]

f. Avoid extreme hemodilution on CPB. Studies have suggested that there is a correlation between the lowest hematocrit on pump (usually <21%, but <24% in one study)[14] and the incidence of AKI, especially in obese patients.[12,13] However, the hematocrit is only one factor in oxygen delivery. Since AKI is more common below a critical level for oxygen delivery (272 mL/min/m²), lower hematocrits may be acceptable as long as oxygen delivery is maintained above the critical level with increased pump flow rates.[146] There is a delicate balance between tolerating a lower hematocrit and administering blood transfusions, as administration of >2 units of blood has been associated with an increased risk of AKI.[114] It has been suggested that patients who are chronically anemic tend to tolerate lower hematocrits on pump, and this might reduce the need to transfuse.[147]

g. Avoid excessive use of cardioplegia to minimize the potassium load. Use low-K+ reinfusions of standard blood cardioplegia, consider del Nido cardioplegia, which requires less frequent administration, and substitute intermittent cold blood (without cardioplegia) to minimize the risk of hyperkalemia.

h. Prevent hyperglycemia or large variations in blood glucose levels during the pump run with intravenous (IV) insulin.[148] Despite some concerns that a very strict hyperglycemia protocol may be associated with episodes of hypoglycemia, it has been shown that maintaining a blood sugar (BS) between 80 and 110 mg/dL is associated with a significant reduction in AKI and the need for dialysis in nondiabetic patients.[149] There may be additional potential benefits of insulin administration related to its anti-inflammatory and antioxidant properties.

i. Initiate hemofiltration towards the end of the pump run to reduce the positive fluid balance and increase the hematocrit. This is especially helpful in patients with preoperative HF and hypoxemia who require urgent surgery.[150]

j. One study suggested that the use of sodium nitroprusside during rewarming on pump improved renal function in patients undergoing elective CABG, although this must not be allowed to occur at the expense of unacceptable hypotension.[151] In addition, any hemolysis and free hemoglobin release during CPB may accelerate the release of free cyanide from SNP.[152]

7. **Considerations upon termination of CPB**

    a. Use Swan-Ganz monitoring and frequent evaluations of transesophageal echocardiography to determine optimal filling pressures and the use of inotropes, vasopressors, or an IABP to support hemodynamics.

    b. Carefully monitor serum potassium in patients with preexisting CKD. Levels greater than 6 mEq/L may need to be treated with dextrose/insulin before coming off pump.

    c. Use dexmedetomidine for sedation post-pump and during the early ICU stay.

    d. Desmopressin may be considered in uremic patients who manifest platelet dysfunction.[153] In patients with coagulopathic bleeding after CPB, consider using factor concentrates (prothrombin complex concentrate or fibrinogen concentrate), rather than plasma, to minimize volume infusions.

    e. Consider placement of a central double-lumen dialysis catheter if concerned about the possibility of needing dialysis in the early postoperative period.

VI. Postoperative Oliguria and Acute Kidney Injury

A. The use of hemodilution during CPB expands the extracellular volume and usually produces an excellent urine output in the immediate postoperative period. Oliguria is considered present in the postoperative cardiac surgical patient when the urine output is **less than 0.5 mL/kg/h.** Transient oliguria is commonly noted in the first 12 hours after surgery and usually responds to a volume infusion or low-dose inotropic support. However, the persistence of oliguria is usually a manifestation of an acute renal insult caused by a prolonged pump run, prolonged hypotension, or a low cardiac output state. The SCr will frequently be lower immediately after CPB and the following morning due to hemodilution, and may have a delayed rise despite a marked reduction in GFR, as it takes time for SCr to accumulate in the bloodstream. Thus, it is important to recognize that AKI may be associated with an abrupt and sustained decrease in urine output and/or a decline in GFR, prior to noting an increase in SCr. Measurement of kidney biomarkers may be the most sensitive means of early detection of AKI.[23-26]

B. **Definition of acute kidney injury.** The incidence of postoperative AKI depends on its definition, but it is estimated to occur in 30–50% of patients and is associated with a fourfold increase in mortality.[73,86,154] Even very slight increases in postoperative SCr contribute to increased mortality.[155]

C. The RIFLE system was devised in 2004 to classify progressively worsening degrees of renal dysfunction (Table 12.3).[156] Since the function of the kidneys is both elimination of nitrogenous waste products and the production of urine, either the SCr level/GFR criteria **or** the urine output criteria were used for classification in this model as well as in two additional models noted below. It should be noted that urine output is determined by the difference between the GFR and the rate of tubular reabsorption. Therefore, if the GFR is low from CKD in association with poor tubular absorption, the patient can have good urine output initially. With AKI, tubular absorption is initially normal with a low GFR and then falls.

    1. In the RIFLE system (Table 12.3), there is a seven-day window to assess changes in SCr. As the degree of AKI worsens, the risk of dialysis increases and short- and intermediate-term mortality rates increase.[157] In fact, once RRT is necessary, the mortality rate is usually about 50%.

Table 12.3 • The RIFLE Criteria for Classification of Renal Failure

Severity Class	SCr/GFR Criteria	Urine Output	Overall Incidence[157, 159,160]	Need for dialysis	Estimated 90-day mortality[157]
Risk	Increase in SCr × 1.5 *or* Decrease in GFR >25%	<0.5 mL/kg/h × 6h	9–30%	1%	8%
Injury	Increase in SCr × 2 *or* Decrease in GFR >50%	<0.5 mL/kg/h × 12 h	3.5–12%	7%	21%
Failure	Increase in SCr × 3 *or* Decrease in GFR >75% or if baseline SCr >4 mg/dL, an acute rise in SCr of >0.5 mg/dL)	<0.3 mL/kg/h × 24h *or* anuria for 12 h	3.5–5%	55%	33%
Clinical Outcomes					
Loss	Persistent acute renal failure with complete loss of kidney function >4 weeks				
ESKD	End-stage kidney disease >3 months				

2. In 2007, a slight modification of the RIFLE system was devised by the Acute Kidney Injury Network (AKIN) (Table 12.4).[158] This did not utilize the GFR, did not require a baseline SCr, but did require two SCr determinations within 48 hours. It provided a fairly comparable assessment of AKI, but would not recognize AKI developing after 48 hours.[159,160]

3. In 2012, another classification system was proposed, termed the Kidney Disease Improving Global Outcomes (KDIGO) criteria.[161] Acute kidney injury was defined as a 0.3 mg/dL increase in SCr from baseline within 48 hours of surgery, a 50% increase in SCr within seven days of surgery, or a decrease in urine output below 0.5 mg/kg/h for six hours.

4. Using each of these systems, the prognosis was worse if both the elevated SCr and oliguria criteria were met.[8,162]

5. The STS definition of AKI (version 2.42, available in 2020) was an increase in SCr to three times greater than baseline, or to >4 mg/dL with an acute rise

Table 12.4 • AKIN Classification System of Acute Kidney Injury		
	SCr	Urine Output
Stage 1	Increased Scr × 1.5 or an increase ≥0.3 mg/dL	<0.5 mL/kg/h × >6 h
Stage 2	Increased Scr × 2	<0.5 mL/kg/h × >12 h
Stage 3	Increased Scr × 3 or Scr ≥4 mg/dL with an acute rise >0.5 mg/dL	<0.3 mL/kg/h × >24 h or anuria >12 h

>0.5 mg/dL, or the requirement for dialysis. This essentially corresponds to the "failure" category of RIFLE and stage 3 of the AKIN. However, oliguria was not taken into consideration.

D. **Diagnosis of AKI.** The early diagnosis of AKI can be difficult to make because of the delay in elevation of SCr and the maintenance of urine output despite nephron damage.

1. The SCr is influenced not just by glomerular function but also by tubular function and the generation of SCr. It is also influenced by patient gender, age, and muscle mass. Thus, it tends to underestimate the degree of renal dysfunction because, as the GFR falls, SCr secretion increases, minimizing the rise in SCr, upon which the GFR calculation is based. Although the SCr may not rise for several days after tubular injury has occurred, the eventual elevation in SCr does reflect changes in GFR, and is therefore valuable in confirming the diagnosis of AKI. A fall in SCr is an indicator of renal recovery from AKI, with the percentage decrease in SCr within 24 hours having the strongest correlation with long-term outcomes.[163]

2. Elevation in plasma and urinary levels of kidney-specific biomarkers, such as NGAL, cystatin C, KIM-1, and IL-18, may be noted within 2–6 hours of surgery and correlates with the extent and duration of AKI.[23-26] These are valuable early indicators of AKI that precede elevation in SCr levels. Although cystatin concentration reflects baseline GFR more accurately than SCr and is independent of muscle mass, NGAL is rapidly induced in renal tubular cells in response to ischemic injury, and although its early appearance is independent of GFR, it is generally predictive of a subsequent decline in GFR. Because elevated NGAL levels may provide for earlier diagnosis and intervention of incipient AKI than elevations in SCr, some authors have recommended that all patients have baseline NGAL levels obtained for comparison with serial postoperative values.[164]

3. **Nonoliguric renal failure,** defined as a rise in SCr with a urine output >400 mL/day, is the most common form of AKI and may occur after an uneventful operation in a patient with preexisting renal dysfunction or risk factors for its development, and occasionally without any precipitating factors. This condition usually reflects less renal damage and is associated with a mortality rate of about 5–10%. Most patients can be managed by judicious fluid administration, hemodynamic support as indicated, and high-dose diuretics to optimize urine output while awaiting recovery of renal function. Patients experiencing AKI have a higher rate of hospital readmission, which is more frequent with more advanced levels of AKI.[165]

4. **Oliguric renal failure** may occur in patients with varying degrees of reduction in GFR, but, when the urine output is <0.3–0.5 mL/kg/h for 12–24 hours and there is a twofold increase in SCr, significant AKI is present with a higher likelihood of requiring RRT and a high mortality rate. It is estimated that the mortality of patients requiring dialysis is three times higher than those with nonoliguric AKI.[166] This high mortality rate has not changed much over the past 10–15 years despite the early institution of various forms of RRT and general improvements in postoperative care. This reflects the higher-risk population undergoing surgery and the morbidity of conditions frequently associated with renal failure, such as low cardiac output states, respiratory failure, infection, and stroke.

E. **Etiology and pathophysiology of postoperative AKI**[8–11,167]

1. In patients with preexisting renal dysfunction, the complex effects of extracorporeal circulation will often induce some degree of AKI. Mechanisms include renal hypoperfusion from low-flow, low-pressure nonpulsatile perfusion with hemodilution and hypothermia, as well as an inflammatory response that may maintain afferent arteriolar constriction. The duration of CPB is therefore a major risk factor for the development of AKI.[3,75–77] Using most of the recommendations delineated in Table 12.2, it may be possible to minimize the intraoperative insult and allow renal function to return to baseline within a few days if no additional insult occurs. However, the most common cause of a prolonged renal insult is a low cardiac output syndrome which may be present at the termination of CPB and may extend well into the early postoperative period in the ICU. An additional contributing factor is intense peripheral vasoconstriction, often related to use of α-agents. Oliguria occurring as a consequence of reduced GFR is most clinically significant early after surgery when fluid overload and hyperkalemia can lead to pulmonary and myocardial complications and impair recovery from surgery.

2. The kidneys have a tremendous capacity to autoregulate and maintain RBF, GFR, filtration fraction, and tubular reabsorption in the face of reduced renal perfusion pressure. Intrinsic renal mechanisms that maintain autoregulation include a reduction in afferent arteriolar resistance and an increase in efferent arteriolar resistance. However, when a low cardiac output state or hypotension persists or potent vasopressor medications are used, these compensatory reserves gradually become exhausted, filtration reserve is exceeded, and endogenous and/or exogenous vasoconstrictors increase afferent arteriolar resistance, resulting in a fall in GFR. At this point of prerenal azotemia, oliguria may occur, but tubular function may still be intact. Aggressive management to optimize renal perfusion at this time is essential to try to avoid tubular damage.

3. However, a more protracted period of ischemia will eventually cause structural tubular injury with sloughing of cells that may obstruct the tubules with back leakage of fluid into the circulation. Impaired sodium absorption and increased sodium concentration in the distal tubules polymerizes proteins, contributing to cast formation. Oxidant injury and inflammatory phenomena result in further hypoperfusion and damage to tubular cells. Some of this damage is reversible and some results in apoptotic cell death. The term "acute tubular necrosis" (ATN) has commonly been applied to this condition, although it is a somewhat misleading term; therefore it is more commonly referred to as "acute kidney injury" (AKI). Thus, what usually originates as a prerenal "hypoperfusion" picture soon causes intrinsic renal damage.

4. It should be noted that an acute ischemic renal insult is a hypoperfusion injury that may be undetected in a normotensive patient.[168] If autoregulation is impaired, the kidney may be more susceptible to lesser degrees of hypoperfusion. Factors to consider are:

   a. Renal arteriolar disease, notably in elderly patients and those with hypertension, CKD, or renal artery stenosis.

   b. Failure of afferent arterioles to dilate appropriately. NSAIDs and Cox-2 inhibitors decrease prostaglandin synthesis and allow endogenous vasoconstrictors to act unopposed; sepsis and liver failure increase afferent arteriolar vasoconstriction.

   c. Use of vasoconstrictors during a low output state, which tend to reduce RBF despite achieving systemic normotension.

   d. Failure of efferent arterioles to constrict, noted with ACE inhibitors, ARBs, or direct renin inhibitors, such as aliskiren (Tekturna).

   e. Systemic venous hypertension, often as a result of right ventricular failure, tamponade, or an abdominal compartment syndrome, which may reduce renal perfusion.[169]

5. The acute development of oliguria and a rising SCr several days after surgery should always raise the specter of **cardiac tamponade**. The combination of systemic venous hypertension and a low output state can compromise renal perfusion even if hypotension is not evident. The patient may have nonspecific systemic symptoms, and a compensatory tachycardia may be absent with the use of β-blockers.

6. Conditions of impaired oxygen delivery (profound anemia from bleeding, hypoxemia from respiratory failure) may contribute to renal ischemia if there is borderline hypoperfusion.

F. Three patterns of acute renal failure were described following open-heart surgery over 30 years ago and in principle still hold true today (Figure 12.5).[170] In the first, termed **"abbreviated ARF"**, a transient intraoperative insult occurs that causes renal ischemia without tubular damage. The SCr peaks on the fourth postoperative day and then returns to normal. In the second pattern, termed **"overt ARF"**, the acute insult is followed by a more prolonged period of cardiac dysfunction and is associated with mild tubular damage. The SCr usually rises to a higher level and gradually returns towards baseline over the course of 1–2 weeks once hemodynamics improve and tubular cell regenerate. The third pattern ("**protracted ARF**") is characterized by an initial insult followed by a period of cardiac dysfunction that resolves. Just as the SCr begins to fall, another insult, often from sepsis or a period of hypoperfusion or hypotension, occurs that triggers a progressive, often irreversible, rise in SCr. A fourth pattern of "protracted ARF" that may be added to this description is that of acute AKI that results from a very severe initial insult that may occur intraoperatively and/or during the early postoperative period that causes extensive tubular damage from the outset and does not improve for quite some time, if at all.

G. **Assessment** (Table 12.5)

1. Assess cardiac hemodynamics (filling pressures, cardiac output). If the patient is no longer being intensively monitored, insertion of a Foley catheter is helpful in assessing urine output. Evidence of jugular venous distention or orthostatic vital

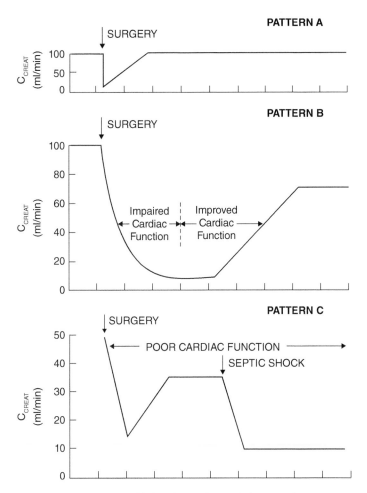

Figure 12.5 • Patterns of acute renal failure (ARF) observed after open-heart surgery. (A) Abbreviated ARF. (B) Overt ARF. (C) Protracted ARF. The reduction in creatinine clearance noted here is paralleled by a rise in SCr. (Reproduced with permission from Myers et al. *N Engl J Med* 1986;314(2):97–105. doi:10.1056/nejm198601093140207.)[170]

signs raise the specter of tamponade. An echocardiogram may be considered to assess ventricular function and the presence of a significant hemopericardium.

2. Identify any drugs being prescribed with potential adverse effects on renal function (ACE inhibitors, ARBs, NSAIDs, nephrotoxic antibiotics).

3. Obtain a serum BUN, SCr, and electrolytes. **Note:** an elevation in SCr with minimal or parallel rise in BUN is frequently noted with AKI. In contrast, a disproportionate rise in BUN with little rise in SCr may reflect a prerenal process or increased protein intake, total parenteral nutrition (TPN), GI bleeding (often associated with prerenal azotemia), hypercatabolism, or steroid administration, which increase urea production.

Table 12.5 • Evaluation of the Etiology of Oliguria

	Prerenal	Renal
BUN/Cr	>20:1	<10:1
U/P creatinine	>40	<20
U_{osm}	>500	<400
U/P osmolality	>1.3	<1.1
Urine specific gravity	>1.016	<1.010
U_{Na} (mEq/L)	<20	>40
FE_{Na}	<1%	>2%
Urinary sediment	Hyaline casts	Tubular epithelial cells Granular casts

4. Examine the urinary sediment. Tubular epithelial or granular ("muddy brown") casts are indicative of tubular injury, whereas hyaline casts are seen in low perfusion states. The sediment is important to examine because tests of tubular function, such as the urine sodium and osmolality, may be inaccurate with use of diuretics.

5. Measure the urine sodium (U_{Na}) and creatinine (U_{Cr}) concentrations. These tests can differentiate prerenal from renal causes, but their interpretation will be influenced by the use of diuretics. A U_{Na} <20 mEq/L is strongly suggestive of prerenal disease, but it could be elevated if the urine output is low. The fractional excretion of sodium (FE_{Na}) is a better marker of renal sodium handling because it normalizes sodium handling against the secretion of creatinine, thus being independent of urine concentration. This is calculated as:

$$FE_{Na} = \frac{U_{Na} \times P_{Cr}}{P_{Na} \times U_{Cr}} \times 100$$

where U and P refer to the urinary and plasma concentrations, respectively, of sodium and creatinine.

a. In the oliguric patient, an FE_{Na} <1% reflects retained tubular function with absorption of sodium and water, consistent with a prerenal problem, except in some cases of contrast nephrotoxicity, HF, and hepatorenal syndrome. In contrast, an FE_{Na} >2% is usually caused by ATN with tubular damage. However, this may also be noted when a prerenal process is superimposed on CKD, with which the kidneys at baseline cannot conserve water and sodium appropriately. A rise in FE_{Na} may be noted during recovery of renal function due to sodium mobilization.

6. Monitor other electrolytes (especially potassium), blood glucose, and acid–base balance frequently.

7. Obtain a renal ultrasound to assess kidney size and rule out obstruction. A renal scan may be performed if a renal embolus is suspected.

H. **Management of oliguria and AKI** (Table 12.6).[171–173] Early aggressive intervention in patients with oliguria and early evidence of AKI may prevent progressive tubular injury and worsening of renal function. However, once AKI is established, very little can be done to promote recovery of renal function except to prevent additional insults. There is little evidence that strategies that increase RBF or increase urine flow to reduce tubular obstruction have any impact on enhancing tubular epithelial cell proliferation and recovery of function. Generally, attention should be directed towards maintaining urine output to reduce tissue edema and treating electrolyte or metabolic problems as they arise.

1. Ensure that the Foley catheter is within the bladder and is patent (this may rule out an obstructive uropathy). Irrigate with saline if necessary or consider changing the catheter empirically. If the Foley catheter has been removed, a bladder scan may indicate whether oliguria is real or spurious. Significant urinary retention may provide evidence of a post-obstructive uropathy as the cause of an elevated SCr. Either way, replacement of the catheter may be helpful in further assessing the urine output.

2. Discontinue all potentially nephrotoxic drugs (ACE inhibitors, ARBs, NSAIDs, nephrotoxic antibiotics) and avoid any diagnostic studies requiring IV contrast.

Table 12.6 • Management of Low Urine Output

1. Ensure that Foley catheter is in the bladder and is patent
2. Optimize cardiac function
   - Treat hypovolemia: minimize use of chloride-liberal solutions
   - Control arrhythmias and pace for slow rhythms
   - Improve contractility
   - Reduce elevated afterload, but allow BP to drift up to 130–140 mm Hg
3. Diuretics or other medications
   - Give increasing doses of furosemide (up to 500 mg IV) or a continuous infusion of 10–20 mg/h
   - Add chlorothiazide 500 mg IV to the loop diuretic
   - Consider bumetanide 4–10 mg or 1 mg bolus, then a 0.5–2 mg/h infusion
   - Consider use of fenoldopam 0.1 µg/kg/min, especially if hypertensive
4. If above fail
   - Limit fluid to insensible losses
   - Readjust drug doses
   - Avoid potassium supplements
   - Nutrition: essential amino acid diet
     → High nitrogen tube feeds if on dialysis
     → Total parenteral nutrition with 4.25% amino acid/35% dextrose
5. Consider early renal replacement therapy

3. Optimize hemodynamics. Although augmenting the cardiac output may not be able to expedite recovery of renal function, it is clear that any additional insult that causes hypotension or hypoperfusion may contribute to a state of "protracted ARF". These insults include hypovolemia (often GI bleeding), low cardiac output states (tamponade), arrhythmias (rapid atrial fibrillation, ventricular tachycardia), antihypertensive medications, or sepsis. Thus, there is little downside to optimizing hemodynamics to increase urine output even if the rate of renal recovery is not hastened.

a. Hemodynamic monitoring with a Swan-Ganz catheter may be indicated if a low cardiac output state is suspected. If the diagnosis is not clear, echocardiography can differentiate ventricular failure from tamponade or significant hypervolemia. Otherwise, assessment of fluid balance, strict I & O's, and/or a careful physical examination may give an overall assessment of the patient's fluid balance and intravascular volume.

b. Optimize preload without being overzealous with fluid administration. Remember that, in a state of capillary leak (often seen following surgery with a long duration of CPB, with a persistent low output state, or with sepsis) or with reduced oncotic pressure (as noted from hemodilution or poor nutritional condition), excessive fluid administration may produce noncardiogenic pulmonary edema. Fluid administration with solutions with high chloride content (5% albumin, normal saline, Hespan, Volvuven) should be minimized as they may increase the risk of AKI.[42,49–51]

c. Optimize heart rate and treat arrhythmias. Increasing the heart rate with atrial or AV pacing (V pacing only if there is no atrial capture) above 80/min to augment the cardiac output might prove beneficial in improving renal perfusion and GFR. Successful electrical or pharmacologic conversion of atrial fibrillation will improve cardiac output.

d. Improve contractility with inotropes if a low cardiac output state is present.

e. Reduce afterload with vasodilators to improve cardiac function, but do so carefully; eliminate drugs that can cause renal vasoconstriction; avoid ACE inhibitors and ARBs.

   i. Do not be overly aggressive in the reduction of systemic blood pressure in patients with preexisting hypertension and CKD. They usually require a higher blood pressure (130–140 mm Hg systolic) to maintain renal perfusion. In fact, while the patient is in the ICU, adding an α-agent to increase the blood pressure to that range often results in a significant improvement in urine output.

   ii. If inotropic drugs with vasodilator properties are used, such as milrinone or dobutamine, an α-agent may be necessary to maintain systemic blood pressure. Vasopressin can be used in vasodilated states with a good cardiac output ("vasoplegia"). Norepinephrine is preferable if the cardiac output is borderline because it will also provide some inotropic support. Use of a pure α-agent, such as phenylephrine, is more likely to cause renal vasoconstriction unless the cardiac output is excellent.

f. If the cardiac output remains marginal despite the use of multiple inotropes, consider the placement of an IABP. This may result in an abrupt and dramatic increase in urine output.

4. If oliguria persists despite optimization of hemodynamics, the next step is selection of a **diuretic**, conditional upon the patient's volume status. The majority of studies have shown that loop diuretics do not prevent AKI, do not improve renal functional recovery or alter the natural history of AKI, do not decrease the need for renal replacement therapy, and in fact may increase operative mortality and delay recovery of renal function.[174-177] If the patient is euvolemic or mildly fluid overloaded, use of diuretics to simply improve urine output is not indicated. However, loop diuretics may improve urine output and can often convert oliguric to nonoliguric renal failure if administered early after the onset of renal failure. An improvement in urine output (diuretic-responsive AKI) suggests that the extent of renal injury is less severe, coincidentally leading to an earlier decrease in SCr. Thus, it is potentially beneficially to administer diuretics to reduce fluid overload, primarily to optimize pulmonary function, although this will not hasten recovery of renal function.

   a. **Furosemide** is given in incremental doses starting at 10 mg IV. However, once acute renal failure is established, a dose of 100 mg IV is commonly required and should be given over 20–30 minutes to minimize ototoxicity. If urine output fails to increase within a few hours, the following steps can be taken:

      i. Increase the dose of furosemide up to 200 mg IV (limiting the cumulative daily dose to 1 g).

      ii. Use a continuous infusion of IV furosemide. Give a loading dose of 40–100 mg, and then initiate an infusion of 10–20 mg/h. Rebolus before an increase in the infusion rate. This may be the best means of maintaining an adequate urine output.

      iii. Alternatively, bumetanide can be given either as a bolus dose of 4–10 mg IV or as a 1 mg load followed by a continuous infusion of 0.5–2 mg/h depending on the estimated creatinine clearance. There is little evidence that one loop diuretic is better than any other, but some patients respond better to one than the other.

   b. Various **combinations** of medications may be effective in improving diuresis.

      i. Add a **thiazide** diuretic to the loop diuretic. These include chlorothiazide 500 mg IV, metolazone (Zaroxolyn) 5–10 mg PO or via a nasogastric tube, or hydrochlorothiazide 50–200 mg PO qd. Thiazides block distal nephron sites and act synergistically with the loop diuretics to increase exposure of the distal tubules to solute. This combination is particularly effective in patients who tend to be diuretic-resistant.[178] The thiazide should be given 20 minutes before the loop diuretic to prime the distal tubules; otherwise, there may be compensatory sodium reabsorption in the distal tubules.

      ii. Although dopamine has not been shown to be effective in preventing AKI, reducing its severity and duration, or lowering the risk of dialysis, one study found that the combination of mannitol (500 mL of 20% Osmitrol) + furosemide (1 g) + dopamine (2–3 µg/kg/min) started within the first six hours of oliguria produced a significant diuresis with early restoration of renal function.[179]

5. **Fenoldopam** has shown equivocal results in the treatment of established AKI after cardiac surgery. One study of patients receiving a 72-hour infusion for early

acute AKI (a 50% rise in SCr) showed a trend towards reduction in mortality and the need for dialysis in nondiabetic patients, but other studies have not shown much benefit.[180,181]

6. **Diltiazem** given intra- and postoperatively (primarily to prevent radial artery graft spasm) has shown an insignificant improvement in creatinine clearance, so whether it has any role in the management of AKI is not clear.[182]

7. **Note: mannitol** is an osmotic diuretic that is frequently used during surgery to increase serum osmolality during hemodilution to minimize tissue edema. It improves renal tubular flow, reduces tubular cell swelling, and also improves urine output. In patients with early postoperative AKI, it increases RBF by decreasing renal vascular resistance, but does not affect filtration fraction or renal oxygenation.[183] Nonetheless, it is best avoided in the postoperative period because its oncotic effect mobilizes fluid into the intravascular space. This could theoretically lead to pulmonary edema if fluid overload is present and urine output does not improve. In fact, a significant increase in serum osmolality can cause renal vasoconstriction and induce renal failure.

I. **Management of established renal failure**

1. Once oliguric renal failure is established, treatment should be directed towards optimizing hemodynamics while minimizing excessive fluid administration, providing appropriate nutrition, and initiating early renal replacement therapy to hopefully reduce morbidity and improve survival. The blood pressure should be maintained at a higher level than usual in hypertensive patients whose kidneys may require higher perfusion pressures.

2. Restrict fluids with mL/mL of fluid replacement (i.e. input = output) plus 500 mL D5W/0.2% normal saline/day (about 200 mL/m²/day). Daily weights are helpful in assessing changes in day-to-day fluid status, but must also take into consideration the influence of nutritional status on body mass.

3. Monitor electrolytes and blood glucose

   a. Avoid potassium supplements and medications that increase potassium levels (β-blockers, ACE inhibitors). Correct hyperkalemia as described on pages 709–711.

   b. Hyponatremia, if associated with inappropriate ADH (SIADH), should be treated with fluid restriction. The hypovolemic patient with hyponatremia may need isotonic saline.

   c. Metabolic acidosis is common with acute/chronic kidney injury and does not need to be corrected if the serum bicarbonate is >15 mEq/L. If it is lower, a potential contributing cause to a hypoperfusion issue should be sought and corrected.

   d. Correct hyperglycemia and abnormalities of calcium, phosphate, or magnesium metabolism.

4. Medications

   a. Eliminate drugs that impair renal perfusion or are nephrotoxic (ACE inhibitors, ARBs, aminoglycosides, NSAIDs).

   b. Avoid or adjust doses of medications that are excreted or metabolized by the kidneys (particularly low-molecular-weight heparin, and renally excreted antibiotics) (see Appendices 12 and 13). Unfractionated heparin may be used for patients with mechanical heart valves until the INR becomes therapeutic on warfarin. NOACs (especially apixaban) can be used in reduced dosage for other patients with indications for anticoagulation other than mechanical heart valves.

c. Give antacid medications (proton pump inhibitors [PPIs]) to minimize the risk of GI bleeding, but avoid magnesium-containing antacids and laxatives. However, PPIs have been linked to hypomagnesemia, interstitial nephritis, and other renal issues when used for more than one week.[184]

5. Remove the Foley catheter and catheterize daily or prn depending on the urine output. Culture the urine if clinically indicated.

6. Improve the patient's nutritional state with enteral nutrition if possible.[185,186] If the patient is able to eat, an essential amino acid diet should be used. Protein should not be restricted if the patient is on hemodialysis, which can result in the loss of 3–5 g/h of protein. Patients on dialysis should receive approximately 25–30 Kcal/kg of nutrition with a minimum of 1.5 g/kg/day of protein.

a. If a patient on dialysis is unable to eat but has a functional GI tract, a high nitrogen tube feeding can be used. For most patients with acute renal failure, there is no need to alter the amount of protein, and standard tube feedings can be used unless hyperkalemia is present. In patients with CKD who do not require dialysis, a low-protein supplement can be used to provide 0.5–0.8 g/kg/day of protein.

b. If the patient is unable to tolerate enteral feedings, total parenteral nutrition using a 4.25% amino acid/35% dextrose solution that contains no potassium, magnesium, or phosphate is recommended.

7. Consider the prompt initiation of renal replacement therapy.

VII. Renal Replacement Therapy

A. Various forms of renal replacement therapy (RRT) can be used to remove excessive fluid and solute to improve electrolyte balance and remove other nitrogenous waste products (Table 12.7).[187]

1. **Indications.** The most important indications for initiation of RRT are fluid overload, hyperkalemia, and metabolic acidosis. Other signs of uremia, such as a change in mental status, pericarditis, or GI bleeding, should also prompt initiation of RRT, although these are uncommon in the acute setting. However, a very important and sometimes difficult decision to make is whether RRT should be initiated at the first sign of persistent oliguria or a rising SCr, especially since the latter tends to lag behind the extent of renal dysfunction. Some studies of cardiac surgical patients have shown that early and aggressive dialysis, before the patient develops signs and symptoms of renal failure and before a marked elevation in SCr occurs, improves outcomes.[188,189] Other studies in ICU patients have shown conflicting results.[190,191] Certainly, when marked oliguria is present early after surgery in a patient with significant fluid overload, and when there is a poor response to diuretics, a delay in initiating RRT may lead to respiratory compromise and prolonged ventilation with its attendant risks. On the other hand, some patients may recover renal function without the need for dialysis, which has numerous risks, including hypotension, which can prolong renal failure.

If the Patient Has	HD	SCUF	CVVH	CVVHD
Unstable hemodynamics	–	+ + +	+ + +	+ + +
Contraindication to heparin	+ +	+	+	+
Vascular access problems	+ + +	+ + +	+ + +	+ + +
Volume overload	+ +	+ + +	+ + +	+ + +
Hyperkalemia	+ + +	0	+ +	+ + +
Severe uremia	+ + +	0	+	+ +
Respiratory compromise	+ +	+ + +	+ + +	+ + +

Table 12.7 • Techniques of Renal Replacement Therapy (Hemofiltration and Hemodialysis)

HD, hemodialysis; SCUF, slow continuous ultrafiltration; CVVH, continuous veno-venous hemofiltration; CVVHD, continuous veno-venous hemofiltration with dialysis
– avoid; 0 minimal effect; + useful; + + better; + + + even better

2. An additional consideration in patients with moderate renal dysfunction (SCr >2–2.5 mg/dL) is use of "prophylactic" preoperative dialysis. Several studies have demonstrated that this reduces the need for postoperative RRT, with a reduction in overall morbidity and mortality.[117–119]

3. RRT involves several processes to remove volume, solute, or waste products. A transmembrane gradient (basically hydrostatic pressure) drives plasma water (ultrafiltration) and solute (convection) across a semipermeable membrane. Solute removal by diffusion is driven by the difference in the solute concentration between plasma and an electrolyte solution on the other side of the membrane.

4. The most common forms of RRT used in cardiac surgery patients are those of intermittent hemodialysis and continuous veno-venous hemofiltration. Selection of the appropriate modality depends on the indications for its use (whether primarily for volume or solute removal), and the hemodynamic stability of the patient. Both of these approaches are associated with comparable outcomes, such as recovery of renal function and survival.[189–191]

B. **Intermittent hemodialysis (HD)**

1. **Principle.** Solute passes by diffusion down a concentration gradient from the blood, across a hollow-fiber semipermeable membrane, and into a dialysate bath. Fluid removal by ultrafiltration and solute transport by convection also occur due to the differences in hydrostatic pressure on either side of the membrane.

2. **Indications.** HD is indicated for the management of hyperkalemia, acid–base imbalances, fluid overload, or a hypercatabolic state in the hemodynamically stable patient. It is the most efficient means of removing solute (urea, creatinine) and

correcting severe acid–base abnormalities. It can be combined with ultrafiltration to remove excess volume.

3. **Access.** Standard intermittent HD is performed using a single 12 Fr double-lumen catheter (such as the Mahurkar [Medtronic] or Niagara, DuoGlide and Power-Trialysis catheters [Bard]) preferentially placed in the internal jugular vein for short-term dialysis. Placement in the subclavian vein can cause venous thrombosis, which could impair ipsilateral fistula maturation if that is required in the future and should be avoided. Femoral venous access is feasible but impairs patient mobility. To reduce the risk of infection in patients requiring more extended periods of dialysis, a double-lumen Permcath (Medtronic) or HemoGlide (Bard) long-term hemodialysis catheter can be placed into the internal jugular vein and brought through a subcutaneous tunnel as a "midline" catheter. Subsequently, a fistula can be created for permanent dialysis. When recovery appears unlikely and a fistula is being considered, the arm vessels on one side should be protected from use as much as possible.

4. **Technique.** Intermittent HD is performed over a three- to four-hour period and is usually performed at least three times per week until renal function recovers. The blood is pumped into the dialysis cartridge at a rate of 300–400 mL/min, while the dialysate solution is infused at a rate of 500–700 mL/min in a direction countercurrent to blood flow. Although heparin is commonly used, heparin-free HD is possible in patients with bleeding problems or heparin-induced thrombocytopenia.

5. **Limitations**

   a. Circulatory instability with hypotension from a blunted sympathetic reflex response to hypovolemia is the most common complication of HD, especially if large volumes are being removed in a short period of time. Rapid removal of volume can cause myocardial stunning, and ultrafiltration exceeding 13 mL/kg/h is associated with increased cardiovascular mortality.[192] Too high a blood flow during initiation of dialysis will reduce plasma osmolality, prompting water movement into cells, exacerbating the depletion of extracellular volume. This problem has been mitigated to some degree by use of biocompatible membranes, bicarbonate baths, initial high dialysate sodium, cool temperatures, and volumetric control during dialysis. Colloid or blood transfusions and hemodynamic support (usually with α-agents or PO midodrine) are frequently necessary. About 20–30% of patients develop hypotension during HD, and about 10% of patients cannot tolerate it because of hemodynamic instability. This is probably more common in patients early in the postoperative period, especially if hemodynamic compromise was a major contributing factor to their developing AKI. Therefore, HD is best avoided in the hemodynamically unstable patient.

   b. Dialysis machines are complex and costly, and require special expertise.

C. **Continuous veno-venous systems** can be used in a variety of ways, including slow continuous ultrafiltration (SCUF), continuous veno-venous hemofiltration (CVVH), and continuous veno-venous hemodialysis or hemodiafiltration (CVVHD).

   1. **Principle.** An occlusive pump is included in a circuit that actively withdraws blood at a designated rate from the venous system, pumps it with hydrostatic pressure through the membrane of a hemofilter, and then returns the blood to the

venous system. This circuit achieves filtration or convection of plasma water. For CVVHD, dialysis fluid runs countercurrent to the direction of blood flow within the ultrafiltration membrane. Solute then passes by diffusion down a concentration gradient across a hemofilter into the dialysate solution.

2. **Indications.** These systems are indicated for the management of fluid overload, especially in the hemodynamically unstable or hypotensive patient. Slow correction of electrolyte imbalance can be achieved with CVVH using a crystalloid solution of different composition for replacement fluid. Severe electrolyte imbalance and hypercatabolic state are better managed with CVVHD.

3. **Access** is obtained using a 12 Fr double-lumen catheter (12 gauge for each lumen) placed in the internal jugular or femoral vein.

4. **Technique** (Figure 12.6)

    a. Most continuous veno-venous circuits are "integrated" systems that include a blood pump, pressure monitors, air detector with shut-off controls, and fluid balancing systems for ultrafiltrate control. A high-efficiency biocompatible hemodialysis cartridge is attached downstream to an occlusive pump and heparin is infused into the inflow portion of the circuit to maintain a dialyzer output (venous) PTT of 45–60 seconds. Alternatively, regional citrate anticoagulation

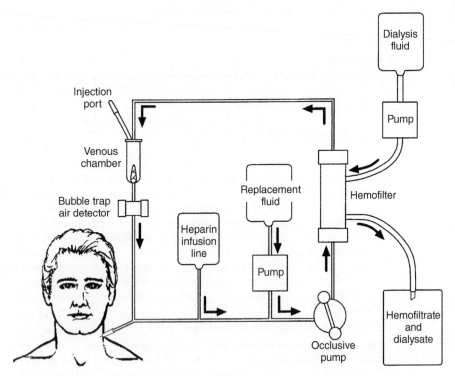

Figure 12.6 • Continuous veno-venous hemofiltration (CVVH). An occlusive pump withdraws blood from the venous circuit, pumps it through a ultrafiltration membrane, and returns it to the venous system through a double-lumen catheter placed in the internal jugular vein.

can be infused into the inflow limb instead of heparin, especially in patients with bleeding or heparin-induced thrombocytopenia.[193,194] When citrate is used, steps must be taken to avoid hypocalcemia and metabolic alkalosis. Calcium should be infused in the venous return line postfilter and alkaline buffers must be reduced in replacement fluids for CVVH or in the dialysate solution for CVVHD.

b. **SCUF** removes fluid by ultrafiltration, but does not remove much solute. The blood flow rate is set at 50–80 mL/min and the ultrafiltrate rate is set at the desired amount (about 5 mL/min), which can potentially achieve a net negative fluid balance of up to 7 L/day. The filter is more prone to clotting due to the slow flow and because the postfilter hematocrit is high. Since no replacement fluid is given and minimal solute is removed, SCUF is used primarily to treat volume overload since it is ineffective for uremia or hyperkalemia.

c. With **CVVH**, fluid and solute are transported by ultrafiltration and convection, respectively, and no dialysate solution is used. The pump is usually set to deliver blood at a rate of 50–300 mL/min and the ultrafiltrate rate is usually set at a preselected rate around 16.7 mL/min or 1 L/h (range of 0.5–4 L/h). The blood then passes through a bubble trap air detector and is returned to the patient. Replacement fluid (alternating 1 L of 0.9% NS plus 1 ampoule [10 mL of a 10% solution] of calcium gluconate with 1 L of 0.45% NS plus 1 ampoule [50 mEq/50 mL] of 8.4% $NaHCO_3$) is infused into the outflow (return) circuit or into the venous chamber to correct electrolyte and acid–base imbalances. The amount administered is dictated by the desired negative fluid balance per hour. This technique can achieve a moderate amount of solute and fluid removal due to the high ultrafiltration rate. Clotting of the system is less likely because the dialyzer can be prediluted with a large volume of fluid.

d. **CVV hemodialysis (CVVHD)** transports solute by diffusion with variable degrees of ultrafiltration to remove fluid, whereas **CVV hemodiafiltration** combines the convective solute removal of CVVH with the diffusive solute removal of hemodialysis, along with ultrafiltration. The blood flow is set at 50–300 mL/min and the dialysate (Dianeal 1.5% with 4 mL of 23% NaCl per 2 L bag) is infused into the dialysis cartridge at a rate of 1–2 L/h or even higher for hemodiafiltration. These techniques are most useful in the highly catabolic patient to remove a large solute load. The effluent flow rate (hemofiltration rate + the dialysate flow rate) should be about 20–25 mL/kg to achieve adequate solute clearance.

5. **Advantages and limitations**

a. Citrate anticoagulation eliminates concerns about use of heparin.

b. High flow rates of CVVH/CVVHD reduce the potential for clotting of the filter noted with SCUF.

c. Use of the blood pump enables CVVH to be performed when the patient is hypotensive or hemodynamically unstable.

d. Because CVVH removes so much fluid, it is essential to carefully monitor electrolytes and modify the replacement solutions as necessary to maintain electrolyte balance.

e. The pump adds some complexity and cost to the system compared with arteriovenous hemofiltration.

D. **Continuous arteriovenous hemofiltration (CAVH)** is used during surgery to remove excessive fluid before terminating CPB. It is beneficial in improving hemodynamics, hemostasis, and pulmonary function in higher-risk patients. Postoperatively, its use is limited by the need for arterial access, heparinization to minimize clotting of the hemofilter, and the requirement for satisfactory arterial pressure to provide the hydrostatic pressure to achieve hemofiltration. Because of these drawbacks, CAVH has been replaced by CVVH in most units.

E. **Peritoneal dialysis (PD)** is rarely used in cardiac surgical patients, because it produces abdominal distention and glucose absorption that can compromise respiratory status, and it carries the risk of peritonitis. Its use is usually limited to patients on chronic peritoneal dialysis.

VIII. Hyperkalemia

A. **Etiology** in cardiac surgery patients

1. High-volume, high-potassium cardioplegia solutions used in the operating room. The potassium load is usually eliminated promptly by normally functioning kidneys, but hyperkalemia can be problematic in patients with acute or chronic renal dysfunction or oliguria from other causes.

2. Low cardiac output states associated with oliguria. Potassium levels may rise with alarming and life-threatening rapidity.

3. Severe tissue ischemia, whether peripheral (from severe peripheral vascular disease or complication of an IABP) or intra-abdominal (mesenteric ischemia). Hyperkalemia is often the first clue to the existence of these problems.

4. Acute and chronic renal insufficiency

5. Medications that impair potassium excretion or increase potassium levels (ACE inhibitors, ARBs, potassium-sparing diuretics [triamterene, spironolactone, amiloride, eplerenone], NSAIDs, β-blockers)

6. Severe hyperglycemia, which increases potassium release from cells into the extracellular fluid

7. **Note:** remember that hyperkalemia is exacerbated by acidosis, which often accompanies low-output or ischemic syndromes. A 0.2 unit change in pH produces about a 1 mEq/L change in serum potassium concentration. However, in conditions of organic acidosis, the potassium is more likely to rise from tissue breakdown and release of potassium from cells (lactic acidosis) or from insulin deficiency and hyperglycemia (ketoacidosis), than from a change in pH.

B. **Manifestations** are predominantly electrocardiographic due to depolarization of cardiac cell resting membrane potentials, which decreases membrane excitability. An asystolic arrest may occur when the potassium rises rapidly to a level exceeding 6.5 mEq/L. The ECG changes of hyperkalemia do not always develop in classic progressive fashion and are more related to the rate of rise of serum potassium than to the absolute level. These changes include:

1. Peaked T waves

2. ST depression

3. Smaller R waves

4. Prolonged PR interval

5. Loss of P waves

6. QRS widening, bradycardia, ventricular fibrillation, and asystole. When the heart is being paced, hyperkalemia may result in failure to respond to the pacemaker stimulus.

C. **Treatment** entails stabilizing the cell membrane, shifting potassium into cells, and increasing its excretion from the body (Table 12.8).[195,196] A hyperkalemic emergency is present when there are ECG changes, a serum potassium >6.5 mEq/L, or a level >5.5 mEq/L with acute renal impairment and ongoing tissue breakdown or potassium absorption (GI bleeding). These patients need an emergency reduction in their potassium levels. In other patients, a slower reduction is feasible.

1. It is essential to identify and remove any potential source of potassium intake or medications that may increase the potassium level (as above); use a low-potassium diet in patients with renal dysfunction and persistent hyperkalemia.

2. Address cardiac toxicity:

a. If there is evidence of advanced cardiac toxicity or ECG changes, usually when the potassium is >6.5 mEq/L, administer **calcium gluconate** 10 mL of a 10% solution (1 g) IV over 2–3 minutes to stabilize the cell membranes. The beneficial effect should be noted within minutes, but lasts only about 30 minutes. Note that calcium potentiates the cardiotoxic effects of digoxin, so hyperkalemia in patients on digoxin should preferentially be treated with digoxin-specific antibody fragments (Digibind), although a slow infusion of calcium gluconate can safely be given over 30 minutes.

Table 12.8 • Acute Treatment of Hyperkalemia

Medication	Dosage	Onset of Action	Duration of Action
Calcium gluconate*	10 mL of 10% solution over 2–3 min	Immediate	30 min
Insulin*	10 units regular insulin IV in 50 mL of 50% dextrose	10–20 min	4–6 h
Sodium bicarbonate	1 amp 7.5% (44.6 mEq)	30 min	1–2 h
Albuterol	10–20 mg by nebulizer	90 min (peak effect)	2–3 h
Furosemide*	20–40 mg IV	15–60 min	4 h
Sodium polystyrene sulfonate (Kayexalate)	Oral: 30 g in 60–120 mL sorbitol PR: 50 g in retention enema	1–2 h	4–6 h

* indicated for hyperkalemic emergencies

b. Alternatively, calcium chloride 5–10 mL of a 10% solution (0.5–1 g) can be infused through a central line over several minutes. This may produce hemodynamic changes, but provides four times more elemental calcium than calcium gluconate.

3. Shift potassium into cells:

a. **Regular insulin** 10 units in 50 mL of a 50% dextrose solution IV. This should lower the potassium about 0.5–1.5 mEq/L within 15 minutes and last for several hours. Another regimen is 10–20 units in 500 mL of 10% dextrose given over 60 minutes. This can be considered first if there is marked hyperkalemia but no ECG changes.

b. **Sodium bicarbonate** ($NaHCO_3$) administration in patients with acidosis results in hydrogen release from cells in exchange for potassium movement into cells. Thus, correction of acidosis should lower potassium levels. Bicarbonate also has a direct effect on hyperkalemia independent of a change in pH.[197] However, boluses of bicarbonate are not that effective in reducing serum potassium, so in hyperkalemic emergencies, an infusion (150 mEq in one liter of D5W given over 2–4 hours) is recommended. In hyponatremic patients, the sodium load may reverse some of the ECG changes of hyperkalemia.

c. β_2-agonists activate the Na^+–K^+–ATPase system to drive potassium into cells and can lower the potassium level by 0.5–1.5 mEq/L. The only recommended drug is **albuterol** 10–20 mg in 4 mL NS by nebulizer over 10 minutes, which has a peak effect in about 90 minutes. Epinephrine (0.05 µg/kg/min) may also be effective, but it is best avoided in the cardiac patient unless there is an inotropic requirement.

4. Enhance potassium excretion because the effects of calcium and glucose-insulin infusions are short-lived.

a. **Furosemide** 20–40 mg IV is very effective in reducing serum potassium in patients without significant renal impairment. Diuretics may be given alone in patients with hypervolemia, but should be combined with a saline infusion in patients who are euvolemic or hypovolemic. Continuous infusions may also be used. In patients with impaired renal function, IV saline or isotonic bicarbonate should be given along with the diuretic, usually in higher doses, since sodium delivery to the distal tubules is essential to promote potassium excretion.

b. **Hemodialysis** is indicated in patients with hyperkalemia and severe renal dysfunction. It can remove up to 50 mEq of potassium per hour.

c. Sodium polystyrene sulfonate (**Kayexalate**) is a cation-exchange resin that may be given orally (15–30 g in 60–120 mL of 20% sorbitol) or as an enema (50 g in 150 mL of tap water, but **NOT** with sorbitol). Each gram may bind up to 1 mEq of potassium. It may be considered if the other measures have failed to reduce the potassium or are not immediately available. However, it should not be given to patients with an ileus or receiving narcotics, which includes most postoperative patients. Kayexalate has been associated with the occurrence of colonic necrosis which may be related to decreased colonic motility, and may occur with or without use of sorbitol.[198]

    d. Sodium zirconium cyclosilicate (ZC-9) is a selective cation-exchanger that entraps potassium in the intestinal tract in exchange for sodium and hydrogen. It is given in doses starting at 2.5 g three times a day and produces a rapid and dose-dependent reduction in potassium levels within 48 hours.[199,200]

    e. Patiromer (8.4 g orally) is a GI cation-exchanger that binds potassium ions in the GI tract in exchange for calcium ions, so less potassium is absorbed and more is excreted in the stool. Potassium starts falling in seven hours and continues to decrease for 48 hours. It should be considered if hemodialysis is not immediately available in a patient with severe renal impairment, but is usually used for the chronic, rather than acute, treatment of hyperkalemia.[200]

IX. Hypokalemia

A. Etiology

1. Profound diuresis without adequate potassium replacement. Potassium excretion parallels the urine output after CPB, which tends to be copious because of hemodilution. The use of potent diuretics may produce a significant diuresis and kaliuresis in the early postoperative period.

2. Insulin to treat hyperglycemia, which redistributes potassium from the extracellular fluid into cells ("redistributive hypokalemia")

3. Hypomagnesemia (usually from diuresis) which can cause refractory hypokalemia

4. Alkalosis (metabolic or respiratory) (the "L" in alkalosis tells you the potassium is "lowered")

5. Significant nasogastric tube drainage

B. Manifestations.
The primary concern with hypokalemia in the cardiac patient is the induction of cardiac reentrant arrhythmias due to enhanced cardiac automaticity and delayed ventricular repolarization. Hypokalemia may produce atrial, junctional, or ventricular ectopy (PACs, PVCs), paroxysmal atrial and junctional tachycardias, AV block, and VT/VF. The ECG may demonstrate flattened ST segments, decreased T-wave amplitude, and the presence of "u" waves. Factors that may promote the development of hypokalemic arrhythmias include myocardial ischemia, enhanced sympathetic tone (often from epinephrine or β_2-agonists), digoxin, and low magnesium levels (commonly seen after CPB). Hypokalemia can also result in weakness involving the respiratory muscles, the GI tract (producing an ileus), or the skeletal muscles.

C. Treatment
is indicated for any potassium level below the normal range, although ECG changes do not become evident until the level is <3 mEq/L.[201,202] Most patients with diuretic-induced hypokalemia have a metabolic alkalosis associated with chloride depletion. Low chloride levels enhance bicarbonate reabsorption in the kidneys, and sodium is exchanged for potassium rather than excreted with chloride. Thus, failure to replenish chloride leads to more potassium wasting.

1. It is essential that renal function and urine output be evaluated before a potassium chloride (KCl) drip is started, because acute hyperkalemia can develop very rapidly when oliguria or renal dysfunction is present. A slower infusion rate is advisable in this situation, with frequent rechecking of the serum potassium level. Particular attention should be paid to sources of urinary or GI loss of potassium that may require more aggressive replacement.

2. Serum magnesium levels should be checked because hypomagnesemia can make the hypokalemia refractory to treatment; if low, magnesium should be replaced.

3. In the ICU setting, KCl is administered through a central line at a rate of 10–20 mEq/h (mix of 20–40 mEq/100 mL in 0.45% NS). An infusion pump should always be considered when the IV bag contains more than 40 mEq or the infusion rate exceeds 10 mEq/h, to avoid a catastrophic hyperkalemic event. A dextrose carrier should be avoided because it may lower the potassium level by stimulating secretion of insulin. The serum potassium rises approximately 0.1 mEq/L for each 2 mEq of KCl administered. Repeat potassium levels should guide therapy.

4. When a central line is not present, a concentrated potassium drip cannot be administered peripherally because it scleroses veins. The maximum concentration of KCl that can be administered peripherally is 60 mEq/L. IV bags containing 60 mEq/L or 10 mEq in a 100–200 mL bag are commonly used.

5. Once the patient is extubated, oral potassium (10–20 mEq tablets up to three to four times a day) will usually suffice to treat potassium levels of 3–4 mEq/L. However, doses of 40–60 mEq three to four times a day may be necessary to maintain normal potassium levels when the potassium is <3 mEq/L.

6. Potassium-sparing diuretics should be considered in the chronic management of HF, but not acutely to raise serum potassium. The preferred drug is amiloride, which is an epithelial sodium channel blocker in cortical collecting ducts. The mineralocorticoid receptor antagonists (spironolactone and eplerenone) can be considered in HF patients with normal or mildly abnormal renal function (SCr <2.5 mg/dL).

7. Note that patients with uncontrolled diabetes may have movement of potassium out of cells due to insulin deficiency and hyperosmolality. Thus, the serum potassium may be elevated despite a marked potassium deficit. Aggressive treatment with insulin will lower the potassium, so potassium levels must be carefully evaluated to determine when to start replenishing potassium. If the patient has severe hyperglycemia and hypokalemia, potassium should be given prior to giving insulin, which will lower potassium levels.

X. Hypocalcemia

A. Calcium plays a complex role in myocardial energetics and reperfusion damage. Ionized calcium (normal = 1.1–1.3 mmol/L) should be measured because total calcium levels, which are affected by protein binding, usually decrease during surgery because of hemodilution, hypothermia, shifts in pH, hypomagnesemia, and the use of citrated blood. Hypocalcemia is usually associated with prolongation of the QT interval on the ECG tracing. It reduces cardiac sensitivity to digoxin.

B. **Treatment**

1. It is common practice to empirically administer a 500 mg bolus of calcium chloride at the termination of CPB to support systemic vascular resistance and possibly increase myocardial contractility.[203] It may be given with protamine to offset its vasodilatory effects.[204]

2. It is questionable whether treatment of hypocalcemia identified in the ICU is of any value in improving cardiovascular function. In fact, calcium salts may attenuate the cardiotonic effects of catecholamines, such as dobutamine or epinephrine,

although they have little effect on the efficacy of milrinone.[205] Nonetheless, if the ionized calcium level is measured and found to be <1 mmol/L, calcium gluconate (10 mL of 10% solution in 50 mL D5W) may be given over 10–20 minutes, although there is no clear benefit to doing so. It may also be given as an infusion of 50 mL/h of a 10% solution (placing 100 mL in 1 L of D5W). Calcium chloride is best avoided for "asymptomatic" hypocalcemia to minimize any acute hemodynamic effects, but similar dosing is used. Because hypocalcemia can be difficult to correct if the serum magnesium level is low, an infusion of magnesium sulfate 2 g (16 mEq) of a 10% solution over 10–20 minutes may be given, with a subsequent infusion of 1 g (8 mEq) in 100 mL of fluid per hour.[206]

3. Calcium chloride (0.5–1 g IV) may be given in emergency situations to provide temporary circulatory support when a low cardiac output syndrome or profound hypotension develops suddenly. The transient improvement in hemodynamics allows time for analysis of causative factors and the institution of other pharmacologic support. It should not be given routinely during a cardiac arrest.

XI. Hypomagnesemia

A. Magnesium plays a role in energy metabolism and cardiac impulse generation. Low levels have been associated with coronary spasm, low cardiac output syndromes, prolonged ventilatory support, a higher incidence of postoperative atrial and ventricular arrhythmias, perioperative infarction, and a higher mortality rate.[207–210]

B. Magnesium levels (normal = 1.5–2 mEq/L) are usually not measured during surgery, but are reduced in the majority of patients. This is usually the result of hemodilution during CPB as well as urinary excretion, but it is also very common in patients undergoing off-pump surgery.[211] Medications contributing to low magnesium levels include diuretics and PPIs.

C. Administration of magnesium sulfate ($MgSO_4$) 2 g in 100 mL solution given over an hour to raise the serum level to 2 mEq/L is effective in reducing the incidence of postoperative atrial fibrillation and ventricular arrhythmias after both on-pump and off-pump surgery.[211] Notably, magnesium has been found to inhibit the vasoconstrictive response to epinephrine, but not its cardiotonic effects.[212] Administering 1–2 g of $MgSO_4$ at the conclusion of bypass and on the first postoperative morning can be recommended.

D. Magnesium may be helpful in the treatment of torsades de pointes.

XII. Metabolic Acidosis

A. Etiology

1. A low cardiac output state causing tissue hypoperfusion is usually the primary cause of metabolic (lactic) acidosis in the cardiac surgery patient. Poor peripheral and visceral perfusion will be exacerbated by use of vasopressors.

2. Intra-abdominal catastrophes, such as mesenteric ischemia from a low-flow state, should always be considered when progressive metabolic acidosis occurs.

3. Low-dose epinephrine occasionally causes a metabolic acidosis out of proportion to its α effects when the cardiac output is satisfactory. This may reflect a metabolic type B lactic acidosis (not associated with tissue hypoxia) caused by metabolic factors that increase lactic acid production, such as hyperglycemia and lipolysis.[213,214]

4. Sepsis
5. High doses of sodium nitroprusside
6. Renal failure (which reduces acid excretion)
7. Acute hepatic dysfunction
8. Diabetic ketoacidosis
9. Aggressive crystalloid infusions with high chloride content (normal saline)

B. **Effects**

1. Adverse effects of metabolic acidosis usually do not occur until the pH is less than 7.20.[215,216] A primary metabolic acidosis (low serum bicarbonate with acidemic pH) may be noted in the heavily sedated patient in whom there is no respiratory compensation. However, compensatory hyperventilation to neutralize the acidosis will occur when the patient can breathe spontaneously, and for every 1 mEq/L fall in bicarbonate, the PCO_2 is generally reduced about 1.2 torr. However, it is not uncommon to see incomplete compensation with a mixed respiratory/metabolic acidosis. Notably, some of the deleterious effects of metabolic acidosis may be related to the metabolic products associated with the acidosis, rather than the absolute level of pH, although they may be reversed by administration of sodium bicarbonate.

2. The presence of a progressive or significant metabolic acidosis (as assessed by the serum bicarbonate level) is often an indication of a serious ongoing problem that must be corrected before adverse consequences occur. Occasionally, this may be identified surreptitiously. For example, after the patient is extubated and the arterial line has been removed, the patient may develop tachypnea of unknown etiology. An ABG or basic metabolic panel may reveal that the patient is compensating for a profound metabolic acidosis. Some adverse consequences of a metabolic acidosis include:

   a. Cardiovascular effects
      • Decreased contractility and cardiac output; reduction in hepatic and renal blood flow
      • Attenuation of the positive inotropic effects of catecholamines
      • Venoconstriction and arteriolar dilatation which increase filling pressures and decrease systemic pressures
      • Increased pulmonary vascular resistance
      • Sensitization to reentrant arrhythmias and reduction in the threshold for ventricular fibrillation
   b. Respiratory effects
      • Dyspnea and tachypnea
      • Decreased respiratory muscle strength
   c. Metabolic changes
      • Increased metabolic demands
      • Hyperglycemia caused by tissue insulin resistance and inhibition of anaerobic glycolysis
      • Decreased hepatic update and increased hepatic production of lactate
      • Hyperkalemia
      • Increased protein catabolism

d. Cerebral function
- Inhibition of brain metabolism and cell volume regulation
- Obtundation and coma

3. Type A lactic acidosis reflects impaired tissue oxygenation and anaerobic metabolism resulting from circulatory failure. The acidosis is self-perpetuating in that excess lactate is being produced at a time when there is suppression of hepatic lactate utilization. The lactate ion, probably more than the acidosis, contributes to potential cardiovascular dysfunction. An elevated lactate level (>3 mmol/L) upon arrival in the ICU is associated with a worse outcome.[217] This is more commonly noted in patients with preexisting renal dysfunction, after long pump runs, and with use of intraoperative vasopressors. It is likely that this reflects inadequate oxygen delivery during bypass that has contributed to splanchnic and renal ischemia, with the acidosis perpetuated by a low cardiac output syndrome. Needless to say, the presence of elevated lactate levels during bypass or upon arrival in the ICU requires prompt attention. The development of a metabolic acidosis several days after surgery raises the specter of mesenteric ischemia, especially in patients requiring additional days of ICU care.

4. Type B lactic acidosis occurs in the absence of tissue hypoxia.[213,214] It may be a catecholamine-induced metabolic effect (especially with epinephrine) caused by hyperglycemia and alterations in fatty acid metabolism that cause pyruvate accumulation and elevated levels of lactic acid. Acute hepatic failure may also be present with severe lactic acidosis due to failure to clear lactic acid. Metformin is associated with lactic acidosis in patients with renal insufficiency, low cardiac output states, and liver disease, and with use of contrast agents.

C. Assessment

1. Measurement of the anion gap (AG) is important is sorting out the etiology of acidosis (AG = $Na^+ - [Cl^- + HCO_3^-]$, with normal range being 10–12 mEq/L).

2. Although there are a number of factors that can influence the AG, an increase in AG generally reflects additional acid production, and high AG metabolic acidosis from lactic acid accumulation is most commonly noted after cardiac surgery. It may also be elevated in diabetic ketoacidosis due to production of hydroxybutyrate, in renal failure from decreased acid excretion and increased bicarbonate excretion, and from excessive ingestion of aspirin/methanol/ethylene glycol.

3. A normal or low AG represents loss of bicarbonate (diarrhea) or inability to excrete an acid load (renal tubular acidosis).

D. Treatment

should be directed primarily towards reversal of the underlying cause. This will allow for oxidation of lactate and regeneration of bicarbonate to correct the acidosis. Whether correction of a primary metabolic acidosis (not one that compensates for a primary respiratory alkalosis) should be considered when the serum bicarbonate is less than 15 mEq/L (base deficit greater than 8–10 mmol/L) is controversial.[218-222]

1. Proponents of bicarbonate administration suggest that severe metabolic acidosis does have significant deleterious effects on cardiovascular function that can be corrected with a more normal pH. Furthermore, more responsiveness to catecholamines does seem to occur with a more normal pH. Thus, correction of the

acidosis may be important when the etiology of the acidosis is unclear or not imminently remediable.

2. Others argue that the use of bicarbonate can cause metabolic derangements with little evidence of hemodynamic improvement.[219,220] Sodium bicarbonate can cause fluid overload, hypernatremia, and hyperosmolarity, increased affinity of hemoglobin for oxygen (and thus less tissue release), and reduced ionized calcium, which may reduce cardiac contractility. It is proposed that bicarbonate may correct only the blood pH, not the intracellular pH, and that the increased production of CO_2 that may not be eliminated in low output states may impair lactate utilization, perpetuating the elevated lactate levels.

3. A randomized study of ICU patients with severe metabolic acidosis found that use of sodium bicarbonate reduced one-month mortality only in patients with acute kidney injury, and did cause more hypernatremia and hypocalcemia.[221] A clinical literature review suggested that there was little documented clinical benefit of using bicarbonate in critically ill patients with metabolic acidosis.[222]

4. Nonetheless, if one elects to correct the pH, sodium bicarbonate is most commonly used. Tromethamine (THAM) is a good alternative in patients with hypernatremia with mixed metabolic/respiratory acidosis, but is no longer available in the USA.

   a. **Sodium bicarbonate** is administered in a dose calculated from the following equation:

   $$0.5 \times \text{body weight in kg} \times \text{base deficit} = \text{mEq NaHCO}_3$$

   This can be given either with bolus doses of 8.4% $NaHCO_3$ (50 mEq/50 mL) or 7.5% $NaHCO_3$ (44.6 mEq/50 mL), or preferably as an IV infusion over several hours (3 amps/1 L D5W, which provides approximately 150 mEq/L) with careful monitoring of the serum sodium concentration. Because the bicarbonate is metabolized to CO_2, this can worsen a respiratory acidosis in a patient with compromised pulmonary function.

   b. **Tromethamine** 0.3 M (THAM or Tris buffer) limits CO_2 generation and will not raise the serum sodium. In contrast to $NaHCO_3$, it does not lower serum potassium, but it can produce hypoglycemia and respiratory depression. It is usually given as a continuous infusion and is contraindicated in renal failure.[223] It is still available outside of the USA and remains an essential component of Buckberg cardioplegia solutions (see Chapter 6). It may be given in a dose up to 0.5 g/kg/h.

   $$\text{kg} \times \text{base deficit} = \text{mL of } 0.3 \text{ M THAM}$$

5. In a mechanically ventilated patient, it is not unreasonable to hyperventilate the patient to lower the PCO_2, which will increase the intracellular and extracellular pH.

6. Critically ill patients with thiamine deficiency can develop lactic acidosis, which is rapidly reversed with thiamine 300 mg IV.[224]

XIII. Metabolic Alkalosis

A. Etiology

1. Excessive diuresis, especially from the loop diuretics, which promotes hypovolemia and depletion of hydrogen ions and chloride

2. Nasogastric drainage and inadequate electrolyte replacement by IV solutions

3. Total parenteral nutrition with inappropriate solute composition

4. Secondary as compensation for respiratory acidosis

B. Pathophysiology

1. A reduction in effective circulating volume (hypovolemia) stimulates aldosterone secretion, which causes sodium retention, which then prevents excretion of sodium bicarbonate. Aldosterone also increases hydrogen secretion into the tubules, increasing bicarbonate reabsorption.

2. Decreased available chloride delivered to the distal tubules results in less chloride–bicarbonate exchange and thus less bicarbonate excretion.

3. Potassium depletion directly increases bicarbonate reabsorption. This shifts hydrogen into the cells in exchange for potassium, raising the plasma bicarbonate concentration, and the lower intracellular pH stimulates hydrogen secretion and bicarbonate reabsorption.

C. Adverse effects

1. Lowers the serum potassium level, potentially leading to atrial and ventricular arrhythmias (especially digoxin-induced arrhythmias) and to neuromuscular weakness.

2. Has an adverse effect on the cardiovascular response to catecholamines that is comparable to that of acidosis.[216]

3. Shifts the oxygen–hemoglobin dissociation curve to the left, impairing oxygen delivery to the tissues. This effect is offset in chronic metabolic alkalosis by an increase of 2,3-DPG in red cells.

4. Produces arteriolar constriction which can compromise cerebral and coronary perfusion. Neurologic abnormalities including headache, seizures, tetany, and lethargy may occur, probably because of the associated hypocalcemia induced by alkalosis. These effects are usually seen with a pH >7.60.

5. Decreases the central respiratory drive, leading to hypoventilation, CO_2 retention, and potentially hypoxemia.

D. Treatment[225]

1. Metabolic alkalosis is sustained by volume depletion ("contraction alkalosis"), as well as by potassium and chloride depletion. Thus, therapy should be directed towards correction of these factors to improve renal excretion of bicarbonate.

2. Potential contributors to alkalosis should be identified and addressed.

   a. Reduce doses of loop diuretics or thiazides to avoid volume depletion. Use PPIs to minimize loss of gastric acid through a nasogastric tube.

   b. Avoid lactated Ringer's solution and acetate (common in parenteral nutrition solutions) that are metabolized to bicarbonate.

3. The administration of chloride, usually as potassium (KCl) or sodium (NaCl), is the primary treatment for metabolic alkalosis. The appropriate solution depends on the patient's volume status and potassium level.

    a. In hypovolemic patients, 0.9% NaCl is the primary replacement fluid, and KCl may also be given for hypokalemia. Volume repletion removes the stimulus for sodium reabsorption, allowing for more bicarbonate excretion. Chloride repletion increases chloride delivery to the distal tubules and augments the chloride–bicarbonate exchange mechanism. Potassium moves into cells in exchange for hydrogen ions which buffer the bicarbonate. The reduction in intracellular pH in renal tubular cells reduces hydrogen secretion and bicarbonate reabsorption.

    b. In patients with total body water overload, typical in the postoperative state or with HF, infusion of NaCl may exacerbate the edema. A KCl infusion is beneficial if the serum K^+ is not elevated, but it can only be given at a limited rate (20 mEq/L). However, during a profound diuresis with significant potassium loss, a faster infusion rate can be used.

  4. Alternative means of treating alkalosis in fluid overloaded patients include the following:

    a. **Amiloride** (5 mg daily) is a potassium-sparing diuretic that may be helpful in improving a metabolic alkalosis. **Spironolactone** 25 mg PO qd or **eplerenone** 50 mg PO qd may also be considered, but they can quickly cause hyperkalemia in patients with HF.

    b. **Acetazolamide** (Diamox) 250–500 mg IV can be given in conjunction with a loop diuretic to increase urine output while increasing bicarbonate excretion. Acetazolamide is a carbonic anhydrase inhibitor that inhibits proximal bicarbonate reabsorption by the kidneys, but it is a weak diuretic when used alone. It can lead to potassium depletion, so normokalemia should be present before it is started.

    c. **Hydrochloric acid** 0.1 N (100 mEq/L) may be administered through a central line at a rate of 10–20 mEq/h. It is rarely required in cardiac surgical patients. The total dose can be calculated based on a bicarbonate space of 50% body weight from either of the two following methods:

      • Chloride-deficit method:

$$\text{mEq HCl} = 0.5 \times \text{kg(IBW)} \times (103 - \text{measured chloride})$$

    where IBW is ideal body weight.

      • Base-excess method:

$$\text{mEq HCl} = 0.5 \times \text{kg(IBW)} \times (\text{serum } HCO_3^- - 24)$$

    where (serum HCO_3^- – 24) represents the base excess. If a profound alkalosis is present, these doses should be given over 12 hours with intermittent reevaluation.

XIV. Hyperglycemia

A. Etiology

  1. The hormonal stress response to surgery induces insulin resistance in both diabetics (who also have impaired insulin production) and nondiabetics.[226] This is associated with elevated levels of the counterregulatory hormones, including cortisol, epinephrine, and growth hormone.

2. Epinephrine, more so than norepinephrine, can exacerbate postoperative hyperglycemia.[227]

3. Total parenteral nutrition with inadequate insulin response

4. Sepsis (often the first manifestation of an occult sternal wound infection or an intra-abdominal process)

B. **Manifestations.** Intraoperative and postoperative hyperglycemia are associated with an increase in morbidity and mortality in both diabetic and nondiabetic patients.[228-231] Protocols to control hyperglycemia can reduce those risks, although this benefit may be less evident in insulin-dependent diabetics.[232-235] Some of the problems associated with poorly controlled hyperglycemia include:

1. Increased urine output from an osmotic diuresis. Although the hypotonic fluid loss may cause hypernatremia, the glucose-induced shift of water from cells into the extracellular fluid compartment may cause hyponatremia. In this situation, the plasma osmolality is elevated despite the low serum sodium, a condition treated by fluid administration, rather than restriction.

2. Impaired wound healing and increased risk of sternal wound infection. This is noted in diabetics and nondiabetics with hyperglycemia, indicating that the blood glucose level itself is an independent risk factor.[236,237]

3. Increased risk of atrial fibrillation, cardiac, respiratory, and renal complications.[228-230]

4. Worsened cognitive function, which has been noted in nondiabetics, but not in diabetics.[238] However, one study found that control of hyperglycemia had no impact on neurologic or neurocognitive outcomes in nondiabetics.[239]

5. Postoperative delirium, which has been noted more commonly in diabetics with elevated preoperative HbA1c levels.[240] Tight glucose control might actually increase the risk, but not the severity, of postoperative delirium.[241]

C. **Treatment**[242-245]

1. Prevention of intraoperative hyperglycemia lowers the risk of infection, may lower the risk of AKI and the development of neurologic complications, and may lower mortality. Thus, it should be considered an integral component of perioperative glucose management. At the very least, IV insulin should be given during surgery to keep the blood sugar (BS) less than 180 mg/dL. Studies evaluating very stringent intra- and postoperative BS controls (keeping BS <100–130 mg/dL vs. <160 mg/dL) have not shown significant differences in outcomes.[246,247] Although stringent BS control might lower the risk of AKI, this must be tempered with the potential for developing hypoglycemia.[149] One study suggested that adverse outcomes correlated more with the preoperative HbA1c than the intraoperative blood glucose, although the latter is often more difficult to get into the target range in patients with elevated HbA1c levels.[248] Another study found that elevated HbA1c levels were predictive of reduced intraoperative insulin sensitivity in diabetes.[249]

2. In the intensive care unit, maintaining a blood glucose <180 mg/dL during the first 48 hours after surgery has been shown to reduce the risk of wound infection and mortality. This benefit has generally been shown in both diabetics and nondiabetics, although some have suggested this benefit is less in insulin-dependent diabetics.[235] It has been suggested that the percentage of time spent out of the

target range correlates best with the risk of wound infection.[250] Therefore, a hyperglycemia protocol should be followed with careful monitoring of blood glucose (Appendix 6). Novolin R is the usual preparation used for IV boluses and infusions. An intravenous bolus of insulin is rapidly cleared from the blood and may lower the potassium level without affecting the blood glucose. Therefore, a bolus followed by an infusion (using a mix of 100 units of regular insulin/100 mL normal saline) is recommended. Excessively stringent control (keeping glucose <120 mg/dL) is potentially dangerous and probably not necessary.

3. All diabetic patients should have a fingerstick blood glucose drawn before meals and at bedtime once they are started on an oral diet. The glucose level may be higher than suspected from the patient's oral intake because of the residual elevation of counterregulatory hormones from the operation. On the other hand, the blood glucose may remain acceptable without medications in some patients with poor oral intake.

4. Patients with type I diabetes mellitus should have their insulin doses gradually increased back to preoperative levels depending on blood glucose levels and early postoperative insulin requirements. It is preferable to use a lower dose of intermediate or long-acting insulin initially (usually one-half of the usual dose) and supplement it with regular insulin as necessary (Table 12.9). Insulin doses may be increased when the patient becomes more active and has an improved caloric intake.

5. In type II diabetics, oral hypoglycemic medications should be restarted once the patient is taking a normal diet, with frequent checking of fingersticks to assess the adequacy of blood glucose control. Additional coverage may be given with regular insulin (Novolin R). If blood glucose is not well controlled postoperatively, or in patients with preoperative HbA1c levels >7, an endocrine consultation should be considered to initiate the patient on insulin therapy.

D. **Hyperosmolar, hyperglycemic, nonketotic coma** has been reported in type II diabetics following surgery. It commonly develops 4–7 days after surgery and is manifested by polyuria in association with a rising BUN or serum sodium. The resultant dehydration, often exacerbated by GI bleeding or use of high-nitrogen, hyperosmolar tube feedings, results in the hyperosmolar state.[251] Gradual correction of hypovolemia, hyperglycemia, hypokalemia, and hypernatremia is indicated. Consultation with an endocrinologist is important in the assessment and management of these patients.

E. **Diabetic ketoacidosis** is rarely seen following cardiac surgery, but may be noted in type I diabetics. An endocrine consultation and standard management with saline infusions, an insulin drip, and correction of potassium and acid–base abnormalities should be followed.

F. **Note: hypoglycemia** is extremely uncommon after open-heart surgery. Possible causes include:

1. Administration of excessive doses of insulin (either SC or as a continuous infusion). Repeating a blood glucose level every two hours is essential in patients on a continuous infusion, especially at high rates.

2. Premature resumption of preoperative insulin or oral hypoglycemic drug doses in patients with poor oral food intake

3. Residual effects of oral hypoglycemic agents in patients with renal dysfunction

4. A severe hepatic insult with impaired glucose production

Table 12.9 • Commonly Used Insulin Products in Postoperative Patients

Preparation	Brand	Onset	Peak	Average Duration
Very fast-acting (give 15 min prior to meals)				
Insulin lispro	Humalog	<15 min	30–90 min	2–4 h
Insulin aspart	Novolog	5–10 min	1–3 h	3–5 h
Short (fast)-acting				
Regular insulin	Humulin R	30–60 min	2–3 h	5–8 h
Regular insulin	Novolin R	30–60 min	2.5–5 h	5–8 h
Intermediate-acting				
NPH insulin	Humulin N	60–90 min	6–12 h	16–24 h
NPH insulin	Novolin N	60–90 min	4–12 h	16–24 h
Long-acting				
Insulin glargine	Lantus	60 min	none	24 h

[1]Combinations of insulin lispro protamine/insulin lispro (Humalog 75/25), insulin aspart protamine/insulin aspart (Novolog mix 70/30), and NPH/regular (Humulin 70/30, Novolin 70/30, Humulin 50/50) provide rapid onset of action with two peaks (the first at 1–3 h and the second at 4–10 h) with durations of effect of 10–16 h for each preparation
[2]Onset, peak, and duration may vary depending in part on dose and patient activity. Humulin products made by Lilly; Novolin products made by Novo Nordisk; Lantus made by Sanofi Aventis

XV. Hypothyroidism

A. Hypothyroidism is difficult to treat preoperatively in the patient with ischemic heart disease because thyroid hormone replacement may precipitate ischemic symptoms. Even so, it may be present more often than realized even in patients taking thyroid hormone. One study showed a significantly greater operative mortality in patients taking thyroxine preoperatively, perhaps for this reason.[252] Nonetheless, cardiac surgery is well tolerated in most patients with mild–moderate hypothyroidism.

B. Serum total and free triiodothyronine (T_3 and free T_3) are significantly reduced after both on- and off-pump surgery and remain low for up to six days, whereas thyroxine (T_4) is low immediately after surgery, but returns to normal within 24 hours.[253–255] There is some evidence that patients with low T_3 levels preoperatively are more prone to the "nonthyroidal illness syndrome" and to a low cardiac output state after surgery. Furthermore, a prolonged reduction in the conversion of T_4 to T_3 may account for the slower recovery of some patients after surgery. Patients with this syndrome may not feel that well, but there is generally little physiologic impact on cardiac function.[256,257]

C. Patients with significant hypothyroidism may be somewhat lethargic and hypotensive from decreased myocardial contractility and bradycardia. They may occasionally have difficulty weaning from the ventilator.[258]

D. Note that amiodarone is associated with thyroid dysfunction in 15–20% of patients. It can cause iodine-induced hyperthyroidism or destructive thyroiditis and hypothyroidism.[259] Therefore, it is essential that thyroid function tests be obtained in any patient taking amiodarone prior to surgery. For patients who will be given short-term amiodarone for atrial fibrillation prophylaxis (<1 month), it is not unreasonable to check thyroid function tests prior to surgery, although it is probably not necessary in the absence of known thyroid disease.

E. **Treatment**

1. Should postcardiotomy ventricular dysfunction occur, triiodothyronine (T_3) in a dose of 10–20 µg can be given in conjunction with an inotrope, such as milrinone, which does not depend on β-receptors for its action.[260]

2. For the hypothyroid patient who has tolerated surgery uneventfully, treatment is initiated postoperatively with levothyroxine (Synthroid) 50 µg PO qd and subsequently increased depending on TSH and T_4 levels. If the patient is unable to take oral medications, one-half of the oral dose can be given intravenously.

3. If the patient is severely hypothyroid, consultation with an endocrinologist is imperative. Doses of T_4 that have been recommended include an initial IV dose of 0.4 mg, followed by three days of 0.1–0.2 mg IV daily, and then a maintenance dose of 50 µg PO qd.

XVI. Adrenal Insufficiency

A. CPB causes an elevation in adrenocorticotropic hormone (ACTH) which returns to baseline soon thereafter. However, cortisol levels tend to remain elevated and this has been linked to an increased risk of cognitive dysfunction.[261,262]

B. Adrenal insufficiency is a rare complication of cardiac surgery that may result from adrenal hemorrhage associated with heparinization (or other anticoagulation) and the hormonal stress response in an elderly patient.

C. Manifestations include flank pain, nonspecific GI complaints (anorexia, nausea, vomiting, ileus, abdominal pain, or distention), fever, and delirium. Late signs include hyperkalemia, hyponatremia, and hypotension with poor response to vasopressors. The clinical scenario can be confused with sepsis. One study suggested that persistent vasopressor-dependent hypotension was in fact associated with "relative adrenal insufficiency" and was present in more than 50% of patients following cardiac surgery performed on-pump.[263]

D. Diagnosis is confirmed by a low serum cortisol level and failure of cortisol levels to rise one hour after a 0.25 mg IV dose of cosyntropin (a synthetic ACTH analog). The level should rise fourfold or to a level greater than 20 mg/mL.

E. Treatment is with 100 mg of hydrocortisone IV every eight hours along with administration of glucose and normal saline. If an additional mineralocorticoid is needed, fludrocortisone 0.05–0.2 mg qd can be given.

XVII. Pituitary Abnormalities

A. Pituitary apoplexy[264-267]

1. **Etiology.** This rare phenomenon results from infarction of a pituitary tumor due to ischemia, edema, or hemorrhage. The risk is exacerbated by use of CPB with heparinization and reduced cerebral blood flow. If the patient has a pituitary adenoma, off-pump surgery should be considered.[266]

2. **Presentation.** Compression of the optic chiasm and parasellar structures results in ophthalmoplegia, a third nerve palsy, visual loss, and headache. An Addisonian crisis may be precipitated by the hypopituitarism.[267]

3. **Treatment**

   a. Decrease intracerebral edema with hyperventilation, mannitol, and steroids (dexamethasone 10 mg q6h).

   b. Consider urgent hypophysectomy if no improvement.

B. Diabetes insipidus (DI) is a rare complication of cardiac surgery caused by diminished production of antidiuretic hormone (ADH). It has been noted in patients taking lithium preoperatively for depression.[268] The presence of polyuria, a urine osmolarity of 50–100 mOsm/L, and hypernatremia should raise suspicion of the diagnosis. Treatment of central DI involves use of desmopressin, administered either intranasally (1–2 sprays = 10–20 µg) at bedtime or 0.05–0.4 mg PO bid. This is not effective in nephrogenic DI, which is usually treated with nonhormonal therapy.

References

1. Cooper WA, O'Brien SM, Thourani VH, et al. Impact of renal dysfunction on outcomes of coronary artery bypass surgery: results from the Society of Thoracic Surgeons National Adult Cardiac Database. *Circulation* 2006;113:1063–70.

2. Corredor C, Thomson R, Al-Subaie N. Long-term consequences of acute kidney injury after cardiac surgery: a systematic review and meta-analysis. *J Cardiothorac Vasc Anesth* 2016;30:69–75.

3. Lopez-Delgado JC, Esteve F, et al. Influence of acute kidney injury on short- and long-term outcomes in patients undergoing cardiac surgery: risk factors and prognostic value of a modified RIFLE classification. *Crit Care* 2013;17:R293.

4. Miceli A, Bruno VD, Capoun R, Romeo F, Angelini GD, Caputo M. Occult renal dysfunction: a mortality and morbidity risk factor in coronary artery bypass grafting. *J Thorac Cardiovasc Surg* 2011;141:771–6.

5. Elmistekawy E, McDonald B, Hudson C, et al. Clinical impact of mild acute kidney injury after cardiac surgery. *Ann Thorac Surg* 2014;98:815–22.

6. Karkouti K, Wijeysundera DN, Yau TM, et al. Acute kidney injury after cardiac surgery: focus on modifiable risk factors. *Circulation* 2009;119:495–502.

7. Lema G, Meneses G, Urzua J, et al. Effects of extracorporeal circulation on renal function in coronary surgical patients. *Anesth Analg* 1995;81:446–51.

8. O'Neal JB, Shaw AD, Billings FT IV. Acute kidney injury following cardiac surgery: current understanding and future directions. *Crit Care* 2016;20:187.

9. Mariscalco G, Lorusso R, Dominici C, Renzulli A, Sala A. Acute kidney injury: a relevant complication after cardiac surgery. *Ann Thorac Surg* 2011;92:1539–47.

10. Vives M, Wijeysundera D, Marczin N, Monedero P, Rao V. Cardiac-surgery associated acute kidney injury. *Interact Cardiovasc Thorac Surg* 2014;18:637–45.

11. Olivero JJ, Olivero JJ, Nguyen PT, Kagan A. Acute kidney injury after cardiovascular surgery: an overview. *Methodist Cardiovasc J* 2012;8:31–6.

12. Ranucci M, Aloisio T, Carboni G, et al. Acute kidney injury and hemodilution during cardiopulmonary bypass: a changing scenario. *Ann Thorac Surg* 2015;100:95–100.

13. Karkouti K, Beattie WS, Wijeysundera DN, et al. Hemodilution during cardiopulmonary bypass is an independent risk factor for acute renal failure in adult cardiac surgery. *J Thorac Cardiovasc Surg* 2005;129:391–400.

14. Habib RH, Zacharias A, Schwann TA, et al. Role of hemodilutional anemia and transfusion during cardiopulmonary bypass in renal injury after coronary revascularization: implications on operative outcome. *Crit Care Med* 2005;33:1749–56.

15. Mehta RH, Castelvecchio S, Ballotta A, Frigiola A, Bossone E, Ranucci M. Association of gender and lowest hematocrit on cardiopulmonary bypass with acute kidney injury and operative mortality in patients undergoing cardiac surgery. *Ann Thorac Surg* 2013;96:133–40.

16. Benedetto U, Sciarretta S, Roscitano A, et al. Preoperative angiotensin-converting enzyme inhibitors and acute kidney injury after coronary artery bypass grafting. *Ann Thorac Surg* 2008;86:1160–6.

17. van Diepen S, Norris CM, Zheng Y, et al. Comparison of angiotensin-converting enzyme inhibitor and angiotensin receptor blocker management strategies before cardiac surgery: a pilot randomized controlled registry trial. *J Am Heart Assoc* 2018;7:e009917.

18. Bhatia M, Arora H, Kumar PA. PRO: ACE inhibitors should be continued perioperatively and prior to cardiovascular operations. *J Cardiothorac Vasc Anesth* 2016;30:816–9.

19. Disque A, Neelankavil J. Con: ACE inhibitors should be stopped prior to cardiovascular surgery. *J Cardiothorac Vasc Anesth* 2016;30:820–2.

20. Coca SG, Garg AX, Swaminathan M, et al. Preoperative angiotensin-converting enzyme inhibitors and angiotensin receptor blocker use and acute kidney injury in patients undergoing cardiac surgery. *Nephrol Dial Transplant* 2013;28:2787–99.

21. Licker M, Neidhart P, Lustenberger S, et al. Long-term angiotensin-converting enzyme inhibitor treatment attenuates adrenergic responsiveness without altering hemodynamic control in patients undergoing cardiac surgery. *Anesthesiology* 1996;84:789–800.

22. Haase M, Haase-Fielitz A, Bellomo R. Cardiopulmonary bypass, hemolysis, free iron, acute kidney injury and the impact of bicarbonate. *Contrib Nephrol* 2010;165:29–32.

23. Boldt J, Wolf M. Identification of renal injury in cardiac surgery: the role of kidney-specific proteins. *J Cardiothorac Vasc Anesth* 2008;22:122–32.

24. Haase M, Bellomo R, Devarajan P, et al. Novel biomarkers early predict the severity of acute kidney injury after cardiac surgery in adults. *Ann Thorac Surg* 2009;88:124–30.

25. Perrotti A, Miltgen G, Chevet-Noel A, et al. Neutrophil gelatinase-associated lipocalin as early predictor of acute kidney injury after cardiac surgery in adults with chronic kidney failure. *Ann Thorac Surg* 2015;99:864–9.

26. Parikh CR, Coca SG, Thiessen-Philbrook H, et al. Postoperative biomarkers predict acute kidney injury and poor outcomes after adult cardiac surgery. *J Am Soc Nephrol* 2011;22:1748–57.

27. Nigwekar U, Kandula P, Hix JK, Thakar CV. Off-pump coronary artery bypass surgery and acute kidney injury: a meta-analysis of randomized and observational studies. *Am J Kidney Dis* 2009;54:413–23.

28. Cheungpasitporn W, Thongprayoon C, Kittanamongkolchai W, et al. Comparison of renal outcomes in off-pump versus on-pump coronary artery bypass grafting: a systematic review and meta-analysis of randomized controlled trials. *Nephrology (Carlton)* 2015;20:727–35.

29. Seabra VF, Alobaidi S, Balk EM, Poon AH, Jaber BL. Off-pump coronary artery bypass surgery and acute kidney injury: a meta-analysis of randomized controlled trials. *J Am Soc Nephr* 2010;5:1734–44.

30. Weerasinghe A, Athanasiou T, Al-Ruzzeh S, et al. Functional renal outcome in on-pump and off-pump coronary revascularization: a propensity-based analysis. *Ann Thorac Surg* 2005;79:1577–83.

31. Sajja LR, Mannam G, Chakravarthi RM, et al. Coronary artery bypass grafting with or without cardiopulmonary bypass in patients with preoperative non-dialysis dependent renal insufficiency: a randomized study. *J Thorac Cardiovasc Surg* 2007;133:378–88.

32. Di Mauro M, Gagliardi M, Iacò AL, et al. Does off-pump coronary surgery reduce postoperative renal failure? The importance of preoperative renal function. *Ann Thorac Surg* 2007;84:1496–503.

33. Chukwuemeka A, Weisel A, Maganti M, et al. Renal dysfunction in high-risk patients after on-pump and off-pump coronary artery bypass surgery: a propensity score analysis. *Ann Thorac Surg* 2005;80:2148–54.

34. Deininger S, Hoenicka M, Müller-Eising K, et al. Renal function and urinary biomarkers in cardiac bypass surgery: a prospective randomized trial comparing three surgical techniques. *Thorac Cardiovasc Surg* 2016;64:561–8.

35. Shaw A, Raghunathan K. Fluid management in cardiac surgery: colloid or crystalloid? *Anesthesiology Clin* 2013;31:269–80.

36. Gallagher JD, Moore RA, Kerns D, et al. Effects of colloid or crystalloid administration on pulmonary extravascular water in the postoperative period after coronary artery bypass grafting. *Anesth Analg* 1985;64:753–8.

37. Boldt J. Pro: use of colloids in cardiac surgery. *J Cardiothorac Vasc Anesth* 2007;21:453–6.

38. Nuttall GA, Oliver WC. Con: use of colloids in cardiac surgery. *J Cardiothorac Vasc Anesth* 2007;21:457–9.

39. McIlroy DR, Kharasch ED. Acute intravascular volume expansion with rapidly administered crystalloid or colloid in the setting of moderate hypovolemia. *Anesth Analg* 2003;96:1572–7.

40. Ernest D, Belzberg AS, Dodek PM. Distribution of normal saline and 5% albumin infusions in cardiac surgical patients. *Crit Care Med* 2001;29:2299–302.

41. Groeneveld AB, Navickis RJ, Wilkes MM. Update on the comparative safety of colloids: a systematic review of clinical studies. *Ann Surg* 2011;253:470–83.

42. Frenette AJ, Bouchard J, Bernier P, et al. Albumin administration is associated with acute kidney injury in cardiac surgery: a propensity score analysis. *Crit Care* 2014;18:602.

43. Davidson IJ. Renal impact of fluid management with colloids: a comparative review. *Eur J Anaesthesiol* 2006;23:721–38.

44. Dailey SE, Dysart CB, Langan DR, et al. An in vitro study comparing the effects of Hextend, Hespan, normal saline, and lactated Ringer's solution on thromboelastography and the activated partial thromboplastin time. *J Cardiothorac Vasc Anesth* 2005;19:358–61.

45. Roche AM, James MF, Bennett-Guerrero E, Mythen MG. A head-to-head comparison of the in vitro coagulation effects of saline-based and balanced electrolyte crystalloid and colloid intravenous fluids. *Anesth Analg* 2006;102:1274–9.

46. Moskowitz DM, Shander A, Javidroozi M, et al. Postoperative blood loss and transfusion associated with use of Hextend in cardiac surgery patients at a blood conservation center. *Transfusion* 2008;48:768–75.

47. Lagny MG, Roediger L, Koch JN, et al. Hydroxyethyl starch 130/0.4 and the risk of acute kidney injury after cardiopulmonary bypass: a single-center retrospective study. *J Cardiothorac Vasc Anesth* 2016;30:869–75.

48. Zarbock A, Milles K. Novel therapy for renal protection. *Curr Opin Anaesthesiol* 2015;28:431–8.

49. Krajewski ML, Raghunathan K, Paluszkiewicz SM, Schermer CR, Shaw AD. Meta-analysis of high-versus low-chloride content in perioperative and critical care fluid resuscitation. *Br J Surg* 2015;102:24–36.

50. Yunos NM, Bellomo R, Hegarty C, Story D, Ho L, Bailey M. Association between a chloride-liberal vs chloride-restrictive intravenous fluid administration strategy and kidney injury in critically ill adults. *JAMA* 2012;308:1566–72.

51. Bhaskaran K, Arumugam G, Vinay Kumar PV. A prospective, randomized, comparison study on effect of perioperative use of chloride liberal intravenous fluids versus chloride restricted intravenous fluids on postoperative acute kidney injury in patients undergoing off-pump coronary artery bypass grafting surgeries. *Ann Card Anaesth* 2018;21:413–8.

52. Järvelä K, Koskinen M, Kaukinen S, Kööbi T. Effects of hypertonic saline (7.5%) on extracellular fluid volumes compared with normal saline (0.9%) and 6% hydroxyethyl starch after aortocoronary bypass graft surgery. *J Cardiothorac Vasc Anesth* 2001;15:210–5.

53. Jahr JS, Weeks DL, Desai P, et al. Does OxyVita, a new-generation hemoglobin-based oxygen carrier, or oxyglobin acutely interfere with coagulation compared with normal saline or 6% hetastarch? An ex vivo thromboelastography study. *J Cardiothorac Vasc Anesth* 2008;22:34–9.

54. Morton AP, Moore EE, Moore HB, et al. Hemoglobin-based oxygen carriers promote systemic hyperfibrinolysis that is both dependent and independent of plasmin. *J Surg Res* 2017;213:166–70.

55. Morimatsu H, Uchino S, Chung J, Bellomo R, Raman J, Buxton B. Norepinephrine for hypotensive vasodilatation after cardiac surgery: impact on renal function. *Intensive Care Med* 2003;29:1106–12.

56. Bellomo R, Wan L, May C. Vasoactive drugs and acute kidney injury. *Crit Care Med* 2008;36(Suppl): S179–86.

57. Dünser MW, Bouvet O, Knotzer H, et al. Vasopressin in cardiac surgery: a meta-analysis of randomized controlled trials. *J Cardiothorac Vasc Anesth* 2018;32:2225–32.

58. Hajjar LA, Vincent JL, Barbosa Gomes Galas FR, et al. Vasopressin versus norepinephrine in patients with vasoplegic shock after cardiac surgery: the VANCS randomized controlled trial. *Anesthesiology* 2017;126:85–93.

59. Roush GC, Kaur R, Ernst ME. Diuretics: a review and update. *J Cardiovasc Pharmacol Ther* 2014;19:5–13.

60. Brater CD. Diuretic therapy. *N Engl J Med* 1998;339:387–95.

61. Algahtani F, Koulouridis I, Susantitaphong P, Dahal K, Jaber BL. A meta-analysis of continuous vs intermittent infusion of loop diuretics in hospitalized patients. *J Crit Care* 2014;29:10–7.

62. Lim E, Ali ZA, Attaran R, Cooper G. Evaluating routine diuretics after coronary surgery: a prospective randomized controlled trial. *Ann Thorac Surg* 2002;73:153–5.

63. Parolari A, Pesce LL, Pacini D, et al. Risk factors for perioperative acute kidney injury after adult cardiac surgery: role of perioperative management. *Ann Thorac Surg* 2012;93:584–91.

64. Yavuz S, Ayabakan N, Dilek K, Ozdemir A. Renal dose dopamine in open heart surgery: does it protect renal tubular function? *J Cardiovasc Surg (Torino)* 2002;43:25–30.

65. Friedrich JO, Adhikari N, Herridge MS, Beyene J. Meta-analysis: low-dose dopamine increases urine output but does not prevent renal dysfunction or death. *Ann Intern Med* 2005;142:510–24.

66. Lassnigg A, Donner E, Grubhofer G, Presterl E, Druml W, Hiesmayr M. Lack of renoprotective effects of dopamine and furosemide during cardiac surgery. *J Am Soc Nephrol* 2000;11:97–104.

67. Soliman R, Hussein M. Comparison of the renoprotective effect of dexmedetomidine and dopamine in high-risk renal patients undergoing cardiac surgery: a double-blind randomized study. *Ann Card Anaesth* 2017;20:408–15.

68. Lin Y, Zheng Z, Li Y, et al. Impact of renal dysfunction on long-term mortality after isolated coronary artery bypass surgery. *Ann Thorac Surg* 2009;87:1079–84.

69. Kangasniemi OK, Mahar M, Rasinaho E, et al. Impact of estimated glomerular filtration rate on the 15-year outcome after coronary artery bypass surgery. *Eur J Cardiothorac Surg* 2008;33:198–202.

70. Husain-Syed F, Ferrari F, Sharma A, et al. Preoperative renal functional reserve predicts risk of acute kidney injury after cardiac operation. *Ann Thorac Surg* 2018;105:1094–101.

71. Levey AS, Bosch JP, Lewis JB, Greene T, Rogers N, Roth D. A more accurate method to estimate glomerular filtration rate from serum creatinine: a new prediction equation: Modification of Diet in Renal Disease Study Group. *Ann Intern Med* 1999;130:461–70.

72. Levey AS, Stevens LA, Schmid CH, et al. A new equation to estimate glomerular filtration rate. *Ann Intern Med* 2009;150:604–12.

73. Huen SC, Parikh CR. Predicting acute kidney injury after cardiac surgery: a systematic review. *Ann Thorac Surg* 2012;93:337–47.

74. Curiel-Balsera E, van de Kroft MD, Macias-Guarasa I, et al. Relation between preoperative use of diuretics and renal replacement therapy after cardiac surgery: a propensity score analysis. *Crit Care* 2014;18(Suppl 1):P390.

75. Perez-Valdivieso J, Monedero P, Vives M, Garcia-Fernandez N, Bes-Rastrollo M. Cardiac surgery associated acute kidney injury requiring renal replacement therapy: a Spanish retrospective case-cohort study. *BMC Nephrol* 2009;10:27.

76. Boldt J, Brenner T, Lehmann A, Suttner SW, Kumle B, Isgro F. Is kidney function altered by the duration of cardiopulmonary bypass? *Ann Thorac Surg* 2003;75:906–12.

77. Sirvinskas E, Andrejaitiene J, Raliene L, et al. Cardiopulmonary bypass management and acute renal failure: risk factors and prognosis. *Perfusion* 2008;23:323–7.

78. Ranucci M, Ballotta A, Agnelli B, Frigiola A, Menicanti L, Castelvecchio S, for the Surgical and Clinical Outcome Research (SCORE) Group. Acute kidney injury in patients undergoing cardiac surgery and coronary angiography on the same day. *Ann Thorac Surg* 2013;95:513–9.

79. Young EW, Diab A, Kirsh MM. Intravenous diltiazem and acute renal failure after cardiac operations. *Ann Thorac Surg* 1998;65:1316–9.

80. Legouis D, Jamme M, Galichon P, et al. Development of a practical prediction score for chronic kidney disease after cardiac surgery. *Br J Anaesth* 2018;121:1025–33.

81. Brown JR, Cochran RP, Leavitt BJ, et al. Multivariable prediction of renal insufficiency developing after cardiac surgery. *Circulation* 2007;116(11 Suppl):I-139–43.

82. Palomba H, de Castro I, Neto AL, Lage S, Yu L. Acute kidney injury prediction following elective cardiac surgery: AKICS score. *Kidney Int* 2007;72:624–31.

83. Thakar CV, Arrigain S, Worley S, Yared JP, Paganini EP. A clinical score to predict acute renal failure after cardiac surgery. *Am J Soc Nephrol* 2005;16:162–8.

84. Mehta RH, Grab JD, O'Brien SM, et al. Bedside tool for predicting the risk of postoperative dialysis in patients undergoing cardiac surgery. *Circulation* 2006;114:2208–16.

85. Engoren M, Maile MD, Heung M, et al. The association between urine output, creatinine elevation, and death. *Ann Thorac Surg* 2017;103:1229–38.

86. Pickering JW, James MT, Palmer SC. Acute kidney injury and prognosis after cardiopulmonary bypass: a meta-analysis of cohort studies. *Am J Kidney Dis* 2015;65:283–93.

87. Leontyev S, Davierwala PM, Gaube LM, et al. Outcome of dialysis-dependent patients after cardiac operations in a single-center experience of 483 patients. *Ann Thorac Surg* 2017;103:1270–6.

88. Rahmanian PB, Adams DH, Castillo JG, Vassalotti J, Filsoufi F. Early and late outcome of cardiac surgery in dialysis-dependent patients: single-center experience with 245 consecutive patients. *J Thorac Cardiovasc Surg* 2008;135:915–22.

89. Durmaz I, Büket S, Atay Y, et al. Cardiac surgery with cardiopulmonary bypass in patients with chronic renal failure. *J Thorac Cardiovasc Surg* 1999;118:306–15.

90. Filsoufi F, Rahmanian PB, Castillo JG, Silvay G, Carpentier A, Adams DH. Predictors and early and late outcomes of dialysis-dependent patients in contemporary cardiac surgery. *J Cardiothorac Vasc Anesth* 2008;22:522–9.

91. Leacche M, Winkelmayer WC, Paul S, et al. Predicting survival in patients requiring renal replacement therapy after cardiac surgery. *Ann Thorac Surg* 2006;81:1385–92.

92. Ivert T, Holzmann MJ, Sartipy U. Survival in patients with acute kidney injury requiring dialysis after coronary artery bypass grafting. *Eur J Cardiothorac Surg* 2014;45:312–7.

93. Garcia S, Ko B, Adabag S. Contrast-induced nephropathy and risk of acute kidney injury and mortality after cardiac operations. *Ann Thorac Surg* 2012;94:772–7.

94. Xu R, Tao A, Bai Y, Deng Y, Chen G. Effectiveness of N-acetylcysteine for the prevention of contrast-induced nephropathy: a systematic review and meta-analysis of randomized controlled trials. *J Am Heart Assoc* 2016;5:e003968.

95. Ma WQ, Zhao Y, Wang Y, Han XQ, Zhu Y, Liu NF. Comparative efficacy of pharmacological interventions for contrast-induced nephropathy prevention after coronary angiography: a network meta-analysis from randomized trials. *Int Urol Nephrol* 2018;50:1085–95.

96. McCullough PA, Choi JP, Feghali GA, et al. Contrast-induced acute kidney injury. *J Am Coll Cardiol* 2016;68:1465–73.

97. Hu Y, Li Z, Chen J, Shen C, Song Y, Zhong Q. The effect of the time interval between coronary angiography and on-pump cardiac surgery on risk of postoperative acute kidney injury: a meta-analysis. *J Cardiothorac Surg* 2013;8:178.

98. Hennessy SA, LaPar DJ, Stukenborg GJ, et al. Cardiac catheterization within 24 hours of valve surgery is significantly associated with acute renal failure. *J Thorac Cardiovasc Surg* 2010;140:1011–7.

99. Lee EH, Chin JH, Joung KW, et al. Impact of the time of coronary angiography on acute kidney injury after elective off-pump coronary artery bypass surgery. *Ann Thorac Surg* 2013;96:1635–42.

100. Ranucci M, Ballotta A, Kunkl A, et al. Influence of timing of cardiac catheterization and the amount of contrast media on acute renal failure after cardiac surgery. *Am J Cardiol* 2008;101:1112–8.

101. Medalion B, Cohen H, Assali A, et al. The effect of coronary angiography timing, contrast media dose, and preoperative renal function on acute renal failure after coronary artery bypass grafting. *J Thorac Cardiovasc Surg* 2010;139:1539–44.

102. Del Duca D, Iqbal S, Rahme E, Goldberg P, de Varennes B. Renal failure after cardiac surgery: timing of cardiac catheterization and other perioperative risk factors. *Ann Thorac Surg* 2007;84:1264–71.

103. Haase-Fielitz A, Haase M, Bellomo R, et al. Preoperative hemodynamic instability and fluid over-load are associated with increasing acute kidney injury severity and worse outcome after cardiac surgery. *Blood Purif* 2017;43:298–308.

104. Marathias KP, Vassili M, Robola A, et al. Preoperative intravenous hydration confers renoprotection in patients with chronic kidney disease undergoing cardiac surgery. *Artif Organs* 2006;30:615–21.

105. Molnar AO, Parikh CR, Coca SG, et al. Association between preoperative statin use and acute kid-ney injury biomarkers in cardiac surgical procedures. *Ann Thorac Surg* 2014;97:2081–8.

106. Billings FT 4th, Pretorius M, Siew ED, Yu C, Brown NJ. Early postoperative statin therapy is associated with a lower incidence of acute kidney injury after cardiac surgery. *J Cardiothorac Vasc Anesth* 2010;24:913–20.

107. Kuhn EW, Liakopoulos OJ, Stange S, et al. Preoperative statin therapy in cardiac surgery: a meta-analysis of 90,000 patients. *Eur J Cardiothorac Surg* 2014;45:17–26.

108. Billings FT 4th, Hendricks PA, Schildcrout JS, et al. High-dose perioperative atorvastatin and acute kidney injury following cardiac surgery: a randomized clinical trial. *JAMA* 2016;315:877–88.

109. Zheng Z, Jayaram R, Jiang L, et al. Perioperative rosuvastatin in cardiac surgery. *N Engl J Med* 2016;374:1744–53.

110. Singh I, Rajagopalan S, Srinivasan A, et al. Preoperative statin therapy is associated with lower requirement of renal replacement therapy in patients undergoing cardiac surgery: a meta-analysis of observational studies. *Interact Cardiovasc Thorac Surg* 2013;17:345–52.

111. Romagnoli S, Ricci Z. Statins and acute kidney injury following cardiac surgery: has the last word been told? *J Thorac Dis* 2016;8:E451–4.

112. Williams ML, He X, Rankin JS, Slaughter MS, Gammie JS. Preoperative hematocrit is a powerful predictor of adverse outcomes in coronary artery bypass graft surgery: a report from the Society of Thoracic Surgeons adult cardiac surgery database. *Ann Thorac Surg* 2013;96:1628–34.

113. Karkouti K, Wijeysundera DN, Yau TM, et al. Influence of erythrocyte transfusion on the risk of acute kidney injury after cardiac surgery differs in anemic and nonanemic patients. *Anesthesiology* 2011;115:523–30.

114. Khan UA, Coca SG, Hong K, et al. Blood transfusions are associated with urinary biomarkers of kidney injury in cardiac surgery. *J Thorac Cardiovasc Surg* 2014;148:726–32.

115. Song YR, Lee T, You SJ, et al. Prevention of acute kidney injury by erythropoietin in patients under-going coronary artery bypass grafting: a pilot study. *Am J Nephrol* 2009;30:253–60.

116. Karkouti K, Wijeysundera DN, Yau TM, et al. Advanced targeted transfusion in anemic cardiac surgical patients for kidney protection: an unblinded randomized pilot clinical trial. *Anesthesiology* 2012;116:613–21.

117. Durmaz I, Yagdi T, Calkavur T, et al. Prophylactic dialysis in patients with renal dysfunction under-going on-pump coronary artery bypass surgery. *Ann Thorac Surg* 2003;75:859–64.

118. Bingol H, Akay HT, Iyem H, et al. Prophylactic dialysis in elderly patients undergoing coronary bypass surgery. *Ther Apher Dial* 2007;11:30–5.

119. Borji R, Ahmadi SH, Barkhordari K, et al. Effect of prophylactic dialysis on morbidity and mortality in non-dialysis-dependent patients after coronary artery bypass grafting: a pilot study. *Nephron* 2017;136:226–32.

120. Cho JS, Shim JK, Soh S, Kim MK, Kwak YL. Perioperative dexmedetomidine reduces the incidence and severity of acute kidney injury following valvular heart surgery. *Kidney Int* 2016;89:693–700.

121. Chen X, Huang T, Cao X, Xu G. Comparative efficacy of drugs for preventing acute kidney injury after cardiac surgery: a network meta-analysis. *Am J Cardiovasc Drugs* 2018;18:49–58.

122. Stafford-Smith M, Phillips-Bute B, Reddan DN, Black J, Newman MF. The association of epsilon-aminocaproic acid with postoperative decrease in creatinine clearance in 1502 coronary bypass patients. *Anesth Analg* 2000;91:1085–90.

123. Patel NN, Angelini GD. Pharmacological strategies for the prevention of acute kidney injury follow-ing cardiac surgery: an overview of systematic reviews. *Curr Pharm Des* 2014;20:5484–8.

124. Zangrillo A, Biondi-Zoccai GG, Frati E, et al. Fenoldopam and acute renal failure in cardiac surgery: a meta-analysis of randomized placebo-controlled trials. *J Cardiothorac Vasc Anesth* 2012;26:407–13.

125. Bergman AS, Odar-Cerderlöf I, Westman L, Bjellerup P, Höglund P, Ohqvist G. Diltiazem infusion for renal protection in cardiac surgical patients with preexisting renal dysfunction. *J Cardiothorac Vasc Anesth* 2002;16:294–9.

126. Ortega-Loubon C, Fernández-Molina M, Pañeda-Delgado L, Jorge-Monjas P, Carrascal Y. Predictors of postoperative acute kidney injury after coronary artery bypass graft surgery. *Braz J Cardiovasc Surg* 2018;33:323–9.

127. Yavuz S, Ayabakan N, Goncu MT, Ozdemir IA. Effect of combined dopamine and diltiazem on renal function after cardiac surgery. *Med Sci Monit* 2002;8:PI45–50.

128. Haase M, Haase-Fielitz A, Plass M, et al. Prophylactic perioperative sodium bicarbonate to prevent acute kidney injury following open heart surgery: a multicenter double-blinded randomized controlled trial. *PLoS Med* 2013;10:e1001426.

129. Tie HT, Luo MZ, Luo MJ, Zhang M, Wu QC, Wan JY. Sodium bicarbonate in the prevention of cardiac surgery-associated acute kidney injury: a systematic review and meta-analysis. *Crit Care* 2014;18:517.

130. Barba-Navarro R, Tapia-Silva M, Garza-Garcia C, et al. The effect of spironolactone on acute kidney injury after cardiac surgery: a randomized, placebo-controlled trial. *Am J Kidney Dis* 2017;69:192–9.

131. Yallop KG, Sheppard SV, Smith DC. The effect of mannitol on renal function following cardio-pulmonary bypass in patients with normal pre-operative creatinine. *Anaesthesia* 2008;63:576–82.

132. Smith MN, Best D, Sheppard SV, Smith DC. The effect of mannitol on renal function after cardiopulmonary bypass in patients with established renal dysfunction. *Anaesthesia* 2008;63:701–4.

133. Lombardi R, Ferreiro A, Servetto C. Renal function after cardiac surgery: adverse effects of furosemide. *Ren Fail* 2003;25:775–86.

134. Bayat F, Faritous Z, Aghdaei N, Dabbagh A. A study of the efficacy of furosemide as a prophylaxis of acute renal failure in coronary artery bypass grafting patients: a clinical trial. *ARYA Atheroscler* 2015;11:173–8.

135. Mahesh B, Yim B, Robson D, Pillai R, Ratnatunga C, Pigott D. Does furosemide prevent renal dysfunction in high-risk cardiac surgical patients? Results of a double-blinded prospective randomised trial. *Eur J Cardiothorac Surg* 2008;33:370–6.

136. Fakhari S, Bavil FM, Bilehjani E, Abolhasani S, Mirinazhad M, Naghipour B. Prophylactic furosemide infusion decreasing early major postoperative renal dysfunction in on-pump adult cardiac surgery: a randomized clinical trial. *Res Rep Urol* 2017;9:5–13.

137. Yilmaz M, Aksoy R, Yilmaz YK, Balci C, Duzyol C, Kunt AT. Urine output during cardiopulmonary bypass predicts acute kidney injury after coronary artery bypass grafting. *Heart Surg Forum* 2016;19:E289–93.

138. Suehiro S, Shibata T, Sasaki Y, et al. Heparin-coated circuits prevent renal dysfunction after open heart surgery. *Osaka City Med J* 1999;45:149–57.

139. Benedetto U, Luciani R, Goracci M, et al. Miniaturized cardiopulmonary bypass and acute kidney injury in coronary artery bypass graft surgery. *Ann Thorac Surg* 2009;88:529–36.

140. Bolcal C, Akay HT, Bingol H, et al. Leukodepletion improves renal function in patients with renal dysfunction undergoing on-pump coronary bypass surgery: a prospective randomized study. *Thorac Cardiovasc Surg* 2007;55:89–93.

141. Ono N, Arnaoutakis GJ, Fine DM, et al. Blood pressure excursions below the cerebral autoregulation threshold during cardiac surgery are associated with acute kidney injury. *Crit Care* 2013;41:464–71.

142. Engelman R, Baker RA, Likosky, et al. The Society of Thoracic Surgeons, the Society of Cardiovascular Anesthesiologists, and the American Society of ExtraCorporeal Technology: clinical practice guidelines for cardiopulmonary bypass–temperature management during adult cardiopulmonary bypass. *Ann Thorac Surg* 2015;100:748–57.

143. Boodhwani M, Rubens FD, Wozny D, Nathan HJ. Effects of mild hypothermia and rewarming on renal function after coronary artery bypass grafting. *Ann Thorac Surg* 2009;87:489–95.

144. Newland RF, Baker RA, Mazzone AL, Quinn SS, Chew DP, Perfusion Downunder Collaboration. Rewarming temperature during cardiopulmonary bypass and acute kidney injury: a multicenter analysis. *Ann Thorac Surg* 2016;101:1655–62.

145. Mori Y, Sato N, Kobayashi Y, Ochiai R. Acute kidney injury during aortic arch surgery under deep hypothermic circulatory arrest. *J Anesth* 2011;25:799–804.

146. Ranucci M, Romitti F, Isgrò G, et al. Oxygen delivery during cardiopulmonary bypass and acute renal failure after coronary operations. *Ann Thorac Surg* 2005;80:2213–20.

147. Karkouti K, Wijeysundera DN, Yau TM, McCluskey AA, van Rensburg A, Beattie WS. The influence of baseline hemoglobin concentration on tolerance of anemia in cardiac surgery. *Transfusion* 2008;48:666–72.

148. Nam K, Jeon Y, Kim WH, et al. Intraoperative glucose variability but not average glucose concentration may be a risk factor for acute kidney injury after cardiac surgery: a retrospective study. *Can J Anaesth* 2019;66:921–33.

149. Lecomte P, Van Vlem B, Coddens J, et al. Tight perioperative glucose control is associated with a reduction in renal impairment and renal failure in non-diabetic cardiac surgical patients. *Crit Care* 2008;12:R154.

150. Luciani R, Goracci M, Simon C, et al. Reduction of early postoperative morbidity in cardiac surgery patients treated with continuous veno-venous hemofiltration during cardiopulmonary bypass. *Artif Organs* 2009;33:654–7.

151. Kaya K, Oğuz M, Akar AR, et al. The effect of sodium nitroprusside infusion on renal function during reperfusion period in patients undergoing coronary artery bypass grafting: a prospective randomized clinical trial. *Eur J Cardiothorac Surg* 2007;31:290–7.

152. Cheung AT, Cruz-Shiavone GE, Meng QC, et al. Cardiopulmonary bypass, hemolysis, and nitroprusside-induced cyanide production. *Anesth Analg* 2007;105:29–33.

153. Desborough MJ, Oakland KA, Landoni G, et al. Desmopressin for treatment of platelet dysfunction and reversal of antiplatelet agents: a systematic review and meta-analysis of randomized controlled trials. *J Thromb Haemost* 2017;15:263–72.

154. Lagni MG, Jouret F, Koch JN, et al. Incidence and outcomes of acute kidney injury after cardiac surgery using either criteria of the RIFLE classification. *BMC Nephrol* 2015;16:76.

155. Lassnigg A, Schmidlin D, Mouhieddine M, et al. Minimal changes of serum creatinine predict prognosis in patients after cardiothoracic surgery: a prospective cohort study. *J Am Soc Nephrol* 2004;15:1597–605.

156. Bellomo R, Ronco C, Kellum JA, Mehta RL, Palevsky P. Acute renal failure- definition, outcome measures, animal models, fluid therapy and information technology needs: the Second International Consensus Conference of the Acute Dialysis Quality Initiative (ADQI) Group. *Crit Care* 2004;8:R204–12.

157. Kuitunen A, Vento A, Suojaranta-Ylinen R, Pettilä V. Acute renal failure after cardiac surgery: evaluation of the RIFLE classification. *Ann Thorac Surg* 2006;81:542–6.

158. Mehta RL, Kellum JA, Shah SV, et al. Acute Kidney Injury Network: report of an initiative to improve outcomes in acute kidney injury. *Crit Care* 2007;11:R31.

159. Haase M, Bellomo R, Matalanis G, Calzavacca P, Dragun D, Haase-Fielitz A. A comparison of the RIFLE and Acute Kidney Injury Network classification for cardiac surgery-associated acute kidney injury: a prospective cohort study. *J Thorac Cardiovasc Surg* 2009;138:1370–6.

160. Lopes JA, Jorge S. The RIFLE and AKIN classifications for acute kidney injury: a critical and comprehensive review. *Clin Kidney J* 2013;6:8–14.

161. Khwaja A. KIDGO clinical practice guidelines for acute kidney injury. *Nephron Clin Pract* 2012;20:c179–84.

162. Kellum JA, Sileanu FE, Murugan R, Lucko N, Shaw AD, Clermont G. Classifying AKI by urine output versus serum creatinine level. *J Am Soc Nephrol* 2015;26:2231–8.

163. Swaminathan M, Hudson CCC, Phillips-Bute BG, et al. Impact of early renal recovery on survival after cardiac surgery-associated acute kidney injury. *Ann Thorac Surg* 2010;89:1098–105.

164. Cruz DN, Gaiao S, Maisel A, Ronco C, Devarajan P. Neutrophil gelatinase-associated lipocalin as a biomarker of cardiovascular disease: a systematic review. *Clin Chem Lab Med* 2012;50:1533–45.

165. Brown JR, Parikh CR, Ross CS, et al. Impact of perioperative acute kidney injury severity index for thirty-day readmission after cardiac surgery. *Ann Thorac Surg* 2014;97:111–7.

166. Crawford TD, Magruder JT, Grimm JC, et al. Renal failure after cardiac operations: not all acute kidney injury is the same. *Ann Thorac Surg* 2017;104:760–6.

167. Bellomo R, Auriemma S, Fabbri A, et al. The pathophysiology of cardiac surgery-associated acute kidney injury (CSA-AKI). *Int J Artif Organs* 2008;31:166–78.

168. Abuelo JG. Normotensive ischemic acute renal failure. *N Engl J Med* 2007;357:797–805.

169. Shear W, Rosner MH. Acute kidney dysfunction secondary to the abdominal compartment syndrome. *J Nephrol* 2006;19:556–65.

170. Myers BD, Moran SM. Hemodynamically mediated acute renal failure. *N Engl J Med* 1986;314:97–105.

171. Esson ML, Schrier RW. Diagnosis and treatment of acute tubular necrosis. *Ann Intern Med* 2002;137:744–52.

172. Tolwani A, Paganini E, Joannidis M, et al. Treatment of patients with cardiac surgery associated-acute kidney injury. *Int J Artif Organs* 2008;31:190–6.

173. Liu KD, Brakeman PR. Renal repair and recovery. *Crit Care Med* 2008;36(suppl):S187–92.

174. Nadeau-Fredette AC, Bouchard J. Fluid management and use of diuretics in acute kidney injury. *Advances in Chronic Kidney Disease* 2013;20:45–55.

175. Perner A, Prowle J, Joannidis M, Young P, Hjortrup PB, Pettilä V. Fluid management in acute kidney injury. *Intensive Care Med* 2017;43:807–15.

176. Ejaz AA, Mohandas R. Are diuretics harmful in the management of acute kidney injury? *Curr Opin Nephrol Hypertens* 2014;23:155–60.

177. Karajala V, Mansour W, Kellum JA. Diuretics in acute kidney injury. *Minerva Anestesiol* 2009;75:251–7.

178. Vánky F, Broquist M, Svedjeholm R. Addition of a thiazide: an effective remedy for furosemide resistance after cardiac operations. *Ann Thorac Surg* 1997;63:993–7.

179. Sirivella S, Gielchinsky I, Parsonnet V. Mannitol, furosemide, and dopamine infusion in postoperative renal failure complicating cardiac surgery. *Ann Thorac Surg* 2000;69:501–6.

180. Tumlin LA, Finkel KW, Murray PT, Samuels J, Cotsonis G, Shaw AD. Fenoldopam mesylate in early acute tubular necrosis: a randomized, double-blind, placebo-controlled clinical trial. *Am J Kidney Dis* 2005;46:26–34.

181. Bove T, Zangrillo A, Guarracino F, et al. Effect of fenoldopam on use of renal replacement therapy among patients with acute kidney injury after cardiac surgery: a randomized clinical trial. *JAMA* 2004;312:2244–53.

182. Manabe S, Tanaka H, Yoshizaki T, Tabuchi N, Arai H, Sunamori M. Effects of postoperative administration of diltiazem on renal function after coronary artery bypass grafting. *Ann Thorac Surg* 2005;79:831–6.

183. Bragadottir G, Redfors B, Ricksten SE. Mannitol increases renal blood flow and maintains filtration fraction and oxygenation in postoperative acute kidney injury: a prospective interventional study. *Crit Care* 2012;16:R159.

184. Al-Aly Z, Maddukuri G, Xie Y. Proton pump inhibitors and the kidney: implications of current evidence for clinical practice and when and how to deprescribe. *Am J Kidney Dis* 2020;75:497–507.

185. Valencia E, Marin A, Hardy G. Nutrition therapy for acute renal failure: a new approach based on "risk, injury, failure, loss and end-stage kidney" classification (RIFLE). *Curr Opin Clin Nutr Metab Care* 2009;12:241–4.

186. Berbel MN, Pinto MP, Ponce D, Balbi AL. Nutritional aspects in acute kidney injury. *Rev Assoc Med Bras* 2011;57:600–6.

187. Tolwani A. Continuous renal-replacement therapy for acute kidney injury. *N Engl J Med* 2012;367:2505–14.

188. Liu Y, Davari-Farid S, Arora P, Porhomayon J, Nader ND. Early versus later initiation of renal replacement therapy in critically ill patients with acute kidney injury after cardiac surgery: a systematic review and meta-analysis. *J Cardiothorac Vasc Anesth* 2014;28:557–63.

189. Garcia-Fernández N, Pérez -Valdivieso JR, Bes-Rastrollo M, et al. Timing of renal replacement therapy after cardiac surgery: a retrospective multicenter Spanish cohort study. *Blood Purif* 2011;32:104–11.

190. Meersch M, Küllmar M, Schmidt C, et al. Long-term clinical outcomes after early initiation of RRT in critically ill patients with AKI. *Am Soc Nephrol* 2018;29:1011–9.

191. Gaudry S, Hajage D, Schortgen F, et al. Initiation strategies for renal-replacement therapy in the intensive care unit. *N Engl J Med* 2016;375:122–33.

192. Flythe JE, Kimmel SE, Brunelli SM. Rapid fluid removal during dialysis is associated with cardiovascular morbidity and mortality. *Kidney Int* 2011;79:250–7.

193. Kutsogiannis DJ, Gibney RT, Stollery D, Gao J. Regional citrate versus systemic heparin anticoagulation for continuous renal replacement in critically ill patients. *Kidney Int* 2005;67:2361–7.

194. Bihorac A, Ross EA. Continuous venovenous hemofiltration with citrate-based replacement fluid: efficacy, safety, and impact on nutrition. *Am J Kidney Dis* 2005;46:908–18.

195. Hollander-Rodriguez JC, Calvert JF Jr. Hyperkalemia. *Am Fam Physician* 2006;73:283–90.

196. Mount DB. Treatment and prevention of hyperkalemia in adults. www.uptodate.com 2019.

197. Fraley DS, Adler S. Correction of hyperkalemia by bicarbonate despite constant blood pH. *Kidney Int* 1977;12:354–60.

198. Sterns RH, Rojas M, Bernstein P, Chennupati S. Ion-exchange resins for the treatment of hyperkalemia: are they safe and effective? *J Am Soc Nephrol* 2010;21:733–5.

199. Packham DK, Rasmussen HS, Lavin PT, et al. Sodium zirconium cyclosilicate in hyperkalemia. *N Engl J Med* 2015;372:222–31.

200. Meaney CJ, Beccari MV, Yang Y, Zhao J. Systematic review and meta-analysis of patiromer and sodium zirconium cyclosilicate: a new armamentarium for the treatment of hyperkalemia. *Pharmacotherapy* 2017;37:401–11.

201. Gennari FJ. Hypokalemia. *N Engl J Med* 1998;339:451–8.

202. Mount DB. Clinical manifestations and treatment of hypokalemia in adults. www.uptodate.com 2020.

203. Dinardo JA. Pro: calcium is routinely indicated during separation from cardiopulmonary bypass. *J Cardiothorac Vasc Anesth* 1997;11:905–7.

204. Kim SJ, Jeong CY, Chung SS, Ha IH, Yoo KY. Effect of calcium chloride on protamine-induced systemic hypotension in adult open-heart patients. *Korean J Anesthesiology* 2002;43:157–64.

205. Butterworth JF, Zaloga GP, Prielipp RC, Tucker WY Jr, Royster RL. Calcium inhibits the cardiac stimulating properties of dobutamine but not of amrinone. *Chest* 1992;101:174–80.

206. Cooper MS, Gittoes NJ. Diagnosis and management of hypocalcaemia. *BMJ* 2008;336:1298–302.

207. Fairley JL, Zhang L, Glassford NJ, Bellomo R. Magnesium status and magnesium therapy in cardiac surgery: a systematic review and meta-analysis focusing on arrhythmia prevention. *J Crit Care* 2017;42:69–77.

208. Booth JV, Phillips-Bute B, McCants CB, et al. Low serum magnesium level predicts adverse cardiac events after coronary artery bypass graft surgery. *Am Heart J* 2003;145:1108–13.

209. Minato N, Katayama Y, Sakaguchi M, Itoh M. Perioperative coronary artery spasm in off-pump coronary artery bypass grafting and its possible relation with perioperative hypomagnesemia. *Ann Thorac Cardiovasc Surg* 2006;12:32–6.

210. Inoue S, Akazawa S, Nakaigawa Y, Shimizu R, Seo N. Changes in plasma total and ionized magnesium concentrations and factors affecting magnesium concentrations during cardiac surgery. *J Anesth* 2004;18:216–9.

211. Maslow AD, Regan MM, Heindle S, Panzica P, Cohn WE, Johnson RG. Postoperative atrial tachyarrhythmias in patients undergoing coronary artery bypass graft surgery without cardiopulmonary bypass: a role for intraoperative magnesium supplementation. *J Cardiothorac Vasc Anesth* 2000;14:524–30.

212. Prielipp RC, Zaloga GP, Butterworth JF IV, et al. Magnesium inhibits the hypertensive but not the cardiotonic actions of low-dose epinephrine. *Anesthesiology* 1991;74:973–9.

213. Maillet JM, Le Besnerais P, Cantoni M, et al. Frequency, risk factors, and outcome of hyperlactatemia after cardiac surgery. *Chest* 2003;123:1361–6.

214. Totaro RJ, Raper RF. Epinephrine-induced lactic acidosis following cardiopulmonary bypass. *Crit Care Med* 1997;25:1693–9.

215. Adrogué HJ, Madias NE. Management of life-threatening acid–base disorders: first of two parts. *N Engl J Med* 1998;338:26–34.

216. Kaplan JA, Guffin AV, Yin A. The effects of metabolic acidosis and alkalosis on the response to sympathomimetic drugs in dogs. *J Cardiothorac Anesth* 1988;2:481–7.

217. Ranucci M, De Toffol B, Isgrò G, Romitti F, Conti D, Vicentini M. Hyperlactatemia during cardiopulmonary bypass: determinants and impact on postoperative outcome. *Crit Care* 2006;10:R167.

218. Adeva-Andany MM, Fernández-Fernández C, Mourino-Bayolo D, Castro-Quintela E, Dominguez-Montero A. Sodium bicarbonate therapy in patients with metabolic acidosis. *Scientific World Journal* 2014;article ID 627673. https://doi.org/10.1155/2014/627673.

219. Forsythe SM, Schmidt GA. Sodium bicarbonate for the treatment of lactic acidosis. *Chest* 2000;117:260–7.

220. Cooper DJ, Walley KR, Wiggs BR, Russell JA. Bicarbonate does not improve hemodynamics in critically ill patients who have lactic acidosis: a prospective, controlled clinical study. *Ann Intern Med* 1990;112:492–8.

221. Jaber S, Paugam C, Futier E, et al. Sodium bicarbonate therapy for patients with severe metabolic acidaemia in the intensive care unit (BICAR-ICU): a multicentre, open-label randomised controlled, phase 3 trial. *Lancet* 2018;392:31–40.

222. Fujii T, Udy A, Licari E, Romero L, Bellomo R. Sodium bicarbonate therapy for critically ill patients with metabolic acidosis: a scoping and a systematic review. *J Crit Care* 2019;51:184–91.

223. Hoste EA, Colpaert K, Vanholder RC, et al. Sodium bicarbonate versus THAM in ICU patients with mild metabolic acidosis. *J Nephrol* 2005;18:303–7.

224. Amrein K, Ribitsch W, Otto R, Worm HC, Stauber RE. Severe lactic acidosis reversed by thiamine within 24 hours. *Crit Care* 2011;15:457.

225. Androgué HJ, Madias NE. Management of life-threatening acid–base disorders: second of two parts. *N Engl J Med* 1998;338:107–11.

226. Liao P, DeSantis AJ, Schmeltz LR, et al. Insulin resistance following cardiothoracic surgery in patients with and without a preoperative diagnosis of type 2 diabetes during treatment with intravenous insulin therapy for postoperative hyperglycemia. *J Diabetes Complications* 2008;22:229–34.

227. Phadke D, Beller JP, Tribble C. The disparate effects of epinephrine and norepinephrine on hyperglycemia in cardiovascular surgery. *Heart Surg Forum* 2018;21:E522–6.

228. Jones KW, Cain AS, Mitchell JH, et al. Hyperglycemia predicts mortality after CABG: postoperative hyperglycemia predicts dramatic increases in mortality after coronary artery bypass graft surgery. *J Diabetes Complications* 2008;22:365–70.

229. Ascione R, Rogers CA, Rajakaruna C, Angelini GD. Inadequate blood glucose control is associated with in-hospital mortality and morbidity in diabetic and nondiabetic patients undergoing cardiac surgery. *Circulation* 2008;118:113–23.

230. Ouattara A, Lecomte P, Le Manach Y, et al. Poor intraoperative blood glucose control is associated with worsened hospital outcome after cardiac surgery in diabetic patients. *Anesthesiology* 2005;103:687–94.

231. Pezzella AT, Holmes SD, Pritchard G, Speir AM, Ad N. Impact of perioperative glycemic control on patient survival after coronary bypass surgery. *Ann Thorac Surg* 2014;98:1281–5.

232. Schmeltz LR, DeSantis AJ, Thiyagarajan V, et al. Reduction of surgical mortality and morbidity in diabetic patients undergoing cardiac surgery with a combined intravenous and subcutaneous insulin glucose management strategy. *Diabetes Care* 2007;30:823–8.

233. Furnary AP, Gao G, Grunkemeier GL, et al. Continuous insulin infusion reduces mortality in patients with diabetes undergoing coronary artery bypass grafting. *J Thorac Cardiovasc Surg* 2003;125:1007–21.

234. Bláha J, Mráz M, Kopecký P, et al. Perioperative tight glucose control reduces postoperative adverse events in nondiabetic cardiac surgery patients. *J Clin Endocrinol Metab* 2015;100:3081–9.

235. Greco G, Ferket BS, D'Alessandro DA, et al. Diabetes and the association of postoperative hyperglycemia with clinical and economic outcomes in cardiac surgery. *Diabetes Care* 2016;39:408–17.

236. Swenne CL, Lindholm C, Borowiec J, Schnell AE, Carlsson M. Peri-operative glucose control and development of surgical wound infections in patients undergoing coronary artery bypass graft. *J Hosp Infect* 2005;61:201–12.

237. Järvelä KM, Khan NK, Loisa EL, Sutinen JA, Laurikka JO, Khan JA. Hyperglycemic episodes are associated with postoperative infections after cardiac surgery. *Scand J Surg* 2018;107:138–44.

238. Puskas F, Grocott HP, White WD, Mathew JP, Newman MF, Bar-Yosef S. Intraoperative hyperglycemia and cognitive decline after CABG. *Ann Thorac Surg* 2007;84:1467–73.

239. Butterworth J, Wagenknecht LE, Legault C, et al. Attempted control of hyperglycemia during cardiopulmonary bypass fails to improve neurologic or neurobehavioral outcomes in patients without diabetes mellitus undergoing coronary artery bypass grafting. *J Thorac Cardiovasc Surg* 2005;130:1319–25.

240. Kotfis K, Szylińska A, Listewnik M, Brykcyzński M, Ely EW, Rotter I. Diabetes and elevated preoperative HbA1c level as risk factors for postoperative delirium after cardiac surgery: an observational cohort study. *Neuropsychiatr Dis Treat* 2019;15:511–21.

241. Saager L, Duncan AE, Yared JP, et al. Intraoperative tight glucose control using hyperinsulinemic normoglycemia increases delirium after cardiac surgery. *Anesthesiology* 2015;122:1214–23.

242. Galindo RJ, Fayfman M, Umpierrez GE. Perioperative management of hyperglycemia and diabetes in cardiac surgery patients. *Endocrinol Metab Clin North Am* 2018;47:203–22.

243. Arthur CPS, Mejia OAV, Lapenna GA, et al. Perioperative management of the diabetic patient referred to cardiac surgery. *Braz J Cardiovasc Surg* 2018;33:618–25.

244. Lazar HL, McDonnell M, Chipkin SR, et al. The Society of Thoracic Surgeons practice guidelines series: blood glucose management during adult cardiac surgery. *Ann Thorac Surg* 2009;87:663–9.

245. Rassias AJ. Intraoperative management of hyperglycemia in the cardiac surgical patient. *Semin Thorac Cardiovasc Surg* 2006;18:330–8.

246. Gandhi GY, Nuttall GA, Abel MD, et al. Intensive intraoperative insulin therapy versus conventional glucose management during cardiac surgery: a randomized trial. *Ann Intern Med* 2007;146:233–43.

247. Chan RP, Galas FR, Hajjar LA, Bello CN, Piccioni MA, Auler JO Jr. Intensive perioperative glucose control does not improve outcomes of patients submitted to open-heart surgery: a randomized controlled trial. *Clinics (Sao Paulo)* 2009;64:51–60.

248. Kim HJ, Shim JK, Youn YN, Song JW, Lee H, Kwak YL. Influence of preoperative hemoglobin A1c on early outcomes in patients with diabetes mellitus undergoing off-pump coronary artery bypass surgery. *J Thorac Cardiovasc Surg* 2020;159:568–76.

249. Tennyson C, Lee R, Attia R. Is there a role for HbA1c in predicting mortality and morbidity outcomes after coronary artery bypass graft surgery? *Interact Cardiovasc Thorac Surg* 2013;17:1000–8.

250. Omar AS, Salama A, Allam M, et al. Association of time in blood glucose range with outcomes following cardiac surgery. *BMC Anesthesiol* 2015;15:14.

251. Seki S. Clinical features of hyperosmolar hyperglycemic nonketotic diabetic coma associated with cardiac operations. *J Thorac Cardiovasc Surg* 1986;91:867–73.

252. Zindrou D, Taylor KM, Bagger JP. Excess coronary artery bypass graft mortality among women with hypothyroidism. *Ann Thorac Surg* 2002;74:2121–5.

253. Velissaris T, Tang AT, Wood PJ, Hett DA, Ohri SK. Thyroid function during coronary surgery with or without cardiopulmonary bypass. *Eur J Cardiothorac Surg* 2009;36:148–54.

254. Sabatino L, Cerillo AG, Ripoli A, Pilo A, Glauber M, Iervasi G. Is the low tri-iodothyronine state a crucial factor in determining the outcome of coronary artery bypass patients? Evidence from a clinical pilot study. *J Endocrinol* 2002;175:577–86.

255. Reinhardt W, Mocker V, Jockenhövel F, et al. Influence of coronary artery bypass surgery on thyroid hormone parameters. *Horm Res* 1997;47:1–8.

256. Cerillo AG, Storti S, Mariani M, et al. The non-thyroidal illness syndrome after coronary artery bypass grafting: a 6-month follow-up study. *Clin Chem Lab Med* 2005;43:289–93.

257. Spratt DI, Frohnauer M, Cyr-Alves H, et al. Physiological effects of nonthyroidal illness syndrome in patients after cardiac surgery. *Am J Physiol Endocrinol Metab* 2007;293:E310–5.

258. Sarma AK, Krisna M, Karunakaran J, Neema PK Neelakandhan KS. Severe hypothyroidism after coronary artery bypass grafting. *Ann Thorac Surg* 2005;80:714–6.

259. Jabrocka-Hybel A, Bednarczuk T, Bartalena L, et al. Amiodarone and the thyroid. *Endokrynol Pol* 2015;66:176–86.

260. Klemperer JD. Thyroid hormone and cardiac surgery. *Thyroid* 2002;12:517–21.

261. Mu DL, Li LH, Wang DX, et al. High postoperative serum cortisol level is associated with increased risk of cognitive dysfunction early after coronary artery bypass graft surgery: a prospective cohort study. *PLoS One* 2013;8:e77637.

262. Gibbison B, Spiga F, Walker JJ, et al. Dynamic pituitary-adrenal interactions in response to cardiac surgery. *Crit Care Med* 2015;43:791–800.

263. Mazine A, Bouhout I, Saydy N, et al. Relative adrenal insufficiency is associated with prolonged postoperative hemodynamic instability. *Ann Thorac Surg* 2018;106:702–7.

264. Mattke AF, Vender JR, Anstadt MR. Pituitary apoplexy presenting as Addisonian crisis after coronary artery bypass grafting. *Tex Heart Inst J* 2002;29:193–9.

265. Hidiroglu M, Kucuker A, Ucaroglu E, Kucuker SA, Sener E. Pituitary apoplexy after cardiac surgery. *Ann Thorac Surg* 2010;89:1635–7.

266. Levy E, Korach A, Merin G, Feinsod M, Glenville B. Pituitary apoplexy and CABG: should we change our strategy? *Ann Thorac Surg* 2007;84:1388–90.

267. Zayour DH, Azar ST. Silent pituitary infarction after coronary artery bypass grafting procedure: case report and review of the literature. *Endocr Pract* 2006;12:59–62.

268. Leeman MF, Vuylsteke A, Ritchie AJ. Lithium-induced nephrogenic diabetes insipidus after coronary artery bypass. *Ann Thorac Surg* 2007;84:656–7.

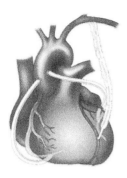

CHAPTER 13

Post-ICU Care and Other Complications

CHAPTER 19

Post-ACT Care and Other Complications

♡ 13 Post-ICU Care and Other Complications

I. General Comments

A. Following a brief stay in the intensive care unit, most patients undergoing cardiac surgical procedures follow a routine pattern of recovery. The use of fast-track protocols and critical care pathways ensures that the healthcare team and the patient have a clear understanding of what to expect at different junctures during recovery. These pathways are designed to standardize care and identify variances from the expected. However, they are not a substitute for careful patient evaluation, which may identify problems that might otherwise be ignored by rigid adherence to protocols.

B. Most patients are transferred to an intermediate care unit or the postoperative cardiac surgical floor on the first postoperative day. Invasive monitoring is no longer utilized, although bedside telemetry should be considered for several days to identify arrhythmias. It should be remembered that patients are still in an early phase of recovery from surgery with many physiologic derangements still present. Restoring the patient to a normal physiologic state requires careful attention to the prevention, identification, and treatment of complications that may develop at any time during the hospital stay. A detailed daily examination of the patient must be performed, with particular attention paid to each organ system. Although pre-printed or computerized order sets are available upon transfer, orders must be thought out carefully and individualized to ensure the best possible postoperative care.

C. Although postoperative complications are more common in elderly patients and those with comorbidities, they may still develop unpredictably in low-risk, healthy patients despite an uneventful surgical procedure and early postoperative course. Problems such as atrial arrhythmias are very common and quite benign, with little influence on the patient's hospital course or long-term prognosis. In contrast, less common complications, such as stroke, mediastinitis, tamponade, renal failure, or an acute abdomen, may be devastating, resulting in early death or prolonged hospitalization with multisystem organ failure.

II. Transfer from the ICU and Postoperative Routines

The patient recovering uneventfully from open-heart surgery is usually extubated within 6–8 hours and off all inotropic support by the first postoperative morning. The following interventions represent standardized steps in a critical care pathway which are applicable to most patients (Table 13.1). In more critically ill patients who may require an additional period of ventilatory or pharmacologic support, adherence to these time-related recommendations may need to be modified, and withdrawal of "intensive care" must be carefully

Table 13.1 • Critical Pathway for Coronary Artery Bypass Grafting

	Preop Day or Office Visit	Day of Surgery	POD #1	POD #2–3	POD #4–5
Cardiovascular	Bilateral BP Height & weight O_2 saturation	Monitor & treat: shivering bleeding arrhythmias hemodynamics Meds (start 8 h postop): aspirin metoprolol	VS q2h Telemetry D/C neck & arterial lines Meds: 2 g MgSO4	VS q4–8h Telemetry	VS before D/C Remove pacing wires
Respiratory	RA O_2 saturation; ABGs if <90% PFTs if COPD	Wean to extubate within 6–8 h IS when awake q1h	40% face mask or nasal cannula IS when awake q1h Splinted cough	Nasal cannula at 2–4 L/min for O_2 sat <95% IS when awake q1h Splinted cough	Room air
Fluids and electrolytes		I & O q1h Keep u/o >1 mL/kg/h	Weight I & O q2h Furosemide IV	Weight I & O qshift Furosemide IV	Weight Furosemide IV/PO until at preop weight

Wounds and drains	Hibiclens shower	OR dressing × 12 h unless Dermabond is used; Monitor/manage CT drainage	DSD with betadine wipe to wounds (unless Dermabond used) & pacing wire sites; D/C CT when total drainage <100 mL/last 8 h	DSD with betadine wipe to wounds (unless Dermabond used) & pacing wire sites	Wounds open to air
Pain control		Continuous or low dose IV MS bolus; NSAID; IV acetaminophen	IV → PCA MS; IV ketorolac	Oxycodone with acetaminophen; Acetaminophen	Oxycodone with acetaminophen; Acetaminophen
Nutrition/GI	NPO after MN	NPO; NG tube to low suction	D/C NG tube; Clear liquids	Advance to hi cal, hi protein, NAS diet; ADA for diabetics; Metamucil/Colace	Progress on diet
Activity	Ambulatory	OOB to chair × 1 after extubation	OOB to chair q8h; Ambulate as tolerated	Ambulate × 3 in room with assist, then in hallway × 4	Ambulate × 6 in hallway; Stair climb 12 stairs × 1

evaluated and not rushed. Typical orders for transfer to the postoperative floor are noted in Table 13.2 and Appendix 5.

A. Postoperative day and night
1. Wean vasoactive medications
2. Wean from ventilator and extubate
3. Remove nasogastric tube
4. Remove Swan-Ganz and arterial lines
5. Get patient out of bed (OOB) in a chair
6. Initiate β-blocker therapy and aspirin
7. Start warfarin for valve patients if minimal chest tube drainage

B. POD #1
1. Remove chest tubes if minimal drainage
2. Transfer to floor; place on telemetry and pulse oximetry × 72 hours
3. Get patient out of bed and ambulating
4. Advance diet
5. Remove Foley catheter
6. Start warfarin for valve patients if not started night before

C. POD #2–3
1. Remove chest tubes if minimal drainage
2. Stop antibiotics (after 48 hours maximum)
3. Advance diet to achieve satisfactory nutrition
4. Increase activity level
5. Continue diuresis to preoperative weight
6. Consider heparin for patients receiving mechanical valves
7. Commence planning for home services or rehabilitation

D. POD #3–4
1. Obtain predischarge laboratory data (hematocrit, electrolytes, BUN, creatinine, chest x-ray, ECG)
2. Remove pacing wires
3. Assess potential discharge location (home vs. rehab)
4. Initiate discharge teaching

E. POD #4–5
1. Carefully review discharge medications and instructions with patient and family
2. Discharge home or to rehab facility

III. Differential Diagnosis of Common Postoperative Symptoms

The development of chest pain, shortness of breath, fever, or just feeling "plain lousy" with a poor appetite and fatigue during the early convalescent period is not unusual, especially in elderly patients. Although the cause of these signs and symptoms may be benign, they should

Table 13.2 • Typical Transfer Orders from the ICU

ALLERGIES: _____
1. Transfer to: _____
2. Procedure: _____
3. Condition: _____
4. Nursing
   - ☐ Vital signs q4h × 2 days, then qshift
   - ☐ ECG telemetry
   - ☐ I & O q8h
   - ☐ Daily weights
   - ☐ Foley catheter to gravity drainage; D/C on __/__ at __; due to void in 8 h
   - ☐ Chest tubes to –20 cm H_2O suction
   - ☐ Ambulate in hall with cardiac rehab
   - ☐ T.E.D. stockings
   - ☐ SpO_2 q8h and 1 time before and after ambulation
   - ☐ Wire and wound care per protocol
   - ☐ Wean oxygen via nasal prongs from 6 L/min to 2 L/min to keep SpO_2 >92%
   - ☐ Incentive spirometry q1h when awake
   - ☐ Glucose via fingerstick/glucometer AC and qhs in diabetics
   - ☐ Notify house staff for:
     - ○ Heart rate <60 or >110
     - ○ Systolic BP <90 or >150 mm Hg
     - ○ Oxygen saturation <90% on room air
     - ○ Temperature >38.5 °C (>101 °F)
   - ☐ Saline lock, flush q8h and prn
5. Diet
   - ☐ NPO
   - ☐ Clear liquids/no added salt (NAS)
   - ☐ Full liquids/NAS
   - ☐ NAS, low fat, low cholesterol diet
   - ☐ _____ cal ADA, NAS low cholesterol diet, if diabetic
   - ☐ Fluid restriction ____ mL per 24 h (IV + PO)
6. Temporary pacemaker settings
   - ☐ Pacemaker on: Mode: ☐ Atrial ☐ VVI ☐ DVI ☐ DDD
        Atrial output: __ mA   Ventricular output: __ mA
        Rate: __/min   AV interval: __ msec
   - ☐ Pacer attached but off
   - ☐ Detach pacer but keep at bedside
7. Laboratory studies
   - ☐ Chest x-ray after chest tube removal
   - ☐ In AM after transfer: CBC, electrolytes, BUN, creatinine, blood glucose
   - ☐ Daily PT/INR if on warfarin
   - ☐ Daily PTT and platelet count if on heparin (see Appendix 7)
   - ☐ On day prior to discharge: chest x-ray, ECG, CBC, electrolytes, BUN, creatinine
8. Consults
   - ☐ Cardiac rehabilitation
   - ☐ Social services
   - ☐ Physical therapy
   - ☐ Occupational therapy
   - ☐ Nutrition

(continued)

Table 13.2 • (Continued)

9. Medications
   a. Antibiotics
      - ☐ Cefazolin 1 g IV q8h for __ more doses (6 doses total); last dose on__/__ at ____ hours
      - ☐ Vancomycin 1 g IV q12h for __ more doses (4 doses total); last dose on__/__ at _____ hours
      - ☐ Mupirocin 2% (Bactroban ointment) via Q-tip nasal swab the evening after surgery and bid × 3 days total
   b. Cardiovascular medications
      - ☐ Metoprolol __ mg PO q12h. Hold for HR <60 or SBP <100
      - ☐ Carvedilol __ mg PO q12h. Hold for HR <60 or SBP <100
      - ☐ Amiodarone ____ mg PO q12h
      - ☐ Lisinopril __ mg PO qd
      - ☐ Diltiazem 30 mg PO q6h (radial artery grafts)
      - ☐ Amlodipine 5 mg PO qd (radial artery grafts)
      - ☐ Imdur (sustained release) 20 mg PO qd (radial artery grafts)
      - ☐ Simvastatin __ mg qd hs (no more than 20 mg if on amiodarone)
   c. Anticoagulants/antiplatelet agents
      - ☐ Aspirin ☐ 81 mg ☐ 325 mg PO qd (hold for platelet count <60,000)
      - ☐ Clopidogrel 75 mg PO qd
      - ☐ Ticagrelor 90 mg PO bid
      - ☐ Low-molecular-weight heparin (Lovenox) ___ mg SC___
      - ☐ Heparin 5000 units SC bid
      - ☐ Heparin 25,000 units/500 mL D5W at ___ units/h starting on___ (per protocol – see Appendix 7)
      - ☐ Warfarin ___ mg PO qd starting on___; daily dose check with HO (per protocol – see page 773 and Appendix 8)
   d. Pain medications
      - ☐ Morphine sulfate via PCA pump or 10 mg IM q3h prn severe pain
      - ☐ Ketorolac 15–30 mg IV q6h prn moderate–severe pain (4–10 on pain scale); D/C after 72 hours
      - ☐ Acetaminophen with oxycodone (Percocet) 2 tabs PO q4h for severe pain (6–10)
      - ☐ Acetaminophen with oxycodone (Percocet) 1 tabs PO q4h for moderate pain; give additional tab if no change in pain after one hour
      - ☐ Acetaminophen 650 mg PO q4h prn mild pain
   e. GI medications
      - ☐ Pantoprazole (Protonix) 40 mg PO qd
      - ☐ For nausea:
         - ☐ Metoclopramide 10 mg IV/PO q6h prn
         - ☐ Ondansetron 4–8 mg IV/PO q4h prn
         - ☐ Prochlorperazine 10 mg PO/IM/IV q6h prn
      - ☐ Milk of magnesia 30 mL PO qhs prn
      - ☐ Docusate (Colace) 100 mg PO bid
      - ☐ Bisacodyl (Dulcolax) 10 mg suppository prn constipation

Table 13.2 • (Continued)

f. Diabetes medications
  - ☐ Oral hypoglycemic: _____
  - ☐ ____ units regular insulin (Novolin R or Humulin R) SC ____ qAM ____ qPM
  - ☐ ____ units NPH insulin (Novolin N or Humulin N) SC ____ qAM ___ qPM
  - ☐ Sliding scale: treat fingerstick/glucometer glucose according to the following scale at 06:00 AM, 11:00 AM, 3:00 PM, and 8:00 PM
    150–160, give 2 units regular insulin SC (Novolin R or Humulin R)
    161–200, give 4 units regular insulin SC
    201–250, give 6 units regular insulin SC
    251–300, give 8 units regular insulin SC
    301–350, give 10 units regular insulin SC
    >350, call house officer

g. Other medications
  - ☐ Acetaminophen 650 mg PO q3h prn temp >38.5 °C
  - ☐ Ascorbic acid 1 g PO qd × 5 days
  - ☐ Zolpidem 2.5–5 mg PO qhs prn sleep
  - ☐ Melatonin ____mg PO qhs prn sleep (1.5–3 mg usual dose)
  - ☐ Furosemide ___ mg IV/PO q _ h
  - ☐ Potassium chloride ___ mEq PO bid (while on furosemide)
  - ☐ Albuterol 2.5 mg/5 mL NS via nebulizer q4h prn
  - ☐ Levalbuterol (Xopenex) 0.63 mg in 3 mL NS q8h via nebulizer or two inhalations q4–6h through a pressured MDI
  - ☐ Duoneb inhaler q6h
  - ☐ Other: _____

not be taken lightly because they may indicate the presence of potentially serious problems that warrant investigation. Careful questioning and examination of the patient on a daily or more frequent basis can prioritize diagnoses, direct the evaluation, and lead to prompt and appropriate treatment.

A. Chest pain

1. **Differential diagnosis.** The development of chest pain following cardiac surgery often raises the suspicion of myocardial ischemia, but the differential diagnosis must include several other potential causes. The greatest fear to a patient is that the recurrence of chest pain indicates a failed operation; the surgeon meanwhile may purposely try to provide an alternative explanation. Although musculoskeletal pain is the most common cause of chest discomfort, significant problems that must be considered include:

- Myocardial ischemia
- Pericarditis

- Arrhythmias
- Pneumothorax
- Pneumonia
- Pulmonary embolism
- Sternal wound infection
- Aortic dissection
- Gastroesophageal reflux

2. **Evaluation.** Careful physical examination (breath sounds, pericardial rub, sternal wound), a chest x-ray, and 12-lead ECG will usually provide the appropriate diagnosis and direct additional testing. Differentiation of ST-segment elevation related to ischemia vs. pericarditis is important and can be difficult to make (Figures 8.2 and 8.3, pages 384 and 385). Consultation with the cardiology service is essential in managing patients with a suspected cardiac origin to their chest pain. Stress imaging or even coronary angiography may be warranted. Other diagnostic modalities include echocardiography, computed tomography (CT) pulmonary angiography to rule out pulmonary embolism, and sternal wound aspiration.

B. **Shortness of breath**

1. **Differential diagnosis.** Shortness of breath is usually caused by splinting from chest wall discomfort and is not uncommon in the anemic patient with underlying lung disease. However, significant shortness of breath, its acute onset, or deterioration in pulmonary status should raise awareness of a significant problem. The source may be of a primary pulmonary nature, but it may also be the consequence of cardiac dysfunction or oliguric acute kidney injury (AKI). Diagnoses to be considered include:

    a. Pleuropulmonary problems
    - Atelectasis and hypoxia from mucus plugging or poor inspiratory effort
    - Pneumothorax
    - Pneumonia (possibly aspiration)
    - Bronchospasm
    - An enlarging pleural effusion
    - Pulmonary embolism

    b. Cardiopulmonary problems – low cardiac output states or acute pulmonary edema caused by:
    - Acute myocardial ischemia or infarction
    - Cardiac tamponade
    - Residual or new-onset mitral regurgitation (ischemic, associated with systemic hypertension) or a recurrent ventricular septal defect
    - Fluid overload from surgery or heart failure, often associated with oliguric AKI
    - Severe diastolic dysfunction
    - Atrial or ventricular tachyarrhythmias

    c. Compensatory response to metabolic acidosis (low cardiac output state)
    d. Sepsis

2. **Evaluation.** Careful lung examination may reveal absent breath sounds or diffuse rales/rhonchi, suggesting a parenchymal process, a pneumothorax, or pulmonary edema. Clinical evidence of cardiac tamponade (muffled heart sounds, orthostatic blood pressure changes, pulsus paradoxus) should be sought. An arterial blood gas (ABG), chest x-ray, and ECG should be obtained. An echocardiogram gives an assessment of ventricular function, detects valve dysfunction or recurrent shunting, and may also identify a large left pleural or pericardial effusion or tamponade. A CT pulmonary angiogram should be performed if pulmonary embolism is suspected.

C. **Fever**

1. **Differential diagnosis.** Fever is very common during the first 48–72 hours after surgery. Initially, it may be related to the systemic inflammatory response or cytokine release from cardiopulmonary bypass (CPB), but subsequently is usually ascribed to atelectasis from poor inspiratory effort after extubation. Thorough evaluation of recurrent fevers is warranted after the first 72 hours.[1,2] Potential causes of postoperative fever include:

- Atelectasis or pneumonia
- Urinary tract infection (UTI)
- Wound infections: sternum or leg
- *Clostridium difficile* colitis or other intra-abdominal process
- Sinusitis (usually in patients with indwelling endotracheal or nasogastric tubes)
- Catheter sepsis
- Endocarditis (especially on a prosthetic valve)
- Decubitus ulcer
- Drug fever
- Deep venous thrombosis (DVT) and pulmonary embolism
- Postpericardiotomy syndrome (PPS)

2. **Evaluation.** The lungs, chest, and leg incisions should be examined carefully. A CBC with differential, chest x-ray, urinalysis, and appropriate cultures should be performed. A stool sample for *C. difficile* should be obtained if the patient has abdominal pain or diarrhea. Indwelling central and arterial lines should be cultured and removed if in place for more than five days or if cultures return positive. If the WBC is normal or there is an eosinophilia, a drug fever may be present. Occult sternal infections may be investigated with a chest CT scan, but results are usually nonspecific; needle aspiration may be performed if suspicion is high. Head CT scans can identify sinusitis. A transesophageal echocardiogram can evaluate the heart valves for vegetations consistent with endocarditis.

3. **Treatment.** It is best to defer antibiotic therapy until an organism has been identified. However, a broad-spectrum antibiotic may be initiated based on the presumed source and organisms involved as soon as cultures have been obtained. This is especially important in patients who have received prosthetic material (valves, grafts). A more narrow-spectrum antibiotic may be substituted subsequently. Empiric oral

vancomycin (125 mg four times a day) may be started for suspected *C. difficile* colitis. Occasionally a patient will have a fever and elevated WBC with no evident source, but will respond to a brief course of antibiotics. Further comments on nosocomial infections and sepsis can be found on pages 776–778.

IV. Respiratory Care and Complications[3,4]

A. Respiratory function is still impaired when the patient is transferred to the postoperative floor, with many patients exhibiting shortness of breath with some splinting from chest wall discomfort. Arterial desaturation is not uncommon, and all patients should have an arterial saturation measured several times daily by pulse oximetry until the SaO_2 remains above 90%. It is not uncommon to see significant desaturation when the patient becomes more ambulatory. Most patients have some degree of fluid overload and require diuresis, and steps must be taken to overcome a poor inspiratory effort and atelectasis. Potential complications, such as pneumonia, bronchospasm, pleural effusions, or pneumothorax, can be identified by examination and a chest x-ray (Table 13.3). Standard orders should include:

1. Supplemental oxygen via nasal cannula at 2–6 L/min on the postoperative floor. In the ICU, high flow oxygen systems or BPAP are useful for hypoxemia, but after transfer to the floor, if the patient requires more than supplemental oxygen by nasal cannula or facemask to achieve an acceptable oxygen saturation, they should probably be transferred back to an ICU setting for more intensive respiratory care.

2. Frequent use of incentive spirometry to encourage deep breathing

3. Progressive mobilization

4. Provision of adequate, but not excessive, analgesia. Patient-controlled analgesia (usually morphine) is particularly beneficial for one or two days following surgery, and may be supplemented with other pain medications, such as ketorolac (Toradol) 15–30 mg IV q6h for a few days. In patients with abnormal renal function, IV acetaminophen is beneficial in the ICU. Most patients obtain adequate analgesia with oral medications 2–3 days after surgery and seem to do better with regular, rather than prn, pain medications.

Table 13.3 • Postoperative Respiratory Complications

- Atelectasis
- Pleural effusions
- Pneumothorax
- Pneumonia (possibly aspiration)
- Bronchospasm
- Pulmonary edema (noncardiogenic or cardiogenic)
- Hypoxemic/hypercapneic respiratory failure/ARDS
- Pulmonary embolism
- Diaphragmatic dysfunction (phrenic nerve paresis)
- Chylothorax

5. Bronchodilators administered via nebulizers should be used if copious secretions or bronchospasm are present (see pages 503–504). These commonly include albuterol, levalbuterol (Xopenex), or a combination of albuterol and ipratropium (Duoneb). Chest physical therapy may benefit patients having difficulty raising secretions.

6. Measures to reduce the risk of venous thromboembolism (antiembolism stockings, sequential compression devices, subcutaneous heparin or low-molecular-weight heparin [LMWH]) should be considered depending on the patient's mobility and risk (see section E on pages 750–752).

7. Patients with a history of obstructive sleep apnea should utilize CPAP machines at night or any other device that has been helpful to them prior to surgery.

B. Patients with preexisting lung disease and a history of heavy smoking often have a tenuous respiratory status postoperatively with borderline oxygenation, and acute decompensation can occur with little provocation, including ambulation. Mucus plugging, atelectasis from poor inspiratory effort, mobilization of "third space" fluid, or even a minor cardiac event can cause arterial desaturation and respiratory distress. In patients without significant underlying lung disease, acute decompensation usually indicates the presence of a significant process, such as a pleuropulmonary event (significant pneumothorax, pneumonia, pulmonary embolism), myocardial ischemia, worsening mitral regurgitation, cardiac tamponade, or acute fluid overload from AKI with oliguria.

C. The management of respiratory insufficiency, pneumothorax, pleural effusions, and bronchospasm is discussed in Chapter 10. Other complications, including diaphragmatic dysfunction from phrenic nerve paresis and pulmonary embolism, are discussed below.

D. **Diaphragmatic dysfunction** from phrenic nerve injury has been noted in 10–20% of patients following open-heart surgery.[5]

1. **Etiology and prevention**

   a. Cold injury to the phrenic nerve from use of iced saline slush in the pericardial well is the primary cause of this problem. Systemic hypothermia may also be contributory. Use of insulation cooling pads that protect the phrenic nerve from cold solutions, minimizing systemic hypothermia, intermittently pouring cold saline over the heart (the "shallow technique"), and avoiding iced slush reduce the incidence of phrenic nerve paresis.[6–8]

   b. The phrenic nerve may be injured directly during dissection of the internal thoracic artery (ITA) in the upper mediastinum, especially on the right side. It may also be damaged when making a V-incision in the pericardium to allow for better lie of the ITA pedicle. Phrenic nerve devascularization with compromise of the pericardiophrenic artery may also be contributory, especially in patients with diabetes.[9]

2. **Presentation**

   a. Most patients with unilateral phrenic nerve paresis have few respiratory symptoms and are extubated uneventfully. Difficulty weaning, shortness of breath, and the requirement for reintubation may be noted in patients with severe chronic obstructive pulmonary disease (COPD).

   b. Bilateral phrenic nerve palsy usually produces tachypnea, paradoxical abdominal breathing, and CO_2 retention during attempts to wean from mechanical ventilation.

3. Evaluation

  a. A chest x-ray will demonstrate an elevated hemidiaphragm at end-expiration during spontaneous ventilation, most commonly on the left side. This will not be evident during mechanical ventilation. An elevated hemidiaphragm may be difficult to appreciate if basilar atelectasis or a pleural effusion is present. Therefore, when planning a thoracentesis or tube thoracostomy for a pleural effusion, one must always consider the possibility of an obscured, elevated hemidiaphragm. The position of the gastric bubble on chest x-ray should identify the position of the diaphragm on the left. If the diaphragm is elevated, one might inadvertently insert a needle below the diaphragm, risking injury to intra-abdominal structures.

  b. Diaphragmatic fluoroscopy ("sniff test") will demonstrate paradoxical upward motion of the diaphragm during spontaneous inspiration if unilateral paralysis is present.

  c. Ultrasonography will show a hypokinetic, immobile, or paradoxically moving diaphragm during respiration.

  d. Transcutaneous phrenic nerve stimulation in the neck with recording of diaphragmatic potentials over the seventh and eighth intercostal spaces can measure phrenic nerve conduction velocities and latency times.[10] This is helpful in assessing whether phrenic nerve dysfunction may be a contributing factor to a patient's respiratory problems.

  e. Transdiaphragmatic pressure measurements can be used to make the diagnosis in patients with bilateral phrenic nerve palsies.[11]

4. Treatment is supportive until phrenic nerve function recovers, which may take up to two years. One study of patients with COPD found that nearly 25% of patients had persistent pulmonary problems with a decreased quality of life at midterm follow-up.[12] Diaphragmatic plication can provide significant symptomatic and objective improvement in patients with marked dyspnea. This can be performed robotically or via a thoracotomy (video-assisted [VATS] or open) or laparoscopically.[13] Ventilatory support is usually necessary for patients with bilateral involvement. Some patients can be managed at home with a cuirass respirator or a rocking bed.

E. **Venous thromboembolism** (VTE) is a term that describes both deep venous thrombosis (DVT) and **pulmonary embolism** (PE). Screening noninvasive studies have documented a 15–20% incidence of DVT and a 6–20% incidence of PE after cardiac surgical procedures, with both being more common after OPCAB.[14,15] However, symptomatic VTE is noted in only about 1–2% of patients.[16,17] One study of routine CT pulmonary angiography and lower-extremity venous studies in patients undergoing elective CABGs and considered at low risk for VTE reported a 21% incidence of DVT, and in more than half of these patients, PE occurred in the absence of lower-extremity DVT.[18]

  1. It has been presumed, perhaps inappropriately so, that the risk of postoperative VTE is low because of heparinization and hemodilution during surgery and the presence of thrombocytopenia and platelet dysfunction in the early postoperative period. However, platelet activity is increased immediately after surgery, and elevated fibrinogen levels, thrombin generation, tissue factor activation, and reduced fibrinolysis are also noted. Increased platelet reactivity and aspirin resistance are

particularly common after off-pump surgery, although the risk of symptomatic VTE is still only 1%.[19–22] A study of patients undergoing on-pump CABGs found that the absorption of aspirin was reduced early after surgery, leading to reduced antiplatelet effect that could contribute to VTE.[23] Thus low-dose aspirin may not be sufficient to inhibit platelet aggregation early after surgery, although this may impact graft patency more than the risk of VTE.

2. **Risk factors** for VTE in the perioperative period include older age, obesity (BMI >30), right- or left-heart failure, a history of VTE, prolonged bed rest and immobility, prolonged ventilation, multiple blood and blood product transfusions, and the occurrence of significant postoperative complications, including acute kidney injury, infection/sepsis, and neurological complications.[17,24,25] VTE may result from heparin-induced thrombocytopenia (HIT) and may occur several weeks later.

3. **Prevention.** Numerous studies have evaluated the use of mechanical or pharmacologic prophylaxis from which general recommendations can be made.[25–27]

   a. Early mobilization is the most important factor in reducing the risk of VTE. Once the patient is stable, getting them out of bed and ambulating several times a day is very important. Having a patient sit in a chair is the least desirable position.

   b. Elastic graduated compression stockings (GCS), such as T.E.D. stockings, should be placed after the initial leg dressing and ace wraps are removed, and should be placed on both legs. Use of sequential compression devices (SCDs) or intermittent pneumatic compression devices (IPCs) in well-mobilized ambulatory patients provides little additional benefit to use of GCS alone.[26,27]

   c. Although increased platelet reactivity and aggregation are present in postoperative patients, most patients are usually given aspirin 81 mg daily after surgery. This dose is insufficient to inhibit platelet aggregation and probably provides little benefit in reducing the risk of VTE.[20] One study did demonstrate, however, that the addition of low-dose aspirin to heparin 5000 units SC q8h reduced the risk of VTE nearly fivefold in patients undergoing OPCAB.[28]

   d. ICU patients may be maintained at bedrest because of ongoing clinical issues and are usually poorly mobilized. For these patients as well as those with the risk factors listed above in section E.2, pharmacologic prophylaxis should be considered in addition to compression devices. One study found the combination of heparin plus one of these devices reduced the risk of PE by 60% compared with heparin alone,[29] although another study of ICU patients found no added benefit of IPC when the patient was already receiving heparin.[30] Nonetheless, the literature remains controversial on whether early initiation of pharmacologic prophylaxis with either SQ heparin (5000 units SC q12h) or LMWH (40 mg SC daily) should be considered in these patients and when it should be started. Some authors recommend initiating one of these medications on the first postoperative day once mediastinal bleeding has tapered off,[24,25,31] but other guidelines have concluded that the bleeding risk outweighs the early benefits.[32] The risk of developing a hemopericardium leading to cardiac tamponade must always be taken into consideration when deciding whether to initiate heparin early after surgery.

4. **Manifestations.** Pleuritic chest pain and shortness of breath with hypoxemia are usually present. The acute onset of these symptoms distinguishes them from typical postoperative respiratory symptoms. The new onset of atrial fibrillation (AF), sinus tachycardia, or fever of unknown origin may be clues to the diagnosis. Calf tenderness and edema are unreliable signs of DVT, especially in the leg from which the vein has been harvested. However, the new development of such findings several days to weeks after surgery should prompt further evaluation.

5. **Assessment.** ABGs, a chest x-ray, ECG, and CT pulmonary angiography should be obtained. The presence of a low arterial oxygen saturation is nonspecific, but may be compared with values obtained earlier in the postoperative course. A positive venous noninvasive study of the lower extremities in association with respiratory symptoms and hypoxia is suggestive evidence of a pulmonary embolism and should prompt further evaluation. A falling platelet count with VTE mandates evaluation for HIT, for which alternative anticoagulation should be initiated.

6. **Treatment.** Traditionally, IV heparin has been recommended for 1 week (unless HIT is present), followed by warfarin for six months. However, equally effective therapy can be achieved with the use of a non-vitamin K antagonist oral anticoagulant (NOAC), such as apixaban (10 mg bid × 1 week, then 5 mg bid) or rivaroxaban (15 mg bid × 3 weeks, then 20 mg daily) – doses conditional upon renal function – and these medications do not require blood monitoring. Early ambulation has not been shown to increase the risk of extending the DVT or developing pulmonary embolism, although bedrest was traditionally considered part of routine management.[33,34] An inferior vena cava filter should be placed if anticoagulation is contraindicated. Systemic thrombolytic therapy should be avoided because of the recent sternotomy incision, although ultrasound-assisted catheter-directed thrombolysis using the EKOS system might be considered.[35,36] Other interventional methods, including suction embolectomy and fragmentation therapy, may be beneficial in patients with massive PE,[37] reserving surgery for salvage situations to avoid a redo sternotomy and pump run. However, surgical pulmonary embolectomy may be applicable to hemodynamically stable patients with massive PE and may be preferable in the rare patient with massive pulmonary embolism early after cardiac surgery, when thrombolytic therapy is contraindicated.[38,39]

V. Cardiac Care and Complications

A. Upon transfer to the postoperative floor, the patient should be attached to a telemetry system to continuously monitor the heart rate and rhythm for several days. Vital signs are obtained every shift if the patient is stable, but more frequently if the patient's heart rate, rhythm, or blood pressure is abnormal or marginal.

B. The evaluation and management of complications noted most frequently in the intensive care unit are presented in Chapter 11. These include low cardiac output states, perioperative infarction, cardiac arrest, coronary spasm, hypertension, and arrhythmias. This section will discuss several cardiac problems commonly noted during subsequent convalescence (Table 13.4).

C. **Arrhythmias and conduction problems**

1. **Atrial arrhythmias** are the most common complication of open-heart surgery and occur with a peak incidence on the second or third postoperative day. Although

Table 13.4 • Cardiac Complications of Cardiac Surgery

- Atrial and ventricular arrhythmias
- Low cardiac output syndrome: RV dysfunction, LV systolic or diastolic dysfunction
- Myocardial ischemia/infarction
- Coronary vasospasm
- Hypertension
- Hypotension
- Cardiac tamponade: early or delayed
- Acute pericarditis
- Postpericardiotomy syndrome
- Cardiac arrest
- Constrictive pericarditis (late)

some patients become symptomatic with lightheadedness, fatigue, or palpitations, many have no symptoms and are noted to be in AF or flutter on telemetry monitoring. Treatment entails rate control, attempted conversion to sinus rhythm, and anticoagulation if AF persists or recurs. Management protocols are discussed in detail on pages 626–632 and in Table 11.15 (page 627).

2. **Ventricular arrhythmias** are always of concern because they may be attributable to myocardial ischemia or infarction and may herald cardiac arrest. Low-grade ectopy or nonsustained ventricular tachycardia (VT) with normal ventricular function does not require aggressive therapy and may be managed with a ß-blocker. In contrast, VT with impaired LV function requires further evaluation and may benefit from placement of an implantable cardioverter-defibrillator (ICD). An echocardiogram should be considered and may identify new regional wall motion abnormalities attributable to a perioperative infarction, which may account for the arrhythmia. On occasion, when epicardial wires are still connected to a temporary pacemaker, VT may develop due to improper sensing, with inadvertent firing on the T wave triggering the malignant arrhythmias ("R on T" phenomenon).

3. **Conduction abnormalities and heart block** (see pages 614–618). Temporary pacemaker wires are routinely removed by the third postoperative day unless there is evidence of symptomatic sinus bradycardia, lengthy sinus pauses, advanced degrees of heart block, or a slow ventricular response to AF. If these issues are present, medications that reduce atrial automaticity or reduce AV conduction (β-blockers, amiodarone, calcium-channel blockers [CCBs], and digoxin) should be stopped. If they persist, permanent pacemaker implantation should be considered.

    a. New bundle branch or fascicular blocks have been noted in up to 45% of patients after CABG and appear to correlate with longer aortic cross-clamp times. However, they resolve in more than half of the patients before discharge.[40,41]

    b. Patients with sick sinus or tachycardia/bradycardia syndrome may have a rapid ventricular response to AF intermixed with a slow sinus mechanism that limits use of ß-blockers. A permanent pacemaker (PPM) system should be considered if these problems persist beyond three days. Studies have shown, however, that pacemaker dependence usually resolves within a few months, unless the indication was complete heart block.[42]

    c. Patients undergoing aortic valve surgery are more prone to conduction disturbances and heart block because of debridement, edema, hemorrhage, or suturing near the conduction system. The average incidence of PPM is 5–9% after AVR,[43,44] but it is greater in patients receiving rapid deployment valves.[45] Preoperative conduction system disease (first-degree block, left anterior hemiblock, right bundle branch block [RBBB], or left bundle branch block [LBBB]) is generally the major risk factor for the development of heart block using both traditional and rapid deployment valves. Both the development of a new postoperative LBBB and the necessity for a permanent pacemaker early after AVR have adverse prognostic significance with a compromise in long-term survival.[46,47]

    d. When pacemaker wires are removed, there is always the potential for bleeding and the development of tamponade. It is recommended that they be removed when the INR is less than 2, but this does not eliminate the possibility of bleeding. If the INR remains persistently elevated, the wires may be cut and left behind. After removal, the patient should remain at bedrest for one hour and vital signs should be taken every 15 minutes for the first hour and then hourly for a few hours to monitor for orthostatic changes. Tamponade can occur within minutes or hours and can prove fatal unless the possibility is entertained and addressed on an urgent, if not emergent, basis. If concern is raised because of hypotension or a complaint of chest pain, a STAT echocardiogram may be helpful. Emergency thoracotomy at the bedside may be life-saving.

    e. A transfemoral temporary pacing wire may be retained at the conclusion of a TAVR procedure if the heart rate is very slow or there is evidence of advanced heart block. The latter is more likely to develop in patients with a preexisting RBBB and first-degree AV block.

        i. If the heart rate stabilizes above 50–60/min and there is no evidence of complete heart block, the wire may be removed several hours later or the following morning. Despite this common practice, some patients with these preexisting conduction abnormalities may still develop delayed heart block (>48 hours later). If heart block persists, permanent pacemaker implantation may be necessary. Guidelines for management of conduction disturbances after TAVR are noted on page 615.[48] One study found that only 21% of patients receiving a PPM after TAVR were pacer-dependent at one year; however, pacer dependence was more common with use of self-expanding valves and post-balloon dilatation, or when complete heart block was the indication for the PPM.[49]

        ii. When the transvenous pacing wire and the 6 Fr transfemoral sheath are removed from the femoral vein after a TAVR, persistent bleeding may occur despite a short period of manual pressure, because antiplatelet therapy is routinely administered within a few hours of the procedure. If this persists, simply suturing the skin entrance site and applying a sandbag are usually effective in controlling the bleeding.

D. Hypertension. When the patient is transferred to the postoperative floor, oral antihypertensive medications must be substituted for the potent intravenous drugs used in the ICU. Blood pressure tends to return to its preoperative level several days after surgery once myocardial function has returned to baseline, the patient has been mobilized, and chest wall pain improves with moderate analgesia. Aggressive patient-specific management is important to prevent issues related to blood pressure variability. For example, a patient with renal dysfunction may need a slightly higher blood pressure to ensure renal perfusion. In contrast, more strict control of blood pressure may be essential in an elderly patient with fragile tissues or in patients with perioperative bleeding. Not only can hypertension increase cardiac wall stress and cause myocardial ischemia, but it may increase any residual mitral regurgitation and can precipitate an aortic dissection from graft or cannulation sites.

1. A decrease in systolic blood pressure from preoperative levels may be noted in patients who are hypovolemic or anemic, or have experienced a perioperative infarction. In these patients, preoperative antihypertensive medications can be withheld and then restarted at lower doses when the blood pressure increases. In contrast, patients who have ongoing pain issues or have undergone an AVR for aortic stenosis may develop significant systolic hypertension.

2. ß-blockers are recommended for virtually all patients after surgery as prophylaxis against AF and can be titrated up to control the heart rate and blood pressure as well. Resumption of the patient's preoperative medications should then be instituted to optimize blood pressure control. Other considerations when selecting an antihypertensive medication include the following:

   a. Poor ventricular function (EF <40%): use one of the ACE inhibitors or ARBs. A ß-blocker, preferably carvedilol, should also be given in this situation, but must be used cautiously if the patient has decompensated heart failure or a low output syndrome.

   b. Sinus tachycardia with good LV function, or with evidence of residual myocardial ischemia: use higher doses of a ß-blocker (metoprolol) or labetalol.

   c. Coronary spasm or use of a radial artery graft: use a nitrate or CCB (amlodipine, diltiazem, or nicardipine).

   d. Sinus bradycardia with good LV function: if initial use of an ACE inhibitor or ARB is insufficient, amlodipine should be considered.

E. **Hypotension** may develop after transfer to the floor and should be evaluated using the differential diagnosis of shock or a low cardiac output state (see Chapter 11).

   1. **Etiology.** The possibility of a significant clinical condition should always be considered in a patient with hypotension, although transient hypotension is usually of a benign etiology. It is best to correlate the patient's cuff pressure with an arterial line pressure in the ICU before the catheter is removed, because a significant discrepancy can confound interpretation of cuff pressures on the postoperative floor. Concerns must always include the possibility of hypoxemia, myocardial ischemia/infarction with cardiogenic shock, an aortic dissection (if discrepant upper extremity pulses), sepsis, and especially delayed **tamponade** (see section G, pages 757–761). However, the more common causes of hypotension several days after surgery include:

      • Hypovolemia, usually from aggressive diuresis
      • Profound anemia
      • β-blockers or amiodarone used prophylactically to prevent AF
      • Significant bradycardia
      • Arrhythmias, especially a rapid ventricular response to AF/flutter and then the medications used to treat them, which usually lower the blood pressure (β-blockers, CCBs, amiodarone)

- Vasoplegia from the residual effects of the systemic inflammatory response from CPB or from a diabetic autonomic neuropathy
- Initiating too high a dose of the patient's preoperative medications. Often the patient's initial postoperative hypertension is related to pain and sympathetic overactivity, and once these resolve, hypotension may result, necessitating fluid resuscitation and unnecessary transfusions.

2. **Assessment and management**
   a. Review of the patient's medications, fluid status, orthostatic blood pressure measurements, heart rate and rhythm, pulse oximetry reading, 12-lead ECG, and hematocrit should be sufficient to delineate the mechanism for hypotension. If the patient appears warm and well perfused, administration of a moderate amount of volume and modification of the medical regimen should suffice.
   b. Management of hypotension associated with AF can be problematic, in that medications that slow the rate tend to cause vasodilation and lower the blood pressure further (especially metoprolol and diltiazem). Amiodarone is an excellent alternative, and usually causes hypotension only with rapid IV infusion. However, in most patients, rate control will improve left ventricular filling and the blood pressure. If the patient has refractory hypotension with a fast rate that is difficult to control pharmacologically, cardioversion may be indicated.
   c. If the patient has refractory hypotension and does not appear well perfused, the likelihood of tamponade is increased and a STAT echocardiogram should be performed.

F. **Myocardial ischemia.** The development of recurrent angina or new ECG changes (usually ST segment elevation) postoperatively always requires careful evaluation for evidence of ischemia or myocardial infarction. Manifestations may include a low output state, hypotension, heart failure and pulmonary edema, ventricular arrhythmias, or cardiac arrest.

1. **Etiology**
   a. Coronary hypoperfusion from:
      1. Acute thrombosis of a graft after CABG, either from an anastomotic problem, a kinked graft, or occasionally grafting to an incompletely endarterectomized artery
      2. Reduced flow from anastomotic narrowing (technical issue) or hypoperfusion through a small conduit (for example, using a very small ITA graft or replacing a moderately diseased vein graft with a small ITA at reoperation)
      3. Coronary spasm (graft or native vessel)
      4. Nonbypassed, diseased coronary arteries either due to failure to locate the vessel, small vessel size, or severe calcification (incomplete revascularization)
      5. Coronary ostial narrowing, occlusion or kinking after AVR or aortic root procedures with coronary button reimplantation
      6. Circumflex artery compromise during mitral valve surgery
   b. Poor myocardial protection during surgery

2. **Evaluation**
   a. Careful review of the ECG may indicate whether the ECG changes are consistent with ischemia or pericarditis (see Figures 8.2 and 8.3 on pages 384 and 385).

    b. Empiric use of a nitrate and/or CCB may be helpful for ischemia or spasm and can be diagnostic.

    c. Urgent coronary arteriography should be considered when there are significant ECG changes.[50] It may identify a technical problem with a graft or confirm the diagnosis of spasm.

    d. In less urgent situations, a nuclear stress imaging study can be performed to identify the presence of myocardial ischemia and differentiate between ischemic and nonischemic causes of chest pain.

3. Treatment

    a. Intensification of a medical regimen with nitrates and ß-blockers is indicated.

    b. Placement of an intra-aortic balloon pump (IABP) is beneficial for ongoing ischemia or evidence of hemodynamic compromise, especially in the immediate postoperative period. However, it should only be considered a supportive measure until the etiology of the problem is identified.

    c. If a technical problem with a graft is identified by coronary angiography, or on occasion, there is failure to graft the correct artery or the graft is placed proximal to the most significant stenosis, percutaneous coronary intervention (PCI) is often the best treatment because it can be performed most expeditiously.[50,51] If this is not feasible, but a major area of myocardium is in jeopardy and the patient has not suffered a significant perioperative myocardial infarction (PMI), reoperation should be considered. In contrast, medical management may be indicated if the coronary vessels supplying an ischemic zone are small and diffusely diseased, if they were bypassed but graft flow was limited by vessel runoff, or if they were not bypassable. Inability to address small vessels should only leave a minor area of the heart potentially ischemic. PCI of larger, more proximal stenotic segments may provide some benefit by improving inflow. If the patient has sustained an extensive infarction and has a delayed assessment, surgical intervention may not prove beneficial and may be high risk.

    d. The long-term results of coronary bypass surgery are influenced by the development of atherosclerotic disease in bypass conduits, nonbypassed native arteries, or native arteries beyond the bypass sites. Factors that can improve these results include use of arterial grafting (one or both ITAs and a radial artery), aggressive control of risk factors, including abstinence from smoking, statins for dyslipidemia, optimal control of hypertension and diabetes, and use of aspirin for at least one year.[52] Supplemental use of a P2Y12 inhibitor may be beneficial in patients undergoing surgery for acute coronary syndromes or after OPCABs. On rare occasions, the late development of ischemia has been attributed to a coronary steal syndrome, either from a coronary–subclavian steal or an ITA–pulmonary artery fistula.[53]

G. Pericardial effusions and delayed tamponade. Pericardial effusions have been noted in about 60–75% of patients undergoing routine echocardiography in the first 1–2 weeks following surgery but usually resolve completely.[54,55] Several large studies have shown that about 1–2% of patients may develop symptomatic effusions that gradually increase in size, leading to a low cardiac output state and tamponade that requires drainage.[56,57] However, smaller series have suggested that invasive treatment for pre-tamponade or tamponade is indicated in about 5% of patients.[58,59] This problem may be noted within the first week of surgery or weeks later. Suspicion must remain high because symptoms may develop insidiously and can be difficult to differentiate from those noted in patients recovering slowly from surgery. **This is one of the most serious yet most potentially correctable of all postoperative problems.**

1. **Etiology**

   a. Risk factors for development of pericardial effusions and delayed tamponade include:[57-60]

      - Use of perioperative antiplatelet drugs (aspirin, P2Y12 inhibitors) or other anticoagulants (heparin, LMWH, NOACs)
      - Early postoperative bleeding that requires blood product administration or re-exploration
      - Early initiation of anticoagulation for VTE prophylaxis, mechanical valves, or the development of AF: a decision that must be made with caution as slow intrapericardial bleeding may occur despite minimal early postoperative bleeding.
      - Comorbidities including larger body surface area, hypertension, immunosuppression, chronic kidney disease (CKD), hepatic dysfunction
      - More advanced heart failure
      - Urgent surgery, more complex operations requiring longer durations of CPB (more coagulopathy), and surgery for endocarditis

   b. Acute hemorrhage may occur during removal of ventricular pacemaker wires from laceration of a superficial artery or vein overlying the right ventricle or from the right ventricle itself. Some surgeons request that pacing wires be removed prior to chest tube removal, but most commonly they are removed a few days after the chest tubes have been removed. Because bleeding might be exacerbated by anticoagulation, it is advisable to remove pacing wires before the INR becomes therapeutic, by withholding 1–2 doses of a NOAC, or by stopping heparin for a few hours to minimize that risk. If the patient is therapeutically anticoagulated, it may be advisable to cut the wires rather than remove them (see also page 609). Bleeding during withdrawal of atrial pacing wires may occur if the wires are directly attached to the atrial wall rather than placed into a plastic sleeve that is sewn to the heart (the Medtronic model 6500 wires). Rarely, a patient may develop a delayed rupture of an infarct zone or LV rupture from a mitral valve prosthesis.

   c. In patients with the above risk factors, especially those taking pre- or postoperative anticoagulants or antiplatelet drugs, a progressively worsening hemopericardium may develop and the presentation may be insidious. In a large series from the Mayo Clinic, nonspecific symptoms often led to performance of an echocardiogram, but 42% of patients had hemodynamic compromise consistent with tamponade. This report also noted that half of the patients who had insignificant effusions on echo after valve surgery were readmitted with tamponade within two weeks of discharge.[56]

   d. Acute pericarditis is occasionally noted on a postoperative ECG and can be difficult to distinguish from an evolving MI (see Figure 8.3). This may be related to epicardial hemorrhage, undrained blood, or an early inflammatory response, but it is often of unclear etiology. It may be asymptomatic and noted only on an ECG and may contribute to the formation of serous or serosanguineous effusions.

e. Late serous or serosanguineous effusions may develop from PPS, which is considered one type of "postcardiac injury" syndrome.[61]

2. Presentation

a. Acute hemorrhage will present with refractory hypotension and the clinical picture of acute cardiac tamponade.

b. Acute pericarditis may cause chest discomfort, but in the early postoperative period may be indistinguishable from the pain of a sternotomy incision.

c. The classic picture of delayed tamponade is a low output state manifest by malaise, shortness of breath, chest discomfort, anorexia, nausea, or a low-grade fever. These symptoms are frequently ascribed to medications or simply a slow recovery from surgery. Jugular venous distention, a pericardial rub, progressive orthostatic hypotension, tachycardia (often masked by use of β-blockers), and a pulsus paradoxus are often noted. Occasionally, the first sign is a decrease in urine output with a rise in the BUN and creatinine caused by progressive renal dysfunction from the low output state, arterial hypotension, and systemic venous hypertension.

3. Evaluation

a. A chest x-ray may reveal enlargement of the cardiac silhouette, but this may be attributed to obtaining an AP portable film during a poor inspiratory effort. However, the chest x-ray is often normal, depending on the site and rapidity of blood accumulation.

b. Two-dimensional echocardiography can identify the pericardial effusion, confirm tamponade physiology (>40% inspiratory increase in tricuspid valve flow and >25% inspiratory decrease in mitral valve flow), and also assess the status of ventricular function. It is important to recognize that tamponade may be caused by selective compression of individual cardiac chambers, often by small effusions, and not necessarily by large circumferential effusions.[57,62] **A transthoracic echocardiogram often has limitations in obtaining certain acoustic windows**, which may be related to the patient's body habitus. Thus, it will occasionally not identify an effusion.

c. If the clinical suspicion remains high and transthoracic imaging is suboptimal, CT scanning can be used to identify and localize a significant effusion. This is useful in patients who are several days out from surgery, hemodynamically stable, and on the postoperative floor.[63] However, in unstable patients and those in the ICU, a **transesophageal echocardiogram (TEE)** is preferable and is more sensitive than a TTE in detecting posterior fluid collections (Figure 13.1).[64]

4. Prevention

a. Stopping antiplatelet and anticoagulant medications at the appropriate time prior to surgery should not be overlooked.

b. Meticulous attention to obtaining hemostasis at the conclusion of surgery is essential to minimize the risk of bleeding, the use of blood products, and the development of a coagulopathy that may lead to delayed tamponade.

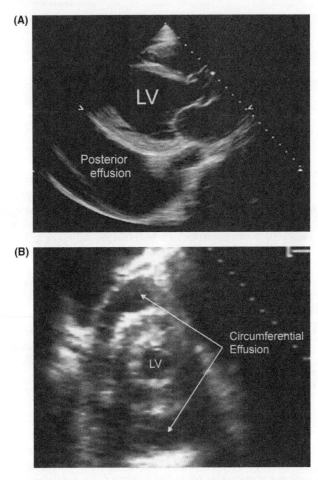

Figure 13.1 • Two-dimensional echocardiograms of significant postoperative pericardial effusions. (A) A transthoracic study in the parasternal long-axis view demonstrating a significant posterior effusion. (B) A transesophageal study in the transgastric short-axis view. Note the circumferential pericardial effusion that prevents adequate ventricular filling. Evidence of diastolic collapse will confirm the hemodynamic significance of the effusion.

    c. Performance of a small posterior pericardiotomy incision at the conclusion of surgery reduces the incidence of posterior pericardial effusions.[65] It is also likely that placing one of the mediastinal tubes below the heart, rather than two tubes anteriorly, might improve drainage and reduce the incidence of residual effusions.

    d. Chest tubes can be removed when drainage for the preceding eight hours is <100 mL. One study found that leaving chest tubes in at least until the second postoperative day and removing them only after the drainage was <50 mL/4h more than halved the incidence of delayed tamponade.[66]

e. Early initiation of anticoagulation following valvular heart surgery, for VTE prophylaxis, or for the management of AF always requires careful judgment as to whether the patient might be at higher risk for mediastinal bleeding and the development of delayed tamponade.

f. Prophylactic use of NSAIDs may reduce the incidence of postoperative pericardial effusions.[67] A number of medications have been successful in reducing the risk of postoperative PPS (see next section), but none can be recommended for routine use for that purpose. However, colchicine, anti-inflammatory medications and/or steroids might be utilized in treating effusions due to pericarditis or PPS which have not produced hemodynamic compromise.

g. Remove pacing wires only in patients who are not therapeutically anticoagulated.

5. **Treatment**

a. Emergency mediastinal exploration is indicated for active bleeding. If the patient is bleeding massively and/or is very unstable, this should be performed in the ICU or even at the bedside on the postoperative floor with equipment available in an "open chest kit". If the patient can be stabilized, but there is suspicion of an active bleeding source, transferring the patient to the operating room for re-exploration is preferable.

b. Pericardiocentesis is the least invasive means of draining a progressively enlarging effusion and is effective in about 50% of cases, usually when the effusion is anterior or circumferential.[56,57] This is usually performed in the cardiac catheterization laboratory under ECG or two-dimensional echocardiographic guidance. This will not be completely effective if the blood has clotted with loculated strands.

c. Subxiphoid exploration should be considered when the echocardiogram suggests that the fluid collection cannot be successfully approached percutaneously (usually a posterior collection) or when it is loculated. If this approach is ineffective in draining the effusion, the entire sternal incision may need to be opened.

d. A pericardial "window" or limited pericardiectomy through a left thoracotomy approach can be considered for loculated posterior effusions or recurrent effusions several weeks after surgery.

H. **Postpericardiotomy syndrome** (PPS) has been reported in 10–20% of patients following open-heart surgery and is considered to represent an autoimmune inflammatory response to injury, often associated with the occurrence of perioperative bleeding and the requirement for blood transfusions.[68,69] It is associated with an elevation in inflammatory markers, including cytokines, markers of neutrophil activation, and oxidative stress mediators.[70] It is one of several forms of "postcardiac injury" syndrome which may also occur after pacemaker implantation, PCI, transmural myocardial infarctions, or radiofrequency arrhythmia ablation, presumably as a response to cardiac injury.[61] It may occur within the first week of surgery or several weeks to months later and appears to have a different etiology than the pericarditis and pericardial effusions noted early after surgery. The development of PPS may contribute to cardiac tamponade, early vein graft closure, or constrictive pericarditis.[71]

1. Risk factors for PPS include younger age, nondiabetics, CKD, lower hematocrits or platelet counts preoperatively (which most likely accounts for more perioperative

bleeding and the need for transfusions), and valve or aortic surgery.[68,69,72] A low preoperative level of interleukin-8 is a high-risk marker for its development.[73]

2. **Presentation.** Fever, pleuritic chest pain, a pericardial friction rub, or a new or worsening pleural or pericardial effusion may be present, with the diagnosis of PPS being made if two or more of these are present. Malaise and arthralgias may also be present.

3. **Prevention.** Colchicine (1 g bid × 1 day, then 0.5 mg bid × 1 month) started after surgery has seen the most promise in preventing PPS.[74,75] The efficacy of prophylactic intraoperative steroids is uncertain[76] – one study showing a benefit of methylprednisolone[77] and another showing no benefit of dexamethasone.[78] Diclofenac (representative of the NSAIDs) has also been effective in reducing the occurrence of postoperative PPS.[79]

4. **Evaluation.** Lymphocytosis, eosinophilia, and an elevated ESR are noted, but a fever work-up is negative. Effusions are usually demonstrable by chest x-ray and echocardiography.

5. **Treatment**

   a. The best initial treatment for PPS is a combination of aspirin (750 mg tid × 2 weeks) and colchicine (0.5 mg bid × 6 months), given with a PPI.[61] If there is minimal symptomatic relief or as an alternative to aspirin, a one- to two-week course of an NSAID, such as ibuprofen 600 mg tid, can be given with cessation of aspirin. It should be noted that the regular use of NSAIDs (especially ibuprofen) may inhibit the cardioprotective antiplatelet effect of aspirin.[80]

   b. For patients with recurrent PPS, a one-month tapering course of prednisolone starting with 0.5 mg/kg daily can be added to the regimen of colchicine and aspirin.[61]

   c. Colchicine (0.5 mg bid × 1 month) is recommended for the treatment of acute and recurrent pericarditis.[75,81]

   d. Pericardiocentesis may be necessary to drain a large symptomatic pericardial effusion.

   e. Pericardiectomy is recommended for recurrent large effusions or constriction, which is more common in younger patients with the early onset of PPS.

I. **Constrictive pericarditis** is a late complication of cardiac surgery that is extremely uncommon despite the development of adhesions that form within the mediastinum following surgery. It has been noted in patients with undrained early postoperative hemopericardium, use of warfarin, early PPS, and previous mediastinal radiation, yet has also developed in the absence of any of these factors. It has been theorized that residual blood and proinflammatory conditions in the pericardium may contribute to the formation of both PPS and later the formation of dense adhesions that more readily cause thickening of the epicardium. This may produce ventricular constriction ("constrictive epicarditis") and also result in graft failure.[70,82]

1. **Presentation.** The patient will note the insidious onset of dyspnea on exertion, chest pain, and fatigue. Signs of right-heart failure (peripheral edema, ascites, and jugular venous distention) are common, but pulsus paradoxus is infrequent.

2. **Evaluation**

   a. The chest x-ray is frequently normal in the absence of a pericardial effusion.

   b. Two-dimensional echocardiography will demonstrate signs of constriction, such as septal bounce and diminished respiratory variation in the inferior vena cava.

    c. A CT or preferably an MRI scan usually documents a thickened pericardium, with delayed enhancement on MRI and occasionally a small pericardial effusion. However, in cases of constrictive epicarditis, pericardial thickening may not be seen.

    d. Right-heart catheterization provides the most definitive information. It will document the equilibration of diastolic pressures and demonstrate a diastolic dip-and-plateau pattern ("square-root" sign) in the right ventricular pressure tracing (see Figure 1.32). On occasion, significant fluid overload will produce hemodynamics consistent with constriction, when in fact there is no anatomic evidence of a thickened pericardium or epicarditis other than standard postoperative scarring.

  3. **Treatment.** If there is no clinical response to diuretics and steroids, a pericardiectomy is indicated to decorticate the heart. This is best performed through a sternotomy incision, which allows for adequate decortication of the right atrium and ventricle and much of the left ventricle. It also allows for the institution of CPB in the event of a difficult or bloody operation. Relief of epicardial constriction is difficult and may result in surgical damage to bypass grafts or significant bleeding. A "waffle" or "turtle shell" procedure is performed with crisscrossing incisions made in the epicardial scar to relieve the constriction.[82] Results are suboptimal when there is poor LV systolic function, higher RV and LV diastolic pressures, persistent impaired diastolic filling, which correlates with the duration of symptoms prior to surgery, and when significant tricuspid regurgitation is present, which usually will not improve with pericardiectomy alone.

VI. Renal, Metabolic, and Fluid Management and Complications

A. **Routine care**

  1. Most patients are still substantially above their preoperative weight when transferred to the postoperative floor. Comparison of the patient's preoperative weight with daily weights obtained postoperatively is a guide to the use of diuretics to eliminate excess fluid. Achievement of dry body weight may require more aggressive diuresis if heart failure (HF) was present before surgery. In the chronically ill patient, preoperative weight may be achieved after several days despite fluid overload, due to poor nutrition.

  2. Dietary restriction (sodium and water) need not be overly strict in most cases. With the availability of potent diuretics to achieve negative fluid balance and the common problem of a poor appetite after surgery, it is more important to provide palatable food without restriction to improve the patient's caloric intake.

  3. If a patient required diuretics before surgery (especially valve patients and those with poor myocardial function), it is advisable to continue them upon discharge from the hospital even if preoperative weight has been attained.

B. **Transient renal failure** (see also Chapter 12). Patients with preoperative renal dysfunction, hypertension and diabetes, prolonged pump runs, postoperative low cardiac output syndromes, or those requiring substantial doses of vasopressors may develop postoperative AKI. Although diuretics are routinely used to reduce the immediate postoperative fluid overload, they have to be used with caution in patients developing

AKI. They do not influence the course of AKI and can in fact exacerbate renal dysfunction by causing prerenal azotemia from intravascular volume depletion. Management can be very difficult on the postoperative floor when methods of monitoring intravascular volume are limited.

1. A common scenario with mild AKI is gradual elevation in serum creatinine (SCr) with or without elevation in the BUN, along with a low serum sodium, reflective of persistent total body water overload. Oliguria may improve and AKI may be transient with adjustment of medications. Antihypertensive medications should be reduced to allow the normally hypertensive patient's blood pressure to rise to higher levels than normal. ACE inhibitors should be withheld, NSAIDs avoided, and diuretics used gently, if at all, to maintain adequate intravascular volume. If the patient was aggressively diuresed and has a poor appetite, additional hydration may be necessary to address prerenal azotemia which will elevate the BUN. In most patients, renal dysfunction is transient as long as the cardiac output remains satisfactory.

2. If a rising SCr is associated with significant fluid retention, compromise of pulmonary function with oxygen desaturation often results. A high dose of diuretics may improve urine output to address this problem even if it does not directly promote renal recovery. If not successful, the patient may need to return to the ICU for more invasive monitoring and possibly use of intravenous inotropic support, more aggressive noninvasive or even mechanical ventilation, and ultrafiltration or dialysis if renal dysfunction is significant. **A rising BUN and creatinine of unclear etiology, especially when associated with new-onset oliguria, should always raise the suspicion of delayed tamponade.** An echocardiogram should be performed to assess myocardial function and look for possible cardiac tamponade.

C. **Hyperkalemia** usually occurs in association with renal dysfunction. Its manifestations and treatment are discussed on pages 708–711. Particular attention should be directed to stopping any exogenous potassium intake, ACE inhibitors ARBs, and NSAIDs, and reevaluating renal function.

D. **Hyperglycemia** in diabetics, and occasionally in nondiabetics, is a common postoperative problem. The blood glucose level may be elevated due to insulin resistance and residual elevation of the counterregulatory hormones (glucagon, cortisol) after surgery.[83] Adequate, but not overly stringent, control of blood glucose during the early postoperative period with an IV insulin protocol has been shown to reduce not only the incidence of wound infection but also other morbidities and operative mortality (see Appendix 6).[84-87] Once the patient is transferred to the floor, frequent fingersticks should be obtained (usually before meals and at bedtime) to assess the adequacy of blood glucose control.

1. Insulin resistance is commonly noted during the early postoperative period. Insulin-dependent diabetics should have their insulin doses gradually increased back to preoperative levels depending on oral intake and blood glucose levels. It is preferable to use a lower dose of intermediate-acting insulin initially and supplement it with regular insulin as necessary (see Table 12.9, page 721, for commonly used insulin preparations).

2. Oral hypoglycemics can be restarted once the patient has an adequate oral intake, usually starting at half the preoperative dose, and increasing the dose depending on oral intake and blood glucose.

E. Other electrolyte and endocrine complications are fairly unusual once the patient has been transferred to the postoperative floor. Chapter 12 discusses the evaluation and management of some of these problems.

VII. Hematologic Complications and Anticoagulation Regimens

A. **Anemia**

1. Despite the obligatory hemodilution associated with use of CPB, effective blood conservation strategies and performance of off-pump surgery have reduced the requirements for perioperative blood transfusions. Although the STS guidelines recommend transfusion for a hemoglobin (Hb) <6 g/dL on CPB in low-risk patients,[88] such a restrictive strategy may increase the risk of renal failure, stroke, and neurocognitive dysfunction, and should not be applied to patients who are elderly, diabetic, have cerebrovascular disease, or are at risk for end-organ ischemia.

2. Most studies recommend maintaining a HCT above 20% on CPB and then at least 22% postoperatively. Multiple studies comparing a liberal (transfuse for a Hb <7 g/dL) and restrictive (transfuse for a Hb <9 g/dL) strategy after cardiac surgery have shown comparable outcomes.[89,90] However, transfusion to a higher hematocrit postoperatively may be considered for elderly patients, those who feel significantly weak and fatigued, and those with ECG changes, hypotension, or significant tachycardia.

3. Although the HCT may rise gradually with postoperative diuresis, it frequently will not as fluid is mobilized into the bloodstream from extracellular tissues. Furthermore, the HCT may be influenced by the shortened red cell lifespan caused by extracorporeal circulation and the loss of 30% of transfused red cells within 24 hours of transfusion. In one study, "hemoglobin drift" was noted in virtually all patients, averaging about 1.1 mg/dL, was greater with longer durations of CPB, but was unrelated to whether the patient received a transfusion.[91] However, with diuresis, the Hb level improved in nearly 80% of patients prior to discharge, and this concept should be taken into consideration when contemplating a transfusion.

4. Any patient with a HCT <30% should be placed on iron therapy (ferrous sulfate or gluconate 300 mg tid for one month) at the time of discharge. Exogenous iron may not be necessary if the patient has received multiple transfusions, because of the storage of iron from hemolyzed cells.

5. Consideration may also be given to use of recombinant erythropoietin (Epogen or Procrit) to stimulate red cell production (50–100 units/kg SC three times a week), especially in patients with CKD with adequate iron stores (transferrin saturation >20% and ferritin >100 ng/mL).

B. **Thrombocytopenia** is caused by platelet destruction and hemodilution during extracorporeal circulation, but platelet counts gradually return to normal within several days. Impaired hemostasis noted in the early postoperative period is caused more commonly by platelet dysfunction induced by CPB or use of antiplatelet medications, although it is attenuated somewhat by the use of the antifibrinolytic drugs.

1. **Etiology**
   - Platelet activation or dilution during CPB
   - Excessive bleeding and multiple blood transfusions without platelet administration

- Use of an intra-aortic balloon pump
- Heparin-induced thrombocytopenia (HIT). **Note:** platelet counts must be monitored on a daily basis in any patient receiving heparin. A falling platelet count after the initial recovery of the platelet count should always raise the specter of HIT and is an indication for *in vitro* aggregation testing to identify HIT.
- Other medications that may reduce the platelet count, such as furosemide, NSAIDs, and ranitidine
- Sepsis
- Thrombotic thrombocytopenic purpura (TTP), which is usually characterized by AKI, thrombocytopenia, and a microangiopathic hemolytic anemia with schistocytes on blood smear. Occasionally, fever and altered mental status may be present.[92]

2. **Treatment.** Platelet transfusions are indicated:
   a. When the platelet count is <20,000–30,000/μL (<20-30 × 10⁹/L).

   a. When the platelet count is <20,000–30,000/μL ($<20\text{-}30 \times 10^9/\text{L}$).
   b. For ongoing bleeding when the platelet count is <100,000/μL and sometimes higher if platelet dysfunction is suspected.
   c. For a planned surgical procedure (such as percutaneous IABP removal) when the platelet count is <60,000/μL ($<60 \times 10^9/\text{L}$).

C. **Heparin-induced thrombocytopenia (HIT)** is a very serious problem that may result in widespread arterial and venous thrombosis, and carries a mortality rate of about 20%. Because of its high risk and the necessity for treatment with direct thrombin inhibitors, early suspicion, identification, and management are essential.[93–96]

1. HIT is an immune-mediated phenomenon caused by the formation of IgG antibodies that bind to the heparin-platelet factor 4 (PF4) complex, producing platelet activation. This results in release of procoagulant microparticles that lead to thrombin generation. This binding causes release of more PF4, promoting more platelet activation. Antibody binding to glycosaminoglycans on the surface of endothelial cells leads to endothelial cell damage and tissue factor expression. This procoagulant milieu promotes arterial and venous thrombosis in 30–50% of patients and may cause a stroke, myocardial infarction, mesenteric thrombosis, or deep venous thrombosis.

2. **Suspicion of the diagnosis**
   a. The diagnosis of HIT requires the presence of heparin antibodies and thrombocytopenia. HIT is more common with use of bovine heparin and is 8–10 times more likely to occur with UFH than LMWH.
   b. The suspicion of HIT is based on the "four Ts", which include the degree of **T**hrombocytopenia, the **T**iming of its occurrence, the occurrence of **T**hrombotic events, and the likelihood of o**T**her potential causes. One scoring system found that independent risk factors for HIT after CPB were a biphasic response to the platelet count, an interval of >5 days since CPB, and a bypass run exceeding about two hours.[97]
      i. Thrombocytopenia is extremely common postoperatively and may be related to hemodilution, platelet damage on pump, clearance of transfused platelets, and sepsis. The platelet count is usually reduced about 40% after surgery on CPB, but begins to rebound by the third or fourth day after

surgery. If the platelet count does not improve after four days or there is a subsequent fall in platelet count >50%, HIT should be suspected.

   ii. Although immediate-onset HIT (occurring within hours of giving heparin) may develop in patients who received heparin within 100 days due to residual circulating HIT antibodies, it is rare for a patient receiving short-term preoperative heparin to develop HIT within the first four days after surgery. The general pattern is for HIT to occur 5–14 days after surgery.

  iii. Delayed-onset HIT (occurring after heparin has been discontinued due to the presence of residual heparin-PF4 platelet-activating antibodies) is often manifested by venous thromboembolism, and is commonly not diagnosed, because platelet counts are rarely checked after heparin is stopped. If there is evidence of a thrombotic event (such as lower extremity VTE), a low platelet count should raise suspicion of this entity.

  iv. It is estimated that 30–50% of patients who develop HIT will develop evidence of thrombosis, mandating additional treatment beyond stopping heparin. Disturbingly, it is estimated that 25% of patients may develop thrombosis before developing thrombocytopenia.[98] Thus, HIT can be a very difficult management problem because of the temptation to administer heparin for a thrombotic event when it might be contraindicated. More commonly, however, patients will develop thrombosis as the platelet count is falling and reaching its nadir, but, as noted, it may occur even after the heparin has been stopped (delayed-onset HIT). Thus, there are clinical scenarios when HIT may be present but the suspicion is low, leading to complications from delayed recognition and management.

  v. Other potential causes, especially medications, use of an IABP, and sepsis should be considered as possible causes of thrombocytopenia.

3. **Diagnostic testing.** ELISA serologic testing for IgG specific heparin-dependent platelet antibodies has replaced prior testing that also detected non-HIT-causing IgM antibodies. Such testing was positive in about 20% of preoperative and in up to 50% of postoperative cardiac surgical patients, but was uncommonly associated with thromboembolic events.[94,99–102] It is estimated that only 1–2% of patients undergoing cardiac surgery will develop HIT. Use of optical densities (ODs) with ELISA testing and antibody titers may be helpful in improving specificity as well, since most cases of HIT are associated with an OD >1.4 units.[95] More specific functional assays of washed platelet activation (serotonin release assay and heparin-induced platelet aggregation studies) are able to more accurately identify antibodies that trigger platelet activation. Preoperative testing for heparin antibodies is not recommended in the absence of thrombocytopenia or thrombosis.

4. **Management**[95,102,103]

  a. If HIT is identified preoperatively with positive testing and thrombocytopenia, an alternative method of anticoagulation (usually bivalirudin) must be used during surgery (see Chapter 4, pages 251–253). Antibodies generally clear within three months of the last heparin administration, and heparinization can be performed safely if HIT testing is negative.

b. With any suspicion of postoperative HIT, even before testing results become available, **all heparin administration must be stopped**. This includes cessation of heparin flushes and removal of heparin-coated pulmonary artery catheters. However, if the likelihood of HIT is low based upon clinical grounds, yet an anticoagulant is indicated for prophylaxis (such as for VTE), fondaparinux 5–10 mg qd SC (weight-based) can be given safely.

c. Platelets should not be routinely administered, because they may promote thrombosis, but may be considered if the patient is bleeding or to prevent bleeding if the platelet count is very low (<30,000). The platelet count generally begins to increase within about a week after cessation of heparin.

d. Warfarin should **not** be started immediately, because tissue necrosis from microvascular thrombosis may occur due to depletion of the vitamin-K-dependent natural anticoagulant protein C. This has been noted in patients who rapidly develop a supratherapeutic INR. Warfarin may be started safely after the platelet count reaches 150×10^9 /L and should overlap the nonheparin anticoagulant for five days, even when the INR is in therapeutic range.

e. Alternative anticoagulation is indicated to minimize the risk of thrombotic events and also to provide protection for the process for which the heparin was originally indicated. This is essential because the risk of symptomatic thrombosis remains greater than 25% if only the heparin is stopped.

  i. **Argatroban** is a synthetic direct thrombin inhibitor that is preferred in patients with renal dysfunction because it undergoes hepatic metabolism. It has a plasma half-life of about 40 minutes. It is given starting at a dose of 2 µg/kg/min once heparin effect has been eliminated (usually four hours for UFH and 12 hours after the last dose of LMWH), and maintained at a rate of 0.5–1.2 µg/kg/min and adjusted to maintain a PTT of 1.5–3 times baseline. Lower doses are recommended in patients with liver disease or heart failure. Conversion from argatroban to warfarin can be somewhat problematic because both affect the INR. Warfarin should be started once the platelet count exceeds 150×10^9 and is given in doses of 2.5–5 mg for five days of overlapping treatment. At that point, the usual protocol is to stop the argatroban if the INR is >4 and recheck an INR in four hours. If the new INR is >2, it does not need to be restarted; if it is <2, the argatroban should be restarted. However, it has been noted that even when the INR is >4, the risk of thrombosis may still exceed the risk of bleeding.[104]

  ii. **Bivalirudin** is a direct thrombin inhibitor that produces reversible binding to thrombin and has a short half-life of only 25 minutes. It can be used for the management of HIT with an initial bolus of 0.75 mg/kg followed by an infusion of 0.15 mg/kg/h to achieve a target PTT of 1.5–2.5 times baseline. Advantages include 80% enzymatic metabolism (although some modification is indicated in patients with a GFR <30 mL/min), non-immunogenicity, and minimal effect on the INR.

  iii. **Danaparoid** is a heparinoid that has a low degree of reactivity with heparin antibodies. It is given in a bolus dose of 2250 anti-Xa units, followed by 400 units/h × 4 hours, then 300 units/h × 4 hours, then a maintenance infusion of 200 units/h. It is monitored by anti-Xa levels, trying to achieve a level of 0.5–0.8 units/mL. It is available from Aspen Pharmacare, but is not available in the USA.

    iv. Non-vitamin K antagonist oral anticoagulants (NOACs) have had limited evaluation in the management of HIT, but may be considered off-label as alternative medications using the doses recommended for acute VTE (see section IV.E, pages 750–752).

    v. Duration of antithrombotic therapy is generally one month without and three months with the occurrence of a thrombotic event.

D. **Coronary bypass surgery.** Postoperative aspirin should be utilized to increase saphenous vein graft patency, although there is no documented benefit in improving the patency of arterial conduits.[52]

    1. Class I recommendations for antiplatelet therapy after CABG in most guidelines (American College of Chest Physicians [ACCP], American College of Cardiology/American Heart Association [ACC/AHA], the European Society of Cardiology [ESC], and the Society of Thoracic Surgeons [STS]) are to start aspirin in doses ranging from 75 mg to 325 mg starting 6–24 hours after surgery and to also prescribe clopidogrel 75 mg after OPCAB.[105-108] The use of higher doses of aspirin may offset the increase in platelet reactivity and the decreased absorption of aspirin noted postoperatively.[23] Non-enteric-coated aspirin has better absorption and is recommended. The timing of initiation of therapy may be influenced by the degree of postoperative mediastinal bleeding. It is recommended to continue aspirin indefinitely due to its benefits in the secondary prevention of coronary disease, although it may not influence graft patency when used beyond one year.

    2. Class IIa recommendations are to prescribe dual antiplatelet therapy (DAPT) with aspirin and a P2Y12 inhibitor (preferably ticagrelor) in patients who have undergone CABG for an acute coronary syndrome (ACS). Several meta-analyses have suggested that DAPT after CABG for stable ischemic heart disease (SIHD) may reduce vein graft occlusion, with the greatest benefit noted following OPCABs (hence the level I recommendation), although it may be associated with more bleeding.[109,110] However, DAPT did not improve cardiovascular outcomes in diabetic patients with multivessel disease undergoing CABG for SIHD or an ACS in the FREEDOM trial.[111] DAPT is only a class IIb indication following on-pump CABG per the ACC/AHA guidelines. If the patient is aspirin-intolerant, clopidogrel should be given with a 300 mg loading dose, followed by 75 mg daily.

    3. DAPT should be resumed after surgery if the patient has received a drug-eluting stent within the past year and it remains patent.

    4. There is no documented superiority in graft patency comparing aspirin to warfarin or to a NOAC (rivaroxaban) whether used alone or in addition to aspirin.[112] Whether one of these might be considered after coronary endarterectomy is not known.

E. **Prosthetic heart valves.** All patients receiving mechanical heart valves must take a vitamin K antagonist (VKA) indefinitely following surgery, but the guidelines regarding the short-term use of a VKA after tissue valve replacement provide differing recommendations.[113] The following recommendations (summarized in Table 13.5) are a general consensus from the 2012 ACCP,[114] 2014/2017 ACC/AHA,[115] and the 2017 ESC guidelines,[116] all of which are updated every few years and are available online. The evolution and comparison of these guidelines are presented in a paper published in 2019.[117]

Table 13.5 • Recommended Anticoagulation Regimens for Prosthetic Heart Valves

	Warfarin	Antiplatelet Drugs
AVR: tissue	INR target 2.5 for 3 months if: • Risk factors (ACCP) • All patients (AHA/ACC IIa) × 3–6 months • All patients (ESC IIb) × 3 months) Possible use of a NOAC after 3 months	Aspirin 75–100 mg alone if no risk factors (ACCP) Aspirin 75–100 indefinitely (AHA/ACC IIa) Aspirin 75–100 mg alone × 3 months (ESC IIa)
AVR: mechanical	INR target 2.5 indefinitely	Aspirin 75–100 mg (ACC/ACCP); only if atherosclerotic disease or history of thromboembolism (ESC)
Mitral valve repair	INR target 2.5 for 3 months (ACC/ESC)	Aspirin 75–100 mg alone (ACCP)
MVR: tissue	INR target 2.5 for 3–6 months (AHA/ACC IIa) or 3 months (ESC IIa) Continue indefinitely if risk factors Possible use of a NOAC after 3 months	Aspirin 75–100 mg with warfarin × 3 months (ACC IIa) Aspirin 75–100 mg after warfarin is stopped
MVR: mechanical	INR target 3.0 indefinitely	Aspirin 75–100 mg (ACC/ACCP); only if atherosclerotic disease or history of thromboembolism (ESC)
AVR-MVR: tissue	INR target 3.0 for 3 months Possible use of a NOAC after 3 months	Aspirin 325 mg after 3 months
AVR-MVR: mechanical	INR 3.0–4.5 indefinitely	Aspirin 75–100 mg
AF with any of above	Continue warfarin indefinitely Possible use of a NOAC if tissue valve after 3 months	

Risk factors: hypercoagulable state, history of systemic thromboembolism, ejection fraction <35%, history of anteroapical infarction, atrial fibrillation
ACCP, American College of Chest Physicians recommendations 2012; ACC/AHA, American College of Cardiology/American Heart Association recommendations 2014; ESC, European Society of Cardiology recommendations 2017
Adapted from Whitlock et al. *Chest* 2012;141(2 Suppl):e576S–600S[114], Nishimura et al., *Circulation* 2017;135:e1159–95 and *J Am Coll Cardiol* 2017;70:252–89[115], Baumgartner et al., *Eur Heart J* 2017;378:2739–91[116].

1. **Tissue valves**

   a. **Aortic valves (surgical).** Some reviews have concluded that use of either aspirin or a VKA provides similar outcomes after bioprosthetic AVR, and the slight decrease in thromboembolism and death from the combination of both is offset by an increased risk of bleeding.[118] Although surgeons and patients often opt for a tissue valve to avoid a VKA, even for a short period of time, there is some evidence that patients not receiving VKAs are more susceptible to thromboembolic complications during the first three months after implantation, with a slightly increased risk of stroke.[119] Furthermore, "subclinical leaflet thrombosis" has been identified on aortic tissue valves implanted surgically or with TAVR and has been associated with an increased risk of stroke after surgical AVR.[120]

      i. The 2012 ACCP guidelines recommend aspirin 75–100 mg (usually 81 mg) indefinitely if the patient is in sinus rhythm, with the addition of warfarin to achieve a target INR of 2.5 if the patient is at higher risk for thromboembolism (AF, hypercoagulable disorder, EF <35%, previous thromboembolism, or a left atrial dimension >50 mm).[114]

      ii. The 2017 AHA/ACC guidelines give level IIa indications to the indefinite use of aspirin and to the use of a VKA for 3–6 months with a target INR level of 2.5 if the patient is at low risk for bleeding. However, the guidelines do not specify whether the recommendation is to use either alone or both together. After 3–6 months, only aspirin is recommended unless there is another indication for warfarin.[115] New guidelines should be available online towards the end of 2020.

      iii. The 2017 ESC guidelines provide a class IIa indication for use of aspirin and a IIb indication for use of an oral anticoagulant (without concomitant use of aspirin), because the addition of a VKA will increase the bleeding risk despite a lower risk of thromboembolism.[116] In contradistinction to the AHA/ACC guidelines, the ESC guidelines do not recommend the indefinite use of aspirin.

      iv. Limited data have shown that a NOAC is noninferior to the use of warfarin in patients with AF and prior bioprosthetic valve replacement or repair. Therefore, it may be feasible to consider use of a NOAC after three months if there is an indication for continuing anticoagulation, such as AF.[121]

   b. **Aortic valves (TAVR).** Standard protocols following TAVR recommend clopidogrel 75 mg daily for six months and aspirin 81 mg daily indefinitely. For patients who are at high risk for bleeding on DAPT, there are data showing that outcomes are comparable with mono and dual antiplatelet therapy.[118,122,123] For a patient in AF, either a VKA or a NOAC is used and may be combined with one antiplatelet medication, but not both.

      i. Concerns about subclinical leaflet thrombosis causing an increased gradient across the valve and an increased risk of stroke have raised the question as to whether a VKA should be used in these patients. This has received an ACC/AHA level IIb indication in patients at low risk for bleeding.[115] This is probably less of an issue in elderly patients in whom anticoagulation is more dangerous, but may be applicable to younger, lower-risk patients undergoing TAVR.

      ii. A NOAC with aspirin cannot be recommended as an alternative approach based on the GALILEO study, which found a higher risk of bleeding, thromboembolism, and death with rivaroxaban + aspirin compared with clopidogrel + aspirin in patients with no other indication for anticoagulation.[124] However, this study did not assess whether use of a NOAC alone might reduce subclinical leaflet thrombosis without increasing risks compared with warfarin or DAPT in patients without AF.

c. **Mitral valves.** Warfarin should be started by the first postoperative day and given along with aspirin (ACC/AHA guidelines level IIa) for 3–6 months to achieve a target INR of 2.5 (range 2.0–3.0). ESC guidelines provide a IIa recommendation for three months of a VKA without aspirin. The initiation of heparin can be considered in the hospital before the INR reaches the target level. The patient can then be discharged on LMWH until the INR reaches the therapeutic range. After three months, warfarin is stopped and aspirin 75–100 mg (usually 81 mg) is given if the patient is in sinus rhythm. However, warfarin should be continued indefinitely in patients at high thromboembolic risk, and aspirin should be added to the regimen. NOACs may be feasible after three months in patients with AF.[113,121]

d. **Mitral rings.** The benefit of using a VKA rather than aspirin after mitral valve repair is not clear. ACCP guidelines recommend aspirin alone if the patient is in sinus rhythm, whereas the ACC/AHA and ESC guidelines recommend use of a VKA for three months. This conclusion is based primarily on evidence that about 30% of patients discharged in sinus rhythm will experience AF shortly thereafter, but is not based upon thromboembolic risk from the prosthetic ring. However, some studies suggest that aspirin alone may be sufficient.[125]

2. **Mechanical valves.** Based on the RE-ALIGN study published in 2013, dabigatran, and inferentially the factor Xa inhibitor NOACs, are contraindicated as anticoagulants in patients receiving mechanical valves.[126]

a. **Aortic valves.** Current-generation bileaflet valves (Abbott St. Jude, Medtronic ATS) should receive warfarin indefinitely starting by the day after surgery to achieve a target INR of 2.5 (range 2.0–3.0). In patients with older valves, which carry higher thromboembolic risk (Starr-Edwards or Bjork-Shiley valves), and in patients with double mechanical valves, the target INR should be 3.0 (range 2.5–3.5). The ESC guidelines recommend increasing the target INR by 0.5 if the risk factors noted in section 1.a.i on page 771 are present. The target INR for On-X aortic valves is also 2.5, but may be lowered to 1.5–2 after three months.

b. **Mitral valves.** Patients should receive warfarin indefinitely starting by the day after surgery to achieve a target INR of 3.0 (range 2.5–3.5).

c. The ACC/AHA and ACCP guidelines recommend the addition of aspirin 75–100 mg daily to warfarin for all patients receiving mechanical valves. Because the evidence supporting this recommendation is weak and the risk of bleeding is unequivocally increased, the ESC recommends the addition of aspirin only if vascular disease, coronary stenting, or recurrent embolism is present.[116,117]

3. In patients receiving mechanical valves or those in AF receiving tissue mitral valves, there is a potentially increased risk of early postoperative thromboembolism when the patient is not therapeutically anticoagulated. Therefore, use of heparin is recommended until the INR becomes therapeutic. However, the timing of initiation of heparin as a bridge is not well defined and must be individualized. Although some groups advocate initiating heparinization as early as the first postoperative day, this may increase the risk of bleeding. A safe approach is to initiate UFH or LMWH on the fourth or fifth postoperative day if the INR is less than 1.8. It is recommended that either of these be continued until the INR has been therapeutic for two days. The ESC recommends anti-factor Xa monitoring if LMWH is used to ensure adequate anticoagulation.

F. **Dosing and overanticoagulation.** Warfarin is a dangerous drug that requires thoughtful administration and careful monitoring to avoid overanticoagulation.[127]

1. Initiation of warfarin results in the more rapid depletion of factors VII, IX, and X than factor II (prothrombin), which has a longer half-life. Thus, it exhibits an antihemostatic effect before it achieves an antithrombotic effect, the latter being attributable primarily to a reduction in factor II. Following cardiac surgery, it is essential that warfarin not be loaded and that doses be carefully individualized to avoid rapid overanticoagulation. An initial dose of 5 mg is given to most patients. However, 2.5 mg should be given to small elderly women, patients with hepatic dysfunction, chronic illness, and those receiving antibiotics or amiodarone (Table 13.6). The INR generally begins to rise in 2–3 days, but often takes 5–7 days to achieve a stable dosing level.

Table 13.6 • Protocol for Initiation of Warfarin Doses

Assess whether patient is at greater risk for sensitivity to warfarin – if so, use low-dose protocol

1. Small, elderly females
2. Over age 75
3. Renal (creatinine >1.5 mg/dL) or hepatic dysfunction
4. Interacting medications (amiodarone, antibiotics)

Day	INR	Standard	Low-Dose
1	WNL	5 mg	2.5 mg
2	<1.5	5 mg	2.5 mg
	1.5–1.9	2.5 mg	1.25 mg
	≥2	HOLD*	HOLD*
3	<1.5	7.5 mg	5 mg
	1.5–1.9	5 mg	2.5 mg
	2–3	2.5 mg	HOLD*
	>3	HOLD*	HOLD*
4	<1.5	10 mg	7.5 mg
	1.5–1.9	7.5 mg	5 mg
	2–3	5 mg	HOLD*
	>3	HOLD*	HOLD*
5	<1.5	10 mg	10 mg
	1.5–1.9	10 mg	5 mg
	2–3	5 mg	HOLD*
	>3	HOLD*	HOLD*
6	<1.5	12.5 mg	10 mg
	1.5–1.9	10 mg	7.5 mg
	2–3	5 mg	2.5 mg
	>3	HOLD*	HOLD*

*Restart warfarin when INR is less than 3.0
WNL, within normal limits

2. Potential dangers of overanticoagulation include cardiac tamponade from intrapericardial bleeding, and gastrointestinal (GI), intracranial, or retroperitoneal hemorrhage. Although there are antithrombotic benefits to the combined use of warfarin and aspirin, which is generally recommended for valve patients, this combination does increase the long-term risk of bleeding for patients with a variety of indications for anticoagulation.[128] An ACC expert consensus pathway was written in 2017 for the management of bleeding related to oral anticoagulation.[127] A brief protocol for the management of overanticoagulation with warfarin is noted in Figure 13.2 and in Appendix 9.

3. If the patient has significant bleeding with a markedly elevated INR, warfarin should be held, and fresh frozen plasma (up to 15 mL/kg) should be given. Vitamin K 5–10 mg IV in 50 mL NS over 30 minutes should be given and may be repeated every 12 hours for persistent INR elevation. Use of four-factor prothrombin complex concentrate (4F-PCC) 25–50 units/kg or recombinant factor VIIa 40 μg/kg may also be considered.

4. If the patient has no evidence of bleeding, general recommendations for management of elevated INRs are as follows, although rapid elevation of the INR in the early postoperative period may warrant more aggressive therapy.

   a. INR ≥9: hold warfarin, give vitamin K 2.5–5 mg orally (INR should fall within 24–48 hours)

   b. INR ≥5 and <9: hold warfarin for 1–2 days and restart when INR is <4; alternatively, omit one dose of warfarin and give 1–2.5 mg of vitamin K orally

   c. INR above therapeutic range but ≤5: lower or omit one dose until at therapeutic range

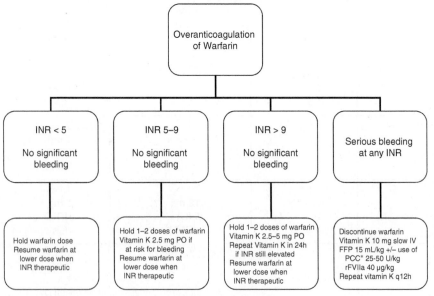

*PCC = 3-factor (Profilnine) or 4-factor (Kcentra) prothrombin complex concentrate

Figure 13.2 • Algorithm for overanticoagulation management

5. Vitamin K given in small oral doses can reduce the INR to a therapeutic level within a few days and is usually the best approach when withholding warfarin does not reduce the INR. Use of large doses of IV vitamin K will produce more rapid reversal of the INR, but it is associated with a small risk of anaphylaxis. It may also lead to warfarin resistance and generally should be avoided. If the INR becomes subtherapeutic (which is usually safer than a markedly elevated INR), heparin can always be given until the INR rises back to the therapeutic range. In patients on long-term warfarin with variable INR responses, concomitant administration of vitamin K 100–200 μg/day orally helps stabilize the INR.[129,130]

6. For patients taking a NOAC, bleeding can be addressed using reversal agents:

   a. For dabigatran, give idarucizumab 5 g IV (Praxbind); if not available, give 4F-PCC 25–50 units/kg.

   b. For factor Xa inhibitors (apixaban, rivaroxaban), give recombinant factor Xa (andexanet alpha [Andexxa]) 400–800 mg at 30 mg/min. If not available, give 4F-PCC 25–50 units/kg.

   c. Prothrombin complex concentrates contains the vitamin-K-dependent coagulation factors II, IX, and X (so-called three-factor PCC [Profilnine]) and may contain variable amounts of factor VII (four-factor PCC [Kcentra].

   d. Another product called FEIBA (anti-inhibitor coagulant complex or activated PCC) may be the best product to control bleeding. This contains nonactivated factors II, IX, and X, activated factor VII, factor VIII inhibitor bypassing activity, and some factor VIII coagulant antigen. It is usually given in a dose of 500–1000 units.

VIII. Wound Care and Infectious Complications

A. General Comments

1. Prophylactic antibiotics are indicated prior to cardiac surgical procedures to minimize the risk of postoperative mediastinitis. A first-generation cephalosporin is usually chosen (cefazolin), although there is some evidence that a second-generation drug (cefuroxime) may be more effective.[131] Vancomycin is substituted if there is a penicillin allergy and is commonly selected for patients undergoing valve or graft placement because of its effectiveness against Gram-positive organisms. The STS guidelines give a level IIb recommendation to give an antibiotic providing Gram-negative coverage (gentamicin) when vancomycin is used, although this is not common practice, and many groups just use cefazolin along with vancomycin to accomplish that. Antibiotics are started within one hour (cephalosporins) or two hours (vancomycin) of surgery and continued for 24–48 hours. They should not be continued any longer even if invasive lines and catheters remain in place.[132,133]

2. Wounds closed with subcuticular sutures and covered with 2-octyl cyanoacrylate adhesive (Dermabond) at the conclusion of surgery do not require dressing coverage. Closed incision negative pressure wound management systems (PREVENA, KCI) applied to a sternotomy wound should be left in place for 5–7 days. If neither of the above is used, the wound should be cleansed and covered with a dressing every day for the first three postoperative days. Subsequent coverage is not necessary unless drainage is noted. All drainage should be cultured and sterile occlusive dressings applied.

B. **Nosocomial infections** develop in 5–10% of patients undergoing cardiac surgery using CPB. Most infections involve the urinary or respiratory tracts, central IV catheters, or the surgical site. Infections are less common in patients undergoing OPCAB, presumably because of the reduced necessity for blood transfusions and the absence of the immunomodulatory effects of extracorporeal circulation.[134,135] A nosocomial infection not only increases the length of stay but also significantly increases operative mortality (to about 20%) because of the frequent development of multisystem organ failure.[135–137] *Staphylococcus* is the most common organism noted in bacteremia and wound infections, whereas Gram-negative infections are more common in the respiratory tract. The high mortality rates of mediastinitis (about 20–25%) and septicemia (30–50%) do not differ much between patients with methicillin-resistant *S. aureus* (MRSA) and other organisms.[138]

1. **Risk factors** have been identified in multiple studies, most of which are included in the STS risk model for major infection shown in Figure 13.3.[139,140] To a large degree, these overlap the risk factors for major mediastinal infections noted on pages 778–779.

   a. Comorbidities: older age, females, diabetes, obesity

   b. Nasal carriage of *S. aureus*, which is associated with a significant incidence of postoperative MRSA infections (about 20%) with a mortality risk of 15–30%.[141,142]

Infection Risk Scores for Major Infection After CABG

Risk Factors	Preop only	Combined
Preoperative variables		
Age (for each 5 years over 55)	1	1
BMI 30 to 40 kg/m²	4	3
BMI 40+ kg/m²	9	8
Diabetes	3	3
Renal failure	4	4
Congestive heart failure	3	3
Peripheral vascular disease	2	2
Female gender	2	2
Chronic lung disease	2	3
Cardiogenic shock	6	N/A
Myocardial infarction	2	N/A
Concomitant surgery	4	N/A
Intraoperative variables		
Perfusion time 100 to 200 minutes	N/A	3
Perfusion time 200 to 300 minutes	N/A	7
Intra-aortic balloon pump	N/A	5

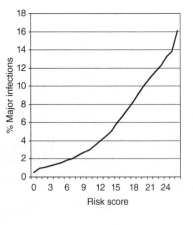

A patient's total risk score is calculated by adding the total points for all risk factors present.

Figure 13.3 • Society of Thoracic Surgeons (STS) risk model for major infections after cardiac surgery. Combined reflects both preoperative patient characteristics and intraoperative variables. (Reproduced with permission from Fowler et al., *Circulation* 2005;112(9 Suppl):I-358–65.)[140]

c. Operative factors: long complex operations, urgent/emergent surgery, reoperations, use of an IABP

d. Postoperative factors (with specific relationships in parentheses)
  - Hyperglycemia (wound infections)
  - Prolonged duration of intubation or need for reintubation (pneumonia). The overall risk of ventilator-associated pneumonia is 5–8%, but it has been estimated to be >50% in patients intubated over 48 hours.[143]
  - Prolonged duration of indwelling Foley catheter (UTI), with the risk of bacteriuria increasing 3–8%/day of catheter usage.[144]
  - Prolonged duration of central venous catheter placement (bacteremia). Central venous catheters with multiple lumens and those changed over guidewires increase the risk of bacteremia.[145,146]
  - Blood transfusions (pneumonia)
  - Reoperation for bleeding
  - Empiric use of broad-spectrum antibiotics
  - Low cardiac output syndromes
  - Postoperative stroke
  - Early development of postoperative renal failure

2. **Preventative measures** that may reduce the incidence of nosocomial infections include:

  a. Perioperative use of intranasal mupirocin to reduce staphylococcal nasal carriage. Although selective use in carriers is most appropriate and can be accomplished using polymerase chain reaction (PCR) assessment, this is not always logistically possible and is not cost-effective, so it is easier to treat all patients as soon as possible before surgery and for 3–5 days postoperatively.[147–149]

  b. Chlorhexidine gluconate 0.12% (Peridex) oral rinse has been shown to reduce the rate of nosocomial respiratory infections, wound infections, and mortality.[150]

  c. Use of a hyperglycemia protocol to maintain early postoperative blood glucose <180 mg/dL.

  d. Early removal of invasive catheters, especially central lines.

  e. Strict adherence to guidelines to avoid prolonged usage of prophylactic antibiotics.[133] One study showed that early postoperative pneumonia was usually caused by organisms that colonized the respiratory tract prior to surgery. However, prolonged use of antibiotics was ineffective in reducing the incidence of pneumonia.[151]

  f. Aggressive ventilatory weaning protocols to reduce the duration of mechanical ventilation and other steps to avoid ventilator-associated pneumonia (see pages 492–493).

  g. Raising the threshold for blood transfusions (transfuse only for a HCT <22% unless clinically indicated).[89,90]

3. The **treatment** of a nosocomial infection requires appropriate antibiotic selection for the organism involved and recognition of the appropriate time course of treatment. Prolonged treatment is often unnecessary and may lead to the development of resistant strains or fungal infections, and not infrequently to hepatic or renal dysfunction. When a Gram-positive bacteremia occurs in a

patient with a prosthetic heart valve, a six-week course of treatment for presumed endocarditis may be indicated. In complex situations, infectious disease consultation is essential.

C. **Sepsis**

1. **Clinical features.** Sepsis resulting in hemodynamic compromise and multisystem organ failure is an uncommon, yet highly lethal, complication of cardiac surgery, with an estimated mortality rate of greater than 30%.[152,153] It is usually noted in critically ill patients who remain in the ICU with multiple invasive monitoring lines, develop respiratory complications, and often have some element of renal dysfunction. It may be the first manifestation of an occult sternal wound infection.

2. **Management.** Basic principles of hemodynamic and ICU management should be initiated early to try to reduce the high mortality rate associated with sepsis. These should include:

   a. Optimization of hemodynamics with fluid resuscitation, inotropic support, and selective use of vasoconstrictors (initially α-agents, and then vasopressin, if necessary). This should be assessed by adequate hemodynamic monitoring (PA catheter and central or mixed venous oxygen saturations), aiming for an oxygen saturation >70%.

   b. Initiation of broad-spectrum antibiotic coverage after panculturing with prompt modification to cover the specific organism isolated

   c. Low tidal volume ventilation if ARDS develops; minimizing sedation to promote early extubation

   d. Early aggressive use of renal replacement therapies (CVVH)

   e. Maintaining the blood glucose <180 mg/dL

   f. Adequate nutrition, preferably by the enteral route

   g. VTE prophylaxis (pneumatic compression devices, possibly SC heparin)

   h. Stress ulcer prophylaxis (sucralfate, proton pump inhibitors)

   i. Low-dose stress steroids to be considered in patients with documented inadequate response to an ACTH challenge

D. **Sternal wound infections (SWI)** complicate about 1% of cardiac surgical procedures performed via a median sternotomy and have been associated with significant hospital mortality (around 20%). Coagulase-negative staphylococcus and *S. aureus* are the most common pathogens encountered despite the use of prophylactic antibiotics specifically directed at these organisms. An incidence of only 1% is amazingly low when one considers that open-heart surgery tends to be performed in the sickest patients with multiple comorbidities, involves the use of CPB, is associated with a high prevalence of transfusions, and entails prolonged wound exposure. Nonetheless, sternal infections remain a major source of physical, emotional, and economic stress when they occur.[154]

1. **Risk factors.** Numerous models have been devised to predict the risk of developing mediastinitis, including that from the STS (available as part of the risk calculator at sts.org). Among the risk factors identified in numerous studies are the following:[135,155,156]

a. Comorbidities: obesity (BMI >40),[157,158] diabetes (elevated HbA1c),[159–161] smoking and COPD,[162] HF, renal dysfunction, peripheral vascular disease (PVD), older age, impaired nutritional status (low serum albumin),[158] use of steroids, and preoperative MRSA colonization[142]

b. Surgical considerations that increase risk include:
- Performing hair removal with razors rather than clippers
- Emergency surgery
- Reoperations
- Bilateral ITA usage in diabetics (controversial)[163]
- Prolonged duration of CPB or surgery
- Need for an IABP
- Use of bone wax[164]
- Contaminated heater/cooler units with mycobacterium chimera, which give rise to latent sternal wound infections[165]

c. Postoperative complications
- Excessive mediastinal bleeding, re-exploration for bleeding, multiple transfusions
- Prolonged ventilatory support (usually in patients with COPD who are actively colonized)
- Low cardiac output states (cardiogenic shock) with use of an IABP
- Refractory hyperglycemia in the ICU, independent of whether the patient has a history of diabetes
- Acute kidney injury
- Central venous line-related bacteremia, which increases the risk fivefold[145]

2. **Prevention.**[154,166] Because of the fairly universal adoption of the basic perioperative measures listed below, the risk of deep SWI in the STS database is about 1% – and this includes a high percentage of patients with multiple risk factors, especially diabetes, obesity, and smoking. The adoption of newer technologies, such as negative pressure management, has generally not been found to be cost-effective, except perhaps in patients at highest risk for infection.[167]

   a. **Preoperative measures**
   - Identify and treat preexisting infections.
   - Advise patients to stop smoking as soon as possible prior to surgery. Although it is suggested that smoking increases the risk of SWI,[162] prominent coughing after surgery in such patients also increases the risk of sternal dehiscence.[168]
   - Optimize diabetic control after initial evaluation of the patient if HbA1C is >7.5.
   - Optimize nutritional status, if possible, in patients with a low serum albumin (<2.5 mg/dL).
   - Chlorhexidine gluconate 0.12% (Peridex) oral rinse.[150]
   - Chlorhexidine chest and leg wash several times the night before and the morning of surgery to reduce the bacterial skin count.

- Intranasal mupirocin (Bactroban) given at a minimum the morning of surgery and continuing for five days to reduce nasal carriage of staphylococcal organisms. This is not beneficial in patients who are MRSA negative, but, unless nasal swabs and PCR testing are performed in advance, it is recommended that all patients be treated with intranasal mupirocin.[149] Although very effective against MSSA, mupirocin is only 50% effective in decolonizing patients with MRSA. One concern of universal decolonization is not just cost but the potential risk of developing antibiotic resistance.[169]

- Hair clipping just prior to surgery

- Appropriate timing and dosage of weight-based prophylactic antibiotics:

  o Cephalosporins should be given within one hour of surgery. Cefazolin is recommended and should be given in a dose of 2 g to patients <120 kg and 3 g if >120 kg. IV bolus injection achieves a peak plasma concentration within 20 minutes and peak interstitial levels within 60 minutes, so ideally it should be given 20–30 minutes before surgery starts.[135] An additional dose should be given on pump or may be repeated in four hours in off-pump cases.

  o Vancomycin is usually selected for patients undergoing valve surgery or placement of prosthetic grafts and may be given as an alternative to cephalosporins in patients who are allergic to penicillin or cephalosporins. It should be started within two hours of surgery and given in a dose of 20 mg/kg. Although not common practice, the 2007 STS guidelines gave a level IIb indication for also giving a single preoperative dose of gentamicin, no more than 4 mg/kg, when vancomycin in used for prophylaxis.[132]

  o If there are contraindications to the above antibiotics, daptomycin (6 mg/kg IV) is usually selected.

b. **Intraoperative measures**

- Careful skin prep with chlorhexidine alcohol may be superior to povidone-iodine (without alcohol).[170–172] Any skin preparation can only reduce the bacterial count but cannot sterilize the skin. One study showed that 89% of subcutaneous wound cultures and 98% of adjacent skin cultures were positive just prior to skin closure after cardiac procedures.[173]

- Consideration may be given to use of a microbial sealant that immobilizes bacteria (InteguSeal, Halyard Health). In some studies, this reduced the risk of SWI, but in others, it did not.[174–176]

- Use of Ioban rather than standard drapes[177]

- Ensure a midline sternotomy and provide a secure sternal closure. Some studies suggest that figure-of-eight wires or rigid fixation systems are superior to simple cerclage wires in producing sternal stability and reducing the incidence of wound infection, although a meta-analysis of closure methods found no difference.[178–182] Use of Robicsek basket-weaving sutures may be considered if the sternum is narrow, osteoporotic, or divided off midline.

- Be selective in the use of bilateral ITAs in diabetic patients. Skeletonizing the ITA may be helpful, but avoidance of bilateral usage in patients with other risk factors, such as severe obesity and COPD, is prudent.[163]
- Use meticulous surgical technique with respect for tissues and obtain adequate hemostasis to minimize mediastinal bleeding.
- Avoid bone wax.
- Use intravenous insulin to maintain intraoperative blood sugar <180 mg/dL.
- Redose cephalosporins after four hours. One study reported that the risk of SWI was greater when the surgical duration approached six hours and there was a low cefazolin plasma concentration (<104 mg/L) during wound closure.[183]
- Tolerate a HCT of 20% on pump; use blood products to help with hemostasis only if absolutely necessary.
- Use subcuticular sutures rather than skin staples and seal wound with a topical adhesive (Dermabond).
- One study suggested that application of bacitracin over the closed wound (if Dermabond is not used) was successful in virtually eliminating the risk of deep SWI.[184]
- Application of platelet-leukocyte rich gel[185] and possibly gentamicin-collagen sponges to the sternal edges may reduce the risk of deep SWI.[171,186–188] Despite remote literature suggesting that vancomycin paste is helpful, a more recent study showed no benefit.[189]
- Consider using a negative pressure wound system in patients at high risk of infection. Studies in patients receiving bilateral ITA grafts had a trend towards a reduced rate of SWI.[190] Universal use of these systems does not appear to be cost-effective.[167]

c. **Postoperative measures**
- Maintain blood glucose <180 mg/dL in the early postoperative course (48 hours) using an IV insulin protocol.
- Use a restrictive transfusion trigger for blood (Hb <8 g/dL) and use blood products sparingly after surgery unless clinically indicated.[191]
- Plan early extubation and removal of invasive catheters as soon as possible as they can cause bacteremia and result in a SWI.
- Discontinue antibiotics after 48 hours.

3. **Presentation** of a mediastinal wound infection can be either overt or occult and often depends on the infectious agent. For example, *S. aureus* infections tend to be virulent and present within the first 10 days of surgery. In contrast, coagulase-negative staphylococcal infections tend to present late with an insidious onset and have a more indolent course.

a. A variety of classification systems for sternal wound infections have been proposed, varying with the time to occurrence, the depth and extent of the infection, and whether prior procedures had been attempted.[192–194] The Centers for Disease Control and Prevention (CDC) and STS definitions (see Appendix 14) differentiate between superficial incisional, deep incisional, and organ/space surgical site infections. However, the latter two categories tend to overlap. This is particularly true since it is difficult to rule out sternal or retrosternal infection when the prepectoral fascia or sternal wires are involved in the infectious process. The eventual approach to management usually depends on operative findings.

b. Minor/superficial infections usually present with local tenderness, erythema, serous drainage, or a localized area of wound breakdown with purulent drainage. The sternum is usually stable.

c. Major/deep incisional infections (deep subcutaneous, osteomyelitis, mediastinitis) may have any of the above, but usually present with significant purulent drainage, often with an unstable sternum. The patient commonly has fever, chills, lethargy, and chest wall pain. Leukocytosis is invariably present. Sternal instability may be noted when mediastinitis is present, but, in the absence of other clinical evidence, it may represent a sterile mechanical dehiscence.

d. Inexplicable chest wall pain or tenderness, fever, Gram-positive bacteremia, or leukocytosis should raise suspicion of a SWI which accounts for more than 50% of postoperative Gram-positive bacteremias. Occult infections are particularly common in diabetic patients, who often mount a very poor inflammatory response and may present several weeks after surgery with extensive purulent mediastinitis but few systemic signs.

e. A chronic draining sinus tract or sternocutaneous fistula is a common delayed presentation of chronic osteomyelitis, and often originates from the sternal wires.[164]

4. **Evaluation**

a. Assessment of the degree of sternal instability is important in deciding how to proceed. If the sternum is unstable, operative exploration is indicated. If it is stable, further diagnostic tests are warranted in an attempt to identify a deep infection.

b. Culture of purulent drainage may identify the organisms and direct appropriate antibiotic therapy.

c. Wound aspiration may diagnose an infection when purulent drainage is not present.[195]

d. Chest CT scanning may be beneficial if the sternum is stable. It may help identify a deep infection if there is loss of the integrity of retrosternal soft tissue fat planes or an undrained retrosternal abscess with air. Although there are reports that CT scanning is quite sensitive and specific for diagnosing wound infections,[196] one must be cautious in its interpretation because hematoma formation and fibrin along the chest tube tracts are commonly present in the retrosternal area and may be interpreted as "consistent with infection". Clinical correlation and occasionally a wound aspirate are necessary before exploring a patient. A chest CT with three-dimensional sternal reconstruction is very helpful in identifying a sternal dehiscence and allows the surgeon to adopt an appropriate strategy for closure, whether for a sterile dehiscence or an infection.

e. White cell scanning, using indium[111] or technetium labeling, and [99mTc]-labeled monoclonal granulocyte antibody scintigraphy are among the radionuclide tests that have been helpful in identifying the presence and/or location of infections.[197,198] FDG-PET/CT scanning has also been helpful.[199]

f. Occasionally, the infection will have to "declare itself" by spontaneous drainage when diagnostic techniques are inconclusive but the clinical suspicion remains high.

5. **Treatment of a sterile sternal dehiscence**

a. When there has been a sterile mechanical dehiscence, the patient usually describes increased chest wall movement and pain with breathing that may have been precipitated by a bout of severe coughing. This problem should be repaired when identified. At the time of exploration, wound cultures should be obtained if there is any suspicion of infection to determine whether long-term antibiotics might be indicated. An attempt should be made to restabilize the sternum. Problems arise primarily when there has been an off-center sternotomy or wires that have pulled through one or both sides of the sternum, producing a "chicklet" sternum. At times, placement of Robicsek basket-weaving sutures on the affected site will allow for standard wire closure. If not, rigid fixation plates (SternaLock Blu, Zimmer Biomet) that extend onto the ribs may be used. If that does not suffice, sternectomy and placement of muscle flaps as described below may be necessary.

b. Use of a rigid fixation system should be considered prophylactically in heavy patients at risk for dehiscence, but should not be used in patients with narrow or osteoporotic sternums. This has been shown to reduce the risk of dehiscence and wound infection.[179–182]

6. **Treatment of minor infections**

a. Minor superficial site infections usually respond to oral antibiotics, opening of the wound, and local wound care. Use of negative pressure wound therapy can be used for larger wounds to expedite closure and may allow for secondary surgical closure, if desired. Persistence of a sinus tract or multiple areas of recurrent breakdown suggest a deeper-seated infection, often involving the sternal sutures. This usually requires surgical exploration rather than repeated dressing changes. It may respond to simple wire removal and curetting of the involved bone with a six-week course of antibiotics. Negative-pressure wound therapy may also be helpful for sternocutaneous fistulas.

b. If the sternal wires or the bone are exposed when the wound is explored, a deeper infection must be ruled out and mediastinal exploration is indicated. This may introduce infection into the mediastinum from the superficial tissues, but may allow for primary reclosure over drains depending on the extent of infection.

7. **Treatment of major infections.**[166,200] Major infections require mediastinal exploration for debridement of infected tissues, removal of foreign bodies (sternal wires or plates), drainage, and elimination of dead space. Antibiotic therapy is generally recommended for six weeks. The approach to achieving wound

closure is conditional upon the time to development of the infection, the extent of mediastinal purulence, and the degree of sternal involvement.

a. When there is a healthy-appearing sternum that requires minimal debridement and minimal purulence in the retrosternal space with pliable mediastinal tissue that can eliminate dead space (usually within 2–3 weeks of surgery), primary sternal closure may be attempted with wires or rigid fixation plates.[201]

b. If there is a large area of dead space behind the sternum or one is worried about exposure of prosthetic material or grafts, placement of omentum may be helpful.[202]

c. Substernal dilute antibiotic (not povidone-iodine) irrigation, suction-irrigation systems, or closed vacuum substernal drainage systems have been used when there is residual mediastinal infection. However, failure to suction out irrigation solutions can lead to cardiac tamponade if more fluid is infused than drained.[203,204]

d. Although skin closure can be performed, it is often advisable to leave the subcutaneous tissue open with use of negative pressure wound therapy (NPWT), such as the V.A.C. Granufoam dressing (KCI, an Acelity Company), rather than continuous wound packing.

e. If there is a very large wound defect, placement of pectoralis flaps with primary skin closure can be performed immediately or days later. Although more chest wall stability and an improvement in respiratory status can be achieved with sternal closure, performing primary sternal closure will predictably fail if the patient has significant mediastinitis or devascularized bone.

f. When there is severe mediastinitis and purulence, marked sternal necrosis (more likely with bilateral ITA usage), or when sternal osteomyelitis requires extensive debridement or has recurred after previous interventions, the sternum should not be or most likely cannot be reapproximated upon first exploration.

   i. Traditionally, the patient was left intubated and sedated for days with dressings applied directly on the heart until purulence improved. Nutrition was optimized, and then the patient would be returned to the OR for placement of muscle flaps over the heart with primary or delayed skin closure. This could include use of one or two pectoralis major flaps based on the thoracoacromial artery to cover the upper 75% of the wound, use of a right rectus flap (the side opposite LITA usage) based on the superior epigastric artery to cover the bottom 25% of the wound, or the use of an omental flap based on the gastroepiploic artery, which could be mobilized laparoscopically and could cover the entire wound.[205] Unless the heart is well mobilized off the sternum at the initial exploration, there is a risk of right ventricular rupture with chest wall distraction, which usually proves fatal.[206] Latissimus dorsi flaps are reserved for patients with very large wound defects.[207]

   ii. To avoid prolonged intubation and potential cardiac damage, an alternative approach is that of immediate coverage after sternal debridement. This is feasible unless there is extensive mediastinitis. Muscle or omental flaps as described are placed over the heart using drains beneath the flaps to remove blood and serous fluid. The subcutaneous tissue can be closed primarily, but with an extensive infection, it should be treated with a NPWT dressing to close by secondary intention or secondary closure.

iii. In the patient with extensive mediastinitis and gross purulence, immediate coverage may be unsuccessful or inadvisable and will lead to persistent infection. NWPT can be used, and a barrier (such as xeroform or petroleum gauze) should be placed between the heart and the NPWT dressing to avoid tissue erosion.[157,208] This stabilizes the chest wall somewhat, but the coverage is not rigid and does not necessarily prevent displacement of the heart into the space between the sternal halves. Thus RV rupture, although rare, is not necessarily prevented.[209] However, NPWT allows for earlier extubation, and will expedite time to eventual closure with muscle or omental flaps or, if there is adequate remaining sternum, to sternal reclosure. This approach of early NPWT dressings over the heart followed a few days later by primary sternal closure or flaps has significantly reduced the mortality associated with deep SWIs.[208,210]

iv. NPWT dressings consist of a polyurethane ether foam with an evacuation tube that drains into an effluent canister connected to negative suction. This will decrease wound edema, reduce bacterial colonization, produce arteriolar dilatation, and improve microcirculatory flow, which encourages granulation tissue formation and accelerates wound healing. It can be used as a bridge to muscle flap coverage, to subsequent sternal rewiring if an adequate amount of sternum remains, or to closure by secondary intention or secondary suture closure of the subcutaneous tissue.

8. The **prognosis** of patients developing a deep SWI is very poor, but has improved with early recognition and appropriate treatment. However, the long-term survival of patients discharged after the treatment of a deep SWI is compromised.[211,212] One of the most significant risk factors for mortality is ventilator-associated pneumonia, so earlier wound coverage or use of NPWT after appropriate mobilization of the heart should allow for earlier weaning from the ventilator. This may reduce the mortality associated with mediastinal wound infections.

E. **Leg wound** complications have become less common with the universal use of endoscopic vein harvesting techniques.[213] This involves a single knee incision and "poke holes" to ligate the vein proximally and distally. Significant bleeding in the endoscopic tract should be addressed surgically, with placement of a drain if there is persistent oozing. Nonetheless, the potential still exists for hematoma formation within the endoscopic tract which causes firmness and ecchymotic changes. Infection may occur at the incision site near the knee, but tract infections are fairly rare. Vein harvesting through one long open incision leads to cellulitis in about 20–30% of patients. This is more likely to occur in patients with severe PVD, diabetes and obesity, and is more common in women. Most complications are related to poor surgical technique with creation of flaps, failure to eliminate dead space, use of excessive suture material, or hematoma formation. With the technique of multiple skip incisions, infections can also occur in a similar fashion to open incisions, especially since this technique may be accompanied by significant tissue trauma from retraction of the tissues for visualization.

1. **Presentation**
   a. Cellulitis
   b. Wound breakdown with purulent drainage
   c. Skin necrosis from thin flaps or a large subcutaneous hematoma; formation of eschar
   d. Warm, indurated wound overlying an endoscopic tract, often with accompanying hematoma or skin ecchymosis and significant leg edema

2. **Prevention**
   a. Use careful surgical technique: avoid tissue trauma, minimize flap formation, obtain meticulous hemostasis, and avoid excessive suture material and tissue strangulation, especially in the small knee incision for endoscopic harvesting.
   b. Use antibiotic wound irrigation prior to closure.
   c. Roll a sponge over the endoscopic tract prior to closure to evacuate any blood that may have accumulated during heparinization. If there is concern about ongoing bleeding, reinspect the wound after protamine administration to ensure hemostasis and then close the wound. If there remains a concern about bleeding, place a suction drain to evacuate blood and eliminate dead space in the endoscopic tract.
   d. Ace wrap the leg fairly tightly at the conclusion of surgery.

3. **Treatment** of minor leg infections after endoscopic harvest requires oral antibiotics, removal of exposed foreign suture material, and drainage. Infections in endoscopic tunnels may require opening of the skin, but often can be managed by opening the skin incision and placing a Blake drain for antibiotic irrigation.[214] If a large hematoma or necrotic skin edges are present after open harvesting, early return to the operating room should be considered to evacuate the hematoma and close the leg primarily. Eschar formation from devitalized flaps may require more aggressive debridement.

F. **Radial artery harvesting.** Obtaining adequate hemostasis during open harvesting and before performing a layered closure that leaves the fascia open should prevent hematoma formation. Cellulitis is the most common manifestation of infection and will respond to antibiotics. Rarely, a purulent infection may occur that requires further drainage. Endoscopic harvesting is usually performed with a tourniquet in place, and blood accumulating in the endoscopic tract after the tourniquet is released should be manually evacuated. A drain is usually placed to evacuate blood and eliminate the dead space.

G. **Antibiotic prophylaxis** for dental procedures is mandatory for all patients with prosthetic valves and grafts. The ACC/AHA guidelines for endocarditis prophylaxis changed significantly in 2007 with the recommendation to use antibiotics for dental procedures only in patients with prosthetic material and other patients at higher risk for infection. These recommendations are available online at www.acc.org and are shown in Table 13.7.[115,215]

Table 13.7 • AHA/ACC Antibiotic Prophylaxis for Dental Procedures to Prevent Endocarditis

Standard regimen	Amoxicillin 2 g PO 1 h before procedure
Unable to take PO medications	Ampicillin 2 g IV/IM within 30 minutes of procedure **or** Cefazolin or ceftriaxone 1 g IV/IM
Penicillin-allergic	Cephalexin 2 g PO **or** Clindamycin 600 mg PO **or** Azithromycin or clarithromycin 500 mg PO
Penicillin-allergic and unable to take PO	Cefazolin or ceftriaxone 1 g IM/IV **or** Clindamycin 600 mg IM/IV

Dental prophylaxis is recommended for patients at high risk:
1. Prosthetic heart valves and grafts, including homografts
2. Prosthetic material used for valve repair (rings, chords)
3. Previous infectious endocarditis
4. Cardiac transplant recipients with valvular regurgitation due to a structurally abnormal valve
5. Unrepaired cyanotic congenital heart disease
6. Repaired congenital heart disease with residual shunts or valvular regurgitation at the site of or adjacent to the site of a prosthetic patch or device

GI/GU procedures do not require prophylaxis, even in patients at high risk
Reproduced with permission from Wilson et al., *Circulation* 2007;116:1736–54[215]; Nishimura et al. Circulation 2017;135:e1159-95.[115]

IX. Neurologic Complications

Neurologic complications following cardiac surgery may involve the central nervous system (CNS) or peripheral nerves. CNS injuries are subdivided into ischemic strokes, delirium (encephalopathy), and neurocognitive deficits. Ischemic strokes are usually attributed to either cerebral embolization or hypoperfusion, whereas the mechanism for delirium and neurocognitive deficits is often multifactorial or of unclear etiology. CPB has been incriminated as the culprit for many neurologic complications, since it is associated with aortic cannulation and clamping, periods of hypotension, production of a systemic inflammatory response, and possibly a disruption of the blood–brain barrier. A meta-analysis did in fact show a 50% reduction in stroke with off-pump surgery, but this was primarily noted in patients with prior TIAs or stroke.[216,217] Otherwise, no difference in neurocognitive function has been shown between on- and off-pump surgery.[218,219]

A. Central nervous system deficits: ischemic stroke

1. Risk factors

a. Preoperative factors. A number of risk factors for postoperative ischemic stroke have been identified.[220–224] A risk model incorporating several of these factors can be used to provide an estimated risk of stroke after surgery (Figure 13.4).[220]

- A prior stroke or transient ischemic attack (TIA) suggests the presence of cerebrovascular disease or risk factors for its development (such as AF). It is likely that CPB can exacerbate preexisting cerebral ischemia or cause cerebral edema in areas where prior damage has caused disruption of the blood–brain barrier. One study reported that 44% of patients with a history of stroke developed a focal neurologic deficit after surgery. Of these, 8.5% were new, 27% represented reappearance of the old deficit, and 8.5% were worsening of the old deficit.[225] Another study reported a fourfold increase in the risk of stroke in patients with prior strokes.[226] Notably, a significant percentage of patients without known clinical strokes (ranging from 4.5 to 54% in various series) have preoperative evidence of silent cerebral infarctions on diffusion-weighted imaging (DWI) MRI scans, which tends to correlate with the occurrence of postoperative strokes.[227–231] These patients tend to be older, have preoperative cognitive impairment, ascending aortic atherosclerosis, and intracranial arterial stenosis.

- Cerebrovascular disease, including intracranial and extracranial cerebral artery disease, in addition to carotid disease.[232] One study found that bilateral carotid disease of any grade increased the risk of stroke.[233]

- Female gender

- Comorbidities, including diabetes, smoking, hypertension, PVD, and renal dysfunction

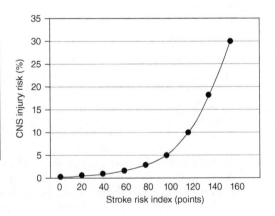

Risk Factors	Weighted Score
Age (years)	(Age-25) × 10/7
Unstable angina	14
Diabetes mellitus	17
Prior stroke/TIA	18
Prior CABG	15
PVD or CVD	18
Pulmonary disease	15

The risk of stroke starts rising exponentially with a score >80.

Figure 13.4 • Risk Model for Neurologic Injury After Cardiac Surgery. (Reproduced with permission from Newman et al., *Lancet* 2006;368:694–703.)[220]

- Atrial fibrillation
- Low ejection fraction or HF; recent MI
- Reoperative surgery[233]
- Urgent/emergent surgery
- Valvular surgery

b. **Intraoperative/postoperative findings/events**
- Ascending aortic and arch atherosclerosis and calcification[234,235]
- Long duration of CPB (>2 hours)
- High transfusion requirement
- Left ventricular mural thrombus
- Opening of a cardiac chamber during surgery with possible air embolization
- Perioperative hypotension or cardiac arrest
- Postoperative AF

2. **Mechanisms[220,236]**

a. Thromboembolic strokes account for about two-thirds of strokes encountered after surgery, usually arise from the aorta, and most commonly affect the right hemiphere.[221,237] Aortic manipulation and/or arch disease commonly account for the development of stroke, and minimizing aortic manipulation can reduce that risk.[238,239] Transcranial Doppler studies have suggested an association between cerebral complications and the number of microemboli detected during surgery.[240] However, despite demonstration that about 45% of patients will have new cerebral infarctions on postoperative DWI, which would be consistent with microembolization, overt manifestations of stroke are not that common.[231,241] Embolic sources may be from:
- Atherosclerotic aorta (during cannulation, cross-clamping or unclamping, application of a sideclamp for proximal anastomoses)
- Solid (lipid) or gaseous microembolism debris from the extracorporeal circuit, which is more significant in patients in whom cardiotomy suction is utilized
- Air embolism from the left heart
- Left atrial or left ventricular thrombus (AF is the most common cause of "delayed" stroke)
- Platelet-fibrin debris from carotid ulcerations
- Multiple blood and blood component transfusions

b. Cerebral hypoperfusion may result from systemic hypotension or impaired cerebral flow from intra- or extracranial carotid disease.
- Systemic hypotension is common during CPB, although cerebral autoregulation can maintain cerebral blood flow down to a mean pressure of 40 mm Hg. This compensatory mechanism is usually inoperative in diabetic, hypertensive patients, and may be impaired by cerebral microembolization.[242] The blood pressure should be maintained at a higher level in these patients to provide adequate cerebral flow independent of the systemic flow rate.[243]

One study showed a fourfold greater incidence of watershed infarcts when there was a 10 mm Hg decrease in intraoperative mean blood pressure compared with preoperative levels.[244]

- The blood pressure may be compromised during off-pump surgery with manipulation of the heart, and is usually reduced pharmacologically during construction of proximal anastomoses when a sideclamp is placed on the ascending aorta.

- Although stroke is more common in patients with symptomatic carotid disease, it is also higher in patients with asymptomatic high-grade unilateral or bilateral disease.[233] Thus, the potential exists in these patients for cerebral hypoperfusion during an episode of perioperative hypotension resulting in a watershed infarct. One study showed that there was a 3.8% risk of stroke after an isolated CABG in asymptomatic patients with 50–99% unilateral disease and a 6.5% risk in patients with bilateral 50–99% lesions.[245]

- Cerebral hypoxemia from a low HCT during CPB may be associated with an increased risk of stroke. One study showed that the risk of stroke increased 10% for every percentage point decrease in HCT, particularly once the HCT was below 21%.[246]

c. Although risk factors may vary depending on when the stroke occurs, cerebral embolization appears to be the dominant mechanism. Consistent with this hypothesis is a study in which postoperative scanning revealed that 77% of patients had large territory embolic infarcts, 16% were watershed, and 7% had a mixed pattern.[247]

3. **Presentation.** The percentage of "early strokes" (noted upon emergence from anesthesia) vs. "delayed strokes" (occurring after a period of normal neurologic recovery) varies in different studies, some indicating that early strokes are more common[248] and some that delayed strokes are more common,[249,250] with a meta-analysis finding there was an equal distribution.[251] Although the clinical presentation depends primarily on the site and extent of the cerebral infarction, the prognosis is better for patients suffering delayed strokes.[248–251] The risk factors also tend to differ depending on the time of occurrence of stroke: early strokes are more common in patients with prior stroke, aortic atherosclerosis, and a long duration of bypass.[248] Delayed strokes are often noted in patients developing AF as well as in those with known cerebrovascular disease and low cardiac output states.[248] However, one study found that AF was a risk factor for delayed stroke only if accompanied by a low cardiac output state.[249]

a. A significant percentage of patients develop silent brain injury during surgery with new DWI MRI abnormalities noted in 25–50% of patients.[231,252] In fact, following TAVR, MRI scans show new "asymptomatic" abnormalities in 77.5–90% of patients![253,254]

b. Focal deficits most commonly produce hemiparesis/hemiplegia, aphasia, or dysarthria. Visual deficits may occur as the result of retinal embolization, occipital lobe infarction, or anterior ischemic optic neuropathy.[255] The latter is more common in patients with long pump runs with extreme hemodilution. One study found that posterior strokes involving the posterior cerebral artery and cerebellum were the most common location, although embolization to the middle cerebral artery (MCA) was also encountered in about 50% of patients since multiple emboli were commonly noted.[256] Another found that the distributions of the MCA and anterior cerebral artery were the most common locations.[221]

   c. TIAs or reversible neurologic deficits (RNDs)

   d. Dysphagia with risk for aspiration

   e. Severe confusion or delirium

4. **Prevention** of neurologic complications requires the identification and appropriate management of potential precipitating factors in the pre-, intra-, and postoperative periods.

   a. Preoperative **evaluation for extracranial carotid disease** should be considered in any patient with current or remote neurologic symptoms or the presence of a carotid bruit. Some centers do this routinely and others do this selectively, with no evidence that neurologic outcomes differ. Noninvasive studies followed by magnetic resonance angiography (MRA), if indicated, may identify significant carotid disease. One study found that the presence of intracranial and extracranial cerebral artery disease detected by MRA was more predictive of stroke risk than extracranial carotid disease.[233]

     i. The approach to symptomatic carotid disease invariably entails either a preliminary carotid endarterectomy (CEA) or stenting or a simultaneous CABG-CEA procedure.[257]

     ii. For patients with asymptomatic carotid disease, management is more controversial. With the hypothesis that hypoperfusion might occur during a period of hypotension during or after coming off CPB when significant carotid disease is present, a concomitant operation is often performed for unilateral carotid disease >80–90% or bilateral high-grade disease or contralateral occlusion (a class IIa indication).[106] Performing a preliminary carotid procedure or simultaneous procedure appears to lower the risk of stroke with comparable results for either approach.[258]

   b. Perioperative use of aspirin has been shown to reduce the risk of stroke by 50%.[259]

   c. Preoperative use of statins may lower not only the risk of stroke but also the risk of delirium.[260,261]

   d. Intraoperative epiaortic echocardiography can be used to identify aortic atherosclerosis that might alter cannulation and clamping techniques to prevent manipulation of a diseased ascending aorta.[262,263] If not used routinely, it should be considered in patients with other markers for aortic atherosclerosis, such as hypertension, PVD, cerebrovascular disease, CKD, and COPD, or when increased thickness of the descending aorta is noted by TEE.[264]

   e. Optimize blood pressure during CPB. Studies have shown that maintaining a mean pressure >80 mm Hg rather than in the 50–60 mm Hg range will reduce neurologic complications.[243]

f. Use of cerebral oximetry may identify a significant decrease in regional cerebral oxygenation that can be improved by various maneuvers, such as maintaining a higher mean arterial pressure during CPB, raising the PCO_2 to increase cerebral blood flow, or transfusing for a profound anemia. Theoretically, these interventions should be able to reduce the incidence of neurologic impairment, especially watershed infarcts caused by low flow.[265–267] Some studies have noted that impaired autoregulation of cerebral blood flow was present in 20% of patients and the amount of time below the lower limit of autoregulation correlated with perioperative neurologic morbidity.[268,269]

g. Minimize aortic manipulation during surgery.[238,239] For on-pump bypass surgery, use of single aortic cross-clamping for construction of both distal and proximal anastomoses, rather than application of a sideclamp for the latter, may reduce the incidence of stroke.[270] For off-pump surgery, use of a proximal anastomotic occluder, such as the Heartstring device (MAQUET) to avoid aortic side-clamping, or avoidance of cross-clamping altogether with use of the ITAs as inflow vessels may be beneficial. In patients with severe aortic calcification requiring CPB, circulatory arrest may be indicated to avoid aortic cross-clamping.

h. Avoidance of hyperglycemia may reduce the risk of neurocognitive dysfunction, especially in nondiabetics.[271] However, excessively strict glucose control may actually increase the risk of stroke.[272]

i. Avoid systemic (and inferentially cerebral) hyperthermia during rewarming, which is associated with a higher risk of stroke and neurocognitive deficits.[273]

j. Maintain a satisfactory HCT on pump. Most studies suggest using a lower limit of 20% since lower levels have been linked to stroke and neurocognitive dysfunction.[274] However, the STS guidelines only recommend transfusions for a Hb <6 g/dL (HCT <18%) unless the patient is at increased risk for decreased cerebral oxygen delivery, such as patients with diabetes, older age, known cerebrovascular disease, or myocardial dysfunction, or considered at risk for end-organ ischemia.[88] However, this includes a large proportion of patients undergoing cardiac surgery.

k. Particulate emboli can be captured by use of the Embol-X intra-aortic filter (Edwards Lifesciences) that is deployed at the time of unclamping and used until the patient is off bypass.

l. Flooding of the operative field with carbon dioxide to evacuate air, especially during valve cases, may reduce the incidence of neurologic impairment.[275]

m. Pharmacologic prevention of AF and initiating anticoagulation when it occurs may reduce the risk of delayed stroke.[223,248,276] Anticoagulation is usually started after 48 hours of continuous AF or for recurrent episodes of AF. Consideration should be given to ligating the left atrial appendage in all patients undergoing surgery with preoperative AF, even if a Maze procedure is not performed. Whether this should be done routinely because of the 25% overall incidence of postoperative AF is debatable.

n. Routine MRI scanning following TAVR has shown new cerebral infarcts in up to 90% of patients.[253,254] However, although cerebral protection devices have been reported to trap debris in 99% of patients,[277] they have not been shown to reduce the total number of new ischemic lesions, despite a slight reduction in new lesion volume, and have not shown any impact on the risk of clinical stroke or neurocognitive changes.[278] Nonetheless, these devices might be considered in patients in whom there is more calcific burden, such as patients undergoing valve-in-valve procedures for prosthetic valve stenosis.

5. **Evaluation** of neurologic deficits requires an assessment of the degree of functional impairment by careful neurologic examination and identification of the anatomic extent of cerebral infarction by CT or DWI MRI scanning. Scanning is most important in assessing whether hemorrhage is present or not, since up to 30% of infarctions may develop hemorrhagic conversion that will contraindicate use of heparin.[247] In nearly 70% of patients with focal deficits, the initial CT scan will not show evidence of an infarction, although abnormalities will usually be evident on subsequent scans.[279] Ideally, a DWI MRI should be obtained because it is more sensitive than CT scanning in identifying ischemic changes, watershed infarcts, or multiple embolic infarcts. However, this procedure can be difficult to obtain in a critically ill patient on a ventilator and multiple infusion pumps. Furthermore, it is important to analyze whether the findings are consistent with an acute perioperative infarct or were preexistent, since preoperative MRI scans are usually not obtained, yet are abnormal in up to 50% of patients.[231] Evaluation should also be undertaken to search for a possible source of the stroke that might require additional attention (echocardiogram, carotid noninvasive studies).

6. **Treatment**
   a. The use of heparin in patients suffering an embolic stroke is controversial. It is recommended for patients with AF, possible valve thrombus, or other sources of intracardiac thrombus, but has unclear benefit in preventing further aortic atheroembolism. It might improve cerebral microcirculatory flow, but the possibility of subsequent hemorrhage into an infarct zone must always be taken into consideration. Some neurologists feel that heparin should be withheld for at least 72 hours to minimize the risk of hemorrhagic conversion.
   b. Use of a clot retrieval device may be considered within 6–8 hours of the development of an ischemic stroke.
   c. Standard measures to reduce intracranial pressure, including diuresis, mannitol, and steroids, may be indicated depending on the extent of cerebral infarction.
   d. A CEA may be considered in patients with severe carotid stenosis and postoperative transient neurologic deficits or small strokes.
   e. Early institution of physical therapy is important.

7. **Prognosis** is favorable for patients with small or temporary deficits, but the operative mortality rate for patients suffering permanent strokes is around 20%.[221,224,280] The outlook for comatose patients is extremely poor, with over 50% dying or remaining in a vegetative state. Five-year survival following a postoperative stroke is only about 50–60%, with most patients continuing to manifest moderate–severe disability.[224,280–282] With such a dismal prognosis, any steps that can possibly be taken to reduce the occurence of stroke must be entertained.

B. **Encephalopathy and delirium** represent an acute change in the patient's mental status that is associated with global impairment of cognitive function.

1. Several risk factors and contributory clinical scenarios for delirium have been identified, and risk models have been developed to predict its occurrence.[283–287] However,

the etiology and pathophysiology are not always clear. The presence of both preexisting and new postoperative cerebral infarcts on MRI are independent risk factors for postoperative delirium, so underlying cerebral damage may leave the brain susceptible to an additional insult from surgery, whether it be microembolization or mild degrees of cerebral hypoperfusion.[286–288] However, some studies suggest that there is no correlation of microembolization with the occurrence of delirium.[289] Therefore, it has been suggested that neuroinflammation associated with the systemic inflammatory response, endothelial dysfunction, and disruption of the blood–brain barrier associated with use of CPB may be the underlying mechanism.[290] However, although some studies have suggested that there is a slightly lower incidence of delirium after OPCABs,[291] others have not found any difference.[286] In general, it appears that various medications and metabolic and clinical issues that prolong the ICU stay are responsible for precipitating delirium in patients with predisposing risk factors.

2. **Predisposing risk factors**[236,285,286,292–296]

    a. Older age (estimated at >20% in patients >age 65 and >30% in patients >age 80)[293]

    b. Recent use of alcohol, opiates, benzodiazepines, or preoperative antipsychotics

    c. Preoperative organic brain diseases

        i. Neurologic diseases: prior stroke, Parkinson's disease, Alzheimer's disease, and other forms of dementia

        ii. Psychiatric disorders: depression, schizophrenia

        iii. Impaired executive or cognitive function with low mini-mental scores[294]

    d. Severe cardiac disease and high-risk status at the time of surgery (cardiogenic shock, urgent status, severe LV dysfunction)

    e. Associated medical problems including AF, smoking, diabetes, cerebrovascular disease, PVD, CKD, and poor nutritional status (low albumin)

    f. Complex and prolonged surgical procedures on CPB

3. **Precipitating factors**

    a. Abnormalities during CPB: low flow rates, low blood pressure, low HCT, low cerebral saturations by cerebral oximetry

    b. Medications: benzodiazepines, propofol, and analgesics[292]

    c. ICU issues: sleep deprivation, too much light at night, physical restraints

    d. Metabolic disturbances

    e. Alcohol withdrawal

    f. Multiple blood transfusions

    g. Postoperative adverse events: low cardiac output, AKI, hypoxia and prolonged ventilation, and stroke

    h. Infections, with or without sepsis

4. **Manifestations**[296]

    a. Hyperactive delirium is manifested by agitation and restlessness.

    b. Hypoactive delirium is associated with lethargy, flat affect, or decreased responsiveness.

    c. Disorientation, confusion, attention deficit, memory loss, disturbed sleep/wake cycle

    d. Paranoia and hallucinations

5. **Evaluation.** Various models have been devised to identify delirium and can be used to ascertain when interventions may be indicated.

   a. The Confusion Assessment Method (CAM-ICU) includes four features required to diagnose delirium: the acute onset of changes or fluctuations in the course of mental status, inattention, and either disorganized thinking or altered level of consciousness.[297]

   b. The Intensive Care Delirium Screening Checklist (ICDSC) includes eight items: altered level of consciousness, inattention, disorientation, hallucinations or delusions, psychomotor agitation or retardation, inappropriate mood or speech, sleep/wake cycle disturbance, and symptom fluctuation. Most patients with delirium have at least four of these features.[298]

   c. Review current medications and drug levels.

   d. Identify possible history of recent alcoholism or substance abuse.

   e. Neurologic examination and brain CT or MRI.

6. **Management**[296,299]

   a. Use soft restraints and keep siderails up to prevent falls out of bed.

   b. Avoid sleep deprivation, encourage early mobilization, use daily interruptions of sedation if on a ventilator.

   c. Correct metabolic abnormalities.

   d. Stop inappropriate medications. Try to avoid benzodiazepines and opiates, which can cause delirium, and if delirium is present, they can exacerbate confusion and produce agitation and stupor, especially in elderly patients. Olanzapine (Zyprexa), a thieno-benzodiazepine, is considered an atypical antipsychotic which has been used successfully in delirious critically ill patients and has been associated with fewer side effects than haloperidol.[300]

   e. Carefully select sedative medications in the ICU to minimize the risk of delirium. Dexmedetomidine is associated with less postoperative delirium than propofol or midazolam when used for immediate postoperative sedation.[301,302] It is also more effective than haloperidol in controlling the agitated, delirious, intubated patient, allowing for earlier extubation.[303]

   f. Select the appropriate medication to control agitation and the delirious state. Generally, most of these medications have equal efficacy, but side effects vary.[304–306]

      i. Haloperidol 2.5–5.0 mg PO/IM/IV q6h is the most commonly prescribed medication for delirium. One should always be aware of the risk of QT prolongation and torsades de pointes in patients receiving IV haloperidol.[307] It can cause extrapyramidal side effects, which may occur within 48 hours of starting the medication.

      ii. Ondansetron (Zofran) is a 5-HT$_3$-receptor antagonist that counteracts activation of the serotoninergic system. It is primarily indicated for the control of postoperative nausea, but is also successful in treating postcardiotomy delirium without major side effects. It is given in a dose of 4–8 mg IV or PO. One study showed equal efficacy to use of haloperidol for treatment of postcardiotomy delirium.[308] A similar medication dolasetron (Anzemet) 12.5–25 mg IV can also be used.

    iii. Several atypical antipsychotics are also beneficial in managing delirium.[304–307]

- Risperidone (0.5 mg PO twice a day) acts by antagonizing dopamine D2 and serotonin 5-HT$_2$ receptors. It is generally well tolerated, but may be associated with extrapyramidal effects. One study showed that administration of 1 mg of risperidone upon regaining consciousness reduced the incidence of delirium by 67%.[309] Another showed that early treatment with risperidone for subsyndromal delirium (a CAM-ICU score positive for 2/4 features or an ICDSC score of 1–3 out of 8) significantly reduced the risk of frank delirium.[310]

- Olanzapine starting at 2.5 mg daily and increasing to 10 mg daily provides comparable benefits to haloperidol, although it is more sedating.[300]

- Quetiapine (Seroquel) using a starting dose of 12.5 mg daily produces even more sedation and can cause hypotension as well as QT prolongation.

  g. Treat suspected alcohol withdrawal[311]

    i. The Clinical Institute Withdrawal Assessment (CIWA) score can be used in assessing the degree of withdrawal. Pharmacologic treatment is indicated for a CIWA score >10.

    ii. Benzodiazepines (lorazepam, diazepam, or chlordiazepoxide) may need to be given for a few days, during which time the patient may require a few additional days of ventilatory support or may require reintubation while being sedated.

    iii. Thiamine 50–100 mg IM/PO bid and folate 1 mg PO qd

    iv. Psychotherapy: reassurance and support

7. Outcomes. Delirium is associated with more postoperative complications, longer ICU stays, increased perioperative mortality, more hospital readmissions, and reduced quality of life. It contributes to cognitive dysfunction, including impaired attention span, memory, perception, and motor function that may persist for up to one year or even longer. It is also associated with greater functional impairment, reducing independence in activities of daily living and affecting mobility for at least six months. It may also increase the long-term risk of death and stroke.[312–315]

C. Neurocognitive dysfunction (NCD) is manifested by problems with memory and executive and cognitive function and is a fairly common complication of cardiac surgery. Depending on the timing and extent of neuropsychiatric testing, the incidence has been reported to be as high as 63%.[316–318] Numerous studies have found that off-pump surgery does not reduce the risk of early or late NCD,[319–322] despite one meta-analysis suggesting it does.[323] In fact, the rate of cognitive decline or impairment in memory after six years appears to be no different in coronary artery disease patients managed medically or surgically.[324–326] Thus, the development of progressive NCD after surgery is probably more related to the patient's baseline cognitive function and comorbidities than to specific precipitating factors postoperatively.

1. Predisposing factors

  a. Risk factors include older age, diabetes, hypertension, preexisting cerebrovascular disease, chronic disabling neurologic illnesses, and lack of social support.[327] Noncoronary atherosclerosis may be a risk factor, but aortic atheroma burden has not been consistently found to be associated with cognitive dysfunction.[328,329]

b. Numerous studies have addressed the relationship between preexisting cognitive abnormalities or abnormal MRI scans and the development of postoperative cognitive decline.

   i. Preoperative cognitive abnormalities have been noted in up to 45% of patients undergoing CABG.[330,331] Patients with less cognitive reserve, dementia, or anxiety/depression are inclined to experience more disabling cognitive dysfunction.

   ii. Although NCD may occur in the absence of demonstrable ischemic lesions on DWI, the presence of pre- or postoperative cerebral infarction, whether symptomatic or not, is likely to be associated with neurocognitive decline. It is estimated that up to 50% of patients have preexisting silent cerebral infarcts and 25–50% develop new postoperative infarcts.[227–230,252,331–333] Although most new infarcts are silent,[252,332] some studies suggest that virtually all patients with abnormal MRIs have evidence of NCD.[317] One study found that two-thirds of patients with multiple cerebral infarctions were asymptomatic, but 25% did develop cognitive decline.[228] Another found that early NCD, but not new ischemic brain lesions, was predictive of late NCD.[333]

2. **Mechanisms** for early and late postoperative cognitive decline appear to be different. Early decline may be related to cerebral microembolization, hypoperfusion, or the systemic inflammatory response to CPB, and may be reversible. Late decline is most likely related to preexisting cerebrovascular disease.[331]

   a. Cerebral microembolization is often thought to be the cause of cognitive decline, but the fairly comparable incidence of NCD with on- and off-pump surgery (despite more embolization during on-pump surgery) and lack of strong evidence correlating embolization and cognitive decline call this hypothesis into question.[335–338] The correlation between aortic atherosclerosis and NCD is also controversial, in contrast to the clear association of atherosclerosis with the occurrence of perioperative stroke. One study did show a slight reduction in early NCD with use of a cell-saving device to reduce lipid embolization, but this benefit was not evident at one year, suggesting that progressive cerebrovascular disease was responsible for late NCD.[339]

   b. Cerebral hypoperfusion is often considered the mechanism causing encephalopathy, delirium, and NCD. This may result from perioperative hypotension, either due to low pressures on CPB or soon thereafter, and may be incriminated if there is a significant or prolonged decrease in cerebral oxygen saturation noted by cerebral oximetry during CPB.[267]

   c. The systemic inflammatory response syndrome (SIRS) may be a contributory factor to neurologic injury, although not a causative mechanism.

   d. Intraoperative hyperglycemia and hyperthermia during rewarming have been associated with NCD.[271,273]

3. **Presentation**

   a. Neurocognitive abnormalities include a deterioration in intellectual function and impaired memory. Forgetfulness, problems with word finding, altered attention span, reduction in psychomotor function, and impaired visual and verbal memory may be present.

   b. In some patients, the degree of cognitive dysfunction is immediately obvious; in others, it can only be detected by a comparison of pre- and postoperative studies.

4. **Prevention.** Steps to reduce cerebral embolization and maintenance of a higher perfusion pressure during surgery may be helpful in patients at high risk. Other recommended strategies include α-stat pH regulation during profound hypothermia cases (see page 302), control of intraoperative glucose levels, and avoidance of cerebral hyperthermia during rewarming. Cerebral oximetry may be useful in identifying cerebral desaturation that has been associated with watershed infarcts, but it has not been shown conclusively to predict the occurrence of cognitive dysfunction.[266]

5. **Evaluation.** MRI scanning often shows multiple infarctions, although such findings are also commonly seen in patients who are asymptomatic and may have been present preoperatively. Brain SPECT studies have shown worse cerebral perfusion at baseline and during surgery in patients with cognitive decline after surgery.

6. **Natural history.** The duration of cognitive decline varies in numerous studies. One seminal study of CABG patients reported that 53% of patients had cognitive decline at hospital discharge, which decreased to 24% at six months but then increased to 42% at five years.[316] Most studies conclude that cognitive function improves from the time of hospital discharge up to one year, and then remains relatively stable or slightly worse during subsequent follow-up.[340] The fact that long-term cognitive function was similar in patients with coronary disease managed surgically or medically suggests that the late decline is most likely due to the presence of poorly controlled risk factors for cerebrovascular disease, including hypertension and diabetes.[324-326]

D. **Psychiatric problems** are fairly common in patients undergoing open-heart surgery. Anxiety and depression occur frequently in patients with known psychiatric disorders, but are also noted in patients who have lost family members due to heart disease. The occurrence of these symptoms after surgery is associated with an unfavorable outcome, including early and late mortality.[341-343] Exacerbation of preexisting disorders, including depression, bipolar disorder, and personality disorders, is also not unusual. A psychiatrist with an interest in postoperative problems is invaluable in helping patients resolve distressing psychiatric symptoms and in providing advice on the appropriate use of psychotropic medications. Cognitive behavioral therapy and stress management support are helpful in alleviating postoperative depression.[344]

E. **Seizures** may accompany cerebral insults from hypoxia, or air and particulate emboli. However, they can also result from medication overdoses (e.g. lidocaine). Contributing factors should be addressed and the patient evaluated by a neurologist. A CT or MRI scan, EEG, or anticonvulsant therapy should be considered upon advice from a neurologist.

F. **Critical illness polyneuropathy** is a syndrome of unknown etiology that complicates the course of sepsis and multisystem organ failure, and is associated with prolonged ventilation, longer ICU stays, and an increased mortality rate that approaches 50%. It usually presents as failure to wean from the ventilator due to weakness of the diaphragm and chest wall muscles. Axonal degeneration of motor and sensory fibers is the underlying pathologic process and is manifested by proximal muscle atrophy and paresis, decreased deep tendon reflexes, and, in some cases, by laryngeal and pharyngeal weakness, producing swallowing difficulties. It may produce motor and sensory deficits and can be diagnosed by electromyography and nerve conduction studies. The syndrome is self-limited and is managed by supportive care (ventilatory support and physical therapy), early mobilization, intensive insulin therapy to control hyperglycemia, and avoidance of neuromuscular blockers and steroids. About half of the patients developing this problem recover completely, but it may take 1–3 months to do so. It must be distinguished from other causes of postoperative muscle weakness, such as medications, nutritional deficiency, disuse atrophy, and other neuromuscular disorders.[345,346]

G. **Brachial plexus injuries**

1. **Etiology and prevention.** Stretch of the inferior cords of the brachial plexus by lateral sternal retraction or asymmetric elevation during ITA harvesting with compression of the brachial plexus between the clavicle and first rib is the most common cause of this injury.[347–349] The incidence may be minimized by cautious and limited asymmetric retraction for ITA takedown, ensuring a midline sternotomy, caudad placement of the retractor, opening it only as much as necessary for adequate exposure, and maintaining a neutral head position.[11] The incidence may also be lessened by positioning the patient in the "hands up" position. Despite taking all of these precautions, a small number of patients will still develop a brachial plexus stretch injury, most likely related to their individual chest wall architecture. Routine electrophysiologic studies identify abnormalities in upwards of 20% of patients, although most patients are asymptomatic.[350] First rib fractures are often noted by bone scan, although they are frequently missed by routine chest x-rays.

2. **Presentation.** Sensory changes, including numbness, paresthesia, and occasionally sharp pains as well as weakness are common in the ulnar nerve distribution (T8–T1), which commonly affects the fourth and fifth fingers. Weakness of the interosseous muscles may also be noted. In more extreme forms, the median or radial nerve distribution may be involved. Radial nerve deficits are more likely to be caused by direct arm compression from retraction bars used for the ITA takedown or from positioning issues.

3. **Evaluation.** Electromyography, motor and sensory conduction velocities, and somatosensory-evoked potentials can be used to assess changes in nerve function, but their significance is not clear. They may be useful in assessing the extent of the deficit and the return of function.

4. **Treatment.** Symptoms resolve in more than 95% of patients within a few months. Rarely, recovery may take up to a year, and some patients may have persistent, bothersome symptoms. Physical therapy is essential to maintain motor tone. If the patient has significant pain, amitriptyline (Elavil) 10–25 mg qhs, gabapentin (Neurontin) starting at 300 mg qd, or carbamazepine (Tegretol) 50–100 mg qid may be helpful.

H. **Paraplegia** is a very rare complication of open-heart surgery caused by spinal cord infarction. It is most common after thoracoabdominal surgery or extensive endovascular stenting. It may also result from an aortic dissection or as a complication of an IABP, presumably on the basis of atherosclerotic plaque shift or rupture, or cholesterol embolism to the spinal cord. There are rare case reports of paraplegia occurring after isolated CABGs, usually caused by a period of hypotension in a patient with preexisting hypertension and severe vascular disease that compromises spinal cord perfusion.[351–353] There is one case report of embolization to bilateral anterior cerebral arteries causing paraplegia.[354]

I. **Common peroneal or sciatic/tibial nerve palsies** are rare complications of surgery that usually have no identifiable contributing factor. Common peroneal nerve injuries cause weakness and sensory changes over the lateral lower leg and foot, whereas tibial nerve problems affect the posterior calf and dorsum of the foot. Direct nerve injury is impossible during vein harvesting, so the suspected mechanism is ischemia caused by direct pressure on the nerves with leg positioning. Older patients with diabetes, PVD, and subnormal body weight with atrophic tissues may be more predisposed to this problem, which is more likely to occur during longer operations involving CPB. However, in most cases, this complication is an unpredictable and unpreventable event. Fortunately, most patients recover satisfactory sensorimotor function and are not limited in their activities.[355]

J. **Compartment syndrome (CS)** may develop following periods of prolonged compromised blood flow to the lower extremities. It may rarely affect the thigh musculature.

1. **Mechanism.** A compartment syndrome develops when the interstitial tissue tension within a confined compartment exceeds the pressure in the microcirculation, resulting in tissue ischemia. A prolonged period of ischemia followed by reperfusion results in cell membrane damage with fluid leakage into the interstitial compartment, which initially compromises the blood supply to nerve tissue and eventually will compress major blood vessels, causing loss of pulses. Thus, loss of pulses is one of the last manifestations of a compartment syndrome, at which time tissue loss has already occurred.

2. **Predisposing factors.** CS is rarely encountered with use of an IABP, most likely because of vigilant attention to leg edema and distal perfusion and the absence of a documented period of prolonged severe leg ischemia. However, CS has been noted in patients requiring prolonged groin cannulation (usually >4–6 hours) for CPB (aortic surgery, minimally invasive or robotic surgery) or for prolonged ECMO support. There are case reports of its occurrence after CABG, following both open and endoscopic vein harvesting.[356–360] With the latter technique, the proposed mechanism is retraction of divided venous or arterial branches, which then bleed into the muscle.

3. **Prevention.** CS can be prevented by using alternative methods of groin cannulation that allow for distal perfusion (sewing a graft to the femoral artery or proximal and distal cannulation).[361,362] However, these are rarely done, because the anticipated duration of CPB may be unpredictable, usually being lengthened when there are technical problems during the surgical procedure. Although placing a femoral arterial cannula via the Seldinger technique avoids the placement of a distal snare, distal flow is quite limited by the size of the cannula and by vasoconstriction during periods of hypothermia during surgery. Distal perfusion with a small cannula or side-arm sheath must be assured when a longer duration of femoral perfusion (such as with femoral cannulation for ECMO) is anticipated. Obtaining adequate hemostasis during endoscopic vein harvesting should avoid development of a CS after CABG.

4. **Monitoring and treatment.** Any patient with a prolonged period of groin cannulation requires careful assessment for the development of a CS. Because patients are anesthetized and sedated for a number of hours, they are unable to complain of severe leg pain, which is one of the first manifestations of a compartment syndrome. Assessment of calf diameter and palpation for tenseness and tenderness, if

possible, are essential. Comparison with the contralateral leg may be beneficial, although less helpful if vein harvesting has been performed. If there is any doubt, obtaining a compartment pressure with a needle attached to a manometer is helpful. A pressure greater than 35 mm Hg or within 20 mm of the diastolic pressure is generally consistent with a compartment syndrome. If suspected, the patient should be returned to the operating room for a four-compartment fasciotomy. The wound can be closed several days later if muscle tissue is still viable once the edema resolves. The muscle becomes nonviable from inside to out, so the superficial muscle may bleed despite ongoing necrosis of deeper muscle, and careful reassessment is important.

5. A compartment syndrome involving the hand and forearm may occur after endoscopic radial artery harvesting, but is more common when there has been inadvertent infiltration of an intravenous line through which large volumes of fluid, especially blood, are given. This is often not recognized until the drapes have been removed, but is immediately obvious because the forearm and hand are pale, mottled, tense, and massively swollen. Removal of the arterial line from that side and an immediate fasciotomy are indicated.[363,364]

K. **Saphenous neuropathy** is caused by damage to small branches of the saphenous nerve that lies adjacent to the saphenous vein in the lower leg.[11,348] This causes sensory changes along the medial side of the calf and foot to the level of the great toe. It is fairly common after open vein harvesting and is more likely with vein harvesting from the ankle up than from the top down. It is proposed that the former is more likely to cause avulsion of the pretibial or infrapatellar branches of the nerve. Neuropathy is also more common when an open incision is closed in two layers, producing neuropraxia from too tight a closure. These symptoms are much less frequent when the vein is harvested endoscopically, but damage to the nerve in the lower leg can still occur.

L. **Forearm neurologic symptoms** following radial artery harvesting are not unusual. In one study comparing open vs. endoscopic harvesting, symptoms occurred in 42% and 64% of patients after open and endoscopic harvesting, respectively. Impaired sensation and paresthesias were more common in the superficial radial nerve distribution with open harvesting, but damage to the lateral antebrachial cutaneous nerve was only seen with open harvests.[365]

M. **Vocal cord paralysis** has been noted in 1–2% of patients after cardiovascular operations and is initially manifested by hoarseness. A number of possible etiologies have been elucidated, but most involve an indirect injury to the recurrent laryngeal nerve producing a reversible neuropraxia.[366,367] A major contributing factor is a longer operation, which is usually associated with a longer period of postoperative intubation. Direct injury may occur during ITA mobilization at the apex of the chest, during central line placement, or during aortic arch surgery. In addition to hoarseness, vocal cord paralysis leads to an ineffective cough, stridor, and the potential for aspiration pneumonia and respiratory failure. Diagnosis can be made by laryngoscopy, which will distinguish it from laryngeal edema. Symptomatic improvement usually occurs within a few months, but if symptoms persist, it is more likely that the injury is permanent. In that situation, vocal cord medialization or thyroplasty may be indicated for unilateral paralysis.

N. **Phrenic nerve palsy.** See pages 749–750.

X. Gastrointestinal Complications

A. Mechanisms and predisposing factors

1. Gastrointestinal (GI) complications develop in approximately 4% of patients undergoing open-heart surgery. Because they frequently occur in critically ill patients, they are often associated with other major adverse postoperative complications, such as low cardiac output syndromes, stroke, and respiratory and renal failure. A US nationwide study of patients undergoing cardiac surgery from 2010–2012 reported a threefold increase in operative mortality (10.8%), with doubling of the length of stay, when GI complications occur.[368]

2. The common pathophysiologic mechanism is sympathetic vasoconstriction, hypoperfusion, and hypoxia of the splanchnic bed.[369–371] This may occur during CPB when there is nonpulsatile flow at low mean pressures with regional redistribution of blood flow away from gut mucosa. However, studies have demonstrated that mesenteric hypoperfusion and gastric mucosal hypoxia are present to a similar extent with OPCAB.[372,373] Postoperative low cardiac output states, hypotension, and use of vasoconstrictors may also result in inadequate tissue perfusion, causing mucosal hypoxia with a reduction in absorptive and barrier functions. This may result in stress ulceration, mucosal atrophy, bacterial overgrowth from stress ulcer prophylaxis, and increased permeability, which in turn may potentially lead to bacterial translocation, the systemic inflammatory response syndrome, sepsis, and multisystem organ failure.[374]

3. Predictive factors for the development of GI complications have been evaluated in multiple studies and include:[375–380]

   a. **Preoperative comorbidities:** older age, CKD, PVD, active smoking, prior GI surgery, use of anticoagulants

   b. **Preoperative cardiac status:** poor LV function or NYHA class IV, preoperative inotropic support, urgent or emergent surgery

   c. **Operative factors:** reoperations, combined valve-CABG cases, long durations of CPB (>120–150 minutes), multiple blood transfusions

   d. **Postoperative issues:** low cardiac output syndrome and hypotension (with use of inotropes, vasoconstrictors, and/or an IABP), bleeding and need for transfusions or re-exploration, use of bicarbonate for a metabolic acidosis, prolonged ventilation, AF, excessive anticoagulation, vascular complications, sepsis, sternal infections

   e. Three of the strongest predictors of GI complications are prolonged mechanical ventilation, AKI, and sepsis, which together contribute to splanchnic hypoperfusion, hypomotility, and mucosal hypoxia.[376]

4. A risk stratification model using a gastrointestinal complication score (GCS) that assessed nine variables has been proposed to predict the risk of developing GI complications (Figure 13.5).[381]

5. **Overall perspective.** The US nationwide survey found that GI complications were statistically more common following off-pump than on-pump CABGs,[368] although other studies concluded that the risk was comparable.[382,383] The risks were higher in patients undergoing valve repair, perhaps related to longer durations of CPB. Paralytic ileus accounted for more than half of the complications

Risk Factors	Score
Age > 80	2.5
Active smoker	2.5
Preoperative inotropes	4.0
NYHA class III–IV	2.0
CPB time >150 minutes	2.5
Postoperative AF	2.5
Postoperative CHF	3.5
Reoperation for bleeding	3.5
Postop vascular complication	9.5

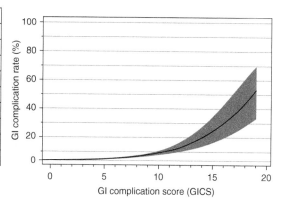

Figure 13.5 • Risk stratification to predict gastrointestinal complications. (Reproduced with permission from Andersson et al., *Interact Cardiovasc Thorac Surg* 2010;10:366–70.)[381]

identified, with no other condition occurring in more than 1% of patients. These included, in descending order of occurrence: GI bleeding, pancreatitis, mesenteric ischemia, bowel obstruction, acute cholecystitis, and intestinal perforation. The mortality rate for any of these conditions was quite high, being 37% for mesenteric ischemia, 32% for intestinal perforation, 18% for GI bleeding, 17% for cholecystitis, and 7% for ileus. Many patients had concomitant conditions that increased the mortality rate, including endocarditis, myocardial infarction, arrhythmias, and COPD. Those who developed GI complications were more prone to develop AKI, AF (which might cause thromboembolic events or require anticoagulation precipitating GI bleeding), or to have sustained a perioperative MI. However, the highest mortalities occurred when the GI complication was associated with shock (31% mortality), a stroke (30%), AKI (21%), or sepsis (20% mortality).

6. Smaller individual studies have shown differing occurrence rates and mortality figures, but all confirm that the development of GI complications, although uncommon, portends high morbidity and mortality.[375–381] Therefore, diligent adherence to common principles of perioperative care is important. These include optimizing the patient's preoperative status, performing an expeditious and complete surgical procedure with good myocardial protection, obtaining careful hemostasis to minimize use of blood transfusions, using sufficient inotropic support for a low cardiac output syndrome, optimizing renal function, achieving early extubation to allow for early mobilization, taking steps to prevent infection, and judiciously anticoagulating the patient when indicated after surgery. Prompt identification and aggressive management are necessary to decrease the mortality associated with GI complications.

B. **Routine care and common complaints.** Most patients have a nasogastric tube inserted in the operating room before heparinization or after its reversal by protamine. This maintains gastric decompression during positive-pressure ventilation, removes gastric contents to minimize the risk of aspiration, decreases gastric acidity, and allows for the administration of oral medications and antacids in the ICU. Sucralfate is often given down the nasogastric tube for initial stress ulcer prophylaxis.[384-386] The tube is usually removed after extubation if bowel sounds are present. An oral diet is then advanced from clear liquids to a regular diet.

1. **Anorexia**, nausea, and a distaste for food are fairly common complaints after surgery and may be attributable to the side effects of medications (narcotics), and possibly to mineral deficiency (especially zinc). However, one must not overlook the possibility of an ileus or other intra-abdominal pathology and should perform a careful physical examination and obtain radiographic studies, if necessary. Bothersome nausea can be treated by a number of medications, which have fairly comparable efficacy.

   a. Metoclopramide (Reglan) 10–20 mg IM qid. This may also stimulate GI motility and decrease the incidence of abdominal distention.

   b. The 5-HT_3 antagonists are powerful antiemetic medications that may be associated with a proarrhythmic effect from QT interval prolongation. The most commonly used medication is ondansetron (Zofran) 4 mg IV.

2. **Pharyngeal dysfunction** with dysphagia and difficulty swallowing liquids or solids has been noted in 1–3% of patients undergoing CABG and can lead to silent or overt aspiration pneumonia.

   a. Predisposing factors include older age, comorbidities (insulin-dependent diabetes, COPD, and renal dysfunction), HF, a history of stroke or new perioperative stroke, or perioperative sepsis.[387-390]

   b. Swallowing dysfunction (dysphagia) and pain with swallowing (odynophagia) are quite common in patients monitored with intraoperative TEE.[390-392] Because TEE is routine in most institutions, one must be alert to this problem in the early postoperative period if the patient has impaired pharyngeal sensation or coughs at the time of initial oral intake. One study found that the risk of dysphagia correlated with the time the probe was in the esophagus. By removing the TEE probe after the initial evaluation and then reinserting it just before weaning from CPB, the risk of dysphagia was reduced from 51 to 29%.[393] Dysphagia has been noted in up to 50% of patients who remain intubated for more than 48 hours, which results in a delay in resumption of oral feeding and a prolongation of the hospital stay.[394] Most hospitals have policies requiring assessment for proper swallowing if the patient is intubated that long.

   c. The occurrence of pharyngeal dysfunction in the absence of common contributing factors (TEE, ventilation) has been ascribed to a new neurologic deficit. Thus, a full neurological evaluation with CT or MRI scanning may be indicated to identify the causative mechanism.

   d. Bedside swallowing tests (usually swallowing 50 mL of water and assessing for a reduction in oxygen saturation by pulse oximetry as well as coughing or choking) can be used as an assessment for aspiration, but they have variable sensitivity in detecting silent aspiration. A modified barium swallow using video fluoroscopy may be indicated before the patient is allowed to eat.[395,396]

e. The management of the patient with pharyngeal dysphagia may include dietary modification, postural adjustments, and working with speech therapists on swallowing maneuvers. Early evaluation of patients with swallowing difficulties by an ENT specialist may identify problems with laryngeal edema or vocal cord paralysis that can be managed to reduce the risk of pneumonia.[397] Persistent dysphagia may require insertion of a feeding tube until satisfactory swallowing can be demonstrated.

3. **Constipation** is a common problem after surgery. Preoperative enemas are usually not given, narcotics are used for analgesia, and elderly patients are often poorly mobilized for several days. Milk of magnesia, bulk laxatives (Metamucil), or stool softeners (Colace) may be helpful in older patients, and rectal suppositories (bisacodyl [Dulcolax]) or enemas may be useful. The possibility of an ileus or bowel obstruction should always be entertained before being too aggressive with medications promoting bowel motility.

C. **Differential diagnosis of acute abdominal pain**

1. **Manifestations.** The presence of an acute intra-abdominal process can be difficult to detect in a critically ill patient in an ICU setting. It is frequently suspected by the presence of fever, an elevation in WBC count, marked tenderness to abdominal palpation, hemodynamic evidence of sepsis, or a positive blood culture. Arriving at the appropriate diagnosis can be even more challenging, but prompt assessment and management are essential because of the high associated mortality.

2. **Etiology**
   - Cholecystitis (acalculous or calculous)
   - Perforated viscus (gastric or duodenal ulceration, diverticulitis)[398]
   - Gastritis
   - Pancreatitis
   - Ischemic bowel (mesenteric ischemia)
   - *C. difficile* colitis
   - Severe paralytic ileus (frequently idiopathic, but occasionally associated with an acute inflammatory process or colitis)
   - Small bowel or colonic obstruction
   - Severe constipation
   - Urinary problems (infection or bladder distention)
   - Retroperitoneal bleeding

3. **Evaluation**
   a. Review of preexisting conditions or prior abdominal surgery
   b. Serial abdominal examinations for tenderness or distention, bowel sounds
   c. Laboratory tests: liver function tests (LFTs), lactic acid, serum amylase and lipase, *C. difficile* titer if diarrhea is present
   d. Radiographic studies
      - KUB (for obstruction or ileus)
      - Semi-upright chest x-ray (for free air under the diaphragm)

- An upper abdominal ultrasound or HIDA scan (if biliary tract obstruction is suspected)
- CT scan of the abdomen with contrast
- Mesenteric arteriography (if mesenteric ischemia is suspected)
- Diagnostic laparoscopy if other tests are unable to provide a diagnosis[399]

4. **Treatment.** General surgery consultation should be obtained from the outset because early exploration may reduce the high mortality associated with the development of GI complications. Laparoscopy is very sensitive in evaluating the nature of the problem, but an exploratory laparotomy may be necessary to further assess and potentially treat the problem. Although many patients with these complications are very ill and often septic, they are usually better able to tolerate exploration after cardiac surgery than they had been before.

D. **Paralytic ileus** occasionally persists for several days after surgery. It is frequently a benign, self-limited problem of unclear etiology and may be more common in diabetics (who may develop gastroparesis), but occasionally may reflect sepsis or a severe intra-abdominal pathologic process. Acute colonic pseudo-obstruction (Ogilvie's syndrome) is a condition of massive colonic dilatation believed to result from autonomic imbalance with either decreased parasympathetic tone or enhanced sympathetic tone. It must be differentiated from mechanical obstruction or toxic megacolon, often related to *C. difficile.*

1. **Contributing factors**
   a. Drugs (catecholamines/cytokine stress response to surgery, opioids, neuromuscular blockade in ventilated patients)
   b. Gastric distention (possibly related to vagal injury)
   c. Congestion of the hepatic or splanchnic bed (from poor venous drainage during surgery or systemic venous hypertension)
   d. Inflammatory processes (e.g. cholecystitis, pancreatitis)
   e. Retroperitoneal bleeding (from groin catheterization, but occasionally spontaneously in an anticoagulated patient)
   f. *C. difficile* colitis
   g. Mesenteric ischemia

2. **Evaluation**
   a. Serial patient examinations for abdominal distention, bowel sounds, and tenderness consistent with an inflammatory process (ischemia or perforation)
   b. Laboratory tests: CBC, amylase, LFTs, *C. difficile* titers if diarrhea
   c. KUB: colonic dilatation to 9 cm is significant, but the risk of perforation increases when the cecal diameter exceeds 12 cm.
   d. CT scan of the abdomen with contrast

3. **Management**
   a. Decompression of the bowel is accomplished by keeping the patient NPO with nasogastric suction. This should prevent gastric distention until peristaltic activity returns. A rectal tube may also be beneficial when colonic distention is marked.
   b. Total parenteral nutrition should be started.

c. Gum chewing may promote bowel motility.[400]

d. Medications that can impair colonic motility must be stopped. These include narcotics, CCBs, and anticholinergic drugs. Although metoclopramide is commonly used to improve GI motility, it has not been shown to be effective in preventing or treating postoperative ileus. Peripheral mu-opioid receptor antagonists (alvimopan and methylnaltrexone) may increase bowel motility in patients treated with narcotics, but they have not been evaluated in the management of ileus after cardiac surgery.[401]

e. All metabolic disturbances must be corrected and therapy directed at any identifiable precipitating problem.

f. Because "pseudo-obstruction" may be caused by a deficiency in cholinergic tone, use of cholinesterase inhibitors may be beneficial in producing rapid colonic decompression. Neostigmine 2 mg IV has proven effective in 90% of patients with this condition, but it is not effective in treating a standard postoperative ileus.[402] Although the initial response to an intermittent bolus or continuous infusion of neostigmine is comparable, a continuous infusion has been noted to give better resolution of colonic dilatation at 24 hours.[403] Side effects include abdominal pain, sialorrhea (excessive salivation), vomiting, and bradycardia. In a patient with recurrent pseudo-obstruction, pyridostigmine 10 mg bid may be beneficial.[404]

g. When colonic distention (>12 cm) persists despite conservative or pharmacologic therapy, decompressive colonoscopy is indicated. If dilatation persists or worsens, urgent surgical intervention, usually by cecostomy or hemicolectomy, is indicated.

h. Abdominal compartment syndrome may develop when there is marked colonic dilatation that produces severe intra-abdominal hypertension (pressure >20 mm Hg). The abdomen is noted to be very tense. This may then produce systemic venous hypertension, impairing splanchnic and renal perfusion, producing hemodynamic and respiratory compromise, and even neurologic symptoms from compression of the inferior vena cava. The release of cytokines, generation of oxygen free radicals, and other factors may lead to bacterial translocation from the gut, interstitial edema, and eventually to multisystem organ failure. If not recognized, it may rapidly lead to progressive metabolic acidosis and death within hours.[405]

E. **Cholecystitis**

1. **Etiology and risk factors.** Cholecystitis is a rare late complication of cardiac surgery with an incidence of 0.1–0.3%. It is noted more commonly in older patients, after surgery requiring prolonged bypass times, and with low cardiac output syndromes requiring inotropes and/or an IABP and continued vasopressor dependence. These risk factors suggest that hypoperfusion is the major mechanism causing cholecystitis, which is more likely to be acalculous than calculous. Other predisposing factors include vascular disease, re-exploration for bleeding or multiple transfusions, prolonged mechanical ventilation, bacteremia, and nosocomial infections. Fasting, parenteral nutrition, and narcotics can decrease gallbladder contractility and produce biliary stasis. If surgery is required because of an inadequate response

to antibiotics, the mortality rate is significant, being 17% in the nationwide survey and 23–43% in three large series.[406–408]

2. **Evaluation**

   a. Serial abdominal examinations may draw attention to an inflammatory process in the right upper quadrant.

   b. LFTs (elevated bilirubin and alkaline phosphatase with minimal change in AST and ALT) may suggest extrahepatic biliary obstruction.

   c. Right upper quadrant ultrasound or HIDA scan can identify a dilated gallbladder and biliary obstruction.

3. **Treatment**

   a. Antibiotic therapy may suffice in patients with acalculous cholecystitis who have no evidence of peritonitis.

   b. If significant clinical improvement does not occur within 24–48 hours, surgical intervention by percutaneous cholecystostomy (especially in critically ill patients) or cholecystectomy (open or laparoscopic) is indicated.

F. **Upper GI bleeding**

1. **Etiology.** Upper GI bleeding is the second most common GI complication after both on- and off-pump surgery with an incidence of 0.5–1%. It usually results from stress ulceration from duodenal ulcers and less commonly from gastric ulcers and esophagogastritis.[409,410] The causative mechanism is usually decreased blood flow, mucosal ischemia, and a hypoperfusion/reperfusion injury that may be exacerbated by increased gastric acidity. A thorough preoperative history and physical examination (stigmata of liver disease, stool guaiac) may identify patients at increased risk of developing postoperative GI bleeding.

2. **Risk factors**

   a. Preoperative: older age, preexisting gastritis or ulcer disease, cirrhosis/portal hypertension/varices, CKD, smoking

   b. Intraoperative: long duration of CPB, valve operations, reoperations, increased lactate level during CPB (suggesting hypoperfusion)

   c. Postoperative: low cardiac output requiring vasopressors, prolonged mechanical ventilation, pulmonary infections, coagulopathy or anticoagulation (antiplatelet agents, heparin preparations, warfarin), blood transfusions

3. **Prophylaxis.** Any patient with a history of ulcer disease or gastritis should receive medications in the ICU to prevent stress-related mucosal damage and, potentially, GI bleeding.[411] In addition, any patient on prolonged ventilatory support, with sepsis, or with a coagulopathy, should receive stress ulcer prophylaxis. Although routine prophylaxis may not be necessary in patients at low risk, there is little downside to initiating a short course of stress prophylaxis routinely during the early postoperative period of intubation when the patient may have a marginal cardiac output, visceral hypoperfusion, and some degree of coagulopathy.[412,413]

   a. Sucralfate 1 g q6h can be given orally or down a nasogastric tube. It does not raise the gastric pH, which will increase gastric bacterial colonization, and thus reduces the incidence of nosocomial pneumonia compared with other medications that raise the gastric pH. However, it has not been shown to reduce the incidence of bleeding or mortality in ICU patients.[385]

   b. Proton pump inhibitors (PPIs) have been shown to be much more effective than histamine H_2 receptor antagonists (H_2 blockers), such as ranitidine, in reducing the incidence of hemorrhagic gastritis and active ulcer formation, although they may increase the risk of pneumonia more than the H$_2$ blockers.[386,413,414] Pantoprazole (Protonix) 40 mg can be given IV or PO, whereas other common preparations, such as omeprazole (Prilosec) 20 mg qd, lansoprazole (Prevacid) 15 mg qd, or rabeprazole (Aciphex) 10 mg qd, can be given orally for prophylaxis. The SUP-ICU study found that use of pantoprazole increased mortality compared with placebo.[415,416] Ranitidine is usually given as an oral dose of 150–300 mg bid.

   c. Patients should be prescribed non-enteric-coated aspirin after CABG or valve surgery because of more antiplatelet efficacy. Studies have not shown that enteric coating reduces the occurrence of GI bleeding or ulceration.[417]

   d. Although clopidogrel may cause fewer GI complications than aspirin in patients with no history of ulceration, either aspirin or clopidogrel (or both) can be used with a PPI if there is a history of a healed ulceration.[418–421]

4. **Manifestations.** Drainage of bright red blood through a nasogastric tube or vomiting of blood is an overt sign of upper GI bleeding. Slow bleeding usually produces melena, but very rapid bleeding may produce bright red bloody stools. Attention should be drawn to potential GI bleeding in the critically ill or heparinized patient with an unexplained fall in HCT or progressive tachycardia or hypotension. If GI bleeding cannot be documented, a retroperitoneal bleed should be entertained as a possible diagnosis and evaluated by an abdominal CT scan.

5. **Evaluation and treatment.** Bleeding that persists despite correction of coagulation abnormalities and intensification of a medical regimen requires further evaluation.[421–423] Bleeding during anticoagulation is commonly associated with some underlying pathology.

   a. It is essential to stop all antiplatelet medications or anticoagulants when there is evidence of GI bleeding, using reversal agents, if necessary, for persistent bleeding. This may entail vitamin K, fresh frozen plasma or prothrombin complex concentrate for high INRs from warfarin (see Figure 13.2 on page 774), or selective antidotes for the NOACs (idarucizumab for dabigatran, recombinant factor Xa for apixaban or rivaroxaban).

   b. PPIs are superior to the H$_2$ blockers in controlling and preventing recurrent bleeding.[421] In the actively bleeding patient, an 80 mg IV bolus of pantoprazole followed by a continuous infusion of 8 mg/h × 72 hours has been recommended, and is able to quickly raise the gastric pH to >6.[422,423] Ranitidine may be given as a 50 mg/h continuous infusion.

   c. Upper GI endoscopy should be performed to identify the site of bleeding and can be used therapeutically with laser bipolar coagulation to control hemorrhage. It can achieve hemostasis in >90% of patients. However, in one series, about 30% of patients required surgery after an initial endoscopic procedure.[424]

   d. Somatostatin 250 μg/h for five days has been shown to be effective in the treatment of severe upper GI bleeding.[425]

   e. Once bleeding is under control, antiplatelet drugs should be restarted when feasible for patients undergoing CABG or valve surgery. Even in patients with a known history of aspirin-induced GI bleeding, resumption of aspirin combined with a PPI is superior to using clopidogrel as an alternative antiplatelet drug.[420] For patients requiring both aspirin and clopidogrel (usually after receiving drug-eluting stents), both can be given safely with a PPI after endoscopic control of a bleeding site. If the patient requires anticoagulation indefinitely following surgery (e.g. for a mechanical prosthetic valve), a definitive procedure must be performed before resuming anticoagulation. The patient should understand that they are at higher thromboembolic risk while the anticoagulation is being held.

6. **Results.** The overall mortality rate for patients developing upper GI bleeding after cardiac surgery is about 15%.[368,424]

G. **Lower GI bleeding** may be manifest by bright-red blood per rectum, blood-streaked stool, or melena, and can usually be differentiated from upper GI bleeding if nasogastric tube drainage is guaiac negative.

1. **Etiology**

   a. Mesenteric ischemia or ischemic colitis caused by periods of prolonged hypoperfusion

   b. Bleeding from colonic lesions (polyps, tumors, diverticular disease) which may be precipitated by anticoagulation

   c. Intestinal angiodysplasia. This is termed "Heyde's syndrome" when associated with aortic stenosis and may be associated with acquired von Willebrand's disease (vWD-IIA). Bleeding usually improves following aortic valve replacement with a tissue valve, but angiodysplasia may persist.[426-428]

   d. Antibiotic-associated colitis (usually *C. difficile*)

2. **Evaluation.** Once an upper GI source has been ruled out, sigmoidoscopy or colonoscopy can be performed. A bleeding scan may identify the bleeding source. Mesenteric arteriography should be considered if bleeding persists.

3. **Treatment** involves correction of any coagulopathy and elimination of precipitating causes.

   a. Antibiotics (vancomycin 125 mg PO qid or fidaxomicin 200 mg twice daily) can be used for *C. difficile* colitis.

   b. Mesenteric angiography with infusion of vasopressin (0.2–0.4 units/min) or selective embolization with microcoils, gelatin sponges, and other particles into the mesenteric arterial branches may be considered.[429-432]

   c. Octreotide (50 μg over 30 minutes) or somatostatin (50 μg bolus followed by an infusion of 250 μg/h) decreases splanchnic blood flow and may be beneficial in patients with GI angiodysplasia.[433]

   d. Surgical intervention is rarely required for persistent bleeding.

H. **Mesenteric ischemia** is a rare (0.2–0.4% incidence) but highly lethal complication of cardiac surgery that is usually noted in elderly patients with generalized atherosclerotic disease. It is often associated with dehydration.

1. **Etiology.** Nonocclusive mesenteric ischemia is the most common etiology, resulting from splanchnic hypoperfusion from a low cardiac output state. This may occur after on- or off-pump surgery, but most commonly after a long pump run.[434,435] Atherosclerotic embolism (usually with use of an IABP) or mesenteric thrombosis (possibly from HIT) occurs less commonly.

2. **Risk factors**[434-438]

   a. Preoperative: older age, poor LV function, more advanced NYHA class, extensive atherosclerosis, CKD

   b. Intraoperative: aortic cross-clamp time >100 minutes

   c. Postoperative: low cardiac output, use of an IABP, inotropic use or use of two or more vasoconstrictor drugs, prolonged mechanical ventilation, AKI, or need for dialysis, blood transfusions, atrial fibrillation

3. **Presentation.** Typical manifestations are a profound ileus or abdominal pain out of proportion to physical findings. The diagnosis can be very difficult to make in the critically ill patient who is frequently ventilated and heavily sedated. Sepsis with hemodynamic instability, lactic acidosis, respiratory distress, GI bleeding, or diarrhea are often present as well. The diagnosis is typically made about 5–10 days after surgery.

4. **Diagnosis** may be suggested by the association of the clinical picture just mentioned with leukocytosis, severe lactic acidosis, and an ileus on KUB or evidence of free abdominal fluid. Endoscopy may be helpful in documenting colonic ischemia. Mesenteric CT angiography may show evidence of pneumatosis intestinalis, venous gas, bowel wall thickening, arterial occlusion, or venous thrombosis.[439] Standard mesenteric arteriography may identify thromboembolism, but most commonly demonstrates vasoconstriction of the peripheral mesenteric vessels. Unfortunately, the diagnosis is frequently made at surgery when irreversible changes have occurred. Early suspicion of mesenteric ischemia, based on a persistent paralytic ileus, absent bowel movements for several days despite laxatives, and a borderline or elevated lactate level may allow for earlier successful intervention with a vasodilator infusion, such as papaverine.[440]

5. **Treatment.** Early diagnosis and treatment are essential to lower the mortality rate of mesenteric ischemia, which was 37% in the US nationwide survey,[368] but in most reports exceeds 65%,[436–438] If mesenteric vasoconstriction is identified, an infusion of papaverine 0.7 mg/kg/h for up to five days may be helpful, especially at an earlier stage of ischemia.[440] When ischemia is prolonged, irreversible intestinal necrosis may occur within hours. Emergency abdominal exploration is indicated if bowel necrosis is suspected. Although a limited bowel resection can be performed, a more likely finding is multiple areas of ischemic bowel that prohibit extensive bowel resection. A second-look operation is indicated if the viability of the bowel is in doubt. The presence of an abdominal compartment syndrome may lead to rapid deterioration of other organ system function and requires emergency exploration.[441]

I. **Diarrhea** developing in a patient in the ICU setting is often an ominous sign because it may result from bowel ischemia caused by a low flow state. However, it is frequently caused by treatable problems including:

1. Antibiotic usage, which can reduce bowel flora and can lead to diarrhea even in the absence of positive titers for *Clostridium difficile*

2. *C. difficile* colitis, which has an overall incidence of 0.8% and is usually, but not always, associated with a prolonged duration of antibiotic therapy. The incidence is similar with use of cephalosporins and fluoroquinolones. *C. difficile* is more common in patients who are older, female, have CKD, and with postoperative acute hyperglycemia. It is also more common in patients taking PPIs and receiving multiple blood products. For a patient with persistent diarrhea or unexplained abdominal pain and a leukocytosis, this diagnosis should be considered, and stool specimens should be sent for *C. difficile* titers. Oral medication may be started immediately upon suspicion of the diagnosis using vancomycin (125 mg PO four times a day) or fidaxomicin (200 mg twice daily) for 10 days for positive titers.[442–444]

3. GI bleeding

4. Intolerance of hyperosmolar tube feedings: dilute with more water and start at a slower infusion rate.

J. **Hepatic dysfunction** manifested by a transient low-grade elevation in LFTs, including ALT, AST, bilirubin, and alkaline phosphatase, is not uncommon after open-heart surgery. About 25% of patients will develop transient hyperbilirubinemia (total bilirubin >3 mg/dL), with a higher incidence noted in patients undergoing valve repair or replacement.[445-447] However, less than 1% of patients will have evidence of significant hepatocellular damage that may progress to chronic hepatitis or liver failure. The elevated bilirubin may be multifactorial, with increased bilirubin production from hemolysis as well as impaired liver function, contributing to both unconjugated and conjugated hyperbilirubinemia.

1. **Predisposing conditions**
   a. Preexisting liver disease. This may be manifest by elevated LFTs, but occasionally will be associated with normal values. However, impaired synthetic function (low serum albumin, high INR) is a marker for hepatic disease. An elevated bilirubin in patients with HF is one of the strongest predictors of the occurrence of postoperative hepatic dysfunction.[448]
   b. Cardiac conditions:
      i. Right-sided HF produces a high right atrial pressure causing passive hepatic congestion
      ii. Preoperative cardiogenic shock (acute MI, papillary muscle rupture, valve thrombosis) may produce elevated LFTs consistent with a "shock liver" before surgery, predisposing the patient to the development of hepatic and multisystem organ failure after salvage open-heart surgery.
      iii. Endocarditis with evidence of sepsis may cause hepatic dysfunction.
   c. Operative factors: prolonged duration of CPB, complex operations (combined CABG–valve, multiple valves), greater number of blood transfusions
   d. Postoperative factors: low cardiac output syndrome, use of multiple inotropes or an IABP, sepsis, blood transfusions
   e. Medications, including statins, acetaminophen, and clopidogrel.[449]

2. **Pathophysiology.** Hepatic dysfunction may result from either reduced hepatic perfusion or systemic congestion.
   a. Hepatocellular necrosis
      • Low cardiac output states usually requiring inotropic and/or vasopressor support
      • Right-heart failure or severe tricuspid regurgitation (chronic passive congestion)
      • Sepsis injures the liver due to inflammatory mediators and other toxins; hepatic dysfunction due to sepsis is a major risk factor for multisystem organ failure and death.[450]
      • Posttransfusion hepatitis C or cytomegalovirus infection (late)
   b. Hyperbilirubinemia
      • Hemolysis (paravalvular leak, long pump run, sepsis, multiple transfusions, drugs)
      • Intrahepatic cholestasis (hepatitis, hepatocellular necrosis, benign postoperative cholestasis, parenteral nutrition, bacterial infections, medications)
      • Extrahepatic obstruction (biliary tract obstruction)

3. **Manifestations** depend on the specific diagnosis. Jaundice is a common accompaniment of hepatocellular damage or cholestasis. Severe liver failure may result in hypotension, coagulopathy, refractory lactic acidosis, hypoglycemia, renal failure, or encephalopathy from hyperammonemia, and sepsis.

4. **Evaluation.** The specific LFT abnormalities usually indicate the nature of the problem. Additional tests may include those that detect hemolysis (LDH, low serum haptoglobin, schistocytes on peripheral blood smear), assess cardiac and valvular function (echocardiography), identify biliary pathology (right upper quadrant ultrasound or HIDA scan), or detect hepatitis (serologies).

5. **Treatment**

   a. An elevated bilirubin is usually a benign and self-limited postoperative occurrence. Bilirubin levels will gradually return to normal when hemodynamics improve unless there is evidence of severe underlying liver pathology. In this situation, progressive and irreversible hepatic dysfunction may result, leading to multisystem organ failure and death.

   b. Coagulopathy with "autoanticoagulation" may occur during a period of hepatic dysfunction because of the impaired capacity of the liver to produce clotting factors. In patients requiring anticoagulation, small doses of warfarin should be used to prevent the INR from becoming elevated to dangerous levels. If this occurs, the patient may develop cardiac tamponade or GI bleeding. In addition, the doses of medications that undergo hepatic metabolism must be altered.

   c. Stress ulcer prophylaxis should be given using one of the PPIs (pantoprazole 40 mg IV/PO qd).

   d. Due to high caloric expenditure and protein catabolism, give 1–1.5 g/kg/day of enteral protein.

   e. Hyperammonemia may cause an encephalopathy, and at levels >150–200 μmol/L may cause intracranial hypertension and cerebral edema.[451,452] This can be treated by:

      i. Control of fever and use of hypothermia protocols

      ii. Intubation and induced hypocarbia

      iii. For intracranial hypertension:
         - Hypertonic saline solutions (20 mL of 30% NaCl or 200 mL of 3% NaCl) keeping the serum sodium <150 mEq/L
         - Mannitol (2 mL/kg of 20% mannitol)

      iv. Medications such as lactulose 30 mL qid with sorbitol and oral neomycin 6 g daily. These may have a role in chronic liver disease but their benefits in acute liver failure are not clear.

      v. Hemodialysis (rarely)

   f. Blood glucose should be carefully monitored to prevent hypoglycemia.

   g. Lactic acidosis may result from impaired lactate metabolism rather than lactate generation from impaired tissue perfusion. Partial correction with sodium bicarbonate should be considered if the base deficit exceeds 10. Thiamine deficiency causing lactic acidosis should be considered and is easily correctable.

K. **Hyperamylasemia** is noted in a substantial number (35–65%) of patients in the early postbypass period, but is associated with clinical pancreatitis in only about 1–3% of patients. Isolated hyperamylasemia in the early postoperative period is usually not associated with clinical symptoms or an elevated lipase level, and most commonly arises from a nonpancreatic source, such as the salivary glands, or results from decreased renal excretion. Transient hyperamylasemia has a comparable incidence after on- or off-pump surgery, so it is not directly related to use of CPB.[453] However, some patients with an amylase level >1000 units/L early after surgery may subsequently develop subclinical pancreatitis about one week later with mild symptoms (anorexia, nausea, ileus) and elevation of serum lipase levels. Late elevations in amylase levels tends to be pancreatic in origin. A brief period of bowel rest may be beneficial for these patients, but no specific treatment is indicated unless there is clinical evidence of overt pancreatitis or GI tract dysfunction.[454]

L. **Overt pancreatitis** is noted in less than 0.5% of patients undergoing cardiac surgery, but is a serious problem associated with a significant mortality rate. Pancreatic necrosis has been noted in 25% of patients dying from multisystem organ failure after cardiac surgery.[455]

　　1. **Etiology.** Pancreatitis usually represents an ischemic, necrotic injury resulting from a low cardiac output state and hypoperfusion. A prolonged duration of CPB may sensitize the pancreas to the subsequent insult of a persistent low output state requiring vasopressors that leads to necrotizing pancreatitis. Additional risks factors include a history of alcohol abuse, hypertension, CKD, and a requirement for norepinephrine support.[456,457]

　　2. **Presentation** is atypical and relatively nonspecific. Fever, elevated WBC, paralytic ileus, and abdominal distention occur first, with abdominal pain, tenderness, and hemodynamic instability representing late manifestations.

　　3. **Diagnosis** is suggested by the association of abdominal pain with elevated lipase levels. An abdominal ultrasound or CT scan may demonstrate a pancreatic phlegmon or abscess.

　　4. **Treatment** should begin with nasogastric drainage and antibiotics. Exploratory laparotomy with debridement and drainage is usually performed as a desperation measure, but it may be the only hope for survival in patients with aggressive necrotizing pancreatitis.

XI. Nutrition

A. Reversal of the catabolic state with adequate nutrition is important during the early phase of postoperative convalescence since malnutrition increases postoperative morbidity and mortality.[458–461] The diet must provide enough calories to allow wounds to heal and to maintain immune competence. Although limitations in salt content, fluids, and cholesterol intake are important, overly strict restrictions should be secondary to providing tasty, high-caloric foods that stimulate the patient's appetite. Too frequently, the combination of anorexia, nausea, and an unpalatable diet prevents the patient from achieving satisfactory nutrition. In non-intubated patients who cannot meet their energy needs with an oral diet, oral supplements with low residue, such as Boost (Nestlé Health Science) or Ensure (Abbott Nutrition), are useful in meeting caloric requirements.

B. **Enteral nutrition.** Patients requiring ventilatory support, those with swallowing difficulties after extubation, and many patients suffering strokes are unable to take oral feedings, but usually have a functional GI tract. If the patient cannot eat within 48 hours of surgery, enteral feeding should be initiated at a consistent hourly rate, not as a bolus feed, and should be increased to goal within 3–7 days. Most patients requiring a tracheostomy after 1–2 weeks of mechanical ventilatory support will benefit from a feeding tube. If there is no evidence of gastroesophageal reflux, a percutaneous endoscopic gastrostomy (PEG) feeding tube can be placed for long-term feeding. If reflux is present, a feeding jejunostomy may be considered at the time of the tracheostomy.

1. General contraindications to enteral feeding include uncontrolled shock, uncontrolled hypoxemia/hypercarbia/acidosis, active upper GI bleeding, bowel ischemia or obstruction, or abdominal compartment syndrome. Enteral feedings can often be started even with absent bowel sounds, unless bowel ischemia or obstruction is suspected. Evidence of distention or high gastric residuals (>500 mL/6h) may indicate temporary intolerance to tube feedings. Despite a reluctance to initiate enteral feeding in hemodynamically unstable patients, especially those on vasopressors, it may be safe to do so as long as the patient has adequate intravascular volume.[462,463] Early enteral nutrition can be used for patients on ECMO, with pancreatitis, and those given neuromuscular blocking drugs to aid with ventilation.

2. A soft nasogastric feeding tube should be placed and tube feedings initiated after confirming the position of the catheter in the stomach. Postpyloric placement may lower the risk of aspiration, but is more difficult to accomplish. This is recommended if there is intolerance to gastric feeding due to gastroparesis or there is a high risk of aspiration. Factors increasing that risk generally include older age, use of mechanical ventilation, altered mental status, neurologic deficits, and gastroesophageal reflux. A three-day course of prokinetic drugs, including erythromycin 200 mg IV in 50 mL NS through a central line or in 200 mL NS peripherally three times a day with or without metoclopramide 10 mg IV q12h, will stimulate gastric motility and increase tolerance to tube feedings.

C. **Parenteral nutrition.** If the GI tract cannot be used, parenteral nutrition provided through a central line may be necessary. Because of the increased risk of infection compared with use of enteral nutrition, it has been recommended that parenteral feedings should be delayed for at least 3–7 days if the patient cannot tolerate any enteral feedings.[459] In addition, if the caloric intake is <60% of the desired level after several days of enteral feedings, adding parenteral nutrition should be considered. Parenteral feedings may be supplemented with a lipid emulsion providing 0.1–0.2 mg/kg of fish oil enriched with docosahexaenoic acid (DHA) and eicosapentanoic acid (EPA) that are immunomodulatory and anti-inflammatory.[459,461]

D. Measures to reduce the risk of aspiration in patients on enteral feedings include the following:[458]

1. Elevate the head of the bed 30–45°.
2. Use chlorhexidine mouthwash twice a day to reduce the risk of pneumonia.
3. Use metoclopramide to promote GI motility.
4. Check the gastric residual volume; if it exceeds 500 mL, the tube feeds should be held for 2–4 hours and then restarted as a continuous infusion at a lower rate.
5. Advance the feeding tube into the small bowel if necessary.

E. Initial enteral feedings should be hypocaloric relative to the patient's energy expenditure and should be increased to a full level by 3–7 days. Thus, one should initiate feeding to provide 8–10 kcal/kg/day and gradually increase feeding to provide a total caloric intake of 25 kcal/kg/day (ideal body weight) within one week. In markedly obese patients, the dosing weight is the ideal body weight (IBW) + 0.4 × (actual body weight – IBW). General nutritional requirements for adult patients include 2–5 g/kg/day of glucose, 1.3 g/kg/day of protein, and 1.2–1.5 g/kg/day of fat provided as an omega-3 enriched formula. A critically ill patient with multisystem organ failure may require 10–20% more calories with a protein requirement of 2–2.5 g/kg/day. A commonly used tube feeding such as Jevity 1.2 (Abbott Nutrition) will provide 1.2 kcal/mL. Thus, for a 70 kg man, 1500 mL/day will provide 1800 calories or 25 kcal/kg/day.

F. Specific considerations in critically ill patients include the following:

1. Blood glucose levels should be monitored several times a day during the initial phase of enteral nutrition. Hyperglycemia must be prevented by use of intravenous insulin infusions.

2. Serum electrolytes, including potassium, magnesium, and phosphate, should be measured daily for the first week, especially looking for "refeeding hypophosphatemia", which may occur when enteral feedings are initiated in a malnourished patient.[464] This is replaced with 0.3–0.6 mmol/kg/day of phosphate.

3. Soluble fiber and fibro-oligosaccharides (FOS) should be included in enteral feedings to optimize bowel function and are indicated if the patient develops diarrhea. These are included in standard tube feeds such as Jevity.

4. Antioxidant vitamins and trace minerals, including vitamin C and selenium, should be provided to critically ill patients receiving parenteral nutrition. Many studies have shown that vitamin C (and fish oils) reduce the incidence of postoperative AF.

5. Patients with hypercarbic respiratory failure might benefit from a feeding that is high-lipid and low-carbohydrate, but this is rarely necessary. If fluid restriction is indicated, a calorie-dense formulation, such as Isosource 1.5 (Nestlé Health Science) or Jevity 1.5, which both provide 1.5 kcal/mL, can be used. In patients with severe acute lung injury, an anti-inflammatory formula containing omega-3 fish oils and antioxidants, such as Impact (Nestlé Health Science) or Oxepa (Abbott Nutrition), may be beneficial.

6. Protein intake should be optimized to promote nitrogen retention while avoiding protein overload. Most patients with AKI can receive standard enteral feedings. Protein intake should be increased to 2.5 g/kg/day for patients on dialysis, which removes about 3–5 g/h of protein. Formulations such as Novasource Renal (Nestlé Health Science) or Nepro (Abbott Nutrition) provide high-protein, low-carbohydrate, and low-potassium loads.

7. Monitoring of visceral protein levels (transferrin and prealbumin) may indicate the adequacy of nutrition, but levels have not been shown to correlate with improved outcomes.

XII. Valve-associated Problems

All patients receiving a prosthetic valve require careful follow-up because of the risk of developing valve-related complications, including thromboembolism, endocarditis, anticoagulant-related hemorrhage, and valve degeneration.[465] It has been aptly stated that when a prosthetic valve is placed, "the patient is exchanging one disease process for another".[466]

A. **Thromboembolism.** The annual risk of thromboembolism averages 1–2% for aortic valves and 2–4% for mitral valves, with a slightly higher incidence in patients with mechanical valves taking warfarin than in those with bioprosthetic valves taking only aspirin. The recommended regimens for tissue and mechanical valves are summarized in Table 13.5 on page 770.

B. **Valve thrombosis** of a mechanical valve may occur despite therapeutic anticoagulation. It is very rare with a bioprosthetic valve, although echocardiographic findings often raise the specter of "subclinical leaflet thrombosis" on both TAVR and surgically implanted tissue valves in patients not taking warfarin, which may increase the risk of stroke.[120,467–471] Suspicion of mechanical valve thrombosis is raised by loss of valve clicks on auscultation and confirmed by fluoroscopy (see Figure 2.10, page 139) or echocardiography. Although thrombolytic therapy can be used in selected circumstances, an immediate operation to replace the valve is usually required.[472]

C. **Pregnancy** poses a serious problem for the woman with a prosthetic valve. The incidence of fetal loss is 60% if warfarin is used during the first trimester, and there is a significant incidence of other congenital defects if pregnancy is completed ("coumadin embryopathy"). Tissue valves have been used for women of childbearing age, acknowledging the limited durability of valves in this age group. Cryopreserved homograft valves or a pulmonary autograft (Ross procedure) can be considered for young women undergoing aortic valve replacement. One anticoagulation regimen recommended by both the ACC/AHA and the ESC for women with mechanical valves who become pregnant is as follows:[473]

1. First trimester (up through 13th week): use warfarin if dose <5 mg/day, or use dose-adjusted LMWH or IV UFH. Doses are usually UFH 10,000 units SC bid to achieve a PTT of twice control or LMWH SC bid (to maintain a four-hour postinjection anti-Xa heparin level >0.5 units/mL).

2. Second and third trimesters: warfarin +/– aspirin

3. Peripartum (or last half of third trimester): dose-adjusted UFH or LMWH (often up to 20,000 units SC q12h) until delivery

4. Resume warfarin after delivery.

D. **Anticoagulant-related hemorrhage** is a major source of morbidity in patients receiving warfarin, especially in patients over the age of 65. In fact, it has been estimated that more than 20% of patients will experience major or minor bleeding episodes. Patient response to warfarin after surgery is quite variable, and may be related to genetic factors. The use of medications that influence INR levels (most commonly amiodarone and antibiotics) must be taken into consideration when dosing warfarin. It is helpful to use an anticoagulation protocol to initiate warfarin therapy (see Table 13.6 and Appendix 8). **It is absolutely critical that careful follow-up be arranged for any patient discharged on warfarin** to avoid under- or overanticoagulation. Home self-testing systems make it easier for patients to check their INRs and have been noted to minimize the fluctuation in the INR levels, resulting in less thromboembolism and improved survival.[474] In patients whose INRs are hard to regulate, concomitant administration of vitamin K 100–200 µg/day orally helps stabilize the INR.[129,130]

E. **Prosthetic valve endocarditis (PVE)** may develop at any time during the lifespan of a prosthetic valve with an annual risk of approximately 1–2%, which appears to be

comparable with surgically implanted and transcatheter valves.[475,476] Early endocarditis (within 60 days of surgery) most commonly results from infection with
staphylococci (coagulase-negative more often than *S. aureus*), fungi, Gram-negative
organisms, and enterococci. This carries a significantly higher mortality than late
PVE, which is most commonly caused by coagulase-negative staphylococci and
Streptococcus viridans. Clinical manifestations may include recurrent fevers, valve dysfunction with regurgitation and heart failure, cerebral or peripheral embolization,
and, most ominously, the development of conduction defects resulting from a periannular abscess. The indications for surgery are noted in Chapter 1 (pages 61–62). It is
critical that the patient understands the need for prophylactic antibiotics when any
dental procedure is performed. The ACC/AHA recommendations detailed in
Table 13.5 should be followed.[215]

F. **Hemolysis** usually indicates the development of a paravalvular leak and is often
worse when the leak is smaller due to increased turbulence. It may also result from
transvalvular leaks resulting from pannus ingrowth or thrombus formation on a
mechanical valve that restricts leaflet movement and may keep one or both leaflets in
a partially open fixed position. Subclinical hemolysis is manifest by elevation in the
LDH and reticulocyte count with a low haptoglobin level. The patient may also
develop mild jaundice or persistent anemia, necessitating transfusion. Valve re-
replacement is indicated for severe hemolysis or a significant paravalvular leak.[477]

G. **Valve failure** is defined as a complication necessitating valve replacement.[465]
Mechanical valve failure is usually caused by thrombosis, thromboembolism, endocarditis, or anticoagulation-related bleeding, and rarely by structural failure. In contrast, primary tissue failure is the most common cause of bioprosthetic valve
dysfunction necessitating valve replacement. This occurs more readily in mitral
valves, which are subject to more leaflet stress than aortic valves. Current-generation
tissue valves (porcine or pericardial) generally have some form of anticalcification
treatment to potentially extend their lifespan. Nonetheless, early and late failures can
occur, so constant vigilance and follow-up echocardiograms are essential.
Bioprosthetic valve failure usually occurs gradually, and valve replacement surgery
can thus be performed on an elective basis either surgically or with a transcatheter
valve-in-valve approach in both aortic and mitral positions. In contrast, high-risk
emergency surgery is usually required for catastrophic mechanical valve failure.

XIII. Discharge Planning

A. As the hospital length of stay continues to decrease, appropriate discharge planning is essential to ensure a smooth convalescence after hospital discharge. Patients
requiring additional subacute care may be transferred to rehabilitation hospitals or
skilled nursing facilities for several days before going home. Even when patients
are well enough to be cared for at home, it is not uncommon for separation anxiety
to develop, with both patients and family members experiencing difficulty handling minor problems.

B. Appropriate discharge planning should involve the patient, family members, case
managers, dietitians, nurses, mid-level providers, and physicians. Patients must be
given explicit instructions as to how they will feel, how fast they should anticipate
recovery, what they must not do, what they should look for, and when to contact
the surgeon's office or the hospital. Several manuals are available that discuss

expectations and the reestablishment of standard routines at home (see www.sts. org and click on the "patients" link for a booklet on "What to Expect After Heart Surgery"). Phone contact from the doctor's office is very beneficial in allaying patients' fears, answering routine questions, and dealing appropriately with potential problems. Since the definition of "operative mortality" extends out to 30 days after surgery, it is imperative that patients be contacted at that time to see whether they have been readmitted and to see how they are faring. This should be done in order to perform appropriate outcomes analysis and submit accurate data to the STS database.

C. Most patients should have an available family member or friend at home for the first week after discharge. This provides reassurance for patients who may not yet be able to care for themselves, and it also provides an objective observer who is able to contact the hospital if serious problems arise.

D. **Medications.**[52,478] The patient should be provided with a list and schedule of all medications. The reason each medication has been prescribed as well as possible side effects and interactions with other medications should be discussed. If the patient is receiving an anticoagulant such as **warfarin**, it is **absolutely imperative that follow-up be arranged** for prothrombin times (INR) and regulation of drug dosage. The adverse influence of alcohol, other medications, and certain foods on the level of anticoagulation must be emphasized (Appendix 11). The most commonly used medications at the time of discharge include the following:

1. **Aspirin** should be given to all CABG patients, not only to improve graft patency but also for the secondary prevention of coronary events. Aspirin has been shown to reduce long-term mortality after CABG. It may be used alone for aortic bioprosthetic valves or combined with warfarin for patients receiving mechanical or bioprosthetic mitral valves.

2. **P2Y12 inhibitors** (clopidogrel, ticagrelor, and prasugrel) are given to patients with recently placed drug-eluting stents and after TAVR or MitraClip procedures. They should be considered along with aspirin in patients undergoing CABG for acute coronary syndromes or after OPCABs.
   a. Drugs that reduce clopidogrel's antiplatelet activity include omeprazole (but not pantoprazole), morphine, and amlodipine (which should not be given with ticagrelor), as well as grapefruit juice.
   b. Drugs that enhance clopidogrel's antiplatelet activity include aspirin and ACE inhibitors.

3. **Warfarin** is prescribed for patients with AF, mechanical valves, and for some patients receiving tissue valves (see Table 13.3). NOACs may be used for AF or with use of tissue valves after three months, but are contraindicated in patients with mechanical valves.

4. **Statins** are indicated for all patients with coronary artery disease because of their lipid-lowering and pleiotropic effects. Statins can stabilize plaque, potentially promote plaque regression, and mitigate the progression of saphenous vein graft disease. They have been shown to improve the short- and long-term results of CABG and even valve surgery. All patients taking statins should have their LFTs checked at baseline and at six-month intervals. High-intensity statins (atorvastatin 40–80 mg or rosuvastatin 20–40 mg) are recommended after CABG in patients <age 75, with moderate-intensity dosing

recommended in older patients. Potential drug–drug interactions may influence whether medications should not be prescribed or whether doses should be modified.

   a. Simvastatin has significant interactions with amiodarone, amlodipine, diltiazem and ticagrelor. No more than 10 mg of simvastatin should be given to patients on verapamil or diltiazem and no more than 20 mg of simvastatin should be given to patients on amiodarone or amlodipine.

   b. Atorvastatin has significant interactions with digoxin, diltiazem, and verapamil. No more than 40 mg of atorvastatin should be given to patients on diltiazem.

5. **β-blockers** are generally prescribed following CABG as prophylaxis against AF in the perioperative period, but they have also provided survival benefits in postinfarction patients treated medically or undergoing CABG, and in other patients with reduced EF or HF. There is some evidence that they may also improve long-term survival in patients without a history of MI or HF.[479] Carvedilol is often used in patients with impaired LV function. Otherwise, metoprolol is the most commonly prescribed β-blocker and is beneficial for control of hypertension as well.

6. **Amiodarone** may be given as prophylaxis for AF, although the optimal duration of therapy is not defined. It can usually be stopped after a couple of weeks if the patient remains in sinus rhythm. It is recommended for several months following a Maze procedure. Amiodarone can affect hepatic, thyroid, and pulmonary function, so any patient in whom therapy is anticipated beyond one month should have LFTs, thyroid function tests, and pulmonary function tests obtained at baseline. There are nearly 600 drugs which interact with amiodarone noted on the www.drugs.com website. Particular concerns in cardiac surgery patients are that amiodarone:

   a. Decreases the metabolism of warfarin, necessitating a 25–50% reduction in warfarin dosing

   b. May rarely reduce platelet inhibition by clopidogrel

   c. Increases QT prolongation when used concurrently with fluoroquinolones (ciprofloxacin, levofloxacin), 5-HT$_3$ antagonists (ondansetron), or haloperidol. These medications are generally contraindicated if amiodarone is being used.

   d. Enhances bradycardia when given with β-blockers or CCBs

7. **ACE inhibitors** (or ARBs if ACE inhibitor intolerant) are recommended as the preferred antihypertensive drug after surgery, and are indicated in all patients with a reduced EF <40%, a history of infarction, diabetes, or CKD. Although short-term mortality benefits have not been demonstrated, ACE inhibitors may provide long-term mortality benefits.

E. **Prophylactic antibiotics.** Any patient who has received prosthetic material (valves or grafts) must be aware of the necessity of taking prophylactic antibiotics if dental work is contemplated. Patients should be told to inform their physician or dentist accordingly and follow the ACC/AHA guidelines for antibiotic prophylaxis delineated in Table 13.5.[215]

F. **Diabetes mellitus** is associated with greater morbidity and mortality after CABG surgery, and poor diabetic control postoperatively may compromise graft patency and contribute to more rapid progression of native vessel disease. Diet and medications should be optimized to achieve a HbA1c <7%.

G. **Diet.** Dieticians should meet with patients before discharge to discuss the particular dietary restrictions for their cardiac disease. This entails discussions of the significance of low-cholesterol or low-salt diets and the provision of appropriate dietary plans.

H. The patient must participate in self-evaluation at home. A daily assessment of pulse rate, oral temperature, and weight should be performed, and all incisions should be inspected for redness, tenderness, or drainage. Visiting nurses are usually recommended for patients discharged home to help with these assessments. Patients should be instructed to contact their physician's office if any abnormalities are noted.

I. Patients should be encouraged to gradually increase their activity as tolerated. Patients with a median sternotomy incision should be discouraged from lifting objects weighing more than 10–15 pounds, because it puts strain on the healing sternum. Driving should be avoided for six weeks. In contrast, there are few physical limitations for patients who have small thoracotomy incisions for minimally invasive surgery or who have undergone TAVR or MitraClip procedures.

J. Lifestyle modification and control of all modifiable risk factors are essential to optimize the long-term results of surgery. These include weight loss, cessation of smoking (with nicotine patches and pharmacologic agents initially), and control of dyslipidemias, diabetes, and hypertension. Postoperative depression is not uncommon and should be identified and treated because it is associated with worse outcomes. Involvement in a cardiac rehabilitation program is an important aspect of long-term care following surgery.

References

1. O'Mara SK. Management of postoperative fever in adult cardiac surgical patients. *Dimens Crit Care Nurs* 2017;36:182–92.

2. Rhee C, Sax PE. Evaluation of fever and infections in cardiac surgery patients. *Semin Cardiothorac Vasc Anesth* 2015;19:143–53.

3. Garcia-Delgado M, Navarette-Sánchez I, Colmenero M. Preventing and managing perioperative pulmonary complications following cardiac surgery. *Curr Opin Anaesthesiol* 2014;27:146–52.

4. Weissman C. Pulmonary complications after cardiac surgery. *Semin Cardiothorac Vasc Anesth* 2004;8:185–211.

5. Tripp HF, Bolton JW. Phrenic nerve injury following cardiac surgery: a review. *J Card Surg* 1998;13:218–23.

6. Dimopoulou I, Daganou M, Dafni U, et al. Phrenic nerve dysfunction after cardiac operations: electrophysiologic evaluation of risk factors. *Chest* 1998;113:8–14.

7. Canbaz S, Turgut N, Halici U, Balci K, Ege T, Duran E. Electrophysiological evaluation of phrenic nerve injury during cardiac surgery: a prospective, controlled, clinical study. *BMC Surg* 2004;4:2.

8. Cassese M, Martinelli G, Nasso G, et al. Topical cooling for myocardial protection: the results of a prospective randomized study of the "shallow technique". *J Card Surg* 2006;21:357–62.

9. Merino-Ramirez MA, Juan G, Ramón M, et al. Electrophysiologic evaluation of phrenic nerve and diaphragm function after coronary bypass surgery: prospective study of diabetes and other risk factors. *J Thorac Cardiovasc Surg* 2006;132:530–6.

10. Cruz-Martinez A, Armijo A, Fermoso A, Moraleda S, Maté I, Marin M. Phrenic nerve conduction study in demyelinating neuropathies and open-heart surgery. *Clin Neurophysiol* 2000;111:821–5.

11. Sharma AD, Parmley CL, Sreeram G, Grocott HP. Peripheral nerve injuries during cardiac surgery: risk factors, diagnosis, prognosis, and prevention. *Anesth Analg* 2000;91:1358–69.

12. Katz MG, Katz R, Schachner A, Cohen AJ. Phrenic nerve injury after coronary artery bypass grafting: will it go away? *Ann Thorac Surg* 1998;65:32–5.

13. Podgaetz E, Garza-Castillon R Jr, Andrade RS. Best approach and benefit of plication for paralyzed diaphragm. *Thorac Surg Clin* 2016;26:333–46.

14. Lee CK, Kim YM, Shim DJ, Na CY, Oh SS. The detection of pulmonary embolisms after a coronary artery bypass graft surgery by the use of 64-slice multidetector CT. *Int J Cardiovasc Imaging* 2011;27:639–45.

15. Beck KS, Cho EK, Moon MH, Kim DY, Song H, Jung JI. Incidental pulmonary embolism after coronary artery bypass surgery: long-term clinical follow-up. *AJR Am J Roentgenol* 2018;210:52–7.

16. Goldhaber SZ, Schoepf UJ. Pulmonary embolism after coronary artery bypass grafting. *Circulation* 2004;109:2712–5.

17. Schwann TA, Kistler L, Engoren MC, Habib RH. Incidence and predictors of postoperative deep vein thrombosis in cardiac surgery in the era of aggressive thromboprophylaxis. *Ann Thorac Surg* 2010;90:760–8.

18. Viana VB, Melo ER, Terra-Filho M, et al. Frequency of deep vein thrombosis and/or pulmonary embolism after coronary artery bypass grafting investigation regardless of clinical suspicion. *Am J Cardiol* 2017;119:237–42.

19. Wang Z, Gao F, Men J, Ren J, Modi P, Wei M. Aspirin resistance in off-pump coronary artery bypass grafting. *Eur J Cardiothorac Surg* 2012;41:108–12.

20. Bednar F, Osmancik P, Hlavicka J, Jedlickova V, Paluch Z, Vanek T. Aspirin is insufficient in inhibition of platelet aggregation and thromboxane formation early after coronary artery bypass surgery. *J Thromb Thrombolysis* 2009;27:394–9.

21. Bednar F, Osmancik P, Vanek T, et al. Platelet activity and aspirin efficacy after off-pump compared with on-pump coronary artery bypass surgery: results from the prospective randomized trial PRAGUE 11-Coronary Artery Bypass and REactivity of Thrombocytes (CABARET). *J Thorac Cardiovasc Surg* 2008;136:1054–60.

22. Cartier RE, Robitaille D. Thrombotic complications in beating heart operations. *J Thorac Cardiovasc Surg* 2001;121:920–2.

23. Hattesen AL, Modrau IS, Nielsen DV, Hvas AM. The absorption of aspirin is reduced after coronary artery bypass grafting. *J Thorac Cardiovasc Surg* 2019;157:1059–68.

24. Ho KM, Bham E, Pavey W. Incidence of venous thromboembolism and benefits and risks of thromboprophylaxis after cardiac surgery: a systematic review and meta-analysis. *J Am Heart Assoc* 2015;4(10): e002652.

25. Ahmed AB, Koster A, Lance M, et al. European guidelines on perioperative venous thromboembolism prophylaxis: cardiovascular and thoracic surgery. *Eur J Anaesthesiology* 2018;3:84–9.

26. Goldhaber SZ, Hirsch DR, MacDougall RC, Polak JF, Creager MA, Cohn LH. Prevention of venous thrombosis after coronary artery bypass surgery (a randomized trial comparing two mechanical prophylaxis strategies). *Am J Cardiol* 1995;76:993–6.

27. Shammas NW. Pulmonary embolus after coronary artery bypass surgery: a review of the literature. *Clin Cardiol* 2000;23:637–44.

28. Mirhosseini SJ, Forouzannia SK, Manshadi SM, Ali-Hasan-Al-Saegh S, Naderi N, Sanatkar M. Comparison of aspirin plus heparin with heparin alone on asymptomatic perioperative deep venous thrombosis in candidates for elective off-pump coronary artery bypass graft: a randomized clinical trial. *Cardiol J* 2013;20:139–43.

29. Ramos R, Salem BI, De Pawlikowski MP, Coordes C, Eisenberg S, Leidenfrost R. The efficacy of pneumatic compression stockings in the prevention of pulmonary embolism after cardiac surgery. *Chest* 1996;109:82–5.

30. Arabi YM, Al-Hameed F, Burns KEA, et al. Adjunctive intermittent pneumatic compression for venous thromboprophylaxis. *N Engl J Med* 2019;380:1305–15.

31. Close V, Purohit M, Tanos M, Hunter S. Should patients post-cardiac surgery be given low molecular weight heparin for deep vein thrombosis prophylaxis? *Interact Cardiovasc Thorac Surg* 2006;5:624–9.

32. Gould MK, Garcia DA, Wren SM, et al. Prevention of VTE in nonorthopedic surgical patients: antithrombotic therapy and prevention of thrombosis, 9th ed: American College of Chest Physicians evidence-based clinical practice guidelines. *Chest* 2012;141:(2 Suppl):e227S–77S.

33. Aissaoui N, Martins E, Mouly S, Weber S, Meune C. A meta-analysis of bed rest versus early ambulation in the management of pulmonary embolism, deep vein thrombosis, or both. *Int J Cardiol* 2009;137:37–41.

34. Liu Z, Tao X, Chen Y, Fan Z, Li Y. Bed rest versus early ambulation with standard anticoagulation in the management of deep vein thrombosis: a meta-analysis. *PLoS One* 2015;10:e0121388.

35. Kolkailah AA, Hirji S, Piazza G, et al. Surgical pulmonary embolectomy and catheter-directed thrombolysis for treatment of submassive pulmonary embolism. *J Card Surg* 2018;33:252–9.

36. Mangi A, Rehman H, Bansal V, Zuberi O. Ultrasound assisted catheter-directed thrombolysis of acute pulmonary embolism: a review of current literature. *Cureus* 2017;9(7):e1492.

37. Eid-Lidt G, Gaspar J, Sandoval J, et al. Combined clot fragmentation and aspiration in patients with acute pulmonary embolism. *Chest* 2008;134:54–60.

38. Akay TH, Sezgin A, Ozkan S, Gultekin B, Aslim E, Aslamaci S. Successful surgical treatment of massive pulmonary embolism after coronary bypass surgery. *Tex Heart Inst J* 2006;33:496–500.

39. Digonnet A, Moya-Plana A, Aubert S, et al. Acute pulmonary embolism: a current surgical approach. *Interact Cardiovasc Thorac Surg* 2007;6:27–9.

40. Baerman JM, Kirsh MM, de Buitleir M, et al. Natural history and determinants of conduction defects following coronary artery bypass surgery. *Ann Thorac Surg* 1987;44:150–3.

41. Cook DJ, Bailon JM, Douglas TT, et al. Changing incidence, type, and natural history of conduction defects after coronary artery bypass grafting. *Ann Thorac Surg* 2005;80:1732–7.

42. Glikson M, Dearani JA, Hyberger LK, Schaff HV, Hammill SC, Hayes DL. Indications, effectiveness, and long-term dependency on permanent pacing after cardiac surgery. *Am J Cardiol* 1997;80: 1309–13.

43. Matthews IG, Fazal IA, Bates MG, Turley AJ. In patients undergoing aortic valve replacement, what factors predict the requirement for permanent pacemaker implantation? *Interact Cardiovasc Thorac Surg* 2011;12:475–9.

44. Dawkins S, Hobson AR, Kalra PR, Tang AT, Monro JL, Dawkins KD. Permanent pacemaker implantation after isolated aortic valve replacement: incidence, implications, and predictors. *Ann Thorac Surg* 2008;85:108–12.

45. Romano MA, Koeckert M, Mumtaz MA, et al. Permanent pacemaker implantation after rapid deployment aortic valve replacement. *Ann Thorac Surg* 2018;106:685–90.

46. Thomas JL, Dickstein RA, Parker FB Jr, et al. Prognostic significance of the development of left bundle conduction defects following aortic valve replacement. *J Thorac Cardiovasc Surg* 1982;84:382–6.

47. Greason KL, Lahr BD, Stulak JM, et al. Long-term mortality effect of early pacemaker implantation after surgical aortic valve replacement. *Ann Thorac Surg* 2017;104:1259–64.

48. Rodés-Abau J, Ellenbogen KA, Krahn AD, et al. Management of conduction disturbances associated with transcatheter aortic valve replacement: JACC Scientific Expert Panel. *J Am Coll Cardiol* 2019;74:1086–106.

49. Kaplan RM, Yadlapat A, Cantey EP, et al. Conduction recovery following pacemaker implantation after transcatheter aortic valve replacement. *PACE* 2019;42:146–52.

50. Gaudino M, Nesta M, Burzotta F, et al. Results of emergency postoperative re-angiography after cardiac surgery procedures. *Ann Thorac Surg* 2015;99:1576–82.

51. Alqahtani F, Ziada KM, Badhwar V, Sandhu G, Rihal CS, Alkhouli M. Incidence, predictors, and outcomes of in-hospital percutaneous coronary intervention following coronary artery bypass grafting. *J Am Coll Cardiol* 2019;73:415–23.

52. Kulik A, Ruel M, Jneid H, et al. Secondary prevention after coronary artery bypass graft surgery: a scientific statement from the American Heart Association. *Circulation* 2015;131:927–64.

53. Kimmelstiel CD, Udelson JE, Salem DN, Bojar R, Rastegar H, Konstam MA. Recurrent angina caused by a left internal mammary artery-to-pulmonary artery fistula. *Am Heart J* 1993; 125:234–6.

54. Pepi M, Muratori M, Barbier P, et al. Pericardial effusion after cardiac surgery: incidence, site, size, and haemodynamic consequences. *Br Heart J* 1994;72:327–31.

55. Ikäheimo MJ, Huikuri HV, Airaksinen KE, et al. Pericardial effusion after cardiac surgery: incidence, relation to the type of surgery, antithrombotic therapy, and early coronary bypass graft patency. *Am Heart J* 1988;116:97–102.

56. Ashikhmina EA, Schaff HV, Sinak LJ, et al. Pericardial effusion after cardiac surgery: risk factors, patient profiles, and contemporary management. *Ann Thorac Surg* 2010;89:112–8.

57. Kuvin JT, Harati NA, Pandian NG, Bojar RM, Khabbaz KR. Postoperative cardiac tamponade in the modern surgical era. *Ann Thorac Surg* 2000;74:1148–53.

58. Khan NK, Järvelä KM, Loisa EL, Sutinen JA, Laurikka JO, Khan JA. Incidence, presentation and risk factors of late pericardial effusions requiring invasive treatment after cardiac surgery. *Interact Cardiovasc Thorac Surg* 2017;24:835–40.

59. You SC, Shim CY, Hong GR, et al. Incidence, predictors, and clinical outcomes of postoperative cardiac tamponade in patients undergoing heart valve surgery. *PLoS One* 2016;11(11):e0165754.

60. Leiva EH, Carreño M, Bucheli FR, Bonfanti AC, Umaña JP, Dennis RJ. Factors associated with delayed cardiac tamponade after cardiac surgery. *Ann Card Anaesth* 2018;21:158–66.

61. Sasse T, Eriksson U. Post-cardiac injury syndrome: aetiology, diagnosis, and treatment. *e-Journal of Cardiology Practice* volume 15 (www.escardio.org).

62. Saito Y, Donohue A, Attai S, et al. The syndrome of cardiac tamponade with "small" pericardial effusion. *Echocardiography* 2008;25:321–7.

63. Floerchinger B, Camboni D, Schopka S, Kolat P, Hilker M, Schmid C. Delayed cardiac tamponade after open heart surgery: is supplemental CT imaging reasonable? *J Cardiothorac Surg* 2013;8:158.

64. Imren Y, Tasoglu I, Oktar GL, et al. The importance of transesophageal echocardiography in diagnosis of pericardial tamponade after cardiac surgery. *J Card Surg* 2008;23:450–3.

65. Bakhshandeh AR, Salehi M, Radmehr F, Sattarzadeh R, Nasr AR, Sadeghpour AH. Postoperative pericardial effusion and posterior pericardiotomy: related or not? *Heart Surg Forum* 2009;12:E113–5.

66. Khan J, Khan N, Mannander A. Lower incidence of late tamponade after cardiac surgery by extended chest tube drainage. *Scand Cardiovasc J* 2019;53:104–9.

67. Inan MB, Yazicioglu L, Eryilmaz S, et al. Effects of prophylactic indomethacin treatment on postoperative pericardial effusion after aortic surgery. *J Thorac Cardiovasc Surg* 2011;141:578–82.

68. van Osch D, Nathoe HM, Jacob KA, et al. Determinants of the postpericardiotomy syndrome: a systematic review. *Eur J Clin Invest* 2017;47:456–67.

69. Lehto J, Gunn J, Karjalainen P, Airaksinen J, Kiviniemi T. Incidence and risk factors of postpericardiotomy syndrome requiring medical attention: the Finland Postpericardiotomy Syndrome Study. *J Thorac Cardiovasc Surg* 2015;149:1324–9.

70. Gaudino M, Anselmi A, Pavone N, Massetti M. Constrictive pericarditis after cardiac surgery. *Ann Thorac Surg* 2013;95:731–6.

71. Alraies MC, AlJaroudi W, Shabrang C, Yarmohammadi H, Klein AL, Tamarappoo BK. Clinical features associated with adverse events in patients with post-pericardiotomy syndrome following cardiac surgery. *Am J Cardiol* 2014;114:1426–30.

72. Lehto J, Kiviniemi T, Gunn J, Airaksinen J, Rautava P, Kytö V. Occurrence of postpericardiotomy syndrome: association with operation type and postoperative mortality after open-heart operations. *J Am Heart Assoc* 2018;7(22):e010269.

73. Jaworska-Wilczynska M, Magalska A, Piwocka K, et al. Low interleukin-8 level predicts the occurrence of the post pericardiotomy syndrome. *PLoS One* 2014;9:1–8.

74. Imazio M, Thrinchero R, Brucato A, et al. COlchicine for the Prevention of the Post-pericardiotomy Syndrome (COPPS): a multicentre, randomized, double-blind placebo-controlled trial. *Eur Heart J* 2010;31:2749–54.

75. Lazaros G, Imazio M, Brucato A, et al. The role of colchicine in pericardial syndromes. *Curr Pharm Des* 2018;24:702–9.

76. Wambolt R, Bisleri G, Glover B, et al. Primary prevention of post-pericardiotomy syndrome using corticosteroids: a systematic review. *Expert Rev Cardiovasc Ther* 2018;16:405–12.

77. Sevuk U, Baysal E, Altindag R, et al. Role of methylprednisolone in the prevention of postpericardiotomy syndrome after cardiac surgery. *Eur Rev Med Pharmacol Sci* 2016;20:514–9.

78. Bunge JJ, van Osch D, Dieleman JM, et al. Dexamethasone for the prevention of postpericardiotomy syndrome: a DExamethasone for Cardiac Surgery Substudy. *Am Heart J* 2014;168:126–31.

79. Sevuk U, Baysal E, Alltindaq R, et al. Role of diclofenac in the prevention of postpericardiotomy syndrome after cardiac surgery. *Vasc Health Risk Manag* 2015;11:373–8.

80. Kurth T, Glynn RJ, Walker AM, et al. Inhibition of clinical benefits of aspirin on first myocardial infarction by nonsteroidal anti-inflammatory drugs. *Circulation* 2003;108:1191–5.

81. Agarwal SK, Vallurupalli S, Uretsky BF, Hakeem A. Effectiveness of colchicine for the prevention of recurrent pericarditis and post-pericardiotomy syndrome: an updated meta-analysis of randomized clinical trials. *Eur Heart J Cardiovasc Pharmacother* 2015;1:117–25.

82. Anderson CA, Rodriguez E, Shammas RL, Kypson AP. Early constrictive epicarditis after coronary artery bypass surgery. *Ann Thorac Surg* 2009;87:642–3.

83. Liao P, DeSantis AJ, Schmeltz LR, et al. Insulin resistance following cardiothoracic surgery in patients with and without a preoperative diagnosis of type 2 diabetes during treatment with intravenous insulin therapy for postoperative hyperglycemia. *J Diabetes Complications* 2008;22:229–34.

84. Ascione R, Rogers CA, Rajakaruna C, Angelini GD. Inadequate blood glucose control is associated with in-hospital mortality and morbidity in diabetic and nondiabetic patients undergoing cardiac surgery. *Circulation* 2008;118:113–23.

85. Galino RJ, Fayfman M, Umpierrez GE. Perioperative management of hyperglycemia and diabetes in cardiac surgery patients. *Endocrinol Metab Clin North Am* 2018;47:203–22.

86. Lazar HL, McDonnell M, Chipkin SR, et al. The Society of Thoracic Surgeons practice guidelines series: blood glucose management during adult cardiac surgery. *Ann Thorac Surg* 2009;87:663–9.

87. Järvelä KM, Khan NK, Loisa EL, Sutinen JA, Laurikka JO, Khan JA. Hyperglycemic episodes are associated with postoperative infections after cardiac surgery. *Scand J Surg* 2018;107:138–44.

88. Society of Thoracic Surgeons Blood Conservation Guideline Task Force, Ferraris VA, Brown JR, Desposits GJ, et al. 2011 update to the Society of Thoracic Surgeons and the Society of Cardiovascular Anesthesiologists blood conservation clinical practice guidelines. *Ann Thorac Surg* 2011;91:944–82.

89. Kheiri B, Abdalla A, Osman M, et al. Restrictive versus liberal red blood cell transfusions for cardiac surgery: a systematic review and meta-analysis of randomized controlled trials. *J Thromb Thrombolysis* 2019;47:179–85.

90. Estcourt LJ, Robert DJ. Six-month outcomes after restrictive or liberal transfusion for cardiac surgery (TRICS III trial). *Transfus Med* 2019;29:77–9.

91. George TJ, Beaty CA, Kilic A, et al. Hemoglobin drift after cardiac surgery. *Ann Thorac Surg* 2012;94:703–9.

92. Saltzman DJ, Chang JC, Jimenez JC, et al. Postoperative thrombotic thrombocytopenic purpura after open heart operations. *Ann Thorac Surg* 2010;89:119–23.

93. Pishko AM, Cuker A. Heparin-induced thrombocytopenia in cardiac surgery patients. *Semin Thromb Hemost* 2017;43:691–8.

94. Arepally GM, Ortel TL. Heparin-induced thrombocytopenia. *N Engl J Med* 2006;355:809–17.

95. Levy JH, Winkler AM. Heparin-induced thrombocytopenia and cardiac surgery. *Curr Opin Anaesthesiol* 2010;23:74–9.

96. Warkentin TE. Heparin-induced thrombocytopenia in critically ill patients. *Semin Thromb Hemost* 2015;41:49–60.

97. Lillo-Le Louët A, Boutouyrie P, Alhenc-Gelas M, et al. Diagnostic score for heparin-induced thrombocytopenia after cardiopulmonary bypass. *J Thromb Haemost* 2004;2:1882–8.

98. Warkentin TE, Greinacher A, Koster A, Lincoff AM. Treatment and prevention of heparin-induced thrombocytopenia: American College of Chest Physicians evidence-based clinical practice guidelines (8th edition). *Chest* 2008;133:340S–80S.

99. Yusuf AM, Warkentin TE, Arsenault KA, Whitlock R, Eikelboom JW. Prognostic importance of preoperative anti-PF4/heparin antibodies in patients undergoing cardiac surgery: a systematic review. *Thromb Haemost* 2012;107:8–14.

100. Bauer TL, Arepally G, Konkle BA, et al. Prevalence of heparin-associated antibodies without thrombosis in patients undergoing cardiopulmonary bypass surgery. *Circulation* 1997;95:1242–6.

101. Everett BM, Yeh R, Foo SY, et al. Prevalence of heparin/platelet factor 4 antibodies before and after cardiac surgery. *Ann Thorac Surg* 2007;83:592–7.

102. Selleng S, Selleng K. Heparin-induced thrombocytopenia in cardiac surgery and critically ill patients. *Thromb Haemost* 2016;116:843–51.

103. Linkins LA, Dans AL, Moores LK, et al. Treatment and prevention of heparin-induced thrombocytopenia: antithrombotic therapy and prevention of thrombosis. 9th ed. American College of Chest Physicians evidence-based clinical practice guidelines. *Chest* 2012;141:e495S–530S.

104. Bartholomew JR, Hursting MJ. Transitioning from argatroban to warfarin in heparin-induced thrombocytopenia: an analysis of outcomes in patients with elevated international normalized ratio (INR). *J Thromb Thrombolysis* 2005;19:183–8.

105. Ferraris VA, Saha SP, Oestreich JH, et al. 2012 update to the Society of Thoracic Surgeons guideline on use of antiplatelet drugs in patients having cardiac and noncardiac operations. *Ann Thorac Surg* 2012;94:1761–81.

106. Hillis LD, Smith PK, Anderson JL, et al. 2011 ACCF/AHA guideline for coronary artery bypass graft surgery: a report of the American College of Cardiology Foundation/American Heart Association task force on practice guidelines. *J Am Coll Cardiol* 2012;58:e123–210.

107. Dunning J, Versteegh M, Fabbri A, et al. Guideline on antiplatelet and anticoagulation management in cardiac surgery. *Eur J Cardiothorac Surg* 2008;34:73–92.

108. Valgimigli M, Bueno H, Byrne RA, et al. 2017 ESC focused update on dual antiplatelet therapy in coronary artery disease developed in collaboration with EACTS: The Task Force for dual antiplatelet therapy in coronary artery disease of the European Society of Cardiology (ESC) and of the European Association for Cardio-Thoracic Surgery (EACTS). *Eur Heart J* 2018;39:213–60.

109. Deo SV, Dunlay SM, Shah IK, et al. Dual anti-platelet therapy after coronary artery bypass grafting: is there any benefit? A systematic review and meta-analysis. *J Card Surg* 2013;28:109–16.

110. Nocerino AG, Achenbach S, Taylor AJ. Meta-analysis of effect of single versus dual antiplatelet therapy on early patency of bypass conduits after coronary artery bypass grafting. *Am J Cardiol* 2013;112:1576–9.

111. Diepen S, Fuster V, Verma S, et al. Dual antiplatelet therapy versus aspirin monotherapy in diabetics with multivessel disease undergoing CABG: FREEDOM insights. *J Am Coll Cardiol* 2017;69:119–27.

112. Lamy A, Eikelboom J, Sheth T, et al. Rivaroxaban, aspirin, or both to prevent early coronary bypass graft occlusion: the COMPASS-CABG Study. *J Am Coll Cardiol* 2019;73:121–30

113. Gaasch WH, Konkle BA. Antithrombotic therapy for prosthetic heart valves: indications. 2020 uptodate.com.

114. Whitlock RP, Sun JC, Fremes SE, Rubens FD, Teoh KH. Antithrombotic and thrombolytic therapy for valvular disease: antithrombotic therapy and prevention of thrombosis. 9th ed. American College of Chest Physicians evidence-based clinical practice guidelines. *Chest* 2012;141(2 Suppl):e576S–600S.

115. Nishimura RA, Otto CM, Bonow RO, et al. 2017 AHA/ACC focused update of the 2014 AHA/ACC guidelines for the management of patients with valvular heart disease: a report of the American College of Cardiology/American Heart Association task force on practice guidelines. *Circulation* 2017;135:e1159–95 and *J Am Coll Cardiol* 2017;70:252–89.

116. Baumgartner H, Falk V, Bax JJ, et al. 2017 ESC/EACTS guidelines for the management of valvular heart disease. *Eur Heart J* 2017;378:2739–91.

117. Singh M, Sporn ZA, Schaff HV, Pellikka PA. ACC/AHA versus ESC guidelines on prosthetic heart management: JACC guideline comparison. *J Am Coll Cardiol* 2019;73:1707–18.

118. Papak JN, Chiovaro JC, Noelck N, et al. Antithrombotic strategies after bioprosthetic aortic valve replacement: a systematic review. *Ann Thorac Surg* 2019;107:1571–81.

119. Chakravarty T, Patel A, Kapadia S, et al. Anticoagulation after surgical or transcatheter bioprosthetic aortic valve replacement. *J Am Coll Cardiol* 2019;74:1190–200.

120. Makki N, Shreenivas S, Kereiakes D, Lilly S. A meta-analysis of reduced leaflet motion for surgical and transcatheter aortic valves: relationship to cerebrovascular events and valve degeneration. *Cardiovasc Revasc Med* 2018;19:868–73.

121. Guimarães PO, Pokorney SD, Lopes RD, et al. Efficacy and safety of apixaban vs warfarin in patients with atrial fibrillation and prior bioprosthetic valve replacement or valve repair: insights from the ARISTOTLE trial. *Clin Cardiol* 2019;42:568–71.

122. Khalil C, Mosleh W, Megaly M, et al. Mono versus dual antiplatelet therapy after transcatheter aortic valve replacement: a systematic review and meta-analysis. *Structural Heart* 2018;2:448–62.

123. Abuzaid A, Ranjan P, Fabrizio C, et al. Single anti-platelet therapy versus dual anti-platelet therapy after transcatheter aortic valve replacement: a meta-analysis. *Structural Heart* 2018;2:408–18.

124. Dangas GD, Tijssen JGP, Wöhrle J, et al. A controlled trial of rivaroxaban after transcatheter aortic valve replacement. *N Engl J Med* 2020;382:120–9.

125. van der Wall SJ, Olsthoorn JR, Huets S, et al. Antithrombotic therapy after mitral valve repair: VKA or aspirin? *J Thromb Thrombolysis* 2018;46:473–81.

126. Eikelboom JW, Connolly RJ, Brueckmann M, et al. Dabigatran versus warfarin in patients with mechanical heart valves. *N Engl J Med* 2013;369:1206–14.

127. Tomaselli GF, Mahaffey KW, Cuker A, et al. 2017 ACC expert consensus decision pathway on management of bleeding in patients with oral anticoagulants. *J Am Coll Cardiol* 2017;70: 3042–67.

128. Johnson SG, Rogers K, Delate T, Witt DM. Outcomes associated with combined antiplatelet and anticoagulant therapy. *Chest* 2008;133:948–54.

129. Reese AM, Farnett LE, Lyons RM, Patel B, Morgan L, Bussey HI. Low-dose vitamin K to augment anticoagulation control. *Pharmacotherapy* 2005;25:1746–51.

130. Sconce E, Avery P, Wynne H, Kamali F. Vitamin K supplementation can improve stability of anticoagulation for patients with unexplained variability in response to warfarin. *Blood* 2007;109:2419–23.

131. Gelijns AC, Moskowitz AJ, Acker MA, et al. Management practices and major infections after cardiac surgery. *J Am Coll Cardiol* 2014;64:372–81.

132. Engelman RM, Shahian DM, Shemin R, et al. The Society of Thoracic Surgeons practice guidelines series: antibiotic prophylaxis in cardiac surgery: part II: antibiotic choice. *Ann Thorac Surg* 2007;83:1569–76.

133. Edwards FH, Engelman RM, Houck P, Shahian DM, Bridges CR. The Society of Thoracic Surgeons practice guideline series: antibiotic prophylaxis in cardiac surgery: part I: duration. *Ann Thorac Surg* 2006;81:397–404.

134. O'Keefe S, Williams K, Legare JF. Hospital-acquired infections after cardiac surgery and current physician practices: a retrospective cohort study. *J Clin Med Res* 2017;9:10–6.

135. Cove ME, Spelman DW, MacLaren G. Infectious complications of cardiac surgery: a clinical review. *J Cardiothorac Vasc Anesth* 2012;26:1094–1100.

136. De Santo LS, Bancone C, Santarpino G, et al. Microbiologically documented nosocomial infections after cardiac surgery: an 18-month prospective tertiary care centre report. *Eur J Cardiothorac Surg* 2008;33:666–72.

137. Michalopoulos A, Geroulanos S, Rosmarakis ES, Falagas ME. Frequency, characteristics, and predictors of microbiologically documented nosocomial infections after cardiac surgery. *Eur J Cardiothorac Surg* 2006;29:456–60.

138. Reddy SL, Grayson AD, Smith G, Warwick R, Chalmers JA. Methicillin resistant *Staphylococcus aureus* infections following cardiac surgery: incidence, impact and identifying adverse outcome traits. *Eur J Cardiothorac Surg* 2007;32:113–7.

139. Rosmarakis ES, Prapas SN, Rellos K, Michalopoulos A, Samonis G, Falagas ME. Nosocomial infections after off-pump coronary artery bypass surgery: frequency, characteristics, and risk factors. *Interact Cardiovasc Thorac Surg* 2007;6:759–67.

140. Fowler VG, O'Brien SM, Muhlbaier LH, Corey GR, Ferguson TB, Peterson ED. Clinical predictors of major infections after cardiac surgery. *Circulation* 2005;112(9 Suppl):I-358–65.

141. Mastoraki A, Kriaras I, Douka E, Mastoraki S, Stravopodis G, Geroulanos S. Methicillin-resistant *Staphylococcus aureus* preventing strategy in cardiac surgery. *Interact Cardiovasc Thorac Surg* 2008;7:452–6.

142. Muñoz P, Hortal J, Giannella M, et al. Nasal carriage of *S. aureus* increases the risk of surgical site infection after major heart surgery. *J Hosp Infect* 2008;68:25–31.

143. Bouva E, Perez A, Munoz P. Ventilator-associated pneumonia after heart surgery: a prospective analysis and the value of surveillance. *Crit Care Med* 2003;35:1518–25.

144. Hooton TM, Bradley SF, Cardenas DD, et al. Diagnosis, prevention, and treatment of catheter-associated urinary tract infection in adults: 2009 International Clinical Practice Guidelines from the Infectious Diseases Society of America. *Clin Infect Dis* 2010;60:625–63.

145. Garnacho-Montero J, Aldabó-Pallás R, Palomar-Martinez M, et al. Risk factors and prognosis of catheter-related bloodstream infection in critically ill patients: a multicenter study. *Intensive Care Med* 2008;34:2185–93.

146. Pawar M, Mehta Y, Kapoor P, Sharma J, Gupta A, Trehan N. Central venous catheter-related blood stream infections: incidence, risk factors, outcome, and associated pathogens. *J Cardiothorac Vasc Anesth* 2004;18:304–8.

147. Jog S, Cunningham R, Cooper S, et al. Impact of preoperative screening for methicillin-resistant *Staphylococcus aureus* by real-time polymerase chain reaction in patients undergoing cardiac surgery. *J Hosp Infect* 2008;69:124–30.

148. Saraswat MK, Magruder JT, Crawford TC, et al. Preoperative *Staphylococcus aureus* screening and targeted decolonization in cardiac surgery. *Ann Thorac Surg* 2017;104:1349–56.

149. Hong JHC, Saraswat MK, Ellison TA, et al. *Staphylococcus aureus* prevention strategies in cardiac surgery: a cost-effectiveness analysis. *Ann Thorac Surg* 2018;105:47–53.

150. Segers P, Speekenbrink RGH, Ubbink DT, van Ogtrop ML, de Mol BA. Prevention of nosocomial infection in cardiac surgery by decontamination of the nasopharynx and oropharynx with chlorhexidine gluconate: a randomized controlled trial. *JAMA* 2006;296:2460–6.

151. Carrel TP, Eisinger E, Vogt M, Turina MI. Pneumonia after cardiac surgery is predictable by tracheal aspirates but cannot be prevented by prolonged antibiotic prophylaxis. *Ann Thorac Surg* 2001;72:143–8.

152. Michalopoulos A, Stavridis G, Geroulanos S. Severe sepsis in cardiac surgical patients. *Eur J Surg* 1998;164:217–22.

153. Paternoster G, Guarracino F. Sepsis after cardiac surgery: from pathophysiology to management. *J Cardiothorac Vasc Anesth* 2016;30:P773–80.

154. Cotogni P, Barbero C, Rinaldi M. Deep sternal wound infection after cardiac surgery: evidences and controversies. *World J Crit Care Med* 2015;4:265–73.

155. Buja A, Zampieron A, Cavalet S, et al. An update review on risk factors and scales for prediction of deep sternal wound infections. *Int Wound J* 2012;9:372–86.

156. Sharif M, Wong CHM, Harky A. Sternal wound infections, risk factors and management: how far are we? A literature review. *Heart Lung Circ* 2019;28:835–43.

157. Kaul P. Sternal reconstruction after post-sternotomy mediastinitis. *J Cardiothorac Surg* 2017;12:94.

158. Engelman DT, Adams DH, Byrne JG, et al. Impact of body mass index and albumin on morbidity and mortality after cardiac surgery. *J Thorac Cardiovasc Surg* 1999;118:866–73.

159. Biancaro F, Giordano S. Glycated hemoglobin and the risk of sternal wound infection after adult cardiac surgery: a systematic review and meta-analysis. *Semin Thorac Cardiovasc Surg* 2019;31:465–7.

160. Kim HJ, Shim JK, Youn YN, Song JW, Lee H, Kwak JL. Influence of preoperative hemoglobin A1c on early outcomes in patients with diabetes mellitus undergoing off-pump coronary artery bypass surgery. *J Thorac Cardiovasc Surg* 2020;159:568–76.

161. Swenne CL, Lindholm C, Borowiec J, Schnell AE, Carlsson M. Peri-operative glucose control and development of surgical wound infections in patients undergoing coronary artery bypass graft. *J Hosp Infect* 2005;61:201–12.

162. Nagachinta T, Stephens M, Reitz B, Polk BF. Risk factors for surgical wound infections following cardiac surgery. *J Infect Dis* 1987;156:967–73.

163. Zhou P, Zhu P, Nie Z, Zheng S. Is the era of bilateral internal thoracic artery grafting coming for diabetic patients? An updated meta-analysis. *J Thorac Cardiovasc Surg* 2019;158:1559–70.

164. Steingrímsson S, Gustafsson R, Gudbjartsson T, Mokhtari A, Ingemansson R, Sjögren J. Sterno-cutaneous fistulas after cardiac surgery: incidence and late outcome during a ten-year follow-up. *Ann Thorac Surg* 2009;88:1910–5.

165. Allen KB, Yuh DD, Schwartz SB, et al. Nontuberculous mycobacterium infections associated with heater-cooler devices. *Ann Thorac Surg* 2017;104:1237–42.

166. Lazar HL, Vander Salm T, Engelman R, Orgill D, Gordon S. Prevention and management of sternal wound infections. *J Thorac Cardiovasc Surg* 2016;152:962–72.

167. Hawkins RB, Mehaffey JH, Charles EJ, et al. Cost-effectiveness of negative pressure incision management system in cardiac surgery. *J Surg Res* 2019;240:227–35.

168. Sharif-Kashani B, Shahabi P, Mandegar MH, et al. Smoking and wound complications after coronary artery bypass grafting. *J Surg Res* 2016;200:732–8.

169. Hong JC, Saraswat MK, Ellison TA. *Staphylococcus aureus* prevention strategies in cardiac surgery: a cost-effectiveness analysis. *Ann Thorac Surg* 2018;105:47–53.

170. Darouiche RO, Wall MJ Jr, Itani KMF, et al. Chlorhexidine-alcohol versus povidone-iodine for surgical-site antisepsis. *N Engl J Med* 2010;362:18–26.

171. Dumville JC, McFarlane E, Edwards P, Lipp A, Holmes A, Liu Z. Preoperative skin antiseptics for preventing surgical wound infections after clean surgery. *Cochrane Database Syst Rev* 2015;21:CD003949. https://doi.org/10.1002/14651858.CD003949.pub3.

172. Raja SG, Rochon M, Mullins C, et al. Impact of choice of skin preparation solution in cardiac surgery on rate of surgical site infection: a propensity score matched analysis. *J Infect Prev* 2018;19:16–21.

173. Kühme T, Isaksson B, Dahlin LG. Wound contamination in cardiac surgery. A systematic quantitative and qualitative study of the bacterial growth in sternal wounds in cardiac surgery patients. *APMIS* 2007;115:1001–7.

174. Dohmen PM, Gabbieri D, Weymann A, Linneweber J, Geyer T, Konertz W. A retrospective nonrandomized study on the impact of INTEGUSEAL, a preoperative microbial skin sealant, on the rate of surgical site infections after cardiac surgery. *Int J Infect Dis* 2011;15:e395–400.

175. Waldow T, Szlapka M, Hensel J, Plötze K, Matschke K, Jatzwauk L. Skin sealant InteguSeal® has no impact on prevention of postoperative mediastinitis after cardiac surgery. *J Hosp Infect* 2012;81:278–82.

176. Konishi Y, Fukunaga N, Abe T, Nakamura K, Usui A, Koyama T. Efficacy of new multimodal preventive measures for post-operative deep sternal wound infection. *Gen Thorac Cardiovasc Surg* 2019;67:934–40.

177. Bejko J, Tarzia V, Carrozzini M, et al. Comparison of efficacy and cost of iodine impregnated drape vs. standard drape in cardiac surgery: study in 5100 patients. *J Cardiovasc Transl Res* 2015;8:431–7.

178. Vos RJ, Van Putte BP, Kloppenburg GTL. Prevention of deep sternal wound infection in cardiac surgery: a literature review. *J Hosp Infect* 2018;100:411–20.

179. Allen KB, Icke KJ, Thourani VH, et al. Sternotomy closure using rigid plate fixation: a paradigm shift from wire cerclage. *Ann Cardiothorac Surg* 2018;7:611–20.

180. Tam DY, Nedadur R, Yu M, Yanagawa B, Fremes SE, Friedrich JO. Rigid plate fixation versus wire cerclage for sternotomy after cardiac surgery: a meta-analysis. *Ann Thorac Surg* 2016;106:298–304.

181. Cataneo DC, Dos Reis TA, Felisberto G, Rodrigues OR, Cataneo AJM. New sternal closure methods versus the standard closure method: systematic review and meta-analysis. *Interact Cardiovasc Thorac Surg* 2019;28:432–40.

182. Marzouk M, Mohammadi S, Baillot B, Kalavrouziotis D. Rigid primary sternal fixation reduces sternal complications among patients at risk. *Ann Thorac Surg* 2019;108:737–43.

183. Zelenitsky SA, Calic D, Arora RC, et al. Antimicrobial prophylaxis for patients undergoing cardiac surgery: intraoperative cefazolin concentrations and sternal wound infections. *Antimicrob Agents Chemother* 2018;62:e01360–18.

184. Chan JL, Diaconescu AC, Horvath KA. Routine use of topical bacitracin to prevent sternal wound infections after cardiac surgery. *Ann Thorac Surg* 2017;104:1496–1500.

185. Vermeer H, Aalders-Bouhuijs SSF, Steinfelder-Visscher J, van der Heide SM, Morshuis WJ. Platelet-leukocyte rich gel application in the prevention of deep sternal wound problems after cardiac surgery in obese diabetic patients. *J Thorac Dis* 2019;11:1124–9.

186. Godbole G, Pai V, Kolvekar S, Wilson AP. Use of gentamicin-collagen sponges in closure of sternal wounds in cardiothoracic surgery to reduce wound infections. *Interact Cardiovasc Thorac Surg* 2012;14:390–4.

187. Sahin M. The role of topical Genta Fleece HD and gentamicin spray in prevention of sternum wound infections after open heart surgery: a comparative study. *Arch Med Sci Atheroscler Dis* 2018;3:e29–34.

188. Kowalewski M, Pawliszak W, Zaborowska K, et al. Gentamicin-collagen sponge reduces the risk of sternal wound infections following heart surgery: meta-analysis. *J Thorac Cardiovasc Surg* 2015;149:1631–40.

189. Lander HL, Ejiofor JI, McGurk S, Tsuyoshi K, Shekar P, Body SC. Vancomycin paste does not reduce the incidence of deep sternal wound infection after cardiac operations. *Ann Thorac Surg* 2017;103:497–503.

190. Ruggieri VG, Olivier ME, Aludaat C, et al. Negative pressure versus conventional sternal wound dressing in coronary surgery using bilateral internal mammary artery grafts. *Heart Surg Forum* 2019;22:E092–6.

191. Horvath KA, Acker MA, Chang H, et al. Blood transfusion and infection after cardiac surgery. *Ann Thorac Surg* 2013;95:2194–201.

192. El Oakley RM, Wright JE. Postoperative mediastinitis: classification and management. *Ann Thorac Surg* 1996;61:1030–6.

193. Jones G, Jurkiewicz MJ, Bostwick J, et al. Management of the infected median sternotomy wound with muscle flaps: the Emory 20-year experience. *Ann Surg* 1997;225:766–76.

194. Greig AV, Geh JL, Khanduja V, Shibu M. Choice of flap for the management of deep sternal wound infection: an anatomical classification. *Plast Reconst Aesthet Surg* 2007;60:372–8.

195. Benlolo S, Matéo J, Raskine L, et al. Sternal puncture allows an early diagnosis of poststernotomy mediastinitis. *J Thorac Cardiovasc Surg* 2003;125:611–7.

196. Misawa Y, Fuse K, Hasegawa T. Infectious mediastinitis after cardiac operations: computed tomographic findings. *Ann Thorac Surg* 1998;65:622–4.

197. Bitkover CY, Gårdlund B, Larsson SA, Åberg B, Jacobsson H. Diagnosing sternal wound infections with 99mTc-labeled monoclonal granulocyte antibody scintigraphy. *Ann Thorac Surg* 1996;62:1412–6.

198. Oates E, Payne DD. Postoperative cardiothoracic infection: diagnostic value of indium-111 white blood cell imaging. *Ann Thorac Surg* 1994;58:1442–6.

199. Zhang R, Feng Z, Zhang Y, Tan H, Wang J, Qi F. Diagnostic value of fluorine-18 deoxyglucose positron emission tomography/computed tomography in deep sternal wound infection. *J Plast Reconstr Aesthet Surg* 2018;71:1768–76.

200. Gudbjartsson T, Jeppsson A, Sjögren J, et al. Sternal wound infections following open heart surgery: a review. *Scand Cardiovasc J* 2016;50:341–8.

201. Douville EC, Asaph JW, Dworkin RJ, et al. Sternal preservation: a better way to treat most sternal wound complications after cardiac surgery. *Ann Thorac Surg* 2004;78:1659–64.

202. Shrager JB, Wain JC, Wright CD, et al. Omentum is highly effective in the management of complex cardiothoracic surgical problems. *J Thorac Cardiovasc Surg* 2003;125:526–32.

203. Berg HF, Brands WGB, van Geldorp TR, Kluytmans-VandenBergh MFQ, Kluytmans JAJW. Comparison between closed drainage techniques for the treatment of postoperative mediastinitis. *Ann Thorac Surg* 2000;70:924–9.

204. Deschka H, Erler S, El-Ayoubi L, Vogel C, Vöhringer L, Wimmer-Greinecker G. Suction-irrigation drainage: an underestimated therapeutic option for surgical treatment of deep sternal wound infections. *Interact Cardiovasc Thorac Surg* 2013;17:85–9.

205. Tewarie L, Moza AK, Khattab MA, Autschbach R, Zayat R. Effective combination of different surgical strategies for deep sternal wound infection and mediastinitis. *Ann Thorac Cardiovasc Surg* 2019;25:102–10.

206. Cartier R, Diaz OS, Carrier M, Leclerc Y, Castonguay Y, Leung TK. Right ventricular rupture: a complication of postoperative mediastinitis. *J Thorac Cardiovasc Surg* 1993;106:1036–9.

207. Bota O, Josten C, Borger MA, Spindler N, Langer S. Standardized musculocutaneous flap for the coverage of deep sternal wounds after cardiac surgery. *Ann Thorac Surg* 2019;107:802–8.

208. Simek M, Chudoba A, Hajek R, Tobbia P, Molitor M, Nemec P. From open packing to negative wound pressure therapy: a critical overview of deep sternal wound infection treatment strategies after cardiac surgery. *Biomed Pap Med Fac Univ Palacky Olomouc Czech Repub* 2018;162:263–71.

209. Sartipy U, Lockowandt U, Gäbel J, Jidéus L, Dellgren G. Cardiac rupture during vacuum-assisted closure therapy. *Ann Thorac Surg* 2006;82:1110–1.

210. Immer FF, Durrer M, Mühlemann KS, Erni D, Gahl B, Carrel TP. Deep sternal wound infection after cardiac surgery: modality of treatment and outcome. *Ann Thorac Surg* 2005;80:957–61.

211. Lu JC, Grayson AD, Jha P, Srinivasan AK, Fabri BM. Risk factors for sternal wound infection and mid-term survival following coronary artery bypass surgery. *Eur J Cardiothorac Surg* 2003;23:943–9.

212. Toumpoulis IK, Anagnostopoulos CE, DeRose JJ Jr, Swistel DG. The impact of deep sternal wound infection on long-term survival after coronary artery bypass grafting. *Chest* 2005;127:464–71.

213. Reed JF III. Leg wound infections following greater saphenous vein harvesting: minimally invasive vein harvesting versus conventional vein harvesting. *Int J Low Extrem Wounds* 2008;7:210–9.

214. Allen KB, Fitzgerald EB, Heimansohn DA, Shaar CJ. Management of closed space infections associated with endoscopic vein harvest. *Ann Thorac Surg* 2000;69:960–1.

215. Wilson W, Taubert KA, Gewitz M, et al. Prevention of infective endocarditis: guidelines from the American Heart Association: a guideline from the American Heart Association Rheumatic Fever,

Endocarditis, and Kawasaki Disease Committee, Council on Cardiovascular Disease in the Young, and the Council on Clinical Cardiology, Council on Cardiovascular Surgery and Anesthesia, and the Quality of Care and Outcomes Research Interdisciplinary Working Group. *Circulation* 2007;116:1736–54 (available at www.acc.org).

216. Sedraykan A, Wu AW, Parashar A, Bass EB, Treasure T. Off-pump surgery is associated with reduced occurrence of stroke and other morbidity as compared with traditional coronary artery bypass grafting: a meta-analysis of systematically reviewed trials. *Stroke* 2006;37:2759–69.

217. Lamy A, Devereaux PJ, Prabhakaran D, et al. Effects of off-pump and on-pump coronary-artery bypass grafting at 1 year. *N Engl J Med* 2013;368:1179–88.

218. Marasco SF, Sharwood LN, Abramson MJ. No improvement in neurocognitive outcomes after off-pump versus on-pump coronary revascularisation: a meta-analysis. *Eur J Cardiothorac Surg* 2008;33:961–70.

219. Dominici C, Salsano A, Nenna A, et al. Neurological outcomes after on-pump vs off-pump CABG in patients with cerebrovascular disease. *J Card Surg* 2019;34:941–7.

220. Newman MF, Mathew JP, Grocott HP, et al. Central nervous system injury associated with cardiac surgery. *Lancet* 2006;368:694–703.

221. Filsoufi F, Rahmanian PB, Castillo JG, Bronster D, Adams DH. Incidence, topography, predictors and long-term survival after stroke in patients undergoing coronary artery bypass grafting. *Ann Thorac Surg* 2008;85:862–71.

222. Bucerius J, Gummert JF, Borger MA, et al. Stroke after cardiac surgery: a risk factor analysis of 16,184 consecutive adult patients. *Ann Thorac Surg* 2003;75:472–8.

223. Likosky DS, Leavitt BJ, Marrin CAS, et al. Intra- and postoperative predictors of stroke after coronary artery bypass grafting. *Ann Thorac Surg* 2003;76:428–35.

224. Baker RA, Hallsworth LJ, Knight JL. Stroke after coronary artery bypass grafting. *Ann Thorac Surg* 2005;80:1746–50.

225. Redmond JM, Greene PS, Goldsborough MA, et al. Neurologic injury in cardiac surgical patients with a history of stroke. *Ann Thorac Surg* 1996;61:42–7.

226. Mérie C, Køber L, Olsen PS, Andersson C, Jensen JS, Torp-Pedersen C. Risk of stroke after coronary artery bypass grafting: effect of age and comorbidities. *Stroke* 2012;43:38–43.

227. Maekawa K, Goto T, Baba T, Yoshitake A, Morishita S, Koshiji T. Abnormalities in the brain before elective cardiac surgery detected by diffusion-weighted magnetic resonance imaging. *Ann Thorac Surg* 2008;86:1563–9.

228. Goto T, Baba T, Honma K, et al. Magnetic resonance imaging findings and postoperative neurologic dysfunction in elderly patients undergoing coronary artery bypass grafting. *Ann Thorac Surg* 2001;72:137–42.

229. Ito A, Goto T, Maekawa K, Baba T, Mishima Y, Ushijima K. Postoperative neurological complications and risk factors for pre-existing silent brain infarction in elderly patients undergoing coronary artery bypass grafting. *J Anesth* 2012;26:405–11.

230. Goto T, Yoshitake A, Baba T, Shibata Y, Sakata R, Ouzumi H. Cerebral ischemic disorders and cerebral oxygen balance during cardiopulmonary bypass: preoperative evaluation using magnetic resonance imaging and angiography. *Anesth Analg* 1997;84:5–11.

231. Knipp SC, Matatko N, Wilhelm H, et al. Evaluation of brain injury after coronary artery bypass grafting: a prospective study using neuropsychological assessment and diffusion-weighted magnetic resonance imaging. *Eur J Cardiothorac Surg* 2004;25:791–800.

232. Raffa GM, Agnello F, Occhipinti G, et al. Neurological complications after cardiac surgery: a retrospective case-control study of risk factors and outcomes. *J Cardiothorac Surg* 2019;14:23.

233. Lee EJ, Choi KH, Ryu JS, et al. Stroke risk after coronary artery bypass graft surgery and extent of cerebral artery atherosclerosis. *J Am Coll Cardiol* 2011;57:1811–8.

234. van der Linden J, Hadjinikolaou L, Bergman P, Lindblom D. Postoperative stroke in cardiac surgery is related to the location and extent of atherosclerotic disease in the ascending aorta. *J Am Coll Cardiol* 2001;38:131–5.

235. Goto T, Baba T, Matsuyma K, Honma K, Ura M, Koshiji T. Aortic atherosclerosis and postoperative neurologic dysfunction in elderly coronary surgical patients. *Ann Thorac Surg* 2003;75:1912–8.

236. McDonagh DL, Berger M, Mathew JP, Graffagnino C, Milano CA, Newman MF. Neurologic complications of cardiac surgery. *Lancet Neurol* 2014;13:490–502.

237. Boivie P, Edström C, Engström KG. Side differences in cerebrovascular accidents after cardiac surgery: a statistical analysis of neurologic symptoms and possible implications for anatomic mechanisms of aortic particle embolization. *J Thorac Cardiovasc Surg* 2005;129:591–8.

238. Kapetanakis EI, Stamou SC, Dullum MKC, et al. The impact of aortic manipulation on neurologic outcomes after coronary artery bypass surgery: a risk-adjusted study. *Ann Thorac Surg* 2004;78:1564–71.

239. Zhao DF, Edelman JJ, Seco M, et al. Coronary artery bypass grafting with and without manipulation of the ascending aorta: a network meta-analysis. *J Am Coll Cardiol* 2017;69:924–36.

240. Clark RE, Brillman J, Davis DA, Lovell MR, Price TR, Magovern GJ. Microemboli during coronary artery bypass grafting: genesis and effect on outcome. *J Thorac Cardiovasc Surg* 1995;109:249–57.

241. Mirow N, Zittermann A, Körperich H, et al. Diffusion-weighted magnetic resonance imaging for the detection of ischemic brain lesions in coronary artery bypass graft surgery: relation to extracorporeal circulation and heparinization. *J Cardiovasc Surg (Torino)* 2011;52:117–26.

242. Sungurtekin H, Boston US, Orszulak TA, Cook DJ. Effect of cerebral embolization on regional autoregulation during cardiopulmonary bypass in dogs. *Ann Thorac Surg* 2000;69:1130–4.

243. Gold JP, Charlson ME, Williams-Russo P, et al. Improvement of outcomes after coronary artery bypass: a randomized trial comparing intraoperative high versus low mean arterial pressure. *J Thorac Cardiovasc Surg* 1995;110:1302–11.

244. Gottesman RF, Sherman PM, Grega MA, et al. Watershed strokes after cardiac surgery: diagnosis, etiology, and outcome. *Stroke* 2006;37:2306–11.

245. Naylor AR, Bown MJ. Stroke after cardiac surgery and its association with asymptomatic carotid disease: an updated systematic review and meta-analysis. *Eur J Vasc Endovasc Surg* 2011;41:607–24.

246. Karkouti K, Djaiani G, Borger MA, et al. Low hematocrit during cardiopulmonary bypass is associated with increased risk of perioperative stroke in cardiac surgery. *Ann Thorac Surg* 2005;80:1381–7.

247. Filsoufi F, Rahmanian PB, Castillo JG, Bronster D, Adams DH. Incidence, imaging analysis, and early and late outcomes of stroke after cardiac valve operation. *Am J Cardiol* 2008;101:1472–8.

248. Hogue CW Jr, Murphy SF, Schechtman KB, Dávila Román VG. Risk factors for early or delayed stroke after cardiac surgery. *Circulation* 1999;100:642–7.

249. Hedberg M, Boivie P, Engström KG. Early and delayed stroke after coronary surgery: an analysis of risk factors and the impact on short- and long-term survival. *Eur J Cardiothorac Surg* 2011;40:379–87.

250. Lisle TC, Barrett KM, Gazoni LM, et al. Timing of stroke after cardiopulmonary bypass determines mortality. *Ann Thorac Surg* 2008;85:1556–63.

251. Gaudino M, Rahouma M, Di Mauro M, et al. Early versus delayed stroke after cardiac surgery: a systematic review and meta-analysis. *J Am Heart Assoc* 2019;8(13):e012447.

252. Sun X, Lindsay J, Monsein LH, Hill PC, Corso PJ. Silent brain injury after cardiac surgery: a review. *J Am Coll Cardiol* 2012;60:791–7.

253. Pagnesi M, Martino EA, Chiarito M, et al. Silent cerebral injury after transcatheter aortic valve implantation and the preventive role of embolic protection devices: a systematic review and meta-analysis. *Int J Cardiol* 2016;221:97–106.

254. Samim M, Hendrikse J, van der Worp HB, et al. Silent ischemic brain lesions after transcatheter aortic valve replacement: lesion distribution and predictors. *Clin Res Cardiol* 2015;104:430–8.

255. Kalyani SD, Miller NR, Dong LM, Baumgartner WA, Alejo DE, Gilbert TB. Incidence of and risk factors for perioperative optic neuropathy after cardiac surgery. *Ann Thorac Surg* 2004;78:34–7.

256. Barbut D, Grassineau D, Lis E, Heier L, Hartman GS, Isom OW. Posterior distribution of infarcts in strokes related to cardiac operations. *Ann Thorac Surg* 1998;65:1656–9.

257. Zacharias A, Schwann TA, Riordan CJ, et al. Operative and 5-year outcomes of combined carotid and coronary revascularization: review of a large contemporary experience. *Ann Thorac Surg* 2002;73:491–8.

258. Gopaldas RR, Chu D, Dao TK, et al. Staged versus synchronous carotid endarterectomy and coronary artery bypass grafting: analysis of 10-year nationwide outcomes. *Ann Thorac Surg* 2011;91:1323–9.

259. Mangano DT. Multicenter Study of Perioperative Ischemia Research Group: aspirin and mortality from coronary bypass surgery. *N Engl J Med* 2002;347:1309–17.

260. Katznelson R, Djaiani GM, Borger MA, et al. Preoperative use of statins is associated with reduced early delirium rates after cardiac surgery. *Anesthesiology* 2009;110:67–73.

261. Kuhn EW, Liakopoulos OJ, Stange S, et al. Preoperative statin therapy in cardiac surgery: a meta-analysis of 90,000 patients. *Eur J Cardiothorac Surg* 2014;45:17–26.

262. Zingone B, Rauber E, Gatti G, et al. The impact of epiaortic ultrasonographic scanning on the risk of perioperative stroke. *Eur J Cardiothorac Surg* 2006;29:720–8.

263. Rosenberger P, Shernan SK, Löffler M, et al. The influence of epiaortic ultrasonography on intraoperative surgical management in 6051 cardiac surgical patients. *Ann Thorac Surg* 2008;85:548–53.

264. Schachner T, Nagele G, Kacani A, Laufer G, Bonatti J. Factors associated with presence of ascending aortic atherosclerosis in CABG patients. *Ann Thorac Surg* 2004;78:2028–32.

265. Slater JP, Guarino T, Stack J, et al. Cerebral oxygen desaturation predicts cognitive decline and longer hospital stay after cardiac surgery. *Ann Thorac Surg* 2009;87:36–44.

266. Murkin JM, Adams SJ, Novick RJ, et al. Monitoring brain oxygen saturation during coronary bypass surgery: a randomized prospective study. *Anesth Analg* 2007;104:51–8.

267. Zorrilla-Vaca A, Healy R, Grant MC, et al. Intraoperative cerebral oximetry-based management for optimizing perioperative outcomes: a meta-analysis of randomized controlled trials. *Can J Anaesth* 2018;65:529–42.

268. Ono M, Brady K, Easley RB, et al. Duration and magnitude of blood pressure below cerebral autoregulation threshold during cardiopulmonary bypass is associated with major morbidity and operative mortality. *J Thorac Cardiovasc Surg* 2014;147:483–9.

269. Hori D, Nomura Y, Ono M, et al. Optimal blood pressure during cardiopulmonary bypass defined by cerebral autoregulation monitoring. *J Thorac Cardiovasc Surg* 2017;154:1590–8.

270. Hammon JW, Stump DA, Butterworth JR, et al. Coronary artery bypass grafting with single cross-clamp results in fewer persistent neuropsychological deficits than multiple clamp or off-pump coronary artery bypass grafting. *Ann Thorac Surg* 2007;84:1174–8.

271. Puskas F, Grocott HP, White WD, Mathew JP, Newman MF, Bar-Yosef S. Intraoperative hyperglycemia and cognitive decline after CABG. *Ann Thorac Surg* 2007;84:1467–73.

272. Gandhi GY, Nuttall GA, Abel MD, et al. Intensive intraoperative insulin therapy versus conventional glucose management during cardiac surgery: a randomized trial. *Ann Intern Med* 2007;146:233–43.

273. Engelman R, Baker RA, Likosky DS, et al. The Society of Thoracic Surgeons, the Society of Cardiovascular Anesthesiologists, and the American Society of ExtraCorporeal Technology: clinical practice guidelines for cardiopulmonary bypass: temperature management during cardiopulmonary bypass. *Ann Thorac Surg* 2015;100:748–57.

274. Mathew JP, Mackensen G, Phillips-Bute B, et al. Effects of extreme hemodilution during cardiac surgery on cognitive function in the elderly. *Anesthesiology* 2007;107:577–84.

275. Martens S, Neumann K, Sodemann C, Deschka H, Wimmer-Greinecker G, Moritz A. Carbon dioxide field flooding reduces neurologic impairment after open heart surgery. *Ann Thorac Surg* 2008;85:543–7.

276. Arsenault KA, Yusuf AM, Crystal E, et al. Interventions for preventing postoperative atrial fibrillation in patients undergoing heart surgery. *Cochrane Database Syst Rev* 2013;(1):CD003611. https://doi.org/10.1002/14651858.CD003611.pub3.

277. Kapadia SR, Kodali S, Makkar R, et al. Protection against cerebral embolism during transcatheter aortic valve replacement. *J Am Coll Cardiol* 2017;69:367–77.

278. Bagur R, Solo K, Alghofaili S, et al. Cerebral embolic protection devices during transcatheter aortic valve implantation: systematic review and meta-analysis. *Stroke* 2017;48:1306–15.

279. Beaty CA, Arnaoutakis GJ, Grega MA, et al. The role of head computed tomography imaging in the evaluation of postoperative neurologic deficits in cardiac surgery patients. *Ann Thorac Surg* 2013;95:548–54.

280. Okada N, Oshima H, Narita Y, et al. Impact of surgical stroke on the early and late outcomes after thoracic aortic operations. *Ann Thorac Surg* 2015;99:2017–23.

281. Salazar JD, Wityk RJ, Grega MA, et al. Stroke after cardiac surgery: short- and long-term outcomes. *Ann Thorac Surg* 2001;72:1195–201.

282. Dacey LJ, Likosky DS, Leavitt BJ, et al. Perioperative stroke and long-term survival after coronary bypass graft surgery. *Ann Thorac Surg* 2005;79:532–7.

283. Koster S, Hensens AG, Schuurmans MJ, van der Palen J. Prediction of delirium after cardiac surgery and the use of a risk checklist. *Eur J Cardiovasc Nurs* 2013;12:284–92.

284. Rudolph JL, Jones RN, Levkoff SE, et al. Derivation and validation of a preoperative prediction rule for delirium after cardiac surgery. *Circulation* 2009;119:229–36.

285. Bakker RC, Osse RJ, Tulen JH, Kappetein AP, Bogers AJ. Preoperative and operative predictors of delirium after cardiac surgery in elderly patients. *Eur J Cardiothorac Surg* 2012;41:544–9.

286. Tse L, Schwarz SK, Bowering JB, Moore RL, Barr AM. Incidence of and risk factors for delirium after cardiac surgery at a quaternary care center: a retrospective cohort study. *J Cardiothorac Vasc Anesth* 2015;29:1472–9.

287. Omiya H, Yoshitani K, Yamada N, et al. Preoperative brain magnetic resonance imaging and postoperative delirium after off-pump coronary artery bypass grafting: a prospective cohort study. *Can J Anaesth* 2015;62:595–602.

288. Otomo S, Maekawa K, Goto T, Baba T, Yoshitake A. Pre-existing cerebral infarcts as a risk factor for delirium after coronary artery bypass graft surgery. *Interact Cardiovasc Thorac Surg* 2013;17:799–804.

289. Rudoph JL, Babikian VL, Treanor P, et al. Microemboli are not associated with delirium after coronary artery bypass graft surgery. *Perfusion* 2009;24:409–15.

290. O'Neal J, Shaw AD. Predicting, preventing, and identifying delirium after cardiac surgery. *Perioperative Medicine* 2016;5:7.

291. Bucerius J, Gummert JF, Borger MA, et al. Predictors of delirium after cardiac surgery: effect of beating-heart (off-pump) surgery. *J Thorac Cardiovasc Surg* 2004;127:57–64.

292. Tse L, Schwarz SK, Bowering JB, Moore RL, et al. Pharmacological risk factors for delirium after cardiac surgery: a review. *Curr Neuropharmacol* 2012;10:181–96.

293. Kotfis K, Szylińska A, Listewnik M, et al. Early delirium after cardiac surgery: an analysis of incidence and risk factors in elderly (≥65 years) and very elderly (≥80 years) patients. *Clin Interv Aging* 2018;13:1061–70.

294. Rudoph JL, Jones RN, Grande LJ, et al. Impaired executive function is associated with delirium after coronary artery bypass grafting. *J Am Geriatr Soc* 2006;54:937–41.

295. Hogan AM, Shipolini A, Brown MM, Hurley R, Cormack F. Fixing hearts and protecting minds: a review of the multiple, interacting factors influencing cognitive function after coronary artery bypass graft surgery. *Circulation* 2013;128:162–71.

296. Evans AS, Weiner MM, Arora RC, et al. Current approach to diagnosis and treatment of delirium after cardiac surgery. *Ann Cardiac Anaesth* 2016;19:328–37.

297. Ely EW, Inouye SK, Bernard GR, et al. Delirium in mechanically ventilated patients: validity and reliability of the confusion assessment method for the intensive care unit (CAM-ICU). *JAMA* 2001;286:2703–10.

298. Bergeron N, Dubois MJ, Dumont M, Dial S, Skrobik Y. Intensive care delirium screening checklist: evaluation of a new screening tool. *Intensive Care Med* 2001;27:859–64.

299. Ibrahim K, McCarthy CP, McCarthy KJ, et al. Delirium in the cardiac intensive care unit. *J Am Heart Assoc* 2018;16;7:e008568.

300. Skrobik YK, Bergeron N, Dumont M, Gottfried SB. Olanzapine vs haloperidol: treating delirium in a critical care setting. *Intensive Care Med* 2004;30:444–9.

301. Riker RR, Shehabi Y, Bokesch PM, et al. Dexmedetomidine vs midazolam for sedation in critically ill patients: a randomized trial. *JAMA* 2009;301:489–99.

302. Maldonado JR, Wysong A, van der Starre PF, Block T, Miller C, Reitz BA. Dexmedetomidine and the reduction of postoperative delirium after cardiac surgery. *Psychosomatics* 2009;50:206–17.

303. Reade MC, O'Sullivan K, Bates S, Goldsmith D, Ainslie WR, Bellomo R. Dexmedetomidine vs. haloperidol in delirious, agitated, intubated patients: a randomised open-label trial. *Crit Care* 2009;13:R75.

304. Tao R, Wang XW, Pang LJ, et al. Pharmacologic prevention of postoperative delirium after on-pump cardiac surgery: a meta-analysis of randomized trials. *Medicine (Baltimore)* 2018;97(43):e12771.

305. Boettger S, Jenewein J, Breitbart W. Haloperidol, risperidone, olanzapine, and aripiprazole in the management of delirium; a comparison of efficacy, safety, and side effects. *Palliat Support Care* 2015;13:1079–85.

306. Marcantonio ER. Delirium in hospitalized older adults. *N Engl J Med* 2017;377:1456–66.

307. Hassaballa HA, Balk RA. Torsade de pointes associated with the administration of intravenous haloperidol: a review of the literature and practical guidelines for use. *Expert Opin Drug Saf* 2003;2:543–7.

308. Tagarakis GI, Voucharas C, Tsolaki F, et al. Ondasetron versus haloperidol for the treatment of postcardiotomy delirium: a prospective, randomized, double-blinded study. *J Cardiothorac Surg* 2012;7:25.

309. Prakanrattana U, Prapaitrakool S. Efficacy of risperidone for prevention of postoperative delirium in cardiac surgery. *Anaesth Intensive Care* 2007;35:714–9.

310. Hakim SM, Othman AI, Naoum DO. Early treatment with risperidone for subsyndromal delirium after on-pump cardiac surgery in the elderly: a randomized trial. *Anesthesiology* 2012;116:987–97.

311. Kosten TR, O'Connor PG. Management of drug and alcohol withdrawal. *N Engl J Med* 2003;348:1786–95.

312. Saczynski JS, Marcantonio ER, Quach L, et al. Cognitive trajectories after postoperative delirium. *N Engl J Med* 2012;367:30–9.

313. Crocker E, Beggs T, Hassan A, et al. Long-term effects of postoperative delirium in patients undergoing cardiac operation: a systematic review. *Ann Thorac Surg* 2016;102:1391–9.

314. Koster S, Hensens AG, Schuurmans MJ, van der Palen J. Consequences of delirium after cardiac operations. *Ann Thorac Surg* 2012;93.705–11.

315. Martin BJ, Buth KR, Arora RC, Baskett RJ. Delirium: a cause for concern beyond the immediate postoperative period. *Ann Thorac Surg* 2012;93:1114–20.

316. Newman MF, Kirschner JL, Phillips-Bute B, et al. Longitudinal assessment of neurocognitive function after coronary-artery bypass surgery. *N Engl J Med* 2001;344:395–402.

317. Barber PA, Hach S, Tippett LJ, Ross L, Merry AF, Milsom P. Cerebral ischemic lesions on diffusion-weighted imaging are associated with neurocognitive decline after cardiac surgery. *Stroke* 2008;39:1427–33.

318. Greaves D, Psaltis PJ, Ross TJ, et al. Cognitive outcomes following coronary artery bypass grafting: a systematic review and meta-analysis of 91,829 patients. *Int J Cardiol* 2019;289:43–8.

319. Hernandez F Jr, Brown JR, Likosky DS, et al. Neurocognitive outcomes of off-pump versus on-pump coronary artery bypass: a prospective randomized controlled trial. *Ann Thorac Surg* 2007;84:1897–903.

320. Ernest CS, Worcester MU, Tatoulis J, et al. Neurocognitive outcomes in off-pump versus on-pump bypass surgery: a randomized controlled trial. *Ann Thorac Surg* 2006;81:2105–14.

321. Jensen BØ, Rasmussen LS, Steinbrüchel DA. Cognitive outcomes in elderly high-risk patients 1 year after off-pump versus on-pump coronary artery bypass grafting. A randomized trial. *Eur J Cardiothorac Surg* 2008;34:1016–21.

322. van Dijk D, Spoor M, Hijman R, et al. Cognitive and cardiac outcomes 5 years after off-pump vs on-pump coronary artery bypass graft surgery. *JAMA* 2007;297:701–8.

323. Sun JH, Wu XY, Wang WJ, Jin LL. Cognitive dysfunction after off-pump versus on-pump coronary artery bypass surgery: a meta-analysis. *J Int Med Res* 2012;40:852–8.

324. Selnes OA, Grega MA, Bailey MM, et al. Do management strategies for coronary artery disease influence 6-year cognitive outcomes? *Ann Thorac Surg* 2009;88:445–54.

325. McKhann GM, Selnes OA, Grega MA, et al. Subjective memory symptoms in surgical and nonsurgical coronary artery patients: 6-year follow-up. *Ann Thorac Surg* 2009;87:27–35.

326. Sauër AMC, Nathoe HM, Hendrikse J, et al. Cognitive outcomes 7.5 years after angioplasty compared with off-pump coronary bypass surgery. *Ann Thorac Surg* 2013;96:1294–1300.

327. Ho PM, Arciniegas DB, Grigsby J, et al. Predictors of cognitive decline following coronary artery bypass graft surgery. *Ann Thorac Surg* 2004;77:597–603.

328. Bar-Yosef S, Anders M, Mackensen GB, et al. Aortic atheroma burden and cognitive dysfunction after coronary artery bypass graft surgery. *Ann Thorac Surg* 2004;78:1556–63.

329. Evered LA, Silbert BS, Scott DA. Postoperative cognitive dysfunction and aortic atheroma. *Ann Thorac Surg* 2010;89:1091–7.

330. Hogue CW Jr, Hershey T, Dixon D, et al. Preexisting cognitive impairment in women before cardiac surgery and its relationship to C-reactive protein concentrations. *Anesth Analg* 2006;102:1602–8.

331. Silbert BS, Scott DA, Evered LA, Lewis MS, Maruff PT. Preexisting cognitive impairment in patients scheduled for elective coronary artery bypass graft surgery. *Anesth Analg* 2007;104:1023–8.

332. Nah HW, Lee JW, Chung CH, et al. New brain infarcts on magnetic resonance imaging after coronary artery bypass graft surgery: lesion patterns, mechanism, and predictors. *Ann Neurol* 2014;76:347–55.

333. Knipp SC, Matako M, Wilhelm H, et al. Cognitive outcomes three years after coronary artery bypass surgery: relation to diffuse-weighed magnetic resonance imaging. *Ann Thorac Surg* 2008;85:872–9.

334. Baumgartner WA. Neurocognitive changes after coronary bypass surgery. *Circulation* 2007;116: 1879–81.

335. Patel N, Minhas JS, Chung EM. Intraoperative embolization and cognitive decline after cardiac surgery: a systematic review. *Semin Cardiotharc Vasc Anesth* 2016;20:225–31.

336. Kruis RW, Vlasveld FA, Van Dijk D. The (un)importance of cerebral microemboli. *Semin Cardiothorac Vasc Anesth* 2010;14;111–8.

337. Motallebzadeh R, Bland JM, Markus HS, Kaski JC, Jahangiri M. Neurocognitive function and cerebral emboli: randomized study of on-pump versus off-pump coronary artery bypass surgery. *Ann Thorac Surg* 2007;83:475–82.

338. Lund C, Hol PK, Lundblad R, et al. Comparison of cerebral embolization during off-pump and on-pump coronary artery bypass surgery. *Ann Thorac Surg* 2003;76:765–70.

339. Dajaini G, Katznelson R, Fedorko L, et al. Early benefit of preserved cognitive function is not sustained at one-year after cardiac surgery: a longitudinal follow-up of the randomized clinical trial. *Can J Anaesth* 2012;59:449–55.

340. Selnes OA, Grega MA, Bailey MM, et al. Neurocognitive outcomes 3 years after coronary artery bypass graft surgery: a controlled study. *Ann Thorac Surg* 2007;84:1885–96.

341. Takagi H, Ando T, Umemoto T, ALICE Group. Perioperative depression or anxiety and postoperative mortality in cardiac surgery: a systematic review and meta-analysis. *Heart Vessels* 2017;32:1458–68.

342. Pignay-Demaria V, Lespérance F, Demaria RG, Frasure-Smith N, Perrault LP. Depression and anxiety and outcomes of coronary artery bypass surgery. *Ann Thorac Surg* 2003;75:314–21.

343. Ho PM, Masoudi FA, Spertus JA, et al. Depression predicts mortality following cardiac valve surgery. *Ann Thorac Surg* 2005;79:1255–9.

344. Freedland KE, Skala JA, Carney RM, et al. Treatment of depression after coronary artery bypass surgery: a randomized controlled trial. *Arch Gen Psychiatry* 2009;66:387–96.

345. Hermans G, De Jonghe B, Bruyninckx F, Van den Berghe G. Interventions for preventing critical illness polyneuropathy and critical illness myopathy. *Cochrane Database Syst Rev* 2014;30:CD006832. https://doi.org/10.1002/14651858.CD006832.pub2.

346. Apostolakis E, Papakonstantinou NA, Baikoussis NG, Papadopoulos G. Intensive care unit-related generalized neuromuscular weakness due to critical illness polyneuropathy/myopathy in critically ill patients. *J Anesth* 2015;29:112–21.

347. Unlü Y, Velioğlu Y, Koçak H, Becit N, Ceviz M. Brachial plexus injury following median sternotomy. *Interact Cardiovasc Thorac Surg* 2007;6:235–7.

348. Jellish WS, Oftadeh M. Peripheral nerve injury in cardiac surgery. *J Cardiothorac Vasc Anesth* 2018;32:495–511.

349. Vahl DF, Carl I, Müller-Vahl H, Struck E. Brachial plexus injury after cardiac surgery. The role of internal mammary artery preparation: a prospective study of 1000 consecutive patients. *J Thorac Cardiovasc Surg* 1991;102:724–9.

350. Canbaz S, Turgut N, Halici U, Sunar H, Balci K, Duran E. Brachial plexus injury during open heart surgery: controlled prospective trial. *Thorac Cardiovasc Surg* 2005;53:295–9.

351. Thomas NJ, Harvey AT. Paraplegia after coronary bypass operations: relationship to severe hypertension and vascular disease. *J Thorac Cardiovasc Surg* 1999;117:834–6.

352. Geyer TE, Naik MJ, Pillai R. Anterior spinal artery syndrome after elective coronary artery bypass grafting. *Ann Thorac Surg* 2002;73:1971–3.

353. Sevuk U, Kaya S, Ayaz F, Aktas U. Paraplegia due to spinal cord infarction after coronary artery bypass graft surgery. *J Card Surg* 2016;31:51–6.

354. Garg A, Bansal A, Bhuyan S, Muniem A. Paraplegia during coronary artery bypass graft surgery caused by bilateral anterior cerebral artery territory infarction. *Ann Transl Med* 2014;2:49.

355. Vazquez-Jimenez JF, Krebs G, Schiefer J, et al. Injury of the common peroneal nerve after cardiothoracic operations. *Ann Thorac Surg* 2002;73:119–22.

356. Tahir M, Galvin S. Acute lower leg compartment syndrome: a rare complication following CABG. *Case Rep Surg* 2016;2016:5268174. doi: 10.1155/2016/5268174.

357. Te Kolste HJ, Balm R, de Mol B. Acute compartment syndrome of the lower leg after coronary artery bypass grafting: a silent but dangerous complication. *Thorac Cardiovasc Surg* 2015;63:300–6.

358. Alameddine AK. Lower limb ischemia with compartment syndrome related to femoral artery cannulas. *Ann Thorac Surg* 1997;64:884–5.

359. Vaidyanathan KR, Sundaramoorthi T, Byalal JR, et al. Lower extremity compartment syndrome after off-pump aortocoronary bypass. *J Thorac Cardiovasc Surg* 2006;131:1173–4.

360. Kolli A, Au JT, Lee DC, Klinoff N, Ko W. Compartment syndrome after endoscopic harvest of the great saphenous vein during coronary artery bypass grafting. *Ann Thorac Surg* 2010; 89:271–3.

361. Vander Salm TJ. Prevention of lower extremity ischemia during cardiopulmonary bypass via femoral cannulation. *Ann Thorac Surg* 1997;63:251–2.

362. Hendrickson SC, Glower DD. A method for perfusion of the leg during cardiopulmonary bypass via femoral cannulation. *Ann Thorac Surg* 1998;65:1807 8.

363. Chandraprakasam T, Kumar RA. Acute compartment syndrome of forearm and hand. *Indian J Plast Surg* 2011;44:212–8.

364. Poullis M, Lawrence D, Ratnatunga C. Forearm fasciotomy post cardiac surgery. *Eur J Cardiothorac Surg* 1999;16:580–1.

365. Bleiziffer S, Hettich I, Eisenhauer B, et al. Neurologic sequelae of the donor arm after endoscopic versus conventional radial artery harvesting. *J Thorac Cardiovasc Surg* 2008;136:681–7.

366. Raut MS, Maheshwari A, Joshi R, et al. Vocal cord paralysis after cardiac surgery and interventions: a review of possible etiologies. *J Cardiothorac Vasc Anesth* 2016;30:1661–7.

367. Itagaki T, Kikura M, Sato S. Incidence and risk factors of postoperative vocal cord paralysis in 987 patients after cardiovascular surgery. *Ann Thorac Surg* 2007;83:2147–52.

368. Chaudhry R, Zaki J, Wegner R, et al. Gastrointestinal complications after cardiac surgery: a nationwide population-based analysis of morbidity and mortality predictors. *J Cardiothorac Vasc Anesth* 2017;31:1268–74.

369. Hessel EA 2nd. Abdominal organ injury after cardiac surgery. *Semin Cardiothorac Vasc Anesth* 2004;8:243–63.

370. Christenson JT, Schmuziger M, Maurice J, Simonet F, Velebit V. Postoperative visceral hypotension the common cause for gastrointestinal complications after cardiac surgery. *Thorac Cardiovasc Surg* 1994;42:152–7.

371. Ohri SK, Velissaris T. Gastrointestinal dysfunction following cardiac surgery. *Perfusion* 2006;21:215–23.

372. Velissaris T, Tang A, Murray M, El-Minshawy A, Hett D, Ohri S. A prospective randomized study to evaluate splanchnic hypoxia during beating-heart and conventional coronary revascularization. *Eur J Cardiothorac Surg* 2003;23:917–24.

373. Fiore G, Brienza N, Cicala P, et al. Superior mesenteric artery blood flow modifications during off-pump coronary surgery. *Ann Thorac Surg* 2006;82:62–7.

374. Baue AE. The role of the gut in the development of multiple organ dysfunction in cardiothoracic patients. *Ann Thorac Surg* 1993;55:822–9.

375. Hashemzadeh K, Hashemzadeh S. Predictors and outcome of gastrointestinal complications after cardiac surgery. *Minerva Chir* 2012;67:327–35.

376. D'Ancona G, Baillot R, Poirier B, et al. Determinants of gastrointestinal complications in cardiac surgery. *Tex Heart Inst J* 2003;30:280–5.

377. Mangi AA, Christison-Lagay ER, Torchiana DF, Warshaw AL, Berger DL. Gastrointestinal complications in patients undergoing heart operation: an analysis of 8709 consecutive cardiac surgical patients. *Ann Surg* 2005;241:895–901.

378. Filsoufi F, Rahmanian PB, Castillo JG, Scurlock C, Legnani PE, Adams DH. Predictors and outcome of gastrointestinal complications in patients undergoing cardiac surgery. *Ann Surg* 2007;246:323–9.

379. Andersson B, Nilsson J, Brandt J, Höglund P, Andersson R. Gastrointestinal complications after cardiac surgery. *Br J Surg* 2005;92:326–33.

380. Marsoner K, Voetsch A, Lierzer C, et al. Gastrointestinal complications following on-pump cardiac surgery: a propensity matched analysis. *PLoS One* 2019;14(6):e0217874.

381. Andersson B, Andersson R, Brandt J, Höglund P, Algotsson L, Nilsson J. Gastrointestinal complications after cardiac surgery: improved risk stratification using a new scoring model. *Interact Cardiovasc Thorac Surg* 2010;10:366–70.

382. Croome KP, Kiaii B, Fox S, Quantz M, McKenzie N, Novick RJ. Comparison of gastrointestinal complications in on-pump versus off-pump coronary artery bypass grafting. *Can J Surg* 2009;52:125–8.

383. Sanisoglu I, Guden M, Bayramoglu Z, et al. Does off-pump CABG reduce gastrointestinal complications? *Ann Thorac Surg* 2004;77:619–25.

384. Toews I, George AT, Peter JV, et al. Interventions for preventing upper gastrointestinal bleeding in people admitted to intensive care units. *Cochrane Database Syst Rev* 2018;6:CD008687. https://doi.org/10.1002/14651858.CD008687.pub2.

385. Alquraini M, Alshamsi F, Møeller MH, et al. Sucralfate versus histamine 2 receptor antagonists for stress ulcer prophylaxis in adult critically ill patients: a meta-analysis and trial sequential analysis of randomized trials. *J Crit Care* 2017;40:21–30.

386. Alhazzani W, Alshamsi F, Belley-Cote E, et al. Efficacy and safety of stress ulcer prophylaxis in critically ill patients: a network meta-analysis of randomized trials. *Intensive Care Med* 2018;44:1–11.

387. Ferraris VA, Ferraris SP, Moritz DM, Welch S. Oropharyngeal dysphagia after cardiac operations. *Ann Thorac Surg* 2001;71:1792–6.

388. Harrington OB, Duckworth JK, Starnes CL, et al. Silent aspiration after coronary artery bypass grafting. *Ann Thorac Surg* 1998;65:1599–603.

389. Werle RW, Steidl EM, Mancopes R. Oropharyngeal dysphagia and related factors in post-cardiac surgery: a systematic review. *Codas* 2016;28:646–52.

390. Hogue CW Jr, Lappas GD, Creswell LL, et al. Swallowing dysfunction after cardiac operations: associated adverse outcomes and risk factors including intraoperative transesophageal echocardiography. *J Thorac Cardiovasc Surg* 1995;110:517–22.

391. Daly E, Miles A, Scott S, Gillham M. Finding the red flags: swallowing difficulties after cardiac surgery in patients with prolonged intubation. *J Crit Care* 2016;31:119–24.

392. Rousou JA, Tighe DA, Garb JL, et al. Risk of dysphagia after transesophageal echocardiography during cardiac operations. *Ann Thorac Surg* 2000;69:486–9.

393. Chin JH, Lee EH, Choi DK, Choi IC. A modification of the trans-oesophageal echocardiography protocol can reduce post-operative dysphagia following cardiac surgery. *J Int Med Res* 2011;39:96–104.

394. Barker J, Martino R, Reichardt B, Hickey EJ, Ralph-Edwards A. Incidence and impact of dysphagia in patients receiving prolonged endotracheal intubation after cardiac surgery. *Can J Surg* 2009;52:119–24.

395. Bours GJ, Speyer R, Lemmens J, Limburg M, de Wit R. Bedside screening tests vs. videofluoroscopy or fiberoptic endoscopic evaluation of swallowing to detect dysphagia in patients with neurological disorders: a systematic review. *J Adv Nurs* 2009;65:477–93.

396. Partik BL, Scharitzer M, Schueller G, et al. Videofluoroscopy of swallowing abnormalities in 22 symptomatic patients after cardiovascular surgery. *AJR Am J Roentgenol* 2003;180:987–92.

397. Miles A, McLellan N, Machan R, et al. Dysphagia and laryngeal pathology in post-surgical cardio-thoracic patients. *J Crit Care* 2018;45:121–7.

398. Alebouyeh N, Toefigh M, Ghasemzadeh N, Mirheydari S, Azargashb E. Predictors of gastrointesti-nal perforation in patients undergoing coronary artery bypass graft (CABG) surgery in Tehran, Iran. *Ann Thorac Cardiovasc Surg* 2007;13:251–3.

399. Hackert T, Keinle P, Weitz J, et al. Accuracy of diagnostic laparoscopy for early diagnosis of abdomi-nal complications after cardiac surgery. *Surg Endosc* 2003;17:1671–4.

400. Leier H. Does gum chewing help prevent impaired gastric motility in the postoperative period? *J Am Acad Nurse Pract* 2007;19:133–6.

401. Zeinali F, Stulberg JJ, Delaney CP. Pharmacological management of postoperative ileus. *Can J Surg* 2009;52:153–7.

402. Valle RG, Godoy FL. Neostigmine for acute colonic pseudo-obstruction: a meta-analysis. *Ann Med Surg (Lond)* 2014;3:60–4.

403. Smedley LW, Foster DB, Barthol CA, Hall R, Gutierrez GC. Safety and efficacy of intermittent bolus and continuous infusion neostigmine for acute colonic pseudo-obstruction. *J Intensive Care Med* 2018;46:241.

404. O'Dea CJ, Brookes JH, Wattchow DA. The efficacy of treatment of patients with severe constipation or recurrent pseudo-obstruction with pyridostigmine. *Colorectal Dis* 2010;12:540–8.

405. Walker J, Criddle LM. Pathophysiology and management of abdominal compartment syndrome. *Am J Crit Care* 2003;12:367–71.

406. Rady MY, Kodavatiganti R, Ryan T. Perioperative predictors of acute cholecystitis after cardiovascu-lar surgery. *Chest* 1998;114:76–84.

407. Passage J, Joshi P, Mullany DV. Acute cholecystitis complicating cardiac surgery: case series involv-ing more than 16,000 patients. *Ann Thorac Surg* 2007;83:1096–101.

408. Mastoraki A, Mastoraki S, Kriaras I, Douka E, Geroulanos S. Complications involving gall bladder and biliary tract in cardiovascular surgery. *Hepatogastroenterology* 2008;55:1233–7.

409. Mahdi A, Noureddine A, Younes M, et al. Upper gastrointestinal bleeding after open heart sur-gery. *J Dig Endosc* 2014;5:101–5.

410. Krawiec F, Maitland A, Duan Q, Faris P, Belletrutti PJ, Kent WDT. Duodenal ulcers are a major cause of gastrointestinal bleeding after cardiac surgery. *J Thorac Cardiovasc Surg* 2017;154:181–8.

411. Buendgens L, Koch A, Tacke F. Prevention of stress-related ulcer bleeding at the intensive care unit: risks and benefits of stress ulcer prophylaxis. *World J Crit Care Med* 2016;5:57–64.

412. Shin JS, Abah U. Is routine stress ulcer prophylaxis of benefit for patients undergoing cardiac sur-gery? *Interact Cardiovasc Thorac Surg* 2012;14:622–8.

413. Bhat M, Larocque M, Amorim M, et al. Prediction and prevention of upper gastrointestinal bleeding after cardiac surgery: a case control study. *Can J Gastroenterol* 2012;26:340–4.

414. Miano TA, Reichert MG, Houle TT, MacGregor DA, Kincaid EH, Bowton DL. Nosocomial pneu-monia risk and stress ulcer prophylaxis: a comparison of pantoprazole vs ranitidine in cardiothoracic surgery patients. *Chest* 2009;136:440–7.

415. Krag M, Marker S, Perner A, et al. Pantoprazole in patients at risk for gastrointestinal bleeding in the ICU. *N Engl J Med* 2018;379:2199–2208.

416. Marker S, Perner A, Wetterslev J, et al. Pantoprazole prophylaxis in ICU patients with high severity of disease: a post hoc analysis of the placebo-controlled SUP-ICU trial. *Intensive Care Med* 2019;45:609–18.

417. Walker J, Robinson J, Stewart J, Jacob S. Does enteric-coated aspirin result in a lower incidence of gastro-intestinal complications compared to normal aspirin? *Interact Cardiovasc Thorac Surg* 2007;6:519–22.

418. Ziegelin M, Hoschtitzky A, Dunning J, Hooper T. Does clopidogrel rather than aspirin plus a pro-ton-pump inhibitor reduce the frequency of gastrointestinal complications after cardiac surgery? *Interact Cardiovasc Thorac Surg* 2007;6:534–7.

419. Chan FK, Ching JYL, Hung LCT, et al. Clopidogrel versus aspirin and esomeprazole to prevent recurrent ulcer bleeding. *N Engl J Med* 2005;352:238–44.

420. Ng FH, Chan P, Kwanching CP, et al. Management and outcome of peptic ulcers or erosions in patients receiving a combination of aspirin plus clopidogrel. *J Gastroenterol* 2008;43:679–86.

421. Laine L. Upper gastrointestinal bleeding due to a peptic ulcer. *N Engl J Med* 2016;374:2367–76.

422. Gralnek IM, Barkun AN, Bardou M. Management of acute bleeding from a peptic ulcer. *N Engl J Med* 2008;359:928–37.

423. Huggins RM, Scates AC, Latour JK. Intravenous proton-pump inhibitors versus H_2-antagonists for treatment of GI bleeding. *Ann Pharmacother* 2003;37:433–7.

424. Jayaprakash A, McGrath C, McCullagh E, Smith F, Angelini G, Probert C. Upper gastrointestinal haemorrhage following cardiac surgery: a comparative study with vascular surgery patients from a single centre. *Eur J Gastroenterol Hepatol* 2004;16:191–4.

425. Torres AJ, Landa I, Hernández F, et al. Somatostatin in the treatment of severe upper gastrointestinal bleeding: a multicentre controlled trial. *Br J Surg* 2005;73:786–9.

426. Horiuchi H, Doman T, Kokame K, Saiki Y, Matsumoto M. Acquired von Willebrand syndrome associated with cardiovascular diseases. *J Atheroscler Thromb* 2019;26:303–14.

427. Tamura T, Horiuchi H, Imai M, et al. Unexpectedly high prevalence of acquired von Willebrand syndrome in patients with severe aortic stenosis as evaluated with a novel large multimer index. *J Atheroscler Thromb* 2015;22:1115–23.

428. Akutagawa T, Shindo T, Yamanouchi K, et al. Persistent gastrointestinal angiodysplasia in Heyde's syndrome after aortic valve replacement. *Intern Med* 2017;56:2431–3.

429. Darcy M. Treatment of lower gastrointestinal bleeding: vasopressin infusion versus embolization. *J Vasc Interv Radiol* 2003;14:535–43.

430. Ramaswamy RS, Choi HW, Mouser HC, et al. Role of interventional radiology in the management of acute gastrointestinal bleeding. *World J Radiol* 2014;6:82–92.

431. Sildiroğlu O, Muasher J, Bloom TA, et al. Acute lower gastrointestinal bleeding: predictive factors and clinical outcome for the patients who needed first-time mesenteric conventional angiography. *Diagn Interv Radiol* 2018;24:23–7.

432. Yi WS, Garg G, Sava JA. Localization and definitive control of lower gastrointestinal bleeding with angiography and embolization. *Am Surg* 2013;79:375–80.

433. Junquera F, Saperas E, Videla S, et al. Long-term efficacy of octreotide in the prevention of recurrent bleeding from gastrointestinal angiodysplasia. *Am J Gastroenterol* 2007;102:254–60.

434. Schütz A, Eichinger W, Breuer M, Gansera B, Kemkes BM. Acute mesenteric ischemia after open heart surgery. *Angiology* 1998;49:267–73.

435. Katz MG, Schachner A, Ezri T, et al. Nonocclusive mesenteric ischemia after off-pump coronary artery bypass surgery: a word of caution. *Am Surg* 2006;72:228–31.

436. Sever K, Ozbek C, Goktas B, et al. Gastrointestinal complications after open heart surgery: incidence and determinants of risk factors. *Angiology* 2014;65:424–9.

437. Goleanu V, Alecu L, Lazar O. Acute mesenteric ischemia after heart surgery. *Chirurgia (Bucur)* 2014;109:402–6.

438. Chaudhuri N, James J, Sheikh A, Grayson AD, Fabri BM. Intestinal ischemia following cardiac surgery: a multivariate risk model. *Eur J Cardiothorac Surg* 2006;29:971–7.

439. Kirkpatrick ID, Kroeker MA, Greenberg HM. Biphasic CT with mesenteric CT angiography in the evaluation of acute mesenteric ischemia: initial experience. *Radiology* 2003;229:91–8.

440. Klotz S, Vestring T, Rötker J, Schmidt C, Scheld HH, Schmid C. Diagnosis and treatment of nonocclusive mesenteric ischemia after open heart surgery. *Ann Thorac Surg* 2001;72:1583–6.

441. Borioni R, Turani F, Fratticci L, Pederzoli A, Binaco I, Garofalo M. Acute mesenteric ischemia after cardiac surgery: role of the abdominal compartment syndrome treatment. *Annali Italiani di Chirurgia* 2015;86:386–9.

442. Crabtree T, Aitchison D, Meyers BF, et al. *Clostridium difficile* in cardiac surgery: risk factors and impact on postoperative outcome. *Ann Thorac Surg* 2007;83:1396–402.

443. Silvetti S, Landoni G. Is *Clostridium difficile* the new bugaboo after cardiac surgery? *J Thorac Dis* 2018;10(Suppl 26):S3278–80.

444. McDonald LC, Gerding DN, Johnson S, et al. Clinical practice guidelines for *Clostridium difficile* infection in Adults and Children: 2017 Update by the Infectious Diseases Society of America (IDSA) and Society for Healthcare Epidemiology of America (SHEA). *Clin Infec Dis* 2018;66:987–94.

445. Sharma P, Ananthanarayanan C, Vaidhya N, Malhotra A, Shah K, Sharma R. Hyperbilirubinemia after cardiac surgery: an observational study. *Asian Cardiovasc Thorac Ann* 2015;23:1039–43.

446. An Y, Xiao YB, Zhong QJ. Hyperbilirubinemia after extracorporeal circulation surgery: a recent and prospective study. *World J Gasroenterol* 2006;12:6722–6.

447. Nishi H, Sakaguchi T, Miyagawa S, et al. Frequency, risk factors and prognosis of postoperative hyperbilirubinemia after heart valve surgery. *Cardiology* 2012;122:12–9.

448. Nishi H, Takahashi T, Ichikawa H, Matsumiya G, Matsuda H, Sawa Y. Prediction of postoperative hepatic dysfunction after cardiac surgery in patients with chronic congestive heart failure. *Gen Thorac Cardiovasc Surg* 2009;57:357–62.

449. Goyal RK, Srivastava D, Lessnau KD. Clopidogrel-induced hepatocellular injury and cholestatic jaundice in an elderly patient: case report and review of the literature. *Pharmacotherapy* 2009;29:608–12.

450. Woźnica EA, Inglot M, Woźnica RK, Lysenko L. Liver dysfunction in sepsis. *Adv Clin Exp Med* 2018;27:547–51.

451. Bernal W, Wendon J. Acute liver failure. *N Engl J Med* 2013;369:2525–34.

452. Wijdicks EFM. Hepatic encephalopathy. *N Engl J Med* 2016;375:1660–70.

453. Wan S, Arifi AA, Chan CS, et al. Is hyperamylasemia after cardiac surgery due to cardiopulmonary bypass? *Asian Cardiovasc Thorac Ann* 2002;10:115–8.

454. Ihaya A, Muraoka R, Chiba Y, et al. Hyperamylasemia and subclinical pancreatitis after cardiac surgery. *World J Surg* 2001;25:862–4.

455. Perez A, Ito H, Farivar RS, et al. Risk factors and outcomes of pancreatitis after open heart surgery. *Am J Surg* 2005;190:401–5.

456. Lonardo A, Grisendi A, Bonilauri S, Rambaldi M, Selmi I, Tondelli E. Ischaemic necrotizing pancreatitis after cardiac surgery: a case report and review of the literature. *Int J Gastroenterol Hepatol* 1999;31:872–5.

457. Chung JW, Ryu SH, Jo JH, et al. Clinical implications and risk factors for acute pancreatitis after cardiac valve surgery. *Yonsei Med J* 2013;54:154–9.

458. Martindale RG, McClave SA, Vanek VW, et al. Guidelines for the provision and assessment of nutrition support therapy in the adult critically ill patient: Society of Critical Care Medicine and American Society for Parenteral and Enteral Nutrition: executive summary. *Crit Care Med* 2009;37:1757–61.

459. Singer P, Blaser AR, Berger MM, et al. ESPEN guideline on clinical nutrition in the intensive care unit. *Clin Nutrition* 2019;38:48–79.

460. Stoppe C, Goetzenich A, Whitman G, et al. Role of nutrition support in adult cardiac surgery: a consensus statement from an International Multidisciplinary Expert Group on Nutrition in Cardiac Surgery. *Crit Care* 2017;21:131.

461. Hill A, Nesterova E, Lomivorotov V, et al. Current evidence about nutrition support in cardiac surgery patients: what do we know? *Nutrients* 2018;10:897.

462. Berger MM, Berger-Gryllaki M, Wiesel PH, et al. Intestinal absorption in patients after cardiac surgery. *Crit Care Med* 2000;28:2217–23.

463. Khalid I, Doshi P, DiGiovine B. Early enteral nutrition and outcomes of critically ill patients treated with vasopressors and mechanical ventilation. *Am J Crit Care* 2010;19:261–8.

464. Mehanna HM, Moledina J, Travis J. Refeeding syndrome: what it is, and how to prevent and treat it. *BMJ* 2008;336:1495–8.

465. Akins CW, Miller DC, Turina MI, et al. Guidelines for reporting mortality and morbidity after cardiac valve interventions. *Ann Thorac Surg* 2008;85:1490–5.

466. Rahimtoola SM. The problem of valve prosthesis-patient mismatch. *Circulation* 1978;58:20–4.

467. Rashid HN, Brown AJ, McCormick LM, et al. Subclinical leaflet thrombosis in transcatheter aortic valve replacement detected by multidetector computed tomography: a review of current evidence. *Circ J* 2018;82:1735–42.

468. Rashid HN, Gooley RP, Nerlekar N, et al. Bioprosthetic aortic valve leaflet thrombosis detected by multidetector computed tomography is associated with adverse cerebrovascular events: a meta-analysis of observational studies. *Eurointervention* 2018;13:e1748–55.

469. Jimenez C, Ohana M, Marchandot B, et al. Impact of antithrombotic regimen and platelet inhibition extent on leaflet thrombosis detected by cardiac MDCT after transcatheter aortic valve replacement. *J Clin Med* 2019;8:E506.

470. Kanjanauthai S, Pirelli L, Nalluri N, Kliger CA. Subclinical leaflet thrombosis following transcatheter aortic valve replacement. *J Interv Cardiol* 2018;31:640–7.

471. D'Ascenzo G, Salizzoni S, Saglietto A, et al. Incidence, predictors and cerebrovascular consequences of leaflet thrombosis after transcatheter aortic valve implantation: a systematic review and meta-analysis. *Eur J Cardiothorac Surg* 2019;56:488–94.

472. Barroso Freitas-Ferraz A, Beaudoin W, Couture C, Perron J, Sénéchal M. Prosthetic aortic valve thrombosis: to fibrinolyse or not to fibrinolyse? That is the question! *Echocardiography* 2019;36:787–90.

473. Alshawabkeh L, Economy KE, Valente AM. Anticoagulation during pregnancy. Evolving strategies with a focus on mechanical valves. *J Am Coll Cardiol* 2016;68:1804–13.

474. Eitz T, Schenk S, Fritzsche D, et al. International normalized ratio self-management lowers the risk of thromboembolic events after prosthetic heart valve replacement. *Ann Thorac Surg* 2008;85: 949–55.

475. Ando T, Ashraf S, Villablanca PA, et al. Meta-analysis comparing the incidence of infective endocarditis following transcatheter aortic valve implantation versus surgical aortic valve replacement. *Am J Cardiol* 2019;123:827–32.

476. Bjursten H, Rasmussen M, Nozohoor S, et al. Infective endocarditis after transcatheter aortic valve implantation: a nationwide study. *Eur Heart J* 2019;40:3263–9.

477. Shapira Y, Vaturi M, Sagie A. Hemolysis associated with prosthetic heart valves: a review. *Cardiol Rev* 2009;17:121–4.

478. Charlson ME, Isom OW. Care after coronary-artery bypass surgery. *N Engl J Med* 2003;348:1456–63.

479. Chan AY, McAlister FA, Norris CM, et al. Effect of β-blocker use on outcomes after discharge in patients who underwent cardiac surgery. *J Thorac Cardiovasc Surg* 2010;140:182–7.

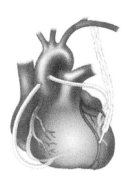

APPENDICES

♡ 1A American College of Cardiology Classes of Recommendation and Levels of Evidence

Class I   Benefit greatly exceeds the risk and the procedure/treatment should be performed/administered (is effective)

Class IIa   Benefit exceeds the risk and it is reasonable to perform procedure or administer treatment (most likely effective)

Class IIb   Benefit probably exceeds the risk and the procedure/treatment may be considered (usefulness/efficacy less well-established)

Class III   The risk may exceed the benefit and the procedure/treatment should not be performed/administered (not recommended)

Level A   Evidence from multiple randomized trials or meta-analyses

Level B   Limited evidence from single randomized trials or nonrandomized studies with some conflicting evidence of benefit

Level C   Expert opinions or case studies

These are general summations of the recommendations for treatment.

1B New York Heart Association Functional Classification

Class I   Patient has cardiac disease but without resulting limitations of ordinary physical activity. Ordinary physical activity (e.g. walking several blocks or climbing stairs) does not cause undue fatigue, palpitation, dyspnea, or anginal pain. Limiting symptoms may occur with marked exertion.

Manual of Perioperative Care in Adult Cardiac Surgery, Sixth Edition. Robert M. Bojar.
© 2021 John Wiley & Sons Ltd. Published 2021 by John Wiley & Sons Ltd.

Class II   Patient has cardiac disease resulting in slight limitation of ordinary physical activity. Patient is comfortable at rest. Ordinary physical activity such as walking more than two blocks or climbing more than one flight of stairs results in limiting symptoms (e.g. fatigue, palpitation, dyspnea, or anginal pain).

Class III   Patient has cardiac disease resulting in marked limitation of physical activity. Patient is comfortable at rest. Less than ordinary physical activity (e.g. walking one to two level blocks or climbing one flight of stairs) causes fatigue, palpitation, dyspnea, or anginal pain.

Class IV   Patient has dyspnea at rest that increases with any physical activity. Patient has cardiac disease resulting in inability to perform any physical activity without discomfort. Symptoms may be present even at rest. If any physical activity is undertaken, discomfort is increased.

1C The Canadian Cardiovascular Society Classification for Grading of Angina

Class I   Ordinary activity does not cause angina. Angina with strenuous, rapid, or prolonged exertion only.

Class II   Slight limitation of ordinary activity. Angina on walking or climbing stairs rapidly, walking or stair climbing after meals, in cold weather, when under emotional stress, during the first few hours of awakening or walking more than two blocks on the level or climbing more than one flight of ordinary stairs at a normal pace under normal conditions.

Class III   Marked limitation of ordinary physical activity. Angina on walking one or two blocks on the level or one flight of stairs at a normal pace under normal conditions.

Class IV   Inability to carry out any physical activity without discomfort or angina at rest.

1D Interagency Registry for Mechanically Assisted Circulatory Support (INTERMACS) Profiles of Advanced Heart Failure

Patients with NYHA class IV and AHA stage D heart failure may be classified as INTERMACS profiles 1–6 indicating the severity of their clinical heart failure. Patients with INTERMACS 7 are those with advanced NYHA class III heart failure.

INTERMACS 1: Critical cardiogenic shock with life-threatening hypotension refractory to rapidly escalating inotropic pressor support, with critical organ hypoperfusion. *"Crash and burn."* Mechanical circulatory support (MCS) is indicated within hours.

INTERMACS 2: Progressive decline with acceptable blood pressure on inotropic support, but worsening renal function, nutritional status, or end-organ function. *"Sliding fast."* MCS is indicated within a few days.

INTERMACS 3: Stable but inotrope-dependent with stable blood pressure and end-organ function, but cannot be weaned from inotropic support without developing hypotension, HF symptoms, or worsening organ system function (usually renal). *"Dependent stability."* MCS may be considered within a few weeks to months.

INTERMACS 4: Resting symptoms at home on oral medications with daily symptoms of HF at rest or with activities of daily living (ADLs). Temporary cessation of inotropic support may be possible, but patient has frequent symptoms of fluid overload requiring very high dose diuretics. Signs and symptoms include orthopnea, dyspnea with ADLs, and lower extremity edema. *"Frequent flyer."* MCS may be indicated within a few months.

INTERMACS 5: Exertion intolerant being comfortable at rest without symptoms of HF, but unable to engage in any other activities; usually have underlying refractory elevated volume status, often with renal dysfunction. *"Housebound."*

INTERMACS 6: Exertion limited patients are comfortable at rest without evidence of fluid overload, and able to do ADLs and minor activities outside of the home. *"Walking wounded."* However, any meaningful physical activity causes fatigue. Symptoms will occasionally worsen, with most patients hospitalized within the past year.

INTERMACS 7: Advanced NYHA Class 3 patients are clinically stable, being comfortable with a reasonable level of mild activity, such as walking a block.

2 Typical Preoperative Order Sheet

1. Admit to: _____
2. Surgery date: _____
3. Planned procedure: _____
4. Diagnostic studies
   - ☐ CBC with differential
   - ☐ PT/INR PTT
   - ☐ Electrolytes, BUN, creatinine, blood glucose
   - ☐ Liver function tests (bilirubin, AST, ALT, alkaline phosphatase, albumin)
   - ☐ TSH level
   - ☐ Lipid profile
   - ☐ Hemoglobin A1c level
   - ☐ Urinalysis and urine culture, if indicated
   - ☐ Electrocardiogram
   - ☐ Chest x-ray PA and lateral
   - ☐ Room air oxygen saturation by pulse oximetry; obtain arterial blood gas if <90%
   - ☐ Antibody ____ screen   ☐ Crossmatch: ____ units packed red blood cells (PRBCs)
   - ☐ Carotid duplex studies
   - ☐ Bilateral digital radial artery studies
   - ☐ Bilateral venous mapping
   - ☐ Pulmonary function tests
   - ☐ Other: _____
5. Treatments/Assessments
   - ☐ Admission vital signs
   - ☐ Measure height and weight
   - ☐ NPO after midnight except sips of water with meds
   - ☐ Surgical clippers to remove hair at 5:00 AM morning of surgery from chest, legs, and both groins
   - ☐ Hibiclens scrub to chest and legs night before and AM of surgery
   - ☐ Incentive spirometry teaching
   - ☐ Smoking cessation education
6. Medications
   - ☐ Mupirocin 2% (Bactroban ointment): apply Q-tip nasal swabs the evening before and the morning of surgery
   - ☐ Chlorhexidine 0.12% (Peridex) gargle on-call to OR
   - ☐ Ascorbic acid 2 g at 9:00 PM night before surgery
   - ☐ Cefazolin ☐ 1 g IV ☐ 2 g IV – send to OR with patient
   - ☐ Vancomycin 20 mg/kg = _____ g IV – send to OR with patient
   - ☐ Discontinue P2Y12 inhibitor immediately (check with surgeon about PRU testing)
   - ☐ Reduce aspirin to 81 mg daily if patient on a higher dose

- ☐ Discontinue NOAC after AM/PM dose on ___ (48 hours in advance of surgery)
- ☐ Discontinue heparin at _____
- ☐ Continue heparin drip into operating room
- ☐ Discontinue low-molecular-weight heparin after AM/PM dose on _____
- ☐ Discontinue IIb/IIIa inhibitor at 4:00 AM prior to surgery
- ☐ Metoprolol ____ mg PO every 12 hours; hold for SBP <100 or HR <60 (CABG patients)
- ☐ Discontinue ACE inhibitor or ARB morning of surgery
- ☐ Discontinue all diabetic medications morning of surgery
- ☐ Discontinue all diuretics morning of surgery

3 Cardiac Surgery Preoperative Assessment Checklist

Planned procedure:_____

Surgery date:_____

☐ Surgical note in chart and consent obtained:_____
☐ Anesthesia preoperative note:_____
☐ Antibiotics ordered:_____
☐ ECG:_____
☐ CXR:_____
☐ Cath report:_____

☐ Echo report:_____

☐ STS risk score (or EuroSCORE):_____
☐ CBC:
☐ Basic metabolic panel:
☐ Liver function tests:
☐ INR/PTT:
☐ Type & cross:
☐ Urinalysis/culture:
☐ Medications:
   ☐ Aspirin dose decreased to 81 mg:_____
   ☐ If patient not on a β-blocker and heart rate >60, initiate metoprolol 12.5–25 mg PO bid (CABG patients)
   ☐ Patient aware not to take ACE inhibitor/ARB, diabetic medications, diuretics the day of surgery
   ☐ Date and time of:
     • Last dose of P2Y12 inhibitor: _____
     • Last dose of warfarin:_____
     • Last dose of low-molecular-weight heparin: _____
     • Last dose of NOAC:_____
☐ Additional studies/Comments:_____
_____
_____
_____
_____

Signature:_____ Date:_____ Time:_____

Manual of Perioperative Care in Adult Cardiac Surgery, Sixth Edition. Robert M. Bojar.
© 2021 John Wiley & Sons Ltd. Published 2021 by John Wiley & Sons Ltd.

4 Typical Orders for Admission to the ICU

1. Admit to ICU on _____ MD service
2. Procedure: _____
3. Vital signs q15 min until stable, then q30 min or per protocol
4. Continuous ECG, arterial, PA tracings, SaO_2 on bedside monitor
5. Cardiac output q15 min × 1 hour, then q1h × 4 hours, then q2–4h when stable
6. IABP 1:1; check distal pulses manually or with Doppler q1h
7. Chest tubes to chest drainage system with –20 cm H_2O suction; record q15 min until <60 mL/h, then q1h until <30 mL/h, then every 2 hours
8. Bair Hugger warming system if core temperature <35 °C
9. Urinary catheter to gravity drainage and record hourly
10. Elevate head of bed 30°
11. Hourly I & O
12. Daily weights
13. Advance activity after extubation (dangle, OOB to chair)
14. VTE prophylaxis
    - ☐ T.E.D. elastic stockings (apply on POD #1)
    - ☐ Sequential or pneumatic compression devices while in bed
    - ☐ Heparin 5000 units SC bid starting on POD #_____
    - ☐ Low-molecular-weight heparin (Lovenox) 40 mg SC daily starting on POD #_____
15. GI/Nutrition:
    - ☐ NPO while intubated
    - ☐ Nasogastric tube to low suction
    - ☐ Clear liquids as tolerated 1h after extubation and removal of NG tube
16. Ventilator settings
    - ☐ FiO_2: _____ in SIMV mode
    - ☐ IMV rate: _____ breaths/min
    - ☐ Tidal volume: _____ mL
    - ☐ PEEP: _____ cm H_2O
17. Respiratory care
    - ☐ Endotracheal suction q4h, then prn
    - ☐ Wean ventilator to extubate per protocol (see Tables 10.3–10.5, pages 475–476)
    - ☐ O_2 via face mask with FiO_2 0.6–1.0 per protocol
    - ☐ O_2 via nasal prongs @ 2–6 liters/min to keep SaO_2 >95%
    - ☐ Incentive spirometer q1h when awake
    - ☐ Cough pillow at bedside
    - ☐ Albuterol 0.5 mL of 0.5% solution (2.5 mg) in 3 mL normal saline q6h via nebulizer or metered dose inhaler 6 puffs via endotracheal tube (90 μg/inhalation)

(continued)

Manual of Perioperative Care in Adult Cardiac Surgery, Sixth Edition. Robert M. Bojar.
© 2021 John Wiley & Sons Ltd. Published 2021 by John Wiley & Sons Ltd.

(continued)

18. Laboratory tests
    ☐ On arrival: STAT ABGs, CBC, electrolytes, glucose
          STAT PT, PTT, platelet count if chest tube output >100/h
          (thromboelastogram if available)
          STAT chest x-ray (if not done in operating room)
          STAT ECG
    ☐ Four and eight hours after arrival and prn: potassium, hematocrit, ABGs (respiratory distress)
    ☐ ABGs per protocol (prior to weaning and prior to extubation)
    ☐ 3:00 AM on POD #1: CBC, lytes, BUN, creatinine, blood glucose, ECG, CXR, INR (if patient to receive warfarin after valve procedure)
19. Pacemaker settings
    Mode: ☐ Atrial ☐ VVI ☐ DVI ☐ DDD
    Atrial output: _____ mA   Ventricular output: _____ mA
    Rate: _____/min   AV interval: _____ msec
    Sensitivity: ☐ Asynchronous ☐ Demand
    ☐ Pacer off but attached
20. Cardiac rehab consult
21. Notify MD/PA/NP for:
    a. Systolic blood pressure <90 or >140 mm Hg
    b. Cardiac index <2.0 L/min/m^2
    c. Urine output <30 mL/h for 2 hours
    d. Chest tube drainage >100 mL/h
    e. Temperature >38.5 °C
22. IV Drips/Medications (with suggested ranges)
    Allergies_____
    a. IV drips:
        ☐ Dextrose 5% in 0.45% NS 250 mL via Cordis/triple lumen to KVO
        ☐ Arterial line and distal Swan-Ganz port: NS flushes at 3 mL/h
        ☐ Epinephrine 1 mg/250 mL D5W: _____ µg/min to maintain cardiac index >2.0 (0.01–0.06 µg/kg/min or 1–4 µg/min)
        ☐ Milrinone 20 mg/100 mL D5W: _____ µg/kg/min (0.25–0.75 µg/kg/min)
        ☐ Dobutamine 250 mg/250 mL D5W: _____ µg/kg/min (5–20 µg/kg/min)
        ☐ Norepinephrine 4–8 mg/250 mL D5W: _____ µg/min to keep systolic BP >100 (0.01–1.0 µg/kg/min)
        ☐ Phenylephrine 20 mg/250 mL NS: _____ µg/min to keep systolic BP >100 (0.1–3.0 µg/kg/min)
        ☐ Vasopressin 100 units/250 mL D5W: _____ units/min (0.01–0.1 units/min)
        ☐ Nitroprusside 50 mg/250 mL D5W: _____ µg/kg/min to keep systolic BP <130 (0.1–8 µg/kg/min)
        ☐ Clevidipine 50 mg/100 mL D5W: _____ mg/h to keep systolic BP <130 (2–21 mg/h)
        ☐ Nicardipine 25 mg/250 mL D5W: _____ mg/h to keep BP <130 (5–15 mg/h)
        ☐ Nitroglycerin 50 mg/250 mL D5W: _____ µg/kg/min (0.1–5 µg/kg/min)
        ☐ Diltiazem: 100 mg/100 mL D5W: _____ mg/h (for radial artery prophylaxis)
        ☐ Esmolol 2.5 g/250 mL NS: _____ µg/kg/min (25–100 µg/kg/min)
        ☐ Amiodarone: after initial IV load in OR, 900 mg/500 mL D5W: 1 mg/min × 6 hours, then decrease to 0.5 mg/min × 18 hours
        ☐ Lidocaine 2 g/250 mL D5W: _____ mg/min IV; wean off at 6:00 AM POD #1

b. Antibiotics
 - ☐ Cefazolin 1 g IV q8h for 6 doses
 - ☐ Vancomycin 1 g IV q12h for 4 doses

c. Sedatives/analgesics
 - ☐ Propofol infusion 10 mg/mL: 25–75 µg/kg/min; wean to off per protocol
 - ☐ Dexmedetomidine: 400 µg (2 vials of 2 mL of 100 µg/mL solution)/100 mL NS: bolus dose of _____ (1 µg/kg) over 10 minutes, then maintenance infusion of _____ µg/kg/h (0.2–1.5 µg/kg/h)
 - ☐ Midazolam 2 mg IV q2h prn agitation; stop after extubation
 - ☐ Morphine sulfate _____ mg IV q2h prn for pain (while intubated)
 - ☐ Meperidine 25–50 mg IV prn shivering
 - ☐ Ketorolac 30–60 mg IV q6h prn for moderate–severe pain (4–10 on pain scale); stop after 72 hours
 - ☐ Acetaminophen 650 mg PO/IV q4h prn pain (maximum 4 g/day)
 - ☐ Oxycodone with acetaminophen (Percocet) 5/325 mg 1–2 tabs PO q4h prn for pain after extubation; start with 1 tab for mild pain (1–3 on pain scale); give additional tab 60 minutes later if no change in pain. Give 2 tabs for moderate–severe pain (4–10 on pain scale)

d. Other medications
 - ☐ β-blocker starting at 8:00 AM on POD #1, then q12 h; hold for HR <60 or SBP <100
   - ☐ Metoprolol _____ mg PO/per NG tube bid (12.5–100 mg bid)
   - ☐ Carvedilol _____ mg PO/per NG tube bid (3.125–25 mg bid)
 - ☐ Amiodarone 400 mg PO bid to start after amiodarone infusion discontinued
 - ☐ Magnesium sulfate 2 g in 50 mL NS IV over 2 hours on POD #1 in AM
 - ☐ Sucralfate 1 g per NG tube q6h until NG tube removed
 - ☐ Pantoprazole (Protonix) 40 mg IV/PO qd
 - ☐ Aspirin ☐ 81 mg ☐ 325 mg PO qd (starting 8 hours after arrival); hold for platelet count <60,000 or chest tube drainage >50 mL/h
 - ☐ Warfarin _____ mg starting _____; check with HO for daily dose (use warfarin protocol) (see Appendix 8)
 - ☐ Ascorbic acid 1 g PO qd × 5 days
 - ☐ Nitroglycerin 50 mg/250 mL D5W at 10–15 µg/min until taking PO (radial artery prophylaxis); then convert to:
   - ☐ Amlodipine 5 mg PO qd ☐ Amlodipine 10 mg PO qd
   - ☐ Isosorbide mononitrate sustained release (Imdur) 20 mg PO qd
 - ☐ Simvastatin _____ mg qd hs (no more than 20 mg if on amiodarone)
 - ☐ Mupirocin 2% (Bactroban ointment) via Q-tip nasal swab the evening after surgery and bid × 3 days
 - ☐ Chlorhexidine 0.12% oral wash (Peridex) 15 mL soft swab and rub oral cavity while intubated q12h

e. Prn medications
 - ☐ Acetaminophen 650 mg PO/PR q4h prn temp >38.5 °C
 - ☐ Metoclopramide 10 mg IV/PO q6h prn nausea
 - ☐ Ondansetron 4–8 mg IV q4h prn nausea
 - ☐ KCl 20 mEq/50 mL D5W via central line to keep K^+ >4.5 mEq/L:
   - ☐ KCl 10 mEq over 30 min for K+ 4.0–4.5
   - ☐ KCl 20 mEq over 60 min for K+ 3.5–3.9
   - ☐ KCl 40 mEq over 90 min for K+ <3.5
 - ☐ Initiate hyperglycemia protocol if blood glucose >150 mg/dL on admission or any time within the first 48 hours (see Appendix 6)
 - ☐ Other

5 Typical Transfer Orders from the ICU

ALLERGIES: _____
1. Transfer to: _____
2. Procedure: _____
3. Condition: _____
4. Nursing
   ☐ Vital signs q4h × 2 days, then qshift
   ☐ ECG telemetry
   ☐ I & O q8h
   ☐ Daily weights
   ☐ Foley catheter to gravity drainage; D/C on __/ __ at __; due to void in 8 hours
   ☐ Chest tubes to −20 cm H_2O suction
   ☐ Ambulate in hall with cardiac rehab
   ☐ T.E.D. stockings
   ☐ SpO_2 q8h and 1 time before and after ambulation
   ☐ Wire and wound care per protocol
   ☐ Wean oxygen via nasal prongs from 6 L/min to 2 L/min to keep SpO_2 >92%
   ☐ Incentive spirometry q1h when awake
   ☐ Glucose via fingerstick/glucometer AC and qhs in diabetics
   ☐ Notify house staff for:
      o Heart rate <60 or >110
      o Systolic BP <90 or >150 mm Hg
      o Oxygen saturation <90% on room air
      o Temperature >38.5 °C (>101 °F)
   ☐ Saline lock, flush q8h, and prn
5. Diet
   ☐ NPO
   ☐ Clear liquids/no added salt (NAS)
   ☐ Full liquids/NAS
   ☐ NAS, low fat, low cholesterol diet
   ☐ _____ cal ADA, NAS low cholesterol diet, if diabetic
   ☐ Fluid restriction _____ mL per 24 h (IV + PO)
6. Temporary pacemaker settings
   ☐ Pacemaker on: Mode: ☐ Atrial ☐ VVI ☐ DVI ☐ DDD
                   Atrial output: __ mA Ventricular output: __ mA
                   Rate: __/min   AV interval: __ msec
   ☐ Pacer attached but off
   ☐ Detach pacer but keep at bedside
7. Laboratory studies
   ☐ Chest x-ray after chest tube removal
   ☐ In AM after transfer: CBC, electrolytes, BUN, creatinine, blood glucose
   ☐ Daily PT/INR if on warfarin

Manual of Perioperative Care in Adult Cardiac Surgery, Sixth Edition. Robert M. Bojar.
© 2021 John Wiley & Sons Ltd. Published 2021 by John Wiley & Sons Ltd.

☐ Daily PTT and platelet count if on heparin (see Appendix 7)
☐ On day prior to discharge: chest x-ray, ECG, CBC, electrolytes, BUN, creatinine
8. Consults
    ☐ Cardiac rehabilitation
    ☐ Social services
    ☐ Physical therapy
    ☐ Occupational therapy
    ☐ Nutrition
9. Medications
    a. Antibiotics
        ☐ Cefazolin 1 g IV q8h for __ more doses (6 doses total); last dose on__/__ at ____ hours
        ☐ Vancomycin 1 g IV q12h for __ more doses (4 doses total); last dose on__/__ at _____ hours
        ☐ Mupirocin 2% (Bactroban ointment) via Q-tip nasal swab the evening after surgery and bid × 3 days total
    b. Cardiovascular medications
        ☐ Metoprolol __ mg PO q12h. Hold for HR <60 or SBP <100
        ☐ Carvedilol __ mg PO q12h. Hold for HR <60 or SBP <100
        ☐ Amiodarone ____ mg PO q12h
        ☐ Lisinopril __ mg PO qd
        ☐ Diltiazem 30 mg PO q6h (radial artery grafts)
        ☐ Amlodipine 5 mg PO qd (radial artery grafts)
        ☐ Imdur (sustained release) 20 mg PO qd (radial artery grafts)
        ☐ Simvastatin __ mg qd hs (no more than 20 mg if on amiodarone)
    c. Anticoagulants/antiplatelet agents
        ☐ Aspirin ☐ 81 mg ☐ 325 mg PO qd (hold for platelet count <60,000)
        ☐ Clopidogrel 75 mg PO qd
        ☐ Ticagrelor 90 mg PO bid
        ☐ Low-molecular-weight heparin (Lovenox) ___ mg SC___
        ☐ Heparin 5000 units SC bid
        ☐ Heparin 25,000 units/500 mL D5W at ___ units/h starting on___ (per protocol – see Appendix 7)
        ☐ Warfarin ___ mg PO qd starting on___; daily dose check with HO (per protocol – see page 773 and Appendix 8)
    d. Pain medications
        ☐ Morphine sulfate via PCA pump or 10 mg IM q3h prn severe pain
        ☐ Ketorolac 15–30 mg IV q6h prn moderate–severe pain (4–10 on pain scale); D/C after 72 hours
        ☐ Acetaminophen with oxycodone (Percocet) 2 tabs PO q4h for severe pain (6–10)
        ☐ Acetaminophen with oxycodone (Percocet) 1 tabs PO q4h for moderate pain; give additional tab if no change in pain after 1 hour
        ☐ Acetaminophen 650 mg PO q4h prn mild pain
    e. GI medications
        ☐ Pantoprazole (Protonix) 40 mg PO qd
        ☐ For nausea:
            ☐ Metoclopramide 10 mg IV/PO q6h prn
            ☐ Ondansetron 4–8 mg IV/PO q4h prn
            ☐ Prochlorperazine 10 mg PO/IM/IV q6h prn

(continued)

(continued)

    ☐ Milk of magnesia 30 mL PO qhs prn
    ☐ Docusate (Colace) 100 mg PO bid
    ☐ Bisacodyl (Dulcolax) 10 mg suppository prn constipation

f. Diabetes medications
    ☐ Oral hypoglycemic: _____
    ☐ ____ units regular insulin (Novolin R or Humulin R) SC ____ qAM ____ qPM
    ☐ ____ units NPH insulin (Novolin N or Humulin N) SC ____ qAM ___ qPM
    ☐ Sliding scale: treat fingerstick/glucometer glucose according to the following
       scale at 06:00 AM, 11:00 AM, 3:00 PM, and 8:00 PM
          150–160, give 2 units regular insulin SC (Novolin R or Humulin R)
          161–200, give 4 units regular insulin SC
          201–250, give 6 units regular insulin SC
          251–300, give 8 units regular insulin SC
          301–350, give 10 units regular insulin SC
          >350, call house officer

g. Other medications
    ☐ Acetaminophen 650 mg PO q3h prn temp >38.5 °C
    ☐ Ascorbic acid 1 g PO qd × 5 days
    ☐ Zolpidem 2.5–5 mg PO qhs prn sleep
    ☐ Melatonin ____mg PO qhs prn sleep (1.5–3 mg usual dose)
    ☐ Furosemide ___ mg IV/PO q _ h
    ☐ Potassium chloride ___ mEq PO bid (while on furosemide)
    ☐ Albuterol 2.5 mg/5 mL NS via nebulizer q4h prn
    ☐ Levalbuterol (Xopenex) 0.63 mg in 3 mL NS q8h via nebulizer or two inhalations
       q4–6h through a pressured MDI
    ☐ Duoneb inhaler q6h
    ☐ Other: _____

♡ 6 Hyperglycemia Protocol for Cardiac Surgery Patients

Goal: to maintain blood sugar (BS) between 110 and 150 mg/dL after surgery

- ☐ Check glucometer BS q1h
- ☐ Decrease to q4h if no changes in insulin drip rate for 6 hours and serum BS <130 on three consecutive measurements.
- ☐ Correlate glucometer BS to serum BS daily
- ☐ Maintain serum potassium between 4.0 and 4.5 mEq/L
- ☐ Page house officer for BS <90 or >320 mg/dL
- ☐ Initiate protocol for BS >150 mg/dL on admission or at any subsequent time with regular insulin 100 units/100 mL NS continuous infusion

Blood Sugar	Regular Insulin IV Bolus	Infusion Rate
151–200	No bolus	2 units/h
201–240	4 units	2 units/h
241–280	6 units	4 units/h
281–320	10 units	6 units/h

IV Insulin Adjustment Protocol

Blood Sugar	Insulin IV Bolus and Infusion Rate
<90	IV bolus with 1/2 amp 50% dextrose and stop infusion
91–110	Stop infusion; restart at 50% of previous rate once BS is <150
111–150	No change in infusion rate
151–200	Increase infusion rate by 2 units/h
201–240	IV bolus with 4 units and increase infusion by 2 units/h
241–280	IV bolus with 6 units and increase infusion by 2 unit/h
281–320	IV bolus with 10 units and increase infusion by 4 units/h
>320	Page house officer

Manual of Perioperative Care in Adult Cardiac Surgery, Sixth Edition. Robert M. Bojar.
© 2021 John Wiley & Sons Ltd. Published 2021 by John Wiley & Sons Ltd.

Transition to Subcutaneous Insulin

☐ units Insulin glargine (Lantus) SC daily

☐ units Insulin aspart (Novolog) SC tid with first dose 30 minutes prior to stopping insulin infusion

1. Take the average hourly requirement for insulin (in units/h) for the past 4 hours and multiply by 24 for the total daily dose of insulin (e.g. 1 unit/h × 24 = 24 units/day)

2. Give 80% of that dose for total daily dose of SC insulin (e.g. 24 units becomes 20 units/day), giving half as insulin glargine (basal) and half as insulin aspart (very fast acting) divided into 3 daily doses. Subsequent requirements may be adjusted based upon response to these initial doses.

3. In this example, for 20 units/day, the patient would receive 10 units of Lantus and approximately 4 units of Novolog tid.

7 Heparinization Protocol for Cardiac Surgery Patients

1. Patient weight: ___ kg
2. PT, PTT, CBC, and platelet count before starting heparin
3. Initial PTT 6 hours after starting infusion (4 hours if a bolus is given)
4. Recheck PTT after changing infusion rate
5. Daily PTT in AM
6. Check platelet count daily if <100,000 and qod if >100,000 while on heparin
7. Guaiac all stools
8. Notify house officer for any bleeding, PTT <35 or >100 seconds
9. Discontinue all previous heparin orders. Do not administer for 12 hours after last dose of low-molecular-weight heparin
10. Heparin bolus
    ☐ No bolus
    ☐ Give IV bolus of 50–75 mg/kg = __ units (round to nearest 100)
11. Heparin infusion 25,000/500 mL of 0.45% NS @ __ units/h (usually 15–18 units/kg)
    ☐ 40–60 kg   600 units/h
    ☐ 61–70 kg   800 units/h
    ☐ 71–80 kg   1000 units/h
    ☐ 81–90 kg   1100 units/h
    ☐ 91–100 kg   1200 units/h
    ☐ >100 kg   1500 units/h
12. Heparin adjustment schedule

PTT (sec)	Infusion Rate	Recheck PTT in
<46	Increase by 4 units/kg/h	4h
46–55	Increase by 2 units/kg/h	4h
56–65	No change	8h
66–75	Reduce by 1 unit/kg/h	6h
76–90	Reduce by 2 units/kg/h	4h
91–100	Stop for 1 hour & reduce by 3 units/kg/h	4h
>100	Stop for 2 hours & reduce by 4 units/kg/h	4h

Manual of Perioperative Care in Adult Cardiac Surgery, Sixth Edition. Robert M. Bojar.
© 2021 John Wiley & Sons Ltd. Published 2021 by John Wiley & Sons Ltd.

8 Protocol for Initiating Warfarin

Assess whether patient is at greater risk for sensitivity to warfarin – if so, use low-dose protocol			
a. Small, elderly females			
b. Over age 75			
c. Renal (creatinine >1.5 mg/dL) or hepatic dysfunction			
d. Interacting medications (amiodarone, antibiotics)			

Day	INR	Standard	Low-dose
1	WNL	5 mg	2.5 mg
2	<1.5	5 mg	2.5 mg
	1.5–1.9	2.5 mg	1.25 mg
	≥2	HOLD*	HOLD*
3	<1.5	7.5 mg	5 mg
	1.5–1.9	5 mg	2.5 mg
	2–3	2.5 mg	HOLD*
	>3	HOLD*	HOLD*
4	<1.5	10 mg	7.5 mg
	1.5–1.9	7.5 mg	5 mg
	2–3	5 mg	HOLD*
	>3	HOLD*	HOLD*
5	<1.5	10 mg	10 mg
	1.5–1.9	10 mg	5 mg
	2–3	5 mg	HOLD*
	>3	HOLD*	HOLD*
6	<1.5	12.5 mg	10 mg
	1.5–1.9	10 mg	7.5 mg
	2–3	5 mg	2.5 mg
	>3	HOLD*	HOLD*
*Restart warfarin when INR is less than 3			

Manual of Perioperative Care in Adult Cardiac Surgery, Sixth Edition. Robert M. Bojar.
© 2021 John Wiley & Sons Ltd. Published 2021 by John Wiley & Sons Ltd.

♡ **9** INR Reversal Protocol

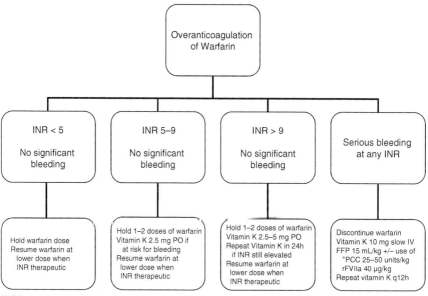

```
                    ┌──────────────────┐
                    │ Overanticoagulation │
                    │   of Warfarin    │
                    └──────────────────┘
```

INR < 5	INR 5–9	INR > 9	Serious bleeding at any INR
No significant bleeding	No significant bleeding	No significant bleeding	

Hold warfarin dose Resume warfarin at lower dose when INR therapeutic	Hold 1–2 doses of warfarin Vitamin K 2.5 mg PO if at risk for bleeding Resume warfarin at lower dose when INR therapeutic	Hold 1–2 doses of warfarin Vitamin K 2.5–5 mg PO Repeat Vitamin K in 24h if INR still elevated Resume warfarin at lower dose when INR therapeutic	Discontinue warfarin Vitamin K 10 mg slow IV FFP 15 mL/kg +/– use of *PCC 25–50 units/kg rFVIIa 40 µg/kg Repeat vitamin K q12h

*PCC = 3-factor (Profilnine) or 4-factor (Kcentra) prothrombin complex concentrate

Manual of Perioperative Care in Adult Cardiac Surgery, Sixth Edition. Robert M. Bojar.
© 2021 John Wiley & Sons Ltd. Published 2021 by John Wiley & Sons Ltd.

♡ 10A The CHA$_2$DS$_2$-VASc Score

The CHA$_2$DS$_2$-VASc score provides a prediction of the risk of stroke in the patient with nonrheumatic atrial fibrillation if not managed with anticoagulation.

Points	Condition
1	C: congestive heart failure (or LV systolic dysfunction)
1	H: hypertension
2	A: age >75
1	D: diabetes mellitus
2	S: prior stroke or TIA
1	V: peripheral vascular disease
1	A: age 65–74
1	Sc: sex category (female)

Annual Stroke Risk

Score	Annual risk of stroke (%)
0	0
1	1.3
2	2.2
3	3.2
4	4.0
5	6.7
6	9.8
7	9.6
8	12.5
9	15.2

General recommendations are:
- No anticoagulation for male with 0 or female with 1 point
- Consider an oral anticoagulant for a male with a score of 1
- Anticoagulation for a score of 2

Manual of Perioperative Care in Adult Cardiac Surgery, Sixth Edition. Robert M. Bojar.
© 2021 John Wiley & Sons Ltd. Published 2021 by John Wiley & Sons Ltd.

10B The HAS-BLED Score

The HAS-BLED score is a predictive model of the one-year risk of major bleeding due to anticoagulation, including intracranial bleeding, hospitalization, hemoglobin decrease >2 g/dL, and/or need for transfusion. A score ≥3 is considered a high risk for bleeding.

Points	Condition
1	H: Uncontrolled hypertension
1 or 2	A: Abnormal renal (dialysis, creatinine >2.26 mg/dL)/hepatic function (cirrhosis, bilirubin 2 × normal, AST/AST/alkaline phosphatase >3 × normal)
1	S: Prior history of stroke
1	B: Prior major bleed or predisposition to bleeding
1	L: Labile INR
1	E: Elderly (age >65)
1	D: Drug usage (concomitant antiplatelet drugs/NSAIDs or consumption of >8 drinks/week of alcohol)

11 Drug, Food, and Dietary Supplement Interactions with Warfarin

Potentiation (increase INR)	Inhibition (decrease INR)	No Effect
Acetaminophen	Azathioprine	Alcohol (if no liver disease)
Alcohol (if liver disease)	Barbiturates	Antacids
Amiodarone	Bosentan	Atenolol
Anabolic steroids	Carbamazepine	Cefazolin
Aspirin	Chlordiazepoxide	Famotidine
Azithromycin	Cholestyramine	Furosemide
Chloral hydrate	Cyclosporine	Ibuprofen
Citalopram	Dicloxacillin	Ketorolac
Clofibrate	Nafcillin	Metoprolol
Diltiazem	Rifampin	Nizatidine
Fenofibrate	Sucralfate	Ranitidine
Floxin antibiotics		Vancomycin
Fluvastatin		
Gemfibrozil		
Lovastatin		
Metronidazole		
Omeprazole		
Phenytoin		
Propafenone		
Propranolol		
Sertraline		
Simvastatin		
Tramadol		
Foods and herbal supplements		
Fish oils	Avocado	Green tea
Grapefruit	Ginseng	
Mango	Green leafy vegetables	
	Multivitamins with vitamin K	
	Soy milk	

This is a partial list of drugs and products that interact with warfarin.
(Adapted from Ansell et al., *Chest* 2008;133:160S–198S.)

12 Doses of Parenteral Medications Commonly Used in the ICU and Their Modifications in Renal Failure

Drug Class	Usual Dosage	Route of Elimination	Adjustment in Moderate Renal Failure
Analgesics			
Fentanyl	50–100 µg IV → 50–200 µg/h	H	no change
Hydromorphone (Dilaudid)	1–2 mg IV/IM q4–6h	H	no change
Ketorolac (Toradol)	15–30 mg IV q6h (× 72 h)	R	reduce
Meperidine (Demerol)	50–100 mg IM q3h	H	use with caution
Morphine	2–10 mg IV/IM q2–4h	H	no change
Antacids			
Pantoprazole (Protonix)	40 mg IV over 15 min	H	no change
Ranitidine (Zantac)	50 mg IV q8h or 6.25 mg/h	R	reduce
Antianginals			
Esmolol	0.25–0.5 mg/kg IV → 0.05–0.2 mg/kg/min IV	M	no change
Metoprolol (Lopressor)	2.5–10 mg IV q15 min × 3	H	no change

Manual of Perioperative Care in Adult Cardiac Surgery, Sixth Edition. Robert M. Bojar.
© 2021 John Wiley & Sons Ltd. Published 2021 by John Wiley & Sons Ltd.

Drug Class	Usual Dosage	Route of Elimination	Adjustment in Moderate Renal Failure
Antiarrhythmics			
Amiodarone (Cordarone)	150 mg IV → 1 mg/min × 6 h → 0.5 mg/min × 18 h, then 1 g/day	H	no change
Lidocaine	1 mg/kg IV → 1–4 mg/min	H	no change
Antibiotics (prophylactic doses)			
Cefazolin (Ancef, Kefzol)	1–2 g IV → 1 g IV q8h	R	reduce
Cefuroxime (Zinacef)	1.5 g IV → 1.5 g IV q8h	R	reduce
Vancomycin	15–20 mg/kg → 1 g IV q12h	R	reduce
Antiemetics			
Dolasetron (Anzemet)	12.5 mg IV	H/R	no change
Droperidol (Inapsine)	0.625–1.25 mg IV	H	no change
Metoclopramide (Reglan)	10–20 mg IM/IV qid	R > H	reduce
Ondansetron (Zofran)	4–8 mg IV	H	no change
Prochlorperazine (Compazine)	5–10 mg IM q4h	H	no change
Antihypertensives (see Table 11.8, page 576)			
Diuretics			
Acetazolamide (Diamox)	250–500 mg IV q6h	R	use with caution
Bumetanide (Bumex)	1–5 mg IV q12h or 0.5–2 mg/h drip	R > H	use with caution
Chlorothiazide (Diuril)	500 mg IV qd	R	use with caution
Ethacrynic acid (Edecrin)	50–100 mg IV q6h	H > R	use with caution
Furosemide (Lasix)	20–200 mg IV q6h or 5–20 mg/h drip	R > H	use with caution

Drug Class	Usual Dosage	Route of Elimination	Adjustment in Moderate Renal Failure
Inotropic agents (see Table 11.6, page 537)			
Paralytic agents (see also Table 4.3, page 246)			
Atracurium (Tracrium)	0.4 mg/kg IV → 8 µg/kg/min	M	no change
Cisatracurium (Nimbex)	0.1–0.2 mg/kg IV → 3 µg/kg/min	M	no change
Doxacurium (Nuromax)	0.06 mg/kg → 0.005 mg/kg q30 min	R	reduce
Pancuronium (Pavulon)	0.1 mg/kg IV → 0.5–1 µg/kg/min	R > H	no change
Rocuronium (Zemuron)	0.6–1.2 mg/kg IV → 10 µg/kg/min	H	no change
Vecuronium (Norcuron)	0.1 mg/kg IV → 0.5–1 µg/kg/min	H	no change
Psychotropics/Sedatives			
Dexmedetomidine (Precedex)	1 µg/kg load, then 0.2–1.5 µg/kg/h	H	no change
Haloperidol (Haldol)	2–10 mg IM/IV q4–6h	H	no change
Lorazepam (Ativan)	1–2 mg IV/2–4 mg IM q6h	H	no change
Midazolam (Versed)	2.5–5 mg IV q1–2h	H	no change
Propofol (Diprivan)	25–75 µg/kg/min	M	no change
Other			
Aminophylline	5 mg/kg IV load → 0.2–0.9 mg/kg/h	H	no change
Flumazenil	0.2 mg q30 sec, then 0.3 mg, then 0.5 mg up to 3 mg max/h	H	no change
Naloxone	0.04–0.08 mg/min IV (postoperative patients) to a total of 0.4 mg	H	no change

Medications metabolized by the liver do not require reduction in dosage for renal failure; medications metabolized by the kidneys must be adjusted according to the serum creatinine, or more precisely by the glomerular filtration rate. The reader should refer to the *Physician's Desk Reference* or online (PDR.net) or other online drug websites, such as Rxlist.com, for complete prescribing information.
H, hepatic metabolism; R, renal elimination; M, metabolized in the bloodstream

♡ **13** Doses of Nonparenteral Drugs Commonly Used After Heart Surgery and Their Modifications in Renal Failure

Drug Class	Usual Dosage	Route of Elimination	Adjustment in Moderate Renal Failure
Analgesics			
Acetaminophen	650 mg PO q4h	R	reduce
Gabapentin (Neurontin)	300–600 mg PO tid	R	reduce
Hydrocodone[a]	5 mg PO q4–6h	H	no change
Hydromorphone (Dilaudid)	2–4 mg PO q4–6h	H	no change
Ibuprofen	400–800 mg PO tid	R	reduce
Ketorolac (Toradol)	20 mg PO → 10 mg q4–6h	R	reduce
Oxycodone[a]	4.5 mg PO q6h	H	no change
[a] usually given with acetaminophen 325 mg (Vicodin or Percocet)			
Antacids/antireflux medications			
Sucralfate (Carafate)	1 g PO qid	R	reduce
H₂ blockers			
Famotidine (Pepcid)	20–40 mg PO qhs	R > M	reduce
Nizatidine (Axid)	150 mg PO bid or 300 qhs	R	reduce
Ranitidine (Zantac)	150 mg PO bid	R	reduce
Proton pump inhibitors			
Lansoprazole (Prevacid)	15 mg PO qd	H	no change

Manual of Perioperative Care in Adult Cardiac Surgery, Sixth Edition. Robert M. Bojar.
© 2021 John Wiley & Sons Ltd. Published 2021 by John Wiley & Sons Ltd.

Drug Class	Usual Dosage	Route of Elimination	Adjustment in Moderate Renal Failure
Omeprazole (Prilosec)	20 mg PO qd	H	no change
Pantoprazole (Protonix)	40 mg PO qd	H	no change
Antianginals (and antihypertensives)			
β-blockers			
Atenolol (Tenormin)	25–50 mg PO qd	R	reduce
Carvedilol (Coreg)	3.125–25 mg PO tid	H	no change
Metoprolol succinate (Toprol XL)	25–200 mg PO qd	H	no change
Metoprolol tartrate (Lopressor)	12.5–100 mg PO bid	H	no change
Calcium channel blockers			
Amlodipine	5–10 mg PO qd	H	no change
Diltiazem	30–60 mg PO tid or 180–360 qd of long-acting preparation	H	no change
Nicardipine	20–40 mg PO tid	H	no change
Nifedipine	10–30 mg PO/SL tid	H	no change
Verapamil	80–160 mg PO tid	H	no change
Nitrates			
Isosorbide dinitrate (Isordil)	5–40 mg PO tid	H	no change
Isosorbide mononitrate (Imdur, Ismo)	20 mg PO qd	—	no change
Nitropaste	1–3" q4h	H	no change
Antiarrhythmics (see Chapter 11, pages 642–650)			
Amiodarone	400 mg PO tid weaned to 200 mg qd	H	no change
Digoxin	0.125–0.25 mg PO qd	R	reduce
Sotalol	80 mg PO bid	R	reduce

Drug Class	Usual Dosage	Route of Elimination	Adjustment in Moderate Renal Failure
Antibiotics			
Cephalexin	500 mg PO bid	R	reduce
Ciprofloxacin	500 mg PO bid	R	reduce
Anticoagulants			
Apixaban (Eliquis)	5–10 mg PO bid	R	reduce
Dabigatran (Pradaxa)	75–150 mg PO bid	R	reduce
Edoxaban (Savaysa)	30–60 mg PO qd	R	reduce
Rivaroxaban (Xarelto)	20 mg PO qd	R	reduce
Antidiabetic drugs (oral hypoglycemics)			
Chlorpropamide (Diabinese)	250 mg PO qd	R	avoid
Glipizide (Glucotrol)	5 mg PO qAM	H	no change
Glyburide (Micronase, Diabeta)	2.5–5 mg PO qAM	H = R	use with caution
Metformin (Glucophage)	500–1000 mg PO bid for regular tablets and qd for extended release tablets	R	avoid
Pioglitazone (Actos)	15–30 mg PO qd	H	no change
Rosiglitazone (Avandia)	4–8 mg PO qd	H	no change
Antiemetics			
Dolasetron (Anzemet)	100 mg PO	H/R	no change
Metoclopramide (Reglan)	10–20 mg PO qid	R > H	reduce
Ondansetron (Zofran)	8–16 mg PO	H	no change
Prochlorperazine (Compazine)	5–10 mg PO q6h	H	no change
Antihypertensives			
Angiotensin-converting enzyme (ACE) inhibitors			
Captopril (Capoten)	6.25–50 mg PO bid	R	avoid
Enalapril (Vasotec)	2.5–5 mg PO qd	R	avoid

Drug Class	Usual Dosage	Route of Elimination	Adjustment in Moderate Renal Failure
Lisinopril (Zestril)	5–40 mg PO qd	R	avoid
Quinapril (Accupril)	10 mg PO qd	R	avoid
Ramipril (Altace)	2.5 mg PO qd	R > H	reduce
Angiotensin II receptor blockers (ARBs)			
Candesartan (Atacand)	8–32 mg PO qd or in 2 divided doses	H	no change
Irbesartan (Avapro)	150–300 mg PO qd	H	no change
Losartan (Cozaar)	25–100 mg PO qd or in 2 divided doses	H	no change
Valsartan (Diovan)	80–160 mg PO qd	H	no change
β-blockers _(see also_ **_Antianginals_**_)_			
Carvedilol (Coreg)	3.125–25 mg PO bid	H	reduce
Labetalol (Trandate, Normodyne)	100–400 mg PO qid	H	no change
Nebivolol (Bystolic)	5–40 mg PO qd	H	no change
Calcium channel blockers _(see also_ **_Antianginals_**_)_			
Amlodipine (Norvasc)	2.5–10 mg PO qd	H	no change
Nicardipine (Cardene)	20–40 mg PO tid	H	no change
Others			
Clonidine (Catapres)	0.1–0.3 mg PO bid	R	reduce
Doxazosin (Cardura)	1.0–8 mg PO qd	H	no change
Prazosin (Minipress)	1.0–7.5 mg PO bid	H	no change
Cholesterol-lowering medications			
Atorvastatin (Lipitor)	10–80 mg PO qd	H	no change
Ezetimibe (Zetia)	10 mg PO qd	—	no change
Pravastatin (Pravachol)	40–80 mg PO qd	H	no change
Rosuvastatin (Crestor)	10–20 mg PO qd	–	no change
Simvastatin (Zocor)	10–80 mg PO qd	H	no change

Drug Class	Usual Dosage	Route of Elimination	Adjustment in Moderate Renal Failure
Diuretics			
Acetazolamide (Diamox)	250–500 mg PO qid	R	reduce
Bumetanide (Bumex)	0.5–2 mg PO qd	H	no change
Furosemide (Lasix)	10–100 mg PO bid	R > H	no change
Hydrochlorothiazide (Hydrodiuril)	50–100 mg PO qd	R	no change
Metolazone (Zaroxolyn)	2.5–10 mg PO qd	R	no change
Torsemide	5–20 mg PO qd	H > R	no change
Diuretics (potassium-sparing)			
Amiloride (Midador)	5–10 mg PO qd	R	avoid
Eplerenone (Inspra)	50 mg PO qd	H	no change
Spironolactone (Aldactone)	25 mg PO qd	R	avoid
Psychotropics/Sedatives/Antidepressants			
Alprazolam (Xanax)	0.25–0.5 mg PO tid	H, R	reduce
Amitriptyline (Elavil)	10–20 mg PO qhs or bid	H	no change
Bupropion (Wellbutrin, Zyban)	100 mg PO bid	H	no change
Buspirone (Buspar)	7.5 mg PO bid	—	no change
Chlordiazepoxide (Librium)	5–25 mg PO tid	H	no change
Citalopram (Celexa)	20 mg PO qd	H	no change
Fluoxetine (Prozac)	20–40 mg PO qd	H	no change
Haloperidol (Haldol)	0.5–2.5 mg PO tid	H	no change
Lorazepam (Ativan)	0.5–2 mg PO bid or hs	H	no change
Olanzapine (Zyprexa)	5–10 mg PO qd	H	no change
Paroxetine (Paxil)	20–50 mg PO qd	H/R	reduce
Quetiapine (Seroquel)	25–100 mg PO bid	H	no change

Drug Class	Usual Dosage	Route of Elimination	Adjustment in Moderate Renal Failure
Risperidone (Risperdal)	2 mg PO qd	H	no change
Sertraline (Zoloft)	50–200 mg PO qd	H	no change
Venlafaxine (Effexor)	25 mg PO bid or tid	R	reduce
Sleep medications			
Chloral hydrate	500–1000 mg PO hs	H	no change
Diphenhydramine (Benadryl)	25–50 mg PO hs	H	no change
Melatonin	0.5–5 mg PO hs	H	no change
Temazepam (Restoril)	15–30 mg PO hs	H	no change
Triazolam (Halcion)	0.125–0.25 mg PO hs	H	no change
Zaleplon (Sonata)	5–10 mg PO hs	H	no change
Zolpidem (Ambien)	5–10 mg PO hs	H	no change
Others			
Carbamazepine (Tegretol)	200 mg PO bid	H	no change
Varenicline (Chantix)	0.5–1.0 mg PO qd	—	no change

Antianginal medications given four times a day (qid) are usually taken four hours apart during the daytime. Other medications should generally be taken at equally spaced intervals.

Medications metabolized by the liver do not require reduction in dosage for renal failure; medications metabolized by the kidneys must be adjusted according to the serum creatinine, or more precisely, by the glomerular filtration rate. The reader should refer to the *Physician's Desk Reference* or online (PDR.net) or other online drug websites, such as Rxlist.com, for complete prescribing information.

H, hepatic metabolism; R, renal elimination; M, metabolized in the bloodstream

14 Definitions from the STS Data Specifications (Version 4.20 2020)

Preoperative Conditions

1. **Chronic lung disease**
   a. Mild: FEV_1 60–75% of predicted, and/or on chronic inhaled or oral bronchodilator therapy
   b. Moderate: FEV_1 50–59% of predicted, and/or on chronic oral/systemic steroid therapy aimed at lung disease
   c. Severe: FEV_1 <50% and/or room air pO_2 <60 or pCO_2 >50

2. **Peripheral arterial disease** (excludes carotid, cerebrovascular disease, or thoracic aorta)
   a. Claudication, either with exertion or at rest
   b. Amputation for arterial vascular insufficiency
   c. Vascular reconstruction, bypass surgery, or percutaneous intervention to the extremities (excluding dialysis fistulas and vein stripping)
   d. Documented abdominal aortic aneurysm with or without repair
   e. Positive noninvasive or invasive test showing > 50% diameter stenosis in any peripheral artery
   f. Documented subclavian artery stenosis

3. **Cerebrovascular disease**
   a. Stroke: an acute episode of focal or global neurological dysfunction caused by brain, spinal cord, or retinal vascular injury as a result of hemorrhage or infarction, where the neurological dysfunction lasts for greater than 24 hours.
   b. TIA: a transient episode of focal neurological dysfunction caused by brain, spinal cord, or retinal ischemia, without acute infarction, where the neurological dysfunction resolves within 24 hours.
   c. Noninvasive or invasive arterial imaging test demonstrating ≥50% stenosis of any of the major extracranial or intracranial vessels of the brain
   d. Vertebral artery, internal carotid or intracranial vessel consistent with atherosclerotic disease with documented presence as cerebrovascular disease
   e. Previous cervical or cerebral artery revascularization surgery or percutaneous intervention
   f. Brain/cerebral aneurysm
   g. Occlusion of vertebral artery, internal carotid artery, or intracranial vessel due to dissection

---

Manual of Perioperative Care in Adult Cardiac Surgery, Sixth Edition. Robert M. Bojar.
© 2021 John Wiley & Sons Ltd. Published 2021 by John Wiley & Sons Ltd.

4. **Diabetes mellitus**
   a. Hemoglobin A1c ≥6.5%; or
   b. A history of diabetes diagnosed and/or treated by a healthcare provider
   c. Definitions in prior specifications included:
      i. Fasting plasma glucose ≥126 mg/dL (7.0 mmol/L); or
      ii. Two-hour plasma glucose ≥200 mg/dL (11.1 mmol/L) during an oral glucose tolerance test; or
      iii. In a patient with classic symptoms of hyperglycemia or hyperglycemic crisis, a random plasma glucose ≥200 mg/dL (11.1 mmol/L)

5. **Renal failure** on dialysis is the only criterion listed on version 4.20 STS entry forms. The serum creatinine is a data entry, and the stage of chronic kidney disease noted below is helpful in assessing the risk of acute kidney injury or the risk of dialysis. GFR is measured in mL/min/1.73 m².
   a. Stage 1   GFR >90
   b. Stage 2   GFR 60–89
   c. Stage 3a   GFR 45–59
   d. Stage 3b   GFR 30–44
   e. Stage 4   GFR 15–30
   f. Stage 5   GFR <15

6. **Hypertension**
   a. A history of hypertension diagnosed and treated with medication, diet, and/or exercise
   b. Currently undergoing pharmacological therapy for treatment of hypertension
   c. Definitions in prior specifications included prior documentation of blood pressure >140 mm Hg systolic and/or >90 mm Hg diastolic for patients without diabetes or chronic kidney disease, or prior documentation of blood pressure >130 mm Hg systolic or >80 mm Hg diastolic on at least two occasions for patients with diabetes or chronic kidney disease (see *J Am Coll Cardiol* 2017;71:e127–248).

7. **Heart failure (HF):** unusual dyspnea on light exertion, recurrent dyspnea occurring in the supine position, fluid retention; or the description of rales, jugular venous distension, pulmonary edema on physical exam, or pulmonary edema on chest x-ray presumed to be cardiac dysfunction. A low ejection fraction alone, without clinical evidence of heart failure, does not qualify as heart failure. An elevated BNP without other supporting documentation should not be coded as HF.
   a. Acute HF: rapid onset of symptoms and signs of HF that may occur with or without previous cardiac disease occurring within 2 weeks of surgery. Acute decompensated HF is a sudden worsening of the signs and symptoms of HF, which typically include difficulty breathing (dyspnea), leg or feet swelling, and fatigue.
   b. Chronic HF develops gradually over time with symptoms of shortness of breath, lower extremity swelling, and fatigue without exacerbation within the 2 weeks prior to admission.
   c. Acute on chronic HF refers to patients with chronic HF who present with acute or worsening symptoms within 2 weeks of surgery.

8. **Stable angina:** angina without a change in frequency or pattern for the six weeks prior. Angina is controlled by rest and/or oral or transcutaneous medications.

9. **Unstable angina**
    a. Rest angina (occurring at rest and prolonged, usually >20 minutes)
    b. New-onset angina (within the past two months, of at least Canadian Cardiovascular Society (CCS) class III severity)
    c. Increasing angina (previously diagnosed angina that has become distinctly more frequent, longer in duration, or increased by one or more CCS classes to at least CCS III severity)

10. **Non-ST-elevation myocardial infarction (non-STEMI):** the patient was hospitalized for a NSTEMI as documented in the medical record. The definition in prior data specifications was the presence of both:
    a. Cardiac biomarkers (creatinine kinase-myocardial band, troponin T or I) that exceed the upper limit of normal. Laboratory confirmation of myocardial necrosis; laboratory parameters with a clinical presentation consistent or suggestive of ischemia. ECG changes and/or ischemic symptoms may or may not be present.
    b. Absence of ECG changes diagnostic of a STEMI.

11. **ST-elevation MI (STEMI):** the patient presented with a STEMI of its equivalent as documented in the medical records. The definition in prior data specifications was the presence of both:
    a. New/presumed new ST segment elevation or new left bundle branch block not documented to be resolved within 20 minutes. ST segment elevation is defined by new or presumed new sustained ST segment elevation at the J-point in two contiguous ECG leads with the cut-off points: ≥ 0.2 mV in men or ≥ 0.15 mV in women in leads V2–V3 and/or ≥ 0.1 mV in other leads and lasting greater than or equal to 20 minutes. ST elevation in the posterior chest leads (V7 through V9), or ST depression that is maximal in V1–V3, without ST segment elevation in other leads, demonstrating posterobasal myocardial infarction, is considered a STEMI equivalent.
    b. Cardiac biomarkers (CK-MB, troponin T or I) exceed the upper limit of normal with a clinical presentation which is consistent or suggestive of ischemia.

12. **Cardiogenic shock:** a sustained (>30 min) episode of hypoperfusion evidenced by systolic blood pressure <90 mm Hg and/or, if available, cardiac index <2.2 L/min/m² secondary to cardiac dysfunction and/or the requirement for parenteral inotropic or vasopressor agents or mechanical support (e.g. IABP, extracorporeal circulation, VADs) to maintain blood pressure and cardiac index above those specified levels.

13. **Resuscitation:** CPR required within 24 hours prior to induction of anesthesia for surgery, which may include use of ECMO or mechanical circulatory support exclusive of an IABP.

14. **Urgency**
    a. Elective: the patient's cardiac function has been stable in the days or weeks prior to the operation. The procedure could be deferred without increased risk of compromised cardiac outcome.
    b. Urgent: procedure required during same hospitalization in order to minimize chance of further clinical deterioration. This includes but is not limited to: worsening or sudden chest pain, HF, acute myocardial infarction (AMI), anatomy, IABP, unstable angina with intravenous nitroglycerin (IV NTG), or rest angina. Any of the conditions that require that the patient remain in the hospital until surgery can take place, but the patient is able to wait for surgery until the next available OR schedule time. Delay in the operation may be necessitated by attempts to improve the patient's

condition, availability of a spouse or parent for informed consent, availability of blood products, or the availability of results of essential laboratory procedures or tests.

c. **Emergent:** surgery is indicated without any delay for ongoing, refractory (difficult, complicated, and/or unmanageable) unrelenting cardiac compromise, with or without hemodynamic instability, and not responsive to any form of therapy except cardiac surgery. Examples include:

    i. Hemodynamic picture of shock that is being chemically or mechanically supported, such as IV inotrope or IABP to maintain cardiac output

    ii. Pulmonary edema requiring intubation and ventilation

    iii. An extending MI

    iv. Signs of ongoing ischemia, i.e. ECG changes

    v. Acute native valve dysfunction (acute papillary muscle rupture or torn leaflet)

    vi. Prosthetic valve dysfunction with structural failure (valve-fractured or torn leaflet, thrombus formation, pannus development which impedes flow through the valve orifice, or valvular dehiscence)

    vii. Acute aortic dissection, rupture or dissection during cardiac cath; perforation, tamponade following cardiac cath

d. **Emergent/Salvage:** the patient is undergoing CPR en route to the OR prior to anesthesia induction or has ongoing ECMO to maintain life.

Postoperative Complications

1. **Operative mortality:** all deaths, regardless of cause, occurring during the hospitalization in which the operation was performed, even if after 30 days (including patients transferred to other acute care facilities) and all deaths, regardless of cause, occurring after discharge from the hospital, but before the end of the 30th postoperative day.

2. **Neurological deficit**

    a. Permanent stroke: any confirmed neurological deficit of abrupt onset caused by a disturbance in blood supply to the brain that did not resolve within 24 hours.

    b. Encephalopathy: altered mental state

    c. New postoperative paralysis, paraparesis, or paraplegia related to spinal cord ischemia and not related to a stroke.

3. **Renal failure**

    a. An increase in serum creatinine level 3.0 × greater than baseline, or serum creatinine level ≥4 mg/dL. Acute rise must be at least 0.5 mg/dL.

    b. A new requirement for dialysis postoperatively.

4. **Prolonged ventilation:** prolonged postoperative pulmonary ventilation >24 hours from time of OR exit plus any additional hours following reintubation.

5. **Superficial wound infection:** an infection that occurs within 30 days after the procedure, **and** involves only skin/subcutaneous tissue of the incision, **and** the patient has at least one of the following:

    a. Purulent drainage from the superficial incision

    b. Organisms isolated from an aseptically obtained culture of fluid or tissue from the superficial incision

    c. Superficial incision that is deliberately opened and is culture positive or not cultured **and** patient has ≥1 of the following: localized pain or tenderness, localized swelling, erythema, or heat. Note that cellulitis alone or a stitch abscess does not qualify as a superficial incisional infection.

6. **Deep sternal wound infection:** an infection that occurs within 30 days after the procedure, **and** involves deep soft tissues of the incision (e.g. fascial and muscle layers) **with** at least one of the following:

   a. Purulent drainage from the deep incision

   b. A deep incision that spontaneously dehisces or is deliberately opened and is culture-positive or not cultured, **and** the patient has at least one of the following signs or symptoms: fever (>38 °C), localized pain or tenderness, an abscess or other evidence of infection involving the deep incision that is detected on direct examination, during invasive procedure, or by histopathologic examination or imaging test.

7. **Organ system infection** that occurs within 30 days after the procedure that involves any part of the body deeper than the fascia or muscle layers that is opened or manipulated during the operative procedure and the patient has at least one of the following:

   a. Purulent drainage from a drain that is placed into the organ/space

   b. Organisms isolated from an aseptically obtained culture of fluid or tissue in the organ/space

   c. An abscess or other evidence of infection involving the organ/space that is detected on direct examination, during invasive procedure, or by histopathologic examination or imaging test, **and** meets at least one of the following criteria for a specific organ/space infection of mediastinitis:

      • Organisms cultured from mediastinal tissue or fluid obtained during an invasive procedure

      • Evidence of mediastinitis seen during an invasive procedure or histopathologic examination; **and**

      • **At least 1** of the following signs or symptoms: fever (>38 °C), chest pain, or sternal instability; **and**

      • **At least 1** of the following: purulent discharge from mediastinal area or organisms cultured from blood or discharge from mediastinal area

15 Body Surface Area Nomogram

Height	Body Surface Area	Weight

Height
cm 200 — 79 in
78
195 — 77
76
190 — 75
74
185 — 73
72
180 — 71
70
175 — 69
68
170 — 67
66
165 — 65
64
160 — 63
62
155 — 61
60
150 — 59
58
145 — 57
56
140 — 55
54
135 — 53
52
130 — 51
50
125 — 49
48
120 — 47
46
115 — 45
44
110 — 43
42
105 — 41
40
cm 100 — 39 in

Body Surface Area
2.80 m^2
2.70
2.60
2.50
2.40
2.30
2.20
2.10
2.00
1.95
1.90
1.85
1.80
1.75
1.70
1.65
1.60
1.55
1.50
1.45
1.40
1.35
1.30
1.25
1.20
1.15
1.10
1.05
1.00
0.95
0.90
0.85 m^2

Weight
kg 150 — 330 lb
145 — 320
140 — 310
135 — 300
130 — 290
280
125 — 270
120 — 260
115 — 250
110 — 240
105 — 230
100 — 220
95 — 210
90 — 200
85 — 190
80 — 180
170
75 — 160
70 — 150
65 — 140
60 — 130
55 — 120
50 — 110
105
45 — 100
95
40 — 90
85
35 — 80
75
70
kg 30 — 66 lb

Manual of Perioperative Care in Adult Cardiac Surgery, Sixth Edition. Robert M. Bojar.
© 2021 John Wiley & Sons Ltd. Published 2021 by John Wiley & Sons Ltd.

♡ 16 Body Mass Index Chart

Weight (in Pounds)

Height (in Inches)	120	130	140	150	160	170	180	190	200	210	220	230	240	250	260
82	13	14	15	16	17	18	19	20	21	22	23	24	25	26	27
80	13	14	15	16	18	19	20	21	22	23	24	25	26	27	29
78	14	15	16	17	18	20	21	22	23	24	25	27	28	29	30
76	15	16	17	18	19	21	22	23	24	26	27	28	29	30	32
74	15	17	18	19	21	22	23	24	26	27	28	30	31	32	33
72	16	18	19	20	22	23	24	26	27	28	30	31	33	34	35
70	17	19	20	22	23	24	26	27	29	30	32	33	34	36	37
68	18	20	21	23	24	26	27	29	30	32	33	35	36	38	40
66	19	21	23	24	26	27	29	31	32	34	36	37	39	40	42
64	21	22	24	26	27	29	31	33	34	36	38	39	41	43	45
62	22	24	26	27	29	31	33	35	37	38	40	42	44	46	48
60	23	25	27	29	31	33	35	37	39	41	43	45	47	49	51
58	25	27	29	31	33	36	38	40	42	44	46	48	50	52	54
56	27	29	31	34	36	38	40	43	45	47	49	52	54	56	58
54	29	31	34	36	39	41	43	46	48	51	53	55	58	60	63

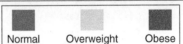

Normal   Overweight   Obese

Manual of Perioperative Care in Adult Cardiac Surgery, Sixth Edition. Robert M. Bojar.
© 2021 John Wiley & Sons Ltd. Published 2021 by John Wiley & Sons Ltd.

♡ 17 Aortic Size Index for Thoracic Aneurysms

BSA (m²)	Aortic Size (cm)									
	3.5	4.0	4.5	5.0	5.5	6.0	6.5	7.0	7.5	8.0
1.30	2.69	3.08	3.46	3.85	4.23	4.62	5.00	5.38	5.77	6.15
1.40	2.50	2.86	3.21	3.57	3.93	4.29	4.64	5.00	5.36	5.71
1.50	2.33	2.67	3.00	3.33	3.67	4.00	4.33	4.67	5.00	5.33
1.60	2.19	2.50	2.80	3.13	3.44	3.75	4.06	4.38	4.69	5.00
1.70	2.05	2.35	2.65	2.94	3.24	3.53	3.82	4.12	4.41	4.71
1.80	1.94	2.22	2.50	2.78	3.06	3.33	3.61	3.89	4.17	4.44
1.90	1.84	2.11	2.37	2.63	2.89	3.16	3.42	3.68	3.95	4.22
2.00	1.75	2.00	2.25	2.50	2.75	3.00	3.25	3.50	3.75	4.00
2.10	1.67	1.90	2.14	2.38	2.62	2.86	2.10	3.33	3.57	3.80
2.20	1.59	1.82	2.05	2.27	2.50	2.72	2.95	3.18	3.41	3.64
2.30	1.52	1.74	1.96	2.17	2.39	2.61	2.83	3.04	3.26	3.48
2.40	1.46	1.67	1.88	2.08	2.29	2.50	2.71	2.92	3.13	3.33
2.50	1.40	1.60	1.80	2.00	2.20	2.40	2.60	2.80	3.00	3.20

= Low risk (~4% per year) = Moderate risk (~7% per year)

= High risk (~12% per year) = Severe risk (~18% per year)

Reproduced with permission from Davies et al., *Ann Thorac Surg* 2006;81:169–77.

Manual of Perioperative Care in Adult Cardiac Surgery, Sixth Edition. Robert M. Bojar.
© 2021 John Wiley & Sons Ltd. Published 2021 by John Wiley & Sons Ltd.

18 Aortic Height Index for Thoracic Aneurysms

Height (inches)	(m)	Aortic Size (cm)									
		3.5	4.0	4.5	5.0	5.5	6.0	6.5	7.0	7.5	8.0
55	1.40	2.50	2.86	3.21	3.57	3.93	4.29	4.64	5.00	5.36	5.71
57	1.45	2.41	2.76	3.10	3.45	3.79	4.14	4.48	4.83	5.17	5.52
59	1.50	2.33	2.67	3.00	3.33	3.67	4.00	4.33	4.67	5.00	5.33
61	1.55	2.26	2.58	2.90	3.23	3.55	3.87	4.19	4.52	4.84	5.16
63	1.60	2.19	2.50	2.81	3.13	3.44	3.75	4.06	4.38	4.69	5.00
65	1.65	2.12	2.42	2.73	3.03	3.33	3.64	3.94	4.24	4.55	4.85
67	1.70	2.06	2.35	2.65	2.94	3.24	3.53	3.82	4.12	4.41	4.71
69	1.75	2.00	2.29	2.57	2.86	3.14	3.43	3.71	4.00	4.29	4.57
71	1.80	1.94	2.22	2.50	2.78	3.06	3.33	3.61	3.89	4.17	4.44
73	1.85	1.89	2.16	2.43	2.70	2.97	3.24	3.51	3.78	4.05	4.32
75	1.90	1.84	2.11	2.37	2.63	2.89	3.16	3.42	3.68	3.95	4.21
77	1.95	1.79	2.05	2.31	2.56	2.82	3.08	3.33	3.59	3.85	4.10
79	2.00	1.75	2.00	2.25	2.50	2.75	3.00	3.25	3.50	3.75	4.00
81	2.05	1.71	1.95	2.20	2.44	2.68	2.93	3.17	3.41	3.66	3.90

■ = Low risk (~4% per year)　　■ = Moderate risk (~7% per year)

■ = High risk (~12% per year)　　■ = Severe risk (~18% per year)

Reproduced with permission from Zafar et al., *J Thorac Cardiovasc Surg* 2018;155: 1938–50.

Manual of Perioperative Care in Adult Cardiac Surgery, Sixth Edition. Robert M. Bojar.
© 2021 John Wiley & Sons Ltd. Published 2021 by John Wiley & Sons Ltd.

19 Aortic Height and Length Index for Thoracic Aneurysms

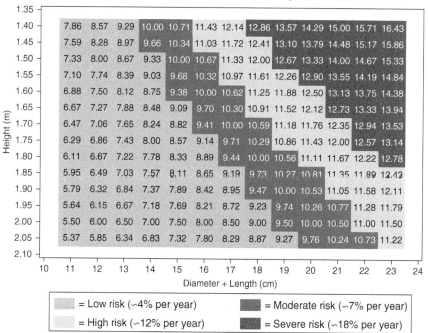

Risk of AAEs by Aortic Size and Height with Aortic-Height Index Given within Chart

Height (m) vs *Diameter + Length (cm)*

= Low risk (~4% per year)
= Moderate risk (~7% per year)
= High risk (~12% per year)
= Severe risk (~18% per year)

Reproduced with permission from Wu et al., *J Thorac Cardiovasc Surg* 2019;74:1883–94.

♡ 20 Technique of Thoracentesis

A. The level of the fluid should be determined on chest x-ray and confirmed by dullness to percussion. The skin is prepped and draped. One percent lidocaine is used for local anesthesia of the skin. A 22-gauge needle is passed to the upper border of the rib and the periosteum is anesthetized. The needle is then passed over the rib into the pleural space.

B. When the pleural space has been entered, fluid should be aspirated to confirm that the effusion has been located. A larger "intracatheter" needle is then passed into the pleural cavity, the plastic catheter advanced, and the metal needle withdrawn to prevent injury to the lung as it expands to appose the parietal pleura. The fluid is then aspirated into collection bottles.

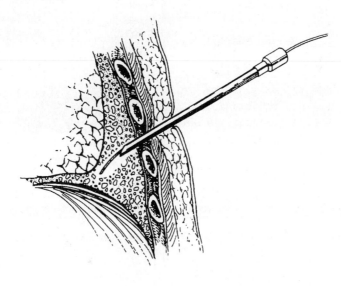

Manual of Perioperative Care in Adult Cardiac Surgery, Sixth Edition. Robert M. Bojar.
© 2021 John Wiley & Sons Ltd. Published 2021 by John Wiley & Sons Ltd.

21 Technique for Tube Thoracostomy

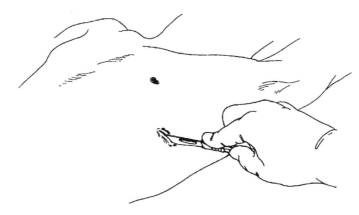

1. Skin incision. One percent lidocaine is used for local anesthesia. A subcutaneous wheal is raised over the fifth or sixth intercostal space in the midaxillary line. The needle is passed to the upper border of the rib and the periosteum is anesthetized. Fluid should be aspirated from an effusion to confirm its location. A 1 cm incision is then made.

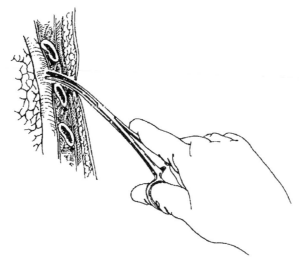

2. Pleural entry. The dissection is carried down to and through the intercostal muscles with a Kelly clamp, the parietal pleura is penetrated, and the pleural cavity is entered. Finger dissection should be used only if loculations are known to be present.

Manual of Perioperative Care in Adult Cardiac Surgery, Sixth Edition. Robert M. Bojar.
© 2021 John Wiley & Sons Ltd. Published 2021 by John Wiley & Sons Ltd.

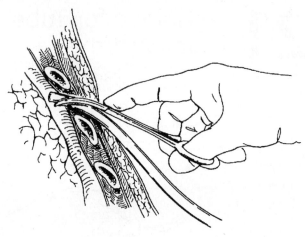

3. Chest tube placement. The chest tube is inserted and directed towards the apex for air and posteriorly for fluid. The tube should be clamped during insertion if fluid is being drained. The tube is then secured with a 2-0 silk suture. A trocar should **never** be used to penetrate the pleura.

Index

Note: page numbers with an *f* indicates figures; those with a *t*, tables; those with an *a*, appendix